Clinical Oncology

A Multidisciplinary Approach for Physicians and Students

7th Edition

Clinical Oncology

A Multidisciplinary Approach for Physicians and Students

7th Edition

Editor **Philip Rubin, M.D.**
Professor and Chairman
Department of Radiation Oncology

Associate Editors **Sandra McDonald, M.B.,Ch.B.**
Assistant Professor
Department of Radiation Oncology

Raman Qazi, M.D.
Associate Professor
Department of Medicine and Oncology

University of Rochester Cancer Center
School of Medicine and Dentistry
Rochester, NY

W.B. SAUNDERS COMPANY
A Division of Harcourt Brace & Company
Philadelphia London Toronto Montreal Sydney Tokyo

W.B. SAUNDERS COMPANY
A Division of Harcourt Brace & Company

The Curtis Center
Independence Square West
Philadelphia, PA 19106

Library of Congress Cataloging-in-Publication Data

Clinical oncology for medical students and physicians: a multi-
  disciplinary approach / [edited by] Philip Rubin. — 7th ed.
        p.   cm.
  Includes bibliographical references and index.
  ISBN 0-7216-3761-2
  1. Cancer.   2. Oncology.   I. Rubin, Philip, 1927–
  [DNLM: 1. Neoplasms.   QZ 200 C6407]
RC261.C652   1993
616.99'4—dc20
DNLM/DLC

                                                    90-7218

Clinical Oncology: A Multidisciplinary Approach for Physicians and Students, 7th Edition   ISBN 0-7216-3761-2

Printed in the United States of America

Last digit is the print number: 9 8 7 6 5 4 3 2 1

in memoriam

Robert A. Cooper, M.D.
August 27, 1932 - April 6, 1992

He brought that sense of challenge to the creation of the University of Rochester Cancer Center, much like the Olympic Games.

He carried the torch.
He lit the way.
He planted the flame high.
Part of the fire in me, in us, the faculty he brought together,
Is his fire.
May that fire—may that flame
Continue to glow and
Be everlasting in its afterglow
In our remembrance of him.

ACKNOWLEDGMENTS

I am deeply indebted to each of the author contributors of this book—the 7th edition of the "orange syllabus." Many have contributed for two or three decades. Each author brought their particular oncology expertise and gave time and effort out of busy schedules to writing and updating their chapters and bibliographies during the long publishing process.

Special thanks to my everwilling, dedicated faculty member—Sandra McDonald, Associate Editor, whose excellence in scholarship and teaching in both radiation and medical oncology is evident in the preparation of many of the tables and figures in the book.

Also, my appreciation to Raman Qazi for his steadfastness in keeping the medical oncology and chemotherapy material up-to-date.

The meticulous organizational and editing skills of Taimi Marple deserve special thanks and acclaim. She assumed responsibility for seeing the book to its completion, working with the authors to update bibliographies, check overall accuracy and fine tune the tables and figures.

Since this edition has been in progress over the past four years, the efforts of other editorial assistants need to be mentioned.

Janette Marshall worked the first round of the book with the many authors in the various oncologic specialties to create the initial versions of the 37 chapters.

Jacqueline Meehan devoted a summer to transferring all the chapters onto an organized floppy disk system, unifying numerous versions and, with Jackie Siwicki, completed the first bibliographic update.

Aimee Miller worked and refined the tables on HyperCard through the many style evolutions and updates. Through her efforts, an electronic computerized version of the book is in development.

Maria Dolor spent hours in the library diligently tracking down permission requests for tables and figures in the book.

Finally, my greatest debt of gratitude is to the publisher, W.B. Saunders Company and especially to Richard Zorab, Senior Medical Editor. As most readers know, *Clinical Oncology for Medical Students and Physicians—A Multidisciplinary Approach* was published for more than two decades by the American Cancer Society whose generous past support made it a companion to the study of oncology for most medical students and general physicians in this country and numerous other countries with translations into Spanish, Portuguese, Russian, and Japanese. When the decision was made to publish this 7th edition independently, of all the publishers contacted only W.B. Saunders had the vision shared by the Editor of this volume. That is, producing the "orange syllabus" so as to assure the widest distribution at an affordable price to students and practitioners in this country and abroad.

The future rests with accurate transfer of past and current experience in the field of oncology—its sciences and clinical investigations—to the next generations of medical students and physicians.

PREFACE

Cancer is curable! In the decades past, since the introduction of a multidisciplinary approach to cancer management, a gradual improvement in local-regional control by surgery and radiation treatment coupled with effective combinations of drugs, particularly as adjuvants, has allowed for ablation of micrometastases. The challenge is to find combined modality approaches that are both effective and non-toxic. The pediatric malignancies treated with conservative surgery, less aggressive irradiation, and reduced cycles of multiagent chemotherapy are the successful models for adult solid cancers, demonstrating that increasing cancer curability is possible without increasing toxicity and complications. As we enter the 1990s, we realize incremental not monumental therapeutic gains have been achieved, survival rates have increased, and mortality rates have decreased for virtually all sites with the exception of lung cancer. The National Cancer Institute goal of a 50% survival rate for all cancer patients by the year 2000 will be reached in this decade.

This volume is organized so that the physician/medical student can rapidly peruse a considerable amount of oncologic data at each major cancer site by the carefully prepared construct of each chapter. The format consists of clear and concise statements with regard to epidemiology (incidence and prevalence) and etiology, offering insight into the biology and cause of the cancer. The *Detection and Diagnosis* section is accompanied with tables providing an abbreviated list of imaging procedures and their relevance to staging. *Anatomic Staging* diagrams and tables assist the physician to define the cancer in its various extensions and spread patterns in the individual patient. Once the anatomic staging process is complete, and the histopathologic grade and type of cancer is known, the "stage" is set for multidisciplinary treatment decision-making. There are numerous treatment possibilities and combinations for surgery, radiation therapy, and chemotherapy and these are succinctly detailed in the text and in tabular form under Principles of Treatment. The *Results*, in figure and tabular form, represent the benchmark works, often based on a randomized clinical trial. The voluminous literature of Results demands an extensive bibliography, but we have culled the references to provide *Recommended Readings*.

In addition to the site-specific chapters, we have provided a series of general introductory chapters on basic concepts in the oncologic sciences of cancer biology, pathology, radiation biology, pathophysiology, and immunobiology. The clinical science of oncology is presented in the chapters on principles of surgery, radiation oncology, medical oncology, psychosocial oncology, nursing oncology, and oncologic emergencies. Concluding chapters cover metastases, general medical and nursing support care, nutrition, pain, and paraneoplastic phenomena.

This new edition emphasizes the increased curability of cancer and optimization of combining modalities to reduce morbidity, decrease complications, and preserve vital, normal structures. More innovative approaches are on the horizon with advances in genetics, biologic response modifiers, and organ and tissue transplantation—all of which are intended to improve cancer curability and the therapeutic ratio.

June 8, 1992

Thomas Anderson, M.D.

Professor of Hematology/Oncology and Chief, Division of Hematology/Oncology, Department of Medicine, Medical College of Wisconsin, Milwaukee, WI

Cynthia Angel, M.D.

Clinical Associate Professor of Oncology in Obstetrics and Gynecology, University of Rochester School of Medicine and Dentistry, Rochester, NY

Robert F. Asbury, M.D.

Associate Professor of Oncology in Medicine, University of Rochester School of Medicine and Dentistry; Associate Attending, The Genesee Hospital, Rochester, NY

Richard F. Bakemeier, M.D.

Professor of Medicine, University of Colorado School of Medicine; Associate Director, University of Colorado Cancer Center, Denver, CO

John M. Bennett, M.D.

Professor of Oncology in Medicine, Pathology and Laboratory Medicine; University of Rochester School of Medicine and Dentistry, Rochester, NY

Thomas A. Bonfiglio, M.D.

Professor and Chairman, Department of Pathology and Laboratory Medicine, University of Rochester School of Medicine and Dentistry, Rochester, NY

Lazlo Boros, M.D.

Associate Professor of Oncology in Medicine, University of Rochester School of Medicine and Dentistry; Associate Attending, The Genesee Hospital, Rochester, NY

David G. Bragg, M.D.

Professor and Chairman of Radiology, University of Utah Medical Center, Salt Lake City, UT

Christopher B. Caldwell, M.D.

Assistant Professor of Surgery, University of Rochester School of Medicine and Dentistry; Attending Surgeon, The Genesee Hospital, Rochester, NY

Elethea H. Caldwell, M.D.

Associate Professor of Plastic Surgery, University of Rochester School of Medicine and Dentistry, Rochester, NY

Alex Yuang-Chi Chang, M.D.

Associate Professor of Oncology in Medicine, University of Rochester School of Medicine and Dentistry; Attending, The Genesee Hospital; Associate Attending, Strong Memorial Hospital, Rochester, NY

George W. Casarett, Ph.D.*

Professor of Radiation Biology and Biophysics, University of Rochester School of Medicine and Dentistry, Rochester, NY

Harvey J. Cohen, M.D.

Professor of Pediatrics, University of Rochester School of Medicine and Dentistry; Chief, Division of Pediatric Hematology/Oncology; Associate Chairman for Research and Development, Department of Pediatrics, Strong Memorial Hospital, Rochester, NY

Louis S. Constine III, M.D.

Associate Professor of Radiation Oncology and Pediatrics, University of Rochester School of Medicine and Dentistry; Attending Radiation Oncologist, Strong Memorial Hospital, Rochester, NY

Robert A. Cooper, M.D.*

Professor of Oncology in Pathology and Director of University of Rochester Cancer Center, School of Medicine and Dentistry, Rochester, NY

William D. DeWys, M.D., F.A.C.P.

Attending Staff, Fairfax Hospital, Falls Church, VA

Brent DuBeshter, M.D.

Director of Gynecologic Oncology, University of Rochester School of Medicine and Dentistry, Rochester, NY

David S. Enterline, M.D.

Associate, Department of Radiology, Duke University Medical Center, Durham, NC; Clinical Assistant Professor, Department of Radiology, University of North Carolina, Chapel Hill, NC

Richard H. Feins, M.D.

Assistant Professor of Surgery and Oncology, University of Rochester School of Medicine and Dentistry; Attending Surgeon, Strong Memorial Hospital, Rochester, NY

Lowell A. Goldsmith, M.D.

Professor and Chair, Department of Dermatology, University of Rochester School of Medicine and Dentistry, Rochester, NY

Thomas C. Hall, M.D., F.A.C.P.

Life Research Professor of the American Cancer Society; Medical Oncologist, Consultants in Medicine, Bellingham, WA

Michael H. Henrichs, Ph.D.

Clinical Associate Professor of Psychiatry, University of Rochester School of Medicine and Dentistry; Clinical Psychologist, Strong Memorial Hospital, Rochester, NY

Edgar C. Henshaw, M.D.*

Professor of Oncology in Medicine and Biochemistry and Associate Director for Basic Science, University of Rochester Cancer Center, School of Medicine and Dentistry, Rochester, NY

Margaret A. Henzler, M.S.

Senior Associate, Department of Radiation Oncology, University of Rochester Cancer Center, School of Medicine and Dentistry, Rochester, NY

LeRoy G. Hoffman, M.D.

Attending Radiation Oncologist, Department of Radiation Oncology, Rex Cancer Center, Raleigh, NC

Jean E. Johnson, Ph.D., R.N.

Professor of Nursing, University of Rochester School of Nursing; Associate Director for Nursing Oncology, University of Rochester Cancer Center, Rochester, NY

Linda S. Jones, M.S., R.N.

Assistant Professor of Clinical Nursing, University of Rochester School of Nursing; Assistant to the Associate Director for Nursing Oncology, University of Rochester Cancer Center, Rochester, NY

James W. Keller, M.D.

Professor of Radiation Oncology, Emory School of Medicine; Associate Chairman for Clinical Affairs, Emory University School of Medicine and The Emory Clinic, Atlanta, GA

Andre Konski, M.D.

Associate Director, Department of Radiation Oncology, The Toledo Hospital; Clinical Assistant Professor, Department of Radiation Therapy, Medical College of Ohio, Toledo, OH

Zachary B. Kramer, M.D.

Assistant Professor of Oncology in Medicine, University of Rochester School of Medicine and Dentistry; Assistant Director of Hematology/Oncology Division, Highland Hospital, Rochester, NY

Hideo Kubo, Ph.D.

Professor and Chief of Physics, University of California Davis Cancer Center, Sacramento, CA

Virginia K. Langmuir, M.D.

Assistant Professor of Surgery, University of Rochester School of Medicine and Dentistry, Rochester, NY

Lowell W. Lapham, M.D.

Professor Emeritus of Neuropathology, University of Rochester School of Medicine and Dentistry, Rochester, NY

Jeffrey Lin, M.D.

Director of Gynecologic Oncology; Assistant Professor of Obstetrics and Gynecology, George Washington University Medical Center, Washington, D.C.

Ahmad Matloubieh, M.S.

Assistant Clinical Physicist, Strong Memorial Hospital; Chief Physicist, Department of Radiation Oncology, Highland Hospital, Rochester, NY

Craig S. McCune, M.D.

Associate Professor of Oncology in Medicine, University of Rochester School of Medicine and Dentistry; Attending Medical Oncologist, Strong Memorial Hospital, Rochester, NY

Joseph V. McDonald, M.D.

Professor Emeritus of Surgery, University of Rochester School of Medicine and Dentistry, Rochester, NY

Sandra McDonald, M.B., Ch.B.

Assistant Professor of Radiation Oncology, University of Rochester School of Medicine and Dentistry; Attending Radiation Oncologist, Strong Memorial Hospital, Rochester, NY

Henry S. Metz, M.D.

Professor of Ophthalmology, University of Rochester School of Medicine and Dentistry; Attending Ophthalmic Surgeon, Strong Memorial Hospital, Rochester, NY

R. Timothy Mulcahy, Ph.D.

Professor of Human Oncology, University of Wisconsin Medical School, Madison, WI

Diana F. Nelson, M.D.

Associate Professor of Radiation Oncology, University of Rochester School of Medicine and Dentistry; Attending Radiation Oncologist, Strong Memorial Hospital, Rochester, NY

John D. Norante, M.D.

Associate Professor of Otolaryngology and Head and Neck Surgery, University of Rochester School of Medicine and Dentistry, Rochester, NY

Robert E. O'Mara, M.D.

Professor of Radiology, University of Rochester School of Medicine and Dentistry; Chief, Division of Nuclear Medicine, Strong Memorial Hospital, Rochester, NY

Robert D. Ornitz, M.D.

Director, Department of Radiation Oncology, Rex Cancer Center, Raleigh, NC

Richard B. Patt, M.D.

Associate Professor of Anesthesiology, Psychiatry, and Oncology, University of Rochester School of Medicine and Dentistry; Medical Director, Pain Treatment Center; Coordinator, Cancer Pain Programs, Strong Memorial Hospital, Rochester, NY

W. Bradford Patterson, M.D.

Consultant, Cancer Epidemiology and Control, Dana Farber Cancer Institute, Boston, MA

James L. Peacock, M.D.
Associate Professor of Surgery and Oncology, University of Rochester School of Medicine and Dentistry; Attending Surgeon, Strong Memorial Hospital, Rochester, NY

Colin A. Poulter, M.D.
Professor of Radiation Oncology, University of Rochester School of Medicine and Dentistry; Attending Radiation Oncolgist, Strong Memorial Hospital, Rochester, NY

Stephen E. Presser, M.D.
Clinical Assistant Professor of Dermatology, Surgery, and Family Medicine, University of Rochester School of Medicine and Dentistry, Rochester, NY

Thomas C. Putnam, M.D.
Clinical Associate Professor of Pediatrics and Surgery, University of Rochester School of Medicine and Dentistry; Attending Surgeon, Strong Memorial Hospital, Rochester, NY

Raman Qazi, M.D., F.A.C.P.
Associate Professor of Oncology in Medicine, University of Rochester School of Medicine and Dentistry; Director, Hematology/Oncology, Highland Hospital, Rochester, NY

Randy N. Rosier, M.D., Ph.D.
Associate Professor of Orthopaedics, Oncology , and Biophysics, University of Rochester School of Medicine and Dentistry; Attending Orthopaedic Surgeon, Strong Memorial Hospital, Rochester, NY

Jacob M. Rowe, M.D.
Professor of Medicine, University of Rochester School of Medicine and Dentistry; Attending Physician, Director of Clinical Services, Hematology Unit, Strong Memorial Hospital, Rochester, NY

Philip Rubin, M.D.
Professor and Chairman, Department of Radiation Oncology, University of Rochester Cancer Center, School of Medicine and Dentistry, Rochester, NY

Deepak M. Sahasrabudhe, M.D.
Associate Professor of Oncology and Medicine, University of Rochester Cancer Center, School of Medicine and Dentistry; Attending Medical Oncologist, Strong Memorial Hospital, Rochester, NY

Omar M. Salazar, M.D., F.A.C.R.
Professor and Chairman, Department of Radiation Oncology, University of Maryland; Chief, Radiation Oncology, University of Maryland Medical System, Baltimore, MD

Edwin D. Savlov, M.D.
Professor of Surgery, University of Nevada; Chief of Surgical Service, Veteran's Administration Hospital, Reno, NV

Charles W. Scarantino, M.D., Ph.D.
Adjunct Professor, Department of Radiation Oncology, East Carolina University School of Medicine, Greenville, NC; Attending Radiation Oncologist, Department of Radiation Oncology, Rex Cancer Center, Raleigh, NC

Paul R. Schloerb, M.D.
Professor of Surgery, University of Kansas Medical Center, Kansas City, KS

Cindy L. Schwartz, M.D.
Associate Professor of Pediatrics, Department of Pediatric Hematology/Oncology, University of Rochester School of Medicine and Dentistry, Rochester, NY

Seymour I. Schwartz, M.D.
Professor and Chair, Department of Surgery, School of Medicine and Dentistry, Rochester, NY; Chief of Surgery, Strong Memorial Hospital, Rochester, NY

Steven S. Searl, M.D.
Clinical Associate Professor of Ophthalmology and Pathology, University of Rochester School of Medicine and Dentistry; Senior Attending Ophthalmologist, Strong Memorial Hospital, The Genesee Hospital, and St. Mary's Hospital, Rochester, NY

George B. Segel, M.D.
Professor of Pediatrics, Medicine, and Genetics, University of Rochester School of Medicine and Dentistry, Rochester, NY

Charles D. Sherman, Jr., M.D.
Clinical Professor of Surgery, University of Rochester School of Medicine and Dentistry; Attending Surgeon, Highland Hospital, Rochester, NY

Dietmar W. Siemann, Ph.D.
Professor and Associate Chair for Research, Department of Radiation Oncology, University of Rochester School of Medicine and Dentistry, Rochester, NY

Julia L. Smith, M.D.
Associate Professor of Oncology and Medicine, University of Rochester School of Medicine and Dentistry; Attending Medical Oncologist, Strong Memorial Hospital; Medical Director, Hospice of Rochester, Rochester, NY

Mark H. Stoler, M.D.
Staff Patholgist, Cleveland Clinic Foundation, Cleveland, OH

Robert M. Sutherland, Ph.D.
Vice President and Executive Director, Life Sciences Division, SRI International, Menlo Park, CA

Alvin L. Ureles, M.D.
Professor of Medicine, University of Rochester School of Medicine and Dentistry; Associate Attending Physician, Strong Memorial Hospital; Senior Attending, Department of Medicine, The Genesee Hospital, Rochester, NY

Paul Van Houtte, M.D.
Professor (U.L.B.), University Libre de Bruxelles, Belgium; Chairman, Department of Radiotherapy, Institut Jules Bordet, Brussels, Belgium

Gunar K. Zagars, M.D.
Associate Professor of Radiotherapy, University of Texas, M.D. Anderson Cancer Center, Houston, TX

* deceased

CONTENTS

Philip Rubin, M.D., Radiation Oncology
Robert A. Cooper, M.D., Pathologic Oncology

Chapter **1**

STATEMENT OF THE CLINICAL ONCOLOGIC PROBLEM

The analysis of many a success or failure (in cancer management) often reveals the important role played by the physician or physicians who dealt with the case in its inception and their decisive influence on the eventual result. Where temporizing guesswork, amateurish approaches, and defeatist attitudes may fail, intelligent understanding, prompt skillful treatment, and a hopeful, compassionate attitude may succeed.

Ackerman and del Regato (1)

PERSPECTIVE

Cancer is curable. This dread disease, which was synonymous with death, has yielded to the advances in modern diagnosis and multimodal treatment as demonstrated in numerous clinical trial investigations and new knowledge in basic science research. Seemingly incurable and devastating cancers are being ablated by a combined modality approach that includes surgery, radiation therapy, and chemotherapy, as illustrated by the outcome of patients with localized cancers given state-of-the-art treatment. Recent analysis of trends in survival (Table 1-1, Fig. 1-1), based upon analysis of Cancer End Results Group data and the National Cancer Institute's (NCI) Surveillance, Epidemiology and End Results (SEER) program (62,71), show a significant improvement for 5-year survival rates by decade, from 39% in the sixties to 43% in the seventies to 50% in the eighties. This gain in survival has occurred at 15 to 20 sites, most of which have reached significance levels. The NCI goal for the year 2000 is to reduce the cancer mortality by one half. In fact, this goal has been reached and promises to be exceeded, since numerous innovations have occurred and newer therapeutic modalities such as monoclonal antibodies or immunotherapy, biologic response modifiers, hyperthermia, chemoprevention, new imaging modalities, and molecular biology diagnosis techniques are becoming effective.

Oncology, the study of neoplastic disease, is generally referred to as the "cancer problem" (1,71,28). It is the study of a large variety of malignant tumors with lethal potential. Cancer cells can arise in any body tissue, at any age. Characteristically, they can invade local tissues by direct extension or they can spread throughout the body through lymphatic or vascular channels. As infectious diseases are brought under control and increased longevity results, the incidence of cancer in a given population rises. In our society, deaths from cancer are exceeded only by those resulting from cardiovascular disease. The number of deaths annually in this country is approaching 500,000 (71) (Fig. 1-2). In addition to the mortality, the associated morbidity demands considerable medical and nursing attention.

The size and scope of the cancer problem are best appreciated with numbers. Almost 56 million Americans now living will be diagnosed as cancer patients — one in every four, according to present rates; it is likely a family member or friend within your acquaintance will be so affected (71). By 1990, approximately one million people annually will be diagnosed as having cancer; this figure does not include nonmelanoma skin cancer (500,000 patients) and cancer *in situ*, which represent another population of hundreds of thousands according to the SEER program (71). Approximately 50% to 60% of those diagnosed as cancer patients will probably die of their disease; in Fig. 1-3 the cancer death rates by site are shown (71). There has been, and continues to be, a steadiness in the age-adjusted deaths, but like the incidence rate, this rate varies with each cancer site. With the exception of lung cancer, which is on the rise, most sites have steadied or are decreasing due to improved diagnosis and treatment.

EPIDEMIOLOGY AND ETIOLOGY

Epidemiology

Approximately one million new cases of cancer are estimated for the United States in 1990 (71). Patterns of incidence and death rates of malignant disease vary with age, sex, race, and geographic location (62). Females are more prone to develop cancer than males, but the gap is closing because of the increase in lung cancer in males and the decrease in cervical cancer in females, and is projected to be equal by the American Cancer Society (71) in 1989. In females, the common cancers by site are breast (28%), rectum (15%), lung (11%), uterus (9%), and hematopoietic and lymphoid (7%), whereas in males, the common sites are prostate (21%), lung (20%), colorectal (14%), urinary tract (10%), and hematopoietic and lymphoid (8%) (Fig. 1-4a). When overall incidence annually

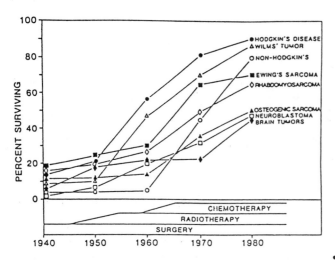

Fig. 1-1. Trends in survival over three decades based upon analysis of Cancer End Results Group data and NCI SEER program results.

Table 1-1. Trends in Survival By Site of Cancer and Cases Diagnosed

	Relative 5-Year Survival Rates (Percent)				
	1960–1963[1]	1970–1973[1]	1974–1976[2]	1977–1979[2]	1980–1985[2]
Site	**W**	**W**	**W**	**W**	**W**
All Sites	39	43	50	50	51**
Thyroid	83	86	92	92	93
Testis	63	72	78	88	91**
Corpus Uteri	73	81	89	87	83**
Melanoma	60	68	79	81	81**
Urinary Bladd	53	61	73	75	78**
Breast-female	63	68	75	75	76**
Hodgkin's Dis.	40	67	72	73	76**
Prostate	50	63	67	71	73**
Larynx	53	62	66	68	68
Cervix Uteri	58	64	69	68	67
Colon	43	49	50	52	55**
Oral Cavity	45	43	55	53	54
Rectum	38	45	48	50	53**
Kidney and Renal Pelvis	37	46	51	50	52
Non-Hodgkin's Lymphoma	31	41	47	48	51**
Ovary	32	36	36	37	38**
Leukemia	14	22	34	36	34
Multiple Myeloma	12	19	24	24	26**
Brain & Central Nervous Sys.	18	20	22	24	24**
Stomach	11	13	14	16	16**
Lung and Bronchus	8	10	12	13	13**
Esophagus	4	4	5	6	8**
Liver	2	3	4	3	4
Pancreas	1	2	3	2	3

[1]Rates are based on End Results Group data from a series of hospital registries and one population-based registry.
[2]Rates are from SEER program, based on data from population-based registries in Connecticut, New Mexico, Utah, Iowa, Hawaii, Atlanta, Detroit, Seattle-Puget Sound, and San Francisco-Oakland. Rates are based on follow-up of patients through 1986.
* The standard error of the survival rate is between 5 and 10 percentage points.
** The difference in rates between 1974-1976 and 1980-1985 is statistically significant (p<0.05).
*** The standard error of the survival rate is greater than 10 percentage points.
— Valid survival rate could not be calculated
Source: Cancer Statistics Branch, National Cancer Institute.
Modified from American Cancer Society (2a).

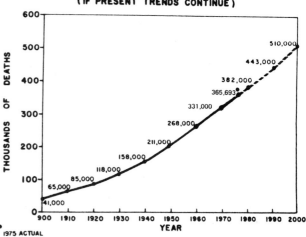

Fig. 1-2. Forecast of cancer deaths if present trends continue. The rise in mortality has been steady since 1900. It is projected that by the year 2000, there will be over one half million deaths from cancer annually if present rates continue. From Epidemiology and Statistics Dept., American Cancer Society, Inc. 6/77, with permission.

of new cases in the United States are considered, the digestive organs are first (227,800 new cases), genital organs are second (181,800), and the respiratory system is third (171,600). New cases of breast cancer (142,900) almost approach the incidence of lung cancer (155,000). Blood disorders, leukemias, and lymphomas together account for almost 80,000 cases annually.

Cancer deaths for all age groups rank either first or second among the leading causes for mortality. The cancer problem in children, however, is growing. Except for accidents, cancer is the leading cause of death for children of both sexes aged 1 to 14 years and young female adolescents and female adults aged 15-34, but for males in these age groups cancer drops to fourth place. From age 35, cancer vies with heart disease for the number one position. For females, cancer leads from ages 35-74 and drops to second place after age 75 years. In males, cancer exceeds heart disease for ages 55-74 when mortality rates are highest. Lung cancer accounts for the highest mortality by far (147,100 cases annually), followed by digestive organs, (123,000). In females, the leading sites of fatal cancers are lung (21%), breast (18%), and rectum (13%), while in males it is lung (35%), prostate (11%), and colorectum (11%) (Fig. 1-4b). The age-adjusted death rates show a steady increase from ages 40-70 for both sexes (75). There has been a 26% increase in cancer in blacks compared with 5% in whites.

The trend toward increasing numbers of cancer deaths results from a variety of factors and should not be viewed as a failure to achieve the goals of the national cancer program. *Improvements in diagnosis and therapy have occurred at many sites; if lung cancer were eliminated, all other sites combined would show a decline in the past decade of mortality attributed to cancer* (16). In pediatric tumors, this is even more evident. However, the continued increase of cancer deaths results from the older age groups in the population, improved diagnosis, complete reporting, and greater incidence because of carcinogenic exposures.

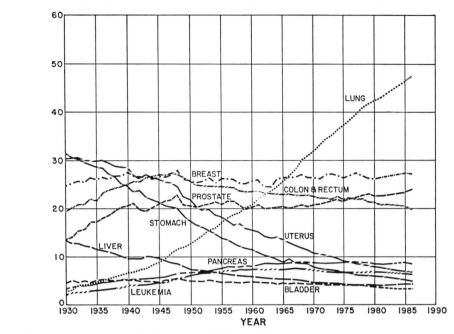

Fig. 1-3. Cancer death rates by site with the rates shown for both sexes combined except for breast, uterus (female population only) and prostate (male population only) in the U.S. by decade from 1930-86. From American Cancer Society (2), with permission.

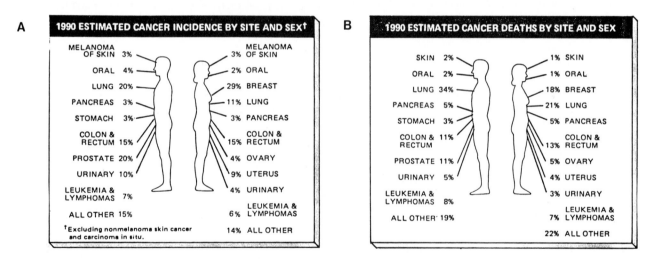

Fig. 1-4. 1989 estimated cancer incidence (a) and death (b) by site and sex. The estimates of the incidence of cancer are based on data from the National Cancer Institute's Surveillance, Epidemiology, and End Results (SEER) program (1983-1985). Nonmelanoma skin cancer and carcinoma *in situ* have not been included in the statistics. The incidence of nonmelanoma skin cancer is estimated to be more than 500,000. From Silverberg (72), with permission.

Etiology (16,49)

The exact cause of cancer remains undetermined. Although there are readily recognizable histopathologic differences between the cancer cell and the normal cell, few metabolic differences have been determined. The biochemical structure of nucleic acids is similar in both types of cells, but some reduction of vital proteins exists in cancer cells, for example, respiratory enzymes, cytochromes, and cytochrome oxidase. According to Warburgh (37), under aerobic conditions in the cancer cell, glycolysis remains a constant and significant difference. There are a number of thorough reviews (8,9) of the biochemical aspects of malignant disease relating the molecular biology of DNA and RNA synthesis, protein and polypeptide synthesis, enzyme activity, and membrane receptions to ultrastructural and cellular components (50,65).

A unified theory of carcinogenesis has been offered by numerous investigators based on study of oncogenes. Evidence exists for conversion of normal cellular genes (c-onc) responsible for cellular metabolism, division, and maturation, often virally induced (v-onc), to malignant oncogenes leading to uncontrolled growth. More than one of these genes could be involved and recently a set of antioncogenes (antionc) has been identified that function as cellular repressors. It is conceptually appealing to envision a network of coordinated gene expression (detailed in Chapter 2, "Pathology of Cancer") where "the target of various carcinogenic stimuli would obviously be the cellular DNA encoding on regulating the 'onc/antionc' products such that lesions produced by radiation, viruses on spontaneous random mutation would activate/unactivate portions of this regulatory network ultimately producing a malignancy" (41,50,52,65).

Chemical Carcinogens (63)

Of the known carcinogenic agents in chemicals, viruses, and radiation, chemicals have emerged as the most important in the induction of human cancers. Their common feature is that they are electrophilic reactants, arising through metabolism. *Carcinogenesis is a multistage process* (8,56,57). The first stage, initiation, occurs rapidly and is irreversible; it affects the genetic apparatus, and results from one or more mutants of cellular DNA. The second stage, promotion, occurs over a longer period; it is epigenetic and is largely reversible in the early stages (60) (Fig. 1-5).

Environmental and Industrial Carcinogens (60)

A substantial list of environmental and occupational agents has been identified through the Occupational Safety and Health Act of 1972. Table 1-1 reviews such agents and factors relating to human cancer (60). Tobacco and alcohol consumption are high on the list for causing lung cancer and upper aerodigestive tract malignancies. Betel nut and tobacco quid chewers are at risk for buccal cavity cancers. Ethylene oxide, a widely used agent for sterilization of animal cages, has shown to be associated with leukemia. Haloethers — especially chlorinated ethers — particularly bis (chloromethyl) ether, is very carcinogenic and has been found to cause lung cancers.

At present, known carcinogenic chemical agents play a small role as *definite overall etiologic factors* (15). The polycyclic hydrocarbons have been studied intensely in animals as inducers of neoplasia; they have been documented as a factor in skin cancers among petroleum product industrial workers.

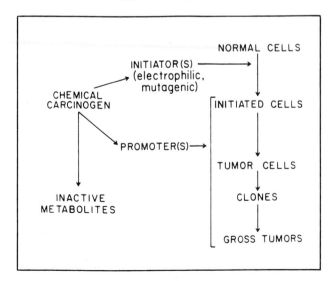

Fig. 1-5. A simplified scheme for the steps in the induction of cancer by a chemical. From Miller and Miller (60), with permission.

Cigarette smoking has come under continual attack since it was implicated as a major causal factor in lung cancer. Use of tobacco has been associated with oral cavity, oropharyngeal and laryngeal cancers, esophageal cancers, and bladder cancer. ß-nephylamine and benzedrine have been implicated as agents in the induction of bladder cancers, although this is rarely a factor in the majority of cases. The concern about radiation exposure as a carcinogenic agent is high, but, once again, this only accounts for the very small fraction of 1% of all cancer patients. Uranium, strontium, nickel, and beryllium have been demonstrated as carcinogenic agents in animals and are probable causes of lung cancer in miners. Asbestos contributes to the development of mesothelioma in asbestos workers.

With the increasing concern over environmental factors, urban air pollution, water contaminants, food processing (including use of nitrites and nitrosamines for meat-curing processes) and saccharin are all being carefully watched as potential carcinogens.

Radiation Carcinogenesis (43)

The concern about radiation exposure is high because of its known carcinogenic action; however, a small fraction — less than 1% — of all cancers is attributable to this cause. This small incidence relates to ongoing efforts to minimize population exposure. Radiation has induced a large variety of cancers with the exception of chronic lymphocytic leukemia. Breast, thyroid, marrow, and bone appear vulnerable, whereas kidney, bladder, and ovary are low in incidence of becoming cancerous. Leukemia is the most radiogenic tumor; the highest incidence occurs 2 to 4 years following exposure and decreases over a period of 25 years. Solid cancers or neoplasms have longer latent periods. There is considerable evidence suggesting that moderate or low radiation doses transform cells genetically and that high doses to small volumes, used clinically, sterilize parenchymal cells and therefore induce fewer tumors despite the larger dose used. Long-term follow-up studies of cervix cancers have not yielded a high incidence of pelvic malignancies, whereas modest sterilizing doses of radiation to the ovary seem to be related to an increase in expected cases of pelvic cancers (43).

Drug-Induced Cancers (22,55)

These are of particular concern to the oncologist, since the induction of a second neoplasm after curing the first is very frustrating (Table 1-2) (2). The use of alkylators (e.g., melphalan and cyclophosphamide) has been known to induce leukemias and bladder cancers. Hormonal agents, such as estrogen-containing compounds, the "pill" in younger women, have been implicated in vaginal adenocarcinomas, endometrial cancer, and more questionably in breast and ovarian cancers. Immunosuppressive agents such as azathioprine have an association with lymphomas, skin cancer, and soft tissue sarcomas. Phenytoin is known to cause lymphoid hyperplasia and, with prolonged administration, lymphoma. Increasingly, the clinician needs to assess the benefits and risks of prolonged drug administration with both the patient and the patient's family. The MOPP program in Hodgkin's disease is associated with second malignancies, particularly when combined with radiation therapy. The combination of multiagent chemotherapy and irradiation, used in treating a variety of cancers, has resulted in secondary leukemias (66).

Table 1-2. Chemicals Generally Recognized as Carcinogenic in Humans

	Exposures	Tumor Formation Sites
Industrial:	2-Naphthylamine	Urinary bladder
	Benzidine	Urinary bladder
	4-Aminobiphenyl	Urinary bladder
	Bis(chloromethyl)ether	Lungs
	Bis(2-chloroethyl)sulfide (mustard gas)	Respiratory tract
	Vinyl chloride	Liver mesenchyme
	Certain tars, soots, oils	Skin, lungs
	Chromium compounds	Lungs
	Nickel compounds	Lungs, nasal sinuses
	Asbestos	Pleura, peritoneum (lungs when combined with cigarette smoking
	Benzene	Lymphoid tissue
Medical:	N,N-bis(2-chloroethyl)-2-naphthylamine (chlornaphazine)	Urinary bladderl
	Diethylstilbestrol	Vagina
	Inorganic arsenic compounds	Skin
	Melphalan	Lymphoid tissue
Societal:	Cigarette smoke	Lungs, urinary tract, other
	Betal nut and tobacco quid	Buccal mucosa

This is a conservative list of human carcinogens for which relatively extensive data are available. Some other chemicals are also suspected of having induced cancer in humans, but the data are more limited.
From Miller and Miller (60), with permission.

Viral and Immunologic Mechanisms (56,70)

The initial intensive studies in avian and murine malignancies indicating that a viral etiology could have a parallel in humans, has not materialized. Considerable data and knowledge about DNA and RNA viruses have resulted, but few true carcinogenic viruses causing human malignancies have been identified (58). The Epstein-Barr virus (EBV) and hepatitis B virus are two agents that chronically infect humans and are associated with neoplasms (53). Burkitt's (46) discovery of an African lymphoma based on its geographic distribution led to identification of a transmissible agent, that is, EBV. The association of nasopharyngeal cancers and EBV has also been extensively studied (58). The association of primary hepatocellular carcinoma and hepatitis B viral infection, a common world-wide malignancy, has been summarized by Blumberg and London (42).

Congenital immunodeficiency states and immunosuppressive therapy in malignancies have been implicated in malignancy induction, particularly in lymphomas and leukemias. With immunosuppression maintenance, patients display a high (8%) yearly risk, with a 100 times greater frequency of developing a tumor than their counterparts in the same age group in the general population (58).

The identification of human immunodeficiency viruses, implicated in causing leukemias, lymphomas, and acquired immune deficiency syndrome (AIDS), has become the major concern in recent years.

DETECTION AND DIAGNOSIS

Typical Clinical Presentations

Changes in normal physiologic functions that persist — alterations in eating habits, loss of appetite, difficulty in swallowing, increased constipation and/or diarrhea — require study (Table 1-3) (2). Typical presentations that demand examination and explanation are a lump or nodule in any site — particularly if it is painless and increasing in size slowly — the appearance of bleeding from orifices, unexplained recurrent pain, recurrent fevers, steady weight loss, and repeated infections that may or may not clear with antibiotics (71). These early signs of cancer have been stressed for different sites and in popular programs for the public, but the fear of the diagnosis of cancer can be an element that delays the patient from seeking advice. Each physician must learn to screen patients, particularly those past 40 years of age, for localized lesions in the skin, uterus, mouth, breast, lungs, rectum, prostate, and thyroid. Only through constant awareness will the asymptomatic patient's occult, localized cancer be found at a stage in which therapy can most often prove successful.

Early Clinical Detection

Early clinical detection means the cancer is localized and has not developed regional extensions or distant spread to nodes and viscera. It is essential to listen carefully for new complaints, some of which the patient may think are unimportant. A complete physical examination for high-risk organ systems and key anatomic sites for cancer development can, in most instances, be performed in a short period (76). If one adds the simple and inexpensive tests recommended, such as the Papanicolaou (Pap) smear, Hemocult slides, urinalysis and blood count, virtually all malignancies detectable by early diagnosis will be evident (Table 1-4) (57). A well-directed history, a well-planned physical examination, and some readily available office procedures will identify early most cancers for which people are at risk.

Screening Procedures

For early detection, it is important to focus on the occult phase, when the lesion is asymptomatic. At some sites, effective screening is possible, e.g., cytology for cervix cancer. This cytologic screening does not apply as readily in many other sites, such as lung, prostate, or bladder. Screening procedures, such as gastric camera and fiber-optic scope, are highly effective for early detection of stomach cancer; however, they are too costly to use in other than specific high-risk groups. Lack of methods and the inaccessibility of some sites often make early recognition impossible. There are two points to remember: First, it is hoped that early clinical detection means the cancer is localized; second, localized small cancers (≤ 2 cm) are highly curable by current treatment

Table 1-3. Cancer's 7 Warning Signals

Change in bowel or bladder habits
A sore that does not heal
Unusual bleeding or discharge
Thickening of lump in breast or elsewhere
Indigestion or difficulty in swallowing
Obvious change in wart or mole
Nagging cough or hoarseness

If you have a warning signal, see your doctor!

From the American Cancer Society (2a), with permission.

Table 1-4. Protocol for Early Detection of Cancer in Asymptomatic Persons

| | New Recommendation | | | |
| | Population | | | Previous |
	Sex	Age/Risk	Frequency	Recommendation
Chest x-ray		Not recommended		High-risk person annually*
Sputum cytology		Not recommended		Not recommended
Sigmoidoscopy	M&F	Over 50	Every 3-5 years†	Persons over 40 annually
Stool guaiac slide test	M&F	Over 50	Every year	Persons over 40
Digital rectal examination	M&F	Over 40	Every year	Same
Pap test	F	20-65‡	Every 3 years§	Annual
Pelvic examination	F	20-40	Every year	Same
Endometrial tissue sample	F	At high risk◊ Menopause	At menopause	Same
Breast self-examination	F	Over 20	Every month	Same
Breast physical examination	F	20-40 Over 40	Every 3 years Every year	Annual Same
Mammography	F	Between 35-40	Baseline	No policy
		40-50	Every year, especially if risk factors exist	Consult personal physician
		Over 50	Every year	
Health counseling and cancer checkup #	M&F	Over 20	Every 3 years	"Periodic"
	M&F	Over 40	Every year	

* Persons over age 40 who smoke or are exposed to other lung carcinogens.
◊ History of infertility, obesity, failure of ovulation, abnormal uterine bleeding, or estrogen therapy.
† After two initial negative examinations a year apart.
# To include examination for cancers of the thyroid, testicles, prostate, ovaries, lymph nodes, oral region, and skin.
‡ Pap test should also be done on women under 20 who are sexually active.
§ After two initial Pap tests done a year apart are negative.
BCDDP = Breast Cancer Detection Demonstration Project..
From Williams (76), with permission.

methods. The literature that attempts to define the role of mammography as a screen for breast cancer (19) best emphasizes the controversy and cost benefit of screening procedures.

A brief review of the common cancer screening procedures follows and will be amplified in chapters dealing with specific sites.

Lung cancer: The results of the Mayo Clinic project (74), in which chest films and sputum cytology were done every 4 months in chronic smokers and in a cohort of randomly assigned patients, have not shown a decrease in mortality as compared with unscreened controls. Some benefits were seen for squamous cell cancer and adenocarcinomas, but not small or large cell cancers; however, the two curves are spreading apart at 4 years with screened patients surviving at a higher rate. This is not statistically significant and no large screens should be undertaken for the older, male, smoking population.

Uterine cancer: Identification of high-risk groups (40) for cytologic studies is possible. Cancer of the cervix occurs more frequently in those who start intercourse in their teens, have multiple sex partners, have many children and/or come from a lower socioeconomic class. In contrast, cancer of the endometrium is a disease of suburbia and occurs in obese, diabetic, infertile women, who often have irregular menses resulting

from failure of ovulation and/or prolonged estrogen administration. Exfoliative cytology is a highly sensitive and inexpensive screening technique for cervical cancer and its precursors, and has led to a significant fall in cancer incidence and death in areas where this was a common disease. Annual Pap smears are still advised for high-risk, sexually active women. However, for other women, after two negative annual Pap smears, 3-year intervals are recommended; it should be noted, however, this is controverted by many experts. For endometrial cancer detection, aspiration curettage taken from the endometrial cavity is advised for those at risk as a quick, relatively painless outpatient method not requiring anesthesia.

Breast cancer: The value of self-examination and mammography has been established in high-risk patients for breast cancer: personal history (5x increased risk), family history (3x), multiparity or first birth after aged 35 years (3x), fibrocystic disease (1.5 to 3.8x). Baseline mammograms are advised for women between the ages of 35 and 40 years; in high-risk women under 50 years, annually; and, after 50 years, on all women annually (47).

Colorectal cancer: The need for early detection is certain if improvement in the 42% 5-year survival rate for late diagnosis is to occur (51). Fecal occult blood testing and sigmoidoscopic examination (rigid or flexible) are advised annually in the 50 years and older group. Colonoscopy and barium enema are reserved for symptomatic patients or to clarify positive tests for occult blood in the stool.

Head and neck cancers: Too often, examinations of rectal and pelvic cancers are done with agility, but careful inspection and palpation of the oral cavity, oropharynx, hypopharynx, and larynx are ignored. Any sore or lump, hoarseness, or dysphagia should be carefully evaluated. Learning how to visualize the larynx and pharynx is a simple, under-used examination.

Tumor Markers (26)

As yet, no simple test(s) are available with sufficient sensitivity and specificity to detect the presence of a cancer before metastasis. Most tumor markers are in the class of immunologic products such as oncofetal antigens (carcino-embryonic antigen); protein or hormonal products such as human growth hormone and adrenocerticotropic hormone; enzymes such as acid and alkaline phosphatases; or metabolic substances such as polyamines or plasma proteins — ferritins, cereplasms, BL immunoglobulin (40). Tumor markers are more useful for monitoring patient response and detecting recurrence than as a definitive diagnostic tool in screening early cancer.

Surgical Biopsy (32)

Once cancer is suspected, a careful work-up is essential and proper consultation is necessary. Questionable findings require periodic follow-up or surgical intervention to establish or exclude the diagnosis. Most importantly, clinical leads should be pursued and investigative studies should not be unduly procrastinated.

Surgical biopsy or excision is the single most important procedure in establishing a firm diagnosis because neoplasms can masquerade as benign or inflammatory conditions. Whenever possible, a histologic diagnosis is essential before undertaking radical treatment. Oncologic imaging can precede or follow the surgical biopsy, depending on clinical circumstances. The tests are necessary in establishing the diagnosis, the stage of the decrease, planning treatment, and in determining prognosis. Once the pathologic diagnosis is made, certain additional tests are advised to determine the anatomic extent or stage of the process.

Oncologic Imaging (7)

An increasing array of medical imaging procedures exists. These include sophisticated radiography, selective arteriography, radioisotopic scanning studies, ultrasound studies and most important, computerized tomography (CT) and magnetic resonance imaging (MRI) (7, 44). The ordering of tests must be done with discrimination to avoid reduplication and huge medical bills. In addition to identification of primary tumors, the search for metastatic disease in regional nodal and distant visceral sites is important. A diagnostic oncologic imaging algorithm shows the disease process as related to cancer management and treatment (Fig. 1-6).

Computerized tomography (CT) scans: Tumor imaging in diagnostic radiology has been revolutionized by CT scanning. The ability to visualize inaccessible structures, as in the mediastinum and retroperitoneal area, has completely changed work-up procedures. The impact and cost of this new technology, and recommendations formulated in decision trees as to sequencing diagnostic studies in a coordinated and noncompetitive fashion, are outlined by Bragg *et al.* (7):

* in suspected brain tumor, CT scan is advised prior to radionuclide scans and only for specific problems is an arteriogram or air study recommended
* in a lung tumor suspected on a chest film, CT scan is not high on the list and its use depends on the problem
* in suspected liver tumor, radioisotopic scans are favored first, then ultrasound, before CT is recommended
* in suspected bone tumor, nuclear imaging should precede and direct the diagnostic radiographic imaging. Although the sensitivity of bone scans is high, the speci-

ficity is not, so that many false-positives exist as a result of inflammatory conditions and degenerative disease. For primary bone tumors, CT adds new dimensions and understanding of tumor spread.

There are newer imaging techniques on the horizon, such as holistic radiographic imaging, nuclear magnetic resonance imaging (MRI), and three-dimensional displays, which will further augment our understanding of tumor behavior and lead to more accurate diagnoses.

Magnetic resonance imaging and magnetic resonance spectroscopy: The use of high intensity magnetic fields to gain images of the anatomy and regional chemistry is one of the most costly and most advanced technologies. This technique has also revolutionized the imaging of tumors by providing beautifully detailed three-dimensional planar views in sagittal, comonal and transverse cuts. The intensity of signals varies with the weighting of T1 or T2* and the strength of the magnet in tests. Specific paramagnetic contrast agents, such as gadolinium can specifically enhance tumors. Many of the images seen with radiography can be reversed, that is, fat is white and blood vessels are black, because of movement of blood. Respiratory and/or cardiovascular gating is required for viewing dynamic structures, such as the heart and lungs.

In addition to MRI, there is the ability to use surface coils and obtain spectral analysis of specific chemical constituents in the region. As spatial resolution improves, research continues to discover unique characteristics or signatures to allow detection of cancer, monitor its response to therapy, and determine if there is tumor volubility. Considerable research is directed to this area.

Nuclear imaging plays an important role in tumor imaging, but more for detecting metastatic disease than primary tumors. It has been displaced by CT for detecting brain metastases, but is still the first line of study for liver and bone deposits. The ultimate goal is specific labelling or targeting of metabolic products, antigens or antibodies with homing characteristics. Gallium-67 has been used in Hodgkin's disease and lung cancer to specifically identify occult deposits in extensions not appreciated on routine filming. Some investigators (54) have reported gallium-67 to have an accuracy of 72-=% to 100%, but Zeman and Gottschalk (77) have not confirmed this level of accuracy and note that hilar and mediastinal spread are detected and confirmed in only half their patients.

Ultrasound remains a less expensive and less hazardous alternative to the aforementioned studies. The hope for tissue or tumor signatures of the "echo" signal has not emerged. For children, ultrasound presents an alternative to CT for tumor imaging since exposures to ionizing irradiation are avoided. However, the images are definitely inferior and less preferable to most nonradiologic physicians.

CLASSIFICATION

It is essential to develop a classification of cancer based on anatomic and histologic considerations. Such a dual classification is the keystone of cancer decision-making as a multidisciplinary process. It is apparent in a review of the literature that differences in classification or language make cross-

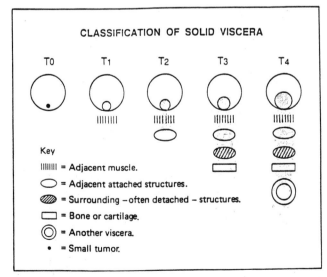

Fig. 1-6. Diagnostic onco-algorithm illustrates diagnostic imaging procedures as a process starting with detection through cancer diagnosis and managment.

---

* relaxation times of MRI, not TNM category

comparisons of different cancers virtually impossible. Thus, a statement referring to early, moderate, and advanced cancers without further description leaves those who are unfamiliar, and even those with experience, uncertain as to where the line is being drawn. Since criteria change for each surgeon with time and the improvement of techniques, terms such as operable, inoperable, resectable, and nonresectable are not illuminating without qualifications.

Many national and international committees are attempting to standardize nomenclature. The main problem is keeping the descriptions from being so complex that they inhibit their clinical use. Simplicity is important, otherwise an experience can be morcellated to the point that it is impossible to have sufficient numbers of patients in any category in the lifetime of an investigator. The two major agencies concerned with the classification of malignant disease are the International Union Against Cancer (UICC) (20) and the American Joint Committee for Cancer Staging and End-Results Reporting (AJC) (3). The objectives of classification are as follows:

- aid the clinician in the planning of treatment
- give some indication of prognosis
- assist in the evaluation of results of treatment
- facilitate the exchange of information
- assist in the continuing investigation of cancer (20)

Histopathologic Classification (14,23)

The histopathologic classification is of equal importance to the anatomic stage in planning treatment and predicting outcome. The need for a standardized nomenclature (13) is evident, and reference to the World Health Organization monographs (38) and the Atlas of Tumor Pathology by the Armed Forces Institute of Pathology (5) provide a basis for uniformity in criteria by illustrative photomicrographs. The two essential features are the histologic grade and type of the tumor.

- The value of *grading* carcinomas [e.g., Broders' (45) classification of squamous cell carcinomas] to express their degree of malignancy is well known. Similar grading systems have been evolved for cancers of the breast bladder. Recently, the sarcomas have been graded. Grading is often more important than type in effecting prognosis, and this is well illustrated for soft tissue sarcomas.
- The need to appreciate the histopathologic *type* of cancer is readily recognized in ovarian and testicular neoplasms. A testicular choriocarcinoma carries a much poorer prognosis and demands different therapy than a similar-stage seminoma. The appreciation of different types of testicular tumors, ovarian cancers, and brain neoplasms is essential to understanding management. The Hodgkin's and non-Hodgkin's lymphomas illustrate this principle most dramatically in the recent literature.
- *Grades (G)* are defined as G1 = well differentiated; G2 = moderately well differentiated; G3 to G4 = poorly to very poorly differentiated.

Dual Classification

Where possible, dual anatomic-histologic classifications should be used, for this is the essence of good reporting. The comparison of one series to another, that is, surgery versus radiation therapy, depends on the presence of a similar group

of cancer patients in each category. True randomization in any series must pass this simple test either retrospectively or prospectively. This is often regulated in prospective studies by stratifying patients into prognostic categories prior to randomization. The only way in which confusion can be eliminated during the next decade is to accept the AJC-UICC classification on a wider basis (3,13,20), and for journal editors to encourage authors to follow these ground rules when reporting end results. The use of tumor grade as the major factor in stage grouping is a new concept in AJC schemas and is reflected in soft tissue sarcomas (3).

Staging Classification

Since Pierre Deniox introduced the tumor, node, metastasis (TNM) system for classification of malignant cancers between the years 1943 and 1952, numerous variations have been introduced by different users (47a). This is the antithesis of standardization, and to correct this deficiency, in 1982 the national committees agreed to formulate a single set allowing for agreements between the UICC and AJC. Throughout this volume these rules for classification will be used and have been published in the fourth edition of the UICC and the third edition of the AJC manuals. A common language is essential for assessing the results of treatment. There is no need to memorize tables but it is important to use them as references.

Anatomic Staging

The essence of a meaningful classification depends on quantifying the extent of disease. This is done in three compartments:

- T for primary tumor
- N for regional lymph nodes
- M for metastases

Most new classifications attempt to define the primary site with a TNM classification (3,20) as follows: T1, T2, T3, or T4 with increasing extent, advancing nodal disease as N0, N1, N2, or N3, and the presence or absence of metastases, respectively, as M0 or M+. These categories may or may not be feasible for all sites and tend to become unwieldy in attempting to maintain complete coverage of all clinical cases. This system allows for considering modes of malignant spread; that is, T for primary or direct extension, N for secondary or lymphatic involvement, and M for vascular dissemination.

"In clinical medicine, the purpose of clinical taxonomy is not merely to classify. The classification must have a purposeful significance in prognosis and therapy" (68). Feinstein (16) has introduced set theory, Boolean algebra, and Venn diagrams to the oncologist and stressed the value of accurate recording of clinical data. In "A unified classification of tumors: An oncotaxonomy with symbols," I have modified Feinstein's thesis to accommodate the TNM classification and have used a symbolic portrayal to unify the variety of classification schema at different organ sites (68).

The basis for oncotaxonomy is that one standard set of TNM definitions, based on a fixed set of criteria, can be provided for all sites. The order of progression of a cancer is reflected in this symbolic cancer language. The criteria are based upon linguistic analysis of the numerous TNM systems in which specific words defining extent of disease have been associated with specific categories such as T1, T2, T3, T4, and N1. A consistent cancer language for all anatomic sites allows for developing a consistent approach to cancer. Generally, the principles of TNM categories are illustrated in the diagrams and tables that follow, with modification at each site.

T Categories

The criterion for categorizing a primary tumor (T) is the apparent anatomic extent of the disease. Extent is commonly based on three features: depth of invasion, surface spread, and size. Following review of existing classifications, an attempt has been made to define the clinical basis for placement of a tumor in T1, T2, T3, or T4 by these criteria in Table 1-5 and Fig. 1-7 (68).

Model Classification

T0: No evidence of a primary lesion found grossly or microscopically. Evidence of malignant change without microinvasion and without a target lesion identifiable clinically.

T1: A lesion confined to the organ of origin. It is mobile, does not invade adjacent or surrounding structures or tissues, and is often superficial.

T2: A localized lesion characterized by deep extension into adjacent structures or tissues. Invasion is into capsules, ligaments, intrinsic muscle, and adjacent attached structures of similar tissue or function. There is some loss of tumor mobility, but it is not complete; therefore, fixation is not present.

T3: An advanced lesion that is confined to the region rather than to the organ of origin, whether solid or hollow. The critical criterion is fixation, which indicates invasion into a fixed structure or past a boundary. These structures are most often bone and cartilage, but invasion of the extrinsic muscle walls, serosa, and skin are also included. Surrounding detached structures of different anatomy or function are in this category; however, this inclusion can be debated because of the varieties of anatomic structures.

T4: A massive lesion extending into another hollow organ, causing a fistula, or into another solid organ, causing a sinus. Invasions into major nerves, arteries, and veins are placed in this category. Destruction of bone in addition to fixation is an advanced sign.

N Categories

The establishment of lymph node categories should be as critical in design as the T or primary categories; however, the criteria currently used are more varied. A unified code should be readily agreed on for grouping of nodes. The criteria consist of size, firmness, capsular versus multiple nodes,

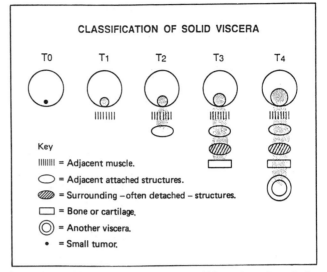

Fig. 1-7. Classification of solid viscera. This series of symbolic diagrams portrays the organ as a large circle and the dotted areas as the cancer. The gravity of cancer spread or progression of the tumor is identified in the sequential spread shown in most sites and is the basis of many classifications. From Rubin (68), with permission.

ipsilateral, contralateral, and bilateral distribution, and distant nodes. These are further defined in Table 1-6 and Fig. 1-8.

Model Classification

N0: No evidence of disease in lymph nodes.

N1: Palpable and movable lymph nodes limited to the first station. A distinction between an uninvolved and an involved palpable node needs to be made. This depends on the firmness and roundness of a node and its size, which is generally greater than 1 cm and usually up to 3 cm in size and solitary.

N2: Firm to hard nodes, palpable and partially movable; they range from 3 to 5 cm. Such nodes show microscopic evidence of capsular invasion; clinically, they may be matted together. Nodes can be contralateral or bilateral.

N3: Fixation is complete. Nodes beyond the capsule with complete fixation to bone, to large blood vessels, to skin, or to nerves — usually greater than 6 cm.

N4: Nodes involved beyond the first station; they are in the second or distant stations. If the first two nodal stations are vertically arranged and both are involved, such double involvement is staged as N4.

Table 1-5. Specific Criteria Related to T Categories

	T1	T2	T3	T4
Depth of invasion				
Solid organs	Confined	Capsule muscle	Bone cartilage	Viscera
Hollow organs	Submucosa	Muscularis	Serosa	
Mobility	Mobile	Partial mobility	Fixed	Fixed and destructive
Neighboring structures	Not invaded	Adjacent (attached)	Surrounding (detached)	Viscera
Surface spread				
Regions (R)	1/2 or R_1	R_1	$R_1 + R_2$	$R_1 + R_2 + R_3$
Circumference	<1/3	1/3 to 1/2	>1/2 to 2/3	>2/3
Size				
Diameter	<2 cm	2 to 4-5 cm	>4-5 cm	>10 cm

From Rubin (68), with permission.

Table 1-6. Specific Criteria Related to N Categories

Station	N1 First	N2 First	N3 First	N4 Second
Drainage				
Unilateral	Ipsilateral	Ipsilateral	Ipsilateral	Contralateral
Bilateral	Ipsilateral	Contralateral or bilateral	Ipsilateral or contralateral	Distant
Number	Solitary	Multiple		
Size	<2-3 cm	>3 cm >5 cm	>10 cm	
Mobility	Mobile	Partial matted muscle invasion	Fixed to vessels, bone, skin	Fixed and destructive

To distinguish N_a from N_1 the specific criteria include: size - between 1-2 cm; firmness — soft to hard; roundness — 1/2 cm to 1 cm.

From Rubin (68), with permission.

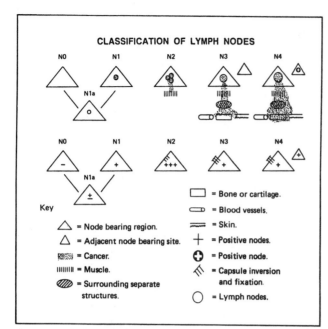

Fig. 1-8. Classification of lymph nodes. From Rubin (68), with permission.

NX: Nodes inaccessible to clinical evaluation.

NL: Nodes evaluated by lymphangiography. L- refers to a negative study and L+ to a positive study. An equivocal finding can be referred to as L ± if equivocally positive and L ∓ if equivocally negative.

N- or N+: Nodes are evaluated by microscopic study and designated as negative or positive depending on findings.

M categories

The lack of a consistent and thorough attempt to categorize an anatomic extent of metastases is conspicuous in the current schema. The important feature is the presence or absence of metastasis, that is, M0 versus M1. The reason for this reflects the poor prognosis if metastases are present. Nevertheless, cure — though rare — is possible for some solitary metastases. As chemotherapy becomes more effective, and results are assessed, there will be a need to categorize and subclassify this group of patients. Classification criteria are further defined in Table 1-7 and Fig. 1-9 (69).

Model Classification

M0: No evidence of metastases.

M1: Solitary, isolated metastasis confined to one organ or anatomic site.

M2: Multiple metastatic foci confined to one organ system or one anatomic site, such as lungs, skeleton, and liver, with no functional to minimal functional impairment of system or site.

M3: Multiple organs involved anatomically, with no or minimal to moderate functional impairment of involved organs.

MX: No metastatic work-up done.

M: Modified to show viscera involved by letter subscript, for example, pulmonary metastases (Mp), hepatic (Mh), osseous (Mo), skin (Mx), and brain (Mb).

M+: Microscopic evidence of suspected metastases, confirmed by pathologic examination.

Principles in Developing an Effective Staging System

It is important to distinguish cancer staging classification. Staging is an attempt to define the true extent of cancer in its

Table 1-7 Specific Criteria Related to M Categories

	M1	M2	M3	M4
No. metastases	1	>1	Multiple	Multiple
No. organs	1	1	Multiple	Multiple
Impairments	0	Minimal	Minimal to moderate	Moderate to severe

M: Modified to show viscera involved by lettered subscript as: pulmonary (M_p), hepatic (M_h), osseous (M_o), skin (M_s), brain (M_b), etc.

M+: Microscopic evidence of suspected metastases, confirmed by pathologic examination

From Rubin (68), with permission.

three compartments (TNM) at a point in time, usually at the time of detection. A classification is a multidimensional and multitemporal frame to include all possibilities of cancer presentations and spread at an organ site. Staging does not imply a regular and predictable progression. Although some cancers proceed in a typical course, advancing from a primary tumor into secondary nodal disease and eventually to remote metastases, many variations exist. Metastases, in fact, can be the first sign of cancer with the primary lesion being smaller and even microscopic in size. The staging is arbitrary and its effectiveness is determined by whether a consensus exists to use it as standard terminology for treatment selection and end stage reporting. A typical type of stage grouping is illustrated in Fig. 1-10.

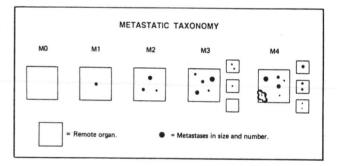

Fig. 1-9. Metastatic taxonomy. From Rubin (68) with permission.

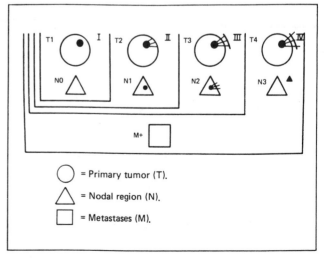

Fig. 1-10. Stage grouping. The stage grouping is based upon clustering TNM categories (see text).

Stage I, T1, N0, M0

Clinical examination reveals a mass limited to organ of origin. The lesion is operable and resectable with only local involvement and there is no nodal or vascular spread. This stage affords the best chance for survival (70% to 90%).

Stage II, T2, N1, M0

Clinical examination shows evidence of local spread into surrounding tissue and first station lymph nodes. The lesion is operable and resectable, but because of greater local extent there is uncertainty about completeness of removal. The specimen shows evidence of microinvasion into capsule and lymphatics. This stage affords a good chance of survival (about 50% ± 5%).

Stage III, T3, N2, M0

Clinical examination reveals an extensive primary tumor with fixation to deeper structures, bone invasion, and lymph nodes of a similar nature. The lesion is operable but not resectable and gross disease is left behind. This stage affords some chance of survival (20% ± 5%).

Stage IV, T4, N3, M +

Evidence of distant metastases beyond the local site or organ. The primary lesion is inoperable. There is little to no chance for survival in most sites (< 5%).

The exact criteria depend on each organ site. These definitions are offered as general guides. The depth of invasion is usually the single most important anatomic factor to quantify the T category, rather than tumor size or surface spread.

There are two approaches with regard to stage grouping. The UICC (20), with few exceptions, does not favor stage grouping but stresses the need for careful definition of each TNM category. The AJC (3) favors stage grouping into four stages since it tends to standardize end-result reporting, which, if derived from a carefully executed protocol, yields excellent data that relate to prognosis. The exact criteria for clustering will vary with each site. A valid system is based on the knowledge of spread and the clinical evolution of the specific cancer and will differ at each anatomic site, depending on the equivalence of T and N categories in terms of prognosis.

Staging Work-Up

Tumor Staging (Fig. 1-6)

A consistent classification of cancer requires a consistent staging or definition work-up. It is now recognized that two phases exist in the use of diagnostic procedures in a cancer patient. The first phase is for diagnosis of the cancer. The second phase is for definition of its anatomic extent in terms of the three compartments.

Primary tumor (T): Clinical examination of accessible lesions is recommended, preferably under anesthesia if the lesion is internal (i.e., cervix or bladder tumors). Radiographs of the site, including special contrast and tomographic techniques, and direct and indirect visualization by endoscopic means are essential studies.

Lymph nodes (N): Clinical examination is important when nodes are accessible. Lymphangiography by means of contrast agents is of value. Needle biopsy, more recently combined with lymphangiography, is being used for confirmation of positive nodes.

Metastases (M): The most common visceral metastases are to lung, liver, bone, bone marrow, and brain. Radiographs of chest and skeletal surveys are often done. Radioisotopic procedures include liver scans (technetium-99m polyphosphate). Laboratory tests include enzyme tests, such as alkaline and acid phosphatases. Liver and bone marrow biopsies are also an aid. Each organ-specific cancer will be discussed in more detail regarding patterns of spread and studies to disclose them.

The major impact of the staging work-up can be seen in Hodgkin's disease, in which the surgical effort, that is, laparotomy, splenectomy, liver and lymph node biopsies, is directed at defining the true extent of the disease, which in turn influences the logical choice and aggressiveness of treatment modalities. This redirection of the surgical effort into staging procedures is the foundation of multidisciplinary conferences for cancer decision-making. Uniform criteria and uniform categories are necessary to make reported series comparable.

Clinical versus Surgical versus Pathologic Criteria for Staging

According to the AJC (3), two different types of evaluative evidence are used for classification of the true extent of disease at different anatomic sites. Check lists and the same anatomic diagrams should be used for careful geographic mapping of cancer extent by clinical oncologists, surgeons, and pathologists.

Clinical-diagnostic staging (cTNM) is noninvasive and relies on careful physical examination and generally available laboratory and radiographic studies (30). This applies to accessible sites such as the head and neck region, especially where more than one modality can be used, and allows for reasonable accuracy in comparison of results.

Surgical pathologic staging (pTNM) is based on information obtained by surgical procedures and is generally useful at inaccessible sites, such as in cancers of the ovary, stomach, colon, and kidney. Biopsies and histopathologic analysis are an essential part of this staging category. Complete resection of organs with drainage of regional lymph nodes is designed for inaccessible sites like the ovaries and pancreas. Correlation of the pathologic findings is important for an evaluation of the accuracy of staging procedures.

It is important to distinguish each type of stage classification, whether clinical-diagnostic, surgical evaluative, or postsurgical pathologic, by the prefix c or p, before TNM categories. A new addition to the postsurgical classification is the concept of residuum disease after surgery.

C-Factor

The C-factor, or certainty factor, reflects the validity of classification according to the diagnostic methods used. Its use is optional. The C-factor definitions are:

C1: Evidence from standard diagnostic means (e.g., inspection, palpation and standard radiography, intraluminal endoscopy for tumors of certain organs).

C2: Evidence obtained by special diagnostic means (e.g., radiographic imaging in special projections, tomography, CT, ultrasonography, lymphography, angiography, scintigraphy, MRI, endoscopy, biopsy, and cytology).

C3: Evidence from surgical exploration, including biopsy and cytology.

C4: Evidence of the extent of disease following definitive surgery and pathologic examination of the resected specimen.

C5: Evidence from autopsy.

Geographic mapping of primary tumor and regional nodes: For many malignancies, accurate mapping of the primary tumor and regional nodes is possible and completes the surgical-pathologic staging process. In addition to the operative note, a series of anatomic diagrams, preferably three-dimensional, should be widely adopted for identification of macroresiduum and microresiduum of tumor. The AJC (3) has check lists and anatomic site diagrams that can be correlated with surgical clips and should allow radiation oncologists to plan treatment more accurately. These same diagrams should be used by pathologists to verify residual diseases. The concept of accurate geographic mapping, so widely adopted in Hodgkin's disease and lymphomas, is being applied to gastrointestinal (GI) tumors, particularly rectal cancers, and is applicable to all sites. *Multimodal treatment requires accurate imaging and mapping of disease, preferably on one set of anatomic forms prior to therapy.*

Residual tumor (R): This information does not enter into establishing stage of tumor but should be recorded on a data form for use in considering additive therapy. When the cancer is treated by definitive surgical procedures, residual cancer, if any is recorded:

- R0 = no residual tumor
- R1 = microscopic residual tumor
- R2 = macroscopic residual tumor

Host classification: Since the widespread acceptance of the Karnofsky Performance Classification (57) and its use by many cooperative groups, the AJC (3) has developed a modification proposal:

- H0 = normal activity
- H1 = symptomatic and ambulatory — cares for self
- H2 = ambulatory more than 50% of time — occasionally needs assistance
- H3 = ambulatory less than 50% of time — requires special nursing and medical assistance
- H4 = bedridden — may need hospitalization

This modification proposal is determined at the time of clinical-diagnostic classification, and recorded at subsequent times of classification as well as at each follow-up examination to measure the quality of life.

The Conversion Rate

Clinical staging is imperfect since it is impossible to detect microscopic extensions or deposits in all potential foci. Despite improvements in diagnosis, a gap in knowledge exists between the apparent clinical stage and the true pathologic stage. This difference may be expressed as a "conversion rate" and is critical to cancer management. In low-conversion rate cancers such as skin cancers, ie, squamous cell or basal cell carcinoma, precise local treatment can be prescribed. In high-conversion rate cancers, such as melanoma or lung cancer, local therapy alone is often ineffective for cure. The concept of conversion rate is illustrated as follows in Fig. 1-11.

The conversion rate is the factor that determines how aggressive or radical a treatment the oncologist should choose. Most cancers are treated at least one stage beyond their clinically defined stage. Very aggressive cancers, such as small cell anaplastic cancer of the lung, Wilm's tumor, and choriocarcinoma, are treated as stage IV or as if they have occult hematogenous metastases, even if they are defined as localized stage I malignancies. Information on conversion

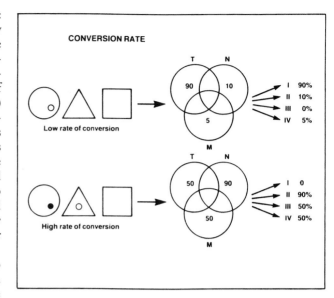

Fig. 1-11. Conversion rate. The low and high conversion rate of a malignancy is illustrated. The low conversion rate cancer is suggested by a squamous cell cancer of the skin 2 cm in diameter. It is identified in the T compartment and 90% of the time is confined in this compartment. If a nodular melanoma of the same size is found clinically, upon a full work-up and follow-up, nodes would be positive 90% and metastases, 50%. This is a high conversion rate. T = tumor; N = node; M = metastases.

rates is sparse but can be collected in well-designed studies. The difference between the clinical stage and the surgical pathologic stages is one kind of information that is being collected for such analysis. The other data needed to establish conversion rates are the incidence and first type of relapse or recurrence after surgical or radiation treatment.

The conversion rate for metastatic disease to distant sites often can be determined for localized and regionalized disease by subtracting the 5-year survival rate from 100. For example, for localized bladder cancer, the conversion rate to metastases is 15% (100-85), whereas for regionalized bladder malignancy, it is as high as 80% (100-20).

PRINCIPLES OF TREATMENT

The finality of treatment in a patient with malignant disease demands that therapy be undertaken only by those who are capable and properly trained (10, 11, 12, 14, 16, 17, 22, 25, 27). There are few situations in medicine where the stakes are as high and the therapeutic procedure as decisive for cure or death. The responsibility is great and the judgment is critical. This is reflected in the emergence of subspecialties in virtually all major disciplines, ie, radiation oncology, medical oncology, surgical oncology, gynecologic oncology, and pediatric oncology. *The first decision is the most important determinant of success in treatment and this should be a multimodal effort.*

The basic principle in therapy is to cure the patient with minimal functional and structural impairment. The decision as to how radical treatment should be is determined by a combination of factors:

- aggressiveness of the cancer
- predictability in regard to its spread
- morbidity and mortality of the therapeutic procedure

- cure rate for the therapeutic procedure under consideration

As the chance for cure decreases, the tendency to be more radical appears justified. In many circumstances, unfortunately, there may not be a decision that will allow for a successful result. A conservative approach may lead to an increased mortality. As in many problems in medicine, the choice is relative. What percentage of survival is acceptable for a debilitating therapeutic modality, be it surgery, radiotherapy or chemotherapy? There is no formula or figure other than personal perspective. If cure is virtually impossible, one must be guided by palliation.

Although there is general agreement on many principles of management (7,11,19, 23), controversy exists over the different procedures that offer limited success. Teamwork between a tumor pathologist, surgeon, radiotherapist, and internist is required for the best effort (11,24,35,36). However, "togetherness" is not a substitute for individual responsibility and judgment on the part of every physician involved. The student will gradually reconcile the differences and assimilate the areas of agreement by carefully following each patient and reading the literature. Maturity of decision rests on clinical experience.

Ideally, each cancer patient should be treated with a highly individual prescription. Optimum treatment is usually designed to treat the defined overt cancer and, where methods are available, suspected occult deposits. Lacking such precision, the selection of treatment should be multidisciplinary because the evidence in many cancers indicates that combinations of treatment are more effective than single modalities in the majority of instances.

The basis for treatment at the time of diagnosis depends upon whether the cancer is localized or metastasizing. The division of patients into these categories is given as 64% localized or regional nodes versus 34% metastatic on presentation (14). For localized disease, 41% are cured after initial treatment (Fig. 1-12). The effectiveness of the standard modalities according to DeVita (48) is displayed in Table 1-8 (14) with surgery curing 43.7%, radiation therapy 18%, and chemotherapy 6.3% as in the initial diagram (Fig. 1-13). Of cancer patients treated by radiation therapy with curative intent, 50% will be controlled, whereas 33% will fail locally and 16% will metastasize (14). The estimated benefit from chemotherapy in cancer patients is that 3.1% will be cured, significant remissions will occur in 5.7% (lasting approximately 2 years), and satisfactory remission will occur in 14.9% (14).

The clinical importance for achieving local regional control of cancer by means of irradiation is given an extra dimension by Fuks and Leibel (49a,57a,57b). They provide compelling evidence at two different anatomic sites that improved local regional control decreases dissemination and metastases and does translate into better overall survival. First in prostate cancer, these authors demonstrate in a large mature series (679 patients) at 15 years, the actuarial distant metastases-free survival (DMFS) for local control is 77% compared to 24% for those who developed local relapses. Virtually every subset analyzed by stage and grade shows this phenomenon. Second, using the large RTOG database in head and neck cancers (57b), they report the incidence of distant metastases only 24% for NED patients versus 36% for patients with persistence of cancer at 5 years and the

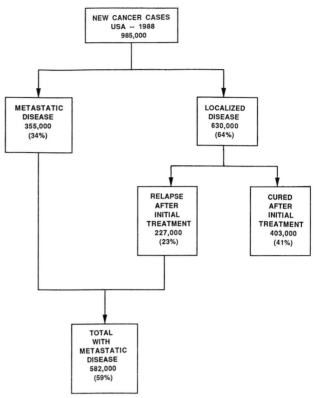

Fig. 1-12. There are a million new cancer cases diagnosed annually of which one-third are metastatic and two-thirds are localized at the time of presentation. Almost half are potentially curable if proper combined modality treatment is applied. Personal communication with Z. Fuks.

Table 1-8. Various Treatment Results With Current Therapies

	No. Patients	(%)
Outcome of Treatment in Patients with Localized Disease Using Current Therapies		
Total New - 1988	985,000	
Total with localized disease	630,000	
Cured with surgery	275,000	(43.7)
Cured with radiation therapy	113,000	(18.0)
Cured (?) with adjuvant chemotherapy	25,000	(3.9)
Cured with chemotherapy	15,000	(2.4)
Will relapse after initial treatment	202,000	(32.0)
local recurrence	133,000	(21.0)
distant metastases	68,000	(11.0)
Estimated Treatment Results of Radiation Therapy in Incurable Patients		
Treated by Radiation with Curative Intent	226,000	
Will be Cured of Cancer	113,000	(50.0)
Will Recur Locally	76,000	(33.4)
Will Relapse with Distant Metastases	34,000	(16.6)
Estimated Benefits from Chemotherapy in Cancer Patients with Metastatic Spread		
Distant metastases	582,000	
Estimated cures with chemotherapy	18,000	(3.1)
Significant remissions (~ 2 yr)	34,000	(5.7)
Satisfactory remissions (~ 1 yr)	87,000	(14.9)
Minimal or no prolongation of life	443,000	(76.3)

Adapted from DeVita (14).

OUTCOME OF TREATMENT IN PATIENTS WITH LOCALIZED DISEASE

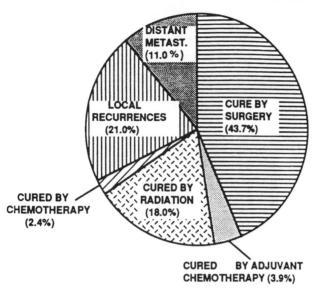

Fig. 1-13. Outcome of treatment in patients with localized disease is portrayed as a function of surgery, radation therapy, and chemotherapy. Local recurrence occurs in 21%, often initial therapy and 11% metastasize.

corresponding 5-year survival is 47% compared to 16%. When analyzed by subgroups, this observation applies to earlier Stage T1-T3N0 patients but not advanced T3-4 N2-3 head and neck cancers; also, this finding holds for all tumor sites, except for hypopharynx and nasopharynx. The explanation for this is that when cancers are very advanced locally with a high degree of nodal involvement, they probably are metastatic at the time of presentation. Most stimulating is the concept put forward to explain these events. Based upon experimental and biological evidence, they explicate that failure to control the primary tumor leads to increased rates of metastatic dissemination because recurrent tumors develop more cell clonogens capable of metastasizing that are phenotypically and genotypically distinct (57a). Based upon these biological considerations, they hypothesize improved local regional control at several anatomic sites is likely to decrease the ultimate rate of metastatic disease.

RESULTS AND PROGNOSIS

Five-Year vs. Ten-Year Survival Rates (Table 1-9, Fig. 1-14)

Survival rates have been used extensively to assess accomplishments of treatment. The most frequently used standard is 5-year survival but as data have matured 10 years and longer survival data have become available, particularly with maturation of the SEER (62,71). Survival rates, however, can be confounded by earlier detection of cancer and improved, more definite staging — both of which may add to and/or appear to lengthen survival. The "Will Rogers" phenomenon, aptly described by Feinstein (16), illustrates how improved staging appears to improve survival for each stage, but not overall survival.

More recently, a better yardstick for measuring overall progress is decreasing the mortality rate. Mortality does have

Table 1-9. Long-Term Survival Rates for Patients Diagnosed in 1973 to 1975, SEER Program, All Races, Males and Females

Primary Site	No. Cases	5-Year Rate Observed	5-Year Rate Relative	10-Year Rate Observed	10-Year Rate Relative	5- to 10-Year Relative Rate for 5-Year Survivors
All sites	160,000	40	48	28	41	84
Oral cavity & pharynx	5,435	43	51	28	41	84
Esophagus	1,690	4	4	2	3	67
Stomach	4,809	11	14	7	11	79
Colon	15,441	38	48	26	44	89
Rectum	7,228	37	46	25	40	84
Liver	950	3	3	2	2	61*
Gallbladder	750	6	8	2	4	58*
Pancreas	4,621	2	3	2	2	79+
Larynx	2,225	55	64	36	51	79
Lung & bronchus	21,474	10	11	6	8	70
Bone	417	48	52	40	46	88
Soft tissue	1,011	52	59	41	53	89
Melanoma	3,009	69	76	56	68	89
Breast	23,289	65	73	47	60	82
Urinary bladder	7,510	55	71	37	63	86
Kidney	2,937	42	49	30	42	84
Brain	2,471	16	18	12	14	73
Thyroid gland	1,933	86	91	81	90	98
Hodgkin's disease	1,665	62	66	50	57	83
Non-Hodgkin's lymphomas	4,416	38	45	23	33	90
Multiple myeloma	1,919	19	23	5	9	36
Leukemias	5,214	27	33	13	20	61
Acute lymphocytic	586	34	36	28	30	82
Chronic lymphocytic	1,656	51	67	23	41	59
Acute granulocytic	1,257	5	6	4	5	74+
Chronic granulocytic	777	16	20	3	5	24

*Standard error is greater than 10%.
+Standard error is 5% to 10%.
SEER = Surveillance, Epidemiology, and End Results.
From Myers and Gloeckler Ries (62) with permission.

the advantage of being a definitive end point, measurable by all investigators. Although overall cancer mortality is tending to rise slightly in recent ACS data (71), it is confounded by death from some cause, which at some time in each life, is unavoidable. Mettlin (59) has introduced the concept of premature mortality — that is, death or curing before the full passage of a normal life span. Evidence will be presented to alert the reader to some pitfalls and pratfalls in cancer statistics but will further emphasize that cancer curability has been increased because of both diagnostic and therapeutic gains that have been made in the past three decades.

The 5-year survival rate is most commonly chosen as a parameter to measure survival, and is indicative of the curability of the cancer (29,33) (Fig. 1-14). It is a simple, convenient parameter but it is based on a complex interplay of many factors. It depends on the accessibility of the cancer, the stage in which the cancer is detected, the effectiveness of treatment, and the type of host harboring the cancer (Table 1-9). Some points of interest follow.

1. Localized cancers are highly curable, ranging from 50% to 80% in most sites.
2. Regionalized lymph node involvement always portends more aggressive disease and is a poor prognostic factor, often reducing survival to 50% or less.

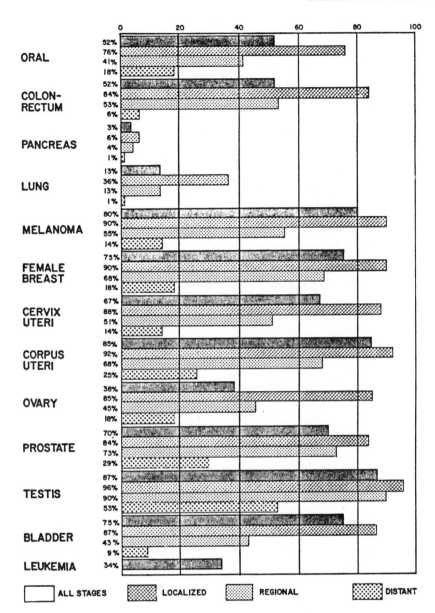

	0	20	40	60	80	100

ORAL
52%
76%
41%
18%

COLON-RECTUM
52%
84%
53%
6%

PANCREAS
3%
6%
4%
1%

LUNG
13%
36%
13%
1%

MELANOMA
80%
90%
55%
14%

FEMALE BREAST
75%
90%
68%
18%

CERVIX UTERI
67%
88%
51%
14%

CORPUS UTERI
85%
92%
68%
25%

OVARY
38%
85%
45%
18%

PROSTATE
70%
84%
73%
29%

TESTIS
87%
96%
90%
53%

BLADDER
75%
87%
43%
9%

LEUKEMIA
34%

☐ ALL STAGES   ▨ LOCALIZED   ▨ REGIONAL   ▨ DISTANT

*Adjusted for normal life expectancy.
This chart is based on cases diagnosed in 1974-1985.

Source: Cancer Statistics Branch,
National Cancer Institute.

Fig. 1-14. Five-year cancer survival rates for selected sites illustrates a large portion of cancers are highly curable if detected in a localized fashion confined to the primary site. Regional nodes and metastasis can be controlled but yield less favorable 5-year survival. From American Cancer Society (2), with permission.

3. Distant metastases are rarely curable but still are compatible, with 5-year survival ranging from 5% to 20%. This survival figure also reflects effective palliation by chemotherapeutic and hormonal agents.
4. Survival is generally better in cancers located in accessible sites than in internal organs because they can be identified while in localized stages. This finding reflects the importance of early detection.

If one examines the trends in survival based upon End Results Group data and the SEER program over the past three decades using the 5-year result, there is evidence for a significant gain in survival for each decade for the majority of

cancer sites (Fig. 1-1 and Table 1-1) (72). The most striking gains (≥ 10%) have been made in colon, rectum, larynx, melanoma, breast (female), uterine (cervix and corpus), prostate, testis, bladder, kidney, thyroid, Hodgkin's, non-Hodgkin's lymphoma, multiple myeloma, and some of the leukemias, e.g., acute lymphocytes.

Ten-Year Follow-Up

Myers and Gloekler Ries (62) provide an in-depth analysis of SEER survival rates for 10 years or longer with important observations as to survival beyond that time. For long-term survival rates, all races, both sexes — the 5- and 10-year rates are 40% and 28% and the relative 5- and 10-year rates are

48% and 41%, respectively. The attrition rate is low and survival averages 84% (70% to 98%), indicating most 5-year survivors live to 10 years, with a few exceptions such as multiple myeloma and chronic lymphocytic and granulocyte leukemias. Table 1-9 (57) provides the 5- and 10-year survival rates for 24 major primary sites and offers relative rates, which is the ratio of observed survival rate to the general population survival rate and is an indirect adjustment for death due to causes other than cancer. The sites with the highest 10-year survival rates are thyroid (90%), melanoma (68%), bladder (63%), breast (60%), and Hodgkin's (51%). In males, favorable sites for 10-year results are testis (74%) and in females corpus cancer (87%). In conclusion, for most cancers the chance for surviving a second 5 years is greater than for the first 5 years.

Mortality (Premature or Cancer-Related Mortality) Rates

In a convincing analysis of years lost to cancer, Mettlin (59) illustrates the advances made through better diagnosis and treatment by age group as a function of decade (Table 1-10). The largest percentage of decrease in mortality rates over the decades is in the pediatric and young adult age group from 0 to 14 and 15 to 24 years of age (44%). The mortality rates have declined for the 25 to 44 year age group to 22% to 23% and even at 45 to 54 years it has fallen 9.4%, the only exception being the 55 to 64 year group, which has risen 3.8% by most sites. A decline in mortality rate has occurred for most major cancer sites except lung cancers, which unfortunately continue to increase in incidence. Mortality rates have lessened for the upper aerodigestive passage, digestive organs, breast, genital organs, primary organs, leukemias, and lymphomas, dropping 11.9% to 38.9% at different sites (Table 1-11) (72).

In summary, standardized rates of years of life lost may be an excellent tool for measuring the success of cancer treatments. The evidence strongly suggests reductions in the cancer burden over the past 3 decades are real.

Lack of Uniformity in End-Stage Reporting (3)

The lack of uniformity in end-stage reporting is a major source of confusion when comparing the results of different treatment modalities. As mentioned, this can be overcome by agreement on a dual anatomic-pathologic classification for each cancer site. Assuming that such a classification exists, the following common errors and points should be looked for:

Table 1-10. Age-Specific and Age-Adjusted Rates of Years of Life Lost to Cancer, 1970 to 1985 (Per 100,000 Population in Category)

Age (yr)	Years of Life Lost				Percent Change from 1970 to 1985
	1970	1975	1980	1985	
0-14	362.25	270.25	258.25	201.25	-44.4
15-24	377.6	304.8	295.8	218.4	-42.2
25-34	585.8	55.2	433.1	450.8	-23.0
35-44	1,517.2	1,326.0	1,241.8	1,783.0	-22.7
45-54	2,828.8	2,833.4	2,777.6	2,563.7	-9.4
55-64	2,376.0	2,391.4	2,374.9	2,465.1	+3.8
Age-Adjusted Rates	1,058.3	988.4	947.7	890.3	-15.9

(1970 Standard Population)
From Mettlin et al. (59), with permission.

Table 1-11. Age-Adjusted Rates*of Years of Life lost by Cancer Type,1970 to 1985

Type of Cancer (ICD Codes)	1970	1985	Percent Change, 1970 to 1985
Lip, oral cavity, & pharynx (140-149)	23.1	19.9	-13.9
Digestive organs & peritoneum (150-159)	185.4	157.9	-14.8
Respiratory & intrathoracic organs (160-165)	199.5	221.2	+10.9
Breast (174-175)	121.1	104.9	-13.4
Genital organs (179-187)	108.1	66.1	-38.9
Urinary organs (188-189)	32.8	27.1	-17.4
All other and unspecified sites (170-173, 190-199)	188.3	165.8	-11.9
Leukemia (204-208)	107.4	71.0	-33.9
Lymphatic & hemapoietic tissues (200-203)	87.0	60.7	-30.2

*Per 100,000 Population.
Ninth International Classification of Disease Three-Digit Codes.
From Silverberg (72), with permission.

1. The starting time for determination of survival recommended by the AJC is the date of treatment initiation or the date tumor-directed treatment was decided on. This definition is used because it usually coincides with the date of clinical staging of the cancer.
2. A probability of less than 5% (P < .05) is generally considered to be of statistical significance in reference to 95% confidence limits.
3. The results should be in terms of absolute survival, that is, patients who are lost to follow-up are included. If they are excluded, the survival rate is inevitably better, and the survival figures are referred to as determinate or relative. Calculation by direct method is the simplest procedure for summarizing patient survival. This is done by calculating the percentage of patients alive at the end of the specified interval, such as 5 years, using only patients exposed to the risk of dying for the last 5 years.
4. The survival may be referred to as, e.g., 3 months to 10 years with an "average" survival of 2.3 years. This is meaningless.
5. The 5-year survival rates should be designated "without recurrence" or, preferably, "symptom-free." For some carcinomas, such as breast cancer and thyroid neoplasm, this is not a long enough follow-up period.
6. Ideally, the presentation of data should be by "actuarial" or "life table" method, corrected for age and sex. This method is described by the AJC (3):
   a. Observed survival (Table 1-9) (73): "The actuarial or life table method uses all survival information accumulated to the closing date of the study and describes the manner in which patient depletion occurred during that period. It presents a survival pattern in which the patients who are lost to follow-up are depleted in a mathematical calculation similar to the patent populations under continued follow-up; it is not a specified point in survival like the 5-year

survival. Such data are often displayed graphically in journals as survival curves ranging from 1 year to 10 years" (3).

  b. Adjusted survival rate: This is usually higher than the observed survival and corrects for deaths from other causes for patients free of cancer at the time of death.

  c. Relative survival rate Table 1-9: The survival rate is adjusted for "normal mortality expectation" in a general population similar to the patient group in the study with respect to race, sex, age, and calendar period of observation.

  d. Projected survival rate: There is a tendency in some of the present literature to project survival curves in investigational studies beyond the median follow-up time. The AJC recommends that "survival rates probably should not be computed for intervals in which fewer than ten patients enter the interval alive" (3). The percentage surviving and the actual number of patients should be shown at the tail end of computerized curves.

The pressure for investigators to publish and to present early and most often projected survival rates has led to false optimism regarding a new form of treatment. Premature survival curves plateau, are horizontal reaching to infinity, or precipitously step vertically to zero depending on the outcome of the first few patients treated. A sobering analysis of the treatment of leukemia by Powles, et al (64), shows how the reported survival rate varies inversely with time from the completion of a study (Fig. 1-15) (64). A statistical value of $P > .05$ for median survival at the completion of a study, or shortly thereafter, does not predict improvement in later overall long-term survival. Only sufficient follow-up of a minimum of 5 years, or better 10 years, is the necessary test of time for true cancer cure.

Patterns of Failure and Corrective Strategies (58)

As important as survival rates are to learn about treatment outcomes such as patterns of failure — that is, the first

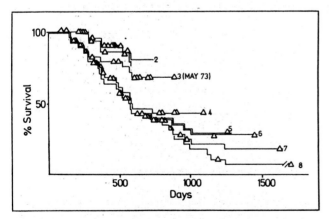

Fig. 1-15. Sequential 6-monthly analysis of the duration of survival (from diagnosis) of 28 patients receiving chemo-immunotherapy. The first analysis (curve 1) was in May 1972, curve 3 (May 1973) corresponds to the entry of the last patient in the group, and curves 4-8 are analyses at 6-monthly intervals thereafter. Triangles denote patients remaining alive and the curves drop each time a patient dies, by an amount proportional to the total number of patients in the study. From Powles *et al.* (64), with permission.

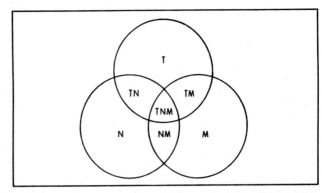

Fig. 1-16. Venn diagram of 7 failure pathways for tumor (T), node (N), metastases (M), and combinations. See the text for an explanation. From Rubin and Carter (69), with permission.

evidence of relapse in recurrence of the cancer. The corrective strategy will depend upon whether the primary tumor, the regional nodes, metastases, or combinations are formed at the time of the work-up of the first relapse. There are seven possible failure pathways, as noted in Fig. 1-16 (69).

Primary (T) Failures

Inability to control primary tumors, particularly in locally advanced stages when invasion of contiguous structures and viscera has occurred, remains a significant obstacle to cancer cure (69). As illustrated in Table 1-12, Suit (73) has estimated the failure rate of advanced cancers at specific sites that are not readily eradicable: cancers of the oral cavity, oropharynx, and nasopharynx (T3, T4, N2, N3); gynecologic cancers of the cervix (stages III and IV), ovary (stage IIB), and vulva; large advanced genitourinary cancers of the bladder (stages B and C) and prostate (stage C) (Table 1-12). GI tumors frequently begin insidiously and can reach advanced stages in the stomach, colon, and inaccessible sites, such as the pancreas. Soft tissue sarcomas are often locally recurrent and invasive prior to metastasizing. Malignant brain tumors, such as glioblastoma multiforme, medulloblastoma, and mixed gliomas, which are locally invasive and rarely disseminate outside the central nervous system, illustrate the problem clearly.

Table 1-12. LOCAL/REGIONAL FAILURE AS PRIMARY CAUSE OF DEATH

Tumor Site	Estimated No. Deaths
Head and neck	4,700
Esophagus	3,763
Breast	4,774
Uterine cervix	4,366
Uterine corpus	1,881
Ovary	6,480
Prostate	12,360
Bladder	4,950
Central nervous system	8,277
Skin	2,240
Lung	8,316
Lymphomas (excluding myeloma)	1,872
Stomach	4,380
Pancreas	12,000
Colon-rectum	20,760
Bone and connective tissue	1,020
Total	102,139

From Suit (73), with permission.

Nodal (N) Failures

Nodal failures can occur at major node-bearing regions that drain the sites of invasive cancers. Metastatic lymph nodes, which can be difficult to control, include cervical nodes in head and neck cancer, axillary and supraclavicular nodes in breast cancer, mediastinal nodes in esophageal and lung cancers, para-aortic and pelvic nodes in gynecologic and genitourinary cancers, and mesenteric nodes in GI cancers. As primary tumors are controlled, the N category is frequently seen as a major failure pathway; this failure has necessitated extended-field radiation treatment at many sites. The introduction of total nodal irradiation techniques for Hodgkin's and non-Hodgkin's lymphomas has focused on the control of nodal extensions, most often in contiguous or adjacent uninvolved nodes, by extending fields below the diaphragm for most presentations above the diaphragm.

Metastatic (M) Failures

The majority of cancer patients fail as a result of disseminated disease. The most common cancers, breast and lung, are aggressive and metastasize in the early stages of growth, often before clinical detection. Undifferentiated and anaplastic cancers generally metastasize aggressively; melanomas, sarcomas of the bone and soft tissue, choriocarcinomas and ovarian cancers can also be widespread at the time of diagnosis. Although metastases affect more than one organ system, the documentation of the first metastatic site may suggest elective treatment to specific organs.

Combinations of TNM

Four additional failure pathways (TN, NM, TM, TNM) represent combinations of the TNM compartments (Fig. 1-13). In many advanced cancers of the breast, lung, head and neck, and gynecologic sites (T3, T4, N2, N3 groupings in stages III and IV), both primary and nodal involvement are difficult to completely resect or eradicate by irradiation. For example, local control of the primary tumor may occur in testicular and ovarian tumors, but nodal and metastatic spread are the main failure pathways (Fig. 1-13). Oat cell cancer, as well as other types of lung cancer, advanced gastric and rectal cancers and pancreatic cancer, can and often do fail in all three compartments. Although the T and N categories may be the overt areas of failure, better local control is certain to unmask occult metastases.

New therapeutic strategies for cancer control should be based on the failure patterns of a given cancer at each stage of presentation. Ideally, all modalities should be optimally combined to achieve the best control possible in the three compartments of TNM. Combined irradiation and chemotherapy will augment each other to control advanced disease in the primary (T) or nodal (N) compartments; in an additive and interactive manner, combined treatments can also be used to control overt or suspected occult metastases in the M compartment. Patients at high risk for recurrence are the optimal target group for clinical trials and protocols investigating the elective addition of treatments.

CLINICAL INVESTIGATIONS

There is an increasing interest in the development of clinical trials (6,69) to reconcile differences in therapeutic claims. This means combined treatment in which surgery and/or radiation therapy and/or chemotherapy can be used. A demonstration of small gains, prospective trials, and detailed protocols is essential for correct conclusions.

The basis of the multidisciplinary approach to cancer management is for all responsible disciplines to be represented in the initial decision making. Unidisciplinary actions can determine a course of events that limit the application of other modalities. The clinical trial and the tumor board offer a means of clinical interaction for patient care that is lacking in consultation by crisis and recurrence.

Cooperative controlled clinical studies (4,18,34) are being developed to answer complex treatment questions. These are multidisciplinary undertakings at the local level, and they involve multiple universities and medical centers at the national and even the international level. Although the hope for rapidly achieving good data lies in cooperative national protocols (34), this ideal will be difficult to achieve. It assumes that clinicians and pathologists at different institutions can agree on classifications, and that treatment selection can be unbiased. These criticisms notwithstanding, this seems to be the only practical solution to the dilemma presented by small series and long time lapses for evaluation of results to be meaningful.

- Decision trees with the option of exercising each of the major modalities (surgery, radiation, and chemotherapy) are good models for protocol design. Models for the multidisciplinary process are shown, indicating many options that exist in developing combinations just by virtue of varying the aggressiveness of a mode or its sequence (Figs. 1-17 and 1-18) (67).
- Vital sources for developing clinical trials are the leads generated by basic research. The integration of the investigation into clinical studies is another essential feature of progress.
- With so many possible therapeutic options (Fig. 1-15) and the development of 25 to 50 effective chemotherapeutic agents that can be used in combinations of 2 to 10, only a few alternatives can be explored. The Cancer Therapy Evaluation Program of the Division of Cancer Treatment at the NCI is responsible for drug development and for monitoring ongoing clinical trials in cooperative groups.

The size and scope of clinical trials in cancer diagnosis and treatment are perhaps the largest such efforts undertaken in modern medicine. New procedures, new agents and new combinations of agents and modalities are being evaluated in a thousand studies worldwide (4). These trials collectively cost hundreds of millions of dollars. Information on these trials is available in abstract form in "Compilation of Experimental Cancer Therapy Protocol Summaries" (34) and include phase I (toxicity), phase II (search for efficacy), and phase III (demonstrate if more effective than standard therapy). Computerized systems exist to provide on-line searching by key terminology of current trends and results.

COMPUTERIZED INFORMATION AND DATABASE SYSTEMS (21')

The BRS Colleague System offers health care professionals, through their computer via telephone lines, access to a number of medical databases. One of the largest is MEDLINE, the National Library of Medicine's (NLM) computer version of *Index Medicus*. It covers over 3800 international journals

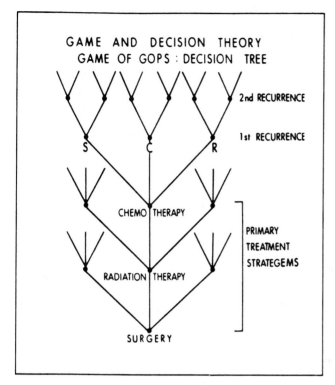

Fig. 1-17. Game and decision theory — game of gops — decision tree. Game of gops refers to the game of pure strategy. Model for this is 3-handed card game in which there is 1 winner. This game can be applied to the cancer management problem when it is seen from a multidisciplinary point of view. For each cancer patient there are 3 players: the surgeon (S), radiotherapist (R), and chemotherapist (C). Each has a primary decision but was made not to use it. Unidisciplinary decision, therefore, has been substituted for what could have been a multidiscipinary decision. From Rubin (67), with permission.

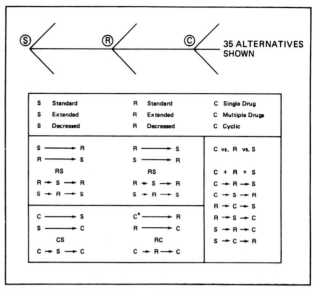

Fig. 1-18. Game of gops model shows three alternatives in cancer management: Surgery (S), radiation therapy (R), and chemotherapy (C). If standard form of treatment is accepted, there are two other possibilities. For each modality they can be extended (made more radical) or decreased (made more conservative). Tabulation below model indicates at least 35 combinations and emphasizes the need for clinical trials. From Rubin (67), with permission.

from 1966 to the present. Of greater use to oncologists is the Oncology Library which consists of:

Cancerlit — produced by the NLM; covers all aspects of cancer research, including therapy, cancer-causing agents, and the biochemistry, immunology, physiology, and other biology of cancer topics.

PDQ Cancer Information — produced by National Cancer Institute (NCI); contains prognostic and state-of-the-art treatment information on 82 major cancers with key citations from the literature.

PDQ Protocole — produced by NCI; contains information on over 1,000 active treatment protocols; includes study objectives, patient entry criteria, special study parameters, details of the treatment regimen, who is performing the trial, and the location of the trial.

PDQ Directory of Physicians and Organizations — produced by NCI; contains names and addresses of physicians and health care organizations who devote a major portion of their clinical practice to treatment of cancer patients.

Cancer Treatment Reports — published monthly by NCI; covers radiotherapy, chemotherapy, immunotherapy, mechanisms of drug action, medicinal chemistry, and summaries of clinical trials.

Journals of the National Cancer Institute — published montly by NCI; contains reports on original observations in laboratory and clinical research on both human and animal subjects.

There is a one-time registration fee to obtain the password, user manual, and customer support services. There is an hourly connect fee and an online and offline document charge for using the databases. To obtain information on BRS Colleague call 1-800-289-4277.

Recommended Reading

There are many excellent general references on the subject of cancer. Our favorite references for the student include *Ackerman's and del Regato's Cancer: Diagnosis, Treatment and Prognosis* (13a) for correlative pathology and clinical presentations, and the AFIP Tumor Fascicles in *Atlas of Tumor Pathology* (5) for detailed pathology at tumor sites, since these are beautifully illustrated. For general principles of cancer treatment, we recommend *Cancer: Principles and Practice of Oncology,* by DeVita, Hellman, and Rosenberg (14); and *Principles and Practice of Radiation Oncology* by Perez and Brady (21). *Clinical Judgment* and *Clinical Epidemiology: The Architecture of Clinical Research* by Feinstein (15a,16) are highly advised as a philosophical approach to the optimal way to obtain, record, and analyze clinical data. For the basic science of oncology, see Tannock's and Hill's *The Basic Science of Oncology* (31). A large number of oncology journals exist entirely devoted to clinical and research reports. These include *Cancer; Seminars in Oncology; Journal of Clinical Oncology; American Journal of Clinical Oncology; International Journal of Radiation Oncology, Biology and Physics; Journal of Gynecologic Oncology;* and *Journal of Surgical Oncology.*

REFERENCES

General References

1. Ackerman, L.V.; del Regato, J.A. Cancer: diagnosis, treatment and prognosis, 5th ed. St. Louis, MO: C.V. Mosby, Co.; 1977.
2. American Cancer Society: Cancer facts and figures. New York: American Cancer Society; 1982.
2a. American Cancer Society. Ca - A Cancer Journal for Clinicians. New York, NY: American Cancer Society; Vol. 40, No. 1, 1990.
3. American Joint Committe on cancer staging and end-results reporting (AJC). Manual for staging of cancer, 3rd ed. Philadelphia, PA: J.B. Lippincott, Co.; 1988.
4. Armitage, P.; Flanant, R.; Gehan, E.A., eds. Controlled therapeutic trials in cancer. International Union Against Cancer (UICC), Technical Report Series, vol. 14, 3rd ed. Geneva, Switzerland: UICC, 1974.
5. Atlas of tumor pathology, second series. Fascicles 1-17. National Research Council Committee on Pathology. Washington, DC: Armed Forces Institute of Pathology; 1950-1980.
6. Atlas of tumor radiology, vols. 1-13. Chicago, IL: Year Book Medical Publishing, 1975-present.
7. Bragg, D.G.; Rubin, P.; Youker, J.E., eds. Oncologic imaging and diagnosis. Elmsford, NY: Pergamon Press; 1985.
8. Busch, H., ed. Methods in cancer research, vols. 1-18. New York, NY: Academic Press; 1979.
9. Busch, H. Molecular biology of cancer. New York, NY: Academic Press; 1974.
10. Calabresi, P.; Schein, P.S.; Rosenberg, S.A., eds. Medical oncology. Basic principles and clinical management of cancer. New York, NY: Macmillan; 1985.
11. Carter, S.K.; Glatstein, E.; Livingston, R.B. Principles of cancer treatment. New York, NY: McGraw-Hill; 1982.
12. Chabner, B.A., ed. Pharmacologic principles of cancer treatment. Philadelphia, PA: WB Saunders Co; 1982.
13. Committee on Tumor Nomenclature, International Union Against Cancer (UICC), 2nd ed. New York, NY: Springer-Verlag; 1969.
13a. del Regato, J.A.; Spjut, H.J.; Cox, J.D. Ackerman and del Regato's Cancer: diagnosis, treatment and prognosis, 6th ed. St. Louis, MO: CV Mosby Co.; 1985.
14. DeVita, V.T.; Hellman, S.; Rosenberg, S.A., eds. Cancer: principles and practice of oncology, 3rd ed. Philadelphia, PA: J.B. Lippincott Co.; 1989.
15. Environment and cancer, 24th symposium on fundamental cancer research, M.D. Anderson Hospital and Tumor Institute, 1971. Baltimore, MD: Williams & Wilkins; 1972.
15a. Feinstein, A.R. Clinical epidemiology: The architecture of clinical research. Philadelphia, PA: WB Saunders Co.; 1985.
16. Feinstein, A.R. Clinical judgement. Huntington, NY: Robert E. Dreiger Publishing Co., Inc.; 1974.
17. Fletcher, G.H. Textbook of radiotherapy, 3rd ed. Philadelphia, PA: Lea & Febiger; 1980.
18. Hellman, K., ed. Interaction of radiation and anti-tumor drugs. Intl. J. Radiat. Oncol. Biol. Phys. 4:1-173; 1978.
19. Holland, J.F.; Frei, E. III, eds. Cancer medicine. Philadelphia, PA: Lea & Febiger; 1973.
20. International Union Against Cancer (UICC). Commission on clinical oncology. TNM classification of malignant tumors. Geneva, Switzerland: UICC; 1968.
21. Perez, C.A.; Brady, L.W., eds. Principles and practice of radiation oncology. 2nd ed. Philadelphia, PA: J.B. Lippincott Co.; 1992.
21'. Physician's Data Query. Cancer. Nat'l Cancer Inst. Bethesda, MD: 1992.
21a. Rhoads, J.E., ed. Cancer. A Journal of the American Cancer Society (supplement). American Cancer Society Workshop on Clinicals Trials held at Naples, Florida, September 14-15, 1989. Philadelphia, PA: J.B. Lippincott Co., Vol. 65, No. 3, February 1990.
21b. Rhoads, J.E., ed. Cancer. A Journal of the American Cancer Society (supplement). Philadelphia, PA: J.B. Lippincott Co., Vol. 65, No. 10, May 1990.
22. Rosenthal, S.; Carignan, J.R.; Smith, B.D., eds. Medical care of the cancer patient. Philadelphia, PA: W.B. Saunders Co.; 1987.
23. Rubin, E.; Farber, J.L., eds. Pathology. Philadelphia, PA: J.B. Lippincott Co.; 1988:140-195.
24. Rubin, P., ed. Current concepts in cancer. Chicago, IL: American Medical Association; 1974.
25. Ruddon, R.W. Cancer biology. New York, NY: Oxford University Press; 1987.
26. Ruddon, R.W., ed. Biological markers of neoplasia: basic and applied aspects. New York, NY: Elsevier, North-Holland; 1978.
27. Skeel, R.T. Handbook of cancer chemotherapy. Boston, MA: Little Brown & Co; 1987.
28. Smithers, D.W. On the nature of neoplasms in man. Edinburgh, Scotland: E. & S. Livingstone; 1964.
29. Staquet, M.J., ed. The design of clinical trials in cancer therapy. Mt. Kisco, NY: Futura Publishing Co.; 1973.
30. Stekel, R.J.; Kagen, A.R. Diagnosis and staging of cancer: a radiological approach. Philadelphia, PA: W.B. Saunders Co.; 1976.
31. Tannock, I.F.; Hill, R.P., eds. The basic science of oncology. Elmsford, NY: Pergamon Press; 1987.
32. Underwood, J.C.E. Introduction to biopsy interpretation and surgical pathology. New York, NY: Springer-Verlag; 1987.
33. End results of cancer therapy. US Dept of Health Education and Welfare, report no. 5. Bethesda, MD: National Cancer Institute; 1976.
34. Summaries of clinical protocols, 5th ed. US Dept of Health and Human Services, Public Health Service. National Institutes of Health, NIH publication #81-1116, May, 1981.
35. Vaeth, J.M., ed. The Interrelationship of chemotherapeutic agents and radiation therapy in the treatment of tancer. In: Frontiers of radiation therapy and oncology, vol. 4. Basel, New York: S. Karger; 1969.
36. Vaeth, J.M., ed. The interrelationship of surgery and radiation therapy and oncology. New York, NY: Karger; 1971.
37. Warburgh, O.H. The metabolism of tumors: investigations from the Kaiser Wilhelm Institute for Biology. London, UK: Constable and Co., Ltd.; 1930.
38. World Health Organization: International histological classification of tumors, Nos. 1-20. Geneva, Switzerland: World Health Organization; 1978.

Specific References

39. Berlin, N.I. Tumor markers in cancer prevention and detection. Cancer 47:1151-1153; 1981.
40. Barger, H.B.K. Uterine cancer (prevention). Cancer 47:1126-1132; 1981.
41. Bishop, J.M. The molecular genetics of cancer. Science 1235:308-311; 1987.
42. Blumberg, G.S.; London, W.T. Hepatitis B virus and primary hepatocellular carcinoma: the relation of "icrons" to cancer. Cold Spring Harbor, NY: 7th Cold Spring Harbor Symposium on Cell Proliferation, 1979; 1983.
43. Boice, J.D.; Hutchison, G.B. Leukemia in women following radiotherapy for cervical cancer: ten-year follow-up of an internation study. J. Natl. Cancer Inst. 65:115-129; 1980.
44. Bragg, D. Tumor imaging in diagnostic radiology. Cancer 47:1159-1163; 1981.
45. Broders, A.C. The grading of carcinoma. Minn. Med. 8:726-730; 1925.
46. Burkitt, D.P. A sarcoma involving the jaws in African children. Br. J. Surg. 46:218-224; 1958-1959.
47. Carlile, T. Breast cancer detection. Cancer 47:1164-1169; 1981.
47a. Denoix, P.F. Bull Inst. Nat. Hyg. (Paris) 1: 1-69 (1944) and 5: 52-82; 1944.
48. DeVita, V.T., Jr. Principles of chemotherapy. In: DeVita, V.T., Jr.; Hellman, S.; Rosenberg, S.A., eds. Cancer: Principles and practice of oncology, 2nd ed. Philadelphia, PA: JB Lippincott Co; 1985:257-285.
49. Fraumeni, J.F., Jr., ed. Persons at high risk of cancer: an approach to cancer etiology and control. New York, NY: Academic Press; 1975.
49a. Fuks, Z.; Leibel, S.A.; Wallner, K.E.; Begg, C.B.; Fair, W.R.; Anderson, L.L.; Hilaris, B.S.; Whitmore, W.F. The effect of local control on metastatic dissemination in carcinoma of the prostate: Long-term results in patients treated with I-125 implantation. Int J Rad Oncol Biol Phys 21:537-547; 1991.
50. Gallo, R.C. The first human retrovirus. Scientific Am. 256(12):89-99; 1986.

51. Gilbertsen, V.A.; Nelms, J.M. The prevention of invasive cancer of the rectum. Cancer 41:1137-1139; 1978.
52. Gordon, H. Oncogenes. Mayo Clinic Proc. 60: 697-713; 1985.
53. Henle, G.; Henle, W.; Diehl, V. Relation of Burkitt's tumor-associated herpes-type virus to infectious mononucleosis. Proc. Natl. Acad. Sci. USA 59:94-101; 1968.
54. Hoffer, P.B.; Beckman, C.; Henkin, R.E., eds. Gallium imaging. New York, NY: John Wiley & Sons; 1978.
55. Hoover, R.; Fraumeni, J.F. Drug-induced cancer. Cancer 47:1071-1080; 1981.
56. Howley, P.M.; Schlegel, R. Papillomavirus transformation. In: Salzman, M.P.; Howley, P.M., eds. The papovaviridae: II. The papillomaviruses. New York: Plenum Publishing Corp.; 1987:141-163.
57. Karnofsky, D.A.; Burchenal, J.H.; Armistead, G.C.; et al. Triethylene melamine in the treatment of neoplastic disease. Arch. Intern. Med. 87:477-516; 1951.
57a. Leibel, S.A.; Ling, C.C.; Kutcher, G.J.; Mohan, R.; Cordon-Cordo, C.; Fuks, Z. The biological basis for conformal three-dimensional radiation therapy. Int J Radiat Oncol Biol Phys 21:805-811; 1991.
57b. Leibel, A.A.; Scott, C.B.; Mohiuddin, M.; Marcial, V.A.; Coia, L.R.; Davis, L.W.; Fuks, Z. The effect of local-regional control on distant metastatic dissemination in carcinoma of the head and neck: Results of an analysis from the RTOG head and neck database. Int J Radiat Oncol Biol Phys 21:549-556; 1991.
58. Merigan, T.C. Virology and immune mechanisms. Cancer 47:1091-1094; 1981.
59. Mettlin, C. Trends in years of life lost to cancer 1970-1985. CA. American Cancer Society, Inc. 39(1):33-39.
60. Miller, E.C.; Miller, J.A. Mechanisms of chemical carcinogenesis. Cancer 47:1055-1064; 1981.
61. Miller, J.A. Carcinogenesis by chemicals: an overview. Cancer Res. 30:559-576; 1970.
62. Myers, M.H.; Gloeckler Ries, L.A. Cancer patient survival rates: SEER program results for 10 years of follow-up. CA. 39(1):21-32; 1989.
63. Pitot, H.C. Drugs as promoters of carcinogenesis. In: Estabrook, R.W.; Lindenlaub, E., eds. The induction of drug metabolism. New York, NY: Schattauer, Verlag; 1979:471.
64. Powles, R.; Russell, J.; Lister, T.A.; et al. Immunotherapy for acute myelogenous leukaemia: a controlled clinical study two and one-half years after entry of the last patient. Br. J. Cancer 35:265-272; 1977.
65. Rapp, F. Current knowledge of mechanisms of viral carcinogenesis. CRC Crit. Rev. Toxicol. 13:197; 1984.
66. Rosner, R.; Grunwald, H.W.; Zarrabi, M.H. Acute leukemia as a complication of cytotoxic chemotherapy. Intl. J. Radiat. Oncol. Biol. Phys. 5:1705-1708; 1979.
67. Rubin, P., ed. Current concepts in cancer: cancer of the urogenital tract, parts I and II. Chicago, IL: American Medical Association; 1969.
68. Rubin, P. A unified classification of tumors: an oncotaxonomy with symbols. Cancer 31:963-982; 1973.
69. Rubin, P.; Carter, S. Combination radiation therapy and chemotherapy: a logical basis for their clinical use. Cancer 26:274-292; 1976.
70. Sarver, N.; Rabson, M.S.; Yang, Y.-C.; Bryne, J.C.; Howley, P.M. Localization and analysis of bovine papillomavirus type 1 transforming functions. J. Virol. 52:377-388; 1984.
71. Silverberg, E.; Boring, C.C.; Squires, T.S. Cancer statistics, 1990. CA. American Cancer Society, Inc. 40:9-26; 1990.
72. Silverberg, E. Cancer statistics, 1989. CA-Cancer J. Clin. 39(1):3-20; 1989.
73. Suit, H.D. Statement of the problem pertaining to the effect of dose fractionation and total treatment on the response to X-irradiation. In: Time and dose relationships in radiation biology as aplied to radiotherapy. Brookhaven National Laboratory Report 50203 (C-57). Upton, NY; 1969.
74. Taylor, W.R.; Fontana, R.S.; Uhlenhopp, M.A.; et al. Some results of screening for early lung cancer. Cancer 47:1114-1120; 1981.
75. Vital Statistics of the United States. US Dept of Health and Human Services, Public Health Service, National Center for Health Statistics, Hyattsville, MD; 1978.
76. Williams, P.A. A productive history and physical examination in prevention and early detection of cancer. Cancer 47:1146-1150; 1981.
77. Zeman, R.K.; Gottschalk, A. Current aspects of nuclear imaging in clinical oncology. Cancer 47:1154-1158; 1981.

Chapter **2**

THE BIOLOGY OF CANCER

The genetic code is the small dictionary which relates the four letter language of the nucleic acids to the twenty letter languaage of proteins.

Francis Crick (2a)

CHARACTERISTICS OF MALIGNANT CELLS

Proliferation

Almost by definition both benign and malignant, cells must proliferate in order to produce a tumor (i.e., a mass) (3).

Autonomy

Tumor cell proliferation is autonomous in the sense that it is inappropriate, and control mechanisms must therefore be abnormal. However, malignant cells may respond to normal control signals (e.g., proliferation of breast cancer cells may be stimulated by low levels of estrogen and inhibited by high levels). The growth of some tumor cells appears to depend upon growth factors that the tumor cells themselves secrete, inappropriately; these cells are not really independent of growth factors (see below).

Cellular Growth Rate

In normal proliferating tissues, such as the intestinal crypt cells, the cell cycle time is generally 24-48 hours; malignant cells do not grow faster than this. Cell cycle times are generally 1-5 days for tumor cells; the abnormal growth of the mass is due to the persistence of cycling rather than a rapid rate of cycling. In normal proliferating tissues, stem cells divide and daughter cells begin to differentiate. After a more or less defined number of divisions, the daughter cells differentiate to terminal cells (for instance mature granulocytes, red blood cells, and squamous cells) and cannot divide again. In tumors arising in stem cell systems, proliferation per se is not abnormal because the normal cell of origin proliferates. Rather, it is differentiation to terminal cells that is abnormal and delayed or absent in cells of the malignant clone. In tumors arising from cells that are normally nonproliferating, such as liver cells, the activation of proliferation is an abnormality, and proliferative signals or the proliferative response are presumed to be altered.

Tumor Growth Rate

Tumor growth rate has been studied extensively in transplantable animal tumors. When the tumor is very small (i.e., consists of only a few cells), the number of cells in the tumor increases exponentially and rapidly as would be predicted from the cell cycle time of 1-2 days. However, as the tumor enlarges the mass ceases to grow exponentially and grows progressively more slowly. More and more tumor cells cease to proliferate (i.e., the growth fraction falls progressively) and more and more tumor cells die. One reason for this is that as the mass grows, many cells become distant from the blood vessels and therefore nutrient-deprived; they stop proliferating and often die (necrosis). Most tumors have areas of necrosis. In addition, in many tumors, a proportion of the cells appear to differentiate to terminal (non-growing) cells. Finally, it is also hypothesized that some cells accumulate so much genetic damage that they die. This S-shaped curve of mass versus time, called a Gompertz growth curve, is obvious clinically: if a 10 gm tumor doubled every 2 days, as an individual cell can, it would weigh over 1 kg in 2 weeks, and over 100 kg in another two weeks.

Invasion and Metastasis (4,5)

The characteristic which distinguishes benign tumor cells, which also can proliferate autonomously, from malignant cells is that the latter invade neighboring tissues and metastasize to distant regions. Invasion is the hallmark of the malignant tumor; the pathologist looks for invasion in the surgical specimen. Cells which can invade sooner or later get into blood or lymph vessels and metastasize to other parts of the body. The ability to invade implies that a multi-faceted program of transcription is activated, so that proteins necessary for motility are expressed, proteins responsible for cell-cell adhesion are altered, and proteins required for basement membrane and extracellular matrix dissolution are secreted (e.g., proteases and collagenases). The regulation of this program is not understood, but invasiveness is a normal characteristic of macrophages, lymphocytes, granulocytes, fibroblasts in a wound, certain migrating embryonal cells, and placental cells, for instance.

Loss of Differentiated Functions (1)

A malignant cell always loses at least some of the functions of the normal cell of origin. When this loss is severe (called anaplasia), the tissue of origin sometimes cannot even be ascertained.

Mutations (2,6)

Cancer is a disease of the genes. It is now clear that tumor cells have mutations which have a critical role in pathogenesis. Certain leukemias and lymphomas which differ minimally from normal cells have only one mutation. These have been studied extensively. Solid tumors have multiple mutations, often a very large number, a specific set of which are important in transforming the cell to malignancy and a large number of which are random and coincidental. The critical mutations in these very complicated tumors are just now becoming identified.

Mutations versus Epigenetic Alterations

In the vast majority of cancers, probably all cancers, mutations (e.g., changes in the sequence of DNA nucleotides) exist and are critical in causation. However, some of the phenotypic differences between the malignant cell and its normal counterpart are almost certainly changes in the differentiation state of the malignant cell rather than mutations in the regulatory region of every gene which is over expressed and every differentiated function which is lost. During the course of embryogenesis and development, enormous phenotypic heterogeneity is generated based on differences in gene expression among cells without any DNA mutations. In theory, generating a cell of any phenotype, including a malignant cell, should be possible solely by epigenetic changes in gene transcription. For instance, there is an embryonal tumor in which the cells grow as a tumor when implanted in the abdomen of an adult mouse, but if a tumor cell is incorporated into the 8-cell embryo, it is converted to normal. This could represent a purely epigenetically generated tumor; such examples, however, are vanishingly rare.

Mutations in the apparatus that is responsible for the epigenetic program are conceivable and may have a profound effect. For instance, one aspect of the epigenetic mechanism is the enzyme system which methylates cytosine in DNA, and there is evidence that this system may be abnormal in some tumors.

Chromosomes

As techniques for analyzing chromosomes under the microscope have improved, karyotypic abnormalities have been recognized in virtually all solid tumors and most hematologic tumors (7)

Translocations: In chronic myelogenous leukemic (CML), a majority of patients have a visible [t(9:22)] translocation in which chromosome 9 is broken in the region of a gene called abl (Abelson) and chromosome 22 is broken at a gene called bcr (breakpoint cluster region). The broken arm of chromosome 9 is translocated to the break site on chromosome 22, so that abl and bcr are fused. In patients lacking a visible translocation, analysis by DNA sequencing still reveals an abl:bcr fusion. The reproducibility of the abl:bcr fusion demonstrates that it is of critical pathogenetic importance. Consistent translocations have been discovered in most hematologic malignancies. Attempts to determine consistent abnormalities in solid tumors have been less successful because the large number of random and irrelevant abnormalities obscures the critical ones, but statistically significant abnormalities are being reported.

Gene amplifications (6): In many animal and human tumors individual genes are found to be duplicated by an abnormal process during DNA replication, so that several copies are now present in the genome. The multiple copies may be situated in a tandem array on the chromosome; these may be visualized by light microscopy as homogeneously staining regions (HSR) of the chromosome if there are sufficient copies. Alternatively, this amplified DNA may be excised from the original chromosome and occur as separate small ("double minute") chromosomes. Often the significance of the amplified genes is not known. However, in tumors which grow out after methotrexate treatment, the cells sometimes contain many copies of the DHFR gene, which confers resistance to methotrexate.

Chromosome loss: Many examples in which specific chromosomes are lost in the malignant cell have also been discovered. In most retinoblastomas, either (1) both copies of chromosome 13 are lost, (2) one copy is lost and a specific region of the other chromosome 13 (known as 13q14) is lost or mutated, or (3) the specific 13q14 region is lost or mutated in both chromosomes (see below).

The Consequences of Genetic Instability — Phenotypic Heterogeneity and Tumor Progression (8,9)

The existence of multiple mutations in tumor cells implies that they are genetically less stable than normal cells. Thus, in most solid tumors, the cells within the tumor do not have identical karyotypes even though they are clonally derived (i.e., all descended from the same ancestral cell). This implies that mutations are occurring at a high rate during the growth of the tumor. When the individual cells of a tumor are separated and each is grown into a cloned line (i.e., individual cells are "cloned"), the cloned lines are not all identical; they may differ in their metastatic potential, growth rate, hormone sensitivity, and morphology among others. And when a given cloned line is expanded to a large number of cells and these are re-cloned, the subclones are also heterogeneous, implying that the genetic instability is a permanent characteristic of the cell. The cause of this genetic mutability in cancer cells is unknown, but the consequences are enormous.

Phenotypic heterogeneity: As is implied by genetic mutability, there is often extensive phenotypic heterogeneity among the cells within a tumor. Some of this heterogeneity is metabolic, caused by the varying distance of the cells from blood vessels. However, the heterogeneity has a major genetic basis as well.

- Antigenic heterogeneity: When a breast cancer tissue section is stained with a monoclonal antibody which has an affinity for a common breast cancer cell surface antigen, there are almost always some cells which do not stain and which therefore have little or none of this antigen on their surface. Thus, if this antibody is used to target specifically tumor cells, there will always be some tumor cells to which the antibody will not bind.
- Hormonal heterogeneity: The response to hormones depends upon tumor cell expression of hormone receptors and receptor pathways. The phenotypic heterogeneity of solid tumors implies that even in a hormone sensitive breast cancer there will be cells which lack the receptor or the pathway and will be hormone independent. In clinical practice even breast cancers which melt away in the presence of high estrogen doses eventually recur and consist of estrogen independent cells.

- Drug sensitivity: The effectiveness of a particular chemotherapeutic drug varies enormously among various tumor types; effectiveness is determined by the metabolism of the drug in the given tumor. However, even with very sensitive tumors, resistant mutants are a serious threat because of the tumor cell mutability, and most solid tumors cannot be cured by chemotherapy even if they initially respond dramatically.

Tumor progression (10): When the growth of a slow-growing, hormone dependent tumor is followed in an individual animal, it is often observed that the tumor will suddenly begin to grow faster, or become hormone independent, or become much more metastatic, etc. When many individual tumors are followed it becomes evident that these changes occur randomly in time, and in random order. Since the rapidly growing cells, or hormone independent cells, have a growth advantage, the tumor will become progressively more malignant. Most solid tumors, with multiple mutations, are probably already in an advanced state of progression, but progression can sometimes be seen clinically in the single-translocation hematologic malignancies noted above. In early CML, when the granulocytes have only the t(9:22) translocation, the tumor cells can be controlled (killed) by a single chemotherapeutic drug and the course is relatively benign. However, eventually immature granulocytes begin appearing with multiple chromosomal abnormalities (the "blast crisis"). These cells grow rapidly and drug-resistant cells quickly become selected.

THE MUTATIONS RESPONSIBLE FOR CANCER: PROTO-ONCOGENES AND ANTI-ONCOGENES

The Normal Proliferation Pathway (11,12)

Cell proliferation and differentiation are regulated by molecules which react with receptors on the cell surface or within the cell. A large group of polypeptide growth factors (such as EGF, FGF, IGF-1, IGF-2, PDGF, and Insulin) bind to specific surface receptors. Steroid hormones (e.g., estrogen, testosterone, and progesterone) bind to intracellular receptors. When PDGF, for instance, binds to a cell surface receptor (a protein of 170,000 molecular weight), it sets in motion a series of reactions: cascades of protein kinases are activated, in which one kinase in a chain phosphorylates the next kinase and activates it, until at the end of the chain some process is turned on or off; ion fluxes change, so that intracellular Na^+ increases, H^+ decreases, Ca^{2+} increases, etc.; other second messengers change, such as cAMP and diacylglycerol; and so forth. As a result of these events, certain metabolic pathways are stimulated (glucose transport, glycolysis, protein synthesis) and the transcription of certain genes is enormously accelerated, while others are decelerated. The transcriptional inductions and repressions are particularly important because they can produce long-lasting changes in multi-component, fundamental cell processes. These transcriptional effects are produced by proteins, often protein complexes, which bind to the DNA of the regulatory region of genes (7). For instance, the protein called jun binds to the sequence -TGAGTCA- in the 5' regulatory region of the DNA of a number of genes, such as thymidine kinase, metallothionine, and collagenase genes, and stimulates the transcription of this set of genes and the synthesis of the proteins these genes code for. Thus, activation of one gene (jun) can activate a whole set of genes, for instance the genes required for proliferation. Furthermore, transcription factors interact. Fos, another transcription factor, binds to jun to form a heterodimer which is more active than either fos or jun alone. Other factors can bind and inactivate transcription. The activity of several transcription factors is controlled by phosphorylation/dephosphorylation.

Proto-oncogenes and Oncogenes (6,8,9)

There have been discovered a number of genes called proto-oncogenes. Cells expressing mutated forms of these genes have a high probability of progressing to malignancy after a limited number of cell divisions. Therefore, the normal genes are called proto-oncogenes and the mutated forms are called oncogenes, and are spoken of as "activated". The genes are denoted by 3-letter names, such as sis. Because many of the oncogenes were first discovered as mutated cellular genes incorporated into the nucleic acid of RNA tumor viruses, the activated forms are denoted v-onc (for instance, v-sis) and the proto-oncogenes are c-onc (c-sis). As the function of various proto-oncogenes has been elucidated, it has become apparent that many of these proto-oncogenes code for proteins involved in the receptor-activated proliferation/differentiation pathways described above.

Function

Growth hormone genes: The proto-oncogene c-sis is the gene for one form of platelet derived growth factor (PDGF) (there are two PDGF genes). The oncogene, v-sis, causes fibroblasts to proliferate because, whereas the normal cellular sis gene, c-sis, is repressed in fibroblasts, the viral copy, v-sis, is under the control of the active viral regulatory region (promoter) and is highly expressed. The cell then makes its own (autocrine) growth factor, PDGF, and grows continuously.

Growth factor receptor genes: c-erb B is the gene for the receptor for the polypeptide growth factor EGF. The normal receptor is a trans-membrane protein, and has an external portion which binds EGF, a hydrophobic trans-membrane domain, and an intracellular domain which is an enzyme, a tyrosine-specific protein kinase which is activated when EGF binds to the extracellular protein. Activation of the receptor triggers the extensive network of reactions which culminate in mitosis. The mutated gene, v-erb B, has a large deletion in the extracellular domain and is activated constitutively, that is, the receptor is active without the presence of EGF. Thus, a cell with this receptor is continuously stimulated to grow.

GTP-binding proteins: There are several related proteins named Kirsten-ras, Harvey-ras, and N-ras which bind GTP and GDP and appear analogous to the G-protein which transmits the signal from a hormone receptor to the adenyl cyclase enzyme. The ras proteins are clearly proteins in proliferation/differentiation pathways. The mutated protein, v-Kirsten-ras, has one amino acid altered from the normal protein, and this mutation causes the protein to affect cellular growth and differentiation dramatically. Presumably it becomes constitutively active in some presently unknown pathway.

Protein kinases: The normal protein c-src is a 60,000 molecular weight enzyme, a tyrosine-specific protein kinase. The function of c-src is unknown and it is not clear why the slightly modified oncogene v-src causes tumors, but the enzyme has the characteristics of a protein kinase in a proliferation pathway.

Nuclear proteins: The c-myc protein is a transcription factor which is increased in amount soon after many different growth stimuli. Thus it probably has a regulatory role in cell growth. Mutations in the regulatory region (promoter/enhancer) of the v-myc gene cause increased expression of the protein and persistent proliferation. Mutations in the coding region are also associated with activation. Jun and fos are other proto-oncogenes similar to myc.

Unknown function: There are several retroviral oncogenes the normal function of which is unknown.

Activation of Proto-oncogenes to Oncogenes:

Oncogenic retroviruses: The retroviruses are single-stranded RNA viruses which carry an enzyme, called "reverse transcriptase", which copies the viral RNA into double-stranded DNA. This viral DNA becomes integrated at random sites in host cell chromosomal DNA. A region of the integrated viral DNA known as the LTR is a strong promoter (i.e., an active regulatory region) in several cell types, so that the viral DNA is transcribed actively in these cells. Occasionally, fragments of host DNA become incorporated into the virus, where they also are actively expressed. A number of altered retroviruses have been discovered, particularly in chickens and mice, which cause tumors rapidly in infected hosts. These viruses, the acutely transforming retroviruses, were found to contain mutated forms of host genes, and it was the host gene which caused the tumor. The host gene is called a proto-oncogene and the mutated ("activated") form an oncogene. Activation of the host gene occurred by two mechanisms: (1) a mutation in the coding sequence made the protein a more potent effector of growth, and (2) modification of the non-coding regulatory region of the gene led to over-expression of a normal stimulatory protein.

Promoter activation by viral insertion: RAV-1 is ordinarily not a transforming retrovirus; it carries no host genes. Occasionally it does transform, however, because it becomes integrated into the control site of a proto-oncogene such as myc and activates it because of the active viral promoter. The mouse mammary tumor virus causes mammary tumors because it occasionally inserts near the int-1 gene. In this way int-1 was discovered as a proto-oncogene.

DNA and RNA tumor viruses with transforming viral proteins: Some DNA viruses (hepatitis B virus, Epstein-Barr virus, human papilloma virus) and some retroviruses (HTLV-l, HIV-1) cause tumors because of a normal viral product. (This is in contrast to the acutely transforming retroviruses discussed above, in which the oncogenes are mutated host genes picked up by the virus.) In adenovirus 2, a DNA tumor virus of mice, a virally-coded protein called E1A which regulates viral transcription can also regulate the transcription of certain proliferation-related host proteins in susceptible cells, through interaction with host transcription factors. Occasionally, such a stimulated host cell progresses to malignancy, presumably through mutations of host genes.

Reproducible translocations: In almost every type of hematological malignancy, one or more consistent translocations affecting specific proto-oncogenes have been identified, as exemplified by CML, described above. In some cases, activation appears to be due simply to an increased transcription of the proto-oncogene in the new position; in other cases the oncogene coding sequence is altered.

Gene amplification: Malignant cells appear abnormally prone to gene amplification. In breast cancer, for instance, the gene known as erbB-2 (probably a hormone receptor) is frequently amplified.

Mutagenesis: U.V. irradiation, x-irradiation, and certain chemicals are proven carcinogens and can activate oncogenes through mutation. For instance, the chemical carcinogen NMU causes hepatomas and causes mutations in which T becomes substituted for A. In the majority of NMU-induced mouse hepatomas, an A to T mutation was found in the codon for the 12th amino acid in ras, causing the normal glycine to be replaced by another amino acid.

Spontaneous mutations: Many oncogenic mutations are probably simply the result of random errors which inevitably occur with a very low frequency during replication.

Mounting evidence indicates that as tumors progress in malignancy, an increasing number of proto-oncogenes are activated to oncogenes and tumor suppressor genes (see below) are mutated or lost. For instance, in a recent study comparing benign colonic adenomas with colonic malignancies (carcinomas) the oncogene ras was mutated in 12% of adenomas and 47% of carcinomas; suspected tumor-suppressive regions of chromosome 5, 17, and 18 were lost or altered in 0, 6, and 13% of adenomas respectively, and 36, 75 and 73% of carcinomas. Among carcinomas, ras was mutated in 9% of those less than 1 cm in size, in 22% of 1-2 cm tumors, and in 70% of tumors larger than 2 cm. Looked at another way, 75% of benign adenomas had none of the above alterations whereas 90% of carcinomas had at least two.

Importance of Activated Oncogenes in Human Cancer (2)

The oncogenes have been discovered primarily in animal tumors; however, their activation is clearly important in human cancer.

- Many of the proto-oncogenes have been found to be amplified with high frequency in specific human cancers. For instance, erbB-2 is amplified in as much as 40% of breast cancers in some series.
- Numerous translocations specific to particular cancers have been found to involve a previously discovered v-oncogene at the break point.
- Specific point mutations have been found with high frequency.

The ras gene is mutated at the 12th, 13th, or 61st amino acid in at least 10% of all human cancers. This was demonstrated initially through a transfection technique. DNA purified from human tumors was transfected into the fibroblast cell line called the NIH 3T3 line. These cells do not grow when implanted in syngeneic mice. However, cells transfected with DNA from certain human tumors were altered (transformed) so that they now grew in syngeneic mice. The human tumor DNA which is responsible for transformation of the 3T3 cells is usually a ras gene with one altered amino acid, as found in certain transforming retroviruses. Thus, this assay reveals proto-oncogenes also found in retroviruses. (However, 3T3 transfection reveals only a limited spectrum of oncogenes, and some of the viral oncogenes do not transform 3T3 cells.)

The one animal mechanism which is unimportant in man is acutely transforming retroviruses. No retroviruses are known in man which carry host derived oncogenes. On the other hand, as noted above, there are several RNA and DNA tumor viruses which transform because of viral proteins. Even so, with the exception of uterine cervical carcinoma, hepatoma, laryngeal and nasopharyngeal carcinomas, and hematologic malignancies, viruses do not appear to be an important cause of human cancer on the basis of present evidence (11).

"Anti-oncogenes:" Recessive Tumor-suppression Genes

For the proto-oncogenes described above, cancer is generated through a mutation which activates one copy of the gene, even though the copy on the other chromosome of the pair remains normal. Thus the mutation is called dominant. There is another very important group of genes for which cancer is generated by the inactivation or loss of the gene, and both copies of the gene must be inactivated. Thus, these genes are called recessive tumor suppressor genes. For instance, in retinoblastoma tumor cells, both copies of a gene called Rb on chromosome 13 are either deleted or mutated so as to be inactive. Certain children are born with a deletion of Rb on one copy of chromosome 13. These children have a much higher than normal probability of developing retinoblastoma because the probability of losing the one remaining good chromosome 13 is much higher than the probability of a cell in a normal person losing both (good) copies. The importance of tumor suppressor genes is further illustrated by cell fusion experiments (3). When malignant mouse fibroblast cell lines are fused with normal mouse fibroblasts, the resulting hybrid cells are not tumorigenic unless they have lost all copies of the normal chromosome 4. This is true even if the malignant parental cell and the resulting hybrid have a mutated ras gene. This was a surprise because when cells transfected with mutant ras are implanted in a syngeneic mouse, a tumor is eventually formed; thus ras was considered to be sufficient for tumorigenesis. However, the tumors that grow out are in fact a selected subpopulation and they have many new chromosomal abnormalities in addition to the original ras mutation.

This model predicts that in human cancers, there will be found both activation of proto-oncogenes and loss or inactivation of tumor suppressor genes. This has proven to be the case, and the list of known tumor-suppressor genes is rapidly growing.

Conclusion

It now seems clear that the pathogenesis of cancer involves somatic mutation and that cells of advanced malignancies are characterized by multiple mutations. Among these are a number of mutation which contribute critically to the malignant phenotype. Some of these critical mutations have been identified; they appear to stimulate pathways leading to proliferation and inhibit pathways leading to terminal differentiation. The oncogenic mutations include "dominant" mutations in which stimulatory genes become abnormally active and "recessive" mutations in which regulatory genes

are lost or inactivated. The detailed mechanisms of the pathways, the mutations responsible for invasiveness, and the mechanisms responsible for the remarkable accumulation of mutations in malignant cells are among the important mysteries which remain to be elucidated.

Recommended Reading

Two excellent reviews were published recently. One is on oncogenic processes in *Cell* (1a) and the other is a review of cancer in *Science* (1b).

REFERENCES

General References

1. Dean, M.; Vande Woude, G.F. Principles of molecular cell biology of cancer: introduction to methods in molecular biology. In: DeVita, V.T., Jr.; Hellman, S.; Rosenberg, S.A., eds. Cancer: Principles & Practice of Oncology, 3rd ed. Philadelphia: J.B. Lippincott Co.; 1989:14-30.
1a. Cell. Reviews on Oncogenic Processes. 64(2):235-363; 1991.
1b. Science. 254 (Nov 22):1131-1177; 1991.

Specific References

2. Callahan, R.; Campbell, G. Mutations in human breast cancer. J. Natl. Cancer Inst. 81:1780-1786; 1989.
2a. Crick, F. Life Itself: Its Origins and Nature. New York, NY: Simon and Schuster; 1981.
3. Harris, H. The analysis of malignancy by cell fusion: the position in 1988. Cancer Res. 48:3302-3306; 1988.
4. Hill, R.P. Metastasis. In: Tannock, I.F., Hill, R.P., eds. The Basic Science of Oncology. New York: Pergamon Press; 1987:160-175.
5. Liotta, L.A.; Stetler-Stevenson, W.G. Principles of moecular cell biology of cancer: cancer metastasis. In: DeVita, V.T., Jr.; Hellman, S.; Rosenberg, S.A., eds. Cancer: Principles & Practice of Oncology, 3rd ed. Philadelphia: J.B. Lippincott Co.; 1989:81-97.
6. Minden, M.D. Oncogenes. In: Tannock, I.F., Hill, R.P., eds. The Basic Science of Oncology. New York: Pergamon Press; 1987:72-88.
7. Mitchell, P.J.; Tjian, R. Transcriptional regulation in mammalian cells by sequence-specific DNA binding proteins. Science 245:371-378; 1989.
8. Park, M.; Vande Woude, G.F. Principles of molecular cell biology of cancer: oncogenes. In: DeVita, V.T., Jr.; Hellman, S.; Rosenberg, S.A., eds. Cancer: Principles & Practice of Oncology, 3rd ed. Philadelphia: J.B. Lippincott Co.; 1989:45-66.
9. Phillips, R.A. The genetic basis of cancer. In: Tannock, I.F., Hill, R.P., eds. The Basic Science of Oncology. New York: Pergamon Press; 1987:24-51.
10. Roberts, A.B.; Sporn, M.B. Principles of molecular cell biology of cancer: growth factors related to transformation. In: DeVita, V.T., Jr.; Hellman, S.; Rosenberg, S.A., eds. Cancer: Principles & Practice of Oncology, 3rd ed. Philadelphia: J.B. Lippincott Co.; 1989:67-80.
11. Sager, R. Tumor suppressor genes: the puzzle and the promise. Science 246: 1406-1412; 1989.
12. Vande Woulde, S.; Vande Woude, G.F. Principles of molecular cell biology of cancer: general aspects of gene regulation. In: DeVita, V.T., Jr.; Hellman, S.; Rosenberg, S.A., eds. Cancer: Principles & Practice of Oncology, 3rd ed. Philadelphia: J.B. Lippincott Co.; 1989:31-44.

Thomas A. Bonfiglio, M.D. Pathologic Oncology
Mark H. Stoler, M.D. Pathologic Oncology

Chapter 3

THE PATHOLOGY OF CANCER

We stand upon the intellectual shoulders of those medical giants of bygone days and, because of the help they afford us, we are able to see a little more clearly than they are able to do.

Claude Bernard (10)

PERSPECTIVE

Various definitions of cancer have been put forth over the years. None is an all encompassing or entirely satisfactory conception of the clinical and pathologic spectrum of entities that comprise this disease. Indeed, cancer is not one disease, but several separate diseases of multiple etiologies that generally, if left untreated, directly or indirectly result in the death of the patient. Conceptually, cancer is considered to be a disease of the cell, in which the normal mechanisms of control of growth and proliferation are disturbed. This results in distinctive morphologic alterations of the cell and aberrations of tissue patterns. These cytologic and histologic alterations are the basis of the diagnosis of cancer.

It must be remembered, however, that the concept of malignancy is clinical rather than morphologic. The pathologist's diagnosis of cancer is an informed opinion based on the knowledge of a correlation between certain cellular or tissue patterns of a tumor and subsequent biologic and, therefore, clinical behavior.

Although of primary importance, diagnosis of malignancy is not the only reason for pathologic evaluation. Consideration of histopathologic features also provides information regarding prognosis, likelihood of metastases, and potential response to therapy.

There are definite limitations to histopathologic and cytopathologic examination, some of which are discussed in this chapter. Technologic advances, however, now permit the acquisition of more information about individual tumors than had been possible previously. Immunocytochemical techniques using antibodies directed against specific tumor antigens or structural proteins permit classification and identification of neoplastic subgroups to a degree that was not possible using standard histologic techniques. In addition, the evaluation of cellular oncogenes and the detection of gene rearrangements are now possible. These techniques have begun to provide additional diagnostic and prognostic information about tumors. Limitations in our ability to evaluate tumors still remain, but it is important to stress that one cannot hope to understand cancer or to treat patients with this disease adequately without understanding its pathology.

DIAGNOSIS OF CANCER

A lesion suspected clinically of being cancer must be definitively diagnosed by pathologic examination (Table 3-1). Many diseases may mimic cancer clinically. These include not only benign neoplasms but many inflammatory and hyperplastic processes as well. Although in rare cases treatment of a supposed malignancy must be started on the basis of clinical impression alone, this is seldom necessary. Such a decision entails the danger of inappropriate and often potentially hazardous therapy for benign disease.

Methods of Definitive Diagnosis

Surgical Biopsy

The traditional and most widely used method of diagnostic verification of suspected carcinoma is histologic examination of tissue removed by excisional or incisional biopsy.

Exfoliative Cytology

This technique, which was fostered by Dr. Papanicoloau (30) in the middle of this century and originally considered primarily a screening technique, has also proven, in experi-

Table 3-1. Summary of Cancer Diagnosis

Definitive diagnosis requires histologic or cytologic examination
Methods of definitive diagnosis
- Surgical biopsy with tissue examination
- Examination of exfoliated tumor cells
- Examination of tissue/cells obtained by needle aspiration or biopsy

Validity of the interpretation depends on both the pathologist and the clinician
- Representative sample must be obtained
- Material must be properly processed
- All pertinent patient data must be available to the pathologist

Important points to remember
- Benign processes can mimic cancer
- Cancer can mimic benign processes
- Histologic or cytologic cancer is not equivalent to clinical cancer
- Cancer, like other diseases, varies in spectrum with individual patients

enced hands, to be a highly accurate diagnostic modality. It is particularly useful in the examination of the cervix and body cavity fluids.

Fine Needle Aspiration Biopsy

Virtually every body organ has been sampled by this diagnostic method, and the technique has gained widespread acceptance in recent years. This procedure produces a sample consisting of both small tissue fragments and isolated cells (Fig. 3-1). When interpreted by expert surgical pathologists and cytopathologists, this technique is a highly accurate and minimally invasive means of obtaining a diagnosis.

Validity of Interpretation

The amount of information obtained from any of these diagnostic modalities depends not only on the knowledge and experience of the pathologist, but also in large part on the clinician.

Representative Sample

The clinician shares with the pathologist the responsibility of insuring that the pathologist receives an adequate representative sample of the lesion for interpretation. An inadequate specimen often results in an inaccurate diagnosis.

Pertinent Data

The clinician and pathologist also must be certain that all the pertinent data regarding the patient are available at the time of interpretation. There are many lesions that can present significant problems if inaccurate or incomplete data are given.

Diagnostic Difficulties

It is important to realize that in certain circumstances a definite diagnosis of benign versus malignant disease cannot be made. If one excludes those instances where a diagnosis is not possible because of technical problems, the cases generally fall into three categories.

1. The morphologic pattern seen may vary so little from normal, either because of the early stage of the process or because of the basic nature of the tumor, that a definitive diagnosis is not possible. Evolving lymphoma

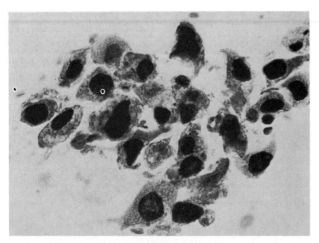

Fig. 3-1. Needle aspiration specimen with malignant tumor cells derived from a well-differentiated squamous cell carcinoma of lung. Note cellular pleomorphism and hyperchromatic nuclei. (800X Pap stain.)

in a lymph node may be an example of a tumor too early in its time course to diagnose. Well-differentiated follicular carcinoma of the thyroid is an example of a tumor that often mimics benign thyroid tissue throughout its course.

2. The second group incorporates those tumors that have some but not all of the features of malignancy. These "borderline tumors" occur in several areas of the body. In some patients, they behave aggressively and in others, innocuously (30). An example is the cellular leiomyoma of the uterus with a moderate mitotic rate (5 to 9 mitoses/10 high power microscopic fields).

3. The third group includes inflammatory or immunologically mediated processes that mimic malignancy so closely that prediction of biologic behavior through routinely available techniques is difficult or impossible. This type of lesion may include some of the atypical lymphoid hyperplastic processes of lymph nodes or atypical alveolar cell proliferations in the lung.

Current knowledge, careful detailed study, and newer diagnostic tools have markedly decreased the number of such problems in the modern pathology laboratory. There remain, however, a few cases in which even the most expert pathologist cannot make a definitive interpretation.

GENERAL HISTOLOGIC AND CYTOLOGIC FEATURES OF MALIGNANCY

Although different malignant tumors vary considerably in their morphologic features, certain features are commonly found and are sufficiently characteristic so as to be considered malignancy criteria. Several important facts must be remembered. First, no single feature is pathognomonic of cancer. Second, while many malignant tumors will demonstrate most of the criteria, some will have very few. Third, some benign tumors will display some of the morphologic features of cancer.

It is possible to summarize the principal histologic and cytologic features of cancer.

Invasiveness

Malignant tumors are not limited by the confines of normal tissue but infiltrate surrounding tissue, often including blood vessels and lymphatic channels.

Destruction of Normal Tissue

This destruction ensues as a result of the invasive infiltrative growth.

Atypical Tissue Structure (Anaplasia)

The growth patterns and resulting tissue architecture are disorderly, with cellular arrangements that often deviate considerably from normal.

Pleomorphism

Tissue patterns vary from area to area in the same tumor. Individual tumor cells also often vary considerably in their morphologic characteristics.

High Mitotic Rate

Malignant tumor cells tend to proliferate at a higher rate than their normal counterparts. This is manifested by increased numbers of mitotic figures in tissue sections.

Aneuploidy

The DNA content of malignant cells is typically abnormal. Whereas normal or hyperplastic cells have diploid or some multiple of the normal diploid content, cancer cells often have irregular and inconstant amounts of DNA. This is reflected by the presence of hyperchromasia and chromatin irregularities within cell nuclei as well as abnormal mitotic figures.

CARCINOGENESIS

Many of the morphologic characteristics of malignancy described above reflect details of nuclear morphology. By implication, the expression of the neoplastic phenotype is intimately associated with the function of the cell nucleus that is, in part, the genetic control of cell growth and differentiation. While many of the other characteristics of a cancer cell may not be morphologically evident, it should be clear that changes such as karyotypic abnormalities, antigenic changes, changes in cell surface, membrane properties, or cellular metabolism are all ultimately mediated through changes in the cell's pattern of gene expression. Furthermore, the common pathway of action of virtually all carcinogenic agents is through an interaction with the host's DNA. These interactions presumably produce mutations that ultimately alter cellular metabolism in such a way as to produce the cancer phenotype.

Tumors can be induced in animals, and cells can be transformed in vitro by the application of a variety of agents. These fall into three broad classes: radiation, chemicals and oncogenic viruses. While a complete discussion of any of these is beyond the scope of this chapter a brief consideration will serve to point out that all act through similar mechanisms and that these same mechanisms are probably also active in the pathogenesis of cancer in humans

Viral Carcinogenesis (18,29,32,36,37, 51)

While there are many examples of viruses that are unequivocally carcinogenic in animals, evidence in humans for a cancer virus(es) has, until recently, been lacking. Table 3-2 lists selected viruses that may be associated with the development of human tumors.

Oncogenic viruses can be separated into two broad classes based on whether their genomes are composed of RNA or DNA. Most of the RNA viruses associated with the production of neoplasms fall into the class of retroviruses, so named because they contain an RNA-dependent DNA polymerase, also called reverse transcriptase. This enzyme mediates the transcription of viral RNA into virus-specific DNA, which is a reversal (hence "retro") of the usual flow of genetic information of DNA to RNA to protein. There are two groups of oncogenic retroviruses: those that transform cells rapidly and those that take a long time to induce cell transformation (acute versus chronic transforming retroviruses). Both types have a similar life cycle; DNA provirus synthesized by the action of reverse transcriptase is incorporated into the host's cellular DNA. The acutely transforming viruses differ, however, in their genetic constitution; that is, they contain a gene that can be shown to be necessary and, in some cases, sufficient for cell transformation [i.e., they contain a viral oncogene (v-onc)]. These viral oncogenes are highly homologous to a family of cellular genes (c-oncs) and these cellular genes have been found to play a central role in the control of cell growth and metabolism. In contrast, the chronic transforming viruses lack an identifiable oncogene, yet still induce neoplastic transformation through an interaction between host and viral genetic information. For example, the process of viral integration may cause disruption or mutation within a host oncogene, within its control region, or in cellular regulatory genes that control the expression of oncogenes.

The DNA tumor associated viruses differ from the RNA viruses both with respect to their genetic organization and to the way they interact with the host cell. For example, there is no reverse transcription, and to transform a cell there can be no viral replication, which, for most DNA viruses, is cytolytic to the host cell. Despite their differences, however, there are some common threads in the apparent mechanisms of viral transformation. These include a surprising frequency of viral integration, usually of only a part of the viral genome. The act of integration may frequently lead to a disruption or dysregulation of viral genes; this abnormal regulation of viral gene expression and its effects on the host may well play a role in cell transformation. Indeed, recently several viral transforming proteins have been shown to interact with host genes which control growth (so-called antioncogenes) proving further mechanistic support for viral carcinogenesis.

Chemical Carcinogenesis (27)

Over the course of this century, it has become clear that hundreds of chemicals have carcinogenic properties in animals and/or humans. While diverse in structure, most chemical carcinogens have in common a highly electrophilic nature that causes them to react with cellular macromolecules with abundant negative charges, mainly DNA, RNA and some proteins. Their main effect seems to be the induction of mutational changes in DNA that cause errors in transcription or replication. Some carcinogenic agents act directly on the cell, whereas others (indirect-acting) require metabolic conversion to become active. Carcinogens vary in the effectiveness with which they initiate the development of a neoplasm, and some chemicals may act additively or synergistically to produce a tumor more effectively. Other chemicals that may be weakly or noncarcinogenic by themselves, if applied after exposure to an initiating agent, may serve to promote the development of a neoplasm. This concept of initiation and promotion and the realization that several chemical carcino-

Table 3-2. Viruses Directly or Indirectly Associated with Development of Human Neoplasia

Virus	Neoplasms
DNA viruses	
Human papillomaviruses	Warts, anogenital carcinomas
Herpes simplex virus-2	Cervix cancer
Epstein-Barr virus	Nasopharyngeal cancer, African Burkitt's lymphoma
Cytomegalovirus	Kaposi's sarcoma
Hepatitis B virus	Hepatocellular carcinoma
Herpes simplex virus -6(HBLV)	Certain B cell lymphomas
RNA viruses	
Human T cell leukemia virus-I	Some T cell leukemia/lymphomas
Human T cell leukemia virus-II	? Some cases of hairy cell leukemia
Human immunodeficiency virus-I	lymphoma /? Kaposi's sarcoma

gens may be more effective in producing a tumor leads one to consider the idea that the production of a cancer is a multistep affair involving multiple genes and perhaps multiple mechanisms, in other words, multistep carcinogenesis.

Radiation Carcinogenesis (47)

Only a few comments will be offered here, since this subject is extensively considered in later chapters. Radiant energy is clearly carcinogenic. There are many sources of potentially carcinogenic radiation in modern life including sunlight, artificial sources of UV light, x-rays, radiochemicals, and nuclear fission. While, as with other carcinogens, the exact mechanism of action is unclear, it is clear that the target of the interaction is the cellular DNA. Radiation-induced mutation in the host cell is the probable mechanism for transmitting irreversible changes in cellular gene expression to cell progeny, and some of these changes may be capable of inducing cell transformation. The more powerful the energy source and the greater the interaction with host macromolecules, the higher the risk of malignant transformation. The long latency period associated with most radiation-induced cancers suggests that long-term exposure or several other steps may be involved in the production of a tumor.

Oncogenes and a Unified Theory of Carcinogenesis (5a,11,12,19,24,43,49, 49a)

As the study of acutely transforming retroviruses revealed the presence of viral oncogenes, probing of eukaryotic DNA revealed cellular homologues of these genes within a diverse range of species, from yeasts to humans. This phylogenetic conservation and a consideration of the life cycle of a retrovirus leads one to conclude that the v-oncs are derived from normal cellular genes (c-oncs) through recombination of the viral genome with the host. The evolutionary conservation of c-onc points out the central role these genes must play in cellular metabolism. More than 30 c-onc have now been characterized. Clearly there is no selective advantage to the host to have genes that predispose it to the development of cancer. However, study of the function of the c-oncs has revealed, as might have been predicted, that these same genes function normally in cells and are involved in the control of cell growth and regulation. Many of them encode growth factors, growth factor receptors, protein kinases, or nucleotide-binding proteins. A detailed comparison of "activated" oncogenes with their normal cellular counterparts has revealed that the mechanism of activation of these genes involves classical genetic mechanisms including point mutation, translocation, amplification, and insertion. More than one of these genes may be activated in a given tumor, providing a molecular basis for multistep carcinogenesis. Recently, another class of genes, so-called anti-oncogenes (antioncs), or tumor supressor genes, has been described. Antionc are genes that seem to function as cellular repressors or regulators of cell growth, and loss of their activity is associated with the development of a cancer.

Given the complementary functions of the oncogenes versus tumor suppressor genes, it is conceptually appealing to envision a network of coordinated gene expression involving these gene products that act to control cell growth within the context of the host. The target of the various carcinogenic stimuli would obviously be the cellular DNA, encoding or regulating the onc/antionc products so that lesions inflicted by radiation, chemicals, viruses, or spontaneous random mutation would activate/inactivate portions of this regulatory network, ultimately producing the malignant phenotype. Note that this unified theory of carcinogenesis also allows the action of more than one of these stimuli, e.g., virus plus chemical carcinogen. Each may act independently to confer stepwise the various abilities a cell must acquire to ultimately become a cancer cell. Note that this multistep process does not occur in isolation. Clearly, certain influences in the host, such as immunologic factors and hormonal influences, may act to enhance or abort the development of a tumor at any step in the process of malignant transformation.

CLASSIFICATION OF NEOPLASIA

Neoplasia has been classified by numerous methods in an attempt to understand its nature. Many of these methods were fanciful, based on incorrect information, or too cumbersome to be of practical value. The best available currently used classification is based on the anatomic site, the tissue or cell type of origin, and the biologic behavior (benign or malignant).

Tumors can arise from virtually all types of normal tissues. The total number of possible different neoplasms is, therefore, quite large. Usually they retain enough of the features of the normal cells and tissue patterns for their origin to be determined.

Consideration of biologic behavior results in the division of tumors into benign and malignant groups. The former are generally innocuous growths which do little harm to the host, while the latter are aggressive neoplasms which, if untreated, generally result in metastases and death.

Using these concepts, benign tumors are usually named by adding the suffix "-oma" to the name of a type of cell or tissue, as in "neuroma" and "osteoma." Malignant tumors are divided into two groups: sarcomas (those of mesenchymal origin), and carcinomas (those of epithelial origin). These terms are then used with the tissue or cell of origin, as in fibrosarcoma and squamous cell carcinoma.

Like most classifications, there are numerous exceptions to the above. Malignancies of hematopoietic and lymphocytic origin are classified separately. In many instances, eponyms are used. This is quite appropriate, particularly when the cell of origin is not established, as with Ewing's sarcoma and Hodgkin's disease. In some instances, all histologic resemblance to any normal tissue is lost and precise classification may be difficult. In the past it was not uncommon to be unable to further characterize these highly undifferentiated neoplasms; however, current technology has markedly diminished the number of cases where this problem persists.

Electron microscopic evaluation of ultrastructural characteristics of tumors, which has been available for many years, permitted both more accurate and more detailed classification of many neoplasms than had been possible previously. In more recent years, the classification of highly undifferentiated neoplasms has been greatly aided by the development of immunocytochemical methods for the evaluation of specific, diagnostically useful tumor markers. These markers are cellular structural characteristics or cell products of the progenitor cell that are maintained by the tumor cell or specific normal or abnormal proteins manufactured by the tumor cells, which can serve to identify them as being of specific origin. Some examples of commonly evaluated markers include intermediate filaments such as cytokeratins, which are present in cells of epithelial origin, and vimentin, which is characteristically found in cells of mesenchymal origin. Neuroendocrine cells contain neuron specific enolase, chromogranin, and often synaptophysin, and tumors derived from these cells can be identified as such by the immunohistochemical demonstration of these proteins within them. Some tumors contain tissue-specific antigens. The cells from adenocarcinoma of the prostate, for example, are characterized by the presence of prostatic specific antigen. The identification of this marker in a metastatic neoplasm essentially confirms that the tumor originated in the prostate gland. Numerous markers are currently available and more are constantly under evaluation. The most commonly used diagnostically valuable markers are listed in Table 3-3 (3,4).

An example of the classification and nomenclature of tumors is seen in Table 3-4. It is beyond the scope of this chapter to provide a comprehensive listing of all the classified neoplasms, but numerous comprehensive works have been devoted to this (7,8,23).

In addition to these categories of tumors, there remains another group, the so-called *preinvasive or in situ malignancies*. These terms are generally limited to lesions of epithelial origin. Many examples can be given, but perhaps the most widely recognized is carcinoma in situ of the cervix. These lesions have most of the cytomorphologic features of malignancy, but lack one cardinal feature — invasiveness. They

Table 3-4. Classification of Neoplasms

Tissue Origin	Benign	Malignant	Examples
Epithelial Glandular	Adenoma	Adenocarcinoma	Thyroid follicular adenoma
			Adenocarcinoma of lung
Squamous and transitional	Polyp, papilloma	Squamous cell	Transitional cell papilloma of bladder
		Transitional cell carcinoma	Squamous cell carcinoma of skin
Connective tissue	Tissue type +	Sarcoma suffix (-oma)	Osteoma
			Osteosarcoma
Hematopoietic and lympho-reticular		Lymphoma	Large cell lymphoma
		Leukemia Hodgkin's disease	Myelocytic leukemia
Neural tissue	Neuroma	Sarcoma	Neurofibrosarcoma
	Neurofibroma	Blastoma	Glioblastoma multiforme
Mixed tissues of origin	Teratoma	Teratocarcinoma	Teratoma of ovary Teratocarcinoma of testis

represent a stage in developing cancer in which the tumor is confined to its epithelium (Fig. 3-2).

The classification of neoplasms has never been a static list. As our knowledge of origins and behavior of tumors has increased and progressed, the names and groupings within our lists have changed. Processes formerly thought to be malignant, for example sclerosing adenosis of the breast, are now known to be benign; lesions that were formerly felt to be innocuous are now known in some instances to be malignant. Tumors once thought to originate from one cell type were later shown to originate from a totally different type of cell.

Table 3-3. Diagnostically Useful Antigens

Antigen	Marker for
Alpha-1-Antitrypsin	Histiocytes and reticulin cells. Not highly specific
Alpha-fetoprotein	Germ cell tumors, hepatocellular carcinoma
Beta- human chorionic gonadotrophin	Trophoblastic tissue and many germ cell tumors
Carcinoembryonic antigen	Adenocarcinomas, particularly GI tract and lung
Chromogranin	Endocrine secretory granules
Common leucocyte antigen	Leucocytes
Cytokeratins	Epithelial cells or mesothelium
Desmin	Smooth or skeletal muscle
Epithelial membrane antigen	Normal and neoplastic epithelium and some other tissues
Factor VIII	Endothelial cells
Glial fibrillary acidic protein	Glial cells and other neural tissues
HMB-45 (monoclonal antibody)	Melanoma, some nevocellular nevi
Kappa & lambda light chains	Immunoglobulin light chains in evaluation of lymphoid proliferations
B72.3 (monoclonal antibody)	Carcinoma cells, particularly adenocarcinoma of lung and breast
Myoglobin	Muscle
Neuron specific enolase	Neuroendocrine cells
Prostatic specific antigen	Prostatic epithelium
Prostatic acid phosphatase	Prostatic epithelium
S-100	Neural tissue, melanoma, chondroid tissue, myoepithelial cells, some other tissues

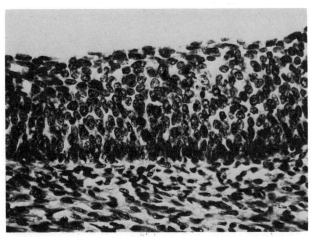

Fig. 3-2. Carcinoma in situ of uterine cervix. The epithelium is replaced by small poorly differentiated cells with many of the cytologic features of malignancy. (160X, H&E.)

Subclassifications have proliferated, changed, and changed again in response to additional knowledge and new methods of examination. In some instances, this has occurred so often and so frequently that it is difficult to avoid confusion. It also resulted in the use, in some cases, of several different names for the same neoplasm. Efforts at standardization, such as those established by World Health Organization (WHO) panels, have done much to solve this problem but changes in these systems remain inevitable. Indeed, these changes are desirable if they are based on increased knowledge that permits more precise treatment and leads to better understanding and outcomes.

The tumor classifications offered throughout this volume are those advocated by WHO.

Grading, Staging and DNA Analysis

In addition to the basic classification discussed above, malignant lesions are also divided according to grade and stage, which serve as useful predictors of prognosis.

Grade

The grade is an evaluation of the degree of differentiation of the tumor and usually, therefore, of the degree of malignancy. Either of two systems are generally used: a numeric grade of 1 to 3 or 1 to 4; or a descriptive grade, such as well, moderately, or poorly differentiated. The low numeric grades or well differentiated tumors are those that cytologically and histologically deviate least from normal, while the high-grade or poorly differentiated tumors are the most anaplastic, or bear the least resemblance to normal cellular and tissue patterns (Figs. 3-3, 3-4, 3-5).

Stage

The stage of the tumor is simply an evaluation of the extent of the tumor at the time of diagnosis and is not necessarily related to its grade. Staging is often a combined clinical and pathologic process, although in some organ sites it is based only on clinical data. The evaluation considers size of the cancer, invasion of adjacent structures, regional lymph node involvement and distant metastases. Several different staging systems are used depending on tumor sites (6). These are discussed in detail in the chapters on specific organs and sites.

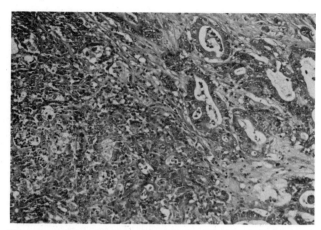

Fig. 3-4. Moderately differentiated adenocarcinoma. The glandular structures are less well-formed, particularly on the left. (200X, H&E.)

The histologic grade and the stage are of value in the prognostic information they imply. In general, the higher the grade and stage, the poorer the prognosis. While grading is subjective and not based entirely on quantitative factors, it is prognostically valuable. The tumor grade correlates with patient outcome. Population studies show that, stage for stage, patients with low-grade tumors have better survival rates than patients with high-grade neoplasms (Fig. 3-6) (20). A staging or grading system that does not correlate well with prognosis is of little clinical use. In an attempt to improve the value, many of the methods of staging and grading have changed over the years.

In some instances, the histologic grade of the tumor is the most important characteristic; for example, in high-grade soft tissue sarcomas (23) and high-grade astrocytomas or glioblastoma multiform, the prognosis is poor regardless of most other factors. In other instances, grading seems to have less bearing on prognosis. Examples exist of tumors that histologically are of low grade but behave very aggressively and other examples can be found of neoplasms that would be classified as high grade histologically but have an excellent prognosis.

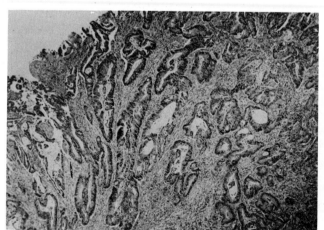

Fig. 3-3. Well-differentiated adenocarcinoma of the colon. Note well-formed glandular structures and resemblance to normal colonic glands. (160X, H&E.)

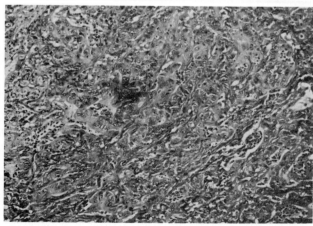

Fig. 3-5. Poorly differentiated adenocarcinoma. There is little resemblance to normal glandular structures with the tumor growing mainly in ill-defined sheets. (200X, H&E.)

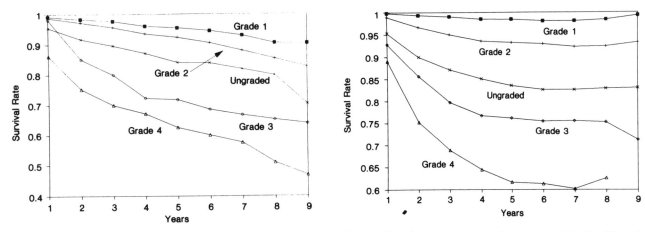

Fig. 3-6. Survival rates as related to neoplastic grade in patients with transitional cell carcinoma of the urinary bladder (A) and adenocarcinoma of the endometrium (B). From Henson, D.E. The histologic grading of neoplasms. Arch. Pathol. Lab .Med. 112: 1091-1096; 1988, with permission.

DNA Analysis

In recent years, pathologic study of tumors has expanded to include other evaluations that provide additional information in regard to specific tumors that may be of value in predicting prognosis and response to treatment. Analysis of the DNA content of tumor cells through the use of flow cytometric or other cell analysis methods is one such methodology. These techniques make use of the fact that certain fluorescent dyes bind stoichiometrically to DNA and that the DNA content can be determined by measurement of the intensity of resulting staining reaction. These measurements are recorded in the form of histograms that depict the DNA distribution in the tumor. Tumors containing normal complements of DNA, diploid neoplasms, are distinguished from those which contain abnormal DNA compliments, aneuploid tumors. In several studies of specific tumor types, the occurrence of aneuploid cell populations has correlated to poorer prognosis when compared with tumors of the same histologic type composed of a diploid cell population. Carcinomas of the urinary bladder, prostate, and colon are examples of neoplasms in which DNA ploidy analysis has provided useful prognostic information (14).

GROWTH AND DISSEMINATION OF CANCER

Although a discussion of etiology and pathogenesis of cancer is beyond the scope of this chapter, a consideration of the growth of cancer and its dissemination is an integral part of its pathology.

Growth Rates

The early growth stages of many tumors in humans are poorly understood because of difficulties inherent in studying them. Several tumors, such as carcinoma of the cervix and some types of carcinoma of the lung, have been extensively studied and the details of the earliest identifiable morphologic stages are well known (9,40).

These studies show that the developmental time for a cancer can be quite long. The length of the preinvasive developmental phase of squamous carcinoma of the cervix, for example, is estimated to average 10 years.

Once a malignant tumor has been established, that is, a cancer with invasive and metastatic potential has developed, we often speak of its growth rate in terms of doubling time (12).

The doubling time is the mean length of time for division of all the tumor cells present. The doubling time varies with different types of tumors and with the same type of tumor in different patients. It depends on a number of interrelated factors, still not well understood (16,45). It has been calculated that approximately 30 doubling times are required for a tumor to reach 1 cm in diameter. A neoplasm of this size contains about 10^9 cells. Most tumors, except perhaps those on the body surface, will have reached this size before being detectable clinically (48). Depending on the doubling time, we see how a cancer can exist for a long period in an occult form prior to its clinical detection (Fig. 3- 7).

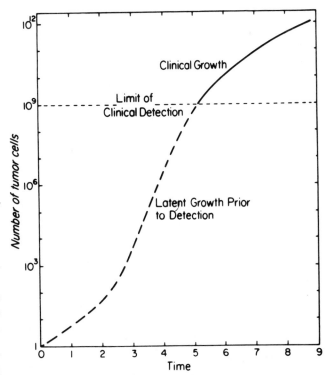

Fig. 3-7. Hypothetical growth curve for a human tumor, showing the long latent period prior to detection. Tumors may show an early lag phase and progressive slowing of growth at large size. From Tannock, I.F.; Hill, R.B. The basic science of oncology. Elmsford, NY: Pergamon Press; 1987, with permission of McGraw-Hill, Inc.

Patterns of Growth

As a tumor grows, it assumes any of a number of forms that usually, but not always, correlate with biologic behavior. Benign tumors generally tend to have a spherical configuration corresponding to their symmetrical, controlled growth (Fig. 3-8). This symmetry can be altered by the location of the tumor and the confines of contiguous structures. These benign growths compress and push normal tissue. They also often demonstrate a capsule. In general, malignant neoplasms expand, invade, and destroy normal adjacent tissue. Their outline is usually irregular and poorly defined. When arising from epithelial-lined surfaces, they often cause ulceration as they destroy and invade underlying tissue (Fig. 3-9). In other instances, they grow as large, fungating, luminal masses. This growth pattern may have a bearing on prognosis, since the infiltrative, more destructive lesions are those most prone to dissemination.

Dissemination

Dissemination of malignant neoplasm occurs through the processes of contiguous spread and metastases. The steps leading to the establishment of metastases are summarized in Fig. 3-10. The most common modes of metastases are through the lymphatic system and by means of the blood stream (Fig. 3-11). Other routes are also possible (e.g., transabdominal spread within the peritoneal cavity or dissemination through the cerebral spinal fluid) but they are much less common. It is by means of its invasive ability that a cancer gains access to the blood and lymphatic vascular systems. Other tumor growths are then established in regional lymph nodes and distant organs. These, in turn, can function as sites from which further metastases may be established (Figs. 3-12, 3-13).

The mechanisms functioning in the invasive process are not completely understood and remain the focus of extensive

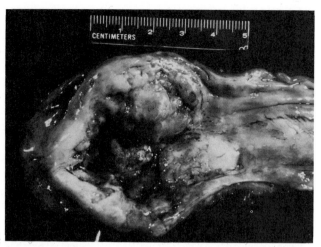

Fig. 3-9. Squamous cell carcinoma of the esophagus. A large, destructive, ulcerative tumor has replaced the esophageal mucosa and wall.

investigation. Numerous theories have been offered to explain the process, and a number of characteristics of tumor cells have been noted which appear to play a role in the process. These include:

- alteration of the surface biochemical structure of tumor cells (20)
- increased motility of tumor cells (50)
- elaboration of lytic substances by tumor cells (26,33,38,44)
- decreased mutual adhesiveness of tumor cells (41)
- loss of "mutual growth restraint" between tumor cells and between tumor cells and normal tissue (15,39)

The currently accepted concepts regarding the initiation of invasion encompass many of these observations. It is thought that the invasive process involves three steps (3,25).

1. The binding of the tumor cells to the basement membrane through the mediation of altered receptors on the cell surface.
2. Dissolution of the basement membrane by lytic enzymes released by the tumor cells.
3. Invasion and movement through the resulting defect.

Although the routes of metastases are well known, the details of the remaining steps in the process are not well explained. Gaining access to vascular spaces does not assure the establishment of metastases. It is well known that tumor cells often circulate in the blood stream and lymphatic channels without the establishment of metastatic foci. It is also known that certain cancers have definite patterns or preferred sites for metastases. There are many theories and suggestions to explain these and other problematic aspects of cancer spread.

Mechanical Theory

This straightforward view states that the incidence and number of metastases are a function of the number of cells and the size of the cells and cell groups gaining access to the circulation. The tumor cells lodge in small capillary and sinusoidal vascular channels due to mechanical factors and interaction with the coagulation system. (Anticoagulants have prevented metastases in experimental systems) (22). Although some or most cancer cells die, some proliferate and invade. If these are the main factors, the selectivity for certain tumors for certain

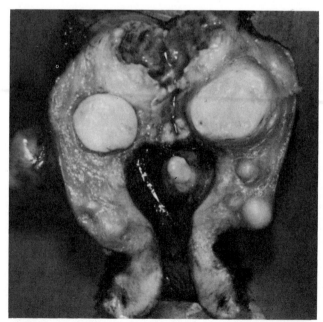

Fig. 3-8. Leiomyomas of the uterus. Note the well-defined nature of these benign tumor nodules. There is cystic degeneration of the nodule at the top.

STEPS IN THE FORMATION OF A METASTASIS

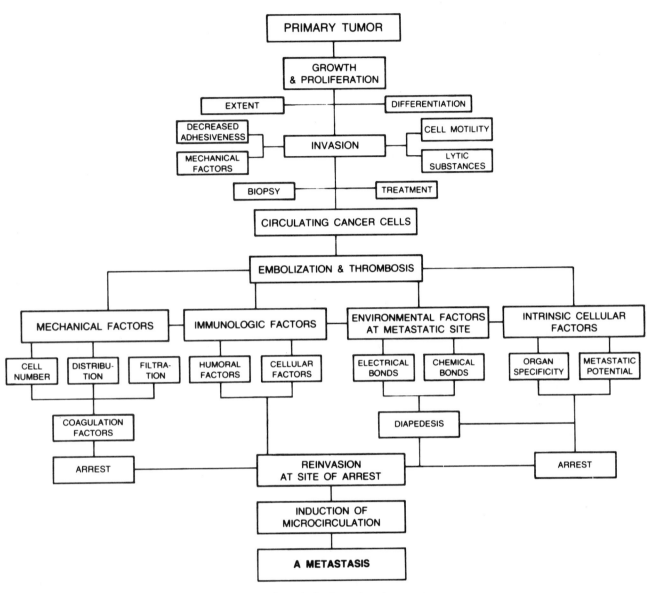

Fig. 3-10 . Steps in the formation of a metastases.

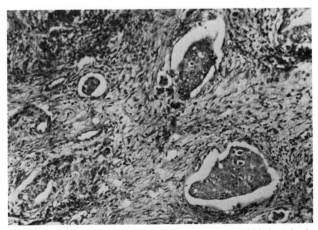

Fig. 3-11. Carcinoma of the breast with tumor cells within lymphatic channels. (400X, H&E.)

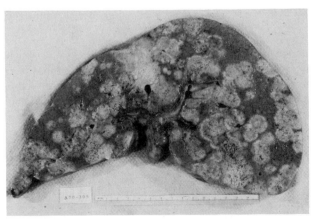

Fig. 3-12. Carcinoma of breast metastatic to liver.

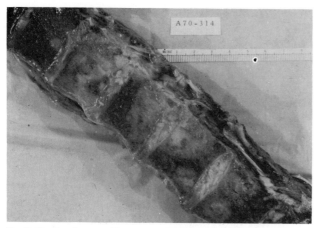

Fig. 3-13. Carcinoma of breast metastatic to vertebral bodies.

body sites is not well explained. This led to the suggestion of *the "soil" theory* (28,46).

"Soil" Theory

This theory holds that metastatic distribution was determined by the environment of the various organs and tissues at which tumor cells arrived. The idea is that certain tumors can thrive only in a particular growing site or "soil." More recently, evidence suggests a third theory.

Intrinsic Cellular Factors Theory (28, 34)

Individual tumor cells have properties that determine their patterns of metastases. The evidence in support of this theory implies that tumor cell populations contain a few subpopulations of cells with a high metastatic potential, and that cells with a propensity to metastasize to a specific body site exist and are selected out during tumor progression.

Immunologic Surveillance (15,17)

In this theory the formation of cancers and their dissemination is a result of a defect in the immunologic defense system of the body. This concept is supported by experimental evidence that circulating tumor cells are destroyed by host macrophages and natural killer lymphocytes. To establish a metastasis, tumor cells must survive these immunologically mediated defenses. Experimental evidence, however, has failed to show consistent correlation between the strength of the immune mechanism and the control of metastases.

No theory so far offered is entirely satisfactory. Indeed, it is clear that many different mechanisms are functioning. The answer to the problem lies within the complex interactions of tumor and host, the subject of much of the current investigative work in oncology. It is most likely that the establishment of metastases is dependent on a large number of factors including those suggested above and some of which we may not yet be aware.

WHAT THE ONCOLOGIST NEEDS TO KNOW ABOUT HISTOPATHOLOGY

Physicians sometimes erroneously assume that pathologists' diagnoses are final and therefore immutable. This is especially true concerning neoplastic disease because the diagnosis of cancer almost always depends on the recognition of a pattern of cellular growth and of deviations of the individual cells from their normal forms as seen by light microscopy. The one physician whose special training enables such decisions is the surgical pathologist, but the ultimate establishment of the diagnosis of cancer sometimes requires more than the examination of a slice of tissue or cells through a microscope. The process of establishing a diagnosis of a tumor and deciding whether it is benign or malignant is not an exact science (42). In spite of the aura of infallibility with which they sometimes are regarded by their clinical colleagues or themselves, pathologists do make mistakes in diagnosis of tumors. Those concerned in the care of patients with tumors should remember several facts.

1. *Pathologists are human and therefore fallible.* In general, the more experienced the pathologist, the greater the likelihood that he or she will be accurate in diagnoses. Occasionally the super-specialist in pathology may be troubled by the "tunnel vision" imposed by concentration on a single organ or tissue in just the same way that the specialty-trained clinical cousins may be led astray by failing to think of the whole patient.

2. *Histologic and cytologic techniques and therefore histopathology and cytopathology are not exact sciences.* A part of the pathologist's fallibility is related to the techniques used. With present methods, it is not practically feasible to separate a group of living cells from a patient and to study them sufficiently well to establish a positive diagnosis while those cells are still alive. When cells or tissues suspected of neoplastic transformation are submitted to a pathologist, they are either frozen or "fixed" with chemicals, producing a variety of artifacts. Although the technologists who help to prepare such specimens for microscopic examination are extremely skillful in the traditional methods of making stained slides of those samples (and pathologists have become quite skillful in interpreting such cell or tissue samples microscopically), there still are many facets of this process to consider:

   a. *Not all technologists are equally skillful.* Unless all conditions are optimum, many artifacts may appear in the final preparation. These artifacts may make accurate diagnosis impossible.

   b. *Although good laboratories have extensive quality-assurance programs to avoid serious errors, mistakes may still occur in processing the tissue.* Possible mistakes may include incorrect identification of the specimen with the proper patient and failure to properly embed the one diagnostic bit of tissue out of several submitted, so that the pathologist never sees it.

   c. *The best possible histologic and cytologic techniques cannot provide an adequate specimen for diagnosis if the biopsy technique is poor or if the sample of tissue selected fails to include the diagnostic part of the lesion.* Pressure or thermal injuries to the tissues during the biopsy may prevent proper diagnostic evaluation.

   d. *Routine histologic and cytologic techniques only produce two-dimensional static samples to be studied by the light microscope.* Many pathologists and clinicians fail to think of the lesion in three dimensions and even more importantly, in terms of the fourth dimension

— time. The cells of a tumor are heterogeneous and change constantly. Most tumors develop after a long latent period following stimulus. Hyperplasia, often long continued, blends imperceptibly with neoplasia.

3. *Pathologists are not omniscient and you should not expect them to be able to predict accurately what will happen in any given patient.* For example, if a pathologist makes a diagnosis of reactive hyperplasia on a lymph node and the patient subsequently develops a nodular malignant lymphoma, you should not necessarily assume that the first diagnosis was incorrect. Disease processes may change with time. Nevertheless, one should request a review of all previous histologic specimens whenever a diagnosis of cancer is made. This will help everyone learn and tends to keep pathologists humble (35)

4. *Avoid becoming trapped by semantics.* Cancer in general sometimes is thought of as a single disease, and a specific kind of cancer, as labeled by the histopathologist, such as a malignant melanoma of the skin, is thought of as a specific neoplastic disease entity. Once the histopathologic diagnosis or label is written on a patient's record, that individual tends to be looked on henceforth as having that specific disease. It should be remembered that individual tumors are as unique as the individual patients in whom they develop. The tumors are composed of living cells and are part of the host. In spite of many definitions of cancers as autonomous, the cells of any malignant tumor, regardless of their degree of anaplasia, are living in and are nourished by the individual host. They are subject to all the complexities of that host including genetic and environmental (both internal and external) influences. The growth potential of many tumors may be modified by changing a variety of host factors (e.g., immunologic, hormonal).

5. *The histologic appearance may vary from area to area within some neoplasms.* In a given tumor, the degree of differentiation of the cancer cells may range from low-grade to high-grade. Obviously, it is hazardous to predict biologic behavior on the basis of limited samples of such tumors and arbitrary numerical grades of carcinomas may be misleading. Furthermore, many cancers undergo necrosis. Samples from necrotic areas usually are impossible to interpret microscopically. The most meaningful evaluations of tumors usually are those in which sufficient samples of the neoplasms have been studied to visualize all possible variations of tumor growth patterns and cytologic changes.

6. *Some tumors appear to be malignant histologically but are benign biologically.* Histopathologists cannot always equate the presence of very bizarre anaplastic and polyploid cells with or without increased mitotic activity with a diagnosis of a malignant tumor. For example, the so-called atypical fibroxanthoma of the sun-exposed skin of elderly patients may look like a sarcoma but almost never metastasizes or gives other evidence of malignant behavior. Other tumors appear to be benign histologically but are malignant biologically. For example, some carcinomas of the thyroid metastatic to bone may look like normal thyroid microscopically.

7. *Virtually identical histologic patterns may represent totally different diseases.* Many pathologists have learned to recognize the histologic pictures they see through the microscope and to identify them with specific labels. Occasionally they forget or are unaware of situations where similar pictures may represent quite different disease processes. For example, a giant cell tumor of bone, an "aneurysmal bone cyst," and the "brown tumor" of hyperparathyroidism are virtually indistinguishable on histologic grounds alone; but they could be separated easily if the pathologist looked at the roentgenograms along with the slides. Such possibilities of misinterpretation when the microscope is the sole tool for diagnosis emphasize the fact that pathologists need to be physicians first and histopathologic experts second. Tumor diagnosis should not be a "guessing game" when patients' lives are at stake. Be sure that the pathologist is made aware of all the data (including historic, laboratory and roentgenographic).

In view of these considerations, it is clear that there are situations where it is prudent not to accept a written report of histopathologic diagnosis as unequivocal. This is especially true when the pathologic diagnosis does not fit with the other clinical data. Histopathologic diagnoses should be considered, as should other laboratory values, and the primary data (the microscopic sections) should be reviewed whenever the interpretation varies from the other clinical aspects of the case. All of the foregoing should be remembered when this review is being done, hopefully as a direct consultation between you and the pathologist. If all the facts still fail to fit the clinical disease as expressed in the unique individual patient, rebiopsy may be indicated. The best interests and welfare of the patient depend on good communication among all the physicians who care for that patient.

Finally, do not act on verbal reports, particularly when it is a secondhand transmission of the pathologist's report. This is doubly true if the patient is referred from another hospital. Check directly with the pathologist and better yet, review the slides with him or her (40).

Recommended Reading

The literature on the pathology of cancer is vast, detailed, and often highly specialized. Numerous journals and textbooks are available relating to basic pathology, histologic, and cytologic diagnosis and research aspects of the disease. The chapter on neoplasia in *Pathology* (3), edited by Rubin and Farber, is an excellent introduction to the pathobiology of cancer. *The Atlas of Tumor Pathology*, published by the Armed Forces Institute of Pathology (8), is a major reference work for tumor morphology and classification and Underwood's *Introduction to Biopsy Interpretation and Surgical Pathology* (5) is a succinct summary of the basic principles related to the formation of accurate histopathologic diagnoses.

ACKNOWLEDGMENTS

The authors wish to express their appreciation to Dr. Roger Terry, a co-author of this chapter in previous editions, for permission to retain sections containing much of what was his original contribution.

REFERENCES

General References

1. DeVita, V.T.; Hellman, S.; Rosenberg, S.A. Cancer: principles and practice of oncology, 3rd ed. Philadelphia, PA: J.B. Lippincott Co.; 1989.
2. Pierce, G.B.; Shikes, R.; Fink, L.M. Cancer: a problem of developmental biology. Englewood Cliffs, NJ: Prentice-Hall; 1978.
3. Rubin, E., Farber, J.L., eds. Pathology. Philadelphia, PA: J.B. Lippincott Co.; 1988:140-195.
4. Tannock, I.F.; Hill, R.B. The basic science of oncology. Elmsford, NY: Pergamon Press; 1987.
5. Underwood, J.C.E. Introduction to biopsy interpretation and surgical pathology. New York: Springer-Verlag; 1987.

Specific References

5a. Aaronson S.A.: Growth factors in cancer. Science: 1146-1152; 1991.
6. American Joint Committee on Cancer. Manual for staging of cancer, 3rd ed. Philadelphia, PA: J.B. Lippincott Co.; 1988.
7. Ashley, D.J.B. Evans histological appearance of tumors, 3rd ed. New York, NY: Churchill Livingstone; 1978.
8. Atlas of tumor pathology, 2nd Series. Sixteen fascicles by various authors. Washington, DC: Armed Forces Institute of Pathology; 1967-1980.
9. Barron, B.A.; Richart, R.M. A statistical model of the natural history of cervical carcinoma based on a prospective study of 557 cases. J. Nat. Cancer Inst. 41:1343-1353; 1968.
10. Bernard, C. Quoted by Krumbhaar, E. B. Pathology. New York, NY: Paul B. Hoeber, Inc.; 1937:VII.
11. Bishop, J.M. The molecular genetics of cancer. Science 1235: 308-311; 1987.
12. Bishop, J.M. Cellular oncogenes and retroviruses. Annual Rev. Biochem. 52: 301-354; 1983.
13. Collins, V.P.; Loeffler, R.K.; Tivey, H. Observations on growth rates of human tumors. Am. J. Roentgenol. Radium Ther. Nucl. Med. 76:988-1000; 1956.
14. Coon, J.S.; Landay, A.L.,;Weinstein, R.S. Biology of disease: advances in flow cytometry for diagnostic pathology. Lab. Invest. 57:453-479; 1987.
15. Fidler, I.J. Inhibition of pulmonary metastases by intravenous injection of specifically activated macrophages. Cancer Res. 34: 1074-1078; 1974.
16. Folkman, J.; Cotran, R. Relation of vascular proliferation to tumor growth. Int. Rev. Exp. Path. 16:207-248; 1976.
17. Frost, P.; Kerbal, R.S. Immunology of metastases: can the immune response cope with dissemination of tumor? Cancer Metastasis Rev. 2:237-256; 1983.
18. Gallo, R.C. The first human retrovirus. Sci. Am. 256 (12): 89- 99; 1986.
19. Gordon, H. Oncogenes. Mayo Clinic Proceedings. 60: 697-713; 1985.
20. Henson, D.E. The histologic grading of neoplasms. Arch. Pathol. Lab .Med. 112: 1091-1096; 1988.
21. Hill, R.B. Metastasis. In: Tannock, I.F.; Hill, R.P., eds. The basic science of oncology. Elmsford, NY: Pergamon Press; 1988:160-175.
22. Honn, K.V.; Cicone, B.; Skoff, A. Protacyclin: a potent antimetastases agent. Science 212:1270-1271;1981.
23. Huntington, R.W. Classification of neoplasia — a critical appraisal. Persp..Biol. and Med. 20:215-222; 1977.
24. Land, H.; Parada, L.F.; Weinberg, R.A. Cellular oncogenes and multistep carcinogenesis. Science 222: 771-778; 1983.
25. Liotta, L.A.; Rao, C.N. Tumor invasion and metastases. In: Fenoglio-Preiser, C.M.; Weinstein, R.S.; Kaufman, N., eds. New concepts in neoplasia as applied to pathology . Baltimore, MD: Williams & Wilkins; 1986:183-192.
26. Liotta, L.A.; Thorgeirsson, U.P.; Garbisa, S. Role of collagenases in tumor cell invasion. Cancer Metastasis Rev. 1:277-297; 1982.
27. Miller, E.C.; Miller, J.A. Mechanisms of chemical carcinogenesis Cancer 47: 1055-1064; 1981.
28. Nicolson, G.I. Cancer metastasis. Sci. Amer. 240:66-76; 1979.
29. Pagano, J.S. Epithelial cell interactions of the Epstein-Barr virus. In: Notkins, A.L.; Oldstone, M.B.A.,eds. Concepts in viral pathogenesis. New York, NY: Springer-Verlag; 1984:307-314.
30. Papanicoloau, G.; Traut, H. F. Diagnosis of uterine cancer by the vaginal smear. New York, NY: The Commonwealth Fund; 1943.
31. Park, W.W. The histology of borderline cancer with notes on prognosis. New York, NY: Springer-Verlag; 1980.
32. Peto, R.; ZurHausen, H., eds. Banbury report 21: viral etiology of cervical cancer. New York, NY: Cold Spring Harbor Laboratory; 1986.
33. Poole, A.R. Tumor hyposomal enzymes and invasive growth. In: Dingle, J.T., ed. Lysosomes in biology and pathology. Amsterdam, Holland: North Holland Pub. Co.; 1973:303-337.
34. Poste, G.; Fidler, I.J. The pathogenesis of cancer metastasis. Nature 283:139-146; 1980.
35. Rambo, O.M. The limitations of histologic diagnosis. In: Buschke, E., ed. Progress in radiation therapy. New York, NY: F. Grune & Stratton; 1962:205.
36. Rapp, F. Current knowledge of mechanisms of viral carcinogenesis. CRC Crit. Rev. Toxicol. 13:197; 1984.
37. Rapp, F.; Howett, M.K. Herpes viruses and cancer. In: Notkins, A L ; Oldstone, M.B.A , eds. Concepts in viral pathogenesis. New York, NY: Springer-Verlag; 300-306; 1984.
38. Recklies, A.D.; Tiltman, K.J.; Stoker, T.A.M.; Poole, A.R. Secretion of proteinases from malignant and nonmalignant human breast tissue. Cancer Research 40:550-555; 1980.
39. Rubin, P.; Green, J.P. Solitary metastases. Springfield, IL: C. C. Thomas; 1967.
40. Saccomano, G.; Archer, U.F.; Auerback, O.; Saunders, R.P.; Brennan, L.M. Development of carcinoma of the lung as reflected in exfoliated cells. Cancer 33:256-270; 1974.
41. Scott RE, Furcht LT: Membrane Pathology of Normal and Malignant Cells: A Review. Human Path; 7:519-532; 1976.
42. Sissons, H.A. Agreement and disagreement between pathologists in histologic diagnosis. Postgrad. Med. J. 51:685-689; 1975.
43. Slamon, D.J. Protooncogenes and human cancers. New Eng. J. Med. 317(15): 955-957:1987.
44. Sloane, B.F. Lysosomal cathepsin B: correlation with metastatic potential. Science 212:1151-1153; 1981.
45. Sommers, S.C. Growth rates, cell kinetics and mathematical models of human cancers. In: Ioachim, H.L., ed. Pathobiology annual. New York, NY: Appleton Century Crofts; 1973:309-340.
46. Southam, C.M.; Babcock, V.I.; Bailey, R.B. Selective localization of human cancer transplants in newborn rats. Transplantation 5:1-10; 1967.
47. Storer, J.B. Radiation carcinogenesis. In: Becker, F.F., ed. Cancer: a comprehensive treatise, 2nd ed. New York, NY: Plenum Publishing; 1982:629-659.
48. Tannock, I.F. Tumor growth and cell kinetics. In: Tannock, I.F.; Hill, R.P., eds. The basic science of oncology. Elmsford, NY: Pergamon Press; 1988:140-159.
49. Weinberg, R.A. Finding the anti-oncogene. Sci. Am. 259(3):44-51; 1988.
49a. Weinberg, R.A. Tumor supressor genes. Science 254: 1139-1145; 1991.
50. Wood, S. Mechanisms of establishment of tumor metastases. In: Ioachim, H.L., ed. Pathobiology annual. New York, NY: Appleton Century Crofts; 1971:281-308.
51. Zurhasen H: Viruses in human cancer. Science 254: 1167-1172; 1991.

Virginia K. Langmuir, M.D., Surgical Oncology   W. Bradford Patterson, M.D., Surgical Oncology
Seymour I. Schwartz, M.D., Surgery

Chapter **4**

PRINCIPLES OF SURGICAL ONCOLOGY

There is no such thing as minor surgery, only minor surgeons.

Anonymous (1)

PERSPECTIVE

In the past, the surgeon often worked independently from other physicians when treating cancer. The surgeon's role was to remove tumors by wide en bloc resection before spread to distant sites had occurred. If metastatic disease developed, the patient was then sent to the medical or radiation oncologist for further therapy. New understandings of the patterns of spread of malignant disease have led surgeons to take a more active role in the multidisciplinary approach to cancer management. It is now believed that cancer does not spread in an orderly fashion from primary site to lymphatics to regional lymph nodes and then into the blood stream to seed distant sites. It is clear that tumor cells can embolize to regional nodes without being trapped in other lymphatics in transit, and hematogenous dissemination can occur independently of lymphatic spread.

In the early years of the twentieth century, it was believed that cancer spread from the primary site, to the regional lymph nodes, and then to the systemic circulation, leading to distant metastases. Wide resection of the primary site in continuity with the regional lymph nodes was performed in the belief that this would prevent distant metastasis in patients who had tumors that had spread to the regional nodes but not yet to the systemic circulation. However, many of these patients still developed distant disease, even if the regional lymph nodes had been negative. Beginning in the 1960s and 1970s, more conservative surgery was used in certain tumors such as breast, colon, and lung cancer, with no evidence that survival was being sacrificed. It is now generally believed that in most cancers, regional lymph node spread occurs independently from systemic metastasis and many surgeons are taking a more conservative approach when resecting the primary tumor.

When treating a patient with a newly diagnosed cancer, the surgeon has several responsibilities: (1) biopsy for tissue diagnosis; (2) adequate staging; (3) consultation with medical and radiation oncologists as to the indications for adjuvant therapy; (4) surgical resection of the tumor when appropriate with attention given to the needs of other consultants, such as marking residual tumor for radiation therapy or removing lymph nodes for staging purposes; and (5) appropriate follow-up.

SURGICAL IMPLICATIONS OF THE BIOLOGY OF CANCER

Predictability of Spread

A few cancers almost always grow in a predictably slow fashion, and can be cured by excision even when advanced, if vital structures are not involved. Other cancers occupy a broad spectrum, with anaplastic sarcomas and carcinomas at the far end, growing at irregular rates, spreading unpredictably, and sometimes being disseminated by treatment.

Undifferentiated cancers with high mitotic rates and rapid cell turnover have a poor prognosis in contrast with the well-differentiated cancers with infrequent mitoses and slow rates of growth. These different growth patterns are associated with a marked difference in 5-year survival rates.

Patterns of Local Invasion

The mechanisms by which cancer cells penetrate basement membranes and infiltrate surrounding tissues are unknown, but this phenomenon of invasiveness is an important characteristic to the surgeon. In the breast, these have been called "pushing" types, as opposed to others called "invading," which expand by sending cells singly and in groups through the surrounding stroma, entering veins, lymphatics, and nerve sheaths. Invasiveness may result from capillaries, which proliferate among the tumor cells in response to an "angiogenesis factor" secreted by the tumor (26).

Invasion of veins of microscopic size is associated with a poor prognosis. In renal cell carcinomas, invasion of the renal vein is not uncommon and usually presages metastases.

Epithelial cancers (e.g., breast, skin, colon, lung) usually incite a fibrous reaction within the tissues they invade. This is called *desmoplasia* and is manifested to the clinician by hardness and rigidity of the invaded tissues. *Tissue texture is thus of great help in distinguishing surgical margins*, and in the differential diagnosis of benign and malignant tumors. (Both acute and chronic inflammatory reactions also may accompany invasive cancers and cause confusing changes in tissue consistency.)

Surgeons commonly determine the margin around a cancer by visible and tactile changes, then try to remove enough surrounding tissue to allow for microscopic invasion.

Margins also are dictated by natural anatomic boundaries, by cosmetic factors, and by experience. There is no survival advantage to excessive removal of surrounding tissue. It has been shown, for example, that no better cure rate is achieved by resecting a whole lung than by taking the involved lobe, as long as there is no gross evidence of involvement of the other lobes noted at the time of operation.

Dysplastic Tissue

If there is evidence of dysplasia (a preneoplastic state) in an organ, removal of the whole organ may be indicated. Examples include total colectomy for a single cancer in the presence of multiple polyposis, total cystectomy for cancer in multiple papillomatosis of the bladder, or excision of mucous membrane if cancer is associated with leukoplakia or a wide area of skin with advanced radiation dermatitis.

Regional Lymph Nodes

Surgeons have debated for many years whether to remove regional lymph nodes during a cancer operation. Little disagreement exists about the management of suspiciously enlarged nodes. All agree they should be excised, if removal can be complete and if they represent the only site of suspected metastasis; however, where nodes are not clinically enlarged or suspicious, some surgeons prefer not to remove them unless they lie close to the primary cancer, as in the colon or lung.

This debate occurs because nodes do have some degree of barrier function. Cells shed from a cancer through lymphatics are often filtered out at the first nodal station and grow there. If this were always true, early removal of lymph nodes could save patients' lives when the cancer had spread to the nodes, but no further. Unfortunately, detached cancer cells may also bypass lymph nodes and lodge only at distant sites. It has been difficult to prove, even in clinical trials, that early elective removal of nodes saves lives (46). Surgeons today are adopting more flexible attitudes toward regional nodes, recognizing that their removal may prevent development of troublesome and painful masses, may reduce the body burden of tumor cells, and is of prognostic importance. However, removal of regional nodes may not be the determining factor in cure or failure (9).

Circulating Cancer Cells

Spread of cancer through veins is common, and when it occurs, surgical cure is much less likely. The surgeon learns of this phenomenon from the pathologist's report describing "blood vessel invasion," or from seeing pulmonary metastases in a patient. Occasionally, with slow-growing tumors, resection of solitary blood-bone metastases is curative.

Cancer cells circulate in the peripheral blood and have been demonstrated by filtration or concentration techniques. The importance of host factors to the fate of these cells is greater than initially supposed, since correlation between the presence of circulating cells and metastases formation and prognosis is lacking. Surgical techniques that minimize handling and attempt to prevent dissemination of tumor cell emboli have long been recommended. However, the initial hope that the "no-touch technique" can lead to improved cure rates has not been substantiated (44). Although biopsy can result in release of tumor cells into the circulation, it has not been demonstrated that metastases increase.

SURGICAL DETECTION AND BIOPSY FOR TISSUE DIAGNOSIS

Several methods can be used to make a tissue diagnosis of cancer. The method to use depends on a number of clinical factors as well as the expertise of the pathologists.

Fine Needle Aspiration (FNA) Cytology

With fine needle aspiration (FNA) cytology, a small gauge needle (usually 22G) is used to aspirate cells and cell clusters from a mass. Multiple passes are made with the needle so that many areas of the tumor are sampled. The contents of the needle are then smeared on a slide, fixed, and stained. The pathologist must make a cytologic interpretation without the benefit of normal tissue architecture as is seen on a regular biopsy. Considerable expertise with this technique is required before it is reliable. With experience, false-positive diagnoses approach zero and false negatives will be minimized (Fig. 4-1).

This technique is commonly used in the diagnosis of thyroid and breast lesions and results are obtained on the same day that the patient is seen, which has obvious psychologic advantages to the patient. There is also the advantage that therapeutic decisions can be made without a preliminary operation. FNA cytology of less accessible organs such as the pancreas can be performed in the radiology department using

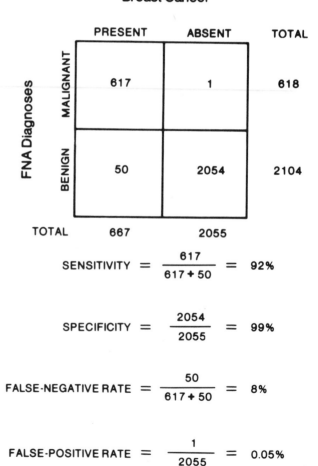

Breast Cancer

	PRESENT	ABSENT	TOTAL
MALIGNANT	617	1	618
BENIGN	50	2054	2104
TOTAL	667	2055	

$$\text{SENSITIVITY} = \frac{617}{617 + 50} = 92\%$$

$$\text{SPECIFICITY} = \frac{2054}{2055} = 99\%$$

$$\text{FALSE-NEGATIVE RATE} = \frac{50}{617 + 50} = 8\%$$

$$\text{FALSE-POSITIVE RATE} = \frac{1}{2055} = 0.05\%$$

Fig. 4-1. Sensitivity and specificity of benign and malignant breast aspirates. From Oertel (41), with permission.

ultrasound or computed tomographic guidance. In patients with unresectable disease, surgery can sometimes be avoided completely by making the diagnosis in this way. Some tumors, such as lymphomas and soft tissue sarcomas, are not easily diagnosed with this technique and open biopsy usually should be performed.

Core Needle Biopsy

This technique uses a large bore needle to take a core of tissue from the tumor. This has the advantage of preserving the histologic architecture so that interpretation is easier. Disadvantages include possible bleeding, seeding of the needle track with tumor cells, and missing the diagnosis because only one small portion of the tumor is sampled. With the advent of FNA, this technique is now used infrequently for palpable lesions; however, it is still a useful technique for intraoperative diagnoses, such as for hepatic lesions and transduodenal biopsy of masses in the head of the pancreas.

Open Biopsy

Open biopsy can be either incisional (partial excision) or excisional (complete excision). In general, excisional biopsy is preferable unless the lesion is very large. With this method, it is possible to examine the whole tumor histologically and thus be sure of an accurate diagnosis. In malignant melanoma, this will allow determination of the maximum depth of invasion, which is important in deciding on definitive therapy. In breast cancer, enough tissue should be taken for measurement of estrogen and progesterone receptors (0.5 mL), as well as for histologic diagnosis. With suspected basal cell and squamous cell carcinomas of the skin, incisional biopsy is adequate. The same is true of endoscopic biopsy of gastrointestinal (GI) and endobronchial malignancies, although multiple biopsies should be taken to increase the likelihood of making the diagnosis. All biopsies (including needle biopsies) should be done with thought given to future therapy. Incisions should be in a line that would be easily excised at the time of definitive surgery.

In some instances, if the margins are adequate, excisional biopsies may suffice as definitive therapy. Such instances include lumpectomy for breast cancer and cone biopsy for carcinoma in situ of the uterine cervix. Marking the margins with India ink is essential to allow the pathologist to state with confidence that the margins are free of tumor. Specimens should also be marked so that their orientation in the patient is clear to the pathologist.

Surgical Staging

Adequate nonoperative staging is essential before definitive surgical therapy for a malignancy because the detection of distant disease may alter the therapeutic approach. Less radical surgery may be performed if the patient is found to have unresectable metastatic disease. On the other hand, a finding of other disease may extend the scope of surgery. For instance, if a second cancer is found in a patient with colorectal cancer, subtotal colectomy may be planned. The appropriate choice of preoperative investigations is determined by the clinical findings and the type of tumor. This is discussed in detail in the chapters on each tumor type.

Operative staging has become important in a number of tumors. The most common staging procedure is lymph node dissection in patients with clinically uninvolved nodes. In

carcinoma of the breast, adjuvant chemotherapy and hormonal therapy may be determined by the pathological status of the regional lymph nodes (47). Recent reports suggest that there is a role for adjuvant therapy in some patients with uninvolved nodes (24,25,36,37,40). If this is proven, lymph node dissection may become unnecessary in certain patient categories. Biopsy of lymph nodes may lead to important therapeutic decisions in other cancers. For instance, in lung cancer the finding of involved nodes at the time of mediastinoscopy may lead to radiation therapy alone rather than thoracotomy and resection.

Staging laparotomy is often performed for Hodgkin's disease (and occasionally for non-Hodgkin's lymphoma) to determine disease extent because the results may alter therapeutic decisions (28,32). It is essential that this operation be done thoroughly. Splenectomy, liver biopsy (core and wedge from both lobes), and biopsy of any enlarged as well as normal-appearing lymph nodes from the celiac axis, upper and lower para-aortic regions, iliac regions, mesentery, porta hepatis, and perisplenic region must be performed (Fig. 4-2) (30). Open iliac crest bone marrow biopsy is also performed. Staging laparotomy should be performed only if positive or negative findings in the abdomen will change the choice of therapy. If a decision has been made to treat with chemotherapy even if the laparotomy

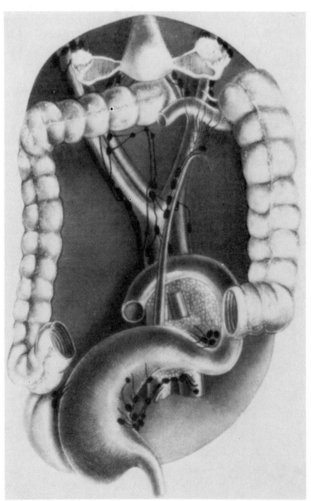

Fig. 4-2. Principal lymph node groups on which biopsies should be done during staging laparotomy for Hodgkin's disease. From Irving (30); by permission of the publishers, Butterworth-Heinemann Ltd.

is negative, then surgery should not be performed. Laparotomy and surgical evaluation are also important in gynecologic cancers such as cancer of the cervix, where pelvic and para-aortic nodes are evaluated, and in the ovary, where the omentum and subdiaphragmatic region are evaluated. With these procedures, GI and colorectal cancers are more precisely defined according to depth and extent of invasion than with current imaging procedures.

PRINCIPLES OF CURATIVE SURGERY

The Primary Tumor

A greater effort is being made in many different sites to provide curative surgery of a more conservative nature, allowing for preservation of normal tissues. This is particularly true now because lesions are being detected at earlier stages and cancers are more readily removed without sacrifice of large portions of the anatomy. The most striking example is the removal of a segment of a breast by lumpectomy in place of radical mastectomy, which involves the removal of the entire breast including the pectoralis muscle (see Figs. 4-3, 4-4, 4-5, and 4-6) (23). In addition, there is a greater tendency for preservation of the anal sphincter in cases of rectal cancer, removal of soft tissue and muscle compartments in limb-sparing procedures for soft tissue sarcoma and nerve-sparing procedures for prostatectomy.

When staging has not detected metastatic disease, there is the possibility that removal of the primary tumor can be

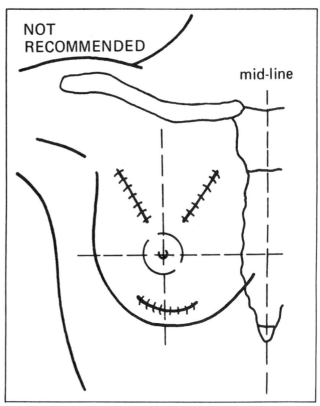

Fig. 4-4. Guidelines in selecting type of operation incision when performing a segmental mastectomy. The radical incisions in the upper half of the breast and continuous incisions shown are to be avoided. Guidelines have evolved from the National Surgical Adjuvant Breast Project's experience with more than 400 patients to date; their implementation will result in improved cosmesis. From Fisher (23), with permission.

curative. For this reason, adequate excision of all visible tumor with histologically free margins is essential. In the past, wide excision, often in continuity with regional lymph nodes, was the norm. In recent years, margins have been reduced substantially in many tumors such as breast cancer, sarcoma, rectal cancer, and malignant melanoma, with no apparent detrimental effect on survival (21). Removal of involved regional lymph nodes may be curative in some tumors, especially squamous cell carcinoma of the head and neck area, so this should be performed when nodes are clinically involved (35).

With certain tumors, it has been shown that adjuvant chemotherapy, hormonal therapy, or radiotherapy of presumed micrometastatic disease improves survival and decreases local recurrences. Therefore, it is important to refer these patients to appropriate consultants. Whenever possible, preoperative consultation should be made. In this way, the patient and the physicians involved are fully informed prior to definitive therapy. This is particularly important now that patients are taking a more active role in treatment decisions. For instance, consultation with the radiation oncologist may lead some women with breast cancer to choose total mastectomy over lumpectomy plus radiation therapy because of the time and effort involved in going for treatments for several weeks.

At the time of definitive surgery, it is important to explore the operative field for evidence of metastatic disease that may have been missed by preoperative staging. Even if evidence of metastases is found, it may be wise to remove the primary unless it is anticipated that the patient will not live long enough to

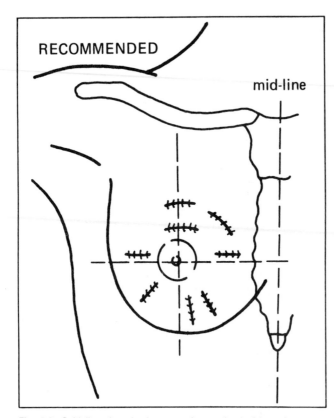

Fig. 4-3. Guidelines in selecting type of operative incision when performing a segmental mastectomy. In lesions located in the upper half of the breast circumferential curvilinear or transverse incisions are recommended. Guidelines have evolved from the National Surgical Adjuvant Breast Project's experience with more than 400 patients to date; their implementation will result in improved cosmesis. From Fisher (23), with permission.

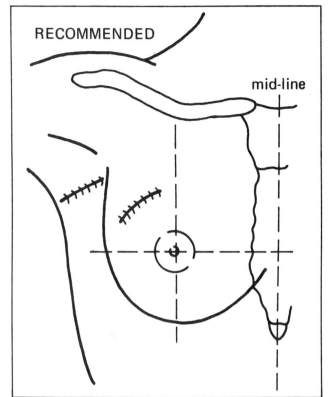

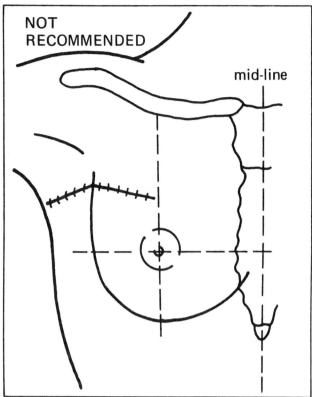

Fig. 4-5. Guidelines in selecting type of operation incision when performing a segmental mastectomy. It is recommended in the majority of instances that the incision for the tumor excision and that for the axillary dissection be separate. A single continuous incision is to be avoided. Guidelines have evolved from the National Surgical Adjuvant Breast Project's experience with more than 400 patients to date; their implementation will result in improved cosmesis. From Fisher (23), with permission.

Fig. 4-6. Guidelines in selecting type of operation incision when performing a segmental mastectomy. An exception to the recommendation to avoid continuous incisions might be for lesions in the axillary tail. Guidelines have evolved from the National Surgical Adjuvant Breast Project's experience with more than 400 patients to date; their implementation will result in improved cosmesis. From Fisher (23), with permission.

make it worthwhile. A good example of this is colorectal cancer with liver metastases. If the patient is expected to live for more than a few months, resection of the primary, particularly if it can be done without a colostomy, may be indicated to relieve symptoms of bleeding, tenesmus, and obstruction, thus improving the quality of the patient's remaining life.

Reconstructive Surgery

The adequate excision of malignant lesions may result in significant deficits of function or appearance and reconstructive surgery often can improve these deficits considerably. Functional deficits such as loss of the stomach or the colon and rectum may require construction of a reservoir to allow adequate nutrition or bowel habit. Extensive head and neck surgery may require reconstruction to improve speech and eating ability as well as for cosmetic reasons. Patients undergoing total mastectomy may desire reconstruction of the breast. The psychologic importance of reconstructive surgery should not be underestimated. If the operative field has not been irradiated extensively, reconstruction may be possible in many of these patients at the time of initial surgery. This will help minimize the inevitable alteration in self-image and can hasten these patients' adjustment to their new appearance.

It is essential that the surgical procedure not be compromised by plans for reconstruction because cure is the most important goal. If the surgeon performing the initial surgery

is not going to do the reconstruction, preoperative consultation between the two surgeons is essential as small changes in the initial procedure that do not compromise the resection planes may markedly enhance the success of the reconstructive procedure (Fig. 4-7) (18).

Regional Lymph Nodes

Regional lymph nodes that are clinically involved with tumor should be removed. Although this may not increase the chance of cure, it will decrease the morbidity of having bulky regional disease. There is little evidence in any tumor that

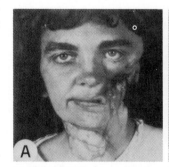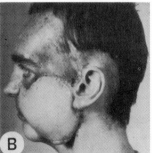

Fig. 4-7. Palliative reconstruction of the face in a patient with recurrent sarcoma of the face. Photograph A is preoperative appearance. Photograph B shows final postoperative appearance. From Bakamjian (18), with permission.

excision of clinically negative lymph nodes will lead to a higher likelihood of cure. In most cancers, however, the presence of pathologically positive lymph nodes predicts a poorer prognosis for the patient. If this will influence the future management of the patient (such as adjuvant chemotherapy in breast cancer), lymph node dissection may be indicated, but it may be a less extensive procedure when done strictly for staging purposes.

Metastatic Cancer

Although the development of metastatic cancer usually indicates incurable disease, in rare instances curative surgical resection may be possible (15). Several criteria must be fulfilled before operating. The primary lesion must be controlled; there must be the potential for complete resection of the metastases; there must be no other equally effective or better antitumor therapy available; metastases should involve only one organ; reasonable postoperative function must be anticipated; expected survival should be better than if left untreated; and the patient must be able to tolerate the surgical procedure.

Pulmonary Metastases

Resection of pulmonary metastases via median sternotomy to allow both lungs to be fully assessed has led to 40% long-term survival rates in patients with osteogenic sarcoma. Lesser but still better-than-untreated survival rates have been obtained in soft tissue sarcoma, urinary tract cancers, and, occasionally, melanoma. In conjunction with chemotherapy, some nonseminomatous testicular cancers have responded well to resection of pulmonary metastases (33).

Hepatic Metastases

Patients with endocrine tumors, e.g., carcinoids, will respond symptomatically if over 90% of the disease in the liver can be removed. This palliation is often long-lasting, since these tumors tend to grow very slowly. A 25% actuarial 5-year disease-free survival has been reported by several groups after resection of liver metastases from colorectal cancer in selected patients (29) (Table 4-1). Results are best if there are fewer than five metastases that are confined to one lobe. With large tumors (> 4 cm diameter), anatomic lobectomy gives better results than local excision. Liver metastases from other primary lesions should probably not be resected because of the poor survival. Possible exceptions include renal cell carcinoma, Wilms' tumor, and intra-abdominal leiomyosarcoma.

Brain Metastases

Most patients with brain metastases are best managed with radiotherapy, although there is a small subset of patients who may do better with surgical excision. These are patients with solitary lesions, minimal neurologic impairment, and a long disease-free interval. Primary tumors most likely to respond well include lung, kidney, thyroid, colon, melanoma, and soft tissue sarcoma (48). Total resection plus postoperative radiotherapy gives the best results.

Palliative Surgery

The purpose of palliative surgery is to improve the patient's quality of remaining life. When undertaking this type of therapy, the potential risks (death, operative complications, prolonged recuperation from surgery, new symptoms) must be weighed against the potential advantages (reduction of pain or other symptoms, cosmesis, prevention of new debilitating symptoms).

Removal of Primary Tumor

Excision of the primary tumor may be indicated in the presence of unresectable metastatic disease. Locally advanced tumor can be very painful and unsightly, can interfere with vital functions such as breathing and swallowing, and can be complicated by bleeding and local infection. Examples of primary cancers that may produce debilitating symptoms if not removed include tumors of the head and neck, esophagus, colon, and rectum. Unless the patient's expected survival is less than the time expected to develop these symptoms, resection of the primary tumor may be indicated and requires careful assessment and multidisciplinary consultation.

Debulking Surgery

In general, there is little to be gained from debulking large, unresectable, solid tumors. In some instances, such as colorectal cancer with retroperitoneal extension, removal of the bowel may eliminate obstruction, bleeding, and tenesmus. Debulking does not offer a survival advantage, however, and should not be performed for the sole purpose of reducing tumor volume. The only exception to this rule is in the few tumors where it has been shown that debulking will enhance the effectiveness of chemotherapy or radiotherapy. This technique has been used in ovarian cancer with some benefit.

Laser Surgery

Although the laser can also be used in curative surgical resections, it has a particularly useful role in palliative surgery (5). The two types of laser used most commonly are the carbon dioxide laser and the neodymium:yttrium aluminum garnet (YAG) laser. The carbon dioxide laser must be used as a direct beam on exposed tissues, and when used with the beam defocused, it can vaporize tissue. The neodymium:YAG laser can be passed through optical fibers and can therefore treat areas not accessible to the carbon dioxide laser. It also has a higher energy; therefore, care must be taken not to penetrate the full thickness of the treated organ. Because of the heat produced by lasers, there is potentially less likelihood of contamination of the wound with bacteria or residual tumor cells.

The neodymium:YAG laser has proved useful in the palliative treatment of unresectable endobronchial lesions (31) that are bleeding significantly or are obstructing the airway. For incomplete airway obstruction, success rates are reported to be as high as 90%. This same technique has been used for esophageal and colorectal tumors. The carbon dioxide laser may be used to vaporize cutaneous lesions, particularly if

Table 4-1. Five-Year Survival After Resection of Liver Metasteses from Colorectal Cancer for Several Investigators

References	No. Patients	5-year Survival (%)
Adson et al.	67	27
Wagner et al.	141	25
Foster	83	21
Morrow et al.	29	27
Butler et al.	62	34
Cobourn et al.	56	25

From Cobourn et al. (20), with permission.

there are many lesions in one area leading to technical difficulties in surgical resection. The systemic injection of hematoporphyrin derivative, which binds preferentially to neoplastic tissue, can be used to sensitize the tumor to light destruction using a dye laser. Clinical trials using this technique are under way and have met with some success in bladder cancer and endobronchial tumors (22,39). The main limitation, however, is the depth of penetration of the laser damage, which is only a few millimeters or less.

Pain Control

When other, simpler methods of pain control have failed, surgical pain management may be necessary. As with all surgery, the potential risks (loss of bladder control, loss of motor power to a limb, poor pain relief) must be weighed against the gains (pain relief, avoidance of sedative effect of narcotics, psychologic well-being of patient). Destructive procedures, in which the afferent fibers from the painful area are interrupted, are most commonly used. If the pain is unilateral, these pain relief procedures are most easily accomplished using techniques such as cordotomy or rhizotomy. In prostatic cancer, bilateral orchiectomy may produce rapid and impressive pain relief from bony metastases. Midline pain, as in advanced cancer of the rectum, is much more difficult to treat and bladder function may have to be sacrificed to attain adequate pain control.

Vascular Access

Adequate vascular access is important in many oncology patients for three main purposes: chemotherapy, antibiotics for opportunistic infections, and intravenous (IV) nutrition when enteral feeding is inadequate.

When peripheral veins are scarce, it may be necessary to insert a central venous catheter. The standard procedure for outpatients has been to use a Hickman catheter inserted via the subclavian vein and then tunneled out onto the anterior chest wall. The distal end of the catheter is external to allow access for injection of medications and blood sampling. However, this also allows an entrance site for microorganisms and leads to some limitations in the patient's activities. In recent years, totally implantable devices have been developed. The infusion port is placed subcutaneously in the infraclavicular region in the same manner as a cardiac pacemaker and is accessed using a special Huber needle (Fig. 4-8) (27). This is much more convenient for the patient since the line does not require daily care and does not have the risk of air embolism during catheter manipulation. Implantable pumps are also available and can be used for the continuous administration of chemotherapy or narcotic analgesics without being attached to an external device.

Prophylactic Surgery

Surgery also has a role in cancer prevention in some patients through the removal of organs that are at high risk of developing cancer. Such surgery includes orchidopexy for undescended testis, excision of large congenital nevi, and colectomy for familial polyposis and ulcerative colitis. In these disorders, in which the risk of developing cancer approaches 100%, the decision for surgery is easy. In patients in whom the risk is less, these decisions become much more difficult, as in patients who are at high risk of developing breast cancer but would prefer not to have bilateral mastec-

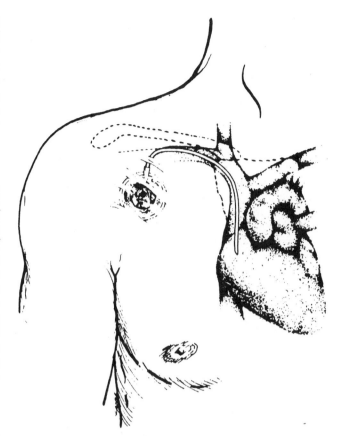

Fig. 4-8. Position of totally implantable vascular device in infraclavicular region. The silastic catheter enters the superior vena cava via the subclavian vein. From Franceschi (27); by permission of Surgery, Gynecology & Obstetrics.

tomy. In these cases, it may be best to present the known facts to the patient, and let the patient make the final decision.

SURGICAL TREATMENT OF THE COMPLICATIONS OF CANCER AND CANCER THERAPY

Surgical Emergencies

Patients with cancer may have surgical emergencies related to their disease and its treatment or completely independent of it (7,16). Because these patients are often higher-than-average surgical risks because of neutropenia, immunosuppression, and nutritional deficiencies, there is the tendency to procrastinate. Lack of the usual signs and symptoms of an acute illness compounds this problem. Unfortunately, when a true surgical emergency exists, these patients are least likely to tolerate a delay in appropriate therapy. It is important, therefore, to be aggressive in making a diagnosis, and if a surgical emergency exists, to operate early. This will produce the highest success rate in these patients. As always, there may be situations in which the patient is in such poor condition that surgery is contraindicated, but the repercussions of nonoperative therapy must be fully appreciated.

Neutropenic patients with an acute abdomen present a particularly vexing problem for the surgeon. A clinical syndrome termed neutropenic enteropathy presents with diffuse abdominal pain and tenderness and diarrhea, and is best managed conservatively with IV antibiotics, fluid replacement, and bowel rest (43). This is a diagnosis of exclusion. Any localizing findings upon clinical or radiologic examination should lead to discarding this disorder as a possible diagnosis and performing early surgery. Although the surgical risk may be high, the mortality of nonoperative therapy of infarcted bowel, a perforated colon, or a large abscess may approach 100%. The development of radiologic techniques for draining abscesses, the biliary tree, and the urinary tract percutaneously has led to some lower-risk methods of dealing with acute problems that could previously be dealt with only by open surgery.

Surgical Complications of Cancer Therapy

All forms of cancer therapy have potential complications, some of which must be dealt with surgically. Cancer surgery itself may lead to complications such as anastomotic leak, wound dehiscence, and postoperative hemorrhage which may require another operation. Re-operation is often a higher risk than the initial procedure and the patient should be prepared carefully and expeditiously prior to the surgery. Extravasation of chemotherapeutic agents, leading to soft tissue necrosis, and bowel perforation from the rapid lysis of lymphoma in the bowel after chemotherapy are two potential surgical complications of chemotherapy.

Patients treated with radiation therapy occasionally present months to years later with surgical problems related to their therapy. The longer the interval from treatment, the less likely that recurrent disease is the cause of the problem. Radiation injuries are more likely to occur in patients who also received chemotherapy or had a previous operation in the radiation field. This is because chemotherapy may sensitize and add to radiation damage and surgery may reduce the blood supply to small vessels, leading to poor healing. Abdominal operations may also produce adhesions which fix tissues, such as the small bowel, in the radiation field so that they receive a higher dose of radiation than they would if they were freely mobile. Possible complications include soft tissue breakdown, intestinal hemorrhage, bowel strictures from fibrotic healing of the mucosal injury, and fistulas. In the surgical management of these conditions it must be remembered that irradiated tissues will not tolerate handling well and have a poor capacity to heal. Therefore, whenever possible, nonoperative therapy should be considered. Normal tissue, such as a skin flap, from nonirradiated areas may need to be brought in. Fortunately, these complications are fairly uncommon. In a series of 1,418 patients treated with radiation therapy for carcinoma of the cervix, 4.3% had significant radiation-induced complications of the intestine (primarily the rectum) which required a surgical opinion (17). Surgery was eventually necessary in 39% of this 4.3%.

Other Surgical Procedures

Surgical procedures unrelated to the tumor may be necessary in some patients. These include open lung biopsy in patients with opportunistic pulmonary infections, liver biopsies for suspected hepatic viral infections, and insertion of inferior vena caval filters or clips for recurrent pulmonary emboli.

PREOPERATIVE AND POSTOPERATIVE CARE

Preoperative Care

Complete preoperative preparation of the patient includes risk assessment and optimization, nutritional evaluation, psychologic preparation, and informed consent.

Operative Risk

The operative risk that the patient and the surgeon will be willing to accept depends on the potential benefits of the surgery. If cure or palliation of debilitating symptoms is likely, a higher risk may be acceptable. Risk is determined by the medical condition of the patient and the extent of the proposed surgery.

The risk of death from general anesthesia alone is low, probably less than one in 4,000 healthy patients. If there are abnormalities of cardiac, pulmonary, renal, or hepatic function, the risk increases. These systems should be normalized as much as possible prior to surgery. If feasible, surgery should be delayed until 6 months after a myocardial infarction. Arrhythmias, congestive heart failure, and hypertension should be controlled. In patients with significant cardiac disease, perioperative monitoring with a Swan-Ganz catheter is helpful in monitoring fluid balance and cardiac function. In some patients with significant coronary lesions, preoperative coronary artery bypass surgery may be indicated.

All smokers should be advised to stop smoking at least 2 weeks before surgery. This will help reduce secretions and improve ciliary function. All patients with underlying pulmonary disease or significant pulmonary symptoms should have preoperative chest x-ray, spirometry, and blood gas determination, especially if thoracic or upper abdominal surgery is planned. This provides a baseline of pulmonary function and will help determine which patients require aggressive preoperative pulmonary therapy with bronchodilators and chest physiotherapy.

Required preoperative laboratory tests include hematocrit, electrolytes, blood urea nitrogen, and urinalysis in most hospitals. Chest x-ray is done much more frequently than actually needed but should be done in most cancer patients to look for pulmonary metastases. Electrocardiogram is indicated in all patients over aged 35 years and in any patient with known or suspected cardiac disease. In patients with suspected liver disease, liver chemistries and clotting parameters should also be checked.

Preoperative nutritional assessment is important in all cancer patients. Often, an adequate history and physical examination are all that are needed. If there is any suspicion of nutritional deficit, further evaluation assessing serum albumin, transferrin, and the presence of cutaneous anergy may be useful in defining which patients are at increased risk. Preoperative alimentation by the enteral or IV route may be indicated in these patients for 1 week or more. If the above indicators improve, it is likely that the risk of operative mortality and major surgical complications will be reduced, particularly in patients with GI cancers (42). A mechanical problem in the GI tract, rather than widespread disease, may be the cause of nutritional deficiency. If possible, the enteral route should be used because the complication rate is much less than with parenteral nutrition. Evidence to support the use of parenteral nutrition in patients receiving chemotherapy or radiation therapy is lacking, since survival, treatment tolerance, treatment toxicity, and tumor response are unchanged with its use. In fact, some papers report an increased infection rate in patients receiving total parenteral nutrition (34). A detailed discussion of nutrition in the cancer patient is presented in Chapter 34, "Nutrition and the Cancer Patient."

With adequate preoperative evaluation, therapy, and careful intraoperative management by the anesthesiologist, the risks of surgery can be minimized. In the case of emergency surgery, time still should be taken to optimize the patient's fluid and electrolyte status unless massive bleeding or some other catastrophe precludes it.

Informed Consent

Informed consent is an essential part of the preoperative management of all patients. In this age of frequent litigation against physicians, it is important not only to inform the patient but to document it well. It is essential that the patient understand the proposed surgical procedure as fully as possible. In patients with a new or suspected diagnosis of cancer, this may be particularly difficult. The patient is in the process of dealing psychologically with a disease that, to many, is synonymous with death. Otherwise attentive patients may misconstrue or completely forget what they are told by the physician.

There are two ways to deal with this problem. One is to have a family member or close friend present for the discussion. The other is to meet with the patient on at least two separate occasions to discuss the diagnosis and the planned surgery. Information in writing and sketches of the proposed surgery allow the patient to review the procedure later in a more relaxed situation and contributes to the adequate psychologic preparation of the patient. Most surgeons agree that a positive mental attitude will often lead to a more rapid recovery.

With the recent increase in patient participation in their own care, there may be a situation in which the patient must choose which operative procedure to have or may choose no surgery. When surgical therapy is known to be superior to other forms of treatment, it is the physician's responsibility to make that clear to the patient and encourage him or her to make that choice. In other instances, the patient may be able to make the best choice, as in breast cancer. In many patients with stage I or stage II breast cancer, lumpectomy plus radiation therapy is as efficacious as total mastectomy. After consultation with the surgeon and the radiation therapist, the patient may then make her own decision. Factors such as daily travel for radiation treatments and cosmesis can best be evaluated by the patient herself.

Postoperative Care

In patients with cancer, postoperative care is lifelong, and is not limited to a few weeks or until the patient has recovered from the operative procedure. Follow-up should be coordinated with the other physicians involved in the patient's care so that services are not duplicated and the patient's time is not wasted. The quality of a particular doctor-patient relationship may partially determine which physician oversees the patient's care.

Immediate postoperative care will not be discussed in detail here, but it is important to remember the psychologic needs of the patient at this time. After potentially curative surgery, patients often feel victorious and do well in the immediate postoperative period, while patients who had only palliative surgery may be discouraged.

After patients are discharged, it is common for them to become depressed, even in cases of benign disease. This depression may be related to the patients' inability to perform their usual activities, loneliness after the attention they received in the hospital, and constant reflection on the possible outcome of the disease. The possibility of depression should be acknowledged in all patients and dealt with appropriately. In the early postoperative period following discharge from hospital, appropriate referrals should be made to therapists (e.g., physical, speech, stomal), support groups (e.g., Reach to Recovery, Lost Chord), and appropriate consultants for postoperative chemotherapy, radiation therapy, psychologic counseling, or other management.

Follow-up (8)

The purpose of periodic follow-up is to detect recurrent disease or new primaries at a time when they may still be cured or at least palliated. History, evaluation, physical examination, and certain laboratory investigations are routinely performed. Unfortunately, in the absence of symptoms, routine screening of chest x-rays, bone scans, blood chemistries, and other tests and procedures are often not productive or cost-effective. A few, such as mammograms and colonoscopy, are necessary and useful. Serum level markers may be useful in detecting recurrent disease when all other tests are negative. Laparotomy for a rising serum carcinoembryonic antigen level in patients with a previous colorectal cancer and an otherwise negative work-up has led to curative resection in 25% to 50% of patients (38).

Recommended Reading

There are three main texts dealing with surgical oncology (1,14,45) that address cancer management from the surgeon's perspective, as well as a third text on pediatric surgical oncology (11). The evolving role of the surgical oncologist is discussed in references 2 and 34. The role of the anaesthesiologist is outline in detail in a manual by Howland et al. (12). Early advanced and more recent recommendations in perioperative nutritional support of cancer patients are discussed in references 5 and 19. Rehabilitation oncology, an important responsibility for the surgeon as well as other specialists, is reviewed by Dietz (3).

REFERENCES

General References

1. Copeland, E.M., ed. Surgical oncology. New York, NY: John Wiley & Sons; 1983.
2. Deitel, M., ed. Nutrition in Clinical Surgery. 2nd ed. Baltimore, MD: Williams and Wilkins; 1985.
3. DeVita, V.T.; Hellman, S.; Rosenberg, S.A., eds. Cancer: principles and practice of oncology, 3rd ed. Philadelphia, PA: J.B. Lippincott Company; 1989.
4. Dietz, J.H., Jr. Adaptive rehabilitation of the cancer patient. Curr. Prob. Cancer 5:1-56; 1980.
5. Dixon, J.A. Surgical application of lasers, 2nd ed. Chicago, IL: Year Book Medical Publishers; 1987.
6. Dudrick, S.F.; MacFadyen, B.V., Jr.; Sonchon, E.A.; et al. Parenteral nutrition techniques in cancer patients. Cancer Res. 37:2440-2450; 1977.
7. Dutcher, J.P. Wiernick, P.H., eds. Handbook of Hematologic and Oncologic Emergencies. New York, NY: Plenum Medical Book Company; 1987.
8. Eiseman, B., Robinson, W.A., Steele, G. Follow-up of the Cancer Patient. Thieme-Stratton; 1982.
9. Fisher, B.; Gebhardt, M.C. The evolution of breast cancer surgery. Semin. Oncol. 5:358-394; 1978.
10. Fraumeni, J.F., Jr., ed. Persons at high risk of cancer: an approach to cancer etiology and control. New York, NY: Academic Press; 1975.

11. Hays, D.M., ed. Pediatric Surgical Oncology. New York, NY: Grune & Stratton, Inc.; 1986.
12. Howland, W.S., Rooney, S.M., Goldiner, P.L. Manual of Anaesthesia in Cancer Care. New York, NY: Churchill Livingston; 1986.
13. McKenna, R.J.; Murphy, G.P., eds. Fundamentals of surgical oncology. New York, NY: Macmillan Publishing Company; 1986.
14. Pilch, Y.H. Surgical Oncology. New York, NY: McGraw Hill Book Co; 1984.
15. Rosenberg, S.A., ed. Surgical treatment of metastatic cancer. Philadelphia, PA: J.B. Lippincott Co.; 1987.
16. Turnbull, A.D.M. Surgical emergencies in the cancer patient. Chicago, IL: Year Book Medical Publishers; 1987.

Specific References

17. Allen-Mersh; T.G.; Wilson, E.J.; Hope-Stone, H.F.; Mann, C.V. The management of late radiation-induced rectal injury after treatment of carcinoma of the uterus. Surg. Gynec. Obstet. 164:521-524; 1987.
18. Bakamjian, V.Y.; Calamel, P.M. Oropharyngo-esophageal reconstructive surgery. In: Bakamian, V.Y.; Calamel, P.M., eds. Reconstructive plastic surgery, 2nd ed., vol. 5. Philadelphia, PA: W.B. Saunders Co.; 1977:2697-2756.
19. Chen, M.K.; Souba, W.W.; Copeland, E.M. 3rd Nutritional support of the surgical oncology patient. Hematol. Oncol. Clin. North Am. 5:125-145; 1991.
20. Cobourn, C.S.; Makowka, L.; Langer, B.; Taylor, B.R.; Falk, R.E. Examination of patient selection and outcome for hepatic resection for metastatic disease. Surg. Gynec. Obstet. 165:239-246; 1987.
21. Day, C.L.; Mihm, M.C.; Sober, A.J.; Fitzpatrick, T.B.; Malt, R.A. Narrower margins for clinical stage I malignant melanoma. New Engl. J. Med. 306:479-482; 1982.
22. Dougherty, T.J. Photoradiation Therapy. Urol (Supple.) 23:61-64; 1984.
23. Fisher, B. (principal investigator) A protocol to compare segmental mastectomy and axillary dissection with and without radiation of the breast and total mastectomy and axillary dissection. National Surgical Adjuvant Breast Project (NSABP) Protocol #B-06. Pittsburgh: University of Pittsburgh; 1980.
24. Fisher, B.; Constantino, J.; Redmond, C.; Poisson, R.; Bowman, D.; Couture, J.; Dimitrov, N.V.; Wolmark, N.; Wickerman, D.L.; Fisher, E.R., et al. A randomized clinical trial evaluating tamoxifen in the treatment of patients with node-negative breast cancer who have estrogen-receptor-positivve tumors. New Engl. J. Med. 320:479-484; 1989.
25. Fisher, B.; Redmond, C.; Fisher, E.R., et al. The contribution of recent NSABP clinical trials of primary breast cancer therapy to an understanding of tumor biology: an overview of findings. Cancer 46:1009-1025; 1980.
26. Folkman, J.; Klagsbrun, M. Angiogenesis factors. Science 1987; 235:442-447.
27. Franceschi, D.; Farrell, C. Simplified technique for placement of implantable vascular devices. Surg Gynec. Obstet. 164:277-279; 1987.
28. Gomez, G.A.; Reese, P.A.; Nava, H.; Panahon, A.M.; Barcos, M.; Stutzman, L.; Han, T.; Henderson, E.S. Staging laparotomy and splenectomy in early Hodgkin's disease. Am. J. Med. 77:205-210; 1984.
29. Hughes, K.S.; Sugarbaker, P.H. Resection of the liver for metastatic solid tumors. In: Rosenberg, S.A., ed. Surgical treatment of metastatic cancer. Philadelphia, PA: J.B. Lippincott Co.; 1987:125-164.
30. Irving, M. The role of surgery in the management of Hodgkin's disease. Br. J. Surg. 62:853-862; 1975.
31. Kaiser, L.R. Tracheobronchial emergencies: use of the neodymium:YAG laser. In: Turnbull, A.D.M. Surgical emergencies in the cancer patient. Chicago, IL: Year Book Medical Publishers; 1987:137-139.
32. Kaplan, H.S.; Dorfman, R.F.; Nelsen, T.S.; Rosenberg, S.A. Staging laparotomy and splenectomy in Hodgkin's disease: analysis of indications and patterns of involvement in 285 consecutive, unselected patients. Natl. Cancer Inst. Monogr. 36:291-301; 1973.
33. Kern, K.A.; Pass, H.I.; Roth, J.A. Surgical treatment of pulmonary metastases. In Rosenberg, S.A., ed. Surgical treatment of metastatic cancer. Philadelphia, PA: J.B. Lippincott Co.; 1987:69-100.
34. Klein, S.; Simes, J.; Blackburn, G.L. Total parenteral nutrition and cancer clinical trials. Cancer 58:1378-1386; 1986.
35. Lotze, M.T. The role of lymph node dissection in the treatment of cancer. In: Rosenberg, S.A., ed. Surgical treatment of metastatic cancer. Philadelphia, PA: J.B. Lippincott Co.; 1987:223-271.
36. Ludwig Breast Cancer Study Group. Prolonged disease-free survival after one course of perioperative adjuvant chemotherapy for node-negative breast cancer. New Engl. J. Med. 320:491-496; 1989.
37. Mansour, E.G.; Gray, R.; Shatila, A.H.; Osborne, C.K.; Tormey, D.C.; Gilchrist, R.W.; Cooper, M.R.; Falkson, G. Efficacy of adjuvant chemotherapy in high-risk node-negative breast cancer. New Engl. J. Med. 320:485-490; 1989.
38. Martin, E.W.; Minton, J.P.; Carey, L.C. CEA-directed second-look surgery in the asymptomatic patient after primary resection of colorectal carcinoma. Ann. Surg. 202:310-317; 1985.
39. McCaughan, J.S.; Hawley, P.C.; Bethel, B.H.; Walker, J. Photodynamic therapy of endobronchial malignancies. Cancer 62:691-701; 1988.
40. McGuire, W.L.; Clark, G.M. Prognostic factors and treatment decisions in axillary-node-negative breast cancer. N. Engl. J. Med. 326:1756-1761; 1992.
41. Oertel, Y.C. Fine needle aspiration of the breast. Boston, MA: Butterworths; 1987.
42. Souba, W.W.; Copeland, E.M. Hyperalimentation in cancer. CA. 1989; 39:105-114.
43. Starnes, H.F.; Moore, F.D.; Mentzer, S.; Osteen, R.T.; Steele, G.D.; Wilson, R.E. Abdominal pain in neutropenic cancer patients. Cancer 57:616-621; 1986.
44. Stearns, M.W. Benign and malignant neoplasms of colon and rectum. Surg. Clin. N. Am. 58:605-618; 1978.
45. Steele, G.D.; Cady, B. eds. General Surgical Oncology. Philadelphia, PA. W.B. Saunders. 1992.
46. Veronesi, U.; Adamus, J.; Bandiera, D.C.; et al. Inefficacy of immediate node dissection in stage I melanoma of the limbs. New Engl. J. Med. 297:627-630; 1977.
47. Wilson, A.J.; Houghton, J.; Baum, M. Adjuvant therapy for breast cancer. In: Slevs, M.L.; Stanet, M.J., eds. Randomized trials in cancer: a critical review by sites. New York, NY: Raven Press; 1986:359-383.
48. Wright, D.C. Surgical treatment of brain metastases. In: Rosenberg, S.A., ed. Surgical treatment of metastatic cancer. Philadelphia, PA: J.B. Lippincott Co.; 1987:165-222.

R. Timothy Mulcahy, Ph.D., Department of Human Oncology
Dietmar W. Siemann, Ph.D., Radiation Oncology and Experimental Therapeutics

Robert M. Sutherland, Ph.D., Biological Sciences

Chapter **5**

BASIC PRINCIPLES OF RADIOBIOLOGY

The most incomprehensible thing about the world is that it is comprehensible.

Albert Einstein (50)

PERSPECTIVE (13,20)

The interaction of ionizing radiation with biologic material proceeds through several stages resulting in a wide variety of biologic end effects. This chapter outlines these effects in systems of increasing biologic complexity and attempts, where possible, to relate these responses to the different stages of interaction. A convenient outline of these interactions follows.

STAGES OF RADIATION ACTION

Physical Stage
Radiation produces activated (excited or ionized) molecules.
- approximate duration = 10^{-18} seconds

Physiochemical Stage
Unstable primary products undergo secondary reactions to produce stable molecules plus chemically reactive free atoms and free radicals (molecules with unpaired electrons).
- approximate duration = 10^{-13} seconds

Chemical Stage
Chemically reactive species react with each other and with the milieu.
- approximate duration = 10^{-6} seconds

Biological Stage
The sequential response of the organism to chemical products of irradiation.
- approximate duration = 10^{-6} seconds, up to many years

A specific scheme has been proposed for inactivation of mammalian cells through these different stages (Fig. 5-1) (20).

Physical Stage (3,27,34,35)

Interaction with Matter
Ionizing radiations of interest include high energy (short wavelength) electromagnetic radiation and high-speed subatomic particles. These interact with molecules through two mechanisms — excitation and ionization of the constituent atoms. In excited atoms, electrons are shifted to different orbits and become more reactive chemically. In ionization, the orbiting electrons are completely ejected from the atoms, leaving free radicals and broken chemical bonds. Charged particles, such as electrons or protons, are directly ionizing; with sufficient kinetic energy they can directly break chemical bonds. Electromagnetic radiations (x- and gamma rays), as well as neutrons, are indirectly ionizing, i.e., they do not themselves disrupt chemical bonds, but produce charged particles with high kinetic energy that do. Neutrons interact with the nuclei of atoms of the absorbing material and impart kinetic energy to fast-recoil protons and other nuclear fragments.

Linear Energy Transfer (LET)
Linear energy transfer (LET) refers to the energy transferred per unit length of the radiation beam track in the absorbing material. The unit usually used for this quantity is KeV per micron of unit density material. Typical LET values for commonly used radiations are: Cobalt-60 x-rays = 0.3 KeV/μ, 250 KeV x-rays = 2.0 KeV/μ, 14 MeV neutrons = 12 KeV/μ heavy charged particles = 100-2,000 KeV/μ.

Differences in LET account for the fact that, although different radiations usually produce qualitatively similar effects initially (ionizations), there are marked quantitative differences as well as different biologic end effects. This results from dissimilarities in spatial proximity (Fig. 5-2) (32) of ionizations and from the influence of secondary processes such as back reactions and chain reactions on the initial physical and chemical events. Biologic modification as a result of structural organization and coupled systems also plays a significant part in the final damage.

High energy photons can penetrate deeply into tissues, giving up their energy gradually as the electrons resulting from ionizations are slowed. This is because the electron has only unit electric charge and a very small mass. On the other hand, in the case of various charged particles with very different charge to mass ratios (for example, protons have about 1,800 times greater mass than electrons), and possibly different velocities as well, there is a maximum release of

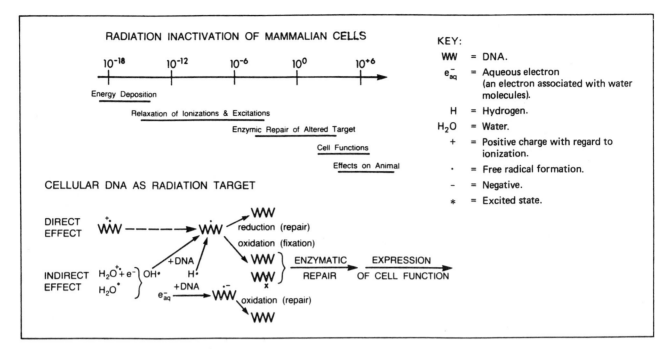

Fig. 5-1. Schematic representation of stages of radiation action involved in inactivation of mammalian cells. The top line drawing represents time scale in seconds. The lower panel shows direct and indirect effects of radiation on cellular DNA. From Chapman (20), with permission.

energy in a relatively short portion of the track — the so-called Bragg peak (14). Since a massive particle travels slower than a light one and is therefore in the vicinity of an ionizable atom longer, the probability is greater that an ionization will occur. Thus, heavily charged particles have relatively short ranges in matter, the range depending significantly on their initial kinetic energy (velocity). The Bragg peak, then, is the

change in LET of a particle with distance along its path, principally because the particle slows down as it transfers its kinetic energy of motion to the surrounding medium (Fig. 5-3).

This release of a large amount of energy in a relatively small localized volume has made various types of particles of considerable interest to therapeutic radiologists. (See Chapter 6, "Principles of Radiation Oncology and Cancer Radiotherapy.")

Relative Biologic Effectiveness

Equal doses of different types of ionizing radiations do not produce equal biologic effects because of differences in LET. It is customary to express the biologic effectiveness of some test radiation compared with 250 KeV x-rays. The relative biologic effectiveness (RBE) is the ratio of the doses of 250 KeV x-rays and the test radiation required for equal biologic

Fig. 5-2. Schematic diagram showing the short tracks (lengths ~70 nm and ~7 nm) produced by the absorption of aluminum K and carbon K ultrasoft x-rays, respectively. Each dot represents about six ionizations. Shown for comparison are a segment of a DNA double helix of diameter about 2 nm and a segment of the track of a fast helium ion of 20 KeV μm⁻¹. The broken circle represents a sphere of diameter 400 nm, which is typical of the distance within which sublesions are assumed to interact within a sensitive site according to the theory of dual radiation action. From Goodhead (31), with permission.

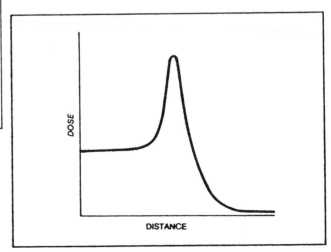

Fig. 5-3. Distribution of energy released for distance traveled by heavily charged particles in an absorbing material.

effect. Note that the RBE varies with the biologic system used and with the level of damage, which is related to the dose delivered in that given system. The RBE for many cellular systems has been shown to increase with increasing LET, peaking at about 100 KeV/μ and then decreasing (Fig. 5-4) (2).

Thus, there appears to be an optimal LET (density of ionizations). Sparsely ionizing radiation is inefficient because more than one particle must pass through the cell to inactivate it. Very densely ionizing radiation is also inefficient because it deposits more than enough energy in the critical sites within the cell, and so energy is wasted.

Physicochemical Stage (17,21,40)

To attempt to understand radiobiologic phenomena in living cells, we must know something about how radiation interacts with molecules and the relative radiosensitivities of these molecules. Methodology has been developed that allows us to sort — from all the numerous and complex radiation-induced interactions — those that are most likely to occur under conditions in which the quality of radiation, biologic material, radiation dose, etc., are specified. It has been most difficult, however, to actually prove molecular mechanisms for cellular radiation effects, and we usually must depend on indirect evidence based on correlations between known molecular effects and biologic effects. This is mainly because, as much as we do know about molecular radiobiology, interpretation of radiobiologic phenomena still depends on a knowledge of how molecules exist in living cells and how they change with time.

Direct and Indirect Effects

Because ionizations produced by radiation are random processes, some molecules will escape ionization, but may undergo radiation-related changes brought about by energy transfer from an ionized molecule or its products to undamaged molecules. Therefore, there are two types of chemical changes in irradiated molecules:

1. Direct effect: The release of energy in the structure of the molecule under discussion.
2. Indirect effect: The initial energy absorbed by one molecule transferred to another molecule being measured.

Metastable states exist in molecules after the direct action of irradiation, and have been demonstrated — along with energy transfer processes — by electron spin resonance and thermoluminescence techniques. Energy is transferred both within and between molecules via special structures, such as tryptophan and benzene rings, alpha-helix and DNA helix, and migration of dissociated small molecular fragments.

Important Physicochemical Reactions

Since cells are at least 70% water, most of the indirect action involves reactive species derived from water molecules. Radiation interacts with water; some of the products formed can then react with other solute molecules and radicals of solute molecules can form final stable products (Fig. 5-5). The relative contributions of direct and indirect damage to radiobiologic effects may be estimated by irradiation in dry or frozen conditions, or by adding chemical protectors that scavenge radicals. The general principle in many of these procedures is to eliminate the production of radicals other than the one under consideration.

Radiation Effects on Important Biologic Macromolecules

The predominant changes that result from irradiation of different classes of macromolecules in solution or dry state can be summarized as follows:

1. *Nucleic acids*: Change or loss of a base, hydrogen bond breakage between strands, single and double strand breakage, formation of cross-links with double helix to other DNA molecules and to chromosomal proteins, and conformation changes.
2. *Proteins*: Damage to side chain groups and changes in secondary and tertiary structure (conformation).
3. *Lipids*: Formation of peroxides of unsaturated fatty acids.

Modifiers of Molecular Radiosensitivity

The complexities of molecular structures and metabolism in living cells will modify radiosensitivities of molecules. Several factors involved are molecular aggregation: presence

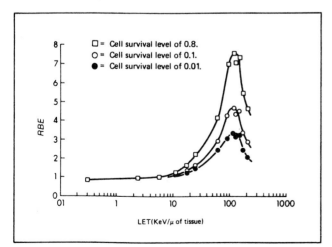

Fig. 5-4. Variation of relative biologic effectiveness (RBE) with linear energy transfer (LET) for survival of mammalian cells of human origin. The RBE rises to a maximum at an LET of about 100KeV/μ, and subsequently falls for higher values of LET. The curves refer to various cell survival levels illustrating that the absolute value of the RBE is not unique, but depends on the level of biological damage, and therefore on the dose level. From Hall (2), with permission.

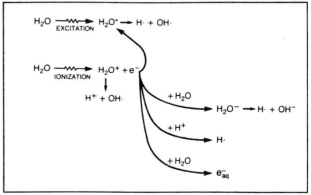

Fig. 5-5. Direct action of ionizing radiation on water molecules, demonstrating the generation of reactive species. From Chapman (20), with permission.

of a high concentration of a second solute medium other than water; molecules absorbed on the surface of subcellular structures; molecules complexed with other molecules; and subcellular distribution of molecules.

There is usually a latent period between damage to the molecules and the final observable radiobiological phenomenon. During this time, further modifications and amplifications of the damage occur via: (a) a coupled reaction in which some types of radiation-damaged molecules can transfer damage to other types of molecules; (b) synthesis of abnormal macromolecules by radiation-damaged templates; (c) structural damage to important molecules; and (d) coupled reactions in multienzyme systems. Other factors, such as the metabolic state, cell age, and repair ability also modify radiation damage and will be discussed later.

Radiation-Sensitive Site in Cells

Nucleus: A variety of experiments over the years have shown that the target site responsible for cell killing is probably within the nucleus. In general, these experiments involve localization of radiation damage to the nucleus versus cytoplasm of cells, using microbeams, low energy electrons, microdissection, nuclear transplantation, and selective incorporation of lethal levels of radioisotopes into macromolecules such as DNA (Fig. 5-6) (42).

DNA: Many studies have indicated positive correlations between DNA content and radiosensitivity in different cellular organisms. In bacteria, alterations in radiosensitivity at the cellular level produce similar variations in DNA radiosensitivity as measured by the functional test of ability of DNA to transform other bacterial strains. Such correlations have been found after altering the LET, the oxygen environment, and different chemical protectors and sensitizers. The relation of DNA damage to cell death has not been easy to evaluate because the chemical yield of products of irradiated DNA is extremely small at biologically effective doses.

However, techniques have been developed to assess damage in DNA from irradiated mammalian cells. These include determination of single- and double-strand breaks, base damage, and formation of dimers. Although these techniques

have been available for some years, they have only recently been developed to a stage that allows assessment of damage at low doses within or near those that kill mammalian cells. Studies using these techniques further implicate DNA as a critical target for ionizing radiation damage.

This relationship between DNA damage and cell killing following irradiation has also been supported by the discovery that cells from patients with certain diseases associated with deficiencies in cellular repair capacities, are particularly sensitive to the cytotoxic action of ionizing radiation. For example, fibroblasts cultured from patients with the disease ataxia telangiectasia are more sensitive to radiation than are fibroblasts from normal individuals (Fig. 5-7) (44). This increased sensitivity is related to a defective excision repair process for the removal of alkali-stabile radioproducts in the DNA of the ataxic fibroblasts (44).

Although the data currently available do not conclusively identify DNA as a critical target, it provides considerable circumstantial evidence. However, even if DNA is the critical target, it should be emphasized that for mammalian cells, the importance of damage to nucleosomal DNA relative to that associated with other chromosomal proteins or with the nuclear membrane is still not clear. In addition, some data suggest that cellular components other than DNA, most notably the cell membrane, play a critical role in cell lethality after irradiation (2). The definitive identification of the critical target for radiation damage has not yet been accomplished.

DNA Repair Processes (21,43)

The considerable progress made in characterizing DNA repair processes is the result of work initially performed with bacterial strains exposed to germicidal ultraviolet (UV) irradiation. Subsequently, several different DNA repair processes identified in bacteria have been demonstrated in mammalian cells as well. These include excision repair, S phase of postreplication repair, photoreactivation, and strand-break repairs.

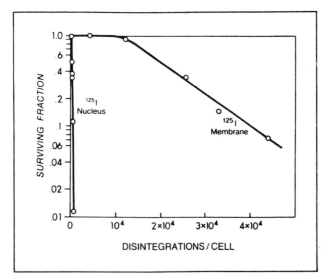

Fig. 5-6. Effects of radioactive iodine (iodine-125) decay in DNA or on the membrane on reproductive integrity of Chinese hamster ovary cells. From Painter (42), with permission.

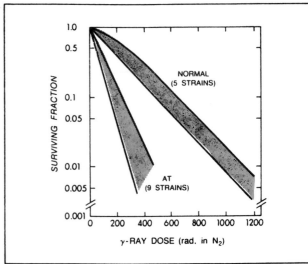

Fig. 5-7. Range of surviving fraction of colony-forming ability of cultured diploid fibroblasts from nine ataxia telangiectasia (AT) patients and five clinically normal subjects as a function of cobalt-60 γ-irradiation delivered under hypoxic conditions. From Paterson *et al.* (44), with permission.

Excision repair: The ability of microbial systems to remove or excise pyrimidine dimers from DNA after UV irradiation was discovered in the 1960s. Excision repair of UV damage goes through a series of biochemical steps that involve the sequential operation of an endonuclease, an exonuclease, a polymerase and a ligase. Similar excision repair processes are active in mammalian cells exposed to ionizing radiation (Fig. 5-8) (22).

Postreplication repair: Repair during the S phase, also called postreplication repair, occurs in bacteria and mammalian cells, although substantial differences exist between these two. Despite the general similarity of gaps detected in nascent DNA strands of both cell types, because of interruption of semiconservative replication at damaged template sites, the damage in bacteria resulting from the gaps can be eliminated by recombination with pieces of parental DNA. However, in mammalian cells, the gaps are filled by a process involving de novo synthesis, and there is no evidence for any involvement of the parental strands. Unlike repair replications, the gap-filling process seems very similar to semiconservative replication.

DNA strand breaks: The most studied and controversial DNA lesion induced by ionizing radiation is the single-strand break. After the introduction of the alkaline sucrose gradient centrifugation technique by McGrath and Williams in 1966 (38), the method was quickly adapted for use with mammalian cells. More recently, the technique of alkaline elution has also been applied to study of radiation-induced DNA single-strand breaks. There is now fairly general agreement that most single strand breaks are repaired. Usually, this repair process consists of two components: a fast component completed within 30 minutes after irradiation, and a slow component requiring several hours. Similar techniques have been adapted for studying double strand break repair. Apparently, many double-strand breaks can also be repaired.

The real question to be resolved in the future is the fidelity of the break repair. This will require more information on the chemical nature of both single- and double-strand breaks.

Photoreactivation: Photoreactivation repair results in the removal of pyrimidine dimers in DNA by a direct enzymatic reversal reaction dependent on energy from light of specific wavelengths. This repair process monomerizes pyrimidine dimers without disrupting the integrity of the involved strand of DNA. Photoreactivation is a particularly important repair pathway used by cells exposed to UV irradiation.

DNA base damage: Another type of DNA lesion produced by ionizing radiation is base damage. Nuclei from HeLa and hamster cells have been shown to remove damaged thymine from irradiated phage DNA. The amount of thymine damage was approximately equal to the single strand-breaks produced, and the kinetics of thymine release by cell repair systems is similar to the kinetics of repair of single-strand breaks. This suggests a common activity that releases damaged bases. The role of base damage in cell killing is unknown, but we know that it is very important for inactivation of phage after both low and high LET irradiation.

Basic replication and unscheduled DNA synthesis: Rasmussen and Painter (1964) (46), first observed unambiguously that ^{3}H thymidine was incorporated into cells at all stages of the cell cycle after irradiation. The process of patching the DNA lesions has been quantified autoradiographically and has been termed unscheduled DNA synthesis. They showed incorporation if tritiated thymidine into cells undergoing regular semiconservative and unscheduled DNA synthesis. Microbeam UV irradiation of a small region of the nucleus indicated that unscheduled synthesis occurred only at the sites actually damaged.

Demonstration that this repair of damaged DNA involved insertion of small patches into parental molecules — that is, repair replication — was achieved by using bromodeoxyuridine labeling and isopyknic gradient analysis. Used initially for Escheria coli by Pettijohn and Hanawalt in 1964 (45), and later for mammalian cells, this analysis has provided much information about excision repair. The average patch size in terms of numbers of bases inserted per UV dimer excised has been estimated in several laboratories to fall in the range of 100 to 200 bases per patch. This immediately raises some interesting questions regarding mechanism. Why is the patch so much larger than the dimer and what determines where repair starts and stops?

Biological Stage (1-4,19,25,53,54)

Cell Life Cycle

The concept of the cell cycle is essential to our understanding of cellular radiobiologic phenomena. Since cell division is a cyclical phenomenon, repeated in each generation of the cells, it is usual to represent it as a circle. It can be divided into four stages beginning with M (mitosis), G_1, (gap 1), S (DNA synthesis), and G_2 (gap 2) (Fig. 5-9) (42). The total circumference of the circle represents the mitotic cycle time. It is also common to identify a G_0 period for cells that may not divide for long periods.

Much is now known about the various events associated with these cycle stages, such as the synthesis of different enzymes and RNA.

The main method of analyzing the life cycle has involved visualizing the cells synthesizing DNA by measuring their uptake of radioactively-labeled thymidine using the technique of autoradiography. The rates at which these cells

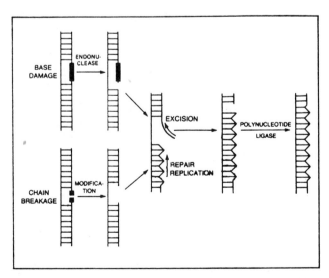

Fig. 5-8. Heuristic scheme for the operational steps in excision repair of damaged bases (e.g., pyrimidine dimers) and broken strands (e.g., ionizing radiation damage) by a common pathway. The initial step for each kind of damage has some unique features, but the excision, replication, and ligase steps can be common. From Cleaver and Trask (22), with permission.

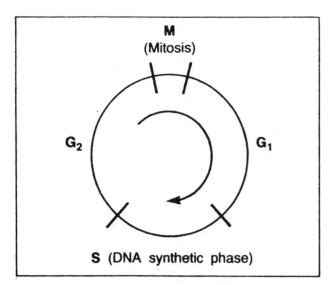

Fig. 5-9. Diagrammatic representation of the different phases of the mammalian cell growth cycle. From Hall (2), with permission.

move into mitosis can be observed microscopically. The study of cell-cycle kinetics has been greatly advanced with the development of a new technique — flow cytometry — with which it is possible to quantitate the percentage of cells in the various stages of the cell cycle using laser activated fluorescent dyes bound to cellular DNA. This rapid quantitation is possible because cells in G_1 have a normal single DNA complement, cells in G_2 and M have twice the normal amount of DNA (parental and newly synthesized), while cells in S have amounts of DNA between the G_1 and G_2 concentrations. For analysis, individual cells are passed through a laser beam that excites the fluorescent dye. The fluorescent intensity for each cell is then measured and recorded for future analysis. The generation time of cell populations ranges from 8 to 30 hours, and the duration of the various stages falls within the following ranges: G_1 = 1.5 to 14 hours, S = 6 to 9 hours, G_2 = 1 to 5 hours, and M = 0.5 to 1 hour.

Effect of Radiation on Cell Cycle Progression

When cells of mixed stages in exponential growth are irradiated, cells in each stage respond differently. Decline of the mitotic index indicates interference with cell progress between stages. This is followed by its rise to or above the pre-

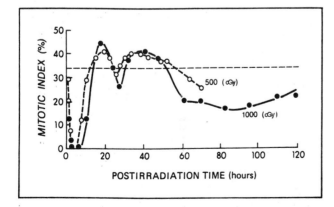

Fig. 5-10. Effect of irradiation on mitotic index of mouse leukemia L5178Y: Dotted line=mitotic index of nonirradiated cells; the dotted line with the open circles = 500 cGy; the solid line with the solid circles=1,000 cGy. From Wantanabe and Okada (55), with permission.

exposure level (Fig. 5-10) (55). In the immediately declining phase of the mitotic index, the rate of decline becomes faster as the radiation dose is increased and reaches a saturation value with doses greater than a few hundred rad. The immediate decline of the mitotic index is accompanied by a cessation of the increase in cell number (Fig. 5-11) (55). The phase of recovery from mitotic delay is heralded by an increase in the mitotic index (Fig. 5-10), which is followed by an increase in cell number (Fig. 5-11). The period from time of irradiation to time when the irradiated cells re-enter mitosis is used to denote the duration of the radiation-induced mitotic delay. The delay time increases linearly as the radiation dose increases (up to about several hundred rad), then flattens out gradually in the high-dose range (Fig. 5-12) (55).

Recent studies show that the main cause of the mitotic delay is a complete — but temporary — block of cell progress in the G_2 stage; this is termed G_2 block. It should be emphasized that the cells entering the M stage after irradiation with low doses (up to several hundred rad for mammalian cells) are probably cells recovering from the G_2 block. Cells entering the M stage after irradiation with high doses, however, are

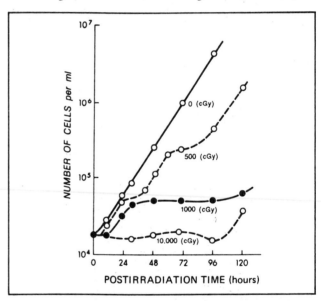

Fig. 5-11. Growth delay caused by radiation exposure of L5178Y mouse leukemia cells. From Wantanabe and Okada (55), with permission.

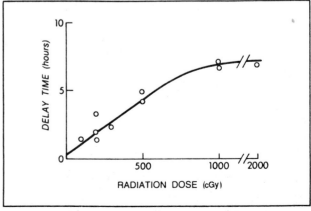

Fig. 5-12. Irradiation-induced mitotic delay in mouse leukemia L5178Y. From Wantanabe and Okada (55), with permission.

probably in G_1 and early S stage at the time of irradiation; these cells, being less responsive than the G_1 cells, overtake the G_2 blocked cells and enter the M stage at the G_2 block. Thus, from studies with cell populations synchronized in different stages, and other experiments on cell cycle kinetics after irradiation, the only other stage that is significantly affected is S (2,54). This results from a depression in the rate of DNA synthesis. Several possible explanations for the mechanism of the G_2 block have been examined. These include chromosome aberrations, uncoiling of condensed chromosomes, and inhibition of the synthesis of proteins necessary for mitosis. The evidence appears to favor the latter. The immediate effects of irradiation on cell cycle progress are summarized in Fig. 5-13 (36).

Following doses up to approximately 1,000 cGy, generally more than 90% of mammalian cells divide at the end of the cycle at which the irradiation occurred (25). However, frequent exceptions to this generality exist. For example, in some experiments with mouse cells, only about 75% divided after 800 cGy, and the probability of division was shown to be dependent on the cell stage at irradiation (0.98 for G_1 versus 0.62 for S and G_2).

The cycle after the one in which irradiation occurred is characterized by prolongation of the generation time, decreased probability of division, and the frequent appearance of dead and nondividing cells and cells with chromosome aberrations. Prolongation of the generation time in this second postirradiation life cycle is usually shorter than that of the cycle in which the irradiation occurred. The decreased probability of division could be attributed to formation of giant cells and to cell death.

Cell-Death Survival Curves

Cell death following radiation exposure can be divided into two classes: *Reproductive death and interphase death.* Reproductive death is limited to cells that are capable of undergoing cell division during their lifetime. In reproductive death, cells that are sufficiently injured by irradiation die during mitosis

or later as a result of faulty mitotic processes. Some cells that ultimately die a reproductive death are capable of completing a small number of postirradiation cell divisions before they die; however, they lose their capacity for sustained proliferation and are, therefore, considered reproductively dead. In general, reproductive death occurs in proliferative cells after exposure to low or moderate doses of radiation.

Unlike reproductive death, interphase death is not restricted to proliferative cells. It can be reproduced in any cell type, but usually requires exposure to relatively large doses of radiation (> 5,000 cGy). Cells dying this type of death do so while still in interphase by a mechanism that is currently unknown. Interphase death represents the sole mode of death for cells, such as neurons, that are not capable of cell division.

Interestingly, small lymphocytes die an interphase death after exposure to extremely low doses (< 100 cGy) of radiation. The reason for this anomalous behavior is not currently understood.

The dose-effect relationship for reproductive death is determined by in vitro colony formation assay techniques. Thus, a known number of cells are "plated," and the colonies formed days later from surviving cells are scored. Using this method, survival curves, which characterize the cell population, can be obtained. Survival curves for mammalian cells are commonly sigmoidal in shape and approximate the curve predicted by one hit, multitarget mode of cell inactivation: $[S = 1 - (1 - e^{-D/D_0})^n]$

This permits us to express survival curves by two parameters, D_0 and n (Fig. 5-14). The shoulder on survival curves for mammalian cells after low LET radiation indicates that damage must be accumulated before lethal damage results. This is characterized by the extrapolation number "n" or the "quasithreshold" dose, D_q, where $D_q = D_0 \ln n$. The slope of the curve is equal to $^{-1}/_{D_0}$ where D_0 is the mean lethal dose, i.e., the dose required to reduce survivors to $1/e$ (0.37) of the initial number.

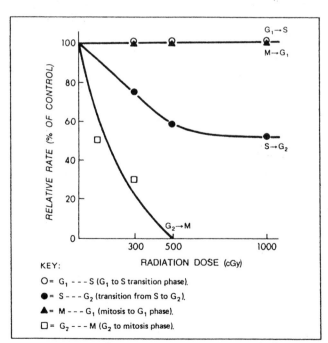

Fig. 5-13. Dose relationships of initial effects of radiation on the rates of cell progression from one phase to the subsequent phase in the cell cycle: mouse Ehrlich ascites tumor in vivo. G_1 = Gap no. 1, G_2 = Gap no. 2, S = DNA synthetic phase. From Kim and Evans (36), with permission.

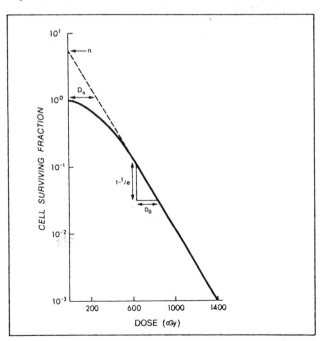

Fig. 5-14. Typical mammalian cell survival curve for low linear energy transfer radiation such as x-rays. D_q = "quasi-threshold" dose; D_0 = mean lethal dose; and n = extrapolation—where $d_q = d_0$ in n. See text for details.

Several ingenious in vivo assays for tumor and normal tissue have also added significantly to our ability to quantitatively determine dose-effect relationships. These include the spleen colony assay for bone marrow cells, lung colonies assays, skin and intestinal crypt cells assays, and transplantation assays for mammary, thyroid, and liver cells. The use of these and other assays for mammalian cells have revealed:

1. The general presence of a shoulder on the survival curves.
2. A comparatively narrow range of D_0 or slopes (50-250 cGy).
3. Modifications of slope and shoulders by radiations of different linear energy transfer.
4. Marked change in sensitivities produced by oxygen and certain chemicals.

Emphasis on dose-effect relationships has shifted to attempts to more accurately assess the low-dose region, not only because of interest in fundamental mechanisms of accumulation of sublethal damage, but also because of applications to estimates of radiation hazards and to radiotherapy, where smaller doses of radiation are pertinent. Based on the work of many groups, most mammalian cell dose-effect curves also appear to fit a linear-quadratic equation (4,5), where the response is directly related to both the dose and the square of the dose ($\ln SF = \alpha D - \beta D^2$). The use of this relationship for mechanistically interpreting radiobiologic effects in terms of energy deposition is still developing. In terms of physical events, it has been suggested that the αD term corresponds to single-event inactivation, or a linear component of cell kill, whereas the βD^2 term represents lethality resulting from an interaction of two individual events. The biologic implications are that the α component represents nonrepairable damage, and that the β component is damage that must be accumulated before becoming lethal and therefore repairable under appropriate conditions. The relative contributions of the α and β components of cellular inactivation differ among tumors and various normal tissues. In radiotherapy, early effects occur in rapidly proliferating tissues and late effects in tissues that proliferate more slowly. Survival curves for tumors and early responding tissues have relatively steep initial slopes (large component) and are characterized by a large ratio of the α and β coefficients coefficients (α/β). In contrast, the dose-response curves for late tissues are curvier, and typified by a reduced α/β ratio. Recognition of this has had profound impact upon the design of contemporary radiation therapy treatment schedules (57) as will be described in greater detail in Chapter 6, "Principles of Radiation Oncology and Cancer Radiotherapy."

Cell Death Versus Cell Cycle Position

Effects of irradiation at different stages in a cell's life can be studied using synchronized populations of cells. There are several available methods to synchronize, such as mitotic selection, addition of drugs that stop cells at a certain cycle stage (e.g., hydroxyurea, colcemid, excess thymidine), temperature shock, centrifugation, elutriation, and cell separation by flow cytometry.

Experiments using synchronized populations of cells in tissue culture (Fig. 5-15) (51) reveal that cell death from ionizing radiation depends on the position of the cell in its growth cycle. Some generalizations based on these studies are:

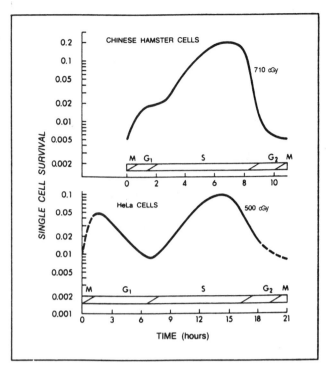

Fig. 5-15. Typical age responses for cells with a short G1 phase (represented by Chinese hamster V79 cells; top panel) or long G1 phase (HeLa cells; lower panel) following irradiation. S = DNA synthetic phase; G_1 = gap no. 1; M = mitosis; G_2 = Gap no. 2. From Sinclair (51), with permission.

1. Cells are generally sensitive at or near mitosis.
2. If G_1 is of appreciable length, a resistant period is usually evident early, followed by a decline in survival toward S. The end of G_1 may be as sensitive as M.
3. In most cell lines, resistance rises during S to a maximum in the later part of S. This is usually the most resistant part of the cycle.
4. In most cell lines, the G_2 period is sensitive, perhaps as sensitive as in mitosis. In some cells, resistance normally seen in S may be delayed until G_2.

Complete Survival Curves Versus Cell Cycle Phase

Both the shoulder and slope may change in different phases of the cell cycle. As shown in Fig. 5-16 (52), the greatest change is in the width of the shoulder for Chinese hamster cells. Other cell lines (e.g., HeLa) may show large slope changes in the survival curves when irradiated at different phases of the cell cycle.

The reasons for the sensitivity changes through the cell cycle are not fully understood. Several mechanisms have been proposed.

1. Since the variation in sensitivity between the most resistant and most sensitive phases of the cell cycle is of the same order of magnitude as the oxygen effect, it was logical to speculate whether oxygen was implicated in the variation of sensitivity through the cell cycle. Experiments have been performed seeking a variation in the oxygen effect at various phases of the cell cycle. In the systems investigated (which include mammalian cells in culture and one simple organized tissue, namely the meristem of the broad bean Vicia faba), no such

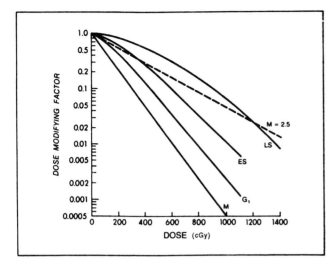

Fig. 5-16. Single-cell survival curves for Chinese hamster cells (V79 line) irradiated at different stages of the cell cycle. M = mitosis; G_1 = Gap no. 1; ES = early S (DNA synthetic) phase; and LS = late S phase. A dose modifying factor of 2.5, which might be expected for anoxic conditions, applied to mitotic cells, is shown by the dotted line. From Sinclair (52), with permission.

variation has been found in the oxygen enhancement ratio (OER) as a function of cell age (2,4,5). The OER appears to have a constant value for all phases of the cell cycle. (See section on oxygen effect for definition of OER.)

2. If DNA is the primary target for radiation-induced cell lethality, as is commonly supposed, then changes in the amount or form of the DNA might be expected to result in variations of sensitivity. During S, the DNA content doubles as the genome is replicated; just prior to mitosis, the chromosome material appears to condense into discrete entities. These two events coincide with the periods of minimum and maximum radiosensitivity, but the exact nature of a cause-effect relationship is not clear.

3. Recent experiments correlate the changed sensitivity through the cycle with varying levels of naturally occurring sulfhydryl compounds in the cell (2,5). These compounds are powerful radiation protectors.

A combination of numbers 2 and 3 above is probably involved in the important and substantial change in radiosensitivity that cells exhibit as they progress through their generation cycle.

Because of the differential cell cycle effect of radiation — both in terms of cell-cycle progression and survival — an asynchronously growing cell population will tend to be synchronized in the most resistant phase (usually late S). If, after a first dose of radiation, the cell population then progresses through the cell cycle, it might be possible to treat the cells during a sensitive phase of the cycle by choosing an appropriate time interval between the first and subsequent doses. It is not understood to what extent this factor is important for radiotherapy of cancer, which is usually given in many fractions. Experiments with tumor model systems to optimize the delivery of the radiation fractions have not been encouraging. In discussing the subject of cell synchronization, there is a great temptation to speculate on the possibility

of inducing synchrony in a tumor by the use of an appropriate drug, and then tailoring the subsequent fractionated treatment regimen so that the tumor cells are always irradiated at the time when they are in the most sensitive phase of the cycle. This is, of course, an attractive possibility, and may one day prove feasible.

Linear Energy Transfer and Relative Biologic Effectiveness

Studies with radiations of different LET have been important in radiobiology because their characteristics give us a different approach to seeking answers, and provide us with more questions than could come from studies with low LET radiation only. During the past 25 years, as variety of high LET radiations — including many accelerated particles and neutrons of different energies — have become available for research. It has been possible, therefore, to obtain a fairly complete picture of the RBE over a wide range of energies.

As LET increases (Fig. 5-17), there is a decrease in the shoulder (Dq) and an increase in the slope (Do) of survival curves. Thus, the RBE increases with increasing LET. It should be noted that the RBE for a given type of radiation varies with the biologic test system and with the level of damage and consequently the dose of radiation (Fig. 5-4) (2). This is due to the comparison of different shapes of the survival curves.

At low LET, oxygen and other modifiers can alter the response to irradiation, but this type of modifications is greatly reduced as LET increases.

Oxygen Effect as Related to Cell Survival

The ability to modify radiation responses has continued to intrigue investigators, both from a mechanistic point of view and because of the obvious applications in radiotherapy and other fields. Probably the most studied modifier has been oxygen. Many biologic responses to radiation have been tested in a variety of cells and the radiation sensitizing properties of oxygen have been firmly established (see also Physicochemical section above).

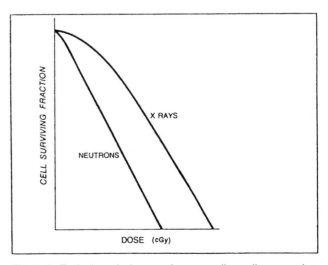

Fig. 5-17. Typical survival curves for mammalian cells exposed to single doses of x-rays and fast neutrons. In the case of x-rays, the survival curve has a large initial shoulder; for fast neutrons the initial shoulder is smaller and the final slope is steeper.

This sensitization is termed the oxygen enhancement ratio (OER), and is the ratio of the doses required to reduce survival to a certain level in hypoxic (N_2) and in oxygenated (O_2) conditions. The OER increases rapidly as oxygen concentration increases (Fig. 5-18) and is maximal at very low oxygen levels. The OER for mammalian cells generally approaches 3.0 (Fig. 5-19) (2). As LET increases, the OER decreases so that, for example, for 14 MeV neutrons, the OER = 1.6. Since tumors may contain radiation resistant hypoxic cells, there is some interest in the use of high LET radiation such as neutrons, both because of the reduced OER and because of the possible RBE advantage.

The oxygen effect has now been characterized kinetically in considerable detail. Using high-dose, pulsed irradiation and oxygen implosion techniques in bacterial systems, the half-life of the oxygen sensitive sites has been estimated to be less than 500 ms. There has also been an accumulation of evidence using rapid-mix techniques with mammalian cells to indicate that the oxygen effect may be divided kinetically into more than one component. Whether this reflects different sites of damage, e.g., outer cell membrane versus DNA in the nucleus, or possible sites with different half-lives, or some other explanation, remains to be elucidated.

Correlations of radiation-chemical with radiobiologic responses, using various sensitizing and protecting chemicals in the presence or absence of oxygen, have provided a useful model within which most of the modifying reactions may be fitted. In this model, cellular DNA is strongly implicated as the sensitive target, because the kinetics of the oxygen effect for single-strand breaks in DNA correlate with the kinetics observed for loss of reproductive capacity. In general, the scheme proposes the production of DNA radicals by both direct and indirect mechanisms. A major part of this damage is attributed to OH• radicals. The outcome of this initial DNA damage is significantly influenced by the oxidation-reduction environment in the cell, particularly near the DNA. Fixed damage, which may or may not involve binding of agents, can possibly be repaired by cellular enzymatic systems. This model provides a framework for much future biochemical investigation of the various pathways proposed.

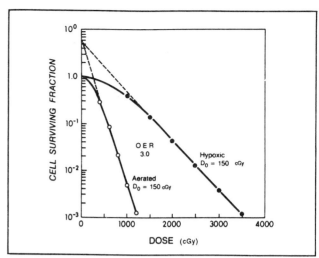

Fig. 5-19. Typical data for survival curves of mammalian cells exposed to x-rays under aerobic and hypoxic conditions illustrating an oxygen enhancement ratio (OER) of 3.0. D_0 = mean, lethal dose. From Hall (2), with permission.

Chemical Radiation Sensitizers (48a)

Hypoxic Cell Sensitizers (54a)

Interest in modification of radiation damage led to the development of radiation-sensitizing chemicals, such as DNA-base analogues and electron affinic agents, useful clinically for tumors. Research in this area has progressed from radiation chemistry to assessment of effectiveness of sensitizing agents in biologic systems in vitro and in vivo, and more recently it has led to biochemical investigations of mechanisms and to determination of physiologic and pharmacologic effects. High concentrations of one class of sensitizing agents, the nitroimidazoles, have proven effective in vitro at producing enhancement ratios approaching those of oxygen (Fig. 5-20) (28). Several nitroimidazoles also have favorable in vivo characteristics and have been shown to sensitize effectively in experimental systems whether assayed by determining tumor cell survival curves or measurements of tumor cure (Fig. 5-21) (49). In contrast, when misonidazole and radiation were combined in animals most normal tissues evaluated indicated little or no enhanced damage, with the possible exceptions of cartilage and esophagus. Consequently, a therapeutic benefit from the combination of radiation and hypoxic cell sensitizers was anticipated. Unfortunately, in humans, the doses of misonidazole that could be administered were limited by neurotoxicity (11). In addition, animal studies demonstrated that in a fractionated radiation dose regimen there was a decrease in the sensitizing ability of misonidazole (2,5,11). This result probably was a consequence of both the reduction in size of the radiation and sensitizer dose and rapid reoxygenation, which can occur in some tumors between subsequent radiation doses. Nevertheless, despite the decrease in sensitizing ability with fractionation and the dose-limiting neurotoxicity, the preclinical investigations appeared sufficiently promising to enter the nitroimidazole compound misonidazole as a radiation sensitizer into phase I-II and phase III clinical trials. While these trials in general have been disappointing, misonidazole has been proven beneficial in a limited number of clinical settings (see Chapter 6, "Principles of Radiation Oncology and Cancer Radiotherapy").

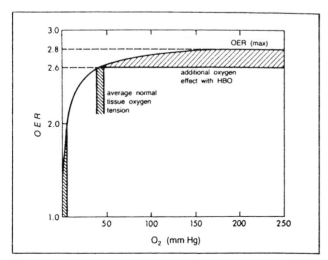

Fig. 5-18. Theoretical curve relating oxygen enhancement ratio (OER) for irradiated mammalian cells to concentration of oxygen. HBO = hyperbaric (i.e., high pressure) oxygen. From Adams (7), with permission.

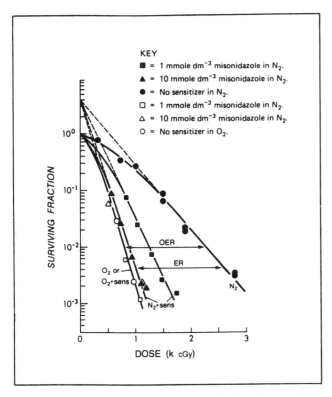

Fig. 5-20. Survival data for oxic and hypoxic Chinese hamster V79-379-A cell x-irradiated in the presence of misonidazole. From Fowler (28), with permission.

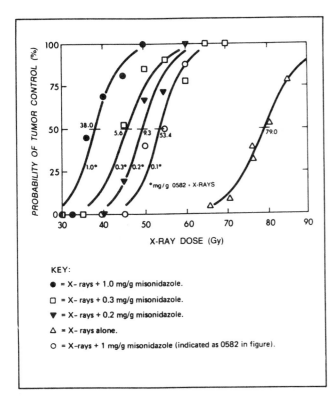

Fig. 5-21. Radiosensitization of the anaplastic MT tumor by the 2-nitroimidazole compared with x-rays alone. One is equal to 100 cGy. From Sheldon and Hill (49), with permission.

Yet clearly misonidazole was not the optimum radiation sensitizer and extensive research to develop better and less neurotoxic compounds has been in progress. These investigations have led to promising new findings with a more hydrophilic 2-nitroimidazole (SR-2508) which was developed at the Standford Research Institute (15,16). This compound has electron affinity and sensitizing ability similar to misonidazole, but is substantially less neurotoxic (15,16). In particular, neurotoxicity assays have indicated that SR-2508 is approximately 3-fold less toxic than misonidazole when given in daily doses. In vitro cell survival and in vivo tumor response studies have demonstrated equivalent radiosensitization of hypoxic cells with misonidazole or SR-2508 (16). Thus these preclinical data indicate that SR-2508 is as effective a radiosensitizer as misonidazole while being substantially less toxic. In addition, a Phase I clinical study has demonstrated that significant doses of SR-2508 can be administered. Consequently, Phase II studies evaluating the efficacy of SR-2508 in combination with radiotherapy have been initiated. In an alternative approach Adams and colleagues (8) have pursued the development of hypoxic cells sensitizers more potent than misonidazole. RSU 1069, the lead compound in a series of nitroimidazole containing an aziridine function, has demonstrated greater radiosensitization than misonidazole both in vitro and in vivo (8). Unfortunately, preliminary clinical studies have revealed a dose-limiting gastrointestinal (GI) toxicity for RSU 1069 (9). However, newly synthesized analogues of RSU 1069 have been developed and some, while less toxic than the parent compound, have retained effective radiosensitization (9).

Nonhypoxic Cell Sensitizers

The halogenated thymidine analogs bromodeoxyuridine (BUdR) and iododeoxyuridine (IUdR) hold considerable promise for use as clinical nonhypoxic radiosensitizers. The rationale for the use of these halogenated deoxyuridines is that they are incorporated selectively into cells undergoing DNA synthesis (30,37). Since, in general, tumors are comprised of a larger proportion of actively dividing cells than are normal tissues having large noncycling cell populations (e.g., liver, lung, brain), it would be anticipated that greater incorporation of these agents would occur in tumors. As a result of this incorporation, the rapidly dividing tumor cells would be more sensitive to radiation because the degree of radiosensitization is directly related to the extent of thymidine replacement in DNA by these analogs (37). Thus, the use of haloperymidines in combination with radiation therapy should lead to increased tumor-cell kill without increasing damage to less rapidly dividing normal tissue. Indeed, preclinical investigations have demonstrated a therapeutic gain in mouse tumor models treated with either BUdR or IUdR and single- or multiple-dose radiation therapy.

A major difficulty with the use of these halogenated thymidine analogs as radiosensitizers has been the need to administer these agents intra-arterially because of rapid degradation of the drugs. In patients, this can result in increased morbidity and potential mortality. However, recent in vivo experiments using rodent-tumor model systems have demonstrated that continuous intravenous infusions can be as effective as intra-arterial exposures at radiosensitizing tumors (30). Consequently, there has been renewed interest in the use of these nonhypoxic cell sensitizers in conjunction with conventional radiotherapy.

Radiation Therapy and Chemotherapy

Recent studies have indicated that the radiation response of cultured cells in vitro, as well as tumor and normal tissue cells in vivo, can be greatly enhanced when radiation therapy is administered in conjunction with certain conventional chemotherapeutic drugs. The magnitude of response enhancement achieved is dependent on the chemotherapeutic agent chosen, the dose used, the sequence and timing of radiation treatment relative to drug administration and the tissue, as well as the biological end point examined. Although a vast amount of experimental data have been accumulated in the past few years, space limitations restrict the current discussion of this promising approach to therapy. The reader is therefore directed to a recent review of work in this area prepared by Bartelink *et al.* (10).

Irradiation and Hyperthermia

Another modality with promising potential for combination with irradiation is hyperthermia. As with combination chemotherapy and radiation therapy, the effectiveness of combined heat and radiation treatment is dependent on many variables — including sequencing, the temperature used, and the tumor or normal tissue examined. The potential of this approach for modifying radiation response results from several important factors including: (1) radioresistant S phase cells are the most sensitive to the cytotoxic and radiosensitizing effect of heat (Fig. 5-22); (2) hyperthermia is particularly effective against hypoxic cells that are resistant to radiation; and (3) hyperthermia can inhibit the repair of irradiation damage. Although much remains to be resolved, heat may

provide a powerful tool for modifying irradiation response in tumors and might also prove to be useful for tumor treatment without combination with other modalities. A review of the combined effects of radiation therapy and hyperthermia has recently been prepared by Overgaard (41).

Effects of Irradiation

Cellular Recovery and Repair

The ability of cells to recover from damage was shown by experiments in the 1930s and 1940s (3,25), where responses decreased as the dose rate decreased and where fractionation or split dose techniques were used to examine end points such as skin erythema and chromosome breaks. Major emphasis in this area developed after 1960 (3,25), when it was shown that mammalian cells exhibited split dose repair or sublethal damage recovery (Fig. 5-23) (24). This increased survival with time between doses is associated with the return of the shoulder on the survival curve.

Another form of recovery — repair of potentially lethal damage (PLD) — has been studied in plateau phase cultures and solid tumors (Fig. 5-24) (33). This recovery, measured by varying the postirradiation incubation conditions, seems to be primarily associated with changes in the slope of the exponential portion of the survival curve. However, it has recently been demonstrated that repair of PLD in normal tissues may be associated with shoulder rather than slope changes (32,39). The significance of PLD repair in the response of human tumors and normal tissues to radiation therapy has not been clearly established.

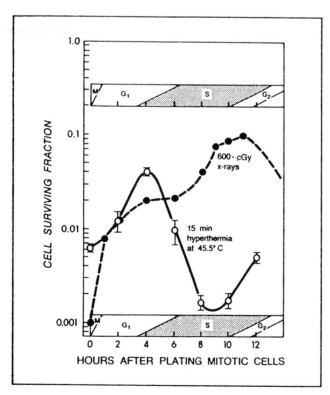

Fig. 5-22. Comparison of the fraction of cells surviving heat or x-irradiation delivered at various phases of the cell cycle. The heat treatment consisted of 15 minutes at 45.5° C, while the x-ray dose was 600 cGy. From Hall (2), with permission.

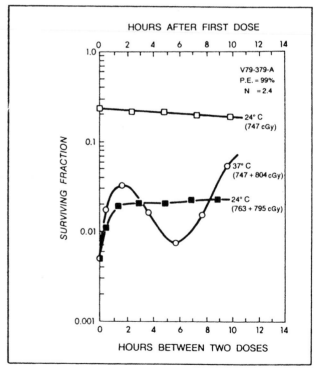

Fig. 5-23. Temperature dependence of two dose survivals. The uppermost curve shows the effect on single-dose survival of storage at 24° C. N stands for cell multiplicity; V-79-379-A is a cell subline name. P.E. = plating efficiency of untreated cells. From Elkind (24), with permission.

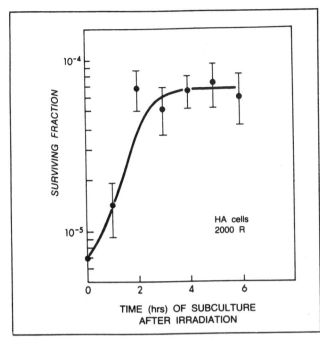

Fig. 5-24. Repair of potentially lethal damage in fed cultures of HA cells exposed to 2,000 R (R = Exposure dose). From Hahn and Little (33), with permission.

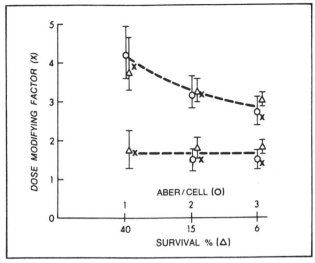

Fig. 5-25. Dose modifying factors for syn-chronized cells. The circles represent the chromosomal data, and the triangles represent survival data; 95% confidence limits on the rations, estimated from a statistical regression analysis, are indicated. The reference survival fractions 40%, 15%, and 6% and corresponding aberration frequencies were observed for cells irradiated in metaphase with 55, 110, and 165 rad, respectively. The dose-modifying factors derived from the x-ray survival curves of Sinclair and Morton (46) for Chinese hamster cells are also indicated by X. From Dewey *et al.* (23), with permission.

Dose Rate

In radiobiology, dose rates of ionizing radiation, extending from a few cGy per day up to thousands of cGy in a fraction of a second, have been used in a variety of organisms. For mammalian cells, the largest effect of changing dose rate is observed between 1 to 100 cGy/min. As the dose rate is lowered, the slope of the survival curve becomes less steep, i.e., the D_0 increases. This is because the lower dose rates allow more time for repair of sublethal radiation damage during irradiation. Below 1 cGy/min there is little effect, because at this level essentially all sublethal damage is repaired during exposure and the residual cell-killing effect results from nonreparable injury.

Cellular Genetic Effects of Radiation Dose

A basic major question is, of course, what are the consequences of DNA damage to the cell? Damage to chromatin material in eukaryotic cells could include chromosomal proteins and perhaps membrane attachment sites. Strong evidence for a relationship between chromosomal aberrations and reproductive death has been obtained. Synchronized Chinese hamster cells were irradiated at different phases in the cell cycle, and chromosomal damage and lethality were compared on the basis of dose-modifying factors that described the changes in radiosensitivity during the cell cycle. The dose-modifying factors based on lethality agreed within 15% of those based on chromosomal aberrations. It was not possible to relate specific chromosomal lesions to lethality or to exclude the possibility that additional unrecognizable chromosome damage or that damage in other cellular organelles was involved (Fig. 5-25) (23).

When cells are irradiated with x-rays, breaks are produced in the chromosomes. The broken ends appear to be "sticky" and can rejoin with any other sticky end. However, it appears that a broken end cannot join with a normal unbroken end of a chromosome. Once breaks are produced, different fragments may behave in a variety of ways.

- the breaks may restitute, i.e., rejoin, to give their original configuration. In this case, of course, nothing amiss will be visible at the next mitosis
- the breaks may fail to rejoin, and give rise to an aberration that will be scored as a deletion at the next mitosis
- broken ends may reassort and rejoin with other broken ends to give rise to chromosomes that appear to be grossly distorted when viewed at the following mitosis

The above is an oversimplified account; whether actual breaks occur in the chromosomes at the time of irradiation is not known, nor is the biologic significance of stickiness understood.

The aberrations seen at metaphase are of two classes, *chromosome* and *chromatid aberrations*. The difference between these two types may be explained as follows:

1. Chromosome aberrations result if a cell is irradiated early in interphase, before DNA and the chromosome material have been duplicated during the DNA synthetic period. In this case, the radiation-induced break will be in a single strand of chromatin; during the DNA synthetic phase that follows, this strand of chromatin will lay down next to itself an identical strand and will also replicate the break that had been produced by the radiation. The chromosome aberration will be visible at the next mitosis, because there will be an identical break in the corresponding points of a pair of chromatin strands.

2. Chromatid aberrations are produced if the dose of radiation is given later in interphase, after the DNA material has doubled and the chromosomes consist of two strands of chromatin. In regions removed from the

centromere, chromatid arms may be fairly well separated; it is reasonable to suppose that the radiation dose might break one chromatid without breaking its sister chromatid, or at least not in the same place. A break that occurs in a single chromatid arm after chromosome replications and leaves the opposite arm of the same chromosome undamaged, leads to chromatid aberrations.

In addition to gross chromosomal aberrations, exposure to ionizing radiation can produce microscopic lesions in DNA, gene or point mutations. These mutations in the genetic code can result from changes at the level of single nucleotides in the DNA base sequence. The mutational effect of ionizing radiation was first demonstrated in the fruit fly, Drosophila, during the early part of the twentieth century. These early studies showed that the production of mutations in the fruit fly increased linearly with radiation dose when administered in a single acute dose, fractionated doses, or protracted over long periods of time (2).

In the late 1940s and early 1950s, similar large-scale genetic studies were initiated in mice by Russell (48). These studies demonstrated significant differences between the mutational effect of radiation on the genetic material of the fruit fly and that of the mouse. These megamouse experiments revealed that: (1) mutation frequently is not linearly related to radiation dose at higher radiation doses (Fig. 5-26); (2) the mutation rate is significantly higher in mice than in *Drosophila* (Table 5-1); and (3) mutation frequency is reduced if the dose rate is reduced. As a result of Russell's megamouse work, the concept that all radiation-induced genetic damage is cumulative and irreversible is no longer held. The cytogenetic response of human cells to ionizing radiation was first described qualitatively and quantitatively by Bender and Gooch in 1962, using short-term cultures of peripheral blood leukocytes (11). Subsequent studies in many laboratories indicate that, in general, human cells respond qualitatively like other biologic materials.

Table 5-1. Mutation Frequencies Induced by Acute X-Ray Doses of 1,000 cGy or Less for a Variey of In Vitro Selection Systems and for the Specific Locus Method with Mouse and Fly Spermatogonia

Cells	Selection Technique	Mutations per cGy
Mouse L5178Y	Alanine auxotrophy to prototrophy	3×10^{-7}
Mouse L5178Y	6-Thioguanine resistance	$1-3 \times 10^{-7}$
Chinese hamster V79	8-Azaguanine resistance	$4-18 \times 10^{-7}$
Chinese hamster CHO	8-Azaguanine resistance	$1-8 \times 10^{-7}$
Human fibroblasts	8-Azaguanine resistance	2.2×10^{-7}
Human lung fibroblasts	6-Thioguanine resistance	3×10^{-7}
Mouse spermatogonia	Specific locus	2.5×10^{-7}
Drosophila spermatogonia	Specific locus	0.1×10^{-7}

From Grosch and Hopwood (32a), with permission.

A recent analysis of published radiation mutation data in several organisms has raised the possibility that we can extract more information and draw more meaningful conclusions about mutational response and genetic hazards than previously expected (Fig. 5-27) (6).

There is a very good correlation between genetic damage and DNA content. Considerable effort has gone into accurately determining dose-effect curves in order to estimate the genetic hazards from low doses. Unfortunately, there is a lower limit to the dose at which genetic effects can be scored. This has necessitated risk estimates based on data that do not clearly indicate whether there is a threshold in the dose-response. Analyses of the yield of specific locus mutations following irradiation of maturing oocytes in female mice were also found to fit the linear-quadratic model described earlier for survival curves. Thus, this model gave predicted values, indicating a mixture of one-hit and two-hit events. It appears that this dose-effect relationship may generally apply for several biologic endpoints after ionizing radiation, and may be useful in the future in more accurately estimating risks at low doses for other late effects of radiation, such as carcinogenesis. However, caution is necessary where multistep carcinogenic processes with mixed-cell populations having different repair capacities could be involved.

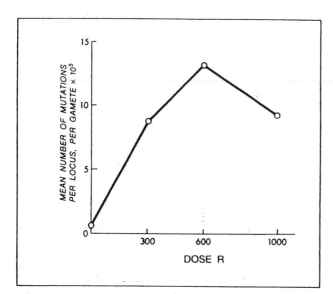

Fig. 5-26. Mutation rates at seven specific loci in the mouse resulting from x-rays delivered at 90 rad/min. Subsequent research using y-ray doses down to a few roentgens per week have provided points that lie much lower. From Grosch and Hopwood (32a), with permission.

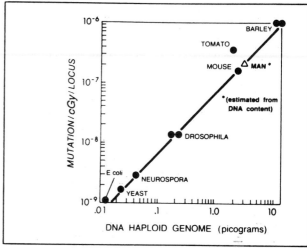

Fig. 5-27. Relation between forward mutation rate per locus per rad and the DNA content per haploid genome. Line drawn with slope of 1 through the mouse point. The point for humans is estimated from DNA content. Reprinted with permission from *Nature* (Abrahamson et al. [6]) Copyright 1973 Macmillian Magazines Limited.

Tissue Effects

Just as detectable cellular injury reflects the cumulative effects of ionizing radiation on cellular molecules, the effects of ionizing radiation on tissues represent the summation of damage to cells within that tissue. Since the functional integrity of many tissues is dependent on the organization of the parenchymal and stromal cells within it, cellular damage in critical tissue components can lead to death of the entire tissue, and even the organism itself. Similarly, many organs and organ systems within animals are linked very closely to other organs; they require normal functioning of these related organs to function properly themselves. It is, therefore, possible to produce functional as well as structural alteration in tissues that are not even included in the exposed area. Any assessment of tissue damage following radiation exposure should also include consideration of these "abscopal" ("ab" — away from, "scopal" — target) effects.

As suggested in the discussion on interphase and reproductive death, cells differ in their sensitivity to radiation. This sensitivity and the time course for expression of damage are, at least in part, directly linked to the reproductive future of the cells. A general classification for cellular sensitivity has been established, based on the proliferative capacity and the degree of differentiation of cell populations within mammalian tissues. The four general categories of cell types used in this classification, their properties and relative radiation sensitivities are shown in Table 5-2. According to this scheme, connective tissue cells — including vascular endothelium — demonstrate radiosensitivity intermediate to differentiating intermitotic cells and reverting postmitotic cells. According to the prevalent theory of tissue damage, the intermediate sensitivity of these cell populations plays a critical role in the time course for expression of radiation damage in certain tissues (18,19,47). As can be seen in Table 5-2 (2), cells that divide regularly are quite sensitive to radiation and die a reproductive death while attempting division shortly after radiation exposure. The acute effects of radiation in tissues of this rapid renewal type therefore results from parenchymal cell depletion. An example of this type of damage is the rapid denudation of the intestinal villi. This occurs when clonogenic stem cells in the intestinal crypts are killed by exposure to radiation and cannot provide differentiated cells that migrate up the villi to replace the cells normally lost from the tips of the villi. This type of damage can occur following low doses of radiation. Following a sufficiently low dose of radiation, cells are frequently capable of recovering from this type of damage if time elapses before the delivery of subsequent doses. This phenomenon is one of the basic principles underlying the use of fractionated doses of radiation in tumor therapy (see Chapter 6).

The pathogenesis of lesions differs in slow renewal and nonrenewal systems. Since in these systems the cells never, or infrequently, divide, and are more resistant than their highly proliferative counterparts, the expression of damage as a result of reproductive death of the parenchymal cells requires longer periods of time and higher doses of radiation. Therefore, because of the intermediate sensitivity of the connective tissue compartment, damage in these tissues is thought to result in part from slowly developing structural and functional alterations in the supporting microvasculature. Evidence of vascular damage, such as endarteritis, fibrosis, and thrombus formation can be found when irradiated tissues are examined histologically (19). These vascular deficits can be responsible for some late damage occurring in rapid renewal systems as well.

However, it has been proposed recently that both acute and chronic damage result from radiation-induced depletion of the parenchymal and/or stromal compartments (56), rather than from vascular damage. According to this theory, the rate of development of injury is dependent on the proliferative rate of the tissue parenchymal cells: acute injury occurs in tissues that divide rapidly, late injury in tissues with a slow cell turnover rate. Therefore, a late effect in slow renewal system is comparable to an acute effect whose expression is delayed until the slowly proliferating cells attempt to divide.

Investigations designed to determine the mechanism of late radiation damage in exposed normal tissues are extremely important because the risk of debilitating late effects ultimately limits the dose of radiation that can be applied for the treatment of tumors. Once potential mechanisms have been elucidated, techniques to modify the pathogenesis of late damage can be developed.

A list of normal tissue end points currently used in radiobiologic studies is included in Table 5-3.

Tumor Effects

For comparison of radiation effects on malignant tissues versus normal tissues, see Chapter 6, "Principles of Radiation Oncology and Cancer Radiotherapy," in which the biologic basis for radiation therapy is discussed.

Whole Body Effects

The total organism is as sensitive as the most vulnerable of vital tissues; the hematopoietic system is the most sensitive of the vital tissues in the human body. It is important to control infection in total-body irradiation since death is usually caused by overwhelming infection. If part of the hematopoietic system is shielded, the tolerance of the individual for radiation is greatly increased, and the next most sensitive vital tissue (the GI tract) determines tolerance.

The tolerance of the organism, or its component collection of normal tissues, varies with the application of radiation depending on four characteristics: dose, time, volume, and

Table 5-2. Categories of Mammalian Cell Sensitivity

Cells	Properties	Examples	Sensitivity*
I Vegetative intermitotic	Divide regularly; no differentiation	Erythroblasts Intestinal crypt cells Germinal cells of epidermis	High
II Differentiating intermitotic Connective tissue cells†	Divide regularly; some differentiation between divisions	Myelocytes	
III Reverting postmitotic cells	Do not divide regularly; variably differentiated	Liver	
IV Fixed postmitotic cells	Do not divide; highly differentiated	Nerve cells Muscle cells	Low

* Sensitivity decreases for each successive group.
† Intermediate in sensitivity between groups II and III.
Based on Casarett (19) and Rubin and Casarett (47).
From Hall (2), with permission.

Table 5-3. Normal Tissue End Points

Tissue	End Point
Central Nervous System	Incidence of paralysis (spinal cord) LD_{50}* (brain) Number of surviving cells in the subependymal plate (brain)
Thyroid	Impairment of stimulated proliferation Survival of clonogenic cells
Heart	Degree of fibrosis

Hemopoietic tissues	Loss of reproductive integrity by stem cells:
	  Spleen colony formation
	  Indirect methods

	Depletion of differentiating cell compartment
	Depletion of mature cells
	LD_{50}
Lung	LD_{50} Breathing frequency
Esophagus	LD_{50}
Gastrointestinal	Microcolony survival
	Macrocolony survival
	Weight loss
	Reduction in DNA content
	Protein leakage
	Reduction in absorptive surface
	LD_{50}
Liver	^{131}Rose bengal uptake
	Mortality
	Survival of clonogenic cells
Kidney	Reduction in organ weight
	LD_{50}
Bladder	Urination frequency
Cartilage	Survival of clonogenic cells
	Stunting of growth
Mammary gland	Survival of clonogenic cells

Skin	Gross reactions:
	  Early
	  Late
	  Deformities

	Survival of clonogenic cells

*LD_{50} = lethal dose for 50% of the population.
Adapted from Field and Michalowski (26).

quality. Too often, radiation effects are described and pharmacopathologic changes are presented without reference to these pertinent radiation factors.

$$BIOLOGICAL\ EFFECT \sim \frac{DOSE \times VOLUME}{TIME}$$

Essentially, the biologic effect of radiation is directly proportional to the dose and volume, and inversely related to the time of administration. Situations that generally occur are described in the next sections.

1. *Large dose, large volume of tissue exposed and high dose rate (radiation accidents or explosions):*
   - *dose:* 450 to 10,000 cGy
   - *time:* Seconds to hours or days
   - *volume:* Total body

   This situation can occur during an atomic bomb explosion or possibly a nuclear reactor accident. The LD_{50} for humans, that is, that dose at which 50 percent of the exposed population would die, is 450 to 550 cGy. Levels of 1,000 to 2,000 cGy are lethal for the entire population (LD_{100}). The syndromes that lead to lethality are dose dependent.

   Bone marrow syndrome: If the patient survives intestinal manifestations with levels of 450 to 1,000 cGy, aplastic anemia and thrombocytopenia will occur in 1 to 3 weeks.

   GI syndrome: Death occurs within days, as a result of electrolyte imbalance and infection, with levels of 1,000 to 2,000 cGy.

   CNS syndrome: Death can occur instantly or in hours, with levels of 6,000 cGy or more.

2. *Small dose, large volume of tissue exposed, and low dose rate (background and occupational exposure):*
   - *dose:* small, but variable
   - *time:* lifetime
   - *volume:* entire population; whole body, but organs of particular concern — gonads, bone marrow, and other tissues especially susceptible to radiation carcinogenesis (breast, thyroid, alimentary tract)

3. *Small dose, small volume of tissue exposed, and high dose rate (diagnostic radiography):*
   - *dose:* small (average individual exposure ~ 91 mrem/year)
   - *time:* intermittent
   - *volume:* variable; organs of particular concern — gonads, bone marrow, and other tissues especially susceptible to radiation carcinogenesis, and the fetus

The average annual total-body exposures for residents of the United States have been estimated to be:

natural background	82 mrem/yr
medical procedures	91 mrem/yr
other (fallout, nuclear power, etc)	~ 10 mrem/yr
Total	~ 184 mrem/yr

For these latter two types of exposure, the genetically significant dose (GSD) is considerably lower than these estimates. For example, the total GSD is estimated to be approximately 110 mrem/yr and approximately 23 mrem/yr for medically-related exposures. This difference reflects the fact that the gonads receive only a fraction of the doses listed above. Furthermore, only exposure to individuals with child-bearing potential are included in GSD estimates.

The major health-related concerns associated with medical and occupational exposure are radiation-induced cancer, genetic damage, and effects on the developing fetus. Genetic risk is considered extremely low at these doses, as is the risk of fetal injury. Carcinogenesis is without a doubt the major somatic effect of exposure of populations to low doses of ionizing radiation. However, as discussed in the following section, the risk is considered to be quite low at these exposure levels.

In the case of medical exposures to radiation, the important questions is, "Does the medical gain outweigh the risks associated with the procedures?" If x-rays are ordered properly there is no question that the immediate and later gains outweigh any theoretic gonadal or carcinogenic hazard. The dose of 0.001 cGy to the gonads during a routine chest film is of no concern in terms of offspring and need not arouse fear in terms of radiation injury. The hazard of not finding an early tuberculous or neoplastic lesion presents a greater risk of morbidity and mortality. We should minimize unnecessary exposure to radiation and use it only when it may benefit health.

4. *Large dose, small volume and high dose rate (radiation therapy)*:
   - *dose*: 4,000 to 10,000 cGy
   - *time*: 4 to 8 wk
   - *volume*: Usually limited to segments of the body or separate organs. Attempts are made to include as little of normal structures as possible in the treatment beams so that segmental damage can be tolerated by the patient. No sensation is felt during irradiation, but after a latent period, a sequence of injurious events may occur as outlined in Chapter 37.

Radiation Carcinogenesis

The ability of radiation to induce cancer and leukemia was appreciated shortly after the discovery of radiation and its application to medicine: pioneer radiologists, ignorant of the hazards, developed skin cancers and leukemias from exposure to radiation sources. Since that time, a great deal of effort has been expended in attempts to elucidate the mechanism(s) of radiation carcinogenesis. Although the overwhelming majority of data currently available are based on animal studies, a considerable amount of human data have been accumulated. Good data relative to tumor induction in humans are available for relatively high dose exposures. This information comes from long-term studies of survivors of the atomic bomb blasts at Hiroshima and Nagasaki, populations accidentally exposed during weapons testing, and patients exposed to large amounts of radiation for diagnostic purposes, or for the treatment of relatively benign diseases. Appropriate epidemiologic assessment and discussion of all the available data are not possible in this format. However, several generalizations about tumor induction resulting from exposure to ionizing radiation can be made (12):

- nearly all tissues in the body are susceptible to tumor induction
- tissues vary considerably with respect to their sensitivity to cancer induction
- major sites of solid tumors induced by total-body exposure to radiation are the breast, thyroid, lung, and digestive organs
- age, both at the time of exposure and at diagnosis, is an important variable relating to cancer induction
- latency period (time from exposure to tumor detection) is frequently long, i.e., years to decades
- interaction between host and environmental factors (i.e., hormonal influences, exposure to other carcinogenic agents) may play a significant role in tumor induction
- dose-response relationships for many animal model systems are qualitatively similar to those for human tumor

induction. However, direct quantitative risk extrapolation from animals to humans would be inappropriate

As already mentioned, most of the available dose-response information is for relatively high doses of radiation. Although many animal studies using lower doses of radiation have been reported, tumor induction information for extremely low doses (those of interest with respect to environmental exposures of large populations) has been difficult to obtain because of the large number of animals that would have to be included to detect statistically significant increases in the rate of tumor induction. To assess risk at low doses and establish protection standards, the shape of the dose-response curve in the low-dose region must be extrapolated from the higher dose regions. However, the dose-response model most appropriate for extrapolation to the low-dose region is the subject of great debate. For a more detailed discussion of this extremely important issue, the reader is advised to read "Health Effects of Exposure to Low Levels of Ionizing Radiation: BEIR V, 1990" prepared for the Environmental Protection Agency by the Biological Effects of Ionizing Radiation Committee of the National Research Council, National Academy of Science (33a).

The biophysical and biological processes that are responsible for tumor induction following radiation exposure have not been clearly identified. Since radiation has been shown to cause damage to DNA, a somatic mutation theory of radiation carcinogenesis is very attractive at first appearance. However, the mechanism of radiation carcinogenesis is clearly more complicated than this. Experimental evidence suggests that radiation induction of neoplasms may be a multistage process in which radiation may induce cellular alterations, rendering cells more susceptible to conditional or promoting factors. The true nature of this induction process is being pursued actively.

Radiation Teratology

The developing fetus is highly susceptible to radiation damage. In animals, radiation exposure during the critical moment in organogenesis, when a specific organ is being induced, can lead to malformation. The most radiosensitive stage in the human fetus is during the period of organogenesis, which is 6 to 12 weeks postconception. A large variety of congenital defects have been induced. The most common reported changes are in the central nervous system (CNS), particularly in the form of microcephaly and mental retardation. Congenital abnormalities in irradiated fetuses have been detected at doses of 5 cGy. Radiation-induced abortion will occur with doses in the LD_{50} range, or 500 cGy.

Again, the reader should refer to a review of the effects of medical radiation on the human embryo by Gaulden and Murry (29) for a more extensive discussion of this issue.

Recommended Reading

The radiobiologic literature is extensive, and therefore, for the convenience of the interested reader we suggest the following textbook material as excellent references to the various areas of radiation biology we have discussed in this chapter. *Radiobiology in Radiotherapy* by Bleehen (1), and *Radiobiology for the Radiologist* by Hall (2) are two excellent general reference texts, the latter being particularly valuable to medical practitioners. *Medical Effects of Ionizing Radiation* by Metler and Moseley (3) is a more advanced, theoretical text but provides enlightening discussions about many current, controversial issues. Finally *Biological Basis of Radiotherapy* by Steel (4) and *The Basic Science of Oncology* by Tannock and Hill (5) provide good current reviews of many of the topics discussed in this chapter.

In addition to these references, we have included current references within many of the chapter subsections. These references provide the detailed discussions that we have frequently been unable to provide because of space limitations. The reader is strongly encouraged to pursue areas of interest by referring to the textbooks and the original material.

REFERENCES

General References

1. Bleehen, N.M., ed. Radiobiology in radiotherapy. London, UK: Springer-Verlag; 1988.
2. Hall, E.J. Radiobiology for the radiologist, 3rd ed. Philadelphia, PA: Harper-Row; 1987.
3. Metler, F.A., Moseley, R.D. Medical effects of ionizing radiation. Orlando, FL: Grune & Stratton; 1985.
4. Steel, G.G.; Adams, G.E.; Peckham, M.J., eds. Biological basis of radiotherapy. Amsterdam, Holland: Elsevier; 1989.
5. Tannock, I.F.; Hill, R.P., eds. The basic science of oncology. Elmsford, NY: Pergamon Press; 1987.

Specific References

6. Abrahamson, S.; Bender, M.A.; Conger, A.D.; *et al.* Uniformity of radiation-induced mutation rates among different species. Nature 245:460-462; 1973.
7. Adams, G.E. Hypoxic cell sensitizers for radiotherapy. In: Becker, F.F., ed. Cancer: a comprehensive treatise, vol 6. New York, NY: Plenum press; 1977:181-223.
8. Adams, G.E.; Ahmed, I.; Sheldon, P.W.; Stratford, I.J. Radiation sensitization and chemopotentiation: RSU 1069 a compound more efficient than misonidazole *in vitro* and *in vivo.* Br. J. Cancer 49:571-577; 1984.
9. Ahmed, I.; Jenkins, T.C.; Walling J.M.; Stratford, I.J.; Sheldon, P.W.; Adams, G.E.; Fielden, E.M. Analogues of RSU 1069: Radiosensitization and toxicity in vitro and in vivo. Int. J. Radiat. Oncol. Biol. Phys. 12:1079-1081; 1986.
10. Bartelink, H.; Begg, A.C.; Dewit, L.; Stewart, F.A. Combined treatment with radiation and anti-cancer drugs: experimental and clinical results. In: Bleehen, M.N., ed. Radiobiology in radiotherapy. London, UK: Springer-Verlag; 1988.
11. Bender, M.A.; Gooch, P.C. Types of rates of X-ray induced chromosome aberrations in human blood irradiated *in vitro.* Proc. Natl. Acad. Sci. USA 48:522-532; 1962.
12. Biological Effects of Ionizing Radiation (BEIR) Committee Report. The effects on populations of exposure to low levels of ionizing radiation. Washington, D.C.: National Academy of Science/National Research Council; 1980.
13. Boag, J.W. The time scale in radiobiology. In: Nygaard, O.F.; Adler, H.I.; Sinclair, W.K., eds. Proceedings of the Fifth International Congress of Radiation Research, Seattle, July 1974. New York, NY: Academic Press; 1975:9-29.
14. Bragg, W.H. Studies in radioactivity. London, UK: Macmillan; 1912.
15. Brown, J.M.; Workman, P. Partition coefficient as a guide to the development of radiosensitizers which are less toxic than misonidazole. Radiat. Res. 82:171-190; 1980.
16. Brown, J.M.; Yu, N.Y.; Brown, D.M.; Lee, W. SR-2508 — a 2-nitroimidazole which should be superior to misonidazole as a radiosensitizer for clinical use. Int. J. Radiat. Oncol. Biol. Phys. 7:695-703; 1981.
17. Casarett, A.P. Radiation biology. Englewood Cliffs, NJ: Prentice Hall; 1968.
18. Casarett, G.W. Concept and criteria of radiologic aging. In: Harris, R.J.C., ed. Cellular bases and aetiology of late somatic effects of ionizing radiation. New York, NY: Academic Press; 1963.
19. Casarett, G.W. Radiation Histopathology, vols, 1 and 11. Boca Raton, FL: Chemical Rubber Co. Press; 1980.
20. Chapman, D.L.; Dugle, D.L.; Reuvers, A.P.; *et al.* Studies on the radiosensitizing effect of oxygen in Chinese hamster cells. Int. J. Radiat. Oncol. Biol. Phys. 26:383-389; 1974.
21. Cleaver, J.E. Repair processes for photochemical damage in mammalian cells. In: Lett, J.T.; Adler, H.; Zellem, eds. Advances in radiation biology, vol. 4. New York, NY: Academic Press; 1974.
22. Cleaver, J.E.; Trosko, J.E. Absence of excision repair in xeroderma pigmentosum. Photochem. Photobiol. 11:547-550; 1970.
23. Dewey, W.C.; Freeman, M.L.; Raaphorst, G.P.; *et al.* Cell biology of hyperthermia and radiation. In: Meyn, R.E.; Withers, H.R, eds. Radiation biology in cancer research. New York: Raven Press; 1980:589-621.
24. Elkind, M.M. Damage and repair processes relative to neutron (and charged particle) irradiation. Curr. Top. Radiat. Res. 7:1-44; 1970.
25. Elkind, M.M.; Whitmore, G.F. The radiobiology of culture mammalian cells. New York, NY: Gordon and Breach Publishers; 1967.
26. Field, S.B.; Michalowski, A. Endpoints for damage to normal tissues. Int. J. Radiat. Oncol. Biol. Phys. 5:1185-1196; 1979.
27. Fowler, J.F. Fundamental aspects of LET in radiobiology. In: Nygaard, O.F.; Adler, I.F.; Sinclair, W.K., eds. Proceedings of the Fifth International Congress of Radiation Research, Seattle, July 1974. New York, NY: Academic Press; 1975:1040-1052.
28. Fowler, J.F.; Adams, G.E.; Denekamp, J. Radiosensitizers of hypoxic cells in solid tumors. Cancer Treat. Rev. 3:227-257; 1976.
29. Gaulden, M.E.; Murry, R.C. Medical radiation and possible adverse effects on the human embryo. In: Meyn, R.E.; Withers, H.R., eds. Radiation biology in cancer research. New York, NY: Raven Press; 1980:227-294.
30. Goffinet, D.R.; Brown, J.M. Comparison of intravenous and intra-arterial pyrimidine infusion as a means of radiosensitizing tumors *in vivo.* Radiology 124:829-822; 1977.
31. Goodhead, D.T. Models of radiation inactivation and mutagenesis. In: Meyn, R.E.; Withers, H.R., eds. Radiation biology in cancer research. New York, NY: Raven Press; 1980:231-247.
32. Gould, M.N.; Clifton, K.H. Evidence for a unique *in situ* component of the repair of radiation damage. Radiat. Res. 77:149-155; 1979.
32a. Grosch, D.S.; Hopwood, L.E. Biological Effects of Radiations. New York, NY: Academic Press; 1979.
33. Hahn, G.M.; Little, J.B. Plateau-phase cultures of mammalian cells: an *in vitro* model for human cancer. Curr. Topics Radiat. Res. 8:39-83; 1972.
33a. Health effects of exposure to low levels of ionizing radiation. BEIR V. Washington, D.C.: National Academy Press; 1990.
34. Johns, G.E. The Physics of Radiology, ed. 3. Springfield, MA: C.C. Thomas; 1969.
35. Kellerer, A.M.; Rossi, H.H. The theory of dual radiation action. Curr. Topics Radiat. REs. 8:85-158; 1972.
36. Kim, J.H.; Evans, T.C. Effects of x-irradiation on the mitotic cycle of Ehrlich ascites tumor cells. Radiat. Res. 21:129-143; 1964.
37. Kinsella, T.J.; Mitchell, J.B.; Russom, A.; Morstyn, G.; Glatstein, E. The use of halogenated thymidine analogs as clinical radiosensitizers: rationale, current status, and future prospects: non-hypoxic cell sensitizers. Int. J. Radiat. Oncol. Biol. Phys. 10:1399-1406; 1984.
38. McGrath, R.A.; Williams, R.W. Reconstruction *in vivo* of irradiated escherichia coli deoxyribonucleic acids; rejoining of broken pieces. Nature 212:534-535; 1966.
39. Mulcahy, R.T.; Gould, M.N.; Clifton, K.H. The survival of thyroid cells: *in vivo* irradiation and *in situ* repair. Radiat. Res. 84:523-528; 1980.
40. Okada, S. Radiation biochemistry, vol. 1. New York, NY: Academic Press; 1970.
41. Overgaard, J. The current and potential role of hyperthermia in radiotherapy. Int. J. Radiat. Oncol. Biol. Phys. 16:535-549; 1989.
42. Painter, R.B. Chemical changes induced in DNA by ionizing radiation and the relationship of their repair to survival of mammalian cells. In: Nygaard, O.F.; Adler, E.F.; Sinclair, W.K., eds. Proceedings of the Fifth International Congress of Radiation Research, Seattle, July 1974. New York, NY: Academic Press; 1975:735-739.
43. Painter, R.B. The role of DNA damage and repair in cell killing induced by ionizing radiation. In: Meyn, R.E.; Withers, H.R., eds.

Radiation biology in cancer research. New York, NY: Raven Press; 1980:59-70.

44. Paterson, M.C.; Smith, P.J.; Bech-Hansen, N.T.; *et al.* Gamma ray hypersensitivity and faulty DNA repair in cultured cells from humans exhibiting familial cancer proneness. In: Okada, S.; Imamura, M.; Terashima, T.; *et al.*, eds. Proceedings of the Sixth International Congress of Radiation Research, Japan, May 1979. Tokyo, Japan: Toppan Printing Company; 1979:484-495.

45. Pettijohn, D.; Hanawalt, P.C. Evidence for repair-replications of ultraviolet damaged DNA in bacteria. J. Molec. Biol. 9:395-401; 1964.

46. Rasmussen, R.E.; Painter, R.B. Evidence for repair of ultraviolet damaged deoxyribonucleaic acid in cultured mammalian cells. Nature 203:1360-1362; 1964.

47. Rubin, P.; Casarett, G.W. Clinical radiation pathology, vol 1. Philadelphia, PA: W.B. Saunders; 1968.

48. Russell, W.L. X-ray-induced mutations in mice. Cold Spring harbor symposium on quantitative biology 16:327-336; 1951.

48a. Seventh International Conference on Chemical Modifiers of Cancer Treatment. Siemann, D., Wasserman, T.H. (eds). Clearwater, FL 2-5 February 1991; Int. J. Radiat. Oncol. Biol. Phys. 22(3)(4):1992.

49. Sheldon, P.W.; Hill, S.A. Hypoxic cell radiosensitizers and local control by X-ray of a transplanted tumor in mice. J. Cancer 35:795-808; 1977.

50. Simpson, J.B. (compiler) Contemporary quotations. New York, NY: Galahad Books; 1964.

51. Sinclair, W.K. Cyclic X-ray responses in mammalian cells *in vitro*. Radiat. Res. 33:620-643; 1968.

52. Sinclair, W.K. Dependence of radiosensitivity upon cell age. In: Time and Dose relationships in radiation biology as applied to radiotherapy. BNL 50203 (C-57), NcCI-AEC Conference, Carmel, California, 1969, U.S. Dept. of Commerce, Washington, DC; 1970.

53. Sinclair, W.K.; Morton, R.A. X-ray sensitivity during the cell generation cycle of cultured Chinese hamster cells. Radiat. Res. 29:450-474; 1966.

54. Steel, G.G. Growth Kinetics of tumors: cell population kinetics in relation to the growth and treatment of cancer. Oxford, UK: Clarendon Press; 1977.

54a. Tumor Hypoxia: Proceedings of a Consensus Meeting organized by the EORTC Cooperative Group for Radiotherapy. Bartelink, H., Overgaard, J. (eds). Leuven, Belgium 7-8 December 1989. Radiother and Oncol. 20(Suppl.1): 1991.

55. Wantanabe, I.; Okada, S. Study of mechanisms of radiation-induced reproductive death of mammalian cells in culture: estimation of stage at death and biological description to cell death. Radiat. Res. 27:290-306; 1966.

56. Withers, H.R.; Peters, L.J.; Kogelnik, H.D. The pathobiology of late effects of irradiation. In: Meyn, R.E.; Withers, H.R., eds. Radiationbiolgoy in cancer research. New York, NY: Raven Press; 1980:439-448.

57. Withers, H.R.; Thames, H.D.; Peter, L.J. A new isoeffect curve for change in dose per fraction. Radiother. Oncol. 1:187-191; 1983.

Philip Rubin, M.D., Radiation Oncology
Dietmar W. Siemann, Ph.D., Radiation Oncology, Tumor
   Biology Division

Chapter **6**

PRINCIPLES OF RADIATION ONCOLOGY AND CANCER RADIOTHERAPY

Improvements in the therapeutic ratio can come from either reduction in normal tissue injury or an increase in the effectiveness of tumor treatment.

Simon Kramer, M. D. (18)

PERSPECTIVE

Cure of cancer, with preservation of structure, function, and aesthetics, has advanced based on modern radiation oncology's technologic gains in radiation physics and insights into radiation biology and pathophysiology. According to Wilson *et al.* (26), more than 37% of all US cancer patients could be treated for cure with organ preservation by irradiation. Using present American Cancer Society statistics (20,21), this figure translates to a favorable outcome for more than 350,000 US cancer patients and pertains to more than 1 million people when applied globally (Table 6-1) (26). Initially, pediatric tumors (6) were ablated without sacrifice of limbs and soft tissues, and then Hodgkin's disease (11) among the lymphomas yielded to extended-radiation-field techniques, eliminating the use of radical neck-node dissections. With early detection techniques, gynecologic malignancies such as cancer of the cervix and uterus are highly curable (14). Head and neck cancers (13) involving the larynx and other upper aerodigestive sites treated by radiotherapy allow for preservation of voice and swallowing. With the dramatic improvements in imaging using computed tomography and magnetic resonance imaging, tumors of the eye and selected brain tumors can be eliminated with preservation of vision and minimal neurologic impairment. Effective screening and routine self-examination for breast cancer allow for long-term survival and conservation of structure and cosmesis. Potency is maintained in both early and relatively advanced prostate cancer through radiation treatment, unlike in radical prostatectomy. Most recently, anal preservation has been achieved in anal cancer patients by supplanting combination chemoradiotherapy for abdomino-perineal surgery. Preoperative irradiation in rectal cancer allows lower-lying lesions to be removed, again with anal sphincter intact.

   The ideal in radiation therapy of malignant disease is achieved when the tumor is completely eradicated and the surrounding normal tissues show minimal evidence of structural or funtional injury. This ideal has been described as the *selective effect* of irradiation. Although this ideal selective effect is being obtained more frequently, in the majority of instances in clinical practice one accepts a certain degree of permanent residual damage as a sequel to the destruction of a lethal tumor. The acceptable extent of such alteration of normal structures varies in different settings, but the integrity of vital tissues always must be maintained. This ability to eradicate the tumor without undue complication or destruction of normal tissues is the essential factor in tumor radiocurability and is referred to as the therapeutic ratio. Therefore, it is necessary to either (a) destroy the tumor cells more readily than vital normal tissues in the treatment field for the same dose absorbed (6a); or (b) focus the radiation beam so that a differential dose between the tumor volume and the normal surrounding tissue is achieved. Such improvements in therapy will result from research advances in biology for the former circumstance and radiation physics in the latter. It is our immediate purpose to elaborate on this concept and to develop its clinical implications, for one of the major frontiers of radiation research is to make radiation more selective and thus approach the ideal situation (3,58).

RADIOCURABILITY OF TUMORS (1,9,19,25,27,46)

Therapeutic Ratio

The relation between radiation dose and the probability of control of a homogeneous group of tumors is sigmoidal; that is, with increasing radiation doses, more and more neoplastic cells are killed, until ultimately all clonogenic cells are destroyed and a cure is achieved. The same principle of radiation killing, however, also applies to normal cells and tissues, and so the probability of normal tissue complications and tumor cure are similar. Because there are approximately 300 varieties of human tumors and 50 different normal organs and tissues, each with different cell types, the overlap in the tolerance dose of normal tissues and the tumor dose for ablation is inevitable. It is this relation between normal tissue tolerance and the tumor lethal dose that determines the therapeutic ratio (Fig. 6-1) (26).

Table 6-1. Cancer Sites Amenable to Conservation Surgery and Radiation Therapy

Site (Type)	No. of Patients
Major	
Breast	108,720
Eye-choroid (melanoma)	1,700
Prostate	39,600
Vocal cord	9,760
Other	
Head and neck	
Esophagus	
Bladder	
Cervix	
Uterus	
Central nervous system	
Soft-tissue (sarcomas)	
Retina (retinoblastoma)	
Anus	
Other	223,320
Total	383,100

From Wilson (26), with permission.

The therapeutic ratio is favorable (i.e., the tumor can be destroyed without excessive normal tissue complication) when the tumor cure curve is to the left of the normal tissue dose effect curve (Fig. 6-2a). When the two curves are identical (Fig. 6-2b), the therapeutic ratio is less favorable, but may be improved by precise radiation physics treatment planning and modern megavoltage techniques, so that greater dose is delivered to the tumor than to the normal surrounding tissue. Finally, if the tumor ablation curve is to the right of the vital normal tissue (Fig. 6-2c), the circumstance is most unfavorable. To reverse this situation, innovations and combined modality approaches are essential to a good outcome.

Tumor Control Dose in Clinical Setting

A dose may be chosen for each type of tumor that will cause destruction of a high proportion of cells and lead in turn to local cure. The prescribed dose for different human tumors is not a fixed dose, but varies with tumor size and extent, tumor type, pathologic grade and differentiation, and its response to irra-

diation. The tumor lethal dose may be defined as the dose that has a 95% probability of achieving tumor control (cure) — TCD_{95}. Practical guides for tumor radiocurability can be developed. Table 6-2 illustrates the TCD_{95} for different tumor types and Table 6-3 (9) shows tumor control probability correlated with radiation dose and volume of cancer.

According to the cell survival theory, tumor size is a critical factor in tumor cure by radiation therapy. Using the tumor, node, metastases (TNM) designation, T0 and N0 refer to *occult* stage or microscopic foci (millimeters), pathologically positive but clinically negative. Localized lesions are T1 and

Table 6-2. Curative Doses of Radiation for Different Tumor Types

2,000-3,000 cGy
Seminoma
Central nervous sytem
Acute lymphocytic leukemia

3,000-4,000 cGy
Seminoma
Wilm's tumor
Neuroblastoma

4,000-4,500 cGy
Hodgkins's disease
Lymphosarcoma
Seminoma
Histiocytic cell sarcoma
Skin cancer (basal and squamous)

5,000-6,000 cGy
Lymph nodes, metastatic
Squamous cell carcinoma, cervix cancer,
  and head and neck cancer
Embryonal cancer
Breast cancer, ovarian cancer
Medulloblsatoma
Retinoblastoma
Ewing's tumor
Dysgerminomas

6,000-6,500 cGy
Larynx (< 1 cm)
Breast cancer, lumpectomy

7,000-7,500 cGy
Oral cavity (< 2 cm, 2-4 cm)
Oro-naso-laryngo-pharyngeal cancers
Bladder cancers
Cervix cancer
Uterine fundal cancer
Ovarian cancer
Lymph nodes, metastatic (1-3 cm)
Lung cancer (< 3 cm)

8,000 cGy or above
Head and neck cancer (> 4 cm)
Breast cancer (> 5 cm)
Glioblastomas (gliomas)
Osteogenic sarcomas (bone sarcomas)
Melanomas
Soft tissue sarcomas (> 5 cm)
Thyroid cancer
Lymph nodes, metastatic (>6 cm)

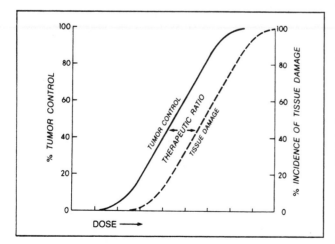

Fig. 6-1. Therapeutic ratio. The response curves of both tumor cure and normal tissue complication are sigmoidal. The differential in dose to achieve these effects is the therapeutic ratio. From Wilson (26), with permission.

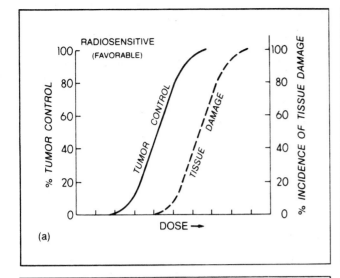

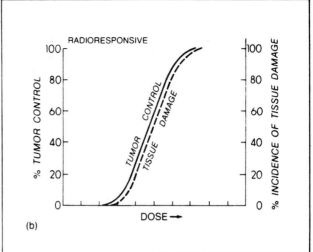

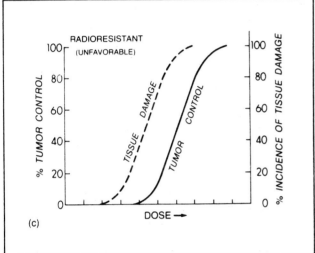

Fig. 6-2. Different therapeutic ratios exist in different clinical circumstances depending on the radiosensitivity (dose-response curves) for tumor versus the critical normal tissue in the treatment field. These figures show (a) a favorable ratio, (b) a less favorable ratio, and (c) an unfavorable ratio.

T2, usually less than 4 cm in diameter, and T3 and T4 are extensive tumors, usually greater than 4 cm.

Highly radiocurable tumors (TCD_{95} range 3,500 to 6,000 cGy), such as seminomas, lymphosarcomas, Hodgkin's disease, neuroblastomas, Wilms' tumors, histiocytic cell sarcomas, medulloblastomas, retinoblastomas, dysgerminomas, and Ewing's sarcomas are treated in this dose range, as are occult cancers — either squamous cell or adenocarcinomas — suspected or residuum after surgery. T1 cancers of the larynx and skin are readily controlled completely. Metastatic lymph nodes with microdeposits are also treated within these dose levels. These doses are well tolerated by normal tissues and complications are minimal.

Radiocurable tumors (TCD_{95} range 6,000 to 7,500 cGy) are those requiring the risk of exceeding normal tissue tolerance to assure a high degree of curability. These are moderate to large tumors (T2 and T3) of the oral cavity, pharynx, bladder, cervix, uterus, ovary, and lung.

Some of the best data available have resulted from thousands of well-documented and well-followed squamous cell cancers in the head and neck region at M.D. Anderson Hospital. Fletcher and colleagues (8) have made careful analyses and built an excellent series of dose-response relationships relating to cancers at different sites in the nasopharynx, oral cavity, oropharynx, hypopharynx, supraglottis, and larynx. Complications are usually modest.

The least radiocurable tumors (TCD_{95} range 8,000 cGy and above) are those large-to-massive squamous cell and adenocarcinomas (T3 and T4) that are less consistently cured by irradiation alone and in which the 95% level is not reached. The lack of tumor control by irradiation may result from shifts in cell cycle kinetics, poor oxygenation, shifts from proliferative to nonproliferative compartments, or inherent radioresistance. Normal tissue tolerance is often exceeded and complications are part of the cost of cure. If interstitial and intracavitary irradiation is applicable in addition to external irradiation, these doses are achievable in some sites within tolerance levels. Some of the recent breast cancer data confirm that tumor control of massive tumors is possible with doses higher than 7,000 cGy, but such radiation doses are associated with a high incidence of late normal tissue effects like fibrosis and atrophy. Tumors arising from mature tissues such as neural, renal, and osseous tissues give rise to radioresistant neoplasms such as glioblastoma multiforme, hypernephroma, and osteogenic sarcomas, respectively (76).

Table 6-3. Tumor Control Probability Correlated to Radiation Dose and Volume of Cancer

	Squamous Cell Carcinoma of the Upper Respiratory and Digestive Tracts	Adenocarcinoma of the Breast
5,000 cGy*	>90% subclinical 60% T1 lesions of nasopharynx 50% 1-3 cm neck nodes	>90% subclinical
6,000 cGy*	90% T1 lesions of pharynx and larynx 50% T3 + T4 lesions of tonsillar fossa	
7,000 cGy* positive	90% 1-3 cm neck nodes 70% 3-5 cm neck nodes 90% T2 lesions of tonsillar fossa and supraglottic larynx 80% T3 + T4 lesions of tonsillar fossa	90% clinically axillary nodes
7,000-8,000 cGy primary (8-9 weeks) primary	............>	65% 2-3 cm 30% > 5 cm
8,000-9,000 cGy primary (8-10 weeks)	............>	56% > 5 cm
8,000-10,000 cGy primary (10-12 weeks)	............>	75% 5-15 cm

*1,000 cGy in five fractions each week.
†The control rate is corrected for the percentage of nodes that would be positive histologically had a dissection of the axilla been done.
Adapted from Fletcher (8).

VARIOUS AIMS OF RADIATION THERAPY (1,9,12,13a,14,25a)

Curative

The patient must be in good physical condition, and general supportive measures of hygiene, nutrition, and blood profile need to be maintained. Radical irradiation is as effective as radical surgery in many of the cancers that have been mentioned; however, it should be recognized that both modalities can be debilitating and can carry a certain morbidity. Generally, the patient will tolerate the course of radiation therapy and most of the untoward acute reactions will clear up within a few weeks after the treatment cessation. Some late effects, such as fibrosis and cellular depletion, may become evident years after treatment, but severe morbid or lethal complications are usually minimal.

Palliative

Palliation often requires curative levels of radiation therapy, although lower doses are also used. Palliative doses must be applied judiciously and might cause some untoward reaction. The aims of palliation are to:
- allow for a symptom-free period appreciably longer than the debilitation caused by the irradiation treatment period

- prolong useful or comfortable survival, increase quality and quantity of life.
- relieve distressing symptoms (e.g., hemorrhage, pain, and obstruction) though survival may not be prolonged
- avert impending symptoms such as hemorrhage, obstruction, and perforation
- make sure that therapy is not debilitating in itself or leads to worse implications than those caused by the neoplastic process itself

TUMOR RADIOSENSITIVITY AND RADIORESISTANCE: CONCEPTS AND CRITERIA

In describing the radiobiologic basis for radiation oncology, two basic concepts will be used in most of the scientific data presented in this chapter. They are the dose-response or dose-effect curve and the clonogenic cell survival fraction.

1. The dose-response or dose-effect curve is sigmoidal and characterizes the relationship between dose and a response on effect, such as tumor control or normal tissue damage, and is plotted on a linear scale. This type of graph refers to the radiation response of in vivo systems (Fig. 6-3).
2. The clonogenic cell survival position represents the fraction or proportion of cells surviving irradiation based on measurements made on cells in tissue culture (in vitro). The data are displayed on a semilog plot (Fig. 6-4) (10).

The R's of Radiobiology (4a,10)

The ability of radiation therapy to cure tumors is established. As the dose increases, more cells are destroyed and, depending on the radiosensitivity of the tumor cells, a cumulative dose can be achieved to completely eradicate the tumor. The resultant dose-response or dose-effect curves in most biologic systems irradiated are sigmoidal. A family of hypothetic dose-response curves, indicating a range of radiation sensitivities, is illustrated in Fig. 6-3.

Different normal tissues and organs in the body have different tolerance doses, depending on whether an early or

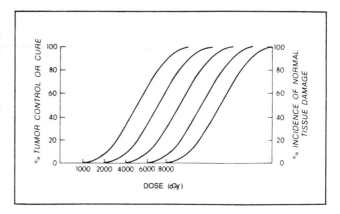

Fig. 6-3. A sigmoidal dose-response curve characterizes the relation between both tumor control and normal tissue damage versus dose. As the radiation dose increases, a threshold is reached beyond which both tumor control and normal tissue injury increase. Several such curves are illustrated, reflecting the variation in radiation sensitivity of the hundreds of varieties of tumors and 50 different normal tissues and organs in the human.

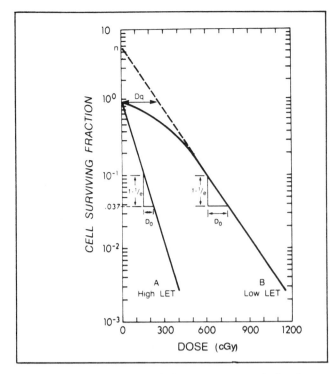

Fig. 6-4. A clonogenic cell survival curve represents the fraction or proportion of cells surviving irradiation. On a semilog plot, after an initial shoulder, the curve bends downward sharply and radiation killing becomes more effective for each cGy absorbed. Cell survival curves are described by their shoulder (Dq) and slope (D0) parameters. These cell survival parameters ultimately contribute to the shape of the therapeutic ratio. LET = linear energy transfer. From Hall (10), with permission.

late effect is studied. From this, it follows that many tumors arising from radiosensitive tissues are radiosensitive, and those arising from radioresistant tissues are often radioresistant (Table 6-4) (19). There is a variation, from the most to the least sensitive, of 20-1 in the sensitivity of human cells and tissues. The testes and ovaries are exquisitely sensitive, as are the lymphoid and bone marrow systems. Proliferating cells and tissues are more sensitive than mature tissues with slow or nondividing cells. Thus, in the adult, neurons, mature bone and cartilage, muscle, and endocrine cells — where they are no longer growing — are more radioresistant. By contrast, in infancy, when neural tissue is rapidly proliferating, it is highly vulnerable to irradiation, particularly in utero and in the first years of life. The same is true of rapidly growing cartilage and bone, muscle, and endocrine glands in the infant and child. Cellular radiosensitivity can be due to a variety of factors, both intrinsic and extrinsic, and their interaction. We will examine each of these factors, beginning with intrinsic radiosensitivity.

Intrinsic Radiosensitivity and Cell Survival Theory (3,14a,18,27,31,48)

Fig. 6-4 illustrates the characteristics of radiation survival curves of mammalian cells following treatment with low (linear energy transfer [LET]) (x and gamma rays) or high LET (neutrons) radiation. The survival curve, plotted on a semilog scale, displays the surviving fraction of cells as a function of dose. Following an initial shoulder region, the radiation killing is essentially logarithmic or exponential. These survival curves can be described by their shoulder (D_q or n) and their slope (D_0). The radiosensitivity is referred to by the D_0, or the dose required to reduce the survival to 37% along with the exponential portion of the curves. Irradiating cells with high LET radiation alters both the slope and shoulder of the survival curve (54). For clinical purposes, the dose required to reduce the surviving fraction to 10% on the exponential portion of the curve, or to provide a log kill, is often a more convenient quantity and is referred to as the $D_{10} = 2.3D_0$.

With this in vitro clonogenic assay for measuring cellular radiosensitivity of animal and human cell lines, various attempts at expressing radiosensitivity have been made. The range of D_0 values typically observed does not explain the variation in response of different human tumors and in recent years the shoulder region of the survival curve has come into greater prominence than the slope. Fertil and Malaise (39,40) suggested cell survival at a dose of 2 Gy to be a measure of

Table 6-4. Various Tumors and Tissues in Decreasing Order of Radiosensitivity

Tumors	Relative Radiosensitivity	Tissues of Origin
Lymphoma, leukemia, seminoma, dysgerminoma	High	Lymphoid, hematopoietic (marrow), spermatogenic epithelium, and ovarian follicular epithelium
Squamous cell cancer of the oropharyngeal, glottis, bladder, skin, and cervical epithelia; and adenocarcinomas of alimentary tract	Fairly high	Oropharyngeal stratified epithelium, sebaceous gland epithelium, urinary bladder epithelium, optic lens epithelium, gastric gland epithelium, colon epithelium, and breast epithelium
Breast, salivary gland tumors, hepatomas, renal cancer, pancreatic cancer, chondrosarcoma, and osteogenic sarcoma	Fairly low	Mature cartilage or bone tissue, salivary gland epithelium, renal epithelium, hepatic epithelium, chondrocytes, and osteocytes
Rhabdomyosarcoma, leiomyosarcoma, and ganglioneurofibrosarcoma	Low	Muscle tissue and neuronal tissue

Adapted from Rubin and Casarett (19).

inherent radiosensitivity. They correlated the data from in vitro survival measurements at 2 Gy with the clinically estimated TCD$_{90}$ values for different histologic types and found a good correlation between the 2 Gy dose and the perceived clinical radioresponsiveness. Deacon *et al.* (34) performed a similar analysis and found a similar relationship, although their data (Fig. 6-5) clearly illustrate a broad range of in vitro responses within each histology group. A similar wide range of individual radiosensitivities for different tumor types also was described by Peters *et al.* (54) when assessing the survival of primary cultures of human histology groups at 2.0 Gy using cumulative frequency histograms.

In addition to the inherent radiation sensitivity, the overall tumor response to radiation therapy will also depend on variations in the capacity of tissues and cells to reoxygenate, reassort in the cell cycle, repair, repopulate, and be recruited from resting to proliferating compartments. These mechanisms and their effect on cellular radioresponsiveness are often referred to as the R's of radiobiology and each will be reviewed briefly.

Reoxygenation: Oxygen Effect (3,7a,10,67) The level of cell killing by low LET radiation is dependent on the degree of oxygenation at the time of irradiation. This effect is directly related to the cellular oxygen tension so that with increasing oxygen concentration, radiation sensitivity usually reaches a

plateau at a partial pressure of oxygen of 20 to 30 mm Hg (Fig. 6-6a) (10). Further increases in oxygen concentration have little additional effect. Cell-survival curves obtained under both oxic and completely hypoxic (absence of oxygen) conditions indicate that the dose required to produce the same biologic effect under hypoxic conditions is approximately 2.5 to 3 times greater than the dose required under fully oxygenated circumstances. Consequently, larger radiation doses would be necessary to eradicate a tumor containing hypoxic cells than one that did not.

Most animal tumors have a hypoxic cell component of 10% to 20% (35,43) and recent evidence suggests that hypoxic cells in at least some human tumors constitute a major limiting factor in cure by conventional radiation therapy (29,36,75). A diagram illustrating how the percentage of hypoxic cells in a tumor affects a single dose survival curve for the tumor as a whole is shown in Fig. 6-6b (10). The data show the survival of fully oxygenated cells as well as the survival of the same cells in the absence of oxygen. When oxygen-deficient cells are present in a tumor, the final slope of the cell-survival curve is seen ultimately to parallel the slope of the fully hypoxic curve. Consequently, even if only 1.0 or 0.1% of the tumor cells are hypoxic, the relative radiation resistance of these cells will limit the curability of the tumor by single-dose radiation therapy.

Fortunately, tumors may reoxygenate during fractionated radiation treatments through a variety of mechanisms (10). For example, as a tumor shrinks, its parenchymal cells are lost and the vasculature collapses, decreasing intercapillary distances, producing a supervascular state, and increasing oxygen diffusion. Reoxygenation can also occur when alternately oxygenated cells die and do not use oxygen, allowing the oxygen to diffuse further to persistent hypoxic cells in tumor cords. Unfortunately, the reoxygenation patterns observed to date vary in a manner strongly dependent on the tumor type (10). In addition, little is known as to whether reoxygenation occurs in human tumors.

Reassortment: Cell Cycle Kinetics and Age Response Function (10,22,24a,50,6a) Mammalian cells replicate by divisional mitosis and the average time between successful mitoses is called a cell cycle (Fig. 6-7a) (10). The phases of the cell cycle, based on labeled thymidine studies, are: mitosis (M); the DNA synthetic phase (S); an interval known as the first gap (G$_1$), before DNA synthesis; and a second gap (G$_2$), before mitosis. The M phase is the only event that can be distinguished through light microscopy, whereas the S phase is identified by the technique of autoradiography. The patterns of radiosensitivity change through the cell cycle (Fig. 6-7b) (10). This change is known as age-response function and varies widely among different cell types. Cells in mitosis are almost always sensitive, followed by cells at the G$_1$/S boundary, while the period of greatest resistance usually is late S. However, in cells having a long G$_1$, a second resistant period in the early G$_1$ phase usually is also seen. Reassortment occurs as cells in the sensitive cycle die and surviving radioresistant cells redistribute into more sensitive phases of cell cycle. Thus, it is conceivable that during fractionated radiation therapy, cells reassort and enter into radiosensitive phases. However, due to the long and varying cell-cycle times, as well as small growth fractions, the impact of favorable cell reassortment on clinical radiotherapy is likely to be small.

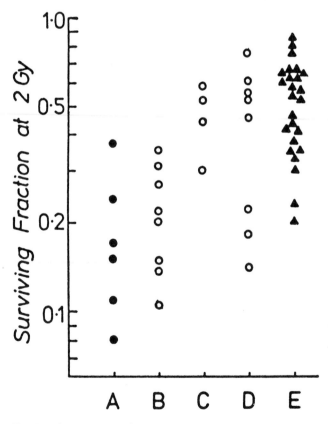

Fig. 6-5. Survival at 2.0 Gy for all lines derived from a variety of human tumor types classified according to clinical radiocurability. Group A are the most sensitive clinically, whereas group E are the most resistant to 2.0 Gy fractions. This illustrates the general correlation between intrinsic cellular radiosensitivity and clinical sensitivity, as well as the large range within each histology class. From Deacon (34), with permission.

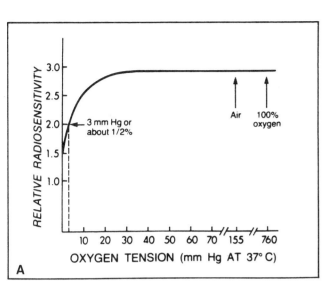

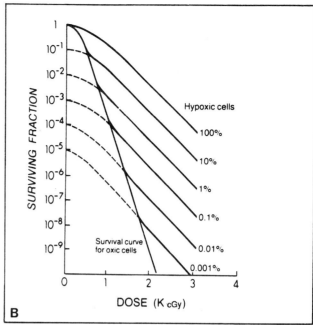

Fig. 6-6. (a) The oxygen effect. The oxygen effect is illustrated as the curve relating relative radiation sensitivity to oxygen tension in tissues. As the oxygen increases, the relative radiosensitivity of cells increases by a factor of approximately 3 for the same dose. (b) the survival curves illustrate the effect of various proportions of oxygen deficient or hypoxic cells on the resultant shape of the survival curve of mixed cell populations of oxic and hypoxic cells. Because of the resistant tail (shallow slope), even a small percentage of hypoxic cells (< 1%) may determine whether irradiation can successfully eradicate a tumor. (K) = thousands. From Hall (10), with permission.

Cell Repair and the Fractionation Effect (7a,10)

The shoulder of the cell survival curve, the D_q (Fig. 6-8) (7a), may represent a minimum number of targets in each cell that must be hit before the target is inactivated, thereby killing the cell. After irradiation, a cell may have received an ionizing event in some, but not all, of its critical sites so that it has been damaged, but not killed. Given time, the cell may be able to repair the effects of this sublethal damage and completely

recover from it. Consequently, if the time interval between successive doses is sufficiently long, each fractional dose will re-establish the shoulder on the survival curve, thus making divided daily doses less effective than a single dose. Fig. 6-8 shows an idealized fractionation experiment by Elkind and Whitmore (7a) using cultured cells in vitro. The survival curve for single acute exposures of x-rays is Curve A; whole Curve S is obtained if the total dose is given as a series of small

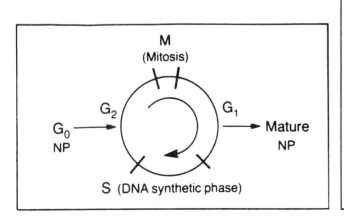

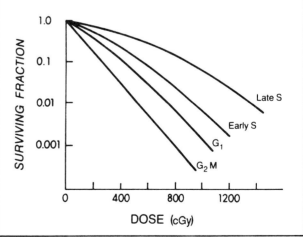

Fig. 6-7. (a) Cell-cycle age: The surviving fraction as function of cell cycle age. The radiosensitivity of a cell changes as it moves through the cell cycle, being most sensitive in G2 and M. (b) Cell cycle "age-response function." The patterns of radiosensitivity change through the cell cycle. This change is known as the "age-function," and varies widely among different cell types. Cells in mitosis are almost always sensitive, followed by cells at the G1/S boundary, while the period of greatest resistance is at late S. G0 = resting (quiescent) cell; G = gaps; G1 = first gap before DNA synthesis; G2 = second gap before mitosis; NP = nonproliferating (mature) cells; M = mitosis; S = early DNA syntheitc phase; late S = late DNA synthetic phase. Adapted from Hall (10).

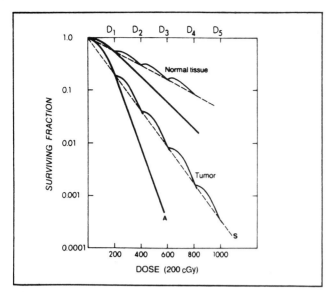

Fig. 6-8. Cell repair and fractionation effect. Each repeated fractional dose allows for cell repair of sublethal damage and is expressed by the recapitulation of the shoulder of the survival curve. If 1,000 cGy is given as a divided fractional dose (D1, D2, D3, D4, D5) of 200 cGy daily, it achieves a similar degree of cell kill (S on the dashed line) as 600 cGy given in one single exposure. The survival curve for single acute exposures of x-rays is curve A. This diagram also shows a differential effect on therapeutic ratio between tumor cells and normal cells that increases with divided or fractional doses of radiaiton. This is displayed by the increasing differences in the slopes of the solid lines (single dose) and dashed lines (fractional dose). Adapted from Elkind and Whitmore (7a).

fractions of the size D_1, with the time interval between fractions sufficient for repair of sublethal damage to take place. From this, it is evident that a much larger total dose of radiation is required to achieve the same degree of killing if it is given in a series of small fractions as compared with a single large exposure. To achieve a clinical advantage, it is important that the D_0 and D_q of the tumor be smaller than that of the normal tissue in the treatment field. The importance of the shoulder region of the tumor cell survival curve also should be noted from the recent interest in and correlation of the survival at 2 Gy and apparent clinical responsiveness described earlier in this chapter.

In addition to sublethal repair, another form of cell recovery, which has been observed when after a dose of radiation cells are held under nonoptimal growth conditions, is referred to as potential lethal damage repair (PLDR). The effect of PLDR is typically to lead to a more shallow slope on the cell survival curve. Weichselbaum *et al.* (76) have implied a correlation with tumor cell PLDR measured in vitro and tumor radioresistance, suggesting this mechanism may be important. Whether PLDR proves to be an important factor in clinical radiotherapy remains to be determined, particularly in light of observations indicating that tumor cells demonstrating significant PLDR in vitro may fail to do so in vivo (28,59).

Repopulation

Another possible means of obtaining a differential effect between normal tissues and tumors occurs if the cellular repopulation between doses is greater in the normal tissue at risk than in the tumor. This is illustrated schematically in Fig. 6-9, where there is regeneration or repopulation of the tissues between each fractional dose. If, as shown, the normal tissue could repopulate itself to a greater extent than the tumor, a differential effect would be established between the tumor and the normal tissue with regard to cell kill per fractional radiation dose. On the other hand, if the tumor repopulates more quickly, the reverse is true. The latter occasionally occurs in highly anaplastic tumors with large growth fractions and short cell cycle times. Such a tumor appears to be radioresistant because it appears to be unchanged, while in fact it is radioresponsive but is repopulating or regrowing between fractions.

Recruitment (10,22)

Recruitment is a special circumstance and applies to the recruitment of nonproliferating G_0 cells into the cell cycle (Fig. 6-10). The assumption is that most cells are more vulnerable to irradiation during mitosis or proliferation than if they are in the nonproliferating compartment. Generally speaking, proliferating cells tend to be more radiosensitive than G_0 cells, which in turn are more sensitive than mature cells. G_0 cells are often stem cells in tissues with a potential for proliferation, whereas mature cells usually, but not always, have lost this capacity. As proliferating cells are ablated, cells are recruited from nonproliferating into proliferating compartments. If tumors behave thus, they become more radiosensitive and curable, producing a favorable therapeutic ratio. The reverse is true for a critical normal tissue.

The R's of radiobiology have been reviewed and an attempt has been made to relate in vivo dose-response curves of normal tissues and tumors with in vitro cell-survival curves. Such a relation between tumor control and cell survival curves is illustrated diagrammatically in Fig. 6-11 (27).

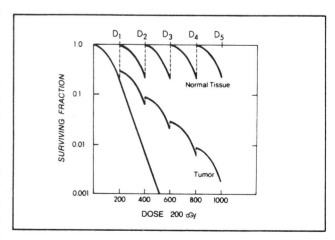

Fig. 6-9. Repopulation. In a rapid renewal system, repopulation or regeneration of cells within the fractional interval occurs. This figure illustrates that, even if the tumor and normal tissue have the same radiation response, the therapeutic ratio is improved through more rapid regeneration of normal tissues than the tumor.

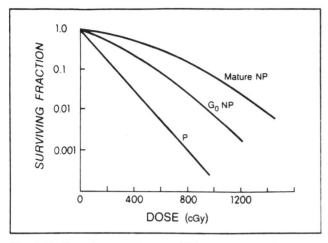

Fig. 6-10. Recruitment. The gap (G0) compartment has non-proliferating cells that can be recruited into cycle and become proliferating cells. Proliferating cells (P) are more radiosensitive than nonproliferating cells (NP).

NORMAL TISSUE TOLERANCE (15,15a,19,61)

Relative Cell Radiosensitivity and Kinetics of Radiation Response:

Radiation acts at a cellular level. Tissue effects represent a summation of cellular effects. Since the key target cells for the survival of a complex organ depend on the organization of all its tissues, cellular damage in a key target cell may result in death of the whole tissue. Small blood vessels are fairly sensitive to irradiation. The effects on the tissue from disruption of the blood supply may be greater than those from the irradiation of the parenchymal cells themselves.

A relative cell radiosensitivity is illustrated in Fig. 6-12 (19) based on Cowdry *et al.* (33) classification schema related to cellular division and differentiation. The uncommitted stem

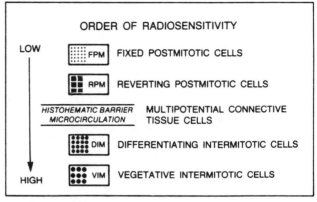

Fig. 6-12. Relative cell radiosensitivity. From Rubin and Casarett (19), with permission.

cell is a vegetative intermitotic cell; the committed stem cell is a differentiating intermitotic cell. Reverting postmitotic cells have the ability to divide when conditioned or challenged as hepatocytes after liver resection. The organization of tissues and organs by these cell types determine their radiosensitivity, which is based on their most radiosensitive cells. Table 6-2 reviews cell and tissue radiosensitivity.

The histologic manifestations in radiation cellular death are pyknosis and karyolysis, swollen vacuolated cells with loss of staining capacity and altered permeability and eventual degeneration and phagocytosis.

The events following exposure to radiation doses are determined, in part, by the radiosensitivity of the cells in the parenchymal compartment as related to the radiosensitivity of vascular stroma and its turnover rate. A *rapid renewal system*. illustrated in Fig. 6-13 (19), consists of vegetative intermitotic cells (VIM), differentiating intermitotic cells (DIM), and fixed postmitotic cells (FPM) as found in skin or mucous membrane of the alimentary tract or in the testes. The initial fractional doses of irradiation destroy the stem cell compartments (VIM and DIM) and reduce the production of cells that normally flow into the postmitotic compartment. The lining or mucous membrane thins and as the dose increases, the connective tissue becomes edematous. With large doses, the parenchymal compartment may be lifted or sloughed as a result of the edema. The ability of the tissue to regenerate depends on the survival of stem cells (VIM), which gradually increase in number, differentiate, and rebuild the postmitotic compartment. The compartments eventually stabilize, but might be relatively reduced as a result of increased fibrosis and increased histohematic barrier. If large doses have been given, the microcirculation might become occluded at a later time, leading to frank delayed necrosis. With lesser degrees of fibrosis, the parenchymal compartment might atrophy, and when stressed, as by infection, might show its limited stem cell reserve capacity or mitotic potential to respond.

The sequence of events differs in a *slow renewal system* or *nonrenewal system* (Fig. 6-14) (19). The parenchymal compartment consists of reverting postmitotic cells or FPM cells. Little or no change occurs in the parenchymal compartment with the fractional dose schemes used clinically. The vascular stromal compartment more often determines the course of events, although there are effects that can be attributed to a

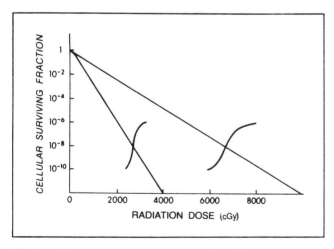

Fig. 6-11. Tumor control and cell survival. The effect on the shape of the tumor control curve of altering the dose (D0) of the cell survival curve by a factor of approximately 2.5 is shown. For a detailed discussion of the relationship between tumor cure and cell survival, see Withers and Peters (27).

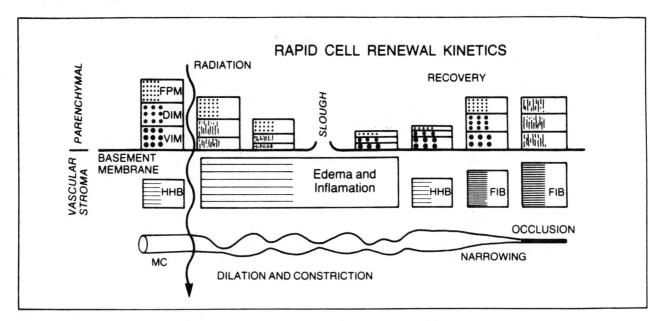

Fig. 6-13. Rapid renewal system illustrating radiation effects on both the parenchyma and microvasculature compartments. VIM = vegetative intermitotic cells; DIM = differentiating intermitotic cells; FPM = fixed postmitotic cells; HHB = histohematic barrier; FIB = increased fibrosis; MC = microcirculation. From Rubin and Casarett (19), with permission.

direct effect on parenchymal cells (57). The late expression of injury of these cells is caused by their slow renewal, hence the slow expression of injury (77).

Clinical Pathologic Course

The sequence of clinical events after the initiation of radiation therapy will be considered in terms of four successive time periods of arbitrary length, as follows: acute clinical period (first 6 months), subacute clinical period (second 6 months), chronic clinical period (second through fifth year), and late clinical period (after 5 years) (Fig. 6-15) (19).

There are two curves illustrating two courses of a potentially infinite number of variations of early and late effect events. The subclinical damage when moderate doses are administered below tissue tolerance and the clinically evident damage that exceeds clinical threshold and result in both early effects and in late effects. Such events as trauma (surgery), infection, or chemotherapy may shift subclinical residual injury to a clinical phase. This is illustrated by the addition of doxorubicin to mediastinal irradiation for Hodgkin's disease patients who later developed cardiac decompensation and a cardomyopathy years after "safe doses" of radiotherapy and/or safe doses of chemotherapy.

Normal Tissue Tolerance Dose (Table 6-5)

The tolerance dose is an attempt to express the minimal and maximal injurious dose acceptable to the clinician. This requires the assignment of an arbitrary — but useful — percentage for the risk of complications. The *minimal tolerance dose* is defined as the $TD_{5/5}$, that is, the dose to which a

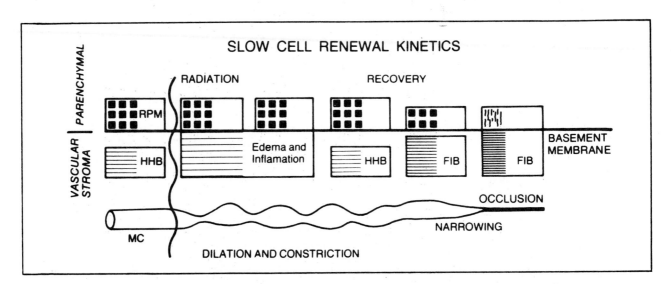

Fig. 6-14. Slow renewal system illustrating effects on the vascular compartment, which in turn produces the late effect in the parenchymal cells as the capillary sclerosis and fibrosis increase. RPM = reverting postmitotic. From Rubin and Casarett (19), with permission.

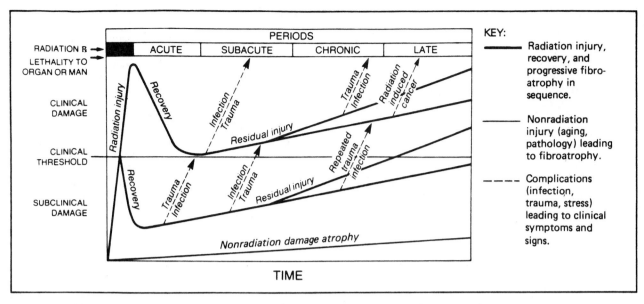

Fig. 6-15. Sequence of clinical events after radiation therapy. From Rubin and Casarett (19), with permission.

Table 6-5. Tolerance Doses for Fractionated Doses to Whole or Partial Organs

Target Cells	Complication End Point	TD5/5-TD50/5 (Gy)
200-1,000 cGy		
Lymphocytes and lymphoid	Lymphopenia	2-10
Testes spermatogonia	Sterility	1-2
Ovarian oocytes	Sterility	6-10
Diseased bone marrow	Severe leukopenia and thrombocytopenia	3-5
1,000-2,000 cGy		
Lens	Cataract	6-12
Bone marrow stem cells	Acute aplasia	15-20
2,000-3,000 cGy		
Kidney: renal glomeruli	Arterionephrosclerosis	23-28
Lung: type II cells, vascular connective tissue stroma	Pneumonitis or fibrosis	20-30
3,000-4,000 cGy		
Liver: central veins	Hepatopathy	35-40
Bone marrow	Hypoplasia	25-35
4,000-5,000 cGy		
Heart (whole organ)	Pericarditis or pancarditis	43-50
Bone marrow micro-environments	Permanent aplasia	45-50
5,000-6,000 cGy		
Gastrointestinal	Infarction necrosis	50-55
Heart (partial organ)	Cardiomyopathy	55-65
Spinal cord	Myelopathy	50-60
6,000-7,000 cGy		
Brain	Encephalopathy	60-70
Mucosa	Ulcer	65-75
Rectum	Ulcer	65-75
Bladder	Ulcer	65-75
Mature bones	Fracture	65-70
Pancreas	Pancreatitis	>70

given population of patients is exposed under a standard set of treatment conditions resulting in no more than a 5% severe complication rate within 5 years after treatment. The *maximal tolerance dose* is defined as the $TD_{50/5}$, that is, the dose to which a given population of patients is exposed under a standard set of treatment conditions resulting in a 50% severe complication rate 5 years after treatment.

The dose-limiting tissues or organs in radiation therapy are based on our inability to define an optimum tumor dose (many biologic factors are unknown clinically) so that the radiation oncologist is often required to treat to tolerance. These dose-limiting tissues/organs are defined according to dose. The dose limits specified are based on the best and most current dose-time date available. These dose limits assume a standard set of conditions:

- supervoltage irradiation (1 to 10 MeV)
- dose delivery of 200 ± 10% cGy per day, five fractions weekly, or 1,000 cGy, 2-day rest intervals
- completion of treatment in 6 to 8 weeks
- doses conditioned by partial-volume organ irradiation

Our longest clinical experience is with limited-field irradiation to part of an organ, and this experience has provided insights into tissue and organ radiation sensitivity (1,2,19). For many dose ranges, only human data or only animal data exist as a guide. Unfortunately, large fractions and shorter intervals are often used in animal experiments, whereas 2 Gy/d and 10 Gy/wk are the standard in conventional clinical schedules.

2 to 10 Gy (200 to 1,000 cGy). With fractionated doses of less than 10 Gy, the testes spermatogonia, ovarian oogonia, and lens epithelium are injured. The testes spermatogonia are very sensitive to smaller fractional doses and are destroyed more efficiently than ovarian tissue. Lymphocytes and lymphoid tissues also will be suppressed with trivial doses.

10 to 20 Gy (1,000 to 2,000 cGy). With fractionated doses of 10 to 20 Gy, the normal bone marrow hematopoetic stem cells will be depressed, but larger doses will be required to achieve suppression with limited volumes. In disease states, unlike in the normal state, smaller fractional doses (<10 Gy) may ablate the bone marrow. Growing cartilage and growing bone will also be arrested within this dose range.

20 to 30 Gy (2,000 to 3,000 cGy). Between 20 and 30 Gy, a number of vital organs reach their radiation threshold and decompensate despite fractionation. This is most apparent when an entire organ is so treated. The kidneys and lungs are both vulnerable to this dose range and demonstrate a combination of injury to the microvasculature and to the epithelial cells.

30 to 40 Gy (3,000 to 4,000 cGy). The liver becomes vulnerable at this level. For many organs, there are limited data on whole-organ fractional therapy schedules, but skin and oropharyngeal mucosa can become acutely reactive. The liver displays a special veno-occlusive event secondary to platelet adhesion to central veins at or somewhat above this dose level.

40 to 50 Gy (4,000 to 5,000 cGy). At this dose level, the heart and gastrointestinal (GI) organs are likely to experience severe and life-threatening injury, particularly with large-volume or whole-organ irradiation.

50 to 60 Gy (5,000 to 6,000 cGy). The majority of organs are vulnerable to fractionated schedules in the 50 to 60 Gy range. GI injury is significant, and the colorectal tissues become vulnerable. The spinal cord and brain may become demyelinated. Vascular connective tissue stroma is affected at this dose range, which has a major effect even with partial-organ irradiation. Long-term fibrosis may occur in lung, liver, kidney, and bone marrow even when smaller volumes are irradiated.

60 to 70 Gy (6,000 to 7,000 cGy). At this range, the brain is more likely to react to irradiation by undergoing demyelination at the TD_{5-50} levels. The rectum and bladder become vulnerable to major injury at the TD_5 level. Mature cartilage and bone are able to withstand these doses as are pancreas, peripheral nerves, and muscle.

Dose Selection

The choice of dose depends on weighing the probability of cure versus the probability of complication (Figs. 6-16a and 6-16b) (50). Models for decision-making include cost-benefit analysis in clinical terms in which negative outcomes are evaluated. The Bayesian model and the ratio operating characteristic (ROC) curves have been suggested for clinical decision-making. (The term ROC is applied to decision-making when there is a negative and a positive outcome.) In these systems, values are assigned to four potential outcomes (35):

- uncomplicated cure } preferred or
- complicated cure } positive outcome

- uncomplicated recurrence } negative outcomes
- complicated recurrence }

When cure rates are similar for different modalities — that is, surgery versus radiation therapy — the negative outcomes, their frequency and severity, often are the basis of the final choice. When results are equivalent for different forms of therapy, the state of the host is also critical to treatment selection. Better survival results for one modality compared with another may be more related to the state of health of the host than the treatment effectiveness.

State of the Host: The associated medical problems of the host, rather than the malignancy, may determine the choice of treatment. For example, when a very elderly patient has bladder cancer, surgery is often contraindicated because of problems such as heart disease. Radiotherapy also places physical demands on a patient, but it is more often better tolerated, with less risk of mortality. The role of natural immunologic factors in radiation therapy is being studied, but at this time, its importance remains clinically undetermined. Vigorous treatment and eradication of primary tumor may allow the host immunologic mechanisms to contain secondary foci. Irradiated tumor, re-injected into the host in

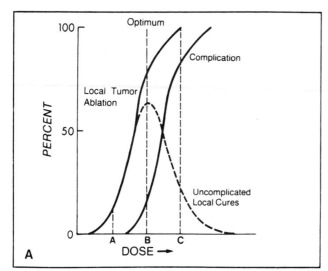

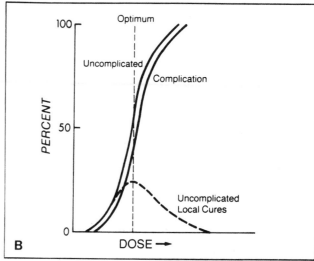

Fig. 6-16. Tumor = treatment outcomes. Uncomplicated curves (dashed line) are the desired results of treatment. This is illustrated as a function of the therapeutic ratio, i.e., the greater the separation between the tumor control curve and the normal tissue complication curve, the greater the number of uncomplicated cures that will result. A, B, and C represent three different dose levels which, if chosen, would lead to three different outcomes. "A" would result result in few tumor cures, but no complications. "C" would lead to complete cure in many cases, but virtually all patients would suffer complications. The optimal choice in this group of dose levels is "B," which would result in the greatest number of cured patients without complications. Compare 16a versus 16b. Adapted from Mendelsohn (50).

experimental systems, increases radioresponsiveness of residual tumor. Nonspecific stimulation with bacille Calmette-Guerin and *Coryn bacterium parvulum* during irradiation remain investigational. To date, this has been a disappointing therapeutic approach and has not substantially improved survival. The most recent series of nonspecific stimulants has been with levamisole, which is reported to be an immunorestorer and would be theoretically useful in lung cancer patients.

Tolerance Volume: The concept of a tolerance volume needs to be defined similar to a tolerance dose. The volume is more critical to complications outcome and also serves as a clinical guide, since it is possible to obliterate or lose a certain volume of a vital organ with large doses, that is, exceeding the TD_{90-100} is akin to surgical resection. Loss of a certain volume does not affect organ survival, because the organ can often compensate for volume loss through regeneration or hypertrophy and remain within functional tolerance for survival, though impaired.

1. Tolerance volume (TV): 5% to 25% of the organ volume irradiated can result in a life threatening or lethal complication.
2. TV 50% to 90%: 50% to 90% of the organ volume irradiated can result in a life-threatening or lethal complication.

There are generally two levels of critical volumes for the dose-limiting or vital organs. Only the GI tract and the central nervous system (CNS) can have disastrous outcomes after small volumes (TV 10% to 25%) are exposed to doses exceeding TD_{5-50}. It is also important to note that necrotic CNS bowel can be resected and on occasion necrotic foci can be resected successfully. For the majority of organs often considered dose-limiting, the bone marrow, lung, kidney, and in all probability the heart and liver can tolerate higher doses to smaller volumes. Such organs may decompensate when more than 50% of the total volume (as applied to paired organs) is exceeded. The time when organ decompensation begins clearly depends on the compensatory regenerative mechanisms that come into play when significant organ volume loss occurs. The dose-response curve is not an absolute or fixed effect, but varies as a function of volume (Fig. 6-17a) (49). This is an important concept since it allows the radiation oncologist to give much larger doses to partial volumes. For TD_5 and T_{50}, the dose increases as the volume decreases (Fig. 6-17b) (49). Note that the slope changes as more than 50% of the whole organ is included. Small increments in dose, i.e., 10% to 20% of the total dose, can be lethal. The dose-volume histogram is being adopted by numerous investigators to predict unfavorable outcomes as a result of volume loss in a critical structure (30,49).

MODIFIERS OF RADIATION RESPONSE (2,4,5,22,27,32,42,56,78)

Response and recovery are as basic to the laws of radiobiologic and radiopathologic mechanisms as are action and reaction to the laws of physical motion. Following the initial interaction of ionizing radiation and biologic matter, a sequence of events begins that may result in a lethal alteration in a living cellular system, be it host tissue or malignant tumor. From the physical event of energy transfer, a chemical reaction occurs with the release of free radicals and the decomposition of water into hydrogen, hydroxyl, and perhydroxyl ionic forms. The biochemical target effects are believed to involve nucleic acids, such as DNA and RNA, and vital enzymes. This results in recognizable biologic injury in the form of mitotic-linked deaths, in which chromosomal aberrations are evident microscopically. Biologic injury in the form of cell death occurs. In radiotherapeutic terms, this cell death results in tumor destruction. Biochemical recovery and biologic repair also can occur; consequently, host tissues may maintain their integrity, allowing successful organ function, thereby preserving the organism or patient. The radiopathologic end effect is the summation of these events, which it is hoped will result in long-term survival of the patient, free from recurrence of the neoplasm.

PHYSICAL MODIFIERS (24)

Classic radiotherapeutic techniques using x-irradiation and radium have been designed to allow for a favorable distribu-

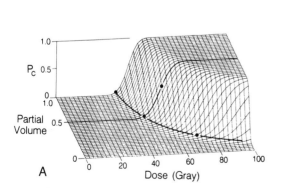

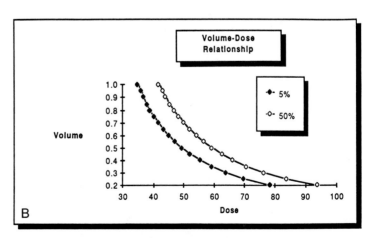

Fig. 6-17. Volume effect: (a) The dose response curve is not an absolute or fixed effect but varies as a function of volume. This important concept allows the radiation oncologist to give much longer doses to partial volumes. (b) For TD5 and T50 the dose increases as the volume decreases. Note that the slope changes as more than 50% of the whole organ is included. Small increments dose, that is 10% to 20%, can prove to be lethal. From Lyman and Wolbarst (49), with permission.

tion of dosage between the tumors and the normal tissues in the treatment beam. That is, one attempts to deliver a maximum dose to the tumor and a minimum dose to the normal tissues.

The major advances in the past decade were telecobalt units and linear accelerators that produce megavoltage irradiation and high energy electrons in the 1 to 25 million MeV range (27). The advantages over orthovoltage are:

- better depth doses — more efficient tumor treatment
- less side scatter — less radiation sickness
- no differential absorption by bone — more uniform dosage
- skin sparing effect — only slight radiation dermatitis

X-irradiation and electron irradiation, even in the 1 to 6 MeV range, are considered low LET irradiation and are less effective in treating hypoxic than oxic cells. However, densely ionizing radiations, such as neutrons, negative pi mesons, and accelerated heavy ions, can reduce the importance of tumor hypoxia (15). The ionizations occur at such close ranges that most hydrogen and hydroxyl radicals tend to combine to form water instead of interacting with organic bases to form organic radicals. Therefore, the absence of oxygen is less influential in determining the quantity of biologic damage. Damage to the important compounds occurs by direct ionization. More detail will be provided in Chapter 7, "Basic Concepts of Radiation Physics."

MODIFICATION OF DOSE-TIME RELATIONSHIPS (17,25,27,37,41,62)

The magnitude of the radiation dose is not the only important variable; of equal importance is the distribution of the dose with respect to time — the fractionation factor. It has been observed that if the interval of time between treatments increases, then the total dose must increase to produce the same effect. This can be explained only on the basis that a certain amount of tissue recovery takes place during the interval. Clinical experience has also shown that normal tissues recover more rapidly than neoplastic tissues. Therefore, by increasing the total dose delivered over a longer period of time, the differential between the tumor lethal dose and tissue tolerance dose can be accentuated in three ways: (1) fractionation — high intensity dosage in short intervals, i.e., external irradiation; (2) *protraction* — low intensity dosage over a long period of time, i.e., interstitial radium; and (3) combinations of low- and high-dose ratio. (See Tables 6-2 and 6-3).

Current Clinical Dose-Time Relationships: The required tumor lethal dose (RTLD) for different human tumors ranges from 2,000 cGy in 2 weeks to 8,000 cGy in 8 weeks, with the vast majority of tumors receiving doses between 4,500 and 7,500 cGy. A daily fractionation schema of $200 \pm 10\%$ cGy is used. The number of daily fractions varies from 3 to 5. Using a standard dose of 6,000 cGy in 6 weeks times five daily doses, the following three major treatment tactics, often using combinations of high-low dose rates, have been selected by radiation therapists.

Higher-than-standard dose, shorter time: When the tumor dose needs to be high, combined internal and external irradiation is preferred over either technique alone. Doses from 6,000 to 10,000 cGy are most often given during combined doses of external and internal irradiation. Because of differ-

ent dose rate or protraction, better total dose-time levels can be achieved. The contrast between dose rate of external and internal irradiation should be noted as intensity of irradiation delivery, that is, low- versus high-dose rate in cGy/hr. When interstitial or intracavitary irradiation is protracted, doses can be given at 1,000 cGy/d and 6,000 to 7,000 cGy/wk.

Higher-than-standard dose, longer time: Longer protracted doses leading to higher levels of irradiation are usually used in tumors occupying large volumes. For large volumes, the 6,000 cGy level may be delivered in 8 to 10 weeks. Doses between 6,000 and 8,000 cGy are often given with booster techniques, using small, coned-down fields with external irradiation or electrons to add another 1,000 to 2,000 cGy. This is referred to as the shrinking field technique. Interstitial implants or intracavitary sources can also add 1,000 to 2,000 cGy to an externally delivered dose of 5,000 to 6,000 cGy. This tactic is often used in split-course techniques, where larger doses are given by interrupting treatment to allow for tumor regression and reduction of volume to be treated. The second course can then be carried to a higher dose level of 7,000 to 8,000 cGy in 8–10 weeks, for a more limited target. Maximum doses used are most often at the 8,000 cGy level in spite of the time factor; some exceptions with levels as high as 9,000 or 10,000 cGy are noted for combined external and interstitial techniques in the cervix to point A, metastatic neck nodes, inoperable breast cancer, and soft tissue sarcomas on limbs.

Lower-than-standard dose, longer time: This tactic is a compromise, often resulting in less than the required tumor dose, and is ineffective with two exceptions: radiosensitive tumors occupying large volumes, or microdeposits or millet size foci in large volumes. Advanced ovarian cancers, with seedings through the abdomen, are treated by this technique.

Low-dose-rate versus high-dose-rate effects: The principle dose rate effect is cell killing occurs between 100 cGy/min to 1 cGy/min. This dose-rate effect is due to repair of sublethal damage that occurs during radiation exposure. At lower dose rates, cell division or repopulation occurs, whereas at higher dose rates, 100 to 1,000 cGy/min, as used with external irradiation, little difference in kill occurs (Figs. 6-18a and 6-18b) (10). Steele introduces the concept of the Regaud dose rate, that is a relatively low dose rate of 1 Gy/hr (1-2 cGy/min) at which dose rate it is approximately isoeffective with fractionated radiotherapy using 2 Gy fractions. At this dose rate, human tumor cell lines show a wide range of radiosensitivity differing by a factor of 7 and may well be the most clinically relevant in the way of describing the radiosensitivity of tumor cells (63).

With intracavitary and interstitial brachytherapy, the commonly used dose rate is 1,000 cGy/24 h or 41.6 cGy/h or 0.69 cGy/min, which, in reference to variations of total dose and total treatment time to produce an equivalent to 6,000 cGy in 7 days (Fig. 6-19) (38), is a dose rate of 35.7 cGy/h. The general shape of Patterson and Parker curves are similar to Ellis and are the basis for dose curves used clinically with some modification.

High dose rate irradiation is comparable to low dose irradiation and is in wide use clinically (44a). The major advantages: the physical placement, the control of dwell-time of single sources, and highly computerized systems rather than the dose rate of irradiation (44b).

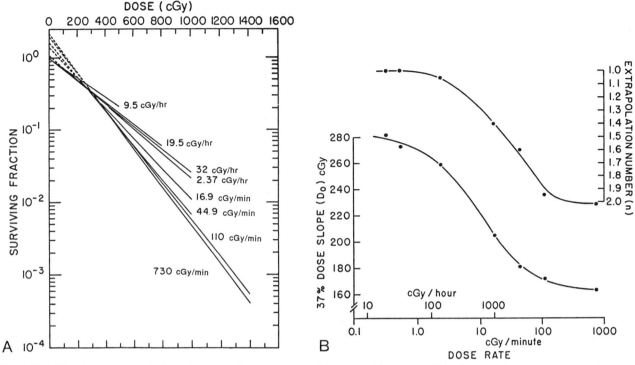

Fig. 6-18. (a) Survival curves for HeLa cells exposed to g rays over a side range of dose rates. (b) Variation with dose rate of the 37% dose slope (D0) and the extrapolation number (n). From Hall (10), with permission.

Altered Fractionation

Table 6-4 shows the different fractionation schemes relative to fraction size, time interval, total dose, and total time. Based on the linear quadratic model, a separation of early and late effects can be demonstrated as a function of fraction size. Four strategies have emerged:

1. *Split-course irradiation* has been widely used and tested in clinical trials as being more or less effective than conventional irradiation. Larger fractions are used daily causing an increased reaction which requires that the course be split with a few weeks rest rather than treating with continuous irradiation on a daily basis as occurs with conventional small fraction doses of 1.5 to 2.0 Gy daily. Generally speaking, the split-course schedules have not proven to be as effective as conventional irradiation fractionation schedules and therefore have been relegated to largely palliative use (49a,50a).

2. *Hyperfractionation*: The basic aim of hyperfractionation is to deliver smaller than standard fractional doses (ie, 100 to 120 cGy), 2 or 3 times daily, at 4- to 6-hour intervals in order to separate early and late normal tissue reactions. The overall treatment time remains 6 to 8 weeks, but the total dose is increased to 75 to 85 Gy. The goal is to keep the late normal tissue reactions the same as those occuring following standard fractionation while accepting somewhat increased acute reactions. Since most tumors appear to behave more like acutely responding normal tissues, the larger dose should obtain greater regressions without increasing late complications. Usually the total dose is increased by 10% to 20%. Clinical trials have demonstrated a gain in locoregional cancer control using this approach.

3. *Accelerated fractionation* involves delivering fractional doses(150 to 200 cGy) multiple times daily with intervals of 4 to 6 hours between fractions. The resulting higher total doses will increase both acute and late normal tissue effects, and consequently split-course regimens, requiring two courses of treatment, are needed. Wang *et al.* (72) has presented large survival and local control gains in head and neck cancer patients when comparing accelerated fractionation schedules to conventional daily irradiation in retrospective,

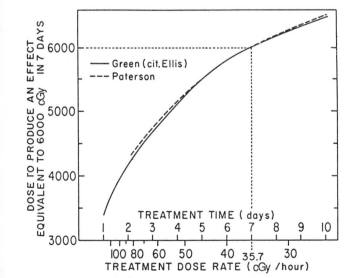

Fig. 6-19. Variation of total dose with treatment time to produce an effect equivalent to 6,000 cGy in 7 days with a radium implant. From (9a) Hall, E.J. Radiol 192: 173-179; 1972., with permission.

nonrandomized studies. The intent of this strategy is to reduce repopulation in rapidly growing tumors. Through the split-course technique, there is the anticipation of keeping the late reactions the same. Thames *et al.* (65) predicted that if conventional overall times are shortened by one third by using 2 to 3 fractions daily, and if the doubling time of clonogenic tumor cells were 5 days or less, there would be large gains in local control. Both clonogenic and nonclonogenic assays to determine whether to use hyperfractionated or accelerated schedule are being developed at a number of institutes (54).

4. *Hypofractionation* has usually been associated with large fractions and has led to increased late effects, unless tumor and target volumes are reduced as the total dose increases. When hypofractionation is combined with chemotherapy and other agents, it may prove more effective and efficient. Large, daily fractional doses are very effective in relieving obstruction and compression, particularly in radiosensitive and radioresponsive tumors such as in spinal cord compression, superior vena caval obstruction, ureteral obstruction, and bronchial or tracheal obstruction. A small field within a large field can also be effective in rapidly growing tumors with large growth fractions requiring large daily doses to be delivered in short time intervals. A once-a-week schedule, or a less-than-daily fractionation (hypofractionation) regimen can be effective for slower growing resistant tumors and tumors with large shouldered (D_q) cell populations.

MATHEMATICAL MODELING (10)

A number of mathematic models have been developed to consider the different treatment fractions of dose-time fractionation based on clinical and experimental data. A variety of formulas exist including normal standard dose (NSD), time-dose fraction (TDF), cumulative radiation effect (CRE), and new computer-based formulations, which are valuable but have limitations. The α / β ratio and the linear quadratic equation are applicable to cellular populations but do not always provide guides to safe doses for in vivo organ tolerances.

Standqvist lines (62): The dose-time isoeffect line introduced by Standqvist (62) is based on the concept that the total dose in the total period of time determines the effects, independent of fractionation (Fig. 6-20) (10). Because of the phenomenon of cell and tissue repair, it is apparent that a greater total dose needs to be given if fractional doses are used that extend the period of time in which the dose is delivered. Using his observations in treating skin cancer and oropharyngeal cancers and comparing this with skin erythema reactions, Standqvist was able to construct a family of curves in which an optimal zone could be found favoring tumor cure with minimal complications.

Normal standard dose (NSD) (37,53): The NSD is a single reference dose developed by Ellis (37) for the biologic effect of a fractionated course radiotherapy regimen. This index facilitates the comparison of treatment plans that have widely different fractionation patterns and overall treatment times. The unit for NSD is *rad equivalent therapy* (ret) and is determined by a formula that converts the cGy dose. The NSD corresponds to the tolerance of the normal tissue at the tumor site and represents the normal connective tissue toler-

ance, which is given as 1,800 ret. The NSD tolerance level varies with different organs and tissues.

The difference between the NSD concept and the Standqvist line is that the NSD formulation allows the separation of the fraction number and time variables. In general, it is the size of the dose per fraction that influences most severely the shape of the isoeffect curves. However, it should be recognized as unlikely that any one isoeffect formulation will hold for all tissues because of the extreme complexities and variations in the responses of different tissues to radiation therapy (38).

Time-dose fraction and cumulative radiation effect: The modification of the NSD concept proposed by Orton (51,52) introduced the concept of partial tolerance and defined a TDF so that one could have guidelines for combining two split courses or continuous irradiation, as in brachytherapy. A standard radium therapy regimen was used in comparison with equivalent techniques (6,000 cGy/168 h). Data derived from different dose-rate effects of different radioisotopes were plotted as isoeffect curves. Ellis's equivalent dose for fractionated external is 1,800 ret, and in a thorough review by Ellis related the NSD-TDF concept to radiotherapy (38).

The CRE concept of Kirk *et al.* (47) was based on the need to assess the biologic effect of various fractionated schemas on the basis of the accumulated subtolerance radiation injury. The application by Turrensen and Notten (68-71) of CRE in predicting late effects in normal tissue gave validity to the concept. However, whatever formulation or computer-generated guidelines are used, caution must be used in selecting safe doses that are unorthodox.

The Linear quadratic survival relationship (α/β Ratio) (44,65): Experiments with isoeffect curves for a variety of acute- and late-responding normal tissues in animals have shown that the isoeffect lines for late responses are steeper than those for early responses (Fig. 6-21). Thames *et al.* (64,66) consequently have suggested a greater capacity for repair of damage that is expressed late than for damage that is expressed early. The observed differences in the slopes of the isoeffect lines between acute- and late-responding normal tissues can be related to differences in the shapes of cell-survival curves. With respect to the linear quadratic survival-curve model, which is represented by the equation,

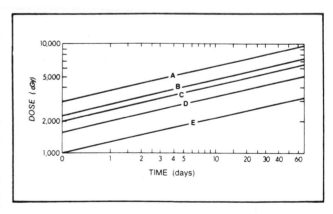

Fig. 6-20. Standqvist lines: The dose-time iso-effect line relates total dose delivered and total time independent of fractionation for different tissue end points: A = skin necrosis; B = cure of skin carcinoma; C = moist desquamation of skin; D = dry desquamation of skin; and E = skin erythema. From Hall (10), with permission.

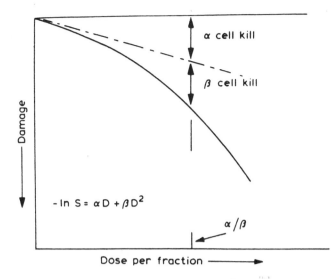

Fig. 6-21. At a dose equal to the ratio a to ß, the log cell-kill due to the a-process (nonreparable) is equal to that due to the ß-process (reparable injury); a/ß is thus a measure of how soon the survival curve begins to bend over significantly. From Perez (14), with permission.

$$Log_e \, S = d + ßd^2$$

a smaller $\alpha/ß$ ratio (14) would be characteristic of a late-responding normal tissue. Consequently, decreasing the fraction size would preferentially spare late-effects tissues (Fig. 6-22). Thus, in hyperfractionation protocols, greater total doses are delivered by giving smaller fractional doses more than once a day. The increased total doses should cause late effects similar to those with standard fractionation but should

give increased tumor responses, since it is thought that tumors respond to fractionated treatments like early responding normal tissues. Thus, with such an approach, a therapeutic benefit is expected (Fig. 6-23).

CHEMICAL MODIFIERS: RADIOSENSITIZERS AND RADIOPROTECTERS (10)

The potential effect of radiation modifiers in radiotherapy is illustrated schematically in Fig. 6-23. This diagram shows that, by protecting the normal tissue or enhancing the radiation damage to the tumor, it is possible to separate further the tumor control and normal tissue complication curves. Such an increased separation will consequently result in an improved therapeutic ratio.

Significant efforts have been expended to overcome the problem of tumor hypoxia, in consideration of the following observations

- the available oxygen tension in and around a cell determines its radiation response. Well-oxygenated cells can be eradicated more efficiently and effectively (factor of 2.5 to 3.0) by the same dose of x-irradiation (10,23)
- since normal tissues are believed to be fully oxygenated, attempts are being made to increase tumor oxygen tension. Means used in the past included atmospheric oxygen breathing with 5% CO_2, hyperbaric oxygen breathing, and hydrogen peroxide perfusion (10,36,75)

Radiosensitizers: Currently, unique agents that act as oxygen substitutes, referred to as hypoxic cell radiosensitizers, are under study (2,5,23). Such electron affinic compounds increase the production of free radicals in a manner similar to that of oxygen. They sensitize only hypoxic cells, not oxygenated cells. Misonidazole (RO-07-0582), a compound that has been widely used in experimentation to overcome tumor cell hypoxia (23,43), had shown much initial promise, but was not substantiated in numerous clinical trials (5,73). New compounds are being developed to test the validity of this approach further (Fig. 6-24) (10).

SR 2508 is more water soluble than misonidazole and is therefore more preferentially excluded from brain and ner-

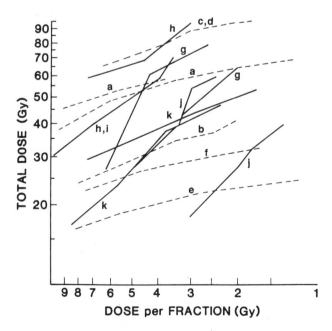

Fig. 6-22. Total dose for isoeffect as a function of dose per fraction. Letters refer to tissue responses as follows: Early response — a = skin; b = colon; c = stomach; d = spleen; e = jejunum; f = testis. Late response — g = skin; h = spinal cord; i = vasculature; j = kidney; k = lung. From Thames *et al.* (80), with permission.

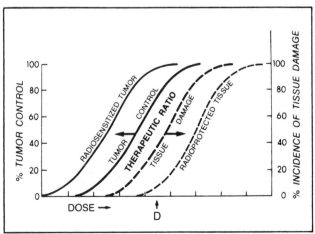

Fig. 6-23. The concept of radiosensitization and radioprotection is based upon the use of agents that can displace either the tumor dose-response curve to the left or the normal tissue damage curve to the right, thereby increasing the therapeutic ratio.

Directions for Development

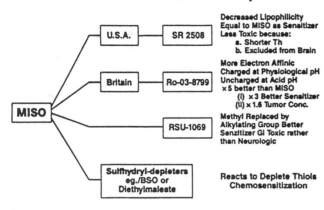

Fig. 6-24. Directions for development. From Hall (10), with permission.

vous tissues. Consequently, three to five times larger quantities of SR 2508 than misonidazole can be given. RO-03-7899 is more electron affinic than is misonidazole and tends to accumulate in tumors because the molecule is uncharged at acid pH. RSU 1069 takes advantage of combining an alkylation moiety and a hypoxic cell sensitizer functional group in the same molecule. Finally, thiol depleters aimed particularly at decreasing glutathione may increase cell response to chemotherapy and/or radiotherapy.

Radioprotectors (74,78,79): Sulfhydryl-containing compounds such as cystine and cysteamine have long been known to be radioprotective. One of the thiophosphate derivatives of cysteamine, WR-2721, has been reported to selectively protect normal tissues, including bone marrow, salivary glands, and intestinal mucosa. It is believed that these sulfhydryl compounds act as radical scavengers that protect from radiation damage by reducing the yield of damaging radiochemical species. Selective protection of normal tissues by WR-2721 has been postulated as a result of the failure of this agent to achieve appreciable concentrations in the tumors. However, some tumor radioprotection by WR-2721 has been reported in preclinical investigations (74,78,79).

Cytoxic agents (32,43,45,55,66a). Because of their spectrum of activities against human neoplasms, cytotoxic chemotherapeutic agents such as doxorubicin and cyclophosphamide are being evaluated in combination with radiotherapy, both in the laboratory and in the clinic. Under certain circumstances, such combinations have been used successfully to improve cancer therapy; but to date, the optimal employment of cytotoxic agents plus radiation therapy to maximize tumor cell kill while minimizing normal tissue toxicity, has not been fully realized. Simultaneous infusion of 5-fluorouracil, mitomycin C, cisplatin — singly or in combination — allow for smaller quantities of chemotherapy to be used, but increase the effect caused by concurrent administration. This has been successfully used in cancers such as anal cancer, esophageal cancer, and bladder cancer. Pilot phase I/II studies indicate toxicity is tolerable and tumor control improved, requiring phase III clinical trials for confirmation.

A recent Third International Conference on the Interaction of Radiation and Systemic Therapy presents the most recent experimental biologic studies relating to combined chemotherapy and radiation therapy and their translation into selected clinical investigations (66a).

Recommended Reading

There is a rich and wide-ranging literature on radiation oncology based on the sciences and advances of radiation biology and radiation physics. *The Principles and Practice of Radiation Oncology* by Perez and Brady (9) is an excellent starting place for an integrated approach to these elements, and an emphasis of the clinical and medical aspects of the cancer at each disease site. The study of late effects is described fully in *Clinical Radiation Pathology* by Rubin and Casarett (19). The radiobiologic basis of radiation oncology is addressed concisely and succinctly in Hall's *Radiobiology for the Radiologist* (10), and Andrews offers a historical perspective on the development of radiation and its integration with other modes of therapy in *The Radiobiology of Human Cancer Radiotherapy* (3). A recent update on normal tissue radiation tolerance can be found in an edited volume by Vaeth and Meyer (15a).

REFERENCES

General References

1. Ackerman, L.V.; del Regato, J.A. Cancer diagnosis treatment and prognosis, 4th ed. St. Louis, MO: C.V. Mosby Co.; 1970.
2. Adams, G.E. Hypoxic cell sensitizers for radiotherapy. In: Becker, F.F., ed. Cancer—a comprehensive treatise, vol. 6. New York, NY: Plenum Press; 1977:181-224.
3. Andrews, J.R. The radiobiology of human cancer radiotherapy, 2nd ed. Baltimore, MD: University Park Press; 1978.
4. Arcangeli, G.; Mauro, F., eds. Hyperthermia in radiation oncology. Milan, Italy: Masson et Cie; 1980.
4a. Bleehen, N.M., ed. Radiobiology in Radiotherapy. Berlin: Springer-Verlag; 1988.
5. Brady, L., ed. Radiation sensitizers. New York, NY: Masson et Cie; 1980.
6. Constine, L.S. Tumors in children. In: Wilson, J.F., ed. Syllabus: a categorical course in radiation therapy: cure with preservation of function and aesthetics. Oak Brook, IL: Radiological Society of North America, Inc.; 1988:75-92.
6a. del Regato, J.A.; Spjut, H.J.; Cox, J.D. Ackerman and del Regato's Cancer: Diagnosis, treatment, and prognosis, 6th ed. St. Louis, MO: The CV Mosby Co; 1985.
7. Electron beam energy. In: Vauth, J.M., ed. Frontiers of radiation therapy and oncology. New York: S. Karger; 1968.
7a. Elkind, M.M.; Whitmore, G. The radiobiology of cultured mammalian cells. New York, NY: Gordon & Breach Publishers; 1967.
8. Fletcher, G.H. Textbook of radiotherapy. Philadelphia, PA: Lea & Febiger; 1980.
9. Glassburn, J.R.; Brady, L.W.; Grisby, P.W. Endometrium. In: Brady, L.W.; Perez, C. eds. Principles and practice of radiation oncology. Philadelphia, PA: J.B. Lippincott Co.; 1992:1203-1220.
9a. Hall, E.J. Radiol 192: 173-179; 1972.
10. Hall, E.J. Radiobiology for the radiologist, 3rd ed. Philadelphia: J.B. Lippincott; 1988.
11. Kaplan, H.S. Hodgkin's Disease, 2nd ed. Cambridge, MA: Harvard University Press; 1980.
12. Mansfield, C.M., ed. Therapeutic Radiology. New York, NY: Elsevier; 1989.
13. Mendenhall, W.; Million, R.; Parsons, J. Tumors of the head and neck: treatment alternatives. RSNA syllabus:13-26.
13a. Moss, W.T.; Cox, J.D., eds. Radiation Oncology: rationale, technique, results, 6th ed. St. Louis, MO: Mosby; 1989.
14. Perez, C. Uterine cervix. In: Perez, C.; Brady, L.W., eds. Principles and practice of radiation oncology. Philadelphia, PA: J.B. Lippincott Co.; 1992:1143-1202.
14a. Peters, L.J.; Chapman, D.J.; Withers, H.R. Conclusions: Prediction of Tumor Treatment Response. In: Prediction of Tumor Treatment Response. Elmsford, NY: Pergamon Press; 1988: 317-320.
15. Radiation effect and tolerance, normal tissue; basic concepts in radiation pathology. In: Vaeth, J.M., ed. Frontiers of radiation

therapy and oncology, vol. 6. Baltimore, MD: University Park Press; 1972.

15a. Radiation Tolerance of Normal Tissues. In: Vaeth, J.M., Meyer, J.L. Frontiers of Radiation Therapy and Oncology. Basel, Switzerland: S. Karger; vol. 23: 1989.

16. Raju, M.R. Heavy particle radiotherapy. New York, NY: Academic Press; 1980:78-81.

17. Relationship of time and dose in the radiation therapy of cancer, vol. 3. In: Vaeth, J.M., ed. Frontiers of radiation therapy and oncology, vol.3. New York, NY: S. Karger; 1968.

18. Research Plan for Radiation Oncology, Committee for Radiation Oncology Studies. Cancer 37 (Suppl 2); 1976:2031-2148.

19. Rubin, P.; Casarett, G.W. Clinical Radiation Pathology, vols. 1 and 2. Philadelphia, PA: W.B. Saunders Co.; 1968.

20. Silverberg, E.; Lubera, J.A. Cancer Statistics. Ca-A Cancer J. for Clinicians 38(1):5-22; 1988.

21. Silverberg, E.; Lubera, J.A. Cancer Statistics. Ca-A Cancer J. for Clinicians 39(1):3-20; 1989.

22. Steel, G.G. Growth kinetics of tumors. Oxford, UK: Clarendon Press; 1977.

23. Sutherland, R.M.; Conroy, P.J.; Siemann, D.W. Potentials and limitations for the use of radiation sensitizers of resistant hypoxic cells in tumors. In: Pediatric oncology, vol. 2. Boston, MA: Martinus Nijhoff; 1983.

24. Tapley, N. du V. Clinical applications of the electron beam. New York, NY: John Wiley & Sons, 1976.

24a. Thames, H.D.; Hendry, J.H. Fractionation in Radiotherapy. Philadelphia, PA: Taylor and Francis; 1987.

25. Time and dose relationships in radiation biology as applied to radiotherapy. Brookhaven National Laboratory (BNL) Report 50203 (C-57). Upton, NY: Brookhaven National Laboratory; 1969.

25a. Wang, C.C., ed. Clinical Radiation Oncology. Indications, Techniques, and Results. Littleton, MA: PSG Publishing Company Inc.; 1988.

26. Wilson, J.F., ed. Syllabus: a categorical course in radiation therapy: cure with preservation of function and aesthetics. Oak Brook, IL: Radiological Society of North America, Inc.; 1988:5-6.

27. Withers, H.R.; Peters, L.J. Biological aspects of radiation therapy. In: Fletcher, G.H., ed. Textbook of radiotherapy. Philadelphia, PA: Lea & Febiger; 1980:103-179.

Specific References

28. Allalunis-Turner, M.J.; Siemann, D.W. Potentially lethal damage (PLD) repair in human epidermoid tumor cells grown *in vivo* and *in vitro*. Proc. Eighth Intl. Congress Radiat. Res. (London, Taylor and Francis). 1:157; 1987.

29. Bush, R.S.; Jenkin, R.D.T.; Allt, W.E.V.; *et al*. Definitive evidence for hypoxic cells influencing cure in cancer therapy. Br. J. Cancer 37:(Suppl III)302-306; 1978.

30. Chen, J.T.Y.; Austin, S.M.; Castro, J.C. *et al*. Dose-volume histograms and treatment planning evaluation of carcinoma of the pancreas. In: Proceedings of the Eighth International Conference on Users of Computers in Radiation Therapy IEEE; 1984:264-268.

31. Cohen, L. Radiosensitivity of tumors and target theory. Br. J. Radiol. 36:226-227; 1963.

32. Conference on Combined Modalities. Chemotherapy/radiotherapy. Intl. J. Radiat. Oncol. Biol. Phys. 5:1139-1721; 1979.

33. Cowdry, E.V. In: Rubin, P.; Cassaret, G. W., eds. Clinical radiation pathology, vol. . Ann Arbor, MI: Books on Demand; 1968.

34. Deacon, J.; Peckham, M.J.; Steel, G.G. The radioresponsiveness of human tumours and the initial slope of the cell survival curve. Radiother. Oncol. 2(4):317-323; 1984.

35. Denekamp, J. Testing of hypoxic cell radiosensitizers *in vivo*. Cancer Clin. Trials 3:139-148; 1980.

36. Dische, S. Hyperbaric oxygen: the medical research council trials and their clinical significance. Br. J. Radiol. 51:888-894; 1979.

37. Ellis, F. Dose, time and fractionation: a clinical hypothesis. Clin. Radiol. 20:1-7; 1969.

38. Ellis, F. Is NST-TDF useful to radiotherapy? Intl. J. Radiat. Oncol. Biol. Phys. 1:1685-1699; 1985.

39. Fertil, B.; Malaise, E.P. Intrinsic radiosensitivity of human cell lines as correlated with radioresponsiveness of human tumors, analysis of 101 published survival curves. Intl. J. Radiat. Oncol. Biol. Phys. 11:1699-1707; 1985.

40. Fertil, B.; Malaise, E.P. Inherent cellular radiosensitivity is a basic concept for human tumor radiobiology. Intl. J. Radiat. Oncol. Biol. Phys. 7:621-629; 1981.

41. Fischer, D.B.; Fischer, J.J. Dose-response relationships in radiotherapy: applications of logistic regression model. Intl. J. Radiat. Oncol. Biol. Phys. 2:773-781; 1977.

42. Fowler, J.F. New horizons in radiation oncology. Br. J. Radiol. 52:523-535; 1979.

43. Fowler, J.F.; Denekamp, J. A review of hypoxic cell radiosensitization in experimental tumors. J. Pharmacol. Exp. Ther. 7:413-444; 1979.

44. Fowler, J.R. Fractionation and therapeutic gain. In: Steel, G.G.; Adams, G.; Peckham, M.J., eds. The biological basis of radiotherapy. Amsterdam, Holland: Elsevier Science Publications; 181-194; 1983.

44a. Fu, K.K.; Phillips, T.L. High-dose-rate versus low-dose-rate intracavitary brachytherapy for carcinoma of the cervix. Int J Radiat Oncol Biol Phys 19: 791-796;1990.

45. Hellman, K., ed. Interaction of radiation and antitumor drugs. Cade Memorial symposium. Intl. J. Radiat. Oncol. Biol. Phys. 4:1-173; 1978.

46. Herring, D.F. Methods for extracting dose-response curves from radiation therapy data, I. A unified approach. Intl. J. Radiat. Oncol. Biol. Phys. 6:225-232; 1980.

47. Kirk, G.; Gray, W.M.; Watson, E.R. Cumulative radiation effect, Part I. Fractionation treatment regimens. Clinical Radiol. 122:145-155; 1971.

48. Little, J.B.; Williams, J.R. Effects of ionizing radiation on mammalian cells. In: Lee, DHK, ed. Handbook of physiology, section 9. Bethesda, MD: American Physiological Society; 1977:127.

49. Lyman, J.T.; Wolbarst, A.B.. Optimization of radiation therapy, III: a method of assessing complication probabilities from dose-volume histograms. Intl. J. Radiat. Oncol. Biol. Phys. 13:103-109; 1987.

49a. Marcial, V.A.; Pajak, T.F.; Kramer, S.; Davis, L.W.; Stetz, J.A.; Laramore, G.E.; Jacobs, J.R.; Al-Sarraf, M.; Brady, W. Radiation Therapy Oncology Group (RTOG) studies in head and neck cancer. Semin. in Oncol 15 (1):39-60;1988.

50. Mendelsohn, M.L. The biology of dose-limiting tissues. In: Time and dose relationships in radiation biolgoy as applied to radiotherapy, Brookhaven National Laboratory (BNL) Report 5023 (C-57). Upton, NY: Brookhaven National Laboratory; 1969:154-173.

50a. Million, R.R.; Cassissi, N.J. eds. Management of Head and Neck Cancer. A Multidisciplinary Approach. Philadelphia, PA: J.B. Lippincott Co; 1984.

51. Orton, C.G.; Colin, L.A. A unified approach to dose-effect relationships and radiotherapy. Modified TDF and linear quadratic equations. Intl. J. Radiat. Oncol. Biol. Phys. 14:549-557; 1988.

52. Orton, C.G.; Colin, L.A. A unified approach to dose-effect relationships and radiotherapy. Inhomogeneous dose distributions. Intl. J. Radiat. Oncol. Biol. Phys. 14:561-565; 1988.

53. Orton, C.G.; Ellis, F. A simplification in the use of the NSD concept in practical radiotherapy. Br. J. Radiol. 46:529-536; 1973.

54. Peters, J.L.; Brock, A.W.; Chapman, J.D.; Wilson, G. Predictive assays of tumor radiocurability. Am. J. Clin. Oncol. 11:275-287; 1988.

55. Pettigrew, R.T.; Ludgate, C.M.; Gee, A.P.; *et al*. Whole body hyperthermia combined with chemotherapy in the treatment of advanced human cancer. In: Streffer, C.; Van Beuningen, D.; Dietzel, F.; *et al*., eds. Cancer therapy by hyperthermia and radiation. Baltimore, MD: Urban and Schwarzenber; 1978:337-339.

56. Phillips, T.L.; Wasserman, T.H.; Johnson, R.J.; *et al*. The hypoxic cell sensitizer programme in the United States. Br. J. Cancer 37(Suppl III):276-280; 1978.

57. Rubin, P. Tolerance doses and volumes: the biology and physiopathologic basis for radiaiton oncology dose/time/volume prescription. In: Wilson, J.F., ed. Syllabus: a categorical course in radiation therapy: cure with preservation of function and aesthetics. Oak Brook, Il: Radiological Society of North America, Inc.; 1988:93-102.

58. Rubin, P.; Rubin, D.; Cowen, R., eds. Radiation oncology research program. Intl. J. Radiat. Oncol. Biol. Phys. 5:593-774; 1979.

59. Siemann, D.W. Do *in vitro* studies of potentially lethal damage repair predict for *in situ* results? Intl. J. Radiat. Oncol. Biol. Phys. 5:567-571; 1989.

60. Sinclair, W.K. Cyclic x ray responses in mammalian cells *in vitro*. Radiat. Res. 33:620-643; 1968.

61. Spanos, W.J.; Montague, E.D.; Fletcher, G.H. Late complications of radiation only for advanced breast cancer. Intl. J. Radiat. Oncol. Biol. Phys. 6:1473-1476; 1980.

62. Standqvist, M. Stubien uber die Kumulative Wirking der Roentgenstrahlen bei Fraktioerrun. Acta Radiol. 55 (Suppl 1):1-300; 1944.

63. Steel, G.G. The ESTRO Breur Lecture: Cellular sensitivity to low dose-rate irradiation focuses the problem of tumour radioresistance Radiother and Oncol 20: 71-83;1991.

64. Thames, H.D.; Hendry, J.H. Fractionation in radiotherapy. Philadelphia, PA: Taylor & Francis; 1987.

65. Thames, H.D.; Withers, H.R.; Mason, K.A.; Reid, B.O. Dose-survival characteristics of mouse jejunal crypt cells. Intl. J. Radiat. Oncol. Biol. Phys. 7:1591-1597; 1981.

66. Thames, H.D.; Withers, H.R.; Peters, L.J.; Fletcher, G.H. Changes in early and late radiation responses with altered fractionation: implications for dose-survival relationships. Intl. J. Radiat. Oncol. Biol. Phys. 8:219-226; 1982.

66a. Third International Conference on the Interaction of Radiation Therapy and Systemic Therapy. Asilomar Conference Center, Monterey, CA; 10-12 Mar 1990. Int J Radiat Oncol Biol Phys 20: 1991.

67. Thomlinson, R.H. Changes of oxygenation in tumors in relation to radiation frontiers in radiation therapy and oncology. 3:109-121; 1968.

68. Turrenson, I.; Notter, G.; The influence of fraction size in radiotherapy on the late normal tissue reaction — II: comparison of the effects of daily and twice-a-week fractionation on human skin. Intl. J. Radiat. Oncol. Biol. Phys. 10:599-606; 1984.

69. Turrenson, I.; Notter, G.; The influence of the overall treatment time in radiotherapy on the acute reaction: comparison of the effects of daily and twice-a-week fractionation on human skin. Intl. J. Radiat. Oncol. Biol. Phys. 10:607-618; 1984.

70. Turrenson, I.; Notter, G.; The influence of fraction size in radiotherapy on late normal tissue reaction — I: comparison of the effects of daily and once-a-week fractionation on human skin. Intl. J. Radiat. Oncol. Biol. Phys. 10:593-598; 1984.

71. Turrenson, I.; Notter, G. The response of pig skin to single and fractionated high dose-rate and continuous low dose-rate 137 Cs irradiation — III. Re-evaluation of CRE system and the TDF system according to present findings. Intl. J. Radiat. Oncol. Biol. Phys. 5:1773-1780; 1979.

72. Wang, C.C.; Blitzer, P.H.; Suit, H.D. Twice-a-day radiation therapy for cancer of the head and neck. Cancerr 55-2100-2104; 1985.

73. Wasserman, T.H.; Phillips, T.L.; Johnson, R.J.; *et al.* Initial United States clinical and pharmacologic evaluaiton of misonidazole (RO-070582), an hypoxic cell radiosensitizer. Intl. J. Radiat. Oncol. Biol. Phys. 5:775-786; 1979.

74. Wasserman, T.H.; Phillips, T.L.; Ross, G.; *et al.* Differential protection against cytotoxic chemotherapeutic effects on bone marrow CFU's and EMT-6 Carcinoma by WR-2721. Cancer Clin. Trials 4:3-6; 1981.

75. Watson, E.R.; Dische, S.; Cade, I.S.; *et al.* Hyperbaric oxygen and radiotherapy: a medical research council trial in carcinoma of the cervix. Br. J. Radiol. 51:879-887; 1978.

76. Wechselbaum, R.R.; Dahlberg, W.; Little, J.B. Inherent radioresistant cells exist in some human tumors. Proceedings National Academy of Science USA 1985. 82:4732-4735.

77. Withers, H.R.; Peters, L.J.; Kogelnick, H.P. The pathobiology of late effects of radiation. In: Meyn, R.E.; Withers, H.R., eds. Radiation biology and cancer research. New York: Raven Press; 1980:439-438.

78. Yuhas, J.M.; Spellman, J.M.; Culo, F. The role of WR-2721 in radiotherapy and/or chemotherapy. Cancer Clin. Trials 3:211-216; 1980.

79. Yuhas, J.M.; Storer, J.B. Differential chemoprotection of normal and malignant tissues. J. Natl. Cancer Instit. 42:331-335; 1969.

Margaret A. Henzler, M.S., Radiation Physics   Ahmad Matloubieh, M.S., Radiation Physics
Hideo Kubo, Ph.D., Radiation Physics

Chapter 7

BASIC CONCEPTS OF RADIATION PHYSICS

The mere formulation of a problem is often far more essential than its solution which may be merely a matter of mathematical or experimental skill. To raise new questions, new possibilities, to regard old problems from a new angle requires creative imagination and marks real advances in science.

Albert Einstein (5)

PERSPECTIVE

The physical act of absorption of x- and gamma-radiation in biologic material takes less than 10^{-7} seconds. Yet the biologic consequences of that absorption may take weeks, months, and even years to occur. These biologic consequences are the subject of radiation biology.

Understanding the quantification of absorption is the first step in appreciating the biologic processes that follow. As an example, consider the absorption of 1,000 cGy in a man weighing 70 kg. This quantity of radiation is roughly 2½ times the lethal dose required to kill 50% of the population (LD_{50}) and will most certainly be lethal to man. One cGy of absorbed dose is 100 erg/gm, so that the man will have absorbed:

$$1,000 \text{ cGy x } 100 \text{ erg/g x } 70,000 \text{ gm} = 7 \text{ x } 10^9 \text{ erg.}$$

The student is not likely to be familiar with an erg, which is a unit of energy; however, he or she can easily convert the erg to its mass equivalent using the expression $E = MC^2$ to get a feeling for the mass or size of a lethal dose of radiation.

$$\text{Mass} = \frac{Energy}{C^2} = \frac{7 \times 10^9 \; erg}{9 \times 10^{20} \; cm^2/sec^2} \sim 10^{-11} \text{ g}$$

Compare this mass of lethal radiation to that mass of botulinus toxin that is considered to be lethal ($\sim 10^{-6}$ g). One interpretation of these numbers is that radiation is 10^5 times more lethal to normal tissue than botulinus toxin, gram for gram. Another simple exercise is to calculate the fraction of the man's atoms that were ionized. The result, approximately one atom in 50 billion, is extremely small, which suggests that there must be biologic rather than physical reasons to explain why this quantity of radiation is so lethal.

The quantification of radiation — both in delivery and absorption within the patient — is the central role of radiation physics in oncology. The precise definition of tumor volume and critical normal tissues allows for accurate treatment planning that maximizes the dose to the tumor and minimizes the dose to normal structures. Physics contributes to the *concept of therapeutic ratio* by using different energies and types of beams in pursuing the aforementioned aim. The areas of physics to be discussed are: (1) production of clinical radiation; (2) absorption of electromagnetic radiation in matter; (3) clinically useful radiation beams; (4) radiation treatment planning; and (5) the optimization of radiation treatment plans.

It is important for the student approaching the subject of radiation oncology to understand the basic tenets of radiologic physics. This complex subject can be simplified to a few fundamental concepts essential to comprehending radiation biology and, consequently, clinical radiation oncology.

PRODUCTION OF CLINICAL RADIATION

Radiation can be defined as the propagation of energy through space or matter. Both particulate and electromagnetic radiation are used in radiology, but historically, radiology, radiation oncology, and nuclear medicine have been concerned with electromagnetic radiation. Beta radiation is the most notable exception; in recent years, heavy particle beams such as neutrons, protons, and negative mesons have been used in radiation oncology to a limited extent.

Particulate Radiation

Particulate radiation consists of traveling particles of matter with a finite rest mass. Although they travel with high speeds, depending on their kinetic energy, it is always less than the speed of light in a vacuum. The rest mass of these particles varies greatly from alpha particles, entire helium nuclei, to electrons or beta particles as does their charge from zero to some multiple of the charge of an electron (Table 7-1) (9). Their interaction with matter and transfer of energy to the medium depends on both their mass and charge.

In radiology, the most common particulate radiation is the electron with a charge of -1 and a mass of only 0.000548

Table 7-1. Properties of Some Subatomic Particles

Name	Symbol	Charge	Mass (Unit)	Clinical Use
Electron	e⁻ or ß⁻	-1	5.5×10^{-4}	6-20 MeV e- in wide use Uniform dose to energy de-pendent depth
Proton	p	+1	1.00728	Favorable dose distribution Biologic prop-erties similar to x-ray
Neutron	n	0	1.00867	Dose fall off similar to photon beams Advantage in biologic effectiveness
Alpha or helium ions		+2	4.00099	Favorable dose distribution Small increase in biologic effectiveness
Negative π-meson	π-	-1	1.5×10^{-1}	Improved dose distribution Modest increase in biologica effectiveness

Adapted from Hall (9).

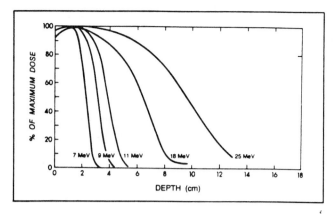

Fig. 7-1. Comparative depths of penetration for electron beams. From Levitt (12), with permission.

atomic mass units. Electrons deposit their energy directly in the medium by excitation or ionization of the atoms or molecules of the medium. As an example, ß particles (electrons) emitted by the nucleus of iodine-131 atoms are used to treat thyroid cancer. If radioactive iodine is ingested the ß particles from atoms within the gland penetrate into the thyroid tissue, losing their kinetic energy through ionization and excitation of atoms and molecules that make up thyroid cells. Cell death occurs as the result of absorption of this energy.

The most common external beam particulate radiation is a beam of high energy electrons produced by a linear accelerator directed at superficial lesions. The electrons lose their kinetic energy over a finite range dependent on their initial kinetic energy. Since their depth of penetration is dependent on energy, by selecting the appropriate energy electron, a uniform dose can be delivered from the surface to the desired depth and yet avoid irradiating critical structures that lie beyond (Fig. 7-1) (12).

Electromagnetic Radiation

Electromagnetic radiation (EMR) consists of the propaga-tion of energy through space or the medium by oscillating electric and magnetic fields traveling at the speed of light in a vacuum. Visible light, radio and radar, infrared and ultra-violet, and x- and -rays are examples of EMR. Although EMR has no rest mass, at times it is convenient in explaining its interactions by considering it as little packets of energy called photons. The energy carried by each of these photons is

directly proportional to its frequency. Photons are classified according to their place of origin.

Gamma rays are emitted from unstable nuclei during nuclear transitions. The nuclei of all atoms are made up of subatomic particles: protons and neutrons. Only certain nuclear ar-rangements of these particles form stable configurations. When unstable arrangements of these particles exist, the atom will decay to a stable configuration.

The decay of cobalt-60 is an example of the generation of useful -radiation. Cobalt-60 undergoes radioactive decay by emitting a ß particle from the nucleus (Fig. 7-2). When this happens, the atom is no longer cobalt-60, but has become an excited state of nickel-60. Nickel-60 will decay almost imme-diately by emitting two high energy γ-rays one after the other of 1.17 and 1.33 MeV. Cobalt-60 has been used for decades to treat cancer patients. For a teletherapy machine, 5,000 to 10,000 Ci of cobalt-60 are encapsulated into a small, sealed cylinder and "stored" in a shielded container with a mecha-nism to move the source from a shielded to exposed position for treating patients.

Some clinically useful radioactive materials are listed in Table 7-2 (13), along with the type of useful radiation, their energy, and their therapeutic value.

X-rays are produced whenever high speed electrons pen-etrate a target material, and are either decelerated by a close approach to the nucleus of an atom or collide with an orbital electron and knock it out of the atom. A typical x-ray spec-trum is a continuous spectrum on which discrete peaks are superimposed (Fig. 7-3) (1).

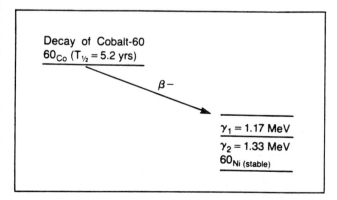

Fig. 7-2. Decay scheme for cobalt-60. T½ = half-life.

Table 7-2. Clinically Useful Radioactive Materials

Radionuclide	Half-life	Useful Type of Radiation	Energy(MeV)	Therapeutic Use
Radium-226	1604 yrs	gamma	principal	Temporary implant 0.61 - 2.09
Cobalt-60	5.26 yrs	gamma	1.17 and 1.33	External beam
Cesium-137	30.0 yrs	gamma	0.662	Temporary implant
Iridium-192	74.2 d	gamma	principal	Temporary implant 0.30-0.61
Iodine-125	60.25 d	gamma	.035 X rays	Permanent Implant .027-.032

Adapted from Medical Physics Data Book (13).

An x-ray tube consists of an evacuated glass envelope in which electrons are boiled off a filament or cathode. A high voltage between the filament (or cathode) and the target (or anode) is used to accelerate the electrons across the gap. The electrons acquire kinetic energy by virtue of their velocity and mass. Once they reach the target, the electrons are decelerated rapidly by interaction with the atoms of the target. If an electron approaches close to the nucleus of one of the target atoms, the electron will be deflected from its path by the strong attraction between the negative electron and the positively charged nucleus, causing it to lose some of its kinetic energy. This energy may be given off in the form of an x-ray photon. If an electron is brought to rest in a single interaction, then all of its kinetic energy will be converted into a single photon. The energy of this photon in kiloelectron volts will be equal to the peak kilovoltage across the x-ray tube. Few of the electrons, however, lose their energy in a single interaction. Most of them undergo many interactions, each resulting in the loss of only a fraction of their kinetic energy, which results in x-rays of lower energy than the maximum. The result is a continuous spectrum of x-rays that has all energies up to the maximum. This radiation produced by decelerating electrons is called *bremsstrahlung* (Fig 7-4a) (3).

An alternate process also generates x-rays in an x-ray tube. It is possible that an incoming electron may collide directly with an orbital electron of one of the target atoms, and if it has sufficient energy, knock that electron completely from the atom, ionizing the atom. The hole created will be filled by an outer orbital electron, and the atom will return to its lowest potential energy by emitting a single x-ray photon. The x-rays produced will have discrete energies characteristic of the binding energies of the orbital electrons of the target material. The x-rays that result from this process are called *characteristic X rays* (Fig. 7-4b) (3).

The fate of a *positron* created in pair production (discussed in the next section) is important because positrons do not usually exist in nature. After losing most of its kinetic energy through collisional interaction, the positron will unite with an electron. In the process, all of the mass of the positron and electron is converted into two photons, each with 0.51 MeV of energy. This process is called *annihilation*, and is useful in nuclear imaging.

ABSORPTION OF ELECTROMAGNETIC RADIATION IN MATTER

When a photon beam enters biological matter, the energy of the beam is eventually converted into biologic damage and heat through a two-step process. The initial step in the sequence is the interaction of the indirectly ionizing photons with the medium to produce high-speed secondary electrons. In traveling through the tissue, these electrons in a second step produce a track of excitation, ionization, and broken molecular bonds resulting in biologic damage. Photons interact with biologic material depending on their energy and the atomic number (Z) of the absorbing medium. Of the 12 possible kinds of interactions, only the following three are of major interest in radiation oncology.

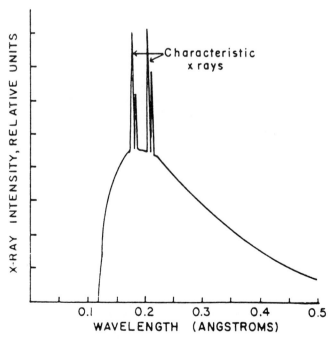

Fig. 7-3. A typical x-ray spectrum illustrating characteristic x-rays superimposed on the continuous bremstrahlung spectrum. From Hendee (1), with permission.

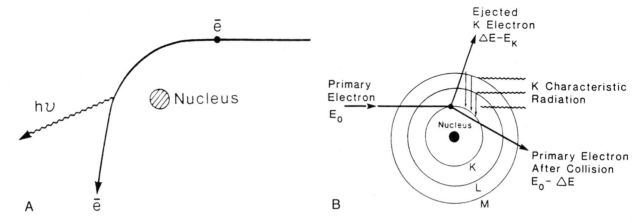

Fig. 7-4. (a) Illustration of a bremsstrahlung process. The x-ray photon, hv, is radiated by the deceleration of an electron, e-, by a nucleus. (b) Diagram of the production of characteristic radiation. An incident electron with energy, E_o, collides with an orbital electron losing energy ΔE, ejecting it with energy $\Delta E- E_k$ (the binding energy of the electron ejected). When an outer shell electron fills the hole, a characteristic x-ray is produced. From Khan (3), with permission.

Photoelectric Effect

The photoelectric effect is the interaction between an incident photon and a bound electron of an atom of the absorbing medium. In this process, the atom acts as a momentum sink and the incident photon is totally absorbed. Usually, a K- or L-shell electron will be ejected from the atom into the surrounding medium with a kinetic energy equal to the difference in energy between the incident photon and the binding energy of the ejected electron. This electron — now called a photoelectron — loses its kinetic energy through excitation and ionization processes with nearby atoms and molecules. The atom is left in an "excited" state since there is a vacancy in the K or L orbital. Therefore, following the photoelectric absorption process, an electron will fill the vacancy with the usual emission of a characteristic x-ray (Fig. 7-5a) (1).

It is important to remember the following about the photoelectric effect (2):
- the process involves bound electrons, and is one of total absorption
- the probability of its occurring is maximal if the photon has just enough energy to eject the electron from its shell
- the process varies with energy approximately as $1/E^3$
- the probability of its occurring per electron or per gram of absorbing material varies with atomic number approximately as Z^3

At low energies, photons are differentially absorbed between biologic materials with even slight differences in

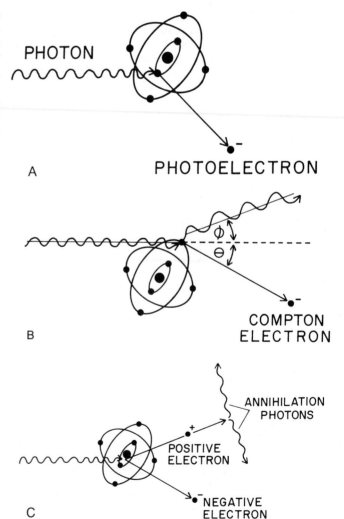

Fig. 7-5. (a) Photoelectric absorption of a photon with energy *hv*. The photon disappears and is replaced by an electron from the atom with kinetic energy $E_k = E_B$, where E_B is the binding energy of the electron. Characteristic radiation and Auger electrons are emitted as electrons cascade to replace the ejected photoelectron. (b) Compton scattering of an x- or gamma-ray photon by a loosely bound electron. Scattering angles theta and phi for the electron and photon are shown. (c) Pair-production interaction of a high-energy photon near a nucleus. Annihilation photons are produced when the positron and an electron annihilate each other. From Hendee (1), with permission.

atomic number such as muscle, fat, and bone. That is why low energy photons — 10 to 200 KVP — are used in diagnostic radiology.

Compton Effect

The Compton effect is an interaction between an incident photon and a loosely bound or "free" electron in the absorbing medium. The incident photon is scattered in a different direction with lower energy and part of its initial energy is given to the recoil electron as kinetic energy. This electron — now called a Compton electron — loses this kinetic energy through excitation and ionization, as mentioned for photoelectrons (Fig. 7-5b) (1).

It is important to remember the following about the Compton effect (2):
- the process involves "free" or loosely bound electrons, and is one of partial absorption
- it is independent of atomic number (Z)
- it generally decreases slowly with increasing energy
- in each collision of the photon, some energy is scattered and some absorbed. The amount depends on the angle of the collision and the energy of the photon

In biologic material in the energy range from about 100 keV to 10 MeV, the Compton absorption process is much more important than either the photoelectric effect or pair production.

Pair Production

Pair production involves the interaction between an incident photon and the electric field of a nucleus of an atom in the absorbing medium. In this interaction, the photon is absorbed completely and two electrons (one positively charged called a positron and one negatively charged) are produced from the energy supplied by the photon. Therefore, this type of interaction can occur only if the photon possesses a minimum of 1.02 MeV of energy, that is, two times the energy equivalent of the rest mass of one electron. These two electrons — now called pair electrons — lose their kinetic energy through excitation and ionization of atoms and molecules in the absorbing medium. In addition, the positron combines with an electron to produce two photons of radiation each with 0.511 MeV of energy, the rest mass of an electron converted into energy (Fig. 7-5c) (1).

It is important to remember the following about the pair production process (2):
- the process involves the nuclear charge, and is one of total absorption
- the threshold for this process is 1.02 MeV
- it increases rapidly with atomic number, depending on Z per gram
- it increases rapidly with energy above the 1.02 MeV level
- the actual energy absorbed is less than the energy of the incident photon by 1.02 MeV

Pair production is of significant interest in radiation oncology only at energies in excess of 10 MeV.

These three processes are involved in the indirect absorption of electromagnetic radiation in matter by producing secondary electrons (photo, Compton, and pair) that lose their kinetic energy through the ionization and excitation of atoms and molecules of the absorbing medium. These secondary electrons are the actual vehicle for the absorption process. Since the range of these electrons may be consider-

able (approximately 6 cm for 25 MV photons) their energy may be deposited away from the site of the initial photon interaction. The energy deposited per unit mass is called the dose. Because the energy of these secondary electrons is not deposited where it is produced, the dose builds up from the surface to an equilibrium depth. Beyond the equilibrium depth, the dose falls off with depth due to attenuation of the photon beam. The depth of the maximum dose increases with photon energy, and the rate of fall-off of dose beyond that depth decreases with energy. The depth dose is defined as the ratio of the dose at a given depth to the maximum dose at the equilibrium depth.

RADIATION BEAMS OF CLINICAL VALUE

Radiation physicists and therapists have searched for a beam of unique physical and biologic characteristics that could selectively affect only cancer cells and spare normal tissues. This ideal has not been reached, but many technical developments have led to improved dose distributions with which the probability of destroying malignant cells increases and normal tissue complications decrease. The major improvements in survival and reduced complications since World War II are due largely to the advent of high energy x-ray and electron beams with the introduction of first the betatron and teletherapy units and then linear accelerators. In addition, improved field shaping techniques and rotational isocentric machines that rotate about a point and always direct their beam at that point, although not as important, have led to improved dose distributions (Fig. 7-6 [11] and Fig. 7-7 [6]).

A variety of clinically useful beams are used in modern radiation oncology facilities. The initial radiation beams

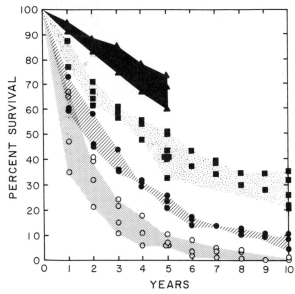

Fig. 7-6. Hodgkin's disease. Improved survival with introduction of megavoltage linear accelerators that allowed large, shaped fields to be used so that better depth doses could be delivered, avoiding irradiation to lungs, liver, spinal cord, and large portions of small intestines. From Kaplan (11), with permission.

were limited by the maximun energies achievable — 200 to 400 kV; they produced "soft" radiation with the maximum dose on the skin and rapid attenuation with depth in tissue causing severe skin reactions in order to achieve reasonable doses to tumors. With the introduction of megavoltage beams from 1 to 25 MeV, high skin doses and other normal tissue reactions could be avoided. These "harder" radiation beams spare superficial tissues by building up to maximal doses well below the skin surface, and have increased depth dose (Fig. 7-8).

Advantages of Megavoltage Radiation (Fig. 7-8) (2)

1. *Skin sparing*: Avoids skin reactions.
2. *Increased depth doses to deep-seated tumors*: Increases tumor control .
3. *Less side scatter and sharper beam edge*: avoids high doses to continguous normal tissues and critical structures.
4. *Predominance of Compton interactions which are independent of atomic number, Z_i*: Results in dose homogeneity and avoids increased dose to bone.

Advantages of Electron Beam Radiation (Fig. 7-1) (12)

1. *Uniform dose from the surface to a depth dependent on electron energy*: approximate useful depth in cm = energy (MeV)/3.
2. *Beyond range of penetration, dose falls rapidly*: avoids irradiation to underlying normal tissues.

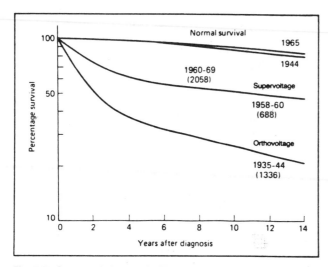

Fig. 7-7. Cancer of the cervix. The rationale for the use of high-energy radiotherapy is based on the concept that a large, more uniform dose of radiation can be concentrated in any tumor in part of the body, and should increase the cure rate. The actuarial survival curves for patients with cancer of the cervix show an improvement in survival between two different time periods. Lower curve: from 1935 to 1944, orthovoltage was used in Ontario. Upper curve: From 1958 through 1969, supervoltage telecobalt and accelerators were employed at Princess Margaret Hospital. The upper two curves represent the survival of normal populations of women in Ontario who had the same age distributions as the patients. Numbers in parentheses indicate the number of patients available for study. From Bush (6), with permission.

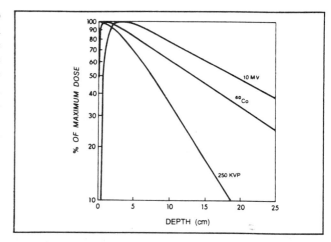

Fig. 7-8. Comparative depths of penetration for x- and -radiation beams. MV = Million volts; KVP = Kilovoltage peak; and ^{60}Co = Cobalt-60. From (2) Johns, H.; Cunningham, J. The physics of radiology, 4th ed. Springfield, IL: Charles C Thomas; 1983. Courtesy of Charles C Thomas, Publisher, Springfield, Illinois.

Advantages of High Linear Energy Transfer Beams (8)

Considerable effort has gone into the development of photon and pi-meson beams since these offer potential for the best distribution of radiation dose due to the physics of the beams. Both of these beams are characterized by having Bragg peaks in which the radiation is delivered deep into the tissues without much loss of energy until the desired depth in the tissue is reached. This is controlled by the level of megavoltage by which the particle is driven into the tissue. By regulating the megagavoltage, the depth of penetration can be controlled as well as using rotational mechanisms. When the beam reaches its desired depth, it releases all of its energy in a Bragg peak. A recent NCI proton workshop (13a) discusses both the theoretical and practical basis for the use of these beams.

1. *Highly focused beams*: π mesons, protons, and heavy ion beams release energy as a peak (Bragg peak) or burst at a certain depth, dependent on energy (Fig. 7-9) (10).

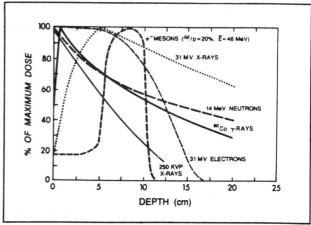

Fig. 7-9. The absorption of radiation as a function of depth. The absorbed dose versus depth for a number of different types of therapeutic beams of radiation is shown. π-mesons = particles; Δp/p = fractional production; and E = average energy. From Horst and Conrad (10), with permission.

2. *Biologically more effective*: Neutrons and charged particles are biologically more effective than low linear energy transfer (x and gamma) radiation. Clinical studies have shown neutrons to be superior for a few specific tumor sites — salivary gland, prostate, and soft tissue sarcomas. Charged particle beams are being explored in investigational studies.

RADIATION TREATMENT PLANNING

Steps in Developing a Radiation Treatment Plan

Treatment planning is a multistep process involving many independent components including staging, multiple diagnostic imaging studies and specialized radiation therapy equipment, such as simulators, linear accelerators, and treatment planning systems, that are not necessarily compatible. Treatment planning is presently undergoing a major transition from mainly a manual input of two-dimensional patient contour data into the treatment planning computer to direct acquisition of multiple cuts of a computed tomography (CT) scan with full three-dimensional treatment planning capabilities. To specify an optimum treatment dose distribution, the target volumes, critical structures, and prescribed dose levels must be defined with great accuracy in three dimensions rather than the single two-dimensional plans of the past. Tools are being developed to judge relative merits of various plans as well as implement them on treatment units.

Cancer staging: The staging of cancer is the first step in the treatment decision. Radiation treatment is usually designed to treat a target volume; this volume is often defined by the tumor site or structure of origin and its local spread to contiguous structures and regional lymph nodes. The extent of metastatic disease also requires definition, as do all fields that extend beyond the sites of obvious involvement. The tumor, node, metastasis system is used and the recommendations of the American Joint Committee (AJC) are followed (4).

Precise definition of the target volume: Planning and delivering treatment has been revolutionized by advances in imaging. Starting in the early 1970s with the advent of CT, and continuing into the 1980s with magnetic resonance imaging (MRI), the tumor extent and surrounding tissues have been increasingly better defined in three dimensions. The delineation of tumor from edema and host reactive changes reduces the risk of complications.

The first step in defining the target volume is the assessment of all relevant diagnostic studies and then correlation of patient anatomic information from one diagnostic study to another. This is essential for the most accurate definition of the target volume. Since CT contains electron density data essential to the radiation dose calculation and bony landmarks visible on plane films, CT is the basic treatment-planning tool. By using either pixel by pixel or bulk density data, corrections can be made for inhomogeneities, producing more accurate dose distributions.

Planning CT must be done with the patient in the exact position that will be used to deliver the treatments. For three-dimensional planning systems, each slice of the CT scan is displayed interactively and selected structures such as the tumor and critical organs are delineated on each slice and then combined to form a three-dimensional representation of the tumor, the target volume, and surrounding critical

structures (Fig. 7-10) (14). On two-dimensional systems only two or three CT images are selected on which to define the tumor and relevant surrounding anatomy giving a much more limited picture. For treatment sites where MRI has been proven to provide superior imaging, e.g., brain and spine, it would be ideal to register the MRI images with corresponding CT images and transfer the tumor locations to the CT. Once the tumor is defined in three dimensions, a margin for suspected microscopic extensions must be added to completely define the target volume or volumes. The target volume may actually be revised at specific prescribed dose levels since microscopic disease does not require the same sterilizing dose as gross tumor and critical organs may reach tolerance and need to be avoided.

The determination of whether involved sites and nodes are truly positive can be augmented by radiographically controlled needle biopsy. Surgical clips left by the surgeon at the time of resection can identify residual disease.

Identification of critical normal structures: Identifying in three-dimensions dose-limiting vital normal tissues that will be included in the treatment fields is an essential part of the treatment plan. The dose to the tumor needs to be given uniformly, but vital tissues and organs should receive as minimal a dose as is consistent with the prescription for the tumor. Table 6-5 in the previous chapter defines complications and tolerance doses for late effects.

Dosimetry: Underlying all treatment planning are computer and display technologies which have progressed rapidly, enabling significant improvements in planning capabilities. True three-dimensional treatment planning must still be developed to allow interactive users, provide access to large data bases, and optimize planning through automated routines rather than the iterative process routinely used. Only a few major institutions have true three-dimensional treatment planning systems due to the high cost, massive software development, and long time required to complete a three-dimensional treatment plan.

Actual treatment plans are developed by having a computer library of isodose distributions of the entire spectrum of beam energies and modalities available in a department for every field size for all open and wedged fields (Fig. 7-11) (2). The beam data can then be added to the three-dimensional

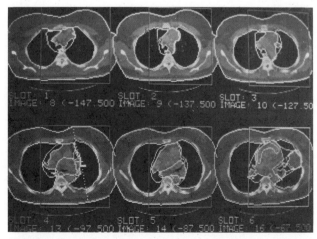

Fig. 7-10. Six computed tomography images simultaneously shown on a monitor with target volumes and critical structures outlined on each contour. From Purdy *et al.* (14) with permission.

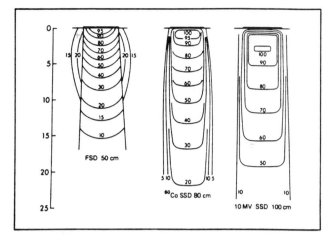

Fig. 7-11. Isodose distributions for 250 KVP and 10 MV X rays and cobalt-60 X rays. FSD = Focal skin distance: The distance from the focal spot in the x-ray tube to the skin of the patient. SSD = Source-surface distance: The distance from the front surface of the source of radiation to the surface of the patient. From Johns, H.; Cunningham, J. The Physics of Radiology, 4th ed. Springfield, IL: Charles C Thomas; 1983. Courtesy of Charles C Thomas, Publisher, Springfield, Illinois.

diagnostic imaging data to develop a treatment plan for the patient. No longer is treatment planning limited to multiple colinear beams, so that, in addition to shaped fixed beam fields and rotations, even conformational therapy is feasible where the multileaf collimators can dynamically vary the field size and shape as the treatment unit rotates around the patient (Fig.7-12) (7). By using multiple fields the actual differences in isodose distributions for different photon energies in the 4 to 18 MV range become negligible. The resulting plan at various levels (usually only one to three levels) can be displayed showing regions of equal dose or isodoses. Different

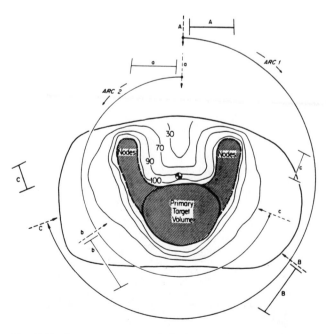

Fig. 7-12. A computer-controlled plan consisting of two arcs irradiates a primary lesion and the inguinal lymph nodes. From Chin *et al.* (7), with permission.

beam arrangements can be calculated and displayed to be assessed for delivering the prescribed dose and minimizing the dose to critical organs and normal tissues.

Traditionally, the "best" individualized plan for each patient is selected in consultation between the radiation physicist and radiation oncologist. Many alternative plans can be computed, but selecting the optimal one from a series of two-dimensional axial isodose plans is inadequate and becomes increasingly more difficult with more complex plans. To quantitatively evaluate dosimetry, one must have a clear understanding of what dose is being delivered in three dimensions.

Dose-volume histograms were developed to provide a more accurate analysis of the merits of competing plans. These histograms are a volumetric analysis of three-dimensional dose distributions which graphically summarizes the uniformity of dose and quickly shows the presence of hot or cold spots. From dose volume histograms of alternative treatment plans, plans that adequately treat the target volume can quickly be selected (Fig. 7-13a) (18). Similarly, these best plans can then be analyzed using dose volume histograms for minimizing the dose to critical organs (Fig. 7-13b,c) (18).

Simulation and Beam's Eye View: A diagnostic x-ray unit, a simulator, with geometric parameters identical to the treatment unit, is used to take radiographs of each of the treatment portals. The patient is immobilzed in the treatment position and fields marked. By drawing areas to be shielded on the simulation films, custom-made diverging blocks can be molded from low melting point alloy that permit only 3% to 5% transmission of the primary beam. Unfortunately, films taken at oblique angles are difficult to read and therefore are seldom shaped to avoid normal tissues.

The three-dimensional treatment planning systems use interactive computer graphics to generate a *beam's eye view* digital image of how the simulation film should look with the target volume and critical structures from that angle delineated, enabling custom shielding from any beam angle. Beam films, short-exposure films taken on the treatment unit to verify proper positioning of the patient and shields, can be matched to the beam's eye view images (Fig. 7-14) (18).

Quality assurance: Quality assurance and reproducibility of daily treatment are essential, since usually 25 to 30 treatments are required for a curative course of radiation therapy. The aim of most treatment is to reduce the variation in dose to less than ±5% at most. Radiation therapy quality control procedures have been developed through cooperative group studies. Weekly chart and beam film reviews are conducted by radiation oncologists, and machine calibrations and phantom and in vivo dosimetry are checked by radiation physicists to assure accuracy and consistency of dose. As both the treatment plans and the dose delivery equipment become more sophisticated, quality assurance becomes more essential for reproducibility and precise treatment.

RADIATION TREATMENT PLANS

Typical Plans

Head and neck tumors: Custom-shaped parallel opposed lateral fields treat the primary and electively treat the cervical nodal chain. At 40 Gy, the spinal cord is blocked, and anterior to the cord an additional 10 Gy is given. The posterior neck is treated with 9 to 13 MeV electrons to another 10 Gy for a

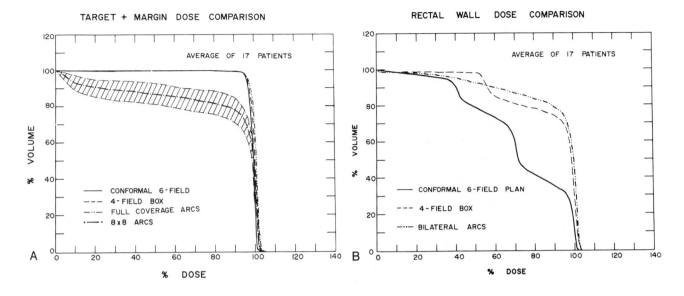

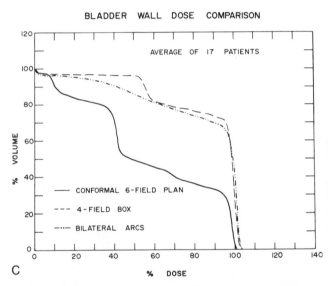

Fig. 7-13. (a) Integral dose-volume histograms (% of volume receiving greater than a given value of % isodose) of the target volume for the various prostate boost treatment techniques. All but the 8 x 8 bilateral arcs fully encompass the cover the target volume to high dose. (b) Integral dose-volume histograms of the rectal wall and bladder wall tissue at risk of receiving high dose for the various full field coverage techniques. The conformal six-field plan treats less normal tissue to high doses. From Ten Haken *et al.* (18), with permission.

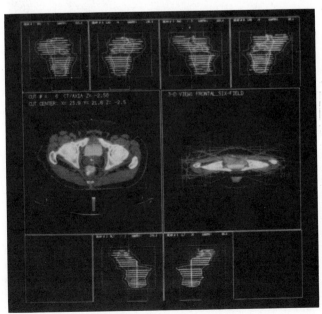

total dose of 50 Gy (Fig. 7-15a). A final boost is given to the primary and ipsilateral J-D node of another 20 Gy using a wedge pair to spare the contralateral parotid (Fig. 7-15b).

Breast cancer: Tangential fields allow for a uniform dose to the breast without excessive radiation to underlying lung. If the internal mammary nodes are treated with a separate photon IMC field the underlying mediastinal structures receive a significant dose (Fig 7-16a). A 12 to 15 MeV internal

Fig. 7-14. Confirmational six-field prostate boost technique. Three sets of opposing fields; laterals and ±45 degrees with respect to the lateral. (Center-left panel) Axial CT image with target volumes outlined. (Center-right panel) Panel perspective view of field arrangement with beam ports. (Outer panels) Beams Eye View displays for each of the six fields showing contours of the target volume and block edges which were automatically generated with a 0.5 cm margin around that volume. Clockwise from upper left, right posterior oblique, left anterior oblique, right anterior oblique, left posterior oblique, right lateral, left lateral. From Ten Haken *et al.* (18), with permission.

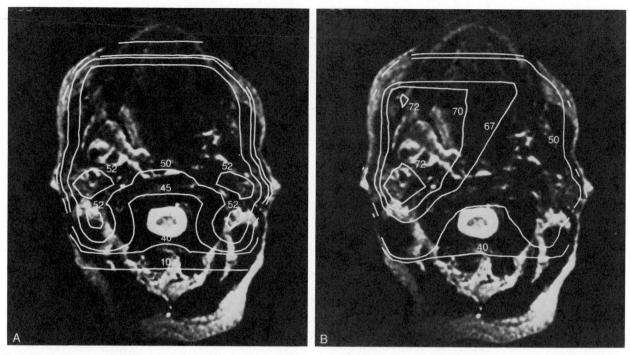

Fig. 7-15. A treatment plan for a carcinoma of the tonsillar region with an ipsilateral J-D node. (a) The primary and cervical nodal chain are treated to 50 Gy. (b) A wedge pair boosts the primary and J-D node to 70 Gy total dose while sparing the opposite parotid.

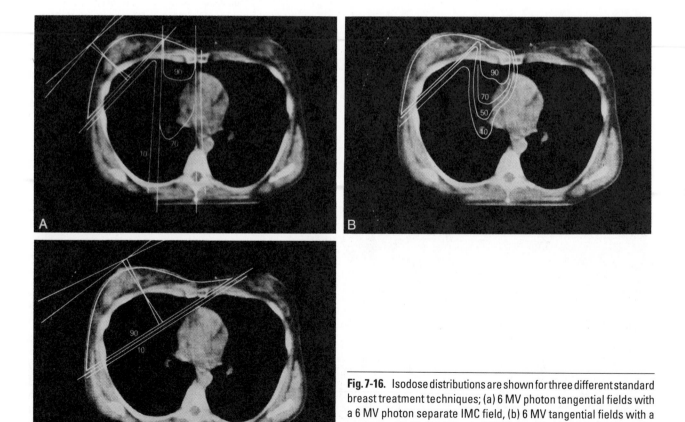

Fig. 7-16. Isodose distributions are shown for three different standard breast treatment techniques; (a) 6 MV photon tangential fields with a 6 MV photon separate IMC field, (b) 6 MV tangential fields with a separate 15 MeV electron IMC field, (c) 6 MV deep tangents encompassing both the IMC nodes and the breast. From Roberson *et al.* (15), with permission.

mammary electron field adequately treats the nodes but avoids the high dose to the underlying normal tissue (Fig.7-16b). To avoid patching of a separate IMC field to treat the internal mammary nodes, deep tangents are used extending across midline to the contralateral breast and treating a larger volume of lung (Fig. 7-16c) (15).

Lung tumor: Large, parallel, opposed custom-shaped lung fields treat both the primary and the mediastinal and hilar nodes. Since these fields include the spinal cord, at 40 Gy an oblique field arrangement will avoid the cord and still treat the primary and anterior mediastinal nodes to an additional 20 Gy for a total dose of 60 Gy, while keeping the cord dose below 45 Gy (Fig. 7-17).

Clinical Investigations Related to Treatment Planning

3-D Conformal/ Dynamic Radiation Therapy: One of the major advances has been the development of a new computer technology for treatment planning and computer-driven treatment systems (11b). The megavoltage linear accelerators have a wide range of energies for their therapeutic beams consisting both of photons and electrons and these can be readily mixed into optimal isodose designs. The multileaf collimators and on-line verification systems allow for highly customized (3D radiation treatment) potentially improving local regional curative cancer treatment. Simply stated, the goal of 3-D treatment planning is to conform the spatial distribution of high radiation dose to the shape of the tumor contour while decreasing the volume of surrounding normal tissue receiving high radiation doses. The essential principles are that volume reduction and exclusion of normal tissue will reduce complications while better targeting the tumor from beam's eye view set-ups which involve multiple fields and should permit tumor dose escalation. Essential to this hypothesis is that local regional control, particularly in early stages of disease where tumor advancement at the primary site and the degree of nodal involvement is either negative or limited to one to three and that metastatic disease can be

prevented. That is, the failure to control the primary tumor at the initial treatment significantly increases the metastatic dissemination. Evidence for this has been illustrated in head and neck, prostate, and cervix cancer sites. This phenomenon, the biological basis for this hypothesis, is that the enhanced mitotic activity associated with the regrowth process of locally recurring primary tumors promotes the multistep transformation of non-metastatic tumors into clonogens with metastatic potential, leading to increased overall rates of metastatic disease. Thus, through the identification of more effective therapeutic strategies designed to eradicate the primary tumor completely at the site at the time of initial therapy a strong rationale for clinical studies using 3-D conformal radiation therapy is provided.

A number of clinical research projects are being pursued at a few institutions. Much of the innovative research is related to the implementation of CT and MRI technologies in the clinic. For example, in 3-D conformational/dynamic radiation therapy, an X ray photon beam is shaped dynamically while it is rotating around the patient to conform to the tumor projection from that angle derived from the CT study. The beam shaping is done by a computer-driven multileaf collimator. Conformational therapy minimizes the dose to the normal tissue while delivering a uniform dose to the tumor volume (8a,11c).

Intraoperative radiation therapy (IORT) is currently used for the treatment of advanced tumors of the pelvis and retroperitoneum, where normal tissue tolerance would limit conventional-beam radiation therapy. At the time of surgery, a single, large fraction of 15 to 20 Gy is delivered to the tumor or the tumor bed. Usually electrons in the 6 to 20 MeV range are used, although orthovoltage is also being tried. The advantage of IORT is that the area to be treated is well-defined at the time of surgery and normal tissues can be excluded from the treatment volume by either moving them out of the way or shielding them.

Investigations are currently being done to study the tolerance of normal tissues that are not normally dose-limiting, such as peripheral nerves and blood vessels, to IORT. Various US centers have reported promising results using IORT, but long-term studies will have to be undertaken to determine whether IORT achieves superior local control without unacceptable morbidity.

Stereotactic radiosurgery: Another new technique being explored is stereotactic radiosurgery (11a). Small photon or heavy charged particle beams are used to deliver single large doses to small intracranial tumors or arterio-venous malformations. Recent advances in brain imaging have allowed intracranial structures to be accurately localized. Once the target volume has been determined, a uniform dose must be delivered with high spatial accuracy and a rapid dose fall-off outside the target volume. To accomplish this, the patient's head is immobilized in a stereotactic frame, imaged for tumor localization, and then treated.

Initially, specially designed multiple cobalt-60 sources or high-energy, heavy charged particle beams were used, but techniques using isocentric linear accelerators as a less expensive and more available alternative are being developed. By using various moving-beam techniques such as single-plane full rotations, noncoplanar converging arcs, and dynamic simultaneous couch and gantry rotations, the desired tumor doses can be delivered with the acceptable dose gradients outside the target volume.

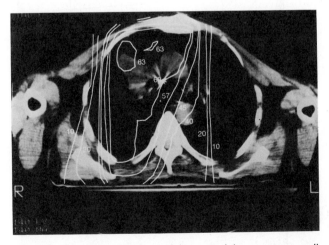

Fig. 7-17. Treatment plan for a right upper lobe squamous cell carcinoma of the lung. Custom shaped parallel opposed fields treat the primary and mediastinal and hilar nodes to 40 Gy. A parallel opposed oblique boost avoids the spinal cord while delivering another 20 Gy to the primary and anterior mediastinal and ipsilateral hilar nodes.

HYPERTHERMIA

Hyperthermia, which means "high temperature" (108°F to 113°F or 42°C to 45°C) is a new adjuvant therapy for cancer treatment. The idea of using heat to treat tumors is not new. There are reports from the late 1800s which noted the surprising remissions or shrinkage of tumors in certain cancer patients who had high fever due to an infection. Other techniques, such as a hot bath of wax or water, were later tried and remained experimental until the mid 1900s.

Physics of Hyperthermia

With the introduction of radio frequency and microwaves combined with new thermometry devices, hyperthermia has been gaining more ground since the mid 1960s. Modern hyperthermia machines are capable of better heat delivery than before to cancerous parts of a body with much reduced risks and complication and a greater degree of comfort to patients. In recent years, these advances have made hyperthermia an acceptable therapy mode. Most of the current machines are microwave or ultrasound in nature. Most microwave machines operate in a fixed mode at 915 MHz. The 915 MHz frequency is approved by the Federal Communication Commission for medical purposes and does not require any special shielding. Microwaves at the 915 MHz frequency have a penetration depth of about 3 cm which makes them easier to apply externally via special wave guides known as applicators with little leakage and exposure to the operating personnel.

An alternative to the 915 MHz microwaves is the use of ultrasound, whose frequency ranges from 0.5 to 3 MHz in frequency. Ultrasound is normally applied externally through high-frequency sound generated by a transducer. The function of a transducer is to convert electrical signals into mechanical signals such as sound waves. Ultrasounds have the ability to penetrate deep (~ 10 cm) and can be focused on the center of a tumor or it can be manipulated so that the focal point can move on the periphery of a tumor. The disadvantage of ultrasound is its high reflection as it passes through one medium into another (e.g., gas cavities or bones). Yet ultrasound has shown great promise in the treatment of head and neck, and solid tumors. Again, the fact that ultrasound transducers can be manipulated mechanically via computers to scan a tumor or a region of a body by focused ultrasound has made this modality a useful tool.

In recent years, a new mode of hyperthermia treatment, interstitial hyperthermia, has also been gaining ground. Interstitial hyperthermia uses microwaves to heat the tumors internally (invasively). For this purpose, special wirelike microwave antennas of various designs are used inside catheters that are placed in the tumor in a prearranged position. By varying the amount of power delivered to each antenna and/or varying their phase shift, one can achieve a desired heating pattern.

Most interstitial antennae available today operate at 915 MHz, which makes them compatible with most hyperthermia systems currently in use. In most cases, these antennae have an active heating length of 7 to 10 cm and can fit in 16-gauge catheters. An important advantage of interstitial hyperthermia is that it can be planned with brachytherapy implants, so that the same catheters can be used for insertion of heating antennae and placement of special radioactive materials. In this procedure, the heat is normally given first, then the radioactive implants are placed. Heat can be applied after the removal of the radioactive materials. Well-planned brachytherapy-interstitial hyperthermia can minimize the risk of complication to a patient by using this invasive procedure only once.

Other hyperthermia treatment techniques, such as capacitative heating, radiofrequency heating, ferromagnetic seed implants, and whole body heating, are being tried, but to date they are considered experimental and have not won any Food and Drug Administration approval. Presently, microwave and ultrasound heating techniques currently are dominant, and are considered an established clinical adjuvant to radiation therapy and chemotherapy.

Biology of Hyperthermia

Although the biology of hyperthermia seems simple, it is yet not fully understood and appreciated. What is known is that heat is effective in killing the cancerous cells in a predictable and repeatable manner. Figure 7-18 (8) shows the most classic effect of heat on cells, which is similar in shape to the effect of radiation on cells.

Another factor in hyperthermia which has been observed experimentally: the complementary effect that heat and irradiation have on cancer cells. This effect is illustrated in Fig. 7-19 (19), which shows the cell survival rate as a function of heat and irradiation during the different cell cycles. The complementary effect of heat and irradiation is emphasized in Fig. 7-20 (16), which shows the optimal effect produced when heat and radiation therapy are given simultaneously, or within short time intervals.

In conclusion, hyperthermia is shown clinically to be effective and beneficial, especially in those patients who have had previous radiation therapy and still have recurrence. In such cases, a short course of radiation therapy combined with hyperthermia is considered the best treatment modality (Table 7-3).

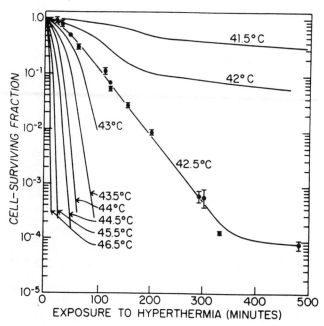

Fig. 7-18. Survival curves for mammalian cells in culture heated at different temperatures for varying lengths of time. From Dewey *et al.* (8), with permission.

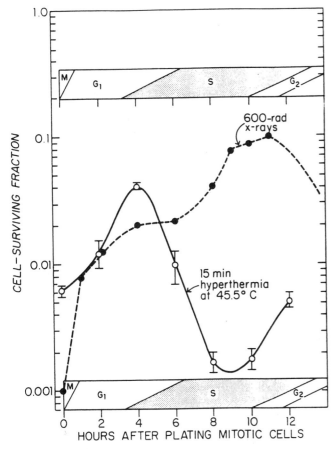

Fig. 7-19. Comparison of the fractions of cells surviving heat or x-irradiation delivered at various phases of the cell cycle. The heat treatment consisted of 15 minutes at 45.5°C, and the x-ray dose was 6 Gy. From Westra and Dewey (19), with permission.

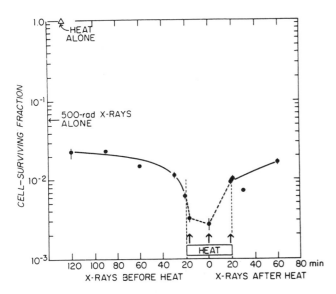

Fig. 7-20. Survival of Chinese hamster cells irradiated with 5 Gy of x-rays before, during, or after a heat treatment of 40 minutes at 42.5°C. No killing was observed with this heat treatment alone (open triangle). The effect of 5 Gy of x-ray alone is shown by the arrow. There is a clear interaction between heat and x-rays, with the maximum effect being produced if the x-rays are delivered midway through the heat treatment. From Sapareto *et al.* (16), with permission.

Table 7-3. The Most Widely Used Schedule for Radiation and Hyperthermia Combined Treatment

	Cure	Palliation
Radiation	60 - 66 Gy, 1.8 Gy/d	32 - 40 Gy, 4 Gy fx 2/wk
Hyperthermia	43°C/60 min, 2/wk	43°C/60 min, 2/wk

Modified from Scott (17).

Recommended Reading

The student will find Hendee's *Medical Radiation Physics* (1), Johns' and Cunningham's *The Physics of Radiology* (2) and Khan's *The Physics of Radiation Therapy* (3) to be good introductions and comprehensive references to the subject of the physics of radiation oncology. Hall's *Radiobiology for the Radiobiologist* (9) has excellent introductions to radiobiology hyperthermia.

REFERENCES

General References

1. Hendee, W.R. Medical radiation physics, 2nd ed. Chicago, IL: Year Book Medical Publishers; 1979.
2. Johns, H.; Cunningham, J. The physics of radiology, 4th ed. Springfield, IL: C. C. Thomas; 1983.
3. Khan, F.M. The Physics of Radiation Therapy. Baltimore, MD: Williams & Wilkins; 1984.

Specific References

4. American Joint Committee on Cancer Staging and End-Results Reporting (AJC). Manual for staging of cancer. Chicago, IL: AJC; 1987.
5. Bartlett, J. Familiar quotations. Boston, MA: Little, Brown and Co.; 1955.
6. Bush, R.S. Malignancies of ovaries, uterus, cervix. London, UK: Edward Arnold; 1979.
7. Chin, L.M.; Kijewski, P.K.; Svensson, G.K.; Bjarngard, B.E. Dose optimization with computer-controlled gantry rotation, collimator motion and dose-rate variation. Int. J. Radiat. Oncol. Biol. Phys. 9:723-729; 1983.
8. Dewey, W.C.; Hopwood, L.E.; Sapareto, S.A.; Geruak, L.E. Cellular response to combination of hyperthermia and radiation. Radiology. 123: 464-477; 1977.
8a. Fagundas, H.; Perez, C.A.; Grigsby, P.W.; Lockett, M.A. Distant metastasis after irradiation alone in carcinoma ofthe uterine cervix. Int J Radiat Oncol Biol Phys. 24(1); 1992.
9. Hall, E J. Radiobiology for the radiobiologist, 3rd ed. Philadelphia, PA: J. B. Lippincott Co.; 1988: 262-291.
10. Horst, W.; Conrad, B. Radiotherapie des Krebses mit negativen Pi-Mesonen. Ein Bericht zum Zuriches. ETH-Isochronzykotron. Fortschr. Rontgenstr. 105:299-321; 1966.
11. Kaplan, H.S. Hodgkin's disease, 2nd ed. Cambridge, MA: Harvard University Press; 1980.
11a. Kooy, H.M; Nedzi, L.A.; Loeffler, J.S.; Alexander III, E.; Cheng, W-w.; Mannarino, E.G.; Holupka, E.J.; Siddon, R.L. Treatment planning for stereotactic radiosurgery of intra-cranial lesions. Int J Radiat Oncol Biol Phys. 21:683-694; 1991.
11b. Leibel, S.A.; Ling, C.C.; Kutcher, G.J.; Mohan, R.; Cordon-Cordo, C.; Fuks, Z. The biological basis for conformal three-dimensional radiation therapy. Int J Radiat Oncol Biol Phys. 21:805-811; 1991.
11c. Leibel, S.A.; Scott, C.B.; Mohiuddin, M.; Marcial, V.A.; Coia, L.R.; Davis, L.W.; Fuks, Z. The effect of local-regional control on distant metastatic dissemination in carcinoma of the head and neck: Results of an analysis from the RTOG head and neck database. Int J Radiat Oncol Biol Phys. 21:549-556; 1991.
12. Levitt, S., ed. Characteristics of megavoltage external radiation beams. Minneapolis, MN: University of Minnesota Press; 1973.
13. Medical Physics Data Book, NBS Handbook 138, Washington, DC: U. S. Government Printing Office; 1982:88.

13a. NCI Proton Workshop: Potential clinical gains by use superior radiation dose distribution. Int J Radiat Oncol Biol Phys. 22(2): 233-383; 1992.

14. Purdy, J. A.; Wong, J.W. ; Harms, W. B.; Emami, B.; Matthews, J. W. State of the art of high energy photon treatment planning. Front. Radiat. Ther. Oncol., 21:4-24; 1987.

15. Roberson, P.L.; Lichter, A,S.; Bodner, A.; Fredrickson, H.A.; Padikal, T.N.; Kelly, B.A.; Van de Geijn, J. Dose to lung in primary breast irradiation . Int.J. Rad. Oncol. Biol. Phys. 9:97-102;1983.

16. Sapareto, S.A.; Hopwood, L.E.; Dewey, W.C. Combined effects of X-irradiation and hyperthermia on CHO cells for various temperatures and orders of application. Radiat. Res. 73(2); 221; 1978.

17. Scott, R.S. Hyperthermia applications. Clinitherm Corp.; 1987.

18. Ten Haken, R.K.; Perez-Tamayo, C.; Tesser, R.J.; McShan, D.L.; Fraass, B.A.; Lichter, A.S. Boost treatment of the prostate using shaped, fixed fields. Intl. J. Rad. Oncol. Biol. Phys. 16:193-200; 1989.

19. Westra, A.; Dewey, W.C. Variation in sensitivity to heat shock during the cell cycle of Chinese hamster cells in vitro. Int. J. Radiat. Oncol. Biol. Phys. 19: 467-477; 1971.

Richard F. Bakemeier, M.D., Medical Oncology
Raman Qazi, M.D., F.A.C.P., Medical Oncology

Chapter **8**

BASIC CONCEPTS OF CANCER CHEMOTHERAPY AND PRINCIPLES OF MEDICAL ONCOLOGY

*Diseases desperate grown
By desperate appliances are relieved
Or not at all*

Hamlet IV.iii 9

PERSPECTIVE

The previously prevalent view that chemotherapy was appropriate only for disseminated stage of cancer is fast becoming obsolete. Since the last edition of this manual, the adjuvant chemotherapy concept of eradicating occult micrometastases through the use of cytotoxic drugs as a complement to local surgery or radiation therapy has been well established. The effectiveness of adjuvant chemotherapy in osteogenic sarcoma and its usefulness in limb salvage has been clearly established (28,29). In high-risk patients with breast cancer, several large randomized studies have confirmed improvement in disease-free and overall survival with adjuvant therapy (16,30,35). Preoperative adjuvant therapy in bladder and head and neck cancer can reduce the need for extensive surgery (40,60). Cure rate with cisplatin-containing chemotherapy is so high in disseminated testicular cancer that need for adjuvant chemotherapy, although effective, is obviated (59).

In the last two decades, medical oncology has also become firmly established as a subspecialty of internal medicine. It encompasses many facets of internal medicine, including infectious diseases and immunology, pulmonary medicine, gastroenterology, hematology, neurology,nephrology, and endocrinology. The major functions of a medical oncologist are the interpretation of the natural history of malignant diseases; the appropriate application of cancer chemotherapeutic techniques, both in the adjuvant setting for primary tumors and for disseminated malignancies; the diagnosis and management of complications of the diseases; and the coordination of emotional, nutritional, and social support. Since approximately two-thirds of the 1,000,000 or more cancer patients diagnosed in the United States annually develop recurrent or disseminated neoplastic disease, a clear need exists for widespread availability of physicians with skills in the discipline (18,19,27).

The medical oncologist should be well informed in the basic principles of the pharmacology of cancer chemotherapy

and pain control; tumor pathobiology, which includes cell kinetics; patterns of metastasis; immunologic aspects of neoplasia; cancer epidemiology; and early detection methods. The development of more effective chemotherapeutic techniques depends on using currently available drugs in optimal ways, as well as in developing new agents. Participation in the clinical trials of cooperative groups is important for progress in this area (see Chapter 9, "Basic Concepts in Investigational Therapeutics and Clinical Trials"). These clinical trials also involve the study of a variety of biologic response modifiers, about which the medical oncologist should stay informed. These will be discussed in Chapter 10, "Basic Concepts of Tumor Immunology and Principles of Immunotherapy."

The history of cancer chemotherapy is relatively brief. The first clinical studies involving nitrogen mustard were undertaken by Gilman, Goodman, Lindskog, and Dougherty in 1942 (although the myelosuppressive and lympholytic properties of mustards were recognized as early as 1919) (1). Another major milestone was the demonstration in 1948 by Farber and associates of a beneficial effect of a folic acid analog in acute lymphoblastic leukemia of childhood. The purine antagonist 6-mercaptopurine was described by Elion and Hitchings in 1952, one of a series of contributions that led to the recent awarding of a Nobel prize. Heidelberger synthesized 5-FU in the early 1950s after reasoning correctly that such an antimetabolite resembling uracil should block the formation of thymine nucleotides and thereby prevent DNA synthesis. This antipyrimidine is still a mainstay of cancer chemotherapy 40 years later.

In the 1960s many new antineoplastic drugs came into clinical use, and in subsequent years the emphasis has been on developing new combinations of available drugs, optimizing their timing and dosage, and modulating their toxicities.

The proper application of new drugs or new combinations of standard agents requires knowledge of the mechanisms of action and metabolism of the drugs involved, as well as their effects on normal tissues. Bone marrow cell kinetics and morphology are particularly important, as is knowledge of drug-induced alterations in renal, gastrointestinal (GI), and pulmonary function. The number and variety of available chemotherapeutic agents, each most useful with a particular group of malignancies, have made true expertise in this field a challenging — even formidable — goal. However, virtually all physicians whose responsibilities involve cancer patient management should have a general appreciation of the principles of cancer chemotherapy. This includes the indications for palliative and adjuvant drug treatment for the common malignancies and the recognition and management of the most frequently experienced side effects of standard chemotherapeutic agents.

It is of primary importance that realistic goals be set for programs of chemotherapy, because these will influence the choice of agents and the intensity of treatment. For example, chemotherapy offers the possibility of complete cure for disseminated Hodgkin's disease, choriocarcinoma in women, metastatic testicular carcinoma, rhabdomyosarcoma, Ewing's sarcoma, and acute lymphoblastic leukemia in children. Currently the most common metastatic human cancers, including those of lung, colon and breast, fail to show satisfactory long-term control or cure, even with intensive chemotherapy programs. However, progress continues toward solutions of these important problems.

The optimal application of antineoplastic drugs requires consideration of:
1. The biologic characteristics of the neoplastic disease.
2. The pharmacology of the agents to be used.
3. The spectrum of drug effectiveness as determined through clinical trials and through currently evolving predictive tests, in vitro and in vivo.
4. The clinical condition of the patient, including nutrition, infections, hematologic status, emotional profile, and general level of activity.

The following discussion will briefly consider these topics, and the reader is referred to more extensive references for additional details (see General References).

TUMOR BIOLOGIC ASPECTS OF CANCER CHEMOTHERAPY

Malignant Transformation

Effective chemotherapeutic control of neoplastic cell growth ideally will be based on knowledge of specific quantitative and qualitative changes in cellular biology resulting from malignant transformation. Such transformation involves a heritable change in a stem cell of virtually any tissue, resulting in the production of daughter cells with absent or imperfect observation of normal homeostatic controls or of normal differentiation. Current knowledge leaves unanswered many relevant questions concerning the genotypic and phenotypic changes involved in the abnormal proliferative, invasive, and metastatic characteristics of cancer cells (see Chapter 2, "The Biology of Cancer").

Some human neoplastic cell genomes have been shown to contain DNA similar to the oncogenes associated with neoplastic transformation in animal tumor systems caused by certain viruses. Furthermore, homologous sequences of DNA have been identified in normal human cells. These cellular

proto-oncogenes function in normal processes of growth and differentiation, and in viral or chemical carcinogenesis they may be activated through mutation, translocation, or gene amplification. Although the mechanisms by which oncogenes contribute to the changes associated with malignancy are still not fully explained, the products of these genes have been identified. They include tyrosine-specific protein kinase activity, growth factors or growth factor receptors, GTP-binding activity, and nuclear proteins which may be involved in chromatin activation (48,52) (see Chapter 2, "The Biology of Cancer").

As these mechanisms are clarified, it seems likely that specific biochemical targets will be identified toward which new chemotherapeutic agents can be directed. The resulting information may permit specific manipulation of the differentiation and proliferation of malignant cells in a manner that spares major alterations in normal cell functions.

Kinetic Basis of Chemotherapy

Tumor cell burden: Fig. 8-1 provides a graphic representation of several concepts important in cancer chemotherapy. One of these concepts is that of the tumor cell burden. The simplified growth curve of the tumor in Fig. 8-1 begins at a hypothetica time-zero. An event occurs from which the first surviving tumor stem cell, or clonogenic cell, results, deviating from its normal counterparts in a manner that permits inappropriate differentiation and proliferation. As tumor cell division occurs, at rates varying from hours to weeks, cells accumulate in one or more sites in numbers that usually must approximate at least 10^9 cells in one location (a mass approximately 1 cm in diameter) for their detection at the so-called clinical horizon. This tumor growth process will involve many cell divisions and tumor size doublings, during which can occur a number of changes important in an eventual interaction of the tumor cells with chemotherapeutic agents. These include changes in:
1. Vascular supply, which eventually may become inadequate, providing poor nutrition of the central zone of the tumor and poor exposure to chemotherapeutic agents.
2. Genetically-determined resistance to chemotherapy, which may result from selective killing of cells in the tumor initially sensitive to the agent, overgrowth of residual chemoresistant cells, (see below), and further development of heterogeneous populations of resistant cells by sequential mutations.

Fig. 8-1 also indicates the various outcomes of tumor therapy. Initial therapy, whether it be surgery, radiation therapy, or cytotoxic chemotherapy, may be curative. If noncurative, the tumor cell burden may be reduced to 10^4 or 10^5 cells. Cytotoxic agents characteristically kill tumor cells according to first-order kinetics, meaning that a constant percentage rather than a constant number of remaining tumor cells is killed by a given exposure to the drug. The killing of 99.999% of the cells when the tumor burden is 10^9 will leave 10^4 cells. Such relatively low tumor cell burdens are usually not detectable without the aid of a biochemical marker such as the beta-subunit of human chorionic gonadotropin (beta-HCG) in gestational trophoblastic disease and certain testicular carcinomas. Despite the appearance of a complete remission, the survival of this reduced number of tumor cells may eventually lead to a clinical recurrence following additional tumor

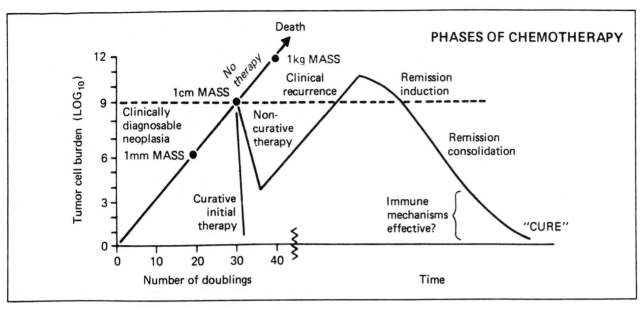

Fig. 8-1. Concept of tumor cell burden and relation to phases of treatment.

doublings, the rate of which depends on the summation of tumor cell divisions and cell death. One of the major roles of chemotherapy is the management of disseminated recurrences with regimens designed for remission induction and consolidation. Such treatment may lead to a significant number of cures, as in testicular carcinoma, Hodgkin's disease, acute lymphoblastic leukemia, and large cell lymphomas. Alternatively, they may lead to effective palliation of symptoms, even without cure.

Cell cycle and growth fraction: The growth and division of cells, both normal and neoplastic, can be diagrammed as in Fig. 8-2 (13). The phases of the cell cycle are termed G1 (G = gap), S (synthesis of DNA), G2 (premitotic interval), and M (mitosis). A prolonged G1 phase or resting phase is com-

monly termed G0. Consideration of the phase(s) in which a given cytotoxic agent has an effect and the time intervals involved are potentially important factors in the choice of agents and the timing of their administration. Since the mechanism of action of most cytotoxic agents involves processes associated with cell division, the response of tumor cells to chemotherapeutic agents is generally enhanced by a large *growth fraction*, i.e., a large percentage of the tumor cells proceeding through the mitotic cycle (i.e., dividing) at any given time. By choosing agents acting in different phases of the cell cycle, combinations of phase-specific drugs, such as those indicated in Fig. 8-2, can be administered with increased tumor cell killing potential. It should also be noted, however, that actively growing *normal* tissues, such as bone marrow, GI epithelium, and hair follicles, are also highly susceptible to the effects of most cytotoxic antineoplastic agents. Toxicity for these normal tissues affects the dose and frequency with which cytotoxic agents safely may be given.

Tumor Cell Resistance to Chemotherapy

Malignant tumors consist of heterogeneous populations of cells depending on their stage in the cell cycle, their distance from the vascular supply of nutrients and drugs, and their genetically-determined resistance to cytotoxic drugs. The latter heterogeneity is illustrated by an initial tumor response to chemotherapy, (representing the killing of chemosensitive cells), followed by progressive regrowth in spite of continued administration of the agent (representing the proliferation of initially chemoresistant cells that attain a selective advantage). Biochemical mechanisms of resistance have been demonstrated in animal or human tumor cells:
- decreased drug uptake
- decreased drug-activating enzymes
- increased drug-inactivating enzymes
- increased levels of the inhibited target enzyme
- altered affinity of the target enzyme for the drug
- increased DNA repair
- increase in an alternative metabolic pathway bypassing the drug inhibition
- increase in drug removal from the cell

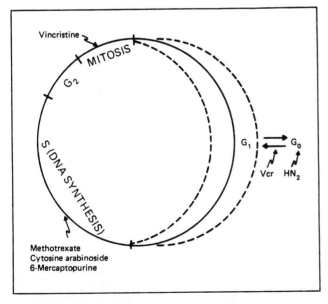

Fig. 8-2. The mitotic cycle with sites of action of certain phase-specific antitumor agents. G_1 = (Gap 1) resting phase; G_2 = (Gap 2) premitotic interval; G_0 = prolonged G_1, or resting phase; Vcr = vincristine; HN_2 = nitrogen mustard.

The last mechanism has been associated with multidrug (pleiotropic) resistance, in which tumor cells become resistant to several structurally unrelated agents. Such cells have been found to be able to pump out these drugs, apparently as a result of high levels of a membrane glycoprotein (P-glycoprotein). Identification of increased levels of P-glycoprotein has the potential of identifying non-responsive tumors. By identifying pleiotrophic resistance, it may be possible to reverse this resistance with other drugs, such as verapamil or quinidine, which increase the intracellular accumulation of the cytotoxic drugs.

Other approaches to preventing the emergence of drug-resistant tumor cell populations include the use of combinations of drugs with independent mechanisms of action (Fig. 8-3). This approach can be extended to the use of two or more alternating non-cross-resistant combinations of several drugs each (21) and using maximal drug doses (42). Much of the approach to this problem is founded on the Goldie-Coldman hypothesis, put forward in 1979, which assumes that drug-resistant cells arise spontaneously at a measurable mutation rate, and that the earlier and more intensively a tumor can be treated, the more the likelihood of fewer drug-resistant cells (22).

Much attention has been devoted over the past decade to the development of predictive assays involving cultured human tumor cells exposed in vitro to cytotoxic drugs (9). A reliable predictive assay would indicate the likelihood of tumor cell chemosensitivity or resistance, and would reduce the need to expose patients to sequential trials of toxic but possibly ineffective drugs. Unfortunately, all tumor specimens cannot be successfully cultured, and when they are the prediction of clinically significant drug sensitivity is correct in only approximately half of patients. However, this tool is potentially important and its investigation continues.

PHARMACOLOGIC ASPECTS OF CANCER CHEMOTHERAPY

Absorption, Distribution, Biotransformation, and Excretion

Optimal application of antineoplastic drugs also requires consideration of general principles of pharmacology, including drug absorption, distribution, biotransformation, and excretion (3).

Absorption: Absorption of drugs determines the route of administration appropriate for a given agent, e.g., oral (PO), intramuscular (IM), intravenous (IV), or intrathecal (IT). The rate of absorption affects the concentration achieved and thus the duration and intensity of the exposure of cancer cells to the drug. The pharmacokinetics, or alterations with time of concentrations of a drug following administration, are important in determining the appropriate dose and intervals between doses. Optimal administration of a given drug may prove to be large, intermittent pulse doses, which will result in periodic high drug gradients across cell membranes, constant infusion for several days, or daily PO dosage on a long-term basis.

Distribution: The concentration and effectiveness of antineoplastic drugs can sometimes be enhanced by local or regional administration, including instillation into a body cavity such as the pleural or intrathecal space, or into an artery, with localization of the drug through infusion. These maneuvers may overcome barriers to the distribution of a drug into "sanctuary sites," such as the central nervous system (CNS). The choice of the agent according to its tissue distribution characteristics also may be important, as is its route of delivery. For example, the nitrosoureas have greater lipid solubility than most other agents, related to their ability to enter the CNS.

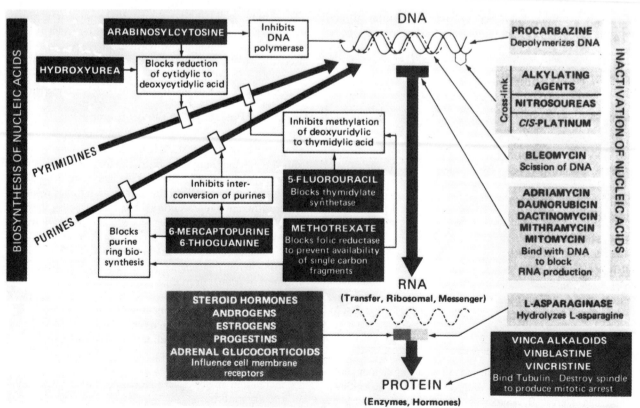

Fig. 8-3. Sites of action of common antineoplastic drugs.

Biotransformation: An example of biotransformation of a cancer chemotherapeutic agent is the activation of the alkylating agent cyclophosphamide by the mixed-function oxidase system of the liver without which the agent is ineffective. Likewise, 5-fluorouracil (5-FU) must be phosphorylated before it is active. The inactivation of an antineoplastic agent must also be kept in mind when considering its use. For example, the purine analogue 6-mercaptopurine (6-MP) is catabolized by the enzyme xanthine oxidase. Its toxicity is increased when it is used concurrently with allopurinol, an inhibitor of the enzyme xanthine oxidase. Since allopurinol is commonly used to prevent hyperuricemia in malignant diseases, the interaction of these two drugs is not a rare occurrence, and 6-MP doses must be reduced in this situation.

Excretion: Excretion patterns of antineoplastic agents are important determinants of toxicity and of the need for alterations in drug dosage, especially when there is impairment of excretory organ function. Since methotrexate, a dihydrofolate reductase inhibitor, is largely excreted by the kidney, doses must be reduced if there is renal impairment. To compound the problem, high doses of methotrexate may also cause increased renal impairment by precipitating in renal tubules, particularly in acid conditions. In the presence of impaired liver function or biliary obstruction, vincristine and doxorubicin doses should be reduced because their excretion in bile is decreased under those circumstances. For a more extensive discussion of these subjects, the reader is referred to other sources (3,4a,21).

Mechanisms of Drug Action

Selection of agents: Understanding the pharmacodynamics of antineoplastic agents is fundamental to their appropriate use. This includes knowledge of the mechanisms of action and physiologic effects of these agents (Fig. 8-3). The majority of current cytotoxic agents act primarily on macromolecular synthesis or function, that is, on the production or function of DNA, RNA, or protein. Thus, although there are approximately 30 available antineoplastic drugs from which to choose, there is considerable overlap in their mechanisms of action. These agents can be grouped into several classes (see Table 8-1 for more details):

- alkylating agents
- antimetabolites
- natural products
  - antibiotics
  - plant alkaloids
  - enzymes
- miscellaneous agents
- hormones and hormone inhibitors

The choice of a chemotherapeutic agent for a given tumor type is generally not a consequence of a priori prediction of antitumor activity by the drug, but is instead the result of empiric clinical trials (see Chapter 9, "Basic Concepts in Investigational Therapeutics and Clinical Trials").

Design of combinations: Since single agents are, with few exceptions, unable to effect cures or even significant remissions, multiple agents are usually administered concurrently or sequentially. This affords the advantages of maximizing the likelihood of tumor cell death by damaging several different biochemical sites, of minimizing the proliferation of resistant tumor cells, and of minimizing the toxicity to normal tissues. Fundamentals to be noted in designing drug combinations are:

- use only drugs that show some activity against the tumor type
- select drugs which differ in their mechanisms of action
- select drugs which differ in the site of their major toxicities (although bone marrow suppression is common to many and is difficult to avoid)
- use optimal doses and timing for each drug (allowing recovery of toxic changes in normal tissues between doses)

An example of the application of these principles is the four-drug CHOP combination for lymphoma. This consists of intermittent doses of cyclophosphamide (an alkylating agent whose major toxicity is marrow suppression); doxorubicin (also termed hydroxydaunorubicin, an antibiotic with DNA-intercalating properties whose major toxicities are marrow suppression and cardiac toxicity at higher doses); vincristine (a vinca alkaloid with peripheral nerve toxicity but very little bone marrow suppression); and prednisone (a synthetic corticosteroid hormone with effects on glucose metabolism and bone matrix). Other non-marrow suppressive drugs, such as bleomycin or methotrexate with leucovorin (folinic acid) rescue, may be used with this combination in the intervals when blood cell counts are low from cyclophosphamide and doxorubicin. The first letters of the drug names are often combined to provide a useful abbreviation, CHOP, MOPP (mechlorethamine/vincristine/procarbazine/prednisone), CMF (cyclophosphamide/methotrexate/5-FU), and CAF (cyclophosphamide/doxorubicin/5-FU).

Synergy and antagonism of drugs: A related phenomenon, which deserves increased attention in its ability to improve the results of combination chemotherapy, is that of *biochemical modulation*, by which two or more drugs interact to enhance their effects (*synergy*) or decrease them (*antagonism*). Knowledge of mechanisms of action of drugs and of intermediary cell metabolism allows the oncologic pharmacologist to predict possible interactions, which may include:

1. *Synergistic inhibition of metabolic pathways.*
   a. Enzyme blockade—cooperative, sequential, or concurrent.
   b. Increased intracellular drug levels from increased influx or decreased efflux (e.g., decreased doxorubicin efflux by verapamil, quinidine).
   c. Increased drug activation (e.g., increased phosphorylation of 5-FU by increased pyrophosphate levels resulting from methotrexate inhibition of synthetic pathways).
2. *Synergistic inhibition of macromolecular synthesis*, repair, or processing.
3. *Synergistic enhancement of cellular toxicity* (without biochemical interaction).
   a. Cell cycle synchronization
4. *Host-selective rescue*: (e.g., leucovorin rescue from methotrexate, diethyldithiocarbamate and thiourea from cisplatin). In the absence of large numbers of new antineoplastic agents greater exploitation of these synergistic effects of two or more drugs should be pursued (23).

CLINICAL ASPECTS OF CANCER CHEMOTHERAPY

Although every potential chemotherapy patient should be approached as an individual, with consideration of a broad range of physiologic and psychologic factors, certain gener-

Table 8-1. Chemotherapeutic Agents and Their Common Abbreviations

Agent	Trade Name	Abbreviation
ALKYLATING AGENTS		
I. NITROGEN MUSTARDS		
Mechlorethamine	Mustargen, nitrogen mustard	HN^2
Cyclophosphamide	Cytoxan, Endoxan	CTX
Ifosfamide	Ifex	IFS
Phenylalanine mustard	Melphalan, Alkeran	L-PAM
Chlorambucil	Leukeran	CLR
II. ETHYLENIMINE DERIVATIVES		
Triethylenethiophos-phoramide	Thiotepa	T-TEPA
III. ALKYL SULFONATES		
Busulfan	Myleran	MYL
IV. NITROSOUREAS		
Cyclohexyl-cholorethyl nitrosourea	Lomustine, CeeNU	CCNU
1, 3 bis-[2-chloroethyl]-1-nitrosourea	Carmustine, BiCNU	BCNU
Streptozotocin	Zanosar	STZC
V. TRIAZENES		
Dimethyl triazeno imidazole carboxamide	Dacarbazine	DTIC
ANTIMETABOLITES		
I. FOLIC ACID ANALOGS		
Methotrexate	Amethopterin	MTX
II. PYRIMIDINE ANALOGS		
5-fluorouracil	Fluorouracil	5-FU
Cytosine arabinoside	Cytarabine, Cytosar	ARA-C
III. PURINE ANALOGS		
6-Mercaptopurine	Purinethol	6-MP
6-Thioguanine	Thioguanine	6-TG
Deoxycoformycin	Pentostatin	VM-26
NATURAL OR SEMISYNTHETIC PRODUCTS		
I. VINCA ALKALOID		
Vinblastine	Velban	VLB
Vincristine	Oncovin	VCR
II. ANTIBIOTICS		
Doxorubicin	Adriamycin	ADR
Mitoxantrone	Novantrone	NOV
Daunorubicin	Daunomycin	DNR
Bleomycin	Blenoxane	BLEO
Dactinomycin	Actinomycin D, Cosmegen	
Mithramycin	Mithracin	
Mitomycin C	Mutamycin	MITO-C
III. ENZYMES		
l-asparaginase	Elspar	L-ASP
IV. EPIPODOPHYLLOTOXINS		
Etoposide	Vepesid	VP-16
Teniposide	Vumon	VM-26
MISCELLANEOUS		
I. PLATINUM COORDINATION COMPLEXES		
Cis-diamminedichloroplatinum II		
Cisplatin, Platinol	DDP	
Carboplatin	Paraplatin	CBP
II. SUBSTITUTED UREA		
Hydroxyurea	Hydrea	HXU

Table 8-1. *(Continued)*

Agent	Trade Name	Abbreviation
III. METHYLHYDRAZINE DERIVATIVE		
Procarbazine	Matulane	PROC
IV. ESTRAMUSTINE PHOSPHATE		Emcyt
V. ACRIDINE DERIVATIVE	Emcyt	
Amsacrine	Amsidyl	m-AMSA
HORMONES AND HORMONE INHIBITORS		
I. ESTROGENS		
Diethylstilbestrol		DES
Conjugated Estrogens	Premarin	
Ethinyl Estradiol	Estinyl	
II. ANDROGENS		
Testosteraone propionate		TES
Fluoxymesterone	Halotestin, Ora-Testryl, Utandren	
III. PROGESTINS		
17-Hydroxyprogester one caproate	Delalutin	
Medroxyprogesterone acetate	Provera	
Megestrol acetate	Megace	
IV. LEUPROLIDE	Lupron	
Goserelin acetate	Zoladex	
V. ADRENOCORTICOSTEROIDS		
VI. ANTIESTROGENS		
Tamoxifen	Nolvadex	
VII. HORMONE SYNTHESIS INHIBITORS		
Aminoglutethimide	Elipten, Cytadren	
VIII. ANTIANDROGENS		
Flutamide	Eulexin	

alizations are useful. Table 8-2 (30) describes criteria for categorizing the performance status of a patient, as described by Karnofsky (43). These categories, based on easily assessed daily activities, permit a functional classification of patients to accompany data from physical examinations and laboratory determinations. A performance status below 40% often predicts an unsatisfactory tumor response and poor tolerance of side effects of drugs. The Eastern Cooperative Oncology Group, a multi-institutional cooperative group for drug studies uses a slightly simpler performance status scale (Table 8-3). It is uncommon for a patient with a performance status below 3 to be given chemotherapy, unless a response of the particular tumor is highly likely and the patient is highly motivated to be treated. At the other end of the clinical spectrum, it may be difficult to justify side effects from chemotherapy in a patient whose tumor-related symptoms are not very severe. However, when major symptoms develop and palliative chemotherapy is elected in the presence of a markedly decreased performance status, the patient's ability to tolerate effective doses of drugs may be significantly limited. The art of chemotherapy involves recognizing the transition between these two phases of the natural history of the malignancy.

Table 8-2. Karnofsky Performance Status Scale

	Percent	
Able to carry on normal activity; no special care is needed	100	Normal; no complaints; no evidence of disease
	90	Able to carry on normal activity; minor signs or symptoms of disease
	80	Normal activity with effort; some signs or symptoms of disease
Unable to work; able to live at home; cares for most personal needs; a varying amount of assistance is needed	70	Cares for self; unable to carry on normal activity or do active work
	60	Requires occasional assistance but is able to care for most needs
	50	Requires considerable assistance and frequent medical care
Unable to care for self; requires equivalent of institutional or hospital care; disease may be progressing rapidly	40	Disabled, requires special care and assistance
	30	Severely disabled; hospitalization is indicated though death not imminent
	20	Very sick; hospitalization is necessary
	10	Moribund; fatal processes progressing rapidly
	0	Dead

From Karnofsky et al. (43), with permission.

Nutritional Status

Related to, but not specifically included in, the performance status criteria is the patient's nutrition. This subject is more fully discussed in Chapter 34, "Nutrition and the Cancer Patient." In general, a cachectic, anorectic patient is less likely to tolerate a meaningful course of chemotherapy and is therefore less likely to attain a good clinical response (see Chapter 8 for definitions of types of responses). Corrective nutritional supplementation may be necessary before beginning cytotoxic chemotherapy, including use of a nasogastric feeding tube, gastrostomy, needle jejunostomy, central venous hyperalimentation, or simply discussing the patient's diet in detail with the patient and family in an attempt to find appetizing and nutritious foods (14,17,56).

Table 8-3. ECOG* Performance Status Scale

Status	Definition
0	Normal activity
1	Symptoms but ambulatory
2	In bed <50% of time
3	In bed >50% of time
4	100% bedridden

* ECOG = Eastern Cooperative Oncology Group

Infections and Bleeding Tendencies

Since many of the antitumor drugs cause bone marrow suppression and immunosuppression (of humoral and cellular immune functions), any preexisting infections should be controlled prior to lowering polymorphonuclear leukocyte counts and inhibiting immune mechanisms. Appropriate use of antibiotics and granulocyte transfusions is important (see Chapter 13, "Oncologic Emergencies"; also see reference 49). Bleeding tendencies should be evaluated and corrected, if possible prior to chemotherapy, with platelet transfusions, vitamin K, or other appropriate therapy. The widespread availability of granulocyte-macrophage colony-stimulating factor may permit more intensive, myelosuppressive chemotherapy in patients whose bone marrow otherwise would not be able to tolerate such therapy (11). The autotransplantation of a large number of undamaged autologous bone marrow stem cells, which have been preserved in vitro during exposure of the remainder of the marrow to cytotoxic chemotherapy, is another innovative technique used to protect the patient from pancytopenic complications (34).

Pain

Uncontrolled pain can markedly lower a patient's performance status and contribute to making tolerance of chemotherapy less satisfactory. Proper use of analgesic agents is an art that all physicians who manage cancer patients should strive to master. The cancer chemotherapy itself may be aimed at pain relief and result in a gradual lessening of narcotic or other analgesic requirements, but in the interval, prior to such a response, adequate pain control may allow a patient to become a candidate for an effective chemotherapy program and to have less difficulty with side effects. Chapters 14, "Principles of Psychosocial Oncology," and 35, "The Nurse and Cancer Care," deal with this subject (31,32).

Emotional Status

The final host factor to be considered, important in assessing a patient's suitability for chemotherapy, can be summarized under the term emotional status. Patients referred for chemotherapy generally are aware, to varying degrees, that they have a malignancy and often that it has spread beyond the possibility of its removal by surgery or local treatment by radiation therapy. Cautious and sympathetic openness on the part of the oncologist is advisable so the patient is made aware that the physician is willing to discuss the disease frankly and that there are treatments available for such a disease. Such communication will permit the oncologist to assess how highly motivated the patient is to undertake therapy. Patient motivation will influence the oncologist's decision to undertake a prolonged, intensive course of chemotherapy with resultant side effects. Concomitantly, the patient is reassured that the physician understands the doubts and anxiety one feels as a result of a diagnosis.

The satisfactory explanation of possible toxic side effects by the oncologist in seeking the patient's informed consent for any investigational chemotherapeutic approach is very important at both an emotional and a medicolegal level. While insufficient explanation puts the patient at a disadvantage in making important decisions, the oncologist can err in the other direction. Hope and optimism that help a patient continue to be active, to maintain nutrition, and to interact with family and friends may be devastated by an overzealous cataloging of major, minor, and rare toxicities and by survival statistics that the patient cannot handle objectively. Therefore, maintaining supportive, trusting rapport between physician and patient will contribute to better patient compliance during chemotherapy. Additional aspects of this subject are discussed in Chapter 14.

Drug Toxicity

Physicians administering antineoplastic drugs have the obligation to understand and anticipate the potential toxic side effects that patients may experience while receiving chemotherapy. While the toxicities of most of these agents for normal tissues are significant, they often assume exaggerated emphasis in the minds of patients and lay public because of anecdotes from acquaintances and from the press and television describing primarily the most severe reactions. The therapeutic index, or relationship between the therapeutic benefit and toxicity, is relatively small for many anticancer drugs. Nevertheless, with astute surveillance for signs of toxicity, and with adequate appreciation of techniques for controlling side effects and for modifying doses when necessary, life-threatening toxicity is generally avoidable.

In general, as noted above in the section on the kinetic basis of chemotherapy, actively dividing cells are more susceptible to the effects of many antineoplastic drugs than nondividing cells. Therefore, toxicity is generally a reflection of varying degrees of damage to actively dividing normal cells in the bone marrow, GI tract, hair follicles, and gonads. Less common toxic reactions such as pulmonary fibrosis (bleomycin, busulfan, and mitomycin C) and cardiotoxicity (doxorubicin, daunomycin, mitoxantrone, and idarubicin) should also be looked for and limited in their severity by restricting total doses to recommended limits and by discontinuing the drug and starting appropriate supportive therapy

if toxicity appears. The toxicity of specific agents has been described in the section on classification of antineoplastic chemotherapeutic agents. General comments are included there, and the reader is referred to other sources for more extensive descriptions (4,8,9).

The screening and development programs for new drugs described in Chapter 9 are designed not only to detect antitumor activity but also to eliminate drugs whose toxicity would be intolerable. Those drugs that enter clinical use usually cause moderate side effects that can be controlled by proper dosage and judicious use of antiemetic agents. Brief comments on bone marrow suppression, immunosuppression, nausea and vomiting, alopecia, sterility, miscellaneous organ toxicities, and second malignancies follow:

1. Bone marrow suppression can be minimized by using intermittent schedules of cell cycle-specific agents that damage dividing hematopoietic stem cells. Most bone marrow stem cells are resting at any given time, and are recruited into the mitotic pool following damage to more mature cells by chemotherapeutic agents. Figure 8-4 indicates the course of the peripheral granulocyte count following a pulse dose of various agents. With most myelosuppressive agents, the lowest peripheral granulocyte counts (the nadir) are reached in about 8 to 10 days. At that point, bone marrow stem cell proliferation is at a maximum. Cycle-specific agents should be avoided at this point to reduce hematopoietic damage, if response of the tumor will permit such a drug-free interval. If the interval between treatments can be extended to 17 to 21 days, most of the stem cells will have returned to the resting state and exposure to the antitumor agents at this time will have minimal effect on the stem cells (13). There are certain exceptions to these generalizations, however, which are important in

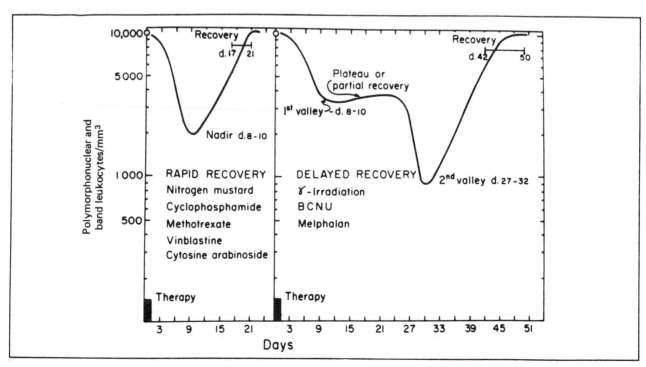

Fig. 8-4. Times to recovery of peripheral granulocyte counts following administration of pulse doses of antitumor drugs. From Bergsagel (13), with permission.

designing drug regimens employing nitrosoureas. These agents produce a biphasic suppression of peripheral granulocytes, the first at 8 to 10 days after a pulse dose, and the second at approximately 27 to 32 days (Fig. 8-4). Re-treatment should be delayed until 6 to 8 weeks have elapsed to permit return of the hematopoietic stem cells to the resting state. Large intermittent doses can be tolerated over many months by observing these intervals. Excessive myelosuppression can also be prevented by using dose adjustments in the presence of decreased blood cell counts.

2. Immunosuppression may not be readily apparent during a course of chemotherapy unless specialized tests of immunologic reactivity are conducted. Antigen-stimulated lymphoid cells undergoing cell division are most susceptible to damage by drugs. Daily treatments are the most damaging to delayed hypersensitivity responses and thus would be most likely to be associated with opportunistic infections such as *Candida albicans*, cytomegalovirus, or herpes zoster. As with bone marrow suppression, intermittent pulse doses appear to be advisable whenever possible to decrease this untoward effect (12).

3. Nausea is widely associated with cancer chemotherapy, especially with cisplatin-based regimens, and may lead to the patient's refusal to continue therapy. Some nausea in chemotherapy patients is clearly psychogenic, since it may occur before a patient is treated, suggesting a conditioned response. Attempts are being made to distract such patients with music or psychotherapy. Nausea and vomiting following the chemotherapy treatment by the usual 3 to 6 hours are more likely the result of physiologic effects on the CNS or the prochlorperazine 5 to 10 mg orally every 4 hours or 25 mg suppositories every 8 hours started before nausea develops. Ondansetron, dexamethasone and metoclopramide have gained wide usage (44,52). Marijuana and tetrahydrocannabinol have been used with limited success for control of nausea and vomiting.

4. *Alopecia* is especially notable with cyclophosphamide, vincristine, doxorubicin, and bleomycin. Patients should be forewarned of this side effect and advised to have a photograph so a realistic wig can be made. Patients should be reassured that their hair usually will return even with continuing therapy, and that regrown hair may be even more attractive than its predecessor. Attempts to reduce hair loss with scalp cooling and tourniquet constriction have met with mixed success (55).

5. *Specific organ toxicity* may involve the kidney, liver, heart, lung, CNS, and gonads.
   a. Renal tubular necrosis can result from the use of cisplatinol without adequate hydration and diuretics to assure a large urine flow. Likewise, high doses of methotrexate can lead to precipitation in the renal tubules, particularly in an acid or concentrated urine. Hydration, alkalinization of the urine with sodium bicarbonate, and diuretics can prevent the renal damage. Creatinine clearance should be checked periodically when these agents are used.
   b. Liver toxicity may occasionally result from L-asparaginase therapy or from prolonged treatment with methotrexate or 6-mercaptopurine. Mithra-

mycin in antitumor doses may cause liver damage, although rarely, if ever, with smaller doses used for controlling hypercalcemia.
   c. Cardiotoxicity has been associated primarily with the anthracycline antibiotics doxorubicin and daunorubicin but it may also be seen with high-dose cyclophosphamide therapy. It may be sudden in onset, irreversible, and associated with a high mortality rate. There may be transient electrocardiographic changes or a delayed cardiomyopathy, with congestive heart failure, particularly with total doses of doxorubicin over 500 mg/m². Histologic examinations of patients dying with this complication have shown degeneration of myocardial cells and interstitial edema. Doxorubicin, daunorubicin, mitoxantrone, and idarubicin should be used with extra caution in patients with pre-existing cardiac disease, particularly if they have also received irradiation to the area of the heart or cyclophosphamide therapy, both of which appear to augment cardiomyopathy. Periodic monitoring of left ventricular ejection fractions should be conducted to detect the cardiotoxicity early enough to avoid serious and irreversible consequences (47,54).
   d. Pulmonary toxicity has been most closely associated with bleomycin, which selectively localizes in the lung. Decrease in diffusion capacity and in total lung capacity may occur in one third to one half of patients who receive bleomycin, with clinically apparent pulmonary fibrosis in approximately 5% of patients. Such fibrosis is usually associated with doses of 300 to 400 U/m² and more, although it may occur with doses of 100 U or less. The toxicity may be reversible on cessation of drug administration and institution of supportive care, including corticosteroids. Pulmonary fibrosis is an uncommon complication of busulfan, BCNU, and mitomycin C therapy (47,54).
   e. Neurotoxicity has been most commonly associated with vincristine, which causes peripheral neuropathy characterized by loss of deep tendon reflexes, paresthesias, motor weakness, and occasionally jaw or other pain. Such changes are usually reversible over several months. Cisplatin neurotoxicity is also characterized by peripheral neuropathy. Ototoxicity is observed in 31% of patients treated with cisplatin. It is usually characterized by tinnitus and/or hearing loss in the high frequency range. Procarbazine and L-asparaginase may cause CNS symptoms, including somnolence, hallucinations, and depression. When given after cranial radiation therapy, methotrexate can lead to increased brain tissue drug concentrations and produce leukoencephalopathy due to white-matter necrosis, particularly in children.
   f. Gonadal damage and consequent sterility have been associated with a number of drugs, including a variety of alkylating agents, vinblastine, procarbazine, cytosine arabinoside, and cisplatin. Combination chemotherapy, such as MOPP chemotherapy for Hodgkin's disease, is particularly damaging, with over 80% of male patients developing azoospermia, testicular atrophy, and elevated gonadotrophin levels. Ovarian failure may occur. Women over aged

40 years are particularly likely to have permanent amenorrhea after adjuvant combination chemotherapy for breast cancer (36).

g. Second malignancies attributable to genetic damage from chemotherapy have been a major concern in recent years as more and more patients have achieved long-term remissions and cures. Since many of the agents used have demonstrable mutagenic properties, this association seems understandable. Studies of patients in complete remission following combination chemotherapy for Hodgkin's disease have indicated the following (15,58):

- chemotherapy alone or chemotherapy plus radiation therapy seems more likely to predispose to secondary acute leukemia than radiation therapy alone
- peak incidence of the onset of secondary acute leukemia is between 3 and 9 years following previous chemotherapy, with a declining frequency thereafter
- certain drugs, including alkylating agents, procarbazine, and nitrosoureas, appear to have more leukemogenic potential than other drugs. This increases expectations that appropriate modifications of current combination chemotherapy may decrease the likelihood of this complication
- risk of secondary leukemia rises with increasing patient age at the time of treatment, especially over 40 years of age

SUMMARY

Increasingly, cancer chemotherapy is being used early in the clinical history of malignant diseases, as in adjuvant therapy for primary breast and colorectal cancers, and as in definitive, potentially curative therapy for certain disseminated malignancies, including Hodgkin's disease, high-grade, non-Hodgkin's lymphomas, testicular carcinoma, choriocarcinoma in women, rhabdomyosarcoma and acute lymphoblastic leukemia of childhood. Medical oncologists also often find themselves in the primary care role of supporting and palliating terminal cancer patients. The doctor-patient relationship engendered during a prolonged chemotherapy program often leads patients to turn primarily to the medical oncologist for help with their problems even after active chemotherapeutic approaches have been exhausted. This supportive role of the medical oncologist is very challenging. It mandates adequate knowledge of not only chemotherapy but also of nutrition, pain control, GI function, treatment of infectious complications, and psychosocial aspects of cancer. Familiarity with community resources for home and institutional care, financial help, nursing support, rehabilitation services, and transportation is also important. A team approach is often highly effective, with oncologists, primary care physicians, nurses, pharmacists, social workers, physical therapists, psychiatrists, and nutritionists complementing each other's functions. The training and personal characteristics of many medical oncologists make them well suited to coordinate such a group in the total care of cancer patients.

New Avenues in Cancer Chemotherapy

In the past, new concepts in cancer treatment have taken a relatively long time to reach clinical acceptance. Combina-

tion chemotherapy, the most important treatment modality capable of curing advanced cancer, was first shown to be more effective therapy than single agents against experimental tumors in the 1950s but its clinical efficacy was not demonstrated until the 1970s (26,45). The concept of applying biochemical modulation to improve combination chemotherapy has already been demonstrated in preclinical studies but clinical trials to reproduce preclinical results are only now under way. In experimental tumor models a sequence of methotrexate followed by 5-FU gives enhanced cell kill; similarly marked improvement in cytotoxic effects is demonstrated when 5-FU is used with leucovorin. The latter predoses excess of intracellular reduced folates necessary for optimal inhibition of thymidylate synthetase by flourinated pyrimidines. Several clinical studies have demonstrated superiority of 5-FU and leukovorin to 5-FU alone in metastatic colon cancer. Encouraged by these results in advanced disease, an intergroup study tests surgery alone against high and low dose leukovorin and 5 FU in patients with Duke's B and C colon cancer (26,44,45).

The observation that several compounds commonly used in cancer therapy can induce cell differentiation in clones of myeloid leukemic cells has made it possible to identify mechanisms that uncouple growth and differentiation signals (51). By inducing differentiation to mature cells, genetic abnormalities that give rise to malignancy can be held in abeyance. This has provided new possibilities for cancer treatment with all-trans retinoic acid in acute promyelocytic leukemia (2a).

Recent demonstration of a clear association between protein phosphorylation and cell transformation offers a number of new avenues with regard to cancer chemotherapy. Since protein kinases show more distinct substrate specificities, designing specific inhibitors should be possible. Alternatively augmenting host-cell protein phosphatases as potential anti-oncogenes could become targets of future chemotherapeutic drug design (33).

The problem of resistence to chemotherapy has also received increasing attention recently. (7). The isolation and characterization of the multidrug resistance gene product as a 170,000 dalton plasma membrane glycoprotein (P-glycoprotein) energy dependent multidrug efflux pump has prompted studies with a variety of agents including verapamil, quinidine, reserpine, to inhibit this multidrug transposter and increase drug accumulation in target cells. The work of Dalton et al. (24) suggests administration of verapamil along with chemotherapy can partially abrogate drug resistance induced by overexpression of P-glycoprotein. Studies using less toxic inhibitors of P-glycoprotien are in progress (39) and may become a useful adjunct in the chemotherapists' armamentarium.

Recommended Reading

The following references allow the reader to pursue this subject in more depth. A comprehensive description of drugs and their pharmacology is found in Calabresi and Parks' chapter in the classic pharmacology text by Gilman et al., *The Pharmacological Basis of Therapeutics*, 7th ed (1). The text by Pratt and Ruddon, *The Anticancer Drugs* (5), is excellent as a well-written, lucid introduction to cancer chemotherapeutic agents. *Medical Oncology: Basic Principles and Clinical Management* (2), *The Chemotherapy Sourcebook* (4a), *Cancer: Principles and Practice of Oncology, ed 3* (4), *Medical Care of the Cancer*

Patient (6), and *Handbook of Cancer Chemotherapy* (8) provide a broad view of malignant diseases and their treatment. Selected specific references provide recent summaries of advances in this field.

REFERENCES

General References

1. Calabresi P, Parks RE, Jr: Chemotherapy of Neoplastic Diseases, in Gilman AG, Goodman LS, Rall TW, Murad F (eds): The Pharmacological Basis of Therapeutics, 7th ed, section XIII. New York, NY: MacMillan, 1985; pp 1240-1306.
2. Calabresi P, Schein PS, Rosenberg SA (eds): Medical Oncology. Basic Principles and Clinical Management of Cancer. New York, NY: MacMillan, 1985.
2a. Castaigne, S.; Chomienne, C.; Therse, D.M.; Ballerene, P.; Berger, R.; Fenaux, P.; Degos, L. All-Trans Retinoic Acid as differentiating therapy for acute promyelocyte Leukemia. 1. Clinical Results Blood. 1990; 76:1704-1709.
3. Chabner, BA (ed): Pharmacologic Principles of Cancer Treatment. Philadelphia, PA: WB Saunders Co, 1982.
4. DeVita VT Jr, Hellman S, Rosenberg SA (eds): Cancer: Principles and Practice of Oncology, 3rd ed. Philadelphia, PA: JB Lippincott Co, 1989.
4a. Perry M.C. (ed): The Chemotherapy Sourcebook. Baltimore, MD: Williams and Wilkens; 1992.
5. Pratt WB, Ruddon RW: The Anti-Cancer Drugs. New York, NY: Oxford University Press, 1979.
6. Rosenthal S, Carignan JR, Smith BD (eds): Medical Care of the Cancer Patient. Philadelphia, PA: W.B. Saunders Co., 1987.
7. Ruddon RW: Cancer Biology. New York, NY: Oxford University Press, 1987.
8. Skeel RT: Handbook of Cancer Chemotherapy. Boston: Little Brown & Co, 1987.
9. Tannock IF, Hill RP (eds): The Basic Science of Oncology. Elmsford, NY: Pergamon Press, 1987.

Specific References

10. Abrams RA, Deisseroth A: Supportive care of the cancer patient. Use of blood and blood products. In DeVita VT Jr, Hellman S, Rosenberg SA (eds): Cancer—Principles and Practice of Oncology, 2nd ed. Philadelphia, PA: JB Lippincott Co, 1985; pp 1920-1940.
11. Antman K, Eder JP, Frei E III: High-dose chemotherapy with bone marrow support for solid tumors. In DeVita VT Jr, Hellman S, Rosenberg SA (eds): Important Advances in Oncology 1987. Philadelphia, PA:, JB Lippincott Co, 1987; pp 221-235.
12. Bast RC: Principles of cancer biology: Tumor immunology. In DeVita VT Jr, Hellman S, Rosenberg SA (eds): Cancer—Principles and Practice of Oncology, 2nd ed. Philadelphia, PA: JB Lippincott Co, 1985; p 142.
13. Bergsagel DE: An assessment of massive-dose chemotherapy of malignant disease. Can Med Assoc J 1971; 104:31-36.
14. Blackburn GL, Miller MM, Bothe A Jr: Nutritional factors in cancer. In Calabresi P, Schein PS, Rosenberg SA (eds): Medical Oncology. Basic Principles and Clinical Management of Cancer. New York, NY: Macmillan, 1985; pp 1406-1432.
15. Blayney DW, Longo DL, Young RC, et al.: Decreasing risk of leukemia with prolonged follow-up after chemotherapy and radiotherapy for Hodgkin's disease. N Engl J Med 1987; 316:710-714.
16. Bonadonna G, Valagusa P: Adjuvant systemic therapy for resectable breast cancer. J Clin Oncol 1985; 3:259-275.
17. Brennan MJ: Supportive care of the cancer patient. Nutritional support. In DeVita VT Jr, Hellman S, Rosenberg SA (eds): Cancer—Principles and Practice of Oncology, 2nd ed. Philadelphia, PA: JB Lippincott Co, 1985; pp 1907-1920.
18. Calabresi P, Carbone PP, Kennedy W, et al.: American Board of Internal Medicine: Medical Oncology Training. Cancer Treat Rev 1977; 4:143-149.
19. Calabresi P, Crosby WH, et al.: American Board of Internal Medicine guidelines for training in hematology and medical oncology. Blood 1977; 49:1011-1017.
20. Chabner BA: The role of drugs in cancer treatment. In Chabner BA (ed): Pharmacologic Principles of Cancer Treatment. Philadelphia, PA: WB Saunders, 1982; pp 3-14.

21. Chabner BA, Myers CE: Clinical Pharmacology of Cancer Chemotherapy. In DeVita VT Jr, Hellman S, Rosenberg SA (eds): Cancer: Principles and Practice of Oncology, ed 3. Philadelphia, PA: JB Lippincott Co, 1989; pp. 349-395.
22. Coldman AJ, Goldie JH: Impact of dose-intense chemotherapy on the development of permanent drug resistance. Semin Oncol 1987; 14 (Suppl 4): 29-33.
23. Damon LE, Cadman EC: The metabolic basis for combination chemotherapy. Pharmac Ther 1988; 38:73-127.
24. Dalton, WS, Grogan, TM, Meltzer, PS et al.: Drug resistance in multiple myeloma and non-Hodgkin's lymphoma: detection of P-glycoprotein. J. Clin. Oncol. 1989; 7:415-424.
24a. Deisseroth A, Wallerstein R: Supportive care of the cancer patient. Use of blood and blood products. In DeVita VT Jr, Hellman S, Rosenberg SA (eds): Cancer: Principles and Practice of Oncology, 3rd ed, Philadelphia, PA: JB Lippincott Co, 1989; pp 2045-2059.
25. DeVita VT Jr: Principles of chemotherapy. In DeVita VT Jr, Hellman S, Rosenberg SA (eds): Cancer: Principles and Practice of Oncology, 3rd ed, Philadelphia, PA: JB Lippincott Co, 1989; pp 276-300.
26. Erlichman C, Fure S, Hong A, et al.: A randomized trial of fluoracil and folinic acid in patients with metastatic colorectal carcinoma. J Clin Oncol 1988; 6:469-475.
27. Edwards MH, Myers WPL, Kennedy BJ, Bakemeier RF, et al.: Graduate education in medical oncology. National Cancer Institute Monoqraph, Bethesda, Md, 1978.
28. Eilber FR, Giulano AE, Eckhardt J, et al.: A randomized prospective trial of adjuvant chemotherapy for osteosarcoma. In Salmon SE (ed): Adjuvant Therapy of Cancer V. Orlando, FL: Grune & Stratton, 1987; pp 691-699.
29. Eilber FR, Mirra JJ, Grant TT et al.: Is amputation necessary for sarcoma? A seven year experience with limb salvage. Ann Surg. 1980; 192:431-437.
30. Fisher B, Redmond CK, Wolmark N, et al.: Long term results from NSABP trials for adjuvant therapy of breast cancer. In Salmon SE (ed): Adjuvant Therapy of Cancer V. Orlando, FL: Grune & Stratton, 1987; pp 285-295.
31. Foley KM: Control of pain in cancer. In Calabresi P, Schein PS, Rosenberg SA (eds): Medical Oncology. Basic Principles and Clinical Management of Cancer. New York, NY: Macmillan, 1985; pp 1385-1405.
32. Foley KM, Arbit, E: Supportive care of the cancer patient. Management of cancer pain. In DeVita VT Jr, Hellman S, Rosenberg SA (eds): Cancer: Principles and Practice of Oncology, 3rd ed, Philadelphia, PA: JB Lippincott Co, 1989; pp 2064-2087.
33. Foulker JG, Rosner RM. Tyrosine-specific protein kinases as mediators of growth control. In Cohen P, Horesley MG (eds): Molecular Aspects of Cellular Regulation, vol. 4. New York, NY: Elsevier North Holland, 1985: 217-252.
34. Gabrilove J, Jakiebowski A, Schieve H, et al.: Effect of granulocyte colon-stimulating factor on neutropenia and associated morbidity due to chemotherapy for transitional cell carcinoma of urothelium. NEJM 1988; 1414-1422.
35. Glic J: Meeting highlights: Adjuvant therapy for breast cancer. JNCI 1988; 20:471-475.
36. Glicksman AS, Schein PS: Acute and late effects of cancer therapy. In Calabresi P, Schein PS, Rosenberg SA (eds): Medical Oncology. Basic Principles and Clinical Management of Cancer. New York, NY: Macmillan, 1985; pp 426-453.
37. Goldie JH, Coldman AJ: The genetic origin of drug resistance in neoplasms: Implications for systemic therapy. Cancer Res 1984; 44:3643-3653.
38. Goldstein LF, Galski H, Fojo A, et al.: Expression of a multidrug resistance gene in human cancers. JNCI 1989; 81:116-124.
39. Gottesman MM, Pastan I. Cinical trials of agents that reverse multidrug resistance. J Clin Oncol 1989; 7:409-411.
40. Hong WK, Dimery IW: Adjuvant chemotherpay in head and neck cancer. Critical review and prospects. In Larson, Ballantyne, Guillamondequi (eds). New York, NY: Macmillan, 1986; pp 195-203.
41. Hong WK, Endicott J, Itric, L, et al.: 13-cisretinoic acid in the treatment of oral leukoplakia. NEJM 1986; 315:1501-1505.
42. Hyrniuk WM: Average relative dose intensity and the impact on design of clinical trials, Semin Oncol 1987; 14:65-74.
43. Karnofsky DA, Abelmann WH, Kraver LF, et al.: The use of

nitrogen mustards in the palliative treatment of carcinoma with particular reference to bronchogenic carcinoma. Cancer 1948; 1:634-669.

44. Kris MG, Gralla RJ, Tyson LB, *et al.*: Controlling delayed vomiting: double-blind, ramdonized trial comparing placebo, dexamethasone alone, and meclopramide plus dexamethasone in patients receiving cisplatin. J Clin Oncol 108-114.

45. Machover D, Goldschmidt E, Choket P. Treatment of advanced colorectal and gastric adenocarcinoma with 5-fluorouracil in high dose folinic acid. J Clin Oncol 1986; 4:685-696.

46. Merkel DE, McGuire WL: Oncogenes and cancer prognosis. In DeVita VT Jr, Hellman 5, Rosenberg SA (eds): Important Advances in Oncology 1988. Philadelphia, PA: JP Lippincott Co, 1988; pp 103- 117.

47. Myers CE, Kinsella TJ: Adverse effects of treatment. Cardiac and pulmonary toxicity. In DeVita VT Jr., Hellman 5, Rosenberg SA (eds): Cancer—Principles and Practice of Oncology, ed 2. Philadelphia, PA: JB Lippincott Co, 1985; pp 2022-2032.

48. Pastan IH, Gottesman MH: Molecular biology of multidrug resistance in human cells. In DeVita VT Jr, Hellman S, Rosenberg SA (eds): Important Advances in Oncology 1988. Philadelphia, PA: JP Lippincott Co, 1988; pp 3-16.

49. Pizzo PA, Myers J: Infections in the cancer patient. In DeVita VT Jr, Hellman S, Rosenberg SA (eds): Cancer: Principles and Practice of Oncology, 3rd ed, Philadelphia, PA: JB Lippincott Co, 1989; pp 2088-2134.

50. Ruddon RW: Causes of cancer: viruses and oncogenes. In Ruddon, RW (ed): Cancer Biology. New York, NY: Oxford University Press, 1987; pp 337-411.

51. Sachs, L. Growth differentiation and the reversal of malignancy. Scientific American 1976; 254:40-47.

52. Sallan SE, Cronin CM: Adverse effects of treatment. Nausea and vomiting. In DeVita VT Jr., Hellman S, Rosenberg SA (eds): Cancer—Principles and Practice of Oncology, ed 2. Philadelphia, PA: JB Lippincott Co, 1985; pp 2008-2013.

53. Schilsky RL, Sherins RJ: Adverse effects of treatment. Gonadal dysfunction. In DeVita VT Jr., Hellman S, Rosenberg SA (eds): Cancer—Principles and Practice of Oncology ed 2. Philadelphia, PA: JB Lippincott Co, 1985; pp 2032-2039.

54. Schwartz RG, McKenzie WB, Alexander J, *et al.*: Congestive heart failure and left ventricular dysfunction complicating doxorubicin therapy. Am J Med 1987; 82:1109-1118.

55. Seipp CA: Adverse effects of treatment. Hair loss. In DeVita VT Jr, Hellman S, Rosenberg SA (eds): Cancer: Principles and Practice of Oncology, 3rd ed, Philadelphia, PA: JB Lippincott Co, 1989; pp 2135-2136.

55a. Sherins RJ, Mulvihill JJ: Adverse effects of treatment. Gonadal dysfunction. In DeVita VT Jr, Hellman S, Rosenberg SA (eds): Cancer: Principles and Practice of Oncology, 3rd ed, Philadelphia, PA: JB Lippincott Co, 1989; pp 2170-2180.

55b. Shike M, Brennan MF: Supportive care of the cancer patient. Nutritional support. In DeVita VT Jr, Hellman S, Rosenberg SA (eds): Cancer: Principles and Practice of Oncology, 3rd ed, Philadelphia, PA: JB Lippincott Co, 1989; pp 2029-2044.

56. Shils ME: Nutrition and diet in cancer. In Shils ME, Young VR (eds): Modern Nutrition in Health and Disease. Philadelphia, PA: Lea & Febiger, 1988; pp 1380-1422.

56a. Stover DE: Adverse effects of treatment. Pulmonary toxicity. In DeVita VT Jr, Hellman S, Rosenberg SA (eds): Cancer: Principles and Practice of Oncology, 3rd ed, Philadelphia, PA: JB Lippincott Co, 1989; pp 2162-2169.

57. Tannock IF: Biologic properties of anticancer drugs. In Tannock IF, Hill RP (eds): The Basic Science of Oncology. New York, NY: Pergamon Press, 1987; pp 278-291.

57a. Torti FM, Lum BL: Adverse Effects of Treatment. Cardiac Toxicity, ed 3. Philadelphia, PA: JB Lippincott Co, 1989; pp 2153-2161.

58. Valagussa P, Santoro A, Fossati-Bellani F, *et al.*: Second acute leukemia and other malignancies following treatment for Hodgkin's disease. J Clin Oncol 1986; 4:830-837.

59. Williams SD, Stablein D, Muggia F, *et al.*: Early stage cancer: the testicular cancer intergroup studies. In Salmon SE (ed): Adjuvant Therapy of Cancer V. Orlando, FL: Grune & Stratton, 1987; pp 587-592.

60. Yagoda A: Neoadjuvant and adjuvant chemotherapy for urothelial tract tumors. In Salmon SE (ed): Adjuvant Therapy for Cancer V. Orlando, FL: Grune & Stratton, 1987; pp 555-563.

61. Zinner SH, Klastensky J: Infectious considerations in cancer. In Calabresi P, Schein PS, Rosenberg SA (eds): Medical Oncology. Basic Principles and Clinical Management of Cancer. New York, NY: Macmillan, 1985; pp 1327-1357.

John M. Bennett, M.D., Medical Oncology

Chapter 9

BASIC CONCEPTS IN INVESTIGATIONAL THERAPEUTICS AND CLINICAL TRIALS

The seeds of great discoveries are constantly floating around us, but they only take root in minds well prepared to receive them.

W. B. Cannon (7)

PERSPECTIVE

The dramatic early successes with nitrogen mustard in Hodgkin's disease, and methotrexate in leukemia and choriocarcinoma, prompted the United States Congress in 1958 to appropriate $5 million to establish a cancer drug development program. The essential activities required to bring a drug into general medical practice involve the so-called linear array, whereby a given agent is acquired and screened, and then undergoes production, formulation, and preclinical toxicology before proceeding into clinical trials (Fig. 9-1) (4).

Drugs for the initial stage of acquisition and selection of new agents are submitted by universities, pharmaceutical houses, and the intramural laboratory programs at the National Cancer Institute (NCI). The second stage—the screening program—involves the evaluation of the new agent in a wide range of experimental tumors that have become standardized over the years. A drug must meet rigid criteria for antitumor activity before it can move to the next stage of large-scale production.

IN VIVO SCREENING PROGRAM

Previously, several animal tumor systems were widely used to screen for anticancer agents. Until 1975, literally thousands of compounds were screened using the L1210 lymphoid leukemia model and other transplantable tumors, such as B16 melanoma and Lewis lung tumors in mice. During the past decade, however, new developments in screening systems, including human tumor xenografts (colon, breast, and lung), grown in immune-deficient athymic or "nude" mice, prompted a revision in the initial drug screening program. In addition to the L1210 system, a more sensitive P388 mouse leukemia screening model is used. A corresponding matching system of mouse solid tumors is also included (e.g., B16 melanoma). From this standard panel, some 500 to 1,000 compounds per year, proven to be active in the P388 prescreen or demonstrated to be positive in other biologic systems, are submitted for mouse and human panel tumors (2,4) (Fig. 9-2).

The first preclinical stage involves toxicologic studies in large animals (dog and monkey). At each key point from production through phase I clinical trials, a multidisciplinary scientific review by the Decision Network Committee takes place. This committee consists of cancer scientists from both intramural programs at the NCI and others from private universities and cancer centers. These toxicology studies are a prerequisite for obtaining an investigational new drug application from the Food and Drug Administration (FDA). Once the application is approved, the clinical evaluation of a new agent can proceed (see "phase I, II, III, and IV studies" that follow).

One example of an agent recently introduced into clinical trials is illustrative of the complexities of bringing drugs into oncologic practice. In 1971, a compound was synthesized as an analog of the enzyme aspartate transcarbamoylase. This drug, called PALA (N-phosphonacetyl, L-aspartic acid, NSC-244131), proved to be a potent inhibitor of pyrimidine biosynthesis. The compound was inactive against L1210 leukemia, a rapid growing tumor, but active against B16 melanoma and the slow-growing Lewis lung and colon tumors (12). Production problems were encountered and it was not until late 1977, 6 years after synthesis, that sufficient material was available to complete toxicology studies. By the time large animal studies were completed and the drug was released for early clinical trials, another year had elapsed. In 1981, trials to determine a spectrum of antitumor activity were completed and, despite the early enthusiasm for this agent, relatively little antitumor activity has been demonstrated with a wide range of cancers (15). Therefore, the agent has been viewed as inactive by the Cancer Therapy Evaluation Program. Of some 83 new drugs tested, 24 (29%) were active in at least one disease during the past 15 years.

Currently there are some 30 drugs available for general use in the treatment of neoplastic disease (see Table 8-1, Chapter 8, "Basic Concepts of Cancer Chemotherapy and Principles of Medical Oncology"); approximately 20 were introduced as a result of NCI sponsorship or as a shared responsibility with private pharmaceutical firms. An additional 80 to 90 agents received initial approval for testing in clinical trials, but were rejected because of either excessive toxicity or low antitumor activity. The process of drug approval by the FDA is lengthy, and approval of active cancer agents has modestly increased in the past 5 years. The doctrine of demonstrating substantial

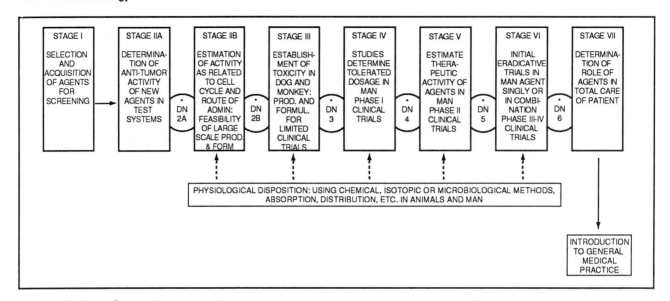

Fig. 9-1. Division of Cancer Treatment (DCT) program linear array: new drug development flow. DN = Decision Network. From National Cancer Institute (16), with permission.

effectiveness is a more difficult one in diseases in which single agents usually produce only modest regressions in a small percentage of patients. Approval for use of today's most active drugs, cisplatin and etoposide, is restricted to only a few malignancies; yet, oncologists have used these agents successfully in many other cancers. It is hoped that new guidelines will be adopted that will improve access for cancer patients to promising new agents similar to those recounted recently by Wittes (19).

CLINICAL TRIALS RESEARCH: TESTING NEW ANTICANCER AGENTS

The NCI has developed multiple resources for the conduct of clinical trials for the testing of new anticancer agents. These include cancer centers, contract supported groups, and the cooperative groups, Eastern Cooperative Oncology Group (ECOG), Cancer and Leukemia Group B (CALGB), Children's Cancer Study Group (CCSG), North Central Oncology Group (NCOG), Gynecologic Oncology Group (GOG), Pediatric Oncology Group (POG), National Surgi-

cal Adjuvant Breast and Bowel Project (NSABP) and Southwest Oncology Group (SWOG). There are several stages of the testing of anticancer drugs in patients. These are referred to as Phases I, II, III, and IV. Each phase has well-defined guidelines that are followed by all clinical investigators (Fig. 9-3) (4,16).

Phase I Studies

Phase I clinical trials are restricted to patients with malignancies that are refractory to all available standard treatments. These studies are designed to determine the maximum tolerated dose of a new agent and to assess toxicity. Several dose schedules are selected. The primary purpose is to establish a dosage schedule; therefore, measurable disease in patients is not a requirement.

The initial dose for human trials is chosen from large animal toxicology studies. One plan is to initiate at one third the minimum toxic dose of a large animal species. Usually three patients are entered at this dosage. Subsequent dose escalations (initial dose n, then 2 x n, 3.3 x n, 7 x n, 9 x n, 12 x n, 16 x n) are initially steep; the percentage then

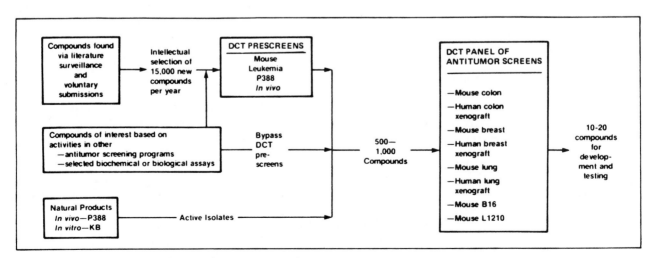

Fig. 9-2. Flow of drugs through Division of Cancer Treatment (DCT) screens. From National Cancer Institute (16), with permission.

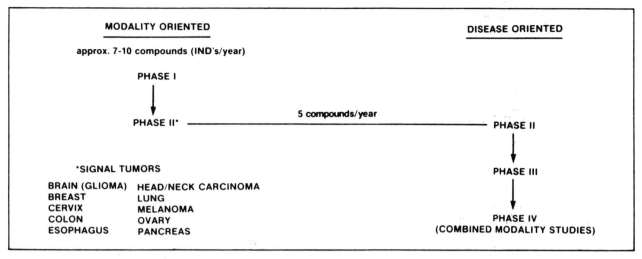

Fig. 9-3. Phases of clinical drug testing in Division of Cancer Treatment (DCT) program. INDs = Investigational new drugs. From National Cancer Institute (16), with permission.

decreases as maximum toxicity is approached, according to a modified Fibonacci search scheme (8). Standard dosage schedules include daily dose times five, repeat every 3 to 4 weeks; single dose, twice daily; and continuous infusion.

It should not be assumed that patients participating in phase I trials will not benefit from the administration of new agents under testing for maximum tolerance. A review of 54 anticancer drugs introduced into phase I trials from 1974 to 1982 resulted in 4% responses (9). The vast majority of these patients had refractory or end-stage disease; therefore, this response rate appears reasonable. Nevertheless, change in the drug-screening programs with more human cell lines, particularly resistant lines, may improve this response rate.

Phase II Studies

Phase II studies are initiated once a new agent proves to be tolerable phamacologically. The question asked is whether the drug has sufficient antitumor activity to consider further clinical evaluation. A clinical panel of human tumors has been selected for initial phase II studies and includes breast, colon, lung, melanoma, acute leukemia, non-Hodgkin's lymphoma, and Hodgkin's disease. Each tumor site is studied by at least three different groups to be certain that unfavorable patient selection (stratification factors) does not result in a new agent being rejected prematurely.

In large groups such as the ECOG, several new agents can be studied simultaneously in individual tumors using the master protocol concept (1). This allows for randomization and prevents investigator bias. In general, patients will have previously received conventional therapy; however, more recently, where no effective chemotherapy exists or the response rate is less than 15% in a given tumor type (e.g., renal cell carcinoma or melanoma), the introduction of new agents in previously untreated patents has been adopted—a policy that appears both reasonable and rational. The practice in these studies has been to obtain 20 to 40 adequately treated and evaluable patients in each category.

A group of 20 evaluable patients showing no response indicates that the maximum response rate, if it exists at all, would be 14% (a one-sided 95% confidence limit). In general, one can quickly assess the upper limit of the uncertainty of an observer response by adding $0.8/\sqrt{n}$ to the observed proportion of response. For example, if one observes four regressions among 40 treatments, then the upper bound is $0.10 + 0.8/\sqrt{40}$ or 0.23 for a maximum response rate of 23% (10).

The most serious error that can occur in phase II trials is the rejection of an effective drug from further clinical study. This rejection error (ß or type II error, false-negative) can occur, despite the best statistical design, if an inadequate dosage is selected, if patients with extensive prior exposure to multiple agents are used exclusively, or if patients with very poor performance status are studied.

The majority of oncologic clinical investigators use the same criteria for evaluation of the response of a patient's tumor to a given program of treatment. Objective tumor response is recorded as follows:

1. Complete response (CR): Disappearance of all measurable tumor. Time factor of at least 2 months' duration.
2. Partial response: Greater or equal to 50% regression of one or more evaluable lesions, with no progression of any lesion.
3. No change: Less than 50% reduction in tumor volume or lack of progression.
4. Progression: The occurrence of any new lesions during treatment or the increase in size by 25% of one or more lesions.

Two types of phase II trials are conducted in the United States. One concerns the assessment of a new agent and can be concluded rather quickly if no responses are observed in the first 12 or so patients. A recent paper (11) concluded that the absence of any responses using a new riboside analog, fludarabine phosphate, indicated that the drug would be unlikely to be active in a large group of patients with advanced bowel cancer with a probability of nonactivity of greater than 95%.

The major purpose of such a trial is to determine biologic activity and to decide whether further evaluation of a new agent that has been developed under considerable expense should or should not be rejected.

In contrast, a large nonrandomized study of "M-VAC" (methotrexate, vinblastine, doxorubicin, and cisplatin) was initiated at Memorial Hospital (18) with an expectation of some success. The drugs were all active in bladder cancer.

Over 90 patients were treated and the results were impressive, with a significant percentage of CR. A phase III trial of M-VAC versus cisplatin by two of the cooperative groups has been completed and confirmed these results. In a sense, this latter trial comes closer to a phase III trial that is of a highly pragmatic nature as defined by Tannock and Warr (17). Some researchers would agree that the randomized trial should have been started initially, but the expense and time frame of such a program would preclude supposition without a hint of significant activity of the new combination.

Phase III Studies

Phase III studies are designed to establish the value of a new treatment relative to what was previously employed. A variety of approaches are used: a new agent may be employed in a previously accepted combination of active drugs; new treatment may be compared with the best standard drug; and combined modality therapy may be employed versus the best single-modality treatment. An example of combined-modality trials is adjuvant therapy in post-operative breast cancer comparing a combination of radiation therapy and chemotherapy versus chemotherapy alone. An example of a single modality study is one conducted by ECOG, comparing phenylalanine mustard versus hexamethylmelamine, cyclophosphamide, doxorubicin, and cisplatin in advanced ovarian carcinoma (EST 2878).

Phase IV Studies

Once a new program is statistically shown to be an improvement over previous treatment for a given disease site and stage of disease, it becomes standard care. This is referred to by some investigators as phase IV. In some instances, community oncologists will be asked to evaluate a new program to ensure that it can be given safely to large numbers of patients and that it demonstrates efficacy.

CLINICAL TRIALS RESEARCH: COOPERATIVE TREATMENT GROUPS

Over the past 25 years, the NCI has provided support for approximately 40 cooperative cancer treatment groups. These groups have consisted of single-disease site, multidisease sites, single-modality (radiation therapy, surgery), and multimodality, multidisease treatment programs. The cooperative groups conduct phases I, II, and III of the clinical trials. Currently, there are 12 programs with almost 30,000 patients entered into some 500 protocols designed to improve the responsiveness and curability of a wide variety of cancers. These studies are supported by research grants to over 190 institutions in the United States at a cost of $35 million in 1980 alone. In addition, a new program, the Community Clinical Oncology Program, was launched by the NCI in 1984 and contributes an additional 3,000 patients each year to the national effort. The total cost of the NCI programs in clinical trials has risen to over $55 million in 1987 (20). An additional 80 centers are supported by contracts for specific projects designed by staff personnel at the NCI. These projects, requests for proposal, are published by the NCI in the Federal Register and sent to universities and cancer centers for their information.

About one third of the studies conducted by the clinical trial groups involve patients with limited or regional disease. The majority, however, are a continuation of traditional

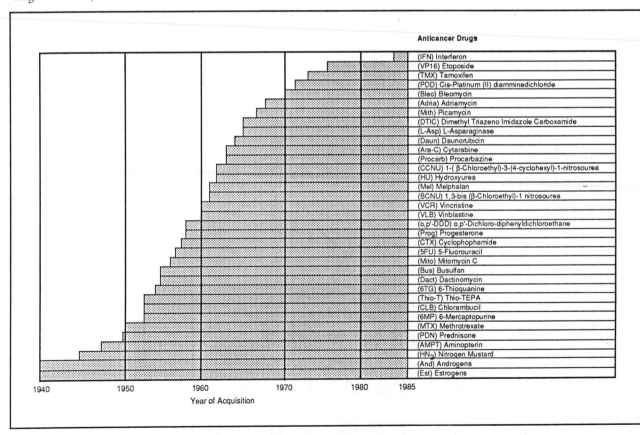

Fig. 9-4. Acquisition of new anticancer drugs since 1940. From Krakoff (13), with permission.

chemotherapy programs in patients with advanced cancers, exploring new agents or combinations of active drugs. Fig. 9-4 illustrates the acquisition of new anticancer drugs since 1940.

The rapid progress in the therapy of a variety of different cancers during the last decade has led to a new era whereby the answers to questions in many clinical trials require the study of large numbers of patients. In adjuvant trials (e.g., breast and colon), the various strata for the number of nodes involved, extent of disease, and other factors demand hundreds of patients to establish potential significance of a program. This may add only a modest gain, yet have a considerable impact if applied to the whole country.

It has been disappointing that only 1% to 3% of the potential number of patients for clinical trials ever enter such programs. Even within the cooperative groups, the percentage of eligible patients who enter trials ranges from 10 to 75%. This is demonstrated by our studies in Rochester (14). Subsequent studies continue to indicate that the vast majority of patients with cancer do not participate in clinical trials (1a).

Improvements in screening and eliminating patients who do not meet eligibility criteria or who cannot be evaluated can improve the programs, but a major communication gap concerning the value of clinical trials continues between academic and community physicians. Moreover, requirements of physician participation and potential problems regarding third-party reimbursement mitigate any significant alteration in the accession patterns in the near future.

Whatever the reasons for the low national accession rates, we must recognize that therapeutic decisions are based on this relatively small sample of patients. Yet, many of us believe that the detailed and elaborate guidelines provided in many of the protocols available for patients with cancer allow for the best care and at least state-of-the-art therapy, if not better treatment than available with conventional care. We have documented this in the treatment of acute leukemia in adults in Rochester, New York (6). More public participation via the news media and discussion about the importance of clinical trials and the necessity to improve the results of particular cancers, including lung, bladder, colorectal and prostate, could be most helpful.

Four thousand investigators receive partial support from the cooperative or contract supported groups, representing six major specialties, gynecology, medicine, pathology, pediatrics, radiation therapy, and surgery.

CLINICAL TRIALS RESEARCH: ETHICAL DILEMMAS

In an editorial, "Randomized Clinical Trials and the Doctor-Patient Relationship: An Ethical Dilemma," Hellman (3) challenged the concept of prospective clinical trials. The basis for this challenge was the contention that a physician's belief or reasoned advice should prevail over objective considerations. It presupposes that, by being in a position of authority and by his or her experience, training, and interest, the oncologist can select the best treatment from a variety of options including unconfirmed but hoped-for improvements in treatment options.

Hellman opposes, as well, the confirmatory clinical trial, wherein a new treatment shows promise in a small number of patients—usually less than 30. In such pilot studies, the false-positive response rate may be close to 25%. To accept such

preliminary reports as standard care without verification would certainly be contrary to the goal of "the greatest good for the greatest number."

No one denies that patient selection for clinical trials exists and that both good and poor candidates are omitted. It is hoped that this practice is balanced throughout participating institutions. Unquestionably, the normal physician-patient relationship is altered by participation of each in prospective clinical trials. The patient should be fully informed about treatment alternatives and available programs if he or she chooses not to participate, and be assured that such refusal would not jeopardize the physician-patient relationship. The prospective clinical trial may not be the ultimate scientific technique for advancing knowledge in therapeutic oncology. However, despite its shortcomings, it provides reasonably impartial data that enable oncologists to reject or accept new programs.

An important aspect of the clinical trials program is the question of reimbursement for the cost of patient participation. Medical insurance agencies have supported the cost of investigative trials whenever this therapy has been viewed as acceptable by the community of peers. However, with spiraling medical costs and the pressure to contain such costs, a closer look at the responsibility for payment may be necessary. A series of meetings between the third-party payers, representatives for the NCI, the Health Care Financing Administration, and clinical investigators should be encouraged. The development of curative strategies, such as those now available for Hodgkin's disease, lymphomas, leukemias, and testicular cancers, can have a positive impact on industrial productivity.

SUMMARY

Despite the advances in the overall, multidisciplinary management of cancer in the United States, 60% of patients diagnosed with cancer will have gross or microscopic metastatic disease. Certainly, several of these advanced malignancies such as acute lymphocytic leukemia, Hodgkin's disease, diffuse histiocytic lymphoma, testicular cancer, Wilms' tumor, Ewing's sarcoma, and Burkitt's lymphoma have yielded to chemotherapeutic regimens. However, the major incident cancers (lung, colon, and breast) continue to be incurable in the macrometastatic setting. A continued search for new agents, including immunoadjuvants, hypoxic sensitizers, and chemoprotectors, is a necessary component of the NCI's long-term plan to reduce the mortality for cancer.

Recommended Reading

The drug development program of NCI (4) is one of the major sources for the introduction of new cancer agents and is well-described in "The Drug Development and Clinical Trials Program of the Division of Cancer Treatment" by DeVita *et al.* (2). The counterpoint to randomized clinical trials can be found in Hellman's statement on the ethical dilemma, "Randomized Clinical Trials and the Doctor-Patient Relationship: An Ethical Dilemma" (3). A good illustration of how pilot agent studies are initiated in a cooperative group is the report by Bennett and Zelen in "Pilot Studies and New Agent Programs of the ECOG" (1). Research strategies in clinical investigative issues for drugs and combined modalities are an active topic in the current literature, "Nonrandomized Clinical Trials of Cancer Chemotherapy" (5) and "Design and Conduct of Clinical Trials" (3a). A good general reference on clinical trials is "New Methodologic Guidelines for Reports of Clinical Trials" (21).

REFERENCES

General References

1. Bennett, J.M.; Zelen, M. Pilot studies and new agent programs of the ECOG. Cancer Treat. Rep. 64:525; 1980.
1a. Benson, A.B. III; Pregler, J.P.; Bean, J.A.; Rademaker, A.W.; Eshler, B.; Anderson, K. Oncologists' reluctance to accrue patients onto clinical trials: an Illinois cancer center study. J. Clin. Onc. 9: (11) 2067-2075, 1991.
2. DeVita, V.T.; Oivero, U.T.; Muggia, F.M.; et al. The drug development and clinical trials program of the division of cancer treatment, National Cancer Institute. Cancer Clin Trials 2:195-217; 1979.
3. Hellman, S. Randomized clinical trials and the doctor-patient relationship: an ethical dilemma. Cancer Clin. Trials 2:189-195; 1979.
3a. Simon, R.M. Design and conduct of clinical trials. In: DeVita, V.T., Jr., Hellman, S., Rosenberg, S.A. (eds.), 3rd ed. Cancer: Principles and Practice of Oncology. Philadelphia, PA: JB Lippincott Co.; 1989:396-422.
4. Summary Report of the Chemotherapy Program. Bethesda, MD: National Cancer Institute; 1972.
5. Tannock, I.; Warr, D. Nonrandomized clinical trials of cancer chemotherapy: phase II or III? J. Ntl. Cancer Inst. 80:800-801; 1988.

Specific References

6. Boros, L.; Chuang, C.; Butler, F.O.; Bennett, J.M. Leukemia in Rochester (NY). A 17-year experience with an analysis of the role of cooperative group (ECOG) participation. Cancer 56:2161-2169; 1985.
7. Cannon, W.B. The way of an investigator. New York, NY: W. W. Norton and Company; 1945.
8. Carter, S.K.; Selawry, O.; Slavik, M. Phase I clinical trials. Natl. Cancer Inst. Monogr. 45:75-80; 1977.
9. Estey, E.; Hoth, D.; Simon, R.; Marsoni, S.; Leyland-Jones, B.; Wittes, R. Therapeutic response in phase I trials of antineoplastic agents. Cancer Treatment Rep. 70:1105-1117; 1986.
10. Gehan, E.A. Early human studies with anti-cancer agents: the question of sample size. J. Chronic Dis. 15:265-268; 1962.
11. Harvey, W.H.; Fleming, T.R.; von Hoff, D.D.; et al. Phase II study of fludarabine phosphate in previously untreated patients with colorectal caricnoma: a Southwest Oncology Group Study. Cancer Treat. Rep. 71:1319-1320; 1987.
12. Johnson, R.K.; Swyryd, E.A.; Stark, G.R. Effects of N (phosphonacetyl) L-aspartate on murine tumors and normal tissues in vivo and in vitro and the relationship of sensitivities to rate of proliferation and level of aspartate transcarbamylase. CancerRes. 33:371-378; 1978.
13. Krakoff, I. Cancer chemotherapeutic agents. In: Ca-a Cancer Journal for Clinicians. New York, NY: American Cancer Society, Inc. Vol. 37, No. 2: 93-105; 1987.
14. McCuster, J.; Wax, A.; Bennett, J.M. Cancer patient accessions into clinical trials. Am. J. Clin. Oncol. 5:227-236; 1982.
15. Marsoni, S.; Holts, D.; Simon, R.; Leyland-Jones, B.; DeRosa, M.; Wittes, R.E.. Clinical drug development: an analysis of phase II trials, 1970-1985. Cancer Treatment Reports 71:71-80; 1987.
16. Radiation Oncology Coordination Subcommittee Organization (ROCS) Prospectus. Int. J. Radiat. Oncol. Biol. 5:595-632; 1978.
17. Rubin, P.; Keys, H.; Salazar, O. New designs for radiation oncology research in clinical trials. Semin. Oncol. 8:453-472; 1981.
18. Sternberg, C.N.; Yagoda, A.; Scher, H.I.; et al. M-VAC for advanced transitional cell carcinoma of the urothelium. J. Urol. 139:461-469; 1988.
19. Wittes, R.E. Antineoplastic agents and FDA regulations: square pegs for round holes? Cancer Treat. Rep. 71:795-806; 1987.
20. Wittes, R.E.; Friedman, M.A. Accrual to clinical trials. J. Natl. Cancer. Inst. 80:884-885; 1988.
21. Wittes, R.E.; Simon, R. New methodologic guidelines for reports of clinical trials. Simon & Wittes Cancer Treatment Report 69:1-3; 1985.

Craig S. McCune, M.D., Medical Oncology
Alex Yuang-Chi Chang, M.D., Medical Oncology

Chapter **10**

BASIC CONCEPTS OF TUMOR IMMUNOLOGY AND PRINCIPLES OF IMMUNOTHERAPY

At the heart of the immune system is the ability to distinguish between self and nonself. Virtually every body cell carries distinctive molecules that identify it as self.

L.W. Schindler (36a)

PERSPECTIVE

Research in immunology has rapidly expanded our knowledge of the cells, cell products, and mechanisms that underlie the normal functions of the immune system. Research in cancer immunology has led to products of the immune system that are being tested as agents for treatment and concepts of treatment involving the immune system. Selected topics in cancer immunology, immune system products, and concepts of therapy will be reviewed in this chapter.

Immune Cells That Can Participate in Killing of Tumor Cells

The T-helper lymphocyte (CD4+) has a central role in the immune response. Although not capable of killing a tumor cell by direct contact, the role of helper lymphocytes in tumor immunity appears to be that these lymphocytes are sensitized by contact with tumor antigens, they circulate in the body, and when they encounter tumor cells, they become activated and release the spectrum of lymphokines that promote cytotoxicity locally by cytotoxic T-lymphocytes (CTL), natural killer (NK) cells, or macrophages. Methods to activate and expand this population of lymphocytes are important areas of investigation.

Cytotoxic cells in humans consist of activated macrophages, activated lymphocytes (CTL), antibody dependent cytotoxic cells (ADCC), NK cells, lymphokine-activated killer lymphocytes (LAK), and tumor-infiltrating lymphocytes (TIL). These cells can be tumor antigen specific (CTL, ADCC, TIL) or nonspecific (macrophage, LAK, NK).

CTLs (CD8+) are sensitized by contact with tumor antigens and circulate. When they encounter a tumor cell bearing the same sensitizing antigen, the CTLs bind to the surface of the tumor cell and cytoplasmic granules migrate to the interface. Cytolytic factors are released that kill the tumor cell.

Circulating and localized macrophages must be activated to be cytotoxic. Activation of macrophages may be multistep and involves mitogen and cytokines (such as interferon (IFN), gamma, and tumor necrosis factor) for macrophages to differentiate to a cytotoxic stage. The mechanism of cytolysis includes generation of free-oxygen radicals, protease, or C3a (10,18).

NK cells are derived from large granular lymphocytes in the peripheral blood (3,18,19). These cells can lyse some tumor cells without prior antigen sensitization and are therefore described as being nonspecific in their cytolytic role. NK cell activity is augmented by IFNs, interleukin-2 (IL-2), and other cytokines. NK cells may also play a role in preventing metastasis from primary tumors.

LAK cells are largely derived from NK cells (3). They can be produced in vitro when peripheral blood lymphocytes are cultured with IL-2. They also may be produced in vivo by administering high doses of IL-2. Like NK cells, they are not dependent on prior antigen stimulation and specificity. The structures they recognize on tumor cell surfaces have not been identified.

TIL are derived from solid tumor samples. In preclinical animal models of therapy, the TIL cells are 50 to 100 times more potent than LAK cells (35). TILs can be expanded by IL-2 and given back to treat the patient from which they were taken. TILs are predominantly T lymphocytes with high antigen specificity in lysing autologous tumor cells, and their activity is restricted by the major histocompatibility complex. In animal studies, the recipient must be pretreated with cyclophosphamide or total body irradiation for TIL cells to function. TILs can pass through capillary vessels and localize to tumor nodules.

Tumor Antigens

The surface of a cell has a variety of molecules such as proteins, glycoproteins, and glycolipids, which project externally. Normally these surface molecules are not antigens; that is, they are not capable of initiating an immune response. These "self" molecules are tolerated by the immune system in contrast to "foreign" molecules that are present on the surface of bacteria or viruses, which function as antigens and provoke an immune response. In the transition from a normal to a malignant cell, marked changes occur in the genetic makeup of cancer cells such that the DNA appears capable of producing new surface molecules, or changes in the frequency and configuration of previous molecules. Some of these changes are sufficiently distinct to be antigenic and recognized as foreign by the immune system. These new molecules are defined as tumor-associated antigens.

Our knowledge of tumor antigens is incomplete and based on indirect evidence such as antibody, cell-mediated, or antitumor responses implying the presence of antigens. Extensive experiments with animal cancers also indicate that tumor antigens are a regular feature of tumors. Three types of immunotherapy are directed at these tumor antigens: monoclonal antibodies, vaccines, and adoptive immunotherapy with tumor specific lymphocytes.

Immune Surveillance

An ongoing surveillance by circulating immune cells has been postulated as the key mechanism in the natural defense against human carcinogenesis (2). It was originally proposed that our immune system can recognize and destroy nascent neoplastic cells. This can easily explain the increased cancer incidence in immune-deficient or immunosuppressed patients and the fact that not everyone develops cancer although we are frequently exposed to carcinogens in the environment. The hypothesis originally had two premises: (l) that tumor cells can elicit immune recognition by expressing tumor specific antigens (i.e., tumor cells are immunogenic) and (2) the host can destroy tumor cells with CTLs specifically reactive to tumor antigens.

It appears that most human tumors are not immunogenic in their natural state; that is, they do not initiate an immune response via cytotoxic T cells. When the human immune system is defective, as in congenital immunodeficiency states or human immunodeficiency virus infection, certain malignancies are more prevalent, particularly lymphomas. It is not clear whether these malignancies are due to a failure of an immune surveillance response or due to basic derangements of the lymphocyte component of immunity.

It has been postulated that macrophages or NK cells may be components of protection against carcinogenesis. The studies suggest NK cells may have a role in preventing metastases but not a significant role in preventing primary tumor development. In summary, immune surveillance continues to be a much discussed concept but lacks firm evidence of a significant role.

ANTIGEN-SPECIFIC IMMUNOTHERAPIES

Monoclonal Antibodies

These highly purified antibodies are produced by cloned hybridoma cell lines. They are selected to produce an antibody that reacts with a single site on an antigen. Extracts from human tumor cells have been used to immunize mice. The mice form antibody-producing B-lymphocytes, which are hybridized to create hybridomas producing murine monoclonal antibodies. Human B-lymphocytes from cancer patients have been used to make hybridomas that produce human monoclonal antibodies. When murine monoclonal antibodies have been administered to patients, a human antimouse antibody response has frequently occurred, which is a major limitation on the use of antibodies of mouse origin. Human monoclonal antibodies are more desirable but much harder to produce (23).

Murine monoclonal antibodies have been used in trials of treatment for melanoma (38,42), chronic lymphocytic leukemia (13), B-cell lymphoma (1,28), and gastrointestinal carcinomas (23,37). Responses have been observed in all of these tumor types (Table 10-1). Methods are being sought to produce more durable responses and higher response rates. One concept is to use the antibody as a carrier for toxins or radioactive isotopes by conjugating these agents to the antibody.

Some of the challenges in this field include: (a) difficulty in achieving a sufficiently high concentration of antibody at the cell surface to deliver the toxin or radioactivity in lethal doses; (b) host antibody responses may block repeated use of the agent; (c) the specificity of the antibodies is frequently not limited to tumor but can be taken up by other tissues; and (d) the tumor antigens being targeted by the antibodies are not constantly expressed by the tumor cells.

Table 10-1. Cancers, Leukemias, and Lymphomas That Have Responded to Immunologic Treatment

	Modality (Response Rate)[l]	(References)
Renal Carcinoma	Vaccines (20%-25%) (15,40)	IFN (16%-17%) (1,29)
	IL-2/LAK (16%-33%) (24,41)	IL-2 (0%-18%) (29)
	Coumarin (33%) (38,39)	
Melanoma	IL-2/TIL (55%) (22)	IL-2/LAK (23%) (24)
	Vaccines (10%-29%) (17,18)	MoAbs (5%-19%) (9,10)
	IFN (11%) (1)	IL-2 (16%-22%) (24,42)
Colon	Vaccines (adjuvant) (16)	IL-2/LAK (12%) (24)
	MoAbs (5%-10%) (13,14)	
Hairy Cell Leukemia	IFN (80%) (25)	
Chronic Myelogenous Leukemia	IFN (70%) (26)	
Lymphomas	MoAbs (55%) (l)	IL-2/LAK (75%) (1)
	IFN (15%-46%) (1)	
Head and Neck	IFN (91%) (1)	IL-2 (80%) (43)
Myeloma	IFN (17%) (1)	
Ovarian Cancer	IFN (19%) (1)	
Kaposi's Sarcoma	IFN (36%) (1,28)	

[l]Complete plus partial responses.

IFN = Interferon; IL-2 = Interleukin-2; LAK = lymphokine activated killer cells; TIL = tumor infiltrating lymphocytes; MoAbs = monoclonal antibodies.

Vaccines for Active Specific Immunotherapy

The vaccines being tested clinically consist of: (a) whole tumor cells irradiated to prevent growth (4,20,36); (b) tumor cells disrupted (lysates) by homogenization, sonication and/ or freezing and thawing (29); (c) virus-infected tumor cell lines disrupted to form a lysate (43); and (d) solubilized surface antigens collected from cultured tumor cell lines (7). These vaccines are administered as injections into the skin along with an adjuvant to make them immunogenic. Animal experiments suggest that vaccines induce cell-mediated responses, especially T-helper lymphocytes and T-cytotoxic lymphocytes, the key elements in killing tumor cells.

Vaccines for malignant melanoma have produced objective remissions in advanced disease (4,29), and vaccines for early melanoma are being studied (7). A randomized study for early colon cancer showed a significant advantage for vaccine-treated patients versus untreated controls (20). Metastatic renal carcinoma patients have undergone regressions lasting longer than 5 years following treatment with vaccines (27,36).

The challenges in this field include: (a) learning to produce vaccines from cultured allogeneic cell lines, which has the practical advantage of not requiring surgical removal of the patient's own tumor; (b) providing multiantigen vaccines to deal with the problem of antigenic heterogeneity; (c) identifying effective, nontoxic local adjuvants; and (d) identifying those cytokines that can augment the inherently weak immunogenicity of these vaccines.

Adoptive Immunotherapy with Tumor-Specific Lymphocytes

This approach refers to methods in which lymphocytes taken from a patient are grown in the laboratory to expand their numbers and acquire a specificity in function by priming them through contact with the target tumor antigens. These tumor-specific lymphocytes are then returned to the patient by transfusion along with the growth factor of the lymphocytes (IL-2). This treatment concept was tested in animal models (8,35), and has shown clinical success in treating melanoma (34). At present, the technique for obtaining tumor-specific lymphocytes is to surgically remove a tumor, dissociate the cells, separate the lymphocytes, and expand them in culture. These cells are the previously mentioned TILs.

There are challenges in this field in that lymphocytes cannot always be grown from a tumor sample; the specificity for tumor cells may not persist during expansion in culture; and the laboratory effort is expensive.

IMMUNOLOGIC AND BIOLOGIC AGENTS FOR IMMUNOTHERAPY

Lymphokine-Activated Killer Cells

While developing the approach of adoptive immunotherapy with tumor-specific lymphocytes, described above, a phenomenon was observed. Lymphocytes taken from patients and grown in vitro with the lymphokine IL-2, developed a subpopulation that acquired a cytotoxic nature (17). These cells do not kill on the basis of antigen specificity, but by a nonspecific mechanism that kills a broad spectrum of tumor cells. For unexplained reasons, these cells do not attack and kill normal cells. The LAK phenomenon has been evaluated in clinical trials that revealed responses in renal carcinoma, melanoma, and colon cancer (33) (Table 10-1).

The challenges in this field include severe side effects from the high doses of IL-2 required, the need for methods to produce higher response rates, and the high costs associated with the extensive laboratory effort.

Interferons

IFNs are a group of proteins produced by a variety of cells, and have many biologic activities. Six are possibly related to the antitumor effects: antiviral, antiproliferative, immunomodulation, alteration of cell membrane, promotion of differentiation, and inhibition of oncogene activation. The mechanisms of action are not clearly understood but appear to involve binding of the IFN molecule to its receptors on the cell membrane, which in turn initiates a second message to synthesize new proteins by gene activation.

There are three major types of IFNs: alpha (leukocyte), beta (fibroblast), and gamma (immune). They differ in physical and chemical properties, and in physiologic functions. Alpha IFN has been studied most extensively in human diseases. IFN-ß is the oldest molecule by evolution and has more antiproliferative activity than either IFNα or IFNγ against solid tumor cell lines. IFNγ is part of the normal immune response to foreign antigens. There is little IFN to be found in the blood of healthy people. However, during a viral infection such as herpes simplex virus, although there is only a small amount of circulating IFN, the fever blister vesicles contain high titers of IFN, which probably mediate many local reactions. It is thought that IFN contributes most of the symptoms and signs we experience during a viral infection such as the flu.

IFN has been shown to inhibit the growth of a variety of normal and malignant cells in vitro. Large-scale clinical trials were only possible when pure recombinant IFNα was made by *E. Coli* with recombinant DNA techniques in 1980. IFN can suppress the passage of cells through the cell cycle, thus increasing the cell cycle length and slowing the cell growth. IFN may affect all phases of the cell cycle and prevent the progression of cells from the G0 to the Gl phase, depending on the kind of cells and its sensitivity to IFN. The antiproliferation effect is one of the major actions of IFN against tumor growth.

IFNs can enhance the cytolytic activity of cytotoxic T lymphocytes, NK lymphocytes, and macrophages against various malignant cells. In addition, in some cases, IFNs increase the expression of the histocompatibility antigens, and tumor-specific antigens, thus making malignant cells more immunogenic. IFNs also alter the cytoskeleton structure of the cell membrane and render malignant cells less mobile.

Recombinant human IFN-alpha is the only kind of IFN approved for use in the United States. Other forms of IFN preparation such as natural IFN-alpha, lymphoblastoid IFN-alpha, a natural IFN-beta, recombinant IFNβ or IFN-gamma are being studied. Interferon-alpha has been found to be highly effective in the treatment of hairy cell leukemia (16) and chronic myelogenous leukemia (CML) (39) (Table 10-1). It is active against nodular lymphoma, cutaneous T-cell lymphoma (12), AIDS-associated Kaposi's sarcoma (22), and the carcinoid syndrome. It also has modest activity in the treatment of renal cell carcinoma (31) and melanoma (1). It has little antitumor activity against common cancers such as lung, colon, or breast.

About 80% of the patients with hairy cell leukemia will respond to low-dose IFN therapy. They may require therapy for 3 to 6 months to show the therapeutic benefits.

One important and interesting finding in the studies of IFN for the treatment of CML is the reduction of Philadelphia-chromosome-positive cells in the bone marrow after therapy. About 70% of the patients will be in remission with IFN treatment and 40% have significant reduction of Philadelphia-chromosome-containing leukemia cells, with 10% becoming negative. Longer observation is required before investigators can determine whether IFN prolongs the survival of CML patients.

The most common side effects of IFN therapy consist of constitutional complaints such as fever, chills, myalgia, headache, nausea, anorexia, and weight loss (so-called flu-like syndrome). This flu-like syndrome is dependent on the dose and is self-limited. However, it is also the most common dose-limiting side effect. Occasionally, patients may develop myelosuppression in the form of leukopenia and, rarely, thrombocytopenia. Myelosuppression is reversible in 24 to 72 hours after discontinuing the IFN. Modest elevation of hepatic enzymes is common and without clinical significance except on rare occasions in which patients' deaths were thought to be due to fulminant hepatic necrosis. Other rare complications include interstitial nephritis with the nephrotic syndrome, confusion, coma, arrhythmia, and hypotension. IFN-ß has been reported to cause more cardiovascular complications and require more attention during therapy. IFN-ß has the least side effects on the basis of antiviral units.

The future investigations of IFN involve combination of IFN with other treatment modalities such as chemotherapy, irradiation, and other biologic agents.

Interleukin-2

IL-2 is produced by T lymphocytes during an immune response after the lymphocyte receives signals from an antigen-presenting cell and IL-1. IL-2 is a T-cell growth factor as well as a differentiation agent. In vitro, high-dose IL-2 expands the lymphocyte numbers with a preference for LAK cells. When adminstered in vivo, the antitumor activity of IL-2 is thought to be caused by the activation and expansion of LAK cells, which can kill the tumor cells directly, although other mechanisms such as induction of tumor necrosis factor and gamma interferon are possible. IL-2 alone at high doses or in combination with LAK cells has been used to treat a variety of cancers. Fifteen to thirty percent of patients with renal cell carcinoma and melanoma have responded. A few patients have long-lasting remissions after a single course of treatment. However, success is at the price of significant side effects such as fever, chills, rash, arthralgia, hypotension, weight gain with edema, oliguria, pulmonary edema, congestive heart failure, and central nervous system (CNS) toxicities. Most of the cardiovascular, renal, and CNS complications can be explained by the capillary leak syndrome caused by IL-2 which simulates endotoxin shock syndrome with peripheral vasodilation and increased demand of cardiac output and oliguria (15,40). Brain edema may also occur and pro-

duce confusion, psychotic behavior, and though rare, coma (9). The side effects of IL-2 are dose and schedule dependent. Lowering the dose and changing the administration to continuous infusion rather than bolus have reduced the frequency and degree of toxicity without compromising the therapeutic results (44). Current clinical investigations focus on the combination of IL-2 with IFN, cyclophosphamide, LAK cells, TIL cells, and cancer vaccines.

Tumor Necrosis Factor

Tumor necrosis factor (TNF) is a nonglycosylated protein of 157 amino acids that can mediate endotoxin shock and induce fever, cachexia, and immunomodulation by activation of neutrophils and macrophages (6). TNF is produced by monocytes, which are part of the immune response. Interest in TNF as an immunotherapeutic agent is based on the fact that TNF is cytotoxic for tumor cells. In addition, TNF also has antiviral activity and can induce and interact with other lymphokines.

Early clinical trials with recombinant TNF have been disappointing, with few objective responses and some severe side effects such as fever, chills, hypotension, CNS toxicity, and coagulopathy. Direct-tumor (intralesional) injection of TNF causes hemorrhagic necrosis and regression of tumor nodules. Trials using combination TNF with other biologic agents, hyperthermia, and chemotherapy are currently under way.

Chemically Defined Immune Modulators

In addition to the biologic products, certain chemical compounds also possess immunomodulatory effects. The agent used in developing such a drug should be orally active without much systemic toxicity to bypass the need for parenteral administration and hospitalization for the patients. Bropirimine (32), levamisole, and coumarin show promising preliminary results in these aspects.

1. *Bropirimine* (2-amino-5-bromo-6-phenyl 4(H)-pyriminone, ABPP) is an orally active biologic response modifier in animals and humans. It can induce elevated IFN levels in the serum, augments NK activity, possesses antiviral properties, and inhibits tumor growth in different animal tumor models. In several ongoing clinical trials, bropirimine causes mild to moderate side effects such as nausea, hypotension, and itching in a small percentage of patients. Clinical responses have been observed in patients with advanced renal cell carcinoma, nodular lymphoma, and melanoma.

2. *Levamisole* is an antihelminthic that can augment and restore macrophage function. In one randomized study it was found to increase the disease-free survival in locally advanced colorectal cancer patients who received levamisole and 5Fu postoperatively (45). In other studies, levamisole failed to show any benefit as an adjuvant therapy in patients with lung cancer and lymphoma. Its benefit for breast cancer patients in the adjuvant setting is controversial (21). Levamisole is also well tolerated by patients—nausea is the most common complaint. Granulocytopenia occurs rarely.

3. *Coumarin* (1,2-benzopyron) is the precursor of warfarin but lacks anticoagulation activity. It has been shown to augment lymphocyte mitogen response to phytohemagglutinin and increase the number of monocytes and

the percentage of DR+ monocytes. Coumarin, when combined with cimetidine, yielded a 33% response in renal cell carcinoma patients in one study (25,26) and caused tumor regression in melanoma patients. Coumarin and cimetidine are well tolerated, with minimal and rare toxicities. Further studies are required to define the immune modulation and the role of coumarin as an immunotherapy agent.

Recommended Reading

Fundamentals of immunology can be reviewed in a variety of texts, including *Textbook of Immunology, 2nd ed.* by Unanue and Benacerraf (41). An overview of tumor immunology and immunotherapy is found in the recent oncologic text, *Principles of Cancer Treatment* (4). A well illustrated, concise text by Schindler provides an excellent primer on "Understanding the Immune System" (36a). Specific references are provided for the reader who wishes to pursue the subject in more depth.

REFERENCES

General References

1. Foon, K.A. Biological response modifiers: the new immunotherapy. Cancer Res. 49:1621-1639;1989.
2. Kripke, M.L. Immunoregulation of carcinogenesis: Past, present, and future. J. Natl. Can. Inst. 80:722-727;1988.
3. Ortaldo, J.R.; Longo, D.L. Human natural lymphocyte effector cells: definition, analysis of activity, and clinical effectiveness. J. Natl. Can. Inst. 80:999-1010;1988.

Specific References

4. Bennett, J.A.; Mitchell, M.S. Principles of tumor immunology. In: Carter, S.K.; Glatstein, E.; Livingston, R.B., eds. Principles of Cancer Treatment. St. Louis, MO: McGraw-Hill; 1982:162-169.
5. Berd, D.; Maguire, H.; Mastrangelo, M. Induction of cell-mediated immunity to autologous melanoma cells and regression of metastases after treatment with a melanoma cell vaccine preceded by cyclophosphamide. Cancer Res. 46:2572;1986.
6. Beutler, B.; Cerami, A. Cachectin: More than a tumor necrosis factor. New Engl. J. Med. 316:379-385; 1987.
7. Bystryn, J.C.; Oratz, R.; Harris, M.N.; Roses, D.F.; Golomb, F.M.; Speyer, J.L. Immunogenicity of a polyvalent melanoma antigen vaccine in humans. Cancer 61:1065-1070; 1988.
8. Cheever, M.A.; Greenberg, P.D., Fefer, A.; Gillis, S. Augmentation of the anti-tumor therapeutic efficacy of long-term cultured T lymphocytes by *in vivo* administration of purified interleukin 2. J. Exp. Med. 155:968-980;1982.
9. Denicoff, K.D.; Rubinow, D.R.; Papa, M.Z.; *et al.* The neuropsychiatric effects of treatment with interleukin-2 and lymphokine-activated killer cells. Ann. Intern. Med. 107:293-300; 1987.
10. Fidler, I.J. Macrophage and metastasis—a biological approach to cancer therapy. Cancer Res. 45:4714-4726; 1985.
11. Fisher, R.I.; Coltman, C.A.; Doroshow, J.H.; Rayner, A.A.; Hawkins, M.J.; Mier, J.W.; Wiernik, P.; McMannis, J.D.; Weiss, G.R.; Margolin, K.A.; Gemlo, B.T.; Hoth, D.F.; Parkinson, D.R.; Paietta, E. Metastatic renal cancer treated with interleukin-2 and lymphokine-activated killer cells. Ann. Intern. Med. 108:518-523; 1988.
12. Foon, K.A.; Roth, M.S., Bunn, P.A., Jr. Interferon therapy of non-Hodgkin's lymphoma. Cancer 59:601-604; 1987.
13. Foon, K.A.; Schroff, R.W.; Bunn, P.A.; *et al.* Effects of monoclonal antibody therapy in patients with chronic lymphocytic leukemia. Blood 64:1085-1094; 1985.
14. Forni, G.; Cavallo, G.P.; Giovarelli, M.; Benetton, G.; Jemma, C.; Barioglio, M.G.; De Stefani, A.; Forni, M.; Santoni, A.; Modesti, A.; Cavallo, G.; Menzio, P.; Cortesina, G. Tumor immunotherapy by local injection of interleukin 2 and non-reactive lymphocytes. Prog. Exp. Tumor Res. 32:187-212;1988.
15. Gaynor, E.R.; Vitek, L.; Sticklin, L.; *et al.* The hemodynamic effects of treatment with interleukin-2 and lymphokine-activated killer cells. Ann. Int. Med. 109:953-958; 1988.
16. Golomb, H.M.; Fefer, A.; Golde, D.W.; *et al.* Report of a multi-institutional study of 193 patients with hairy cell leukemia treated with interferon alfa-2b. Semin. Oncol. 15(Suppl. 5):7-9; 1988.
17. Grimm, E.A.; Mazumder, A.; Zang, H.; Rosenberg, S. The lymphokine-activated killer cell phenomenon: lysis of NK-resistant fresh solid tumor cells by IL-2 activated autologous human peripheral blood lymphocytes. J. Exp. Med. 155:1823;1982.
18. Herberman, R.B. Overview of the role of macrophages, natural killer cells and antibody-dependent cellular cytotoxicity as mediators of biological response modification. In: Chirigos, M.A., ed. Mediation of Cellular Immunity in Cancer by Immune Modifiers. New York, NY: Raven Press; 1981:261-267.
19. Herberman, R.B. Possible role of natural killer cells and other effector cells in immune surveillance against cancer. J. Invest. Dermatol. 83:137s-140s; 1984.
20. Hoover, H.; Surdyke, M.; Dangel, R.; Peters, L.; Hanna, M. Delayed cutaneous hypersensitivity to autologous tumor cells in colorectal cancer patients immunized with an autologous tumor cell: Bacillus Calmette-Guerin vaccine. Cancer Res. 44:1671;1984.
21. Klefstrom, P.; Grohn, P.; Heinonen, E.; Holsti, L.; Holsti, P. Adjuvant postoperative radiotherapy, chemotherapy, and immunotherapy in stage III breast cancer. Cancer 60:936-942; 1987.
22. Krown, S.E. The role of interferon in the therapy of epidemic Kaposi's sarcoma. Semin. Oncol. 14(Suppl. 3):27-33; 1987.
23. Larrick, J.W.; Bourla, J.M. Prospects for the therapeutic use of human monoclonal antibodies. J. Biol. Resp. Mod. 5:379-393;1986.
24. LuBuglio, A.F.; Saleh, M.N.; Lee, J.; Khazaeli, M.B.; Carrano, R.; Holden, H.; Wheeler, R.H. Phase I trial of multiple large doses of murine monoclonal antibody C017-1A. I. Clinical aspects. J. Natl. Can. Inst. 80:932-936;1988.
25. Marshall, E.; Mendelsohn, L.; Butler, K.; *et al.* Treatment of metastatic renal cell carcinoma with coumarin and cimetidine: a pilot study. J. Clin. Oncol. 5:862-866;1987.
26. Marshall, M.E.; Riley, L.K.; Rhoades, J.; *et al.* Effects of coumarin and cimetidine on peripheral blood lymphocytes, a natural killer cell and monocytes in patients with advanced malignancies . J. Biol. Resp. Mod. 8:62-69;1989.
27. McCune, C.S.; Schapira, D.V.; Henshaw, E.C. Specific Immunotherapy of advanced renal carcinoma: Evidence for the polyclonality of metastases. Cancer 47:1984-1987; 1981.
28. Miller, R.A.; Maloney, D.G.; Warnke, R.; Levy, R. Treatment of B-cell lymphoma with monoclonal anti-idiotype antibody. New Engl. J. Med. 306:517-522; 1982.
29. Mitchell, M.S.; Kan-Mitchell, J.; Kempf, R.A.; Harel, W.; Shau, H.; Lind, S. Active specific immunotherapy for melanoma: phase I trial of allogeneic lysates and a novel adjuvant. Can. Res. 48:5883; 1988.
30. Mitchell, M.S.; Kempf, R.A.; Harel, W.; Shau, H.; Boswell, W.D.; Lind, S.; Bradley, E.C. Effectiveness and tolerability of low-dose cyclophosphamide and low-dose intravenous interleukin-2 disseminated melanoma. J. Clin. Oncol. 6:409-424; 1988.
31. Muss, H.B. The role of biological response modifiers in metastatic renal cell carcinoma. Seminars in Oncol. 15:30-34; 1988.
32. Rios, A.; Stringfellow, D.A.; Fitzpatrick, F.A.; *et al.* Phase I study of ABPP, an oral interferon inducer, in cancer patients. J. Biol. Resp. Mod. 5:330-338; 1986.
33. Rosenberg, S.A.; Lotze, M.T., Muul, L.M.; Chang, A.E.; Avis, F.P.; Leitman, S.; Linehan, W.M.; Robertson, C.N.; Lee, R.E.; Rubin, J.T.; Seipp, C.A.; Simpson, C.G.; White, D.E. A progress report on the treatment of 157 patients with advanced cancer using lymphokine-activated killer cells and interleukin-2 or high-dose interleukin-2 alone. New Engl. J. Med. 316:889-897; 1987.
34. Rosenberg, S.A.; Packard, B.S.; Aebersold, P.M.; Solomon, D.; Topalian, S.L.; Toy, S.T.; Simon, P.; Lotze, M.T.; Yang, J.C.; Seipp, C.; Simpson, C.; Carter, C.; Bock, S.; Schwartzentruber, D.; Wei, J.P.; White, D.E. Use of tumor-infiltrating lymphocytes and interleukin-2 in the immunotherapy of patients with metastatic melanoma. New Eng. J. Med. 319:1676-1680; 1988.
35. Rosenberg, S.A.; Spiess, P, Lafreniere, R. A new approach to the adoptive immunotherapy of cancer with tumor-infiltrating lymphocytes. Science 233:1318-1321; 1986.
36. Sahasrabudhe, D.; deKernion, J.; Pontes, J.; Ryan, D.; O'Donnell, R.; Marquis, D.; Mudholkar, G.; McCune, C. Specific immuno-

therapy with suppressor function inhibition for metastatic renal cell carcinoma. J. Biol. Resp. Mod. 5:581; 1986.

36a. Schindler, L.W. Understanding the immune system. U.S. Dept. Health and Human Services. Bethesda, MD: NIH, July 1988.

37. Sears, H.F.; Herlyn, D.; Steplewski,Z.; Koprowski, H. Phase II clinical trial of a murine monoclonal antibody cytotoxic for gastrointestinal adenocarcinoma. Cancer Res. 45:5910-5913; 1985.

38. Spitler, L.E.; del Rio, M.; Khentigan, A.; Wedel, N.I.; Brophy, N.A.; Miller, L.L.; Harkonen, W.S.; Rosendorf, L.L.; Lee, H.M.; Mischak, R.P.; Kawahata, R.T.; Stoudemire, J.B.; Fradkin, L.B.; Bautista, E.E.; Scannon, P.J. Therapy of patients with malignant melanoma using a monoclonal antimelanoma antibody-ricin A chain immunotoxin. Can. Res. 47:1717-1723; 1987.

39. Talpaz, M.; Kantarjian, H.M.; McCredie, K.B.; Keating, M.J.; Trujillo, J.; Gutterman, J. Clinical investigation of human alpha interferon in chronic myelogeneous leukemia. Blood 69:1280-1288; 1987.

40. Textor, S.C.; Margolin, K.; Blayney, D.; Carlson, J.; Doroshow, J. Renal volume, and hormonal changes during therapeutic administration of recombinant interleukin-2 in man. Am. J. Med. 83:1055-1061; 1987.

41. Unanue, E.R.; Benacerraf, B. Textbook of immunology, 2nd ed. Baltimore, MD: Williams and Wilkins; 1984.

42. Vadhan-Raj, S.; Cordon-Cardo, C.; Carswell, E.; Mintzer, D.; Dantis, L; Duteau, C.; Templeton, M.A.; Oettgen, H.F.; Old, L.J.; Houghton, A.N. Phase I trial of a mouse monoclonal antibody against GD3 ganglioside in patients with melanoma: Induction of inflammation responses at tumor sites. J. Clin. Oncol. 6:1636-1648;1988.

43. Wallack, M.E.; Bash, J.A.; Leftheriotis, E. Positive relationship of clinical and serologic responses to vaccinia melanoma oncolysate. Arch. Surg. 122:1460-1463; 1987.

44. West, W.H.; Tauer, K.W.; Yannelli, J.R.; *et al.* Constant-infusion recombinant interleukin-2 in adoptive immunotherapy of advanced cancer. New Engl. J. Med. 316:898-905; 1987.

45. Windle, R.; Bell, P.R.F.; Shaw, D. Five year results of a randomized trial of adjuvant 5-fluorouracil and levamisole in colorectal cancer. Br. J. Surg. 74:569-572; 1987.

Chapter 11

AIDS

It is always darkest before the day dawneth.

Thomas Fuller (1608-1661)

PERSPECTIVE

Acquired immune deficiency syndrome (AIDS) is a fatal disorder characterized by life-threatening opportunistic infections in patients not exposed to immunosuppressive therapy or apparent immunosuppressive diseases. It is now known that the disorder is initiated by human immunodeficiency virus (HIV).

In addition to opportunistic infections, it is recognized that certain malignancies are associated with AIDS (5,10,16,23,32,91) and the Centers for Disease Control (CDC) proposed in 1986 to include certain malignancies—Kaposi's sarcoma (KS), high-grade lymphomas, and primary CNS lymphomas—in the classification system for HIV infection (4). Thus, the clinical spectrum of AIDS was expanded to include not only opportunistic infections, but also opportunistic neoplasia.

MALIGNANCY IN THE IMMUNOCOMPROMISED HOST

The concept of immunological surveillance, as proposed by Burnett and Thomas (3,26), theorizes that malignant clones of cells constantly arise only to be rejected by an intact host immune system. Any impairment of this system may lead to an uncontrolled tumor proliferation. Whatever the ultimate merit of this theory (8,24,27), there is considerable precedent for specific tumors arising in certain immunocompromised states. (Table 11-1). These have increased the understanding of the basic etiologic mechanisms of certain tumors and may enable one to anticipate the proliferation of tumors in immunocompromised states, such as in AIDS patients.

Tumors in Organ Transplant Recipients

With the advent of organ transplantation, there has been a marked increase of neoplasms in recipients of such transplants (15). The most comprehensive data have been collected by the Cincinnati Transplant Tumor Registry, which has reported on over 3,000 malignancies in organ transplant patients (19,20,21). Most of these patients had renal transplants.

The occurrence of certain tumors at constant time periods following transplantation is of interest. KS, for example, presents at a mean of 2 years following transplantation; lymphomas present 3 years following transplantation and tumors of the perineum 8 to 10 years after transplantation. On the other hand, there was no increase noted in the Cincinnati registry in the incidence of common cancers such as lung, prostate, colon and rectum, heart, and cervix.

Cancer of the skin and lips occurs with a 30-fold increase compared with age-matched controls (21). These tend to be mostly squamous cell neoplasia compared with the more common basal cell tumors in the general population. Additionally, these skin cancers often present as multiple tumors and tend to have a more aggressive clinical course that includes lymph node and visceral metastases.

KS, a rare tumor in the general population, occurs with an approximately 500-fold increased frequency in organ transplant recipients (12,21). While the disease may present as an indolent localized tumor similar to classic KS, more than one third of patients have a rapidly progressive clinical course, mainly with pulmonary and gastrointestinal (GI) involvement. The disease is fatal in 30% of these patients. It is interesting that there is response and remission induction in up to 30% of patients when the only treatment is a reduction or cessation of immunosuppressive therapy (42).

Non-Hodgkin's lymphomas occur with 50-fold in renal transplant recipients and account for 13% of malignancies reported to the Cincinnati registry (21). These are mainly B-cell, high-grade lymphomas; extranodal disease is commonly present and there is a marked predilection for central nervous system (CNS) involvement. The association with Epstein-Barr virus (EBV) infection is intriguing; the viral genome is almost always isolated from the lymphomatous tissue (11). The lymphoma may be polyclonal or monoclonal and, as in patients with KS, the disease may spontaneously remit following cessation of the immunosuppressive therapy (11).

Tumors Following Immunosuppressive Therapy (Nontransplant)

Autoimmune disorders and certain chronic inflammatory conditions are associated with an increased incidence of neoplasia (2,14,18). Nonetheless, there also appears to be an increase in malignancies in these conditions due to the immunosuppressive therapy given. In one study (15), non-Hodgkin's lymphomas increased 11-fold in patients treated with immunosuppressive agents (azathioprine, cyclophosphamide, or chlorambucil) for autoimmune disorders such as

Table 11-1. Tumors of the Immunocompromised Patient

Immuno-compromised State	Predominant Malignancy	Special Features
Organ Transplant Recipients	Skin and lips	Aggressive squamous cell.
	Kaposi's sarcoma High-grade lymphoma	May regress with reduced immuno-suppression.
Following Immunosuppressive Therapy	High-grade lymphoma	Similar to transplant recipients but lesser problem.
Following Cytotoxic Therapy	High-grade lymphoma (following Hodgkin's disease)	Must distinguish from the true carcinogenic effect of cytotoxic therapy.
Congenital immune deficiency	High-grade lymphoma Carcinoma Leukemia	Mainly in childhood. No increase in incidence of common cancers for this age group.
Acquired immune deficiency	Kaposi's sarcoma High-grade lymphoma	No evidence for direct involvement by HIV in tumor genome.

rheumatoid arthritis, systemic lupus erythematosus, or Sjogren's syndrome. Fortunately, the problem is small because of the limited use of immunosuppressive agents for nonmalignant conditions.

Tumors Following Cytotoxic Cancer Chemotherapy

Secondary malignancies are a well-recognized complication of cytotoxic therapy, especially alkylating agents. Most of the therapy-related malignancies are myeloid stem cell disorders such as myelodysplasia or frank acute myelogenous leukemia (6). The etiology of these malignancies is thought to be primarily related to the carcinogenic effects of alkylating agents leading to predictable chromosomal abnormalities (13). The contribution, if any, of the immunosuppressive effect of these drugs is unknown.

Of interest, however, is the increased incidence of non-Hodgkin's lymphoma following treatment for Hodgkin's disease, with a latent period as long as 10 to 15 years (20). It is likely that the immunosuppressive therapy given to cure the Hodgkin's disease may play a significant etiologic role in the genesis of the subsequent non-Hodgkin's lymphoma.

Tumors Associated with Congenital Immunodeficiencies

To date, there are 14 genetically determined immunodeficiency states associated with malignancy (7,25). The most comprehensive data have been collected by the Immunodeficiency Cancer Registry at the University of Minnesota, which has reported on malignancies in almost 400 patients (7). These immune deficiencies have a variety of cellular and/or humoral defects. Malignancies in ataxia-telangiectasia account for 35% of those reported to the Immunodeficiency registry; common variable immunodeficiency disease for 23%; Wiskott-Aldrich syndrome for 16%; and severe combined immunodeficiency disease for 6%. However, some of the more severe congenital immunodeficiency states have a low rate of malignancy only because of the poor survival of these patients as a result of their primary immunologic disorder. Approximately one half of the malignancies are non-Hodgkin's lymphomas and a majority of these are B-cell-aggressive lymphomas with frequent extranodal involvement of the brain and GI tract (9,17). Since most of these diseases occur in childhood, it is noteworthy that malignancies usually seen in this age group—nonlymphomatous cancer of the CNS; rhabdomyosarcoma; Wilms' tumor, Ewing's sarcoma, and retinoblastoma—are rarely observed. The rare disorder, x-linked lymphoproliferative syndrome, is of special interest because of the possible role of virus in the etiology of the associated malignancy, and because of the model that this syndrome may provide for other B-cell lymphomas associated with immunodeficiency, such as AIDS (22). In x-linked lymphoproliferative syndrome, there is a recognized impairment of T-cell regulation associated with recurrent EBV infection. What begins as an unregulated B-cell proliferation with polyclonal expansion may terminate as a monoclonal B-cell, high-grade lymphoma (22).

KAPOSI'S SARCOMA IN AIDS

Since the initial description of classic KS over a century ago (40), other types of KS have been recognized. While they all have identical histopathologic features, they differ in their mode of presentation and clinical course. In particular, they have transformed what was a rare disorder into a common neoplasm in certain immunodeficiency states, such as in renal transplants and AIDS (58).

Classic KS affects mainly elderly men, mostly of Jewish or Italian descent (54). It is confined to the lower extremities and has an indolent clinical course with a 10- to 15-year survival rate (56). Of special interest is the association in more than one third of the patients with other malignancies (56).

African KS was recognized early this century as a more aggressive disease than classic KS. Young adults living in Central Africa developed a disease that was often invasive to underlying bones and was fatal within 5 to 8 years (38). An even more virulent form of the disease, presenting with generalized lymphadenopathy and rapidly fatal, was described in children with African KS. The disease often occurred in clusters in Central Africa, usually in the setting of some immunologic compromise (50, 57). The disease also was noted to occur in a region geographically similar to African Burkitt's lymphoma (51). The association of KS with *renal transplants* has been previously described in this chapter. The association with immunodeficiency was confirmed when it was recognized that the disease would often remit, or even resist, as immunosuppressive therapy was withdrawn.

Epidemic KS is the term applied to KS that is associated with HIV infection. Up to 25% of all patients with AIDS have been reported to have KS (28) and in 1986 it was recognized as part of the clinical spectrum of AIDS and included in the CDC's classification (4). Epidemic KS is the commonest neoplasm in AIDS and the risk of developing this is close to 1,000 times that of the general population. Nevertheless, the distribution among AIDS patients is not equal, occurring more commonly in white male homosexuals than in other groups at risk for AIDS, suggesting that other etiologies associated with homosexuality may play a role (35).

While the clinical features are variable, epidemic KS often presents with disseminated mucocutaneous lesions with frequent lymph node and visceral involvement, especially of the GI tract and lungs. While several authors have attempted to deal with the varying clinical presentations by proposing different staging systems for AIDS-related KS (41,47,48) (Table 11-2) (41,47), it is not clear that anatomic classifications are of major prognostic importance in predicting the course of the disease (55). The course of the disease is often fulminant, with only a 20% survival in 2 years if there are associated opportunistic infections at the time of presentation.

Etiology

As with classic KS, the etiology of epidemic KS is unknown. While there is no clear genetic pattern to the disease, studies of histocompatibility antigens have reported an increased frequency of human leukocyte angtigen 5 among epidemic KS patients of Italian or Jewish descent (52). There appears to be an association with cytomegalovirus (CMV) infection. Elevated CMV titers are common in epidemic KS and DNA sequences as well as other viral antigens have been isolated from KS tissue (33). Because CMV is commonly present in AIDS patients (30) and because patients with classic KS do not have an increased frequency of CMV infection, it is likely that CMV is not causally related to KS, but may play a cofactorial role. Similarly, the HIV itself is thought to play no more than a cofactorial role, as there has been no evidence for direct involvement of HIV as the causative agent in epidemic KS (6a).

Treatment

There are no clear-cut guidelines for the therapy of epidemic KS, since there is currently no single, widely accepted staging system (see above). This adds to the difficulty of comparing published results of treatment.

The general basic principles for treatment, outlined in Table 11-3, are based on the extent of disease involvement; rate of progression or adverse prognostic factors such as B-symptoms, opportunistic infections, or cytopenias.

Radiotherapy

Radiotherapy, the primary therapy for classic KS, has also been used for epidemic KS.

It is an effective palliative modality for localized lesions or more extensive lesions that may be cosmetically unpleasant or functionally troublesome, such as lesions on the face, legs, soles of the feet, or any extensive cutaneous lesion that is ulcerated. The tumor itself is highly sensitive to radiation therapy (36) and single doses of 800 cGy can produce dramatic regression (37).

A range of fractionation schedules have been used and are equally effective. Thus, 1.5 to 3 or 5 Gy to levels of 15 to 40 Gy have been explored with a similar response rate of 90%, a median time to progression of 21 months, and actuarial freedom from relapse at 6 months of 69%.

Severe reactions, often in mucosa, occur in less than 20% of patients and can be modified with small fractions. Retreatment occurs in 8% to 23% of the patients.

Chemotherapy

Chemotherapy plays an important role in the treatment of epidemic KS (61). The most widely used single agent is vinblastine, which can produce good responses in up to 50% of patients (60). Other single agents with activity are vincristine and etoposide (VP-16) (41,45). The major advantage of using these single agents is the limited myelosuppression in these immunosuppressed patients.

More extensive disease is often treated with combination chemotherapy, which is most effective if adverse prognostic factors are not present. One combination regimen consists of

Table 11-2. Staging for Epidemic Kaposi's Sarcoma

NYU Staging (41)		UCLA Staging (47)	
Stage		*Stage*	
I	Cutaneous, locally indolent	I	Limited cutaneous (<10 lesions or one anatomic area
II	Cutaneous, locally aggressive with or without regional lymph nodes	II	Disseminated cutaneous (<10 lesions or more than one anatomic area)
III	Generalized mucocutaneous and/or lymph node involvement*	III	Visceral only (GI,LN)
IV	Visceral	IV	Cutaneous and visceral, or pulmonary KS
Subtypes		*Subtypes*	
A	No systemic signs or symptoms	A	No systemic signs or symptoms
B	Systemic signs: weight loss (10%) or fever (100°F orally, unrelated to an identifiable source of infection lasting >2 wks)	B	Fevers >37.8°C unrelated to identifiable infection for >2 wk, or weight loss >10% of body weight.

GI = gastrointestinal; LN = lymph node. Generalized = more than upper or lower extremities alone includes minimal GI disease defined as <S lesions and <2 cm in combined diameters.
Adapted from Kriegel et al. (41) and Mitsuyasu and Groopman (47).

Table 11-3. Basic Principles for Therapy of Epidemic Kaposi's Sarcoma

Clinical Features	Treatment
Localized or "minimal" extent and/or Favorable prognostic factors and/or Slow rate of progression	No treatment Radiotherapy or Single agent chemotherapy or alpha interferon
Extensive disease and/or Adverse prognostic factors and/or Rapid growth	Combination chemotherapy and/or Alpha interferon (Palliative radiotherapy)

alternating vinblastine and vincristine (39). Other regimens include vinblastine plus methotrexate, vinblastine plus bleomycin and the addition of doxorubicin (34,46,62). All of these combinations can induce good initial responses, but the median duration of response in the reported series is only 6 to 8 months.

Interferon

Interferon (IFN) has been used for epidemic KS because of its immunomodulatory activity (31, 7a). Alpha-IFN is known specifically to augment natural-killer cell activity, T-cell mediated cytotoxocity, macrophage function, and to modify antibody response. In addition, it has antiproliferative and potent antiviral activity (29). Various trials used alpha-IFN for epidemic KS (43,44,53). High doses are required (>20 million U/mm^2) for a response rate of 30%. Of great academic interest is the effect of gamma-IFN in epidemic KS. Gamma IFN is a central lymphokine involved in macrophage inhibition. Patients with AIDS have deficient gamma-IFN production by their T cells (49), and it has also been shown that the addition of exogenous gamma-IFN to phagocytes from AIDS patients allowed normal in vitro killing of an intracellular pathogen, *Toxoplasma gondii*. However, preliminary clinical trials have failed to detect significant activity for gamma-IFN in epidemic KS (59).

LYMPHOMAS AND AIDS

Non-Hodgkin's Lymphoma

Like KS, the risk of non-Hodgkin's lymphoma in patients with AIDS is now well established (1a,8a,13a,21a,81,82,91). As a result, the classification of AIDS has been revised by the CDC to include individuals with high-grade B-cell non-Hodgkin's lymphoma in the setting of HIV-positivity and high risk factors for AIDS (4).

Initially, the majority of patients described had high-grade lymphomas, histologically grouped as B-cell immunoblastic or undifferentiated lymphomas of the Burkitt's or non-Burkitt's variety (66,72,78). These high-grade lymphomas were reported in approximately 65% of patients with non-Hodgkin's lymphoma and AIDS (92). Intermediate-grade lymphomas (90), mainly of the diffuse large cell histologic subtype, were reported in 30% of patients. More recently, other reports have described intermediate-grade lymphomas in approximately 40% to 50% of patients diagnosed with non-Hodgkin's lymphoma in the setting of AIDS (65,79).

In the wake of these reports, it is likely that criteria from the CDC for the diagnosis of AIDS (4) will be expanded to include patients with diffuse large cell lymphomas (65).

Etiology

There have been several reports of an association between EBV and lymphomas in AIDS patients (63,75,76,81). EBV is known to activate B lymphocytes and may lead to polyclonal expansion, resulting in both polyclonal and monoclonal B-cell lymphoproliferative disorders in the setting of immuno-suppression after organ transplantation (67,74,83,86). The association of EBV with African Burkitt's lymphoma is established, and viral DNA and nuclear antigens are almost always found in tumor cells of patients with this disease (85). In one detailed study of the pathogenesis of B-cell lymphoma in patients with AIDS using careful serological and molecular analysis, an individual with this disease was found to have: (a)

evidence of HIV infection; (b) monoclonal rearrangement of immunoglobulin and T-cell receptor genes; (c) rearrangement of c-myc oncogenes; (d) evidence for presence of EBV in the B-cell genome; and (e) absence of HIV in the B-cell genome (73). The rearrangement of the c-myc oncogene is of particular significance, as this oncogene is reportedly expressed in Burkitt's lymphoma (69). The bulk of current evidence suggests that the EBV may potentiate the development of B-cell neoplasia in the setting of immunosuppression induced by HIV infection. It appears that HIV does not have a direct causal relation to the lymphoma but may provide the immunosuppressive milieu to allow the initial polyclonal B-cell expansion to develop into an aggressive monoclonal lymphoproliferative disorder (Fig. 11-1).

Clinical Features

At the time of presentation of non-Hodgkin's lymphoma, one third of the patients will have had an opportunistic infection and a similar number will have had preceeding generalized lymphadenopathy (92). Approximately 20% of patients with non-Hodgkin's lymphoma also have KS at some time during the course of their disease (88) and virtually all patients have a T-cell helper: suppressor ratio of less than one.

Presentation at extranodal sites is common, especially the CNS (30% to 45%) and bone marrow (30% to 45%). Other frequent sites of extranodal presentation include the GI tract, lungs, and skin (71,82,92). Overall, at the time of diagnosis approximately 90% of patients will have extranodal involvement (80).

Treatment

The non-Hodgkin's lymphomas associated with AIDS have, by and large, a rapidly progressive clinical course. It appears that the lymphomas are responsive to conventional therapy, but the remission tends to be brief and the relapses are frequent (82). This group of patients is particularly hard to treat because of the concurrent immune deficiency and the risks that further therapy-related marrow suppression may

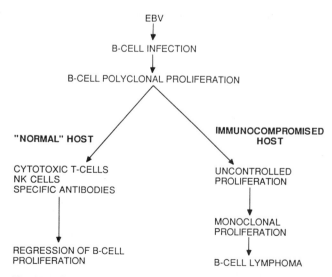

Model for "Opportunistic" Neoplasia

Fig. 11-1. Possible pathogenesis of non-Hodgkin's lymphoma in acquired immune deficiency syndrome (AIDS).

cause. Glucocorticoid, one of the most important agents in the therapy of lymphomas, may be particularly hazardous in patients with AIDS. Consequently, many patients treated for this lymphoma received attenuated treatment courses, both in drug dosage and duration of therapy. Thus, it is difficult to reach unequivocal conclusions about the responsiveness of AIDS patients with non-Hodgkin's lymphoma, when compared with the general population (Table 11-4). Additionally, there is a high early mortality associated with intensive non-Hodgkin's lymphoma treatment regimens in AIDS patients (71). Most treatment regimens have been standard or modifications of standard regimens used for lymphomas such as CHOP or m-BACOD (see Chapter 18," Malignant Lymphomas"). One report used a novel intensive high-dose methotrexate/high-dose cytosine arabinoside regimen (71, 17b).

The most important predictive variable in most reported studies is the performance status of the patient at the time of presentation, which is usually related to the underlying disease and the number, frequency, and severity of opportunistic infections. It would follow, therefore, that patients who present with non-Hodgkin's lymphoma early in their AIDS course may be expected to respond better to therapy. Furthermore, it has been suggested that a short course of an intensive regimen may be preferable for these patients because of the immunosuppression induced by prolonged cytotoxic therapy. A trial using MACOP-B (see Chapter 18), with its relatively short duration of therapy, has yielded a response rate of 65% with a median survival of 20 months for responding patients (65).

HODGKIN'S DISEASE

Recently, Hodgkin's disease has been described in individuals with AIDS (1,17a, 64,68,70,77, 84,87,89). Some authors consider that Hodgkin's disease should be added to the known malignancies associated with AIDS (88). Others have emphasized that the association is difficult to establish due to the expected occurrence of Hodgkin's disease in young males (80). The case reports describing Hodgkin's disease in AIDS have included a description of a patient with both KS and Hodgkin's disease—both diseases associated with T-cell dysfunction. Conceptually, of course, it would not be surprising if Hodgkin's disease would be *facilitated* by HIV infection, with its known T-cell dysfunction. Nonetheless, to date there are no unequivocal epidemiological studies linking Hodgkin's disease with AIDS, despite increasing numbers of case reports describing the two disease entities in the same patients.

Table 11-4. Principles of Treatment for non-Hodgkin's Lymphoma in AIDS

- If only "mild" immunosuppression and/or few, if any, complications

  Use *standard* aggressive therapy with no dose modification. *Definite* potential for prolonged unmaintained remissions.

- In setting of "severe" immunosuppression and/or opportunistic infections . . . especially where chemotherapy is likely to exacerbate underlying condition

  Reasonable to use an attenuated regimen or radiotherapy with primary palliative intent.

AIDS = acquired immune deficiency syndrome.

Recommended Reading

Good general reviews may be found in "Cancer in the Immunosuppressed Host" by Blattner and Hoover in *Cancer: Clinical Principles and Practice of Oncology* (1b) and in the reviews by Safai, "Cancers in HIV Infection," (88) and Levine, "Non-Hodgkin's Lymphomas and Other Malignancies in the Acquired Immune Deficiency Syndrome" (80).

REFERENCES

Malignancy in the Immunocompromised Host

1. Ames ED, Conjalka MS, Goldberg AF, *et al*. Hodgkin's disease and AIDS. 23 new cases and a review of the literature. Hematology-Oncology Clinics of North America 5(2):343-356, 1991.

1a. Beral V, Peterman T, Berkelman R, *et al*. AIDS-associated non-Hodgkin's lymphoma. Lancet 337 (8745):805-809, 1991.

1b. Blattner, W.A.; Hoover, R.N. Cancer in the immunosuppressed host. In: DeVita, V.T.; Hellman, S.; Rosenberg, S.A., eds. Cancer: Principles and Practice of Oncology. Philadelphia: J.P. Lippincott; 1985:1999-2006.

2. Brickner, M.; Wilber, E. The incidence of malignant tumors in patients with respiratory sarcoid. Br. J. Cancer 19:247-251; 1974.

3. Burnett, F.M. The concept of immunological surveillance. Prog. Exp. Tumor Res. 13:1-27; 1970.

4. Classification system for human T-lymphotrophic virus type III/lymphadenopathy-associated virus infections: MMWR. 35:334-338; 1986.

5. Curran, J.W. AIDS — Two Years Later: New Engl. J. Med. 309:609-611; 1983.

6. DeGramont, A.; Louvet, C.; Krulik, M.; *et al*. Preleukemic changes in cases of non-lymphocytic leukemia secondary to cytotoxic therapy. Analysis of 105 cases. Cancer 58:630-634; 1986.

6a. Ensoli B, Barillari G, Gallo RC. Pathogenesis of AIDS-associated Kaposi's Sarcoma. Hematology-Oncology Clinics of North America 5 (2):281-295, 1991.

7. Filipovich, A.; Zebbe, D.; Spector, B.; *et al*. Lymphomas in persons with naturally occurring immunodeficiency disorders. In: McGrath, I.T., O'Conor, G.T., Ramot, B., eds. Pathogenesis of leukemias and lymphomas: environmental influences. New York, NY: Raven Press; 1984:225-234.

7a. Fischl MA. Antiretroviral therapy in combination with interferon for AIDS related Kaposi's Sarcoma. Am J Med April 10, 1991 (4A):2S-7S, 1991.

8. Fraumeni, J.F.; Hoover, R.N. Immunosurveillance and cancer: epidemiologic observations. Natl. Cancer Inst. Monogr. 47:121-126; 1977.

8a. Freter CE. Acquired immunodefieciency syndrome-associated lymphomas. Monographs-National Cancer Institute. 10:43-45, 1990.

9. Frizzera, G.; Rosai, J.; Dehner, L.P.; *et al*. Lymphoreticular disorders in primary immunodeficiencies: new findings as an up-to-date histologic classification of 35 cases. Cancer 46:692-699; 1980.

10. Groopman, J.E. Neoplasms in the acquired immune deficiency syndrome: the multi-disciplinary approach to treatment. Semin. Oncol. 14(2):1-6; 1987.

11. Hanto, D.W.; Gajl-Peczalska, K.J.; Frizzera, G.; *et al*. Epstein-Barr virus (EBV) induced polyclonal B-cell lymphoproliferative diseases occurring after renal transplantation; clinical, pathologic and urologic findings and implications for therapy. Ann. Surg. 193:356-369; 1983.

12. Harwood, A.R.; Asoba, D.; Hofstader, S.L.; *et al*. Kaposi's sarcoma in recipients of renal transplants. Am. J. Med. 67:759-765; 1979.

13. Kantarjian, H.M.; Keating, M.J.; Walters, R.S.; *et al*. The association of specific "favourable" cytogenetic abnormalities with secondary leukemia. Cancer 58:924-927; 1986.

13a. Kaplan LD. AIDS-associated lymphoma. Aids Clinical Review 2:181-195, 1991.

14. Kassan, S.S.; Thomas, T.L.; Moutsopolous, M.M.; *et al*. Increased risk of lymphoma in sicca syndrome. Ann. Intern. Med. 89:888-892; 1978.

15. Kinlen, L.J. Incidence of cancer in rheumatoid arthritis and other disorders after immunosuppressive treatment. Am. J. Med. 78:44-49; 1985.

16. Krown, S.E. Neoplasia in AIDS. Bull. N.Y. Acad. Med. 63(7):679-691; 1987.

17. Louie, S.; Schwartz, R.S. Immunodeficiency and the pathogenesis of lymphoma and leukemia. Semin. Hematol. 15:117-138; 1978.

17a. Monfardini S, Tirelli U, Vaccher E, *et al.* Hodgkin's disease in 63 intravenous drug users infected with human immunodeficiency virus. Gruppo Italiano Cooperativo AIDS and Tumopri (GICAT). Annals of Oncology 2(2):201-205, 1991.

17b. Northfelt DW, Kahn JO, Volberding PA. Treatment of AIDS-related Kaposi's Sarcoma. Hematology-Oncology Clinics of North America 5 (2):297-310, 1991.

18. Penn, I. Malignancies associated with immunosuppressive or cytotoxic therapy. Surgery 83:492-502; 1978.

19. Penn, I. The occurrence of cancer in immune deficiencies. Curr. Probl. Cancer 6:1-64; 1982.

20. Penn, I. Cancer is a complication of severe immunosuppression. Surg. Gynecol. Obstet. 162:603-610; 1986.

21. Penn, I. Tumors of the immunocompromised patient. Ann. Rev. Med. 39:63- 73; 1988.

21a. Pluda JM, Yarchoan R, Broder S. HIV-associated the non-Hodgkin's Lymphomas. Annals of Oncology 2 (4):248-249, 1991.

22. Purtillo, D.T.; Linder, J. Oncological consequences of impaired surveillance against ubiquitous viruses. J. Clin. Immunol. 3:197-206; 1983.

23. Safai, B.; Lynfield, R.; Lowenthal, D.A. Cancers associated with HIV infection. Anti. Cancer Res. 7(5B):105-106; 1987.

24. Schwartz, R.S. Another look at immunologic surveillance. New Engl. J. Med. 293:181-183; 1975.

25. Spector, B.D.; Perry, G.S.; Kersey, J.H.L. Genetically determined immunodeficiency disease (GDID) and malignancy: report from the Immunodeficiency Cancer Registry. Clin. Immunol. Immunopathol. 11:12-39; 1978.

26. Thomas, L. Discussion. In: Lawrence, H.S., ed. Cellular and Tumoral Aspects of Hypersensitive State. New York, NY: Hoeber-Harper; 1959:539.

27. Waldman, T.A.; Strober, W.; Blaese, R.M. Immunodeficiency disease and malignancy: various immunologic deficiencies of man and the role of immune processes in the control of malignant disease. Ann. Intern. Med. 77:605-628; 1972.

Kaposi's Sarcoma in AIDS

28. Centers for disease control update: acquired immunodeficiency syndrome — United States MMWR 35:17-21; 1985.

29. Chessman, S.H.; Rubin, R.H.; Stuart, J.A.; *et al.* Controlled clinical trial of prophylactic human leukocyte interferon in renal transplantation: effect on cytomegalovirus and herpes simplex viral infections. New Engl. J. Med. 300:1345-1349; 1979.

30. Drew, W.L.; Mintz, L.; Miner, R.C.; *et al.* Prevalence of cytomegalovirus infection in homosexual men. J. Infect. Dis. 143:188-192; 1981.

31. Fauci, A.F.; Masur, H.; Gelmann, E.T.; *et al.* The acquired immunodeficiency syndrome: an up-date. Ann. Intern. Med. 102; 800-813; 1985.

32. Friedman-Kien, A.E.; Lauberstein L.J.; Rubenstein, P.; *et al.* Disseminated Kaposi's sarcoma in homosexual men. Ann. Intern. Med. 96:693-700; 1982.

33. Giraldo, G.; Bethe-Huang, E. Kaposi's sarcoma and its relationship to cytomegalovirus. III. CMV, DNA and CMV early antigens in Kaposi's sarcoma. Am. J. Cancer 26:23-29; 1980.

34. Glaspy, J.; Miles, S.; McCarthy, S.; *et al.* Treatment of advanced state Kaposi's sarcoma with vincristine and bleomycin. Proc. Am. Soc. Clin. Oncol. 5(3); 1986 (Abstract).

35. Haverkos, H.W.; Curran, J.W. Recurrent outbreak of Kaposi's sarcoma and opportunistic infections. CA 32:330-332; 1982.

36. Hill, D.R. The role of radiotherapy for epidemic Kaposi's sarcoma. Semin. Oncol. 14(2):19-22; 1987.

37. Holecek, M.J.; Harwood, A.R. Radiotherapy of Kaposi's sarcoma. Cancer 41:1733-1738; 1978.

38. Hutt, M.S. The epidemiology of Kaposi's sarcoma. Antibiot. Chemother. 29:3-8; 1981.

39. Kaplan, L.; Abrams, D.; Volberding, P. Treatment of Kaposi's sarcoma in acquired immunodeficiency syndrome with an alternating vincristine-vinblastine regimen. Cancer Treat. Rep. 70:1121-1122; 1986.

40. Kaposi, M. Idiopathisches multipls Pigmentsarkom der Haut. Arch. Dermato. Syph 4; 265-273, 1872.

41. Kriegel, R.L.; Laubenstein, L.J.; Muggia, F.M. Kaposi's sarcoma: A new staging classification. Cancer Treat. Rep. 67:531-534; 1983.

42. Kriegel, R.L. The natural history and treatment of epidemic Kaposi's sarcoma. Ann. N.Y. Acad. Sci. 437:447-452; 1984.

43. Krown, S.E.; Real, F.X.; Krim, M.; *et al.* Recombinant leukocyte A interferon in Kaposi's sarcoma. Ann. N.Y. Acad. Sci. 437:431-438; 1984.

44. Krown, S.E. The role of interferon in the therapy of epidemic Kaposi's sarcoma. Semin. Oncol. 14(2):27-33; 1987.

45. Laubenstein, L. Post-graduate Course on Epidemic Kaposi's Sarcoma and Opportunistic Infections in Homosexual Men. NYU Medical Center, March 1983. New York, NY: Mason; 1984.

46. Minor, D.R.; Brayer, T. Velban and methotrexate (MTX) combination chemotherapy for epidemic Kaposi's sarcoma. Proc. Am. Soc. Clin. Oncol. 5(1); 1986 (Abstract).

47. Mitsuyasu, R.T.; Groopman, J.W. Biology and therapy of Kaposi's sarcoma. Semin. Oncol. 11:53-59; 1984.

48. Mitsuyasu, R.T. Clinical variance and staging of Kaposi's sarcoma. Semin. Oncol. 14(2); 13-18; 1987.

49. Murray, H.W.; Rubin, B.Y.; Masur, H; *et al.* Impaired cell mediated immune responses in the acquired immune deficiency syndrome: patients with opportunistic infection failed to secrete activating lymphokine and gamma interferon. New Engl. J. Med. 310:883-889; 1984.

50. Oettle, A.G. Geographical and racial differences in the frequency of Kaposi's sarcoma as evidence of environmental or genetic causes. Acta Vir. Int. Cancer 18:330-363; 1962.

51. Olivery, C.L.M. Kaddumukasa, A.; Atine, I; *et al.* Childhood Kaposi's sarcoma: clinical features and therapy. Br. J. Cancer 33:555-563; 1976.

52. Pollack, M.S.; Safai, B.; Myskowski, P.L.; *et al.* Frequency of HLA and Gm immunogenetic markers in Kaposi's sarcoma. Tissue Antigens 21:1-8; 1983.

53. Real, F.X.; Oettgen, H.F.; Krown, S.E. Kaposi's sarcoma and the acquired immunodeficiency syndrome: treatment with high and low doses of recombinant leukocyte A interferon. J. Clin. Oncol. 4:544-551; 1986.

54. Rothman, S. Remarks on sex, age and racial distribution of Kaposi's sarcoma and on possible pathogenetic factors. Acta. Un Int. Cancer 18:326- 329; 1962.

55. Safai, B.; Johnson, K.G.; Myskowski, P.L.; *et al.* The natural history of Kaposi's sarcoma in the acquired immunodeficiency syndrome. Ann. Intern. Med. 103; 744-750; 1985.

56. Safai, B. Pathophysiology and epidemiology of epidemic Kaposi's sarcoma. Semin. Oncol. 14(2); 7-12; 1987.

57. Taylor, J.F.; Templeton, A.C.; Vogel, C.L.; *et al.* Kaposi's sarcoma in Uganda: a clinical pathological study. Intl. J. Cancer 8:122-135; 1971.

58. Urmacher, C.; Myskowski, P.; Ochoa, M.; *et al.* Outbreak of Kaposi's sarcoma in young homosexual men. Am. J. Med. 72:569-575; 1982.

59. Vadhan-Raj, S.; Al-Katib, A.; Pelus, L.; *et al.* Phase I trial of recombinant interferon gamma in cancer patients. J. Clin. Oncol. 4:137-146; 1986.

60. Volberding, P.A.; Abrams, A.I.; Conant, M.; *et al.* Vinblastine therapy for Kaposi's sarcoma in acquired immunodeficiency syndrome. Ann. Intern. Med. 103:335-338; 1985.

61. Volberding, P.A. The role of chemotherapy for epidemic Kaposi's sarcoma. Semin. Oncol. 14(2); 23-26; 1987.

62. Wernz, J.; Laubenstein, L.; Hymes, K.; *et al.* Chemotherapy and assessment of response in epidemic Kaposi's sarcoma (EKS) with bleomycin/velban. Proc. Am. Soc. Clin. Oncol. 5(4); 1986.

Lymphomas in AIDS

63. Andiman, G.; Gradoville, L.; Heston, L.; *et al.* Use of cloned probes to detect Epstein-Barr viral DNA in tissues from patients with neoplastic and lymphoproliferative diseases. J. Infect. Dis. 148:967-977; 1983.

64. Baer, D.M.; Anderson, E.T.; Wilkinson, L.S. Acquired immune deficiency syndrome in homosexual men with Hodgkin's disease. Case Reports. Am. J. Med. 80:738-740; 1986.

65. Bermudez, M.A.; Grant, K.M.; Rodvien, R.; *et al.* Non-Hodgkin's lymphoma in the population with or at risk for acquired immunodeficiency syndrome: indications for intensive chemotherapy. Am. J. Med. 86:71-76; 1989.

66. Centers for Disease Control. Undifferentiated non-Hodgkin's lymphoma among homosexual males — United States. MMWR 31:277-281; 1982.

67. Cleary, M.L.; Warnke, R.; Sklar, J. Monoclonality of lymphoproliferative lesions in cardiac transplant recipients. New Engl. J. Med. 310:477-482; 1984.

68. Coonley, C.J.; Strauss, D.J.; Filippa, D.; et al. Hodgkin's disease presenting with rectal symptoms in a homosexual male. Cancer Invest. 2:279- 284; 1984.

69. Dalla-Favera, R.; Bregni, M.; Erikson, J.; et al. Human c-mic oncogene is located on the region of chromosome 8 that is translocated in Burkitt lymphoma cells. Proc. Natl. Acad. Sci. USA 79:7824-7827; 1982.

70. Dancis, A.; Odajnyk, C.; Triegel, R.L.; et al. Association of Hodgkin's and non-Hodgkin's lymphomas with the acquired immunodeficiency syndrome (AIDS). Proc. Am. Soc. Clin. Oncol. 361a; 1984.

71. Gill, P.S.; Levine, A.M.; Krailo, M.; et al. AIDS-related malignant lymphoma: results of perspective treatment trials. J. Clin. Oncol. 5(9):1322-1328; 1987.

72. Gill, P.S.; Levine, A.M.; Meyer, P.R.; et al. Primary ventral nervous system lymphoma in homosexual men. Clinical, immunologic, pathologic features. Am. J. Med. 78:742-748; 1985.

73. Groopman, J.E.; Sullivan, J.L.; Mulder, C.; et al. Pathogenesis of B cell lymphoma in a patient with AIDS. Blood 67; 612-615; 1986.

74. Hanto, D.W.; Gajl-Peczalska, K.J.; Frizzera, G.; et al. Epstein-Barr virus (EBV)-induced polyclonal and monoclonal B-cell lymphoproliferative diseases occurring after renal transplantation. Ann. Surg. 198:356-359; 1983.

75. Henle, W.; Henle, G.; Lennette, E.T. The Epstein-Barr virus. Sci Am. 241:48059; 1979.

76. Hochberg, F.H.; Miller, G.; Schooley, R.T.; et al. Central nervous system lymphomas related to Epstein-Barr virus. New Engl. J. Med. 309:745-748; 1983.

77. Ioachim, H.L.; Cooper, M.L.; Hellman, G.C. Lymphomas in men at high risk for acquired immune deficiency syndrome (AIDS): a study of 21 cases. Cancer 56:2831-2842; 1985.

78. Jill, P.S.; Levine, A.M.; Meyer, T.R.; et al. Primary central nervous system lymphoma in homosexual men: clinical immunological and pathologic features. Am. J. Med. 78:6742-6748; 1985.

79. Kalter, S.P.; Riggs, S.A.; Cabanillas, F.; et al. Aggressive non-Hodgkin's lymphomas in immunocompromised homosexual males. Blood 66:655-659; 1985.

80. Levine, A.M. Non-Hodgkin's lymphomas and other malignancies in the acquired immune deficiency syndrome. Semin. Oncol. 14(2):34-39; 1987.

80a. Levine, A.M. Acquired immunodeficiency syndrome-related lymphoma. Blood 80:8-20; 1992.

81. Levine, A.M.; Gill, P.S.; Meyer, P.R.; et al. Retrovirus and malignant lymphoma in homosexual men. J. Am. Med. Assoc. 254:3405-3408; 1985.

82. Levine, A.M.; Meyer, T.R.; Begnady, M.K.; et al. Development of B cell lymphoma in homosexual men: clinical and immunologic findings. Ann. Intern. Med. 100; 1984.

83. Marker, S.C.; Ascher, M.L.; Kalis, J.M.; et al. Epstein-Barr virus antibody responses and clinical illness in renal transplant patients. Surgery 85:433-440; 1979.

84. Mitsuyasu, R.T.; Colman, M.F.; Sun, N.C.J. Simultaneous occurrence of Hodgkin's disease and Kaposi's sarcoma in a patient with the acquired immune deficiency syndrome. Am. J. Med. 80:954-958; 1986.

85. Pagano, J.S.; Huang, C.H.; Levine, T.H. Absence of Epstein-Barr viral DNA in American Burkitt's lymphoma. New Engl. J. Med. 289:1395-1399; 1973.

86. Pirsch, J.D.; Stratta, R.J.; Sollinger, H.W.; et al. Treatment of severe Epstein-Barr virus induced lymphoproliferative syndrome with ganciclovir: two cases of the solid organ transplantation. Am. J. Med. 86:241-244; 1989.

87. Robert, N.J.; Schneiderman, H. Hodgkin's disease in the acquired immunodeficiency syndrome. Ann. Intern. Med. 101:142-143; 1984.

88. Safai, B.; Lynfield, R.; Lowenthal, D.A. Cancers associated with HIV infection. Anti Cancer Res. 7:1055-1068; 1987.

89. Schoeppel, S.L.; Hoppe, R.T.; Dorfman, R.F.; et al. Hodgkin's disease in homosexual men with generalized lymphadenopathy. Ann. Intern. Med. 102:68-70; 1985.

90. The non-Hodgkin's lymphoma pathologic classification project: National Cancer Institute, sponsored study of classifications of non-Hodgkin's lymphomas. Summary and description of a working formulation for clinical usage. Cancer 49:2112-2135; 1982.

91. Ziegler, J.L, Drew, W.L.; Miner, R.C.; et al. Outbreak of Burkitt's-like lymphoma in homosexual men. Lancet 2:631-633; 1982.

92. Ziegler, J.L.; Becksead, J.A.; Volderding, P.A.; et al. Non-Hodgkin's lymphoma in 90 homosexual men: relation to generalized lymphadenopathy and the acquired immunodeficiency syndrome. New Engl. J. Med. 311:565-570; 1984.

William D. DeWys, M.D., F.A.C.P., Medical Oncology
Thomas C. Hall, M.D., F.A.C.P., Medical Oncology

Chapter **12**

PARANEOPLASTIC SYNDROMES

It has been estimated that at any given time 20% of a group of cancer patients in all stages of their diseases will be suffering from a "paraneoplastic syndrome" and that 75% of all patients will develop one during the course of their disease.

T.C. Hall (3)

PERSPECTIVE

A paraneoplastic syndrome is defined as a remote or distant effect of a neoplasm not related to the site of the primary or metastatic tumor. Metastatic lesions may cause multiple location-related complications, but these are not generally included in the discussion of paraneoplastic syndromes (see Chapter 33, "Metastases and Disseminated Disease"). Other terms in use before Hall (3) introduced the term paraneoplastic syndrome include ectopic hormone syndromes, metabolic consequences of tumors, systemic effects of malignancy, and remote effects of cancer on the host.

This chapter will discuss selected remote effects of malignancy that may be experienced by cancer patients during the course of their disease (1-5). Paraneoplastic syndromes are of interest to the oncologist for many reasons. For instance, evaluation of the pathophysiology of paraneoplastic syndromes has provided important insights into tumor biology, including histogenesis of tumors and the process of malignant transformation. A paraneoplastic syndrome may be the initial presentation of a neoplasm, and understanding relationships between a specific syndrome and the tumor causing that syndrome may assist in an earlier cancer diagnosis.

If a paraneoplastic syndrome is caused by a measurable circulating factor, selective sampling may provide information as to tumor localization and extent (129).

A paraneoplastic syndrome may provide an important marker of the status of the patient's tumor, including response to treatment and relapse of disease. With the use of antitumor-marker antibodies, it is possible to scan tumors with isotopes and may be possible to deliver radioactive or chemical therapy to the tumor cells.

Paraneoplastic syndromes may be an important factor in morbidity and mortality, and appropriate treatment of the syndrome may improve the quality of the patient's life and survival duration.

The study of the molecular biology of paraneoplastic syndromes may enhance our understanding of the human genome. Mutations or activation of oncogenes that cause malignancy may also activate the gene(s) producing the protein causing the paraneoplastic syndrome. In addition, study of ectopically produced hormones and other molecules may elucidate mechanisms of control of tumor growth, since these molecules may be acting as growth factors for the tumor in an autocrine or paracrine manner.

PATHOGENESIS

The paraneoplastic syndromes result from a number of mechanisms.

Syndromes often are caused by specific mediators (e.g., trophic hormones) that are the products of activation of specific genes. Activation occurs when cells that normally would develop to a differentiated end-stage cell fail to do so, and (as a tumor cell) begin to perform synthetic functions of early stages of the precursor cell.

In other cases, tissue products that normally are excluded from the body circulation achieve systemic release through abnormal tumor vasculature or disrupted basement membranes. Immunologic reactions, inappropriate initiation of normal host physiologic functions, or other manifestations then occur that disrupt normal host tissue function. Such situations have been termed "forbidden contacts." The altered immunologic state of the cancer patient may be related in part to such non-physiologic effects.

Autoimmune disease may evolve as a paraneoplastic syndrome as a result of host recognition and reaction to tumor-related antigens (5-8). Immune complex diseases have been related to tumor-associated antigens, particularly in the kidney, and will be discussed in the section on the kidney herein.

Many paraneoplastic syndromes have obscure or multiple causes. The protean effects of lung (85) and pancreatic neoplasms or just one tumor type (e.g., thymoma) (112) likely depend on multiple mechanisms.

Concluding that a syndrome is a remote effect of a malignancy should be based on the following considerations:

1. The syndrome has been associated with the tumor in published reports.
2. The syndrome has regressed after removal or regression of the tumor.
3. When a circulating factor is known (93), one can demonstrate
   - an arteriovenous gradient across the tumor
   - the factor in tumor tissue in concentrations greater than adjacent normal tissue
   - secretion *in vitro*

Paraneoplastic syndromes involve many different combinations of tumor type and target system. The following discussion is organized both according to site and type of tumor, and according to the target systems for paraneoplastic effects.

RELATIONSHIPS TO SITE AND TYPE OF TUMOR

A paraneoplastic syndrome may arise from neoplasia in virtually any organ of the body. Whether a paraneoplastic effect occurs depends on several aspects of the neoplastic cell.

1. The synthetic potential of the cell based upon the ontogeny of the parent cell (i.e., gene activation), specifically tumors developing from the nephrogenic ridge, may produce erythropoietin, as does the normal kidney.
2. The synthetic capabilities of the neoplastic cell based on its location and degree of differentiation.
3. The possibility that tumor products will be recognized as antigenic by the host immune system.
4. Host factors such as susceptibility, modification by treatment, and length of time needed for a clinical syndrome to become apparent.

Cells of Neural Crest Origin

Tumors derived from cells of neural crest origin frequently cause paraneoplastic syndromes. In the embryo, primitive neuroectoderm differentiates into four classes of cells: neuroganglions, melanocytes, Schwann cells (19), and amine precursor uptake and decarboxylation (APUD) cells (19,48,110). All four groups have malignant counterparts, the first three become neuroblastomas, melanomas, and schwannomas, while the APUD-derived cells in the embryo migrate to become enterochromaffin cells in the lung, the pancreatic islets, and enterochromaffin cells in the gastrointestinal (GI) tract. Tumors arising from these APUD cells produce hormone or hormonelike activity ectopically in tumors arising in the lung (small cell), pancreatic islets, carcinoid tumors, and other sites. A highly malignant APUDoma, small cell carcinoma of the lung (SCLC), can cause multiple paraneoplastic syndromes (110). APUDoma may produce corticotropin (ACTH), antidiuretic hormone (ADH), and other pituitary hormones (reflecting a common embryologic origin for the pituitary and the APUD cells) in addition to the hormones related to their tumor site (e.g., insulin for an islet cell tumor).

Squamous Cell Carcinomas

Squamous cell carcinomas arising from tissues derived from the embryonic foregut are frequently associated with the production of parathormone (PTH) or a parathyroid-like hormone (the ectopic PTH syndrome). Squamous cell carcinoma of the mouth, larynx, esophagus, and lung all have approximately a 10% incidence of hypercalcemia because of PTH or PTH-like substances (35,85a). Parathyroid hormone or PTH-like hormone production is the most common mechanism of hypercalcemia in patients with these categories of squamous cell cancer. This is in contrast to some other tumor types, such as breast cancer, where metastases to bone with local dissolution of bone may be the most frequent mechanism of hypercalcemia. The parathyroid gland is derived embryologically from the same anlage that gives rise to these squamous cell tissues; this may explain this association. Patients with squamous cell cancers of the upper aerodigestive system should be monitored for the development of hypercalcemia. In a patient with a cancer of unknown primary associated with hypercalcemia, this area should receive intensive scrutiny as a possible source of the primary cancer. Squamous cell cancers of other sites such as the gallbladder have also been associated with hypercalcemia.

Lung Cancer

Lung cancer is the malignancy most commonly associated with paraneoplastic syndromes (56). Most of these syndromes can be explained by the production of hormones or hormonelike substances by the tumor (Table 12-1). Ectopic hormone syndromes may be seen clinically in 3% to 6% (55) of lung cancer patients but laboratory evidence of ectopic hormone production may be detected in as many as 21% (40). Elevated serum or plasma levels of one or more peptide hormones or neuron-specific enolase in patients with SCLC can be detected at diagnosis in up to 70% of cases (56).

In patients with lung cancer, one may be able to predict tumor histology by observation of a specific hormonal syndrome (55,56,85). For example, a lung tumor associated with hypercalcemia in the absence of metastases is likely to be a squamous cell carcinoma, while a lung tumor producing ACTH or ADH is likely to be a small cell carcinoma. A myasthenia-like syndrome (Eaton-Lambert), characterized by weakness and fatigue of the proximal muscles, occurs almost exclusively with SCLC. This syndrome is caused by impairment of neuromuscular transmission and manifests decreased signal with repeated muscle contraction on electromyography.

Retroperitoneal Tumors

One may be able to predict the histology of retroperitoneal tumors by searching for tumor by-products or paraneoplastic syndromes. A retroperitoneal tumor that produces polycythemia is likely to be an adenocarcinoma of the kidney producing erythropoietin. A retroperitoneal tumor producing hypertension could be either a pheochromocytoma, an aldosteronoma, or a renin-producing tumor of the kidney.

Endocrine System

A broad range of syndromes is derived from the endocrine system:

1. Syndromes associated with a single tumor of an endocrine organ that produce the hormone of the parent cell (e.g., corticosteroid production by adrenal carcinoma) (49).
2. Syndromes occurring in patients with the multiple endocrine adenomatosis (MEA) syndrome; these have a genetic basis and can be classified into specific types (18,19,20).

Table 12-1. Ectopic Hormone Syndromes in Patients with Lung Cancer

Ectopic Hormone	Clinical and Laboratory Findings
Adrenocorticotropin (ACTH)	Hypokalemia, edema, hypertension, hyperpigmentation, weakness
Antidiuretic hormone (ADH)	Hyponatremia, low serum osmolality, confusion, weakness, incoordination
Parathyroid hormone (PTH)	Hypercalcemia, hypophosphatemia, lethargy, confusion, nausea, vomiting
Serotonin	Flushing, diarrhea
Human chorionic gonadotropin (hCG)	Gynecomastia

3. An MEA syndrome may be combined with ectopic hormone production (98).

In many cases the substance causing the syndrome is the authentic hormone produced in sufficient quantity to permit measurement in a standard radioimmunoassay (RIA) (e.g., ACTH, PTH, melanocyte-stimulating hormone [MSH], thyrotropin [TSH], or human chorionic gonadotropin [B-HCG]). In other cases, a substance nearly identical to the authentic peptide, often a precursor of the hormone may produce an endocrine syndrome or metabolic effect. In some cases, elevated levels of hormone cannot be measured by standard RIA because the tumor product is biologically active but is different enough from the normal hormone so that it is undetectable by RIA. In other cases, a tumor may produce a peptide subunit that is detectable by RIA but is not associated with recognizable pathology (97,99,126). These substances may be useful clinically as tumor markers (see section on tumor markers and clinical use of antigens). Tumors may also produce hormone precursors or prohormones that are subsequently metabolized to an active hormone.

For example, islet cell tumors cause ulcer syndromes, diarrhea, and other metabolic disturbances (39,60). The ulcer disease of the Zollinger-Ellison syndrome may be cured surgically by removal of the stomach, the target organ (46), if removal of the islet tumor is not feasible. Other systemic effects produced by islet cell tumors respond favorably to specific therapy (24,39,101,102).

Hematologic Neoplasms

The acute leukemias cause many neurologic dysfunctions (88). The globulins of macroglobulinemia and occasionally of myeloma may cause hyperviscosity syndromes (17), cryoprecipitation damage (53), and other problems (71).

Prostate

The paraneoplastic syndromes most frequently associated with prostate cancer include diffuse intravascular coagulation, venous thrombosis, nonbacterial thrombotic endocarditis, and anemia (78).

TARGET SYSTEM FOR PARANEOPLASTIC EFFECTS

Endocrine-Metabolic System Effects

A broad range of endocrine-metabolic effects of neoplasms associated with tumors derived from nonendocrine organs that produce hormones or hormonelike substances ectopically has been described (12,14,50,91,109,111). Many syndromes remain unexplained (84), and a full discussion of each syndrome is beyond the scope of this chapter. Ectopic hormone production usually is not a random function of tumors but can be explained by an understanding of the embryology, metabolism, and biochemistry of the tissue of origin.

The metabolic conditions most often seen in cancer patients include hypercalcemia, hyponatremia (inappropriate antidiuretic hormone), hypokalemia (ectopic ACTH), hypoglycemia, lactic acidosis, hyperuricemia, and the tumor lysis syndrome. Most of these conditions are produced by metabolic or hormonal products of the tumor, but others result from or are worsened by antineoplastic therapy, especially the tumor lysis syndrome.

Clinically similar metabolic paraneoplastic syndromes may have different mechanisms in different patients. For example,

hypoglycemia may be caused by elevated levels of insulin, insulin-like growth factors (30,51), or somatomedins; deficiencies of hormones that maintain normal glucose homeostasis; or increased consumption of glucose by a large tumor. Usually one mechanism predominates in each patient. Syndromes also may be produced when a trophic hormone cross-reacts with a gland that is not its usual target. For example, hyperthyroidism, caused by very high levels of hCG, may develop (6,64) because of structural similarities between hCG and TSH (6).

Hypercalcemia occurs in up to 10% of cancer patients, and may be subdivided into three categories: hematologic malignancies, solid tumors with bone metastases (most commonly breast, lung, and kidney), and solid tumors without bone metastases (most commonly squamous cell carcinomas). Hypercalcemia in hematologic malignances is usually due to production of osteoclast-activating factor by tumor cells. Hypercalcemia in patients with solid tumors that have not metastasized to bone results from ectopic production of one or more humoral mediators (11,22,39,42,82,103,114). Hypercalcemia as an effect of a malignancy is more common than hypercalcemia caused by parathyroid adenoma or hyperplasia in hospitalized patients (44). The signs and symptoms of hypercalcemia are protean and include drowsiness, confusion, nausea, and vomiting.

Inappropriate secretion of ADH may occur with a variety of medical conditions, but underlying neoplasia is the most frequent cause. Small cell carcinoma of lung (SCLC) is most often associated with this syndrome. Cyclophosphamide and vincristine chemotherapy have also been associated with inappropriate secretion of ADH (95). Arginine vasopressin secreted by the tumor results in plasma volume expansion, low serum sodium, and high urine osmolality. The syndrome usually causes mental confusion and may progress to coma and death, but it is very treatable (see below).

Cushing's syndrome may be caused by ectopic production of ACTH by a neoplasm or by topic steroid hormone production by adrenal or testicular neoplasms (47). Ectopic ACTH production most commonly occurs with lung cancers; the tumor is usually visible on chest x-ray, and the resultant bilateral adrenal hyperplasia may be seen on computed tomography (CT) scan. Adrenal tumors are usually unilateral on CT scan and testicular tumors are palpable on physical exam.

Virilization is usually caused by adrenal or ovarian neoplasms but may develop as a paraneoplastic syndrome with other tumors. Differentiation between adrenal or ovarian origin can usually be made on the basis of CT and the finding of elevated urinary 17-ketosteroids and plasma dehydroepiandrosterone associated with adrenal neoplasms. Feminization is usually associated with neoplasia of the adrenal or testis and the tumor should be detectable by CT of the adrenal gland or examination of the testes. Acromegaly may develop secondary to paraneoplastic production of growth hormone or of growth hormone releasing factor (57).

Neuromuscular System

Paraneoplastic syndromes involving the neuromuscular system may occur in as many as 2% of all cancer patients (13,115). Subacute sensory neuropathy and subacute cerebellar degeneration may appear before other symptoms of malignancy and evaluation of patients with these syndromes may lead to earlier diagnosis of malignancy (36). A spectrum of degenerative syndromes (cerebellar, spinal cord, or other central nervous system parenchyma) and specific peripheral neuropathies and neuromyopathies may be seen as paraneoplastic effects (89,116). In many syndromes, the mechanism may be unknown but some peripheral neuropathies may be antibody-mediated (73). The extent of the diagnostic evaluation of patients with these syndromes should be guided by knowledge of specific syndrome-tumor associations (86). Myasthenic syndromes (Eaton-Lambert and myasthenia gravis) may be associated with several different carcinomas—most often with SCLC (85)—or thymoma (112) and may respond to symptom-specific treatment (41). The syndrome of progressive multifocal leukoencephalopathy may be associated with Hodgkin's disease, other lymphomas, and leukemia (120), and appears to be at least partially viral etiologically. Some remote effects may improve with successful management of the underlying malignancy (67).

Cutaneous Manifestation

Cutaneous manifestations of malignant disease include purpuras, phlebitis, flushing and erythema, urticarial and bullous states, hyperpigmentation, calcinosis cutis, acquired icthyosis, pruritus, herpes zoster, alopecia mucinosa, acquired pachydermoperiostosis, erythema nodosum, hypertrichosis, acanthosis nigricans or the stigmata of ectopic production of MSH or ACTH (25,62,70,114). A syndrome of fever, neutophilia, and painful cutaneous plaques most often associated with hematologic malignancies is a particularly dramatic cutaneous manifestation of malignancy (28). These syndromes demand proper interpretation when seen in a patient who is not known to have malignancy. These syndromes often respond to appropriate topical or systemic therapy. In addition, one should be aware of premalignant or comorbid dermatologic conditions such as xeroderma pigmentosum (94), hereditary tylosis, multiple mucosal neuromas, and the cutaneous cysts of Gardner's syndrome.

Hematologic Disorders

Hematologic disorders are seen both as a consequence of specific tumors and as a consequence of antitumor therapy. The coagulation and anemia problems of cancer are discussed in Chapters 13 and 33, "Oncologic Emergencies" and "Metastases and Disseminated Disease," respectively. Leukemoid and leukoerythroblastic reactions may herald malignancy (125). Myelophthisic marrow failure may result from metastases to bone marrow, an indirect connective tissue response, or a response to globulins produced by thymomas or lymphomas. Both aplasia (112,121) and erythrocythemia (ectopic erythropoietin) occur. Shortened red cell survival is a frequent concomitant of a variety of malignancies. Patients with lymphomas and chronic lymphocytic leukemia may develop red cell antibodies that cause Coombs-positive hemolytic anemia. Hemolysis may also have a mechanical basis related to abnormal blood vessels in a tumor (92). The hematologic problems associated with malignant disease often require supportive care such as blood component therapy. They may respond dramatically to appropriate measures, such as heparin therapy (20), or epsilon-aminocaproic acid (104), as in the intravascular coagulation-fibrinolysis syndromes.

Gastrointestinal Tract Disorders

The entire gastrointestinal (GI) tract is susceptible to paraneoplastic disease. A myriad of malabsorption and deficiency syndromes affect the absorptive mucosa (123). The GI tract plays a significant role in the anorexia-cachexia syndrome of malignancy. The mechanism of this syndrome is poorly understood but is multifactorial (38) including effects on food-intake-regulating centers of the brain and alteration of metabolism. For example, tumor cell death may release purines that may affect regulation of food intake (74). Tumors may release lipolytic and proteolytic products that alter host metabolism (15). Tumor-associated macrophages may produce cachectin (tumor necrosis factor), which has potent cachexia-inducing properties (117). Decreased liver alanine transferase may be associated with tumors and may result in decreased synthesis of normal host proteins (127). The liver may be a target of systemic malignancy, including nonmetastatic hepatomegaly or hepatic dysfunction, on a paraneoplastic basis (52).

Kidney

The kidneys may be the target of paraneoplastic diseases, including acute renal failure from glomerular or tubular damage from myeloma protein (32), hypercalcemia, hyperuricemia, or amyloid deposition. The kidney is the target organ of ADH in ectopic ADH syndrome. Membranous glomerulopathy has been associated with circulating immune complexes from tumor antigens or products (66). Carcinoembryonic antigen (CEA) has been identified through immunologic methods in glomeruli in nephrotic syndrome in a patient with colonic carcinoma (29). Malignancies may present with minimal-change glomerulopathy (e.g., Hodgkin's disease (105) or colon carcinoma (66)). Therapy of the malignancy may lead to remission of both the tumor and the nephrotic syndrome. Nephrogenic diabetes insipidus has been associated with malignancy without a clearly defined mechanism (43).

Connective Tissue—Collagen-Vascular Diseases

The connective tissue or collagen-vascular diseases have a long history of association with malignancy (27). Dermatomyositis and polymyositis may be associated with neoplasia including adenocarcinomas of the GI tract, lung, breast, and ovary, and occasionally lymphomas (10,18,120). Lymphomas are also associated with rheumatic disease (80,120). One autoimmune disease, Sjogren's syndrome, may be associated with a spectrum of benign to malignant lymphoproliferation (7). A variety of autoimmune phenomena (e.g., systemic lupus erythematosus, rheumatoid arthritis, sarcoid, scleroderma) have been associated with tumors, especially thymoma or parathyroid adenomas (112). Amyloid deposition in several organs has been seen, particularly with Hodgkin's disease, myeloma, and renal cell carcinoma (72). Hypertrophic osteoarthropathy is frequently associated with lung cancer. Palmar fasciitis and polyarthritis have been associated with ovarian cancer (76,87) and may precede the diagnosis of ovarian cancer by 5 to 25 months. Polymyalgia rheumatica has been reported to precede (76) or accompany (68) the clinical diagnosis of malignancy.

Cardiorespiratory System Disorders

The cardiorespiratory system may be the target of paraneoplastic phenomena, including nonbacterial, verrucous, marantic endocarditis, appearing principally in patients with mucin-producing adenocarcinoma unrelated to disease duration, infection or nutrition status (96). This syndrome may produce sudden death or various patterns of infarction resulting from arterial embolism. The carcinoid syndrome may cause valvular heart disease (tricuspid and pulmonary insufficiency), endocardial fibrosis, or bronchospastic pulmonary disease (31,128).

Other Syndromes

Other syndromes cannot be classified by target system. Fever may occur as a systemic effect of malignancy; however, an infectious etiology must always be considered and fully evaluated. Since fever may increase metabolic requirements and may cause malaise and debility, symptomatic therapy is worthwhile. With control of fever there may be relief of malaise and fatigue and improved patient activity.

TUMOR MARKERS AND ANTIGENS—CLINICAL USE

As noted in the endocrine-metabolic system section, tumors often produce assayable hormones, subunits of hormones, or precursors of hormones (12,14,50,91,98,99,102,109,111,126). Tumors also release a spectrum of antigens and other products. Assays for these substances may, in appropriate circumstances, aid in diagnosis, assist in estimating prognosis, monitor response to therapy, and assist in making decisions regarding changes in therapy.

Carcinoembryonic Antigen

CEA (119,122) is a nonspecific tumor-associated antigen that may be elevated in a wide variety of benign and malignant conditions. When CEA is elevated preoperatively in colorectal carcinoma, the level should fall to the normal range if the tumor has been completely resected; persistent elevation suggests occult metastatic disease. A normal postoperative CEA level may become elevated prior to clinical detection of relapse. Generally, the higher the preoperative CEA level, the poorer the prognosis. CEA levels may be elevated significantly in 90% of patients with pancreatic and advanced colon carcinoma, 60% of those with metastatic breast carcinoma, and in varying frequency in patients with other malignancies (77). A positive correlation exists between increased CEA levels and increasing differentiation of tumor cells. However, CEA cannot be used as a diagnostic test or as a screening test for malignancy because of a high incidence of false-positives and false-negatives (119,130). Specifically, there is a high frequency of false-negative readings of CEA in early malignancy. For example, with Duke's A (mucosal level) colorectal cancer, less than one third of patients will have abnormal CEA tests (65,77,122). The application of CEA for cancer detection is also limited by false-positive CEA levels in

nonneoplastic disease such as alcoholic cirrhosis, inflammatory bowel disease, tuberculosis, and in heavy cigarette smoking.

Oncofetal Antigens

Alpha-fetoprotein is a normal globulin produced by differentiating embryonic liver and secreted into fetal serum. Its appearance in the adult is associated primarily with hepatoma, liver regeneration, and germ cell tumors (108). Certain placental proteins and their subunits may be present in neoplasms (99). An oncofetal antigen that may be specific to the pancreas has been described (9).

Hormone Subunit

The ß subunit of hCG (ß-hCG), is a useful marker in germ cell tumors. It is elevated in 90% of patients with nonseminomatous germ cell testicular tumors (63). This marker is useful for monitoring surgical completeness in testicular cancer patients with clinical stage I and II disease, for monitoring completeness of response to chemotherapy in stage III disease, and for detecting relapse in all stages of disease. This marker is also useful for monitoring trophoblastic diseases. It may also be elevated in a small fraction of patients with a variety of other neoplasms.

Other Factors

Other factors have been reported to be useful in monitoring cancer patients, such as an elevated lactic dehydrogenase in many tumors (probably related to anaerobic metabolism in these tumors) (23) and circulating mucin in Wilms' tumor (90). CA-125 is useful for monitoring patients with ovarian cancer and other pelvic malignancies. CA 15-3 has worthwhile sensitivity for breast cancer but lacks specificity (61). CA 549 has a sensitivity in patients with breast cancer that is better than CEA (77% versus 61%) with comparable specificity of 92% (16). Eventually, it may be possible to monitor virtually every tumor by some biologic marker. Tormey *et al.* (118) have reported that 97% of breast cancer patients with metastatic disease and 67% of patients who had positive lymph nodes at mastectomy have an elevated marker if CEA, hCG, and a nucleoside, N-2, N-2, dimethylguanosine, are measured. For further information on markers the reader is referred to references (54,63,100,106,113). As sensitivity and specificity of tumor markers improve, their use in diagnosis, prognostic evaluation, monitoring, and therapy will increase.

DIAGNOSTIC CONSIDERATIONS

When a possible paraneoplastic syndrome appears prior to the diagnosis of a neoplasm, one must consider the diagnostic differentiation between paraneoplastic and other causes of the clinical presentation and the possible tumors associated with the syndrome. This can be illustrated by considering the patient with hypercalcemia. Frequently other symptoms or clinical findings (such as chest x-ray findings in a patient with lung cancer) will permit the clinician to move quickly to the diagnosis.

In other cases, a methodic approach to diagnosis is needed. Compared with hyperparathyroidism, paraneoplastic hypercalcemia may have a more rapid onset, be more severe (calcium >15 mg/dL), and be associated with lower phosphate and serum chloride levels. An RIA is useful diagnostic

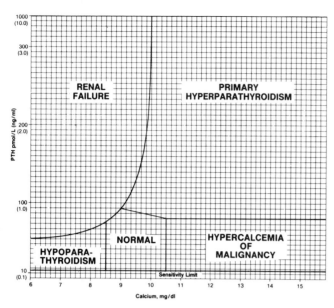

Fig. 12-1. Relationship between serum PTH and serum calcium in several medical conditions.

study for parathormone. When this result is displayed graphically in relation to the calcium level, it is possible to see that the patient may fall into one of several categories (Fig. 12-1). An RIA for parathyroid hormone-related protein may detect elevated levels in two-thirds of patients with hypercalcemia of malignancy (85a). If neoplasia is suspected, one must then consider whether the mechanism is a systemic effect or an effect related to bone metastases. An elevated serum phosphate level suggests bone metastases, and a bone marrow biopsy may help to clarify the diagnosis. If the phosphate is not elevated, one must consider the tumor types frequently associated with hypercalcemia, including lung cancer, esophageal cancer, and head and neck cancer. Other less frequently associated tumors such as kidney, cholangiocarcinoma, and gallbladder cancer must also be considered. Site-related diagnostic studies can then be used to clarify the diagnosis.

In some clinical situations, provocative testing may assist in distinguishing between topic and ectopic hormone production. Calcitonin levels rise significantly after pentagastrin stimulation in patients with medullary carcinoma of the thyroid (topic production) while ectopic production of calcitonin by a neoplasm is usually insensitive to pentagastrin (83).

THERAPEUTIC CONSIDERATIONS

General

When a paraneoplastic syndrome is a cause of symptoms and is life-threatening, medical management of the syndrome often ameliorates the condition (21). Definitive antineoplastic therapy should also be instituted for long-term control (81). During initiation of antineoplastic therapy, it should be anticipated that a paraneoplastic condition may be precipitated (such as the tumor lysis syndrome) or temporarily worsened (hypercalcemia). In selected instances, it may be desirable to phase in the antineoplastic therapy to minimize the severity of such a sequence. For example, when beginning chemotherapy in a case where tumor lysis is anticipated, different chemotherapy drugs could be administered on

successive days instead of giving all drugs on the same day, thus reducing the abruptness of tumor lysis.

Hypercalcemia

Hypercalcemia often constitutes an oncologic emergency, but fortunately therapeutic measures exist (26,35). The incidence of hypercalcemia may be diminished by encouraging ambulation, decreasing calcium intake, and maintaining a normal hydration state. Management of hypercalcemia should include definitive antitumor therapy, including surgery, irradiation, chemotherapy, or hormonal therapy in conjunction with measures aimed at lowering the serum calcium. Since reabsorption of calcium in the renal tubules is linked to sodium reabsorption, serum calcium can often be acutely lowered by administration of a sodium load (to induce loss of sodium and calcium) and/or administration of diuretics affecting the loop of Henle and the distal tubule (furosemide). Other acute measures include use of calcitonin, mithramycin (108), steroids (especially useful in hematologic malignancies because they inhibit the osteoclast-activating factor), diphosphonates (59), and Gallium nitrate (123a). Long-term therapy for the patient who has had hypercalcemia includes restriction of dietary calcium and administration of phosphate.

Inappropriate Anti-diuretic Hormone Secretion Syndrome

Inappropriate secretion of ADH in severe form requires treatment with hypertonic saline (3%) and furosemide to obtain free water clearance (34). Less severe forms may respond to fluid restriction, but patients may have difficulty accepting this on a long-term basis. A useful alternative is demeclocycline 600 to 1200 mg/d in divided doses, which produces a vasopressin-resistant polyuria and permits flexibility in fluid intake (37, 45). However, this drug may cause nephrotoxicity or superinfection. Urea has been used to induce a persistent osmotic diuresis with excellent symptom control (33).

Ectopic Corticotropic Syndrome

The metabolic hallmark of this syndrome, hypokalemic alkalosis, should be treated with potassium chloride orally or intravenously (IV). Spironolactone to antagonize aldosterone also may be useful, and doses up to 400 mg/d may be needed to correct hypokalemia. Hypertension and fluid retention should be treated with diuretics. Adrenal enzyme inhibitors and drugs cytotoxic for the adrenal gland are also useful, and combinations of metyrapone, aminoglutethimide, and mitotane may be superior to each of these drugs used alone. Aggressive cytotoxic therapy of the underlying neoplasm, usually a SCLC, may completely reverse the syndrome.

Hypoglycemia

Hypoglycemia should be treated urgently with IV infusion of glucose. Long-term control may be achieved with frequent feedings and use of glucagon. Diazoxide and strepozotocin may be effective in insulinoma but are not usually effective in hypoglycemia caused by other mechanisms.

Fever of Malignancy

Fever in patients with cancer usually responds to indomethacin (75, 124). Use of this agent in a long-acting form on a fixed schedule may be especially efficacious and avoids the swings of temperature and associated diaphoresis that usually occur when antipyretics are given on an as-necessary basis.

Hyperuricemia

Hyperuricemia may develop during treatment, especially of hematologic malignancies, and is largely preventable by beginning allopurinol several days prior to starting chemotherapy and/or radiation therapy. Hydration with alkaline solutions is also useful and, rarely, hemodialysis may be necessary.

Tumor Lysis Syndrome

Rapid destruction of a sensitive tumor may result in hyperuricemia, hyperkalemia, hyperphosphatemia, and hypocalcemia. Prophylactic measures include allopurinol, alkaline hydration, and phased-in institution of chemotherapy. Therapeutic measures include diuretics to lower serum potassium level, aluminum antacids to bind phosphate in the gut, and, rarely, hemodialysis.

CONCLUSION

The paraneoplastic syndromes are complicated and often confusing disorders. To the researcher, their etiologies have considerable importance in the investigation of oncogenesis. To the clinician, their recognition and appropriate interpretation and management may alter the course of disease in the cancer patient.

Recommended Reading

There is an excellent collection of literature on paraneoplastic syndromes which, though somewhat old, contains well-established observations. *Paraneoplastic Syndromes*, edited by Hall (3), contains 48 original papers on all aspects of the topic. The first five references listed in the reference list provide general background reading. The other references generally are more topic-specific. One should be directed to these by clinical interests.

REFERENCES

General References

1. Bunn P, Ridgway EC: Paraneoplastic syndromes In: DeVita, V.T.Jr, Hellman S, Rosenberg SA, eds. Cancer: Principles and Practice of Oncology, 3rd ed., Philadelphia, PA: JB Lippincott Co.; 1989:1896-1940.
2. Frohman LA: Ectopic Hormone Production. Am J Med. 70:955-997;1981.
3. Hall TC (ed): Paraneoplastic Syndromes. Ann NY Acad Sci. 230:1-577;1974.
4. Trump DL, Baylin SB: Ectopic Hormone Syndromes. In: Abeloff, M.D, ed. Complications of Cancer. Baltimore, MD: Johns Hopkins University Press; 1979:211-241.
5. University of Texas, M.D. Anderson Hospital & Tumor Institute. Endocrine and Nonendocrine Hormone-producing Tumors. Chicago, IL: Year Book Medical Publishers.;1974.

Specific References

6. Amir SM, Sullivan RC, Ingbar SH: *In Vitro* Responses to Crude and Purified HCG in Human Thyroid Membranes. J Clin Endocrinol Metab 51:51-58;1980.
7. Anderson LG, Talai N: The Spectrum of Benign to Malignant Lymphoproliferation in Sjogren's Syndrome. Clin Exp Immunol 9:199-221;1971.
8. Anderson NE, Cunningham JM, Posner JB: Autoimmune pathogenesis of paraneoplastic neurological syndromes. Crit Rev Neurobiol. 3:245-299; 1987.
9. Banwo O, Versey J, Hobbs JR: New Ocofetal Antigen for Human Pancreas. Lancet 1:643-648;1974.
10. Barnes B: Dermatomyositis and Malignancy. Ann Intern Med 84:68-76;1976.
11. Barnes DM: New tumor factor may disrupt calcium levels. Science 237:363-364;1987.
12. Bartuska D: Humoral Manifestations of Neoplasms. Semin Oncol 2:405-409;1975.
13. Bashir R, Hochberg F: Paraneoplastic neurological syndromes. Cancer Investigation 6:117-118;1988.
14. Baylin S: Ectopic Production of Hormones and Other Proteins by Tumors. Hosp Pract.10:117-126;1975.
15. Beck SA, Tisdale MJ: Production of lipolytic and proteolytic factors by a murine tumor producing cachexia in the host. Cancer Res 47:5919-5923;1987.
16. Beveridge RA, Chan DW, Bruzek D, *et al.*: A new biomarker in monitoring breast cancer: CA 549. J Clin Oncol 6:1815-1821;1988.
17. Block K, Maki D: Hyperviscosity Syndromes Associated with Immunoglobulin Abnormalities. Semin Hematol 10:113-124;1973.
18. Bohan A, Peter J: Polymyositis and Dermatomyositis. N Engl J Med 292:344-347;403-407;1975.
19. Bolande R: The Neuralcrestopathies. Human Pathol 5:409-429;1974.
20. Bowie E, Owen C (eds): Symposium on the Intravascular Coagulation Fibrinolysis Syndrome. Mayo Clin Proc 49:643-679;1974.
21. Brennan JT: Oncologic emergencies and paraneoplastic syndromes. Primary care. 14:365-379; 1987.
22. Brereton H, Halushka PV, Alexander RW, *et al.*: Indomethacin Responsive Hypercalcemia in a Patient with Renal Cell Adenocarcinoma. N Engl J Med 291:83-86;1974.
23. Brereton H, Simon R, Pomeroy T: Pretreatment Serum LDH Predicting Metastatic Spread in Ewing's Sarcoma. Ann Intern Med 83:352-354;1975.
24. Broder L, Carter S: Pancreatic Islet Cell Carcinoma. II. Results of Therapy with Streptozotocin. Ann Intern Med 79:108-118;1973.
25. Brown J, Winkelman R: Acanthosis Nigricans. Medicine 47:33-51;1968.
26. Buescu A, Dimich AB, Myers WPL: Cancer Hypercalcemia: A Pragmatic Approach. Clinical Bulletin 5:91-98;1975.
27. Calabro J: Cancer and Arthritis. Arthritis Rheum 10:553-567;1967.
28. Cohen PR, Talpaz M, Kurzock R: Malignancy-associated Sweet's syndrome: Review of the world literature . J Clin Oncol 6:1887-1897;1988.
29. Costanza ME, Pinn V, Schwartz RS *et al.*: CEA Antibody Complexes in a Patient with Colon Carcinoma and Nephrotic Syndrome. N Engl J Med 289:520-522; 1973.
30. Daughaday WH, Emanuele MA, Brooks MH, *et al.*: Synthesis and secretion of insulin-like growth factor II by a leiomyosarcoma with associated hypoglycemia. N Engl J Med 319:1434-1440;1988.
31. Davis Z, Moertel CG, McIrath DC: The Malignant Carcinoid Syndrome. Surg Gynecol Obstet 137:637-644; 1973.
32. De Fronzo R, Humphrey RL, Wright JR, *et al.*: Acute Renal Failure in Multiple Myeloma, Medicine 54:209-224; 1975.
33. Decaux G, Genette F: Urea for Long-term Treatment of Syndrome of Inappropriate Secretion of Antidiuretic Hormone. Br Med J 283:1081-1086; 1981 .
34. Decaux G, Waterlot Y, Genette F, *et al.*: Treatment of the syndrome of inappropriate secretion of antidiuretic hormone with furosemide. N Eng J Med 304:329-330; 1981.
35. Deltos L, Neer R: Medical Management of the Hypercalcemia of Malignancy. Annu Rev Med 25:323-331; 1974.
36. Denny-Brown D: Primary sensory neuropathy with muscular changes associated with carcinoma J Neurol Neurosurg Psychiatr 11:73-87; 1948.
37. DeTroyer A: Demeclocycline: Treatment of Syndrome of Inappropriate Antidiuretic Hormone Secretion. JAMA 237:2723-2736; 1977.
38. DeWys WD: Pathophysiology of Cancer Cachexia: Current Understanding and Areas for Future Research. Cancer Res 42:7215-7265; 1982.
39. DeWys WD, Stoll R, Au WY, *et al.*: Effect of Streptozotocin on islet cell carcinoma with hypercalcemia. Am J Med 55:671-676; 1973.
40. Eagan RT, Maurer LH, Forcier RJ, *et al.*: Small cell carcinoma of the lung: Staging, paraneoplastic syndromes, treatment and survival. Cancer 33:527-532; 1974.

41. Engel AG: Myasthenia Gravis and myasthenic syndromes. Ann Neurol 16:519-534; 1984.
42. Farr H, Fahey TJ, Nash AG, et al.: Primary hyperparathyroidism and cancer. Am J Surg 126:539-543; 1973.
43. Feibusch J, Barbosa-Saldivar JL, Bernstein RS, et al.: Tumor-associated nephrogenic dibetes insipidus. Ann Int Med 92:797-798; 1980 .
44. Fisken RA, Heath DA, Somers S, et al.: Hypercalcemia in hospital patients: Clinical and diagnostic aspects. Lancet 1:20 2-206; 1981.
45. Forrest JN Jr, Cox M, Hong C, et al.: Superiority of Demeclocycline over Lithium in the Treatment of Chronic Syndrome of Inappropriate Secretion of Antidiuretic Hormone. N Engl J Med 298:173-177; 1978.
46. Fox P, Hofman JW, Wilson SD, et al.: Surgical Management of Zollinger-Ellison Syndrome. Surg Clin North Am 54:395-407; 1974.
47. Freeman DA: Steroid hormone-producing tumors in man. Endocrine Rev 7:204-220; 1986.
48. Friesen S, Hermreck AS, Mantz FA: Glucagon, Gastrin, and Carcinoid Tumors of the Duodenum, Pancreas, and Stomach: Polypeptide "APUDomas" of the Foregut. Am J Surg 127:90-101; 1974 .
49. Friesen SR: Update on the diagnosis and treatment of rare neuroendocrine tumors. Surg. Clin. N. Am. 67:379-393; 1987.
50. Gordon GS, Roof BS: Humors from Tumors: Diagnostic Potentials of Peptides. Ann Intern Med 76:501-502; 1972.
51. Gordon P, Hendricks CM, Kahn CR, et al.: Hypoglycemia Associated with Non-Islet Cell Tumor and Insulin-like Growth Factors. N Engl J Med 305:1452-1455; 1981.
52. Greenberg E, Divertie M, Woolner LB: A Review of Unusual Systemic Manifestations Associated with Cancer. Am J Med 36:106-120; 1964.
53. Grey H, Kohler P: Cryoimmunoglobulins. Semin Hemat 10:87-112; 1973.
54. Griffiths K, Meville AM, Pierrepoint CG: Tumor Markers: Determination and Clinical Role. Baltimore, MD: University Park Press; 1978.
55. Gropp C, Havemann K, Scheuer A: Ectopic hormones in lung cancer patients at diagnosis and during therapy. Cancer 46:347-354; 1980.
56. Gropp C, Luster W, Havemann K: Ectopic hormones in lung cancer. In: Ergebnisse der Inneren Medizin und Kinderheilkunde. Bd 53. Berlin Heidelberg: Springer-Verlag; 1984:133-164.
57. Guillemin R, Brazeau P, Bohlen P, et al.: Growth hormone-releasing factor from a human pancreatic tumor that caused acromegaly. Science 218:585-586; 1982.
58. Hall TC: Oncocognitive Autoimmunity and Other Paraneoplastic Syndromes Yet to be Described. Ann NY Acad Sci 230:565-570; 1974.
59. Hasling C, Charles P, Mosekilde L: Etidronate disodium for treatment of hypercalcemia of malignancy: A double blind placebo controlled study. J Clin Invest 16:433-437,1986.
60. Haverback B, Dyce B: Gastrins, MEA's, and Zollinger-Ellison Syndrome. Ann Intern Med 83:307-311; 1975.
61. Hayes DF, Zurawski VR, Kufe DW: Comparison of circulating CA 15-3 and CEA levels in patients with breast cancer. J Clin Oncol 4:1542-1550; 1986.
62. Helm F, Klein E: Cutaneous Clues to Malignant Disease. J Surg Oncol 6:481-499; 1974.
63. Herberman RB, McIntire KR: Immunodiagnosis of Cancer. New York, NY: Mark Dekker; 1979.
64. Higgins H, Hershman JM, Keminer JG, et al.: The Thyrotoxicosis of Hydatidiform Mole. Ann Intern Med 83:307-311; 1975.
65. Holyoke ED: Present and Probable Uses of CEA, CA 25:22-26; 1975.
66. Hopper J: Tumor Related Renal Lesions. Ann Intern Med 81:550-551; 1974.
67. Horenstein S: Distant Effect of Neoplasms on the Nervous System. Post-grad Med 50:85-90; 1971.
68. Kalra L, Delamere JF: Lymphoreticular malignancy and monoclonal gammopathy presenting as polymyalgia rheumatica. Brit J Rheumatol 26:458-459; 1987.
69. Khair M, Dexter RN, Burzynski NJ, et al.: Mucosal Neuroma, Pheochromocytoma, and Medullary Carcinoma of the Thyroid, MEN Type 3. Medicine 54:89-112; 1975.
70. Kierland R: Cutaneous Signs of Internal Cancer. CA 22:364-371; 1972.
71. Kyle R: Subject Review: Multiple Myeloma. Mayo Clin Proc 50:20-40; 1975.
72. Kyle RA, Bayrd ED: Amyloidosis: Review of 236 Cases. Medicine 54:271-299; 1975.
73. Latov N, Sherman WH, Nemni R, et al.: Plasma cell dyscrasia and peripheral neuropathy with a monoclonal antibody to peripheral nerve myelin. N Eng J Med 303:618-621; 1980.
74. Levine AS, Morley JE: Purinergic regulation of food intake. Science 217:77-79; 1982.
75. Lusch CJ, Serpick AA, Slater L: Antipyretic Effect of Indomethacine in Patients with Malignancy. Cancer 21:781-786; 1968 .
76. Maganelli P, Borghi L, Coruzi T, et al.: Paraneoplastic polymyalgia rheumatica. Case contribution. Minerva Med 77:1739-1741; 1986.
77. Martin EW: Carcinoembryonic Antigen: Clinical and Historical Aspects. Cancer 37:62-81; 1976.
78. Matzkin H, Braf Z: Paraneoplastic syndromes associated with prostatic carcinoma. J Urol 138:1129-1133; 1987.
79. Medsger TA, Dixon JA, Garwood VF: Palmar Fascitis and Polyarthritis Associated with Ovarian Carcinoma. Ann Intern Med 96:424-431; 1982.
80. Miller D: The Association of Immune Disease and Malignant Lymphoma. Ann Intern Med 66:507-521; 1967.
81. Moertel CG: An odyssey in the land of small tumors. J Clin Oncol 5:1503-1522; 1987.
82. Muggia F, Heineman H: Hypercalcemia Associated with Neoplastic Disease. Ann Intern Med 73:281-290; 1970.
83. Mulder H, Hackeng WHL: Ectopic secretion of Calcitonin. Acta Med Scand 204:253-256; 1978.
84. Nathanson L, Hall T: Lung Tumors: How They Produce Their Syndromes. Ann NY Acad Sci 230:367-377; 1974.
85. Omenn G, Wilkins E: Hormone Syndromes Associated with Bronchogenic Carcinoma. J Thorac Cardiovasc Surg 59:877-881, 1 975 .
85a. Orloff JJ, Wu TL, Stewart AF: Parathyroid hormone-like proteins: Biochemical responses and receptor interactions. Endocr Res 10:476-495; 1989.
86. Patchell RA, Posner JB: Neurological complications of systemic cancer. Neurol Clin 3:729-750; 1985.
87. Pfinsgraff J, Buckingham RB, Killian PJ, et al.: Palmar fasciitis and arthritis with malignant neoplasms: a paraneoplastic syndrome. Semin Arth Rheum 16:118-15; 1986.
88. Pochealy C: Neurologic Manifestations in Acute Leukemia, HII, NY State J Med 75:575-580; 715-721; 878-881; 1975.
89. Posner J: Neurologic Complication of Systemic Cancer. Med Clin North Amer 55:625-646; 1971.
90. Powars D, Allerton SE, Beierle J, et al.: Wilms' Tumor: Clinical Correlation with Circulation Mucin in 3 Cases. Cancer 29:1597-1606; 1972.
91. Primack A: The Production of Markers by Bronchogenic Carcinoma: A Review. Semin Oncol 1:235-244; 1974.
92. Rauch AE, Tartaglia AP, Kaufman R, et al.: RBC fragmentation and thymoma. Arch Int Med 105:1280-1282; 1984.
93. Rees LH: The biosynthesis of hormones by non-endocrine tumors. J Endocr 67:143-175; 1975.
94. Robbins J, Kraemer KH, Lutzner MA, et al.: Xeroderma Pigmentosum. Ann Intern Med 80:221-248; 1974.
95. Robertson GL, Bhoopalm N, Felkowitz LJ: Vincristine neurotoxicity and abnormal secretion of antidiuretic hormone. Arch Int Med 132:717-720,1973.
96. Rosen P, Armstrong D: Nonbacterial Thrombotic Endocarditis in Patients with Malignant Neoplastic Disease. Am J Med 54:23-29; 1973.
97. Rosen S, Weintraub B: Ectopic Production of the Isolated a subunit of the Glycoproteins. N Engl J Med 290:1441-1447; 1974.
98. Rosen S, Weintraub B: Humors, Tumors and Caveats. Ann Intern Med 82:274-276; 1975.
99. Rosen S, Weintraub BD, Vaitukaitis JL, et al.: Placental Proteins and their Subunits as Tumor Markers. Ann Intern Med 82:71-83; 1975.
100. Ruddon RW: Biological Markers of Neoplasia: Basic and Applied Aspects. New York, NY: Elsevier, North-Holland; 1978.
101. Schein P: Chemotherapy and Management of the Hormone Secreting Endocrine Malignancies. Cancer 30:1616-1626; 1972.

102. Schein P, DeLellis RA, Kahn CR, et al.: Islet Cell Tumors: Current Concepts and Management. Ann Intern Med 79:239-257; 1973.

103. Scholz D, Purnell DC, Goldsmith RS, et al.: Hypercalcemia and Cancer. CA 25:27-30; 1975.

104. Schwartz BS, Williams EC, Conlan MG, et al.: Epsilon-aminocaproic acid in the treatment of patients with acute promyelocytic leukemia and acquired alpha-2 plasmin inhibitor deficiency. Ann Int Med 105:873-876; 1986.

105. Schwartz MK, Young DS: Cancer. In Brown SS, Mitchell FL, Young DS (eds): Chemical Diagnosis of Disease. New York, NY: Elsevier, North-Holland; 1979, pp. 1293-1347.

106. Sherman R, Susin M, Weksler ME, et al.: Lipoid Nephrosis in Hodgkin's Disease. Am J Med 52:699-706; 1972.

107. Slayton R, Shnider BI, Elias E, et al.: New Approach to the Treatment of Hypercalcemia. Clin Pharmacol Ther 12:833-837; 1971.

108. Smith J, O'Neil R: Alpha-Fetoprotein Occurrence in Germinal Cell and Liver Malignancy. Am J Med 51:767-771; 1971.

109. Smith L, Salmon SE, Schrier RW: Endocrine Manifestations of Malignant Disease. California Medicine 116:43-51; 1972.

110. Smith LH: The APUD Cell Concept. J Surg Oncol 8:137-142; 1976.

111. Smith LH: Ectopic Hormone Production. Surg Gynecol Obstet 141:443-453; 1975.

112. Souod jian JV, Enriquez P, Silverstein MN, et al.: The Spectrum of Disease Associated with Thymoma. Arch Intern Med 134:374-379; 1974.

113. Statland BE: Tumor Markers. Diagn Med 4:21-38; 1981.

114. Stone S: Cutaneous Clues to Cancer. Am Fam Prac 12:82-88; 1975.

115. Tagnon JH, Hildebrand J: Paraneoplastic Syndromes. Europ J Cancer Clin Oncol 17:969-990; 1981.

116. Tandon R, Walden M, Falcon S: Catatonia as a manifestation of paraneoplastic encephalopathy. J Clin Psychiatry 49:3-4; 1988.

117. Ternell M, Moldawer LL, Lonnroth C, et al.: Plasma protein synthesis in experimental cancer compared to paraneoplastic conditions, including monokine administration. Cancer Res 47:5825-5829; 1987.

118. Tormey D, Waalkes TP, Ahmann D: Biologic Markers in Breast Cancer. Cancer 35:1095-1100; 1975.

119. Turner M: Carcinoembryonic Antigen. JAMA 231:756-758; 1975.

120. Ultmann JE, Moran E: Clinical Course and Complications in Hodgkin's Disease. Arch Intern Med 131:332-353; 1973.

121. Vasavada P, Prasan J, Bournigal LJ, et al.: Thymoma Associated with Pure Red Cell Aplasia and Hypogammaglobulinemias. Postgrad Med 54:93-98; 1973.

122. Vider M, Kashmiri R, Meeker WR, et al.: Carcinoembryonic Antigen Monitoring and the Management of Radiotherapeutic and Chemotherapeutic Patients. Am J Roentgenol 124:630-635; 1975.

123. Waldmann T, Broder S, Strober W: Protein-losing Enteropathies in Malignancy. Ann NY Acad Sci 230:306-317; 1974.

123a. Warrell RP Jr: Gallium in the treatment of hypercalcemia and bone metastases. Imp Advin Oncol 1:205-220; 1989.

124. Warshaw AL, Carey RW, Robinson DR: Control of Fever Associated with Viscerai Malignancies by Indomethacine. Surgery 89:414-416; 1981.

125. Weick J, Hagedorn AB, Linman JW: Leukoerythroblastosis. Mayo Clin Proc 49:110-113; 1974.

126. Weintraub B, Rosen S: Ectopic Production of the Isolated B subunit of Human Chorionic Gonadotrophin. J Clin Invest 52:3135-3142; 1973.

127. Williams JE: Mechanisms of cachexia, Cancer Forum 21:119-120, 1980.

128. Wilson H, Cheek RC: Carcinoid Tumors: Curr Probl Surg 4-31, (with 3 related articles); 1970.

129. Wolf P, Reid D: Use of radiolabeled antibodies for localization of neoplasms. Arch Int Med 141:1067-1070; 1981.

130. Zamcheck N, Pusztaszevi G: CEA, AFP, and other Potential Tumor Markers. CA 25:204-214; 1975.

Zachary B. Kramer, M.D., Medical Oncology
James W. Keller, M.D., Radiation Oncology

Philip Rubin, M.D., Radiation Oncology

Chapter **13**

ONCOLOGIC EMERGENCIES

In the fields of observation, chance favors only the mind that is prepared.

Louis Pasteur (7)

PERSPECTIVE

The anatomic, metabolic, or immunologic disturbances effected by malignancy create exigent problems for the cancer patient. Anticipation, early recognition, and timely treatment of these oncologic crises avert otherwise morbid consequences. Oncologic emergencies often arise late in the course of known, advanced cancer. In this setting, appropriate management provides significant palliation. Oncologic emergencies also occur as initial presentations or treatment-related complications of curable malignancies. In these settings, optimal therapeutic intervention affords an opportunity for long-term survival.

CARDIOVASCULAR EMERGENCIES

Pericardial Effusion and Cardiac Tamponade

Cardiac tamponade occurs when fluid accumulation in the pericardial sac impairs diastolic filling of the heart, thereby producing hemodynamic compromise. Infiltration of the pericardium by metastatic cancer may create sufficient effusion to cause tamponade (36). Pericardial metastases and effusion, usually late complications of cancer, are most commonly due to metastatic lung or breast cancer.

Diagnosis

1. Symptoms of tamponade include dyspnea, orthopnea, chest pain, and altered mental status. Physical findings include tachycardia, tachypnea, cyanosis, hypotension, pulsus paradoxus, diminished heart sounds, and a pericardial rub.
2. The chest film demonstrates an enlarged globular heart shadow and often a pleural effusion. The electrocardiogram demonstrates sinus tachycardia, low voltage, and atrial arrhythmias.
3. Echocardiography is the diagnostic procedure of choice. Pericardial effusion is readily demonstrated. During tamponade, right atrial and ventricular diastolic collapse may be noted.

Therapy

1. Emergent pericardiocentesis is required for relief of cardiac tamponade. Fluid should be obtained for cytologic, culture, and chemistry studies. Cytology is diagnostic of malignancy in 85% of cases (44).

2. Lasting control of malignant pericardial effusion is achieved by surgical creation of a pericardial window. An alternative treatment involves sclerosis of the pericardial space by tetracycline, using a pericardial catheter (54).
3. Hemodynamically stable patients with small to moderate effusions may be treated with chemotherapy or irradiation. This approach is suitable only for responsive tumors such as breast cancer and lymphoma.

Superior Vena Cava Syndrome

Obstruction of the superior vena cava by mediastinal tumor produces a distinct clinical syndrome. The syndrome is usually caused by lung cancer, especially small cell lung carcinoma (SCLC), but lymphomas and other metastatic tumors are also causal (54). The severity of the superior vena cava syndrome is determined by the rate of caval obstruction and the degree of compensatory venous collateralization. Despite a dramatic presentation, isolated caval obstruction is rarely, if ever, fatal. However, concomitant compromise of other mediastinal structures, such as the trachea or pericardium, may have disastrous consequences (1).

Diagnosis

1. Headache, nausea, vomiting, visual disturbances, and syncope are presenting complaints. Symptoms of hoarseness, dyspnea, dysphagia, or back pain suggest involvement of other mediastinal structures.
2. Upper body venous distention, edema, and cyanosis are prominent physical findings.
3. A chest film usually reveals a right-sided paratracheal or mediastinal mass. Computerized tomography (CT) of the chest is diagnostic and helpful in defining disease extent, guiding biopsy attempts, differentiating extrinsic caval compression from intrinsic obstruction, and planning radiation therapy (47). Radionuclide venography, although rarely necessary since the advent of CT, confirms the diagnosis of superior vena cava obstruction.
4. Tissue diagnosis may be pursued during the treatment of the severely symptomatic patient. In rare cases, attempts at tissue diagnosis must be deferred in favor of urgent therapy.

147

Therapy

1. Emergency treatment usually entails prompt administration of radiation therapy to the obstructing mediastinal mass. Symptoms are ameliorated in 70% of cases by this approach.
2. Initially, high daily doses of radiation (400 cGy x 3) are optimal to achieve rapid tumor volume reduction. Evaluation of comparative groups indicates that the high dose (400 cGy) is superior to standard- or lower-dose treatment (≤ 200 cGy) in relieving obstruction within a week of initiating therapy.
3. Chemotherapy is equally effective for patients with lymphoma or SCLC, and simultaneously treats overt or suspected metastatic disease (39).

HEMATOLOGIC EMERGENCIES

Disseminated Intravascular Coagulation

Disseminated intravascular coagulation (DIC) is a thrombohemorrhagic syndrome characterized pathophysiologically by excessive thrombin activation and effect. This leads to extensive consumption and depletion of circulating clotting factors, and deposition of injurious fibrin-platelet thrombi in the microvasculature.

Thus, the clinical manifestation of DIC is a generalized bleeding disorder accompanied by multiorgan dysfunction (35). The disorder frequently occurs at diagnosis or during cytoreductive therapy of acute promyelocytic leukemia, but may complicate other leukemias as well. The coagulopathy is thought to be initiated by tissue thromboplastins, proteases, or interleukins released from leukemic blasts.

Diagnosis

1. Severe bleeding, often from multiple sites, is characteristic of DIC. Fatal intracranial hemorrhage occurs in a significant number of patients.
2. Laboratory studies demonstrate marked thrombocytopenia, prolongation of the prothrombin, thrombin, and partial thromboplastin times, hypofibrinogenemia, and elevated fibrin degradation products. Red cell fragmentation may be noted on blood smear.

Therapy

1. Patients with acute leukemia and ongoing or anticipated DIC often receive intravenous (IV) heparin (5 to 10 U/kg/h) to inhibit thrombin activity (28).
2. Diligent administration of platelets, plasma, and cryoprecipitate is required to replete hemostatic factors. Clotting studies must be carefully monitored: the platelet count should be maintained above 50,000/μL and the fibrinogen level above 150 mg/dL. Transfusion support and heparin therapy are continued until chemotherapy has reduced the tumor burden and the coagulopathy has resolved (23).

Leukostasis

Leukostasis is a complication of hyperleukocytic leukemia, in which small blood vessels are obstructed and infiltrated by leukemic blasts. This disorder usually occurs when the white blood cell (WBC) count exceeds 100,000/μL. Neurologic and pulmonary dysfunction develops due to sludging in, or hemorrhage from, small blood vessels.

Acute and chronic myelogenous leukemias, acute lymphoblastic leukemia, and, rarely, chronic lymphocytic leukemias produce leukostasis. Patients with monocytic variants of acute leukemia are particularly prone to leukostatic complications (41). This disorder usually presents prior to any therapeutic intervention; it may also occur precipitously during chemotherapy or blood transfusion.

Diagnosis

1. The syndrome should be considered in patients with blast counts greater than 50,000/μL who have central nervous system (CNS) deficits or respiratory distress. Symptoms include dyspnea, stupor, ataxia, visual disturbances, or confusion. Priapism or symptoms of arterial insufficiency may also occur (33).
2. Physical examination may reveal papilledema, retinal venous distention, tachypnea, or diffuse pulmonary rales. Hypoxemia may be documented by measurement of arterial blood gases or oximetry.

Therapy

1. Rapid lowering of the WBC count is indicated to prevent respiratory failure and to avoid devastating intracranial hemorrhage.
2. Leukapheresis used emergently will reduce the WBC count by 30% to 60% and lessen the metabolic effects of chemotherapy-related tumor lysis (15).
3. Hydroxyurea administered orally (PO) at a dose of 3 g/m² for 2 days will rapidly decrease cell counts in leukemia. Definitive antileukemic therapy follows the above measures, as the effects of cytophoresis and hydroxyurea are transient.

Thrombocytopenia

Significant thrombocytopenia in cancer patients is most often related to decreased production of platelets. This may be mediated by the myelosuppressive effects of chemotherapy or radiation therapy, or by infiltration of the bone marrow by malignancy. Spontaneous hemorrhage rarely occurs when the patient's platelet count exceeds 50,000/μL. The risk of bleeding, usually from mucosal surfaces, increases considerably as the count falls below 20,000/μL (29). Intracranial hemorrhage is the most feared complication of thrombocytopenia.

Diagnosis

1. Epistaxis, ecchymoses, menometrorrhagia, hematuria, or gastrointestinal (GI) bleeding may occur. Thrombocytopenia is readily documented by measurement of the platelet count and review of the blood smear.

Therapy

1. Platelet transfusion is indicated when bleeding occurs during severe thrombocytopenia, or as prophylaxis against hemorrhage when the platelet count is less than 20,000/μL.
2. In the absence of concomitant fever, infection, splenomegaly, or alloimmunization, 1 U of platelets per 10 kg body weight (5 to 7 U/m²) is sufficient to raise the platelet count to an adequate level. During an episode of active bleeding, the platelet count should be maintained above 50,000/μL.
3. Any agents that impair platelet function, such as aspirin, should be avoided until thrombocytopenia resolves.

METABOLIC EMERGENCIES

Hypercalcemia

Hypercalcemia is often encountered as a metabolic consequence of uncontrolled malignancy, and is usually, but not invariably, associated with bone metastases. Malignant hypercalcemia may develop suddenly and worsen rapidly, a feature that distinguishes it from other hypercalcemic disorders such as hyperparathyroidism. Hypercalcemia of malignancy arises by various pathogenic mechanisms that may operate concurrently (11). In some cases, cytokines released from metastatic bone deposits stimulate osteoclast activity and local bone resorption, resulting in hypercalcemia (37). Alternatively, tumors may produce peptides with some functional similarities to parathormone, resulting in hypercalcemia even in the absence of bone metastases (17).

Diagnosis

1. Symptoms of hypercalcemia include anorexia, nausea, vomiting, constipation, polyuria, polydipsia, and altered sensorium. Hypercalcemia is documented readily by serum calcium measurement. A variable degree of azotemia is often noted.

Therapy

1. Forced normal saline diuresis, (200 to 250 cc/h), should be initiated promptly to reverse volume contraction and promote calciuresis. Fluid balance and cardiopulmonary status must be monitored closely to avoid volume overload and congestive heart failure in older patients. Furosemide, a diuretic, may be required. Saline hydration significantly reduces the serum calcium level after 1 to 2 days.
2. Plicamycin (mithramycin), 25 µg/kg, may be administered IV. This drug inhibits osteoclasts and a resultant hypocalcemic effect begins 12 hours after a dose. The effect is maximal at 1 to 2 days and persists up to 3 weeks. Its use is relatively contraindicated in patients with severe renal failure or marked thrombocytopenia.
3. Corticosteroids such as prednisone are useful for treatment of the hypercalcemia of lymphoma, myeloma, or breast cancer; their therapeutic benefit is observed after 5 to 10 days' administration.
4. Newer osteoclast inhibitors such as the diphosphonates or gallium nitrate may be used when malignant hypercalcemia is refractory to other measures or other agents are contraindicated. The onset of action of these drugs is somewhat slower than mithramycin (48 to 96 hours), and initial administration is via the IV route (46).
5. The key to lasting control of hypercalcemia is effective antineoplastic therapy; this therapy should be initiated as soon as possible.

Tumor Lysis Syndrome

The tumor lysis syndrome encompasses a group of metabolic derangements that complicate the treatment of bulky and highly proliferative neoplasms. This syndrome typically occurs in patients with Burkitt's lymphoma, lymphoblastic lymphoma, acute lymphoblastic leukemia with hyperleukocytosis, or accelerated chronic myelogenous leukemia. These neoplasms are exquisitely chemosensitive so that marked cytoreduction occurs with treatment. The resultant lysis of tumor cells liberates great quantities of intracellular urate, phosphate, and potassium into the circulation. The sheer excess of these waste products overwhelms the excretory capacity of the kidneys. Consequently, hyperphosphatemia, secondary hypocalcemia, hyperuricemia, and hyperkalemia develop (57b). Precipitation of urate or calcium phosphate in the renal tubules causes acute renal failure and worsening metabolic disarray. Cardiac arrhythmias and encephalopathy occur subsequently (2,56).

Diagnosis

1. Serial blood chemistry measurements document progressive abnormalities as described above. Phosphate crystals may be grossly visible in the urine sediment.

Therapy

1. Preventive measures as described below are initiated 48 hours prior to chemotherapy, and are continued for 3 to 5 days.
2. IV hydration 3000 mL/m²/d promotes excretion of urate and phosphate. Allopurinol 500 mg/m²/d given PO helps reduce uric acid production.
3. If the uric acid level exceeds 7 mg/dL, urinary alkalinization with IV sodium bicarbonate is recommended. Urinary pH is maintained above 7 until hyperuricemia has resolved.
4. Hemodialysis is indicated for severe cases of tumor lysis syndrome.

Hyperuricemia

Marked hyperuricemia as an isolated abnormality may develop abruptly during the treatment of leukemias, myeloproliferative disorders, lymphoma, or myeloma. As tumor cells break down during chemotherapy, purines are released; these are catabolized to uric acid. In overabundance, uric acid precipitates in the renal tubules and collecting system, resulting in renal failure or, rarely, acute urate nephrolithiasis (24).

Diagnosis

1. Symptoms of uremia may develop. Hematuria and flank pain suggest the presence of nephrolithiasis.
2. The serum uric acid exceeds 10 mg/dL and averages 20 mg/dL. Oliguria or anuria with or without uric acid crystalluria is observed. Blood urea nitrogen and serum creatinine levels are elevated.
3. A urine uric acid to creatinine ratio greater than 1.0, measured on a random sample, supports the diagnosis of hyperuricemic nephropathy.

Therapy

1. Allopurinol, hydration, and urinary alkalinization therapy as detailed in the tumor lysis section are used. Generally, allopurinol and moderate hydration are adequate prophylatic measures unless the tumor burden is high or marked hyperuricemia is present.
2. Hemodialysis, if required, rapidly reverses hyperuricemia and ameliorates renal function.

Hyponatremia

Hyponatremia in cancer patients is commonly due to the ectopic or inappropriate secretion of antidiuretic hormone (ADH). Most often it is the autonomous production of ADH by SCLC that accounts for the hyponatremia. Other tumor types, usually of neuroendocrine origin, also produce ADH. Hyponatremia due to ectopic hormone production occasionally antedates the diagnosis of malignancy by months (34), but usually the tumor is clinically overt when hyponatremia is manifest. The syndrome of inappropriate antidiuretic hormone secretion (SIADH) may also occur secondarily in the setting of brain metastases or after treatment with cytotoxic drugs such as cyclophosphamide or vincristine. In these situations, disturbances of hypothalamic-pituitary function are responsible for the syndrome.

Diagnosis

1. Symptoms correlate poorly with the severity of hyponatremia and may depend in part on its rate of development. Anorexia, nausea, vomiting, weakness, and lethargy occur.
2. The serum sodium is 130 mEq/L or less, and a level less than 115 mEq/L is associated with altered mental status or seizures.
3. Other causes of hyponatremia, such as diuretics, hypoadrenalism, hypothyroidism, renal disease, edema states, and volume depletion, must be excluded.
4. Simultaneous measurement of serum and urine osmolality showing inappropriate concentration of the urine (urine osmolality greater than serum osmolality) supports a diagnosis of SIADH. Urinary sodium excretion is not depressed (16).

Therapy

1. Mild to moderate hyponatremia secondary to SIADH is treated with restriction of free water intake to 500 mL/d.
2. Chemotherapy of SCLC will eliminate the ectopic hormone source and correct hyponatremia in a few weeks.
3. Radiation therapy and corticosteroid treatment may reverse SIADH due to brain metastases.
4. Severe hyponatremia, especially if complicated by neurologic symptoms, may warrant careful infusion of hypertonic saline. Resolution of hyponatremia and avoidance of circulatory overload is facilitated by furosemide administration (5).
5. Demeclocycline, an antibiotic that causes nephrogenic diabetes insipidus, may be administered. This drug produces modest results and is contraindicated in patients with renal or hepatic disease. Demeclocycline is usually administered when hyponatremia is resistant to other measures. Urea, administered orally, is also effective for management of resistant hyponatremia.

Lactic Acidosis

Lactic acidosis is a rare sequel of malignancy, and is associated with a large tumor burden and extensive neoplastic infiltration of the liver (21). It has been reported most often as a complication of leukemia or lymphoma. Very rarely, lactic acidosis can occur in patients with solid tumors, such as SCLC or pheochromocytoma (9). Impaired hepatic lactate catabolism, coupled with overproduction of lactate by tumor cells, is the suggested mechanism for malignancy-induced acidosis.

Diagnosis

1. Symptoms are nonspecific but include nausea, vomiting, dyspnea, and somnolence.
2. Arterial pH is less than 7.35. The anion gap is widened and the serum lactate exceeds 5 mEq/L.

3. Other causes of lactic acidosis such as sepsis or toxin ingestion must be excluded.

Therapy

1. IV sodium bicarbonate may be required emergently.
2. The prompt initiation of antineoplastic therapy is essential for resolution of the acidosis.

Hypoglycemia

Severe hypoglycemia as a direct effect of malignancy is an infrequently observed phenomenon. It is a well-described presentation of the rare insulin-producing pancreatic islet cell tumor, the insulinoma. Hypoglycemia is also classically associated with large mesenchymal tumors, such as mesothelioma, fibrosarcoma, and hepatoma and adrenal cortical carcinoma. Non-insulinoma tumor hypoglycemia is apparently mediated by secretion of insulin-like growth factors by the tumor cells. These growth factors promote peripheral use of glucose and may inhibit the effect of other counterregulatory hormones (4). Tumor-induced hypoglycemia is commonly precipitated by fasting or exercise; prolonged hypoglycemia may result in irreversible brain damage.

Diagnosis

1. Neurologic symptoms predominate; irritability, stupor, coma, confusion, agitation, seizures, or visual disturbances occur.
2. A fasting plasma glucose level less than 50 mg/dL or a postprandial level below 40 mg/dL indicates hypoglycemia.
3. Insulinoma patients demonstrate increased insulin levels despite hypoglycemia, and the fasting insulin to glucose ratio is elevated.
4. Other etiologies, including alcoholism, starvation, endocrinopathy, or hepatic and renal failure, must be ruled out.

Therapy

1. Emergent management entails bolus infusion of 50% dextrose followed by continuous infusion of 10% dextrose.
2. Partial or complete surgical ablation of operable tumors will eliminate hypoglycemia (31). Chemotherapy or radiotherapy of unresectable tumors is also effective for responsive cancers.
3. Prolonged administration of corticosteroids, glucagon, or diazoxide may be necessary if other measures are ineffective or unfeasible.

INFECTIOUS EMERGENCIES

Fever in the Neutropenic Host

Neutropenia of variable severity is seen in cancer patients treated with myelosuppressive chemotherapy. Neutropenia may also occur when the bone marrow is infiltrated by metastatic carcinoma or hematopoietic malignancy. An absolute neutrophil count below 1000/μL confers an increased risk of infection (12). This risk is most pronounced at neutrophil counts under 500/μL. The susceptibility of the neutropenic patient to infection may be increased by a concomitant immunodeficiency such as asplenia, hypogammaglobulinemia or monocytopenia (8).

Delay in the evaluation and empiric treatment of the febrile, neutropenic patient is unacceptable, because the potential for rapidly fatal sepsis is considerable. All episodes of fever in these patients are considered to be infection until proven otherwise. Initial infections during neutropenia are usually due to bacterial pathogens; however, in half of all acute febrile episodes no infectious site or pathogen is identified (27). Systemic fungal infections also occur, particularly if neutropenia is protracted.

Diagnosis

1. A temperature above 38.0° C requires evaluation. Thorough examination of the patient is warranted, with attention to the gingiva, pharynx, perirectal region, and to vascular access sites. Clinical signs of infection may be deceptively minimal.
2. Laboratory evaluation includes cultures of blood, urine, pharynx, and other sites as clinically indicated. A chest radiograph should be obtained.

Therapy

1. Prompt initiation of broad-spectrum antibiotics is mandatory. A combination of an aminoglycoside and an antipseudomonal beta-lactam antibiotic (e.g., azlocillin, ceftazidime, pipracillin) is traditionally recommended. The optimal antibiotic combination may vary, depending on the antimicrobial susceptibility pattern at a given institution or the specific clinical findings.
2. Initial use of vancomycin, an antistaphylococcal agent, is warranted if gram-positive bacterial or catheter-related infection is suspected.
3. Persistent, unexplained fever in the neutropenic patient on conventional antibiotics is an indication for empiric antifungal treatment with amphotericin B.

Systemic Mycoses in Immunocompromised Cancer Patient

Granulocytopenia and defective cell-mediated immunity predispose the cancer patient to invasive or disseminated fungal infection. The specific fungal pathogens involved depend on the nature of the immunodeficiency. For example, in leukemia patients who experience prolonged neutropenia, infections with *Candida*, *Aspergillus*, or *Mucor* sp predominate. The risk of these infections is amplified by such conditions as prolonged corticosteroid treatment, central hyperalimentation, mucositis, broad-spectrum antibiotic therapy, or the presence of indwelling catheters. In contrast, lymphoma patients may acquire infection with *Cryptococcus* sp in the absence of neutropenia, because of attendant impairment of cell-mediated immunity.

Invasive candidiasis often produces esophagitis, enteritis or pneumonia, and dissemination to brain, skin, liver, or eye may follow. The syndrome of hepatic candidiasis may present with fever, abdominal pain, elevated alkaline phosphatase, and liver lesions apparent only after recovery from neutropenia (55). *Aspergillus* and *Mucor* sp characteristically produce pulmonary or sinus infections. These organisms are angioinvasive; pulmonary infarction or fulminant necrosis of the sinus, palate, and orbit may result and dissemination is common. Infection with *Cryptococcus* sp is typically meningeal, and affected patients present subacutely with headache, lethargy, fever, and altered mentation (30).

Diagnosis

1. Identification of fungi in biopsy specimens or isolation from cultures of blood or cerebrospinal fluid (CSF) is required. Fungemia is rarely detected despite systemic infection.
2. Serologic testing for cryptococcal antigen in CSF or blood is a sensitive and specific detection method for this pathogen. India ink preparations of CSF demonstrate *Cryptococcus* sp in 50% of cases.

Therapy

1. Prolonged treatment with amphotericin B, a polyene antibiotic, is required for systemic mycoses. Resolution of infection is critically dependent on recovery from neutropenia.
2. Surgical debridement of fungal sinus infections is often recommended.
3. Withdrawal of immunosuppressive medications is beneficial.
4. Catheter-related fungemia requires removal of the infected venous access device.

Disseminated or Severe Viral Infections

Herpes virus infection in immunodeficient cancer patients is characteristically severe, prolonged, and prone to dissemination. The disease-related immunologic dysfunction and heavily immunosuppressive treatment of leukemia and lymphoma patients makes them most susceptible.

Reactivated herpes simplex produces an ulcerative mucositis of the mouth, oropharynx, and esophagus that impairs alimentation and promotes secondary bacterial or fungal infection (51). Viral dissemination, albeit rare, can lead to devastating interstitial pneumonitis, hepatitis, or encephalitis. Primary infection with varicella zoster, (chickenpox virus), causes a severe exanthem and potentially fatal pneumonitis in immunocompromised patients. Recrudescence of latent varicella infection in adults causes shingles; a painful, unilateral vesicular eruption with a dermatomal distribution. Cutaneous or visceral viral dissemination may follow.

Diagnosis

1. Herpes simplex mucositis may be difficult to differentiate from that due to chemotherapy, irradiation, or candidiasis. The cutaneous presentations of chickenpox and shingles are readily recognized.
2. Cytologic study of vesicle scrapings demonstrates multinucleated giant cells with intranuclear inclusions. Herpes is readily cultured from vesicle fluid or mucous membranes.

Prophylaxis

1. Administration of varicella immune globulin up to 72 hours after exposure decreases the likelihood and severity of primary varicella infection.
2. Oral or IV acyclovir, an antiviral drug, decreases the incidence of mucocutaneous herpes simplex infection in seropositive patients receiving antileukemic therapy (52).

Therapy

1. Varicella infections in immunocompromised hosts requires prompt treatment with IV acyclovir. A dose of 500 mg/m^2 every 8 hours is recommended.

2. Mucocutaneous herpes simplex lesions respond to treatment with acyclovir. A regimen of 250 mg/m² IV every 8 hours is suggested for inpatients. Oral acyclovir may be considered for outpatients.

Parasitic Infection in Cancer Patients

Opportunistic parasitic infection produces overwhelming disease in the immunosuppressed cancer patient. Affected patients typically have an underlying hematopoietic malignancy or have received substantial corticosteroid therapy. Pathogens involved may be protozoans (e.g., *Pneumocystis carinii, Toxoplasma gondii*, or nematodes such as *Strongyloides stercoralis*. The principal target organs of these three parasites are lung, CNS, and small intestine, respectively (59).

Pneumocystis pneumonia classically presents after tapering of corticosteroid therapy with symptoms of fever, cough, and dyspnea. The pneumonia appears radiographically as diffuse interstitial/alveolar infiltrates (40). Toxoplasmosis, which may be a primary or reactivated infection, causes encephalitis, intracerebral mass lesions, and meningitis; patients have neurologic deficits and signs of increased intracranial pressure. CT of the brain demonstrates enhancing mass lesions that are indistinguishable from metastatic disease or other infections. *Strongyloides* sp produces a hyperinfection syndrome with unchecked replication of the parasite in the small intestine. The filariform larvae of this parasite invade the intestinal mucosa and spread to lung or other organs. Since the parasite carries enteric flora, secondary bacterial and fungal pneumonia, meningitis, or septicemia develop.

Diagnosis

1. Detection of pneumocystis pneumonia in lung is accomplished by bronchoalveolar lavage and transbronchial biopsy, or open lung biopsy. Organisms are demonstrated by methenamine silver stains.
2. Diagnosis of toxoplasmosis may be confirmed serologically in many cases. However, absence of positive serology in the immunocompromised host does not rule out infection. In some cases, demonstration of the protozoan in tissue sections may be necessary.
3. *Strongyloides* sp is detected by examination of duodenal contents, stool, or fluids from other affected organs.

Therapy

1. Pneumocystis pneumonia is treated with trimethoprim (15-20 mg/kg/d) for 2 weeks. Pentamidine isethionate (4 mg/kg/d) is another effective, albeit more toxic, treatment.
2. Pyrimethamine and sulfadiazine combination therapy is indicated for CNS toxoplasmosis. The antibiotics are continued several weeks beyond clinical resolution of infection, and months of therapy may be required.
3. *Strongyloides* sp hyperinfection syndrome requires therapy with the antihelmintic thiabendazole. Antibiotics are administered for secondary bacterial infections.
4. Ongoing immunosuppressive treatments should be curtailed.

GASTROINTESTINAL EMERGENCIES

Esophageal Obstruction

Primary esophageal carcinoma is the principal cause of malignant esophageal obstruction. Rarely, obstruction may occur when the esophageal lumen is compressed by lymphoma or lung carcinoma in the surrounding mediastinum. Esophageal carcinoma produces a gradual obstruction and presents with progressive dysphagia, odynophagia, weight loss, and ultimately aspiration of oral secretions. Tracheoesophageal fistula formation occurs in more than 10% of cases, and is associated with unrelenting cough and recurrent pneumonia (10).

Diagnosis

1. Irregular narrowing of the esophagus by carcinoma is readily identified on esophogram. Endoscopic visualization and biopsy is indicated for definitive diagnosis.
2. Compressive lesions extrinsic to the esophagus are demonstrated by CT of the chest.
3. Rarely, hematemesis may complicate the course of advanced esophageal cancer and is secondary to a pinhole aortic perforation that communicates with the esophagus. This condition is largely irreversible and death from exsanguination follows within hours.

Therapy

1. Nutritional support with feeding jejunostomy or hyperalimentation is indicated for the minority of patients who have potentially curable disease.
2. Surgical resection of limited disease cures a small fraction of patients with esophageal carcinoma. Nonsurgical approaches using combined chemotherapy and radiation therapy are evolving and may yield equivalent results.
3. The dysphagia of far-advanced esophageal cancer may be palliated by radiation therapy; other alternatives include esophageal intubation, endoscopic laser therapy, or surgery in selected cases (20). A risk of these nonsurgical therapies is esophageal perforation.
4. Esophageal obstruction produced by extrinsic compression by other cancers requires radiation treatment or chemotherapy.
5. Tracheoesophageal fistula may be treated surgically in some instances; creation of an esophageal bypass superiorly and gastrostomy inferiorly is required.

Bowel Obstruction

Intestinal obstruction is observed in patients with advanced intra-abdominal cancer and is attended by fluid and electrolyte disturbances and the risk of bowel perforation. Obstruction may occur at one or multiple sites. The diffuse peritoneal carcinomatosis produced by ovarian, GI, or breast cancer is associated with multifocal small and large bowel obstruction. Small bowel obstructions due to carcinomatosis are often partial (58). Unifocal obstruction is typically produced by a localized but constrictive carcinoma of the colon.

In the absence of overt metastatic disease in patients with a prior history of cancer, benign causes of bowel obstruction (i.e., adhesions, hernia) should also be considered.

Diagnosis

1. Patients report anorexia, vomiting, abdominal bloating, cramping, and the inability to pass bowel movements.
2. Abdominal examination reveals distention, hyperactive bowel sounds, and diffuse tenderness.
3. Flat and upright abdominal films demonstrate multiple air fluid levels or dilated bowel loops.

4. Barium enema studies obtained when the patient has stabilized may disclose the site and cause of obstruction.

Therapy

1. Dehydration and electrolyte imbalance requires correction with IV fluids.
2. Decompressive nasogastric suction should be initiated.
3. Complete bowel obstructions are treated surgically when feasible. Partial small bowel obstructions may resolve with nasogastric suction.
4. Surgery is often inadvisable or inefficacious in patients with extensive abdominal carcinomatosis. Beneficial palliation of vomiting and colic may be achieved with narcotics, antiemetic and anticholinergic drugs, or celiac axis nerve blocks (6).

Bowel Perforation

Bowel perforation may result from erosion of tumor through the intestinal wall, or from rupture of the bowel—typically the thin walled cecum—proximal to a malignant obstruction. Perforation may also follow chemotherapy-induced necrosis of intestinal lymphoma. In addition, during a course of radiation therapy for lymphoma involving stomach or bowel, rapid tumor lysis can occur even with small overall doses or fractions, and perforation is an inherent risk of treatment. Uncontained perforation of the bowel leads to diffuse peritonitis, septicemia, and shock.

Diagnosis

1. Symptoms include generalized severe abdominal pain and fever. The patient's abdomen is rigid and diffusely tender, and bowel sounds are absent. However, patients on corticosteroids often have deceptively minimal findings.
2. Abdominal films demonstrate free air under the diaphragm(s).

Therapy

1. IV fluids and broad-spectrum antibiotics are administered.
2. Emergency exploratory laparotomy is mandatory after initial stabilization; this entails resection of necrotic or perforated bowel, abdominal irrigation, and abscess drainage. In many cases a diverting ileostomy is created and bowel reanastomosis is performed a later (58).

Gastrointestinal Hemorrhage

Acute, severe GI bleeding with consequent hypovolemia and shock is sometimes encountered in patients with active malignancy. Uncommonly, massive hemorrhage is an outcome of a fungating, necrotic tumor of the esophagus, stomach, or intestine. Quite often, other non-neoplastic conditions produce GI bleeding in cancer patients. Upper tract bleeding may result from peptic ulcer disease, drug-induced gastritis, diffuse mucosal hemorrhage secondary to thrombocytopenia, Mallory-Weiss tears, or varices related to the portal hypertension of liver metastases and myeloproliferative disorders. Lower GI bleeding may arise from colonic diverticula or angiodysplasia, as well as from various forms of colitis (45).

Diagnosis

1. Hematemesis suggests a lesion proximal to the ligament of Treitz, while bright-red rectal bleeding usually indicates a large bowel lesion.
2. Upper endoscopy is a highly accurate means of identifying sources of esophageal and gastroduodenal bleeding. Urgent colonoscopy is useful in the evaluation of lower GI bleeding, but may be difficult in the massively bleeding or unstable patient (26).
3. Nuclear bleeding scans (radiolabelled red cell or sulfur colloid studies) may be helpful in the localization of lower tract hemorrhage, particularly in conjunction with colonoscopy or selective angiography.
4. Angiography is the procedure of choice in individuals with ongoing massive colonic bleeding, particularly in the hemodynamically unstable patient (45).

Therapy

1. Initial management to achieve stabilization includes careful hemodynamic monitoring, volume repletion, and transfusion. Coagulopathy or significant thrombocytopenia should be corrected, if possible. Bleeding is often self-limited and resolves with conservative measures.
2. Bleeding gastroduodenal ulcers or gastritis requires therapy with H_2-receptor antagonists (cimetidine, ranitidine) and antacids. Endoscopic electrocautery or laser photocoagulation is an option for patients with a high risk of rebleeding or with stigmata of active hemorrhage.
3. Threatened variceal exsanguination has traditionally been treated with balloon tamponade (Sengstaken-Blakemore tube) and infusion of the splanchnic vasoconstrictor vasopressin. Endoscopic sclerotherapy of varices is subsequently performed; this may be used as initial therapy when bleeding is less massive (49).
4. Selective arteriographic infusion of vasopressin may provide temporary control of persistent colonic hemorrhage; it is usually followed by segmental resection of the identified site of bleeding.
5. Palliation of bleeding from far-advanced rectal cancer may be accomplished by transrectal resection or endoscopic fulguration of the tumor.

Ascites

Malignant ascites is a significant cause of distress for affected cancer patients. Ascites is commonly the result of peritoneal carcinomatosis complicating ovarian, breast, or GI carcinoma; the pathophysiology of ascites in this setting involves obstruction of subdiaphragmatic lymphatics and exudation of intraperitoneal fluid by tumor implants. Occasionally, malignant ascites results from the portal hypertension and hypoalbuminemia that complicates hepatic metastases, or from extensive intra-abdominal lymphoma. Symptoms of anorexia, nausea, abdominal discomfort, and distention predominate; massive ascites may hinder respiration and produce dyspnea.

Diagnosis

1. Physical examination reveals abdominal distention, shifting abdominal dullness, bulging flanks, and a palpable fluid wave.
2. Ascites is readily demonstrated by abdominal ultrasound, plain abdominal films, or CT.
3. In some instances, diagnostic paracentesis is indicated for cytologic confirmation of malignancy or to exclude benign causes.

Therapy

1. Malignant ascites is best managed by treatment of the underlying neoplasm.
2. In the absence of effective antineoplastic therapy, a therapeutic trial of bed rest and diuretics is sometimes beneficial. Spironolactone 100 to 200 mg/d is recommended.
3. Paracentesis of several liters provides immediate symptomatic relief, but fluid reaccumulation is rapid. Repeated paracentesis causes severe protein depletion and is associated with an increased complication rate.
4. In selected patients, peritoneovenous shunting is highly efficacious. However, a favorable outcome of shunting is expected only for patients without marked hyperbilirubinemia, cardiac or renal insufficiency, or bloody, loculated, or highly proteinaceous ascites (32).

UROLOGIC EMERGENCIES

Obstructive Uropathy

Progressive urethral or bilateral ureteral obstruction by tumor results in renal failure. Ureteral obstruction occurs with advanced genitourinary cancers, such as cervical, bladder, or prostate carcinoma; it may also complicate lymphoma or other retroperitoneal tumors. Urethral obstruction is observed in patients with prostate cancer or in the rare patient with urethral carcinoma. The renal failure of obstructive uropathy develops insidiously. Therefore, uropathy may be detected incidentally at a presymptomatic stage, or may present with unheralded florid uremia (22).

Diagnosis

1. Hydronephrosis due to ureteral obstruction is readily demonstrated by renal ultrasound. The etiology and site of obstruction may be further identified by CT scan of the abdomen and pelvis or by cystoscopy and retrograde pyelography.
2. Prostate enlargement producing urethral obstruction is obvious on rectal examination. Inability to catheterize the bladder suggests urethral obstruction.

Therapy

1. Percutaneous nephrostomy relieves ureteral obstruction, and may be followed by anterograde pyelography and ureteral stent placement.
2. Impassable urethral obstruction requires suprapubic cystostomy for bladder decompression.
3. Definitive surgery or radiation therapy of the obstructing tumor may allow restoration of urinary tract continuity. Some cases require permanent urinary tract diversion.

Hematuria

Severe hematuria may be observed in patients with advanced infiltrative bladder cancer, renal cell carcinoma, or, infrequently, with other pelvic neoplasms that invade the bladder. In addition, hemorrhagic cystitis, a complication of cyclophosphamde or ifosfamide chemotherapy, can cause massive vesical hemorrhage in cancer patients. Hemorrhagic cystitis is usually encountered in patients receiving very-high-dose cyclophosphamide (as in the bone marrow transplant setting) but is a limiting toxicity of even standard dose ifosfamide regimens (14). The urothelial toxicity of these agents is mediated by drug metabolites concentrated in the urine.

Diagnosis

1. Patients have suprapubic pain, symptoms of bladder irritability, urinary obstruction, and clot passage. Bleeding may be sufficient to require transfusion.
2. Urinary tract infection should be excluded by urinalysis and culture studies.

Therapy

1. Vigorous IV hydration promotes urinary dilution and lessens the likelihood of obstructing clots. Urethral catheterization is especially beneficial for patients with bladder outlet obstruction.
2. Bleeding from advanced bladder carcinoma is usually managed with transurethral resection and fulguration of the tumor. Other approaches include instillation of intravesical cauterizing agents, embolization of the vesicoarterial circulation, or external beam radiotherapy given in 200 to 500 cGy fractions for a total dose of 3 to 5 Gy (19).
3. Hemorrhagic cystitis related to chemotherapeutic agents is largely preventable by prophylactic hyperhydration and administration of the uroprotectant drug mesna (3).
4. Established chemotherapy-induced cystitis may require cystoscopy, intravesical instillation of formalin, and bladder irrigation, to arrest hemorrhage.
5. Palliation of hematuria in patients with unresectable renal cell carcinoma may be accomplished by transcatheter embolization of the renal artery.

RESPIRATORY EMERGENCIES

Pleural Effusions

Malignant pleural effusions are exudative processes usually related to the presence of tumor cell implants in the visceral or parietal pleura. Infrequently, these effusions develop because of impairment of pleural lymphatic drainage by mediastinal tumor. Metastatic breast and lung cancer and lymphoma account for more than 75% of malignant pleural effusions. A significant fraction of effusions are asymptomatic (50). However, large pleural effusions severely restrict ventilation and contribute to respiratory insufficiency in the cancer patient.

Diagnosis

1. Symptoms of dyspnea, unproductive cough, and dull chest discomfort are reported. Physical findings include decreased breath sounds and percussive dullness in the area of effusion.
2. Significant pleural effusions are visible on chest radiographs. Lateral decubitus films confirm free-flowing fluid.
3. Diagnostic thoracentesis is required to confirm a malignant etiology, and a large volume of fluid should be sent for cytologic analysis. Pleural fluid chemistries (lactate dehydrogenase [LDH], protein, glucose, pH levels), cultures, and blood cell count should also be obtained.
4. Cytologic confirmation of cancer by repeated thoracentesis is accomplished in 75% of cases (36). In the patient with negative cytology and an isolated *exudative* effusion (pleural fluid LDH greater than 200, a pleural

fluid-to-blood LDH ratio greater than 0.6, or a protein ratio greater than 0.5), pleural biopsy may be indicated.

Therapy

1. Large-volume thoracentesis provides immediate relief for the dyspneic patient. In the absence of effective antineoplastic treatment, fluid reaccumulates in a few days. Repeated thoracentesis is not recommended for long-term management because of the risk of infection, protein depletion, or other complications.
2. Persistently symptomatic patients are treated with tube thoracostomy and tetracycline pleurodesis. Lasting control of effusion is achieved in 70% to 85% of cases.
3. Pleural effusions due to lymphoma, breast cancer, and SCLC often respond to chemotherapy. Despite absence of a mediastinal mass, a short course of irradiation (200 cGy x 10) to the mediastinum is effective in relieving chylous effusion due to thoracic duct obstruction.

Upper Airway Obstruction

Tracheal or major bronchial obstruction by tumor may develop anywhere from the larynx to the carina. Recognition of this complication is extremely important because progressive obstruction culminates in fatal asphyxia. External compression of the trachea, carinae or major bronchi by mediastinal malignancies or contiguous nodal metastases is the usual obstructive mechanism. Neoplasms causing upper airway compromise include lymphoma, bronchogenic carcinomas, and, occasionally, thyroid or head and neck cancers. In many patients, tracheal obstruction represents progression of known disease. In others, it is the initial manifestation of their malignancy.

Diagnosis

1. Patients with upper airway obstruction experience severe respiratory distress. Inspiratory crowing, biphasic respiratory stridor, and wheezing are noted. Tachypnea and retraction of the suprasternal and intercostal spaces usually is observed.
2. The chest radiograph almost invariably reveals a superior mediastinal mass or widening, and deviation or compression of the tracheal air column. Although additional anatomic information is provided by CT or magnetic resonance imaging (MRI), patients are often too symptomatic to undergo these procedures.
3. Pathologic diagnosis usually can be made on the basis of sputum cytology, needle aspiration, biopsy of suspicious peripheral nodes, or ventilated bronchoscopy with brushings and biopsy. Patients with tracheal obstruction are poor candidates for general anesthesia. This precludes diagnostic mediastinoscopy, mediastinotomy, or thoracotomy.
4. In the acute situation, conclusive diagnostic procedures may need to be deferred in favor of expeditious treatment.

Therapy

1. Oxygen should be administered. A mixture of oxygen and helium has been used in these situations (57).
2. Corticosteroids are administered to reduce airway edema, although their benefit has not been rigorously proven.
3. The mainstay of treatment has been radiation therapy

to the area of obstruction. Initially, high fractions (300 to 400 cGy) are given, followed by more conventional (180 to 200 cGy) fractions. The total dose administered will vary with the clinical situation. Accelerated fractionation—using a field within a field—allows rapid focused delivery of dose in a short time and may be given twice daily.
4. Intraluminal tracheal obstruction may also be alleviated by bronchoscopic laser or photodynamic therapy. The success rate for this approach in selected patients exceeds 90% (38). In addition, intraluminal radioisotope therapy using high-dose-rate brachytherapy or ^{125}I seeds within bronchial catheters has been used to deliver rapid, short, intense courses of irradiation and has produced successful palliation.
5. If the tumor is chemoresponsive, as with lymphoma, germ cell tumors, and SCLC, chemotherapy should be strongly considered after initial radiotherapy.

CENTRAL NERVOUS SYSTEM EMERGENCIES

Increased Intracranial Pressure

Elevated intracranial pressure (ICP) may complicate primary or metastatic neoplasms of the CNS. The causative tumors are usually located in the brain parenchyma; leptomeningeal metastatic disease also produces increased ICP. As mass lesions within the brain expand, pressure in the semirigid cranial compartment rises. Eventually the autoregulatory mechanisms that preserve cerebral blood flow are defeated and CNS hypoxia develops. More importantly, brain shifts occur, leading to central and uncal tentorial herniation, and to life-threatening brain stem injury. Leptomeningeal metastases interfere with CSF absorption, and thus raise ICP by an indirect mechanism.

In adults, brain tumors are usually metastases from melanoma or lung, breast, kidney, or GI carcinomas, and are characteristically multiple. Primary brain tumors in adults are most commonly gliomas (astrocytoma, ependymoma, or oligodendroglioma) and are solitary lesions. Leptomeningeal metastases are most often associated wtih acute leukemias and lymphomas, but are also seen with solid tumors (especially lung and breast carcinoma) (42,43).

Diagnosis

1. Symptoms of increased ICP include headache, vomiting, visual blurring, diplopia, mental slowness, and unsteadiness. Headache is classically worse in the morning, exacerbated by straining or coughing, and relieved by vomiting.
2. Signs of increased ICP include papilledema (present in only 50% of cases), and nuchal rigidity in patients with meningeal disease. Focal neurologic deficits referrable to the tumor location also are observed. Herniation is accompanied by third cranial nerve palsy and systemic hypertension and bradycardia.
3. CT or MRI of the brain is urgently indicated. Frequent findings include enlarged ventricles, periventricular edema, white matter edema, mass effect, and contrast-enhancing mass lesions. Lumbar puncture is contraindicated in patients with intracranial neoplasms; removal of CSF may precipitate brain shifts and herniation.

4. Cytologic confirmation of suspected leptomeningeal metastases requires lumbar puncture. Repeated sampling may be needed to detect abnormal cells. A brain CT scan should be performed first for the reasons discussed above. MRI with gadolinium contrast appears to be a promising technique for visualization of leptomeningeal tumor.

Therapy

1. Corticosteroids are administered promptly to reduce peritumoral edema. Traditionally, dexamethasone 16 mg/d in divided doses is given and prompt improvement is observed almost invariably.
2. Patients with rapidly evolving herniation requiring intubation and mechanical hyperventilation to maintain the pulmonary arterial pressure of CO_2 around 30 mm Hg. The osmotic diuretic mannitol is administered 1.5 to 2.0 g/kg by bolus injection, repeated every 4 to 6 hours. Monitoring of ICP by ventriculostomy or subarachnoid screw may be required (42,43,48).
3. Radiation therapy is usually used for the patient with brain metastases. Treatment usually consists of 3,000 cGy delivered to the whole brain in ten fractions. Median survival is in the range of 4 to 6 months, with about 25% survival at 1 year.
4. Surgical exploration is indicated for patients with suspected primary brain tumors. Radiation therapy is administered after surgical excision, since residual disease is invariably present (43).
5. Chemotherapy does not have a role in the emergency treatment of intraparenchymal brain lesions. However, intrathecal chemotherapy (methotrexate, cytarabine) is the treatment of choice for leptomeningeal metastases. This is sometimes combined with radiation therapy to the whole brain or areas of bulk meningeal disease.

Spinal Cord Compression

Advanced spinal cord compression by tumor has devastating sequelae, including paraplegia, incontinence, and quadraplegia. Recognition of incipient cord compression is essential, because expeditious treatment at this stage prevents irreversible neurologic injury. Neoplastic cord compression is almost always secondary to extramedullary, extradural metastases (most frequently from breast, lung, prostate,

lymphoma, or kidney); primary spinal cord tumors are unusual. Commonly, compression develops by posterior expansion of vertebral metastatic disease or by extension of paraspinal metastases through the intervertebral foramina. In 70% of cases, the thoracic spinal cord is most often involved. The lumbar and cervical spine are involved in 20% and 10% of cases, respectively (13,17a).

Diagnosis

1. Almost all patients present initially with neck or back pain, which may be central or radicular. Leg weakness, numbness, and parasthesias follow; loss of sphincter control is a late event. Spine tenderness is common and neck flexion or straight leg raising may provoke radicular pain. The specific neurologic findings depend on the level of the cord lesion (Table 13-1).
2. Plain films of the spine frequently demonstrate associated vertebral blastic or lytic lesions. MRI of the spine is the procedure of choice for detection and localization of cord compression. Myelography may be employed if MRI techniques are not available. At the time of myelography, CSF should be obtained for cytology.

Therapy

1. Dexamethasone should be administered as described previously, to reduce cord edema.
2. Decompressive laminectomy is indicated initially if a tissue diagnosis is required, if the cord compression is in a previously irradiated area, or if neurologic deterioration occurs during radiation treatment. Laminectomy may also be considered for patients with radioresistant tumors, or those patients with rapid evolution of paraplegia.
3. Radiation therapy alone is used for patients with the following: (a) radiosensitive tumors; (b) lesions below the conus medullaris; (c) slow onset of compression; (d) medical contraindications to surgery; and (e) surgically unapproachable disease. Patients treated initially with decompressive laminectomy should also receive postoperative radiation therapy. Initially, high doses of radiation should be administered (400 cGy x 3). Subsequently, the daily fractional dose should be reduced to conventional levels and the total dose adjusted appropriately.

Table 13-1. Clinical Findings in Spinal Cord Compression

Sign/Deficit	Spinal Cord	Conus Medullaris	Cauda Equina
Weakness	Symmetrical, profound	Symmetrical, variable	Asymmetrical, may be mild
Deep tendon reflexes	Increased or absent	Increased knee, decreased ankle	Decreased
Plantar reflex	Extensor	Extensor	Plantar
Sensory	Symmetric sensory level	Symmetric saddle	Asymmetric, radicular
Sphincters	Late onset	Early onset	Spared possibily
Progression	Rapid	Variable	Variable

4. Chemotherapy may be considered for patients with chemosensitive tumors who can no longer benefit from surgical intervention or radiation therapy.

5. The results of treatment are best in patients who present with minimal or no neurologic impairment and poorest in those with established paraplegia. About 60% to 70% of patients in the former category are able to walk after treatment, compared to 5% in the latter group (13,25).

OPHTHALMOLOGIC EMERGENCIES

The orbit may be a site of distant metastases of carcinoma (usually lung or breast cancer) or of lymphoma or melanoma. Involvement of the orbit also occurs as a result of direct spread from tumors of the paranasal sinuses or nasopharynx. Primary orbital malignancies are rare in adults. Unchecked tumor growth in the orbit leads to retinal and optic nerve damage and blindness.

Diagnosis

1. Presenting symptoms are diplopia, orbital pain, loss of visual acuity, and proptosis (18).
2. Ophthalmologic examination reveals ocular displacement and ophthalmoplegia.
3. CT or MRI of the orbit provides definitive evidence of tumorous involvement.
·4. Isolated orbital lesions may require biopsy for definitive diagnosis.

Therapy

1. Emergent radiation therapy is indicated to preserve sight and relieve pain. Chemotherapy may be used for treatment of sensitive tumors such as lymphoma.
2. When radiotherapy is administered, shielding of the lens and anterior chamber is done, if feasible. However, late ocular effects of irradiation may not be a consideration in patients with metastatic disease and limited survival.

Recommended Reading

Excellent and relatively current overviews of the oncologic emergencies are presented in *Cancer: Principles and Practice of Oncology*, edited by DeVita *et al.* (16,19a,22,57a,58,61) nd in *Seminars in Oncology*, December 1989 (7a). The interested reader is also directed to the references cited in our chapter. These references were carefully selected because they either provide informative and comprehensive reviews of specific topics, or detail the most current and widely used approaches to the management of the oncologic emergencies.

REFERENCES

1. Ahmann, F.R. A reassessment of the clinical implications of the superior vena cava syndrome. J. Clin. Oncol. 2:961-969; 1984.
2. Allegretta, G.J.; Weisman, S.J.; Altman, A.J. Oncologic emergencies. I. Metabolic and space occupying consequences of cancer and cancer treatment. Pediat. Clin. N. Am. 32:601-611; 1985.
3. Antman, K.H.; Ryan, L.; Elias, A. Response to ifosfamide and mesna: 124 previously treated patients with metastatic or unresectable sarcoma. J. Clin. Oncol. 7:126-131; 1989.
4. Axelrod, L.; Ron, D. Insulin-like growth factor II and the riddle of tumor-induced hypoglycemia. New Engl. J. Med. 319:1477-1488; 1988.
5. Ayus, J.C.; Krothpalli, R.K.; Arieff, A.J. Treatment of symptomatic hyponatremia and its relation to brain damage: a prospective study. New Engl. J. Med. 317:1190-1194; 1987.
6. Baines, M.; Oliver, D.J.; Carter, R.L. Medical management of intestinal obstruction in patients with advanced malignant disease. Lancet 8462:990-993; 1985.
7. Bartlett, J. Familiar Quotations. Boston, MA: Little, Brown and Co.; 1980.
7a. Berger; N.A. (ed). Oncologic Emergencies. Semin. Oncol. 16: 461-587; 1989.
7b. Bilezileian, J.P. Management of acute hypercalcemia. N Engl J Med 326:1196-1203; 1992.
8. Bodey, G.P. Infection in cancer patients: a continuing association. Am. J. Med. 81(Suppl. 1A):11-26; 1986.
9. Bornemann, M.; Hill, S.C.; Kidd, G.S. Lactic acidosis in pheochromocytoma. Ann. Intern. Med. 105:880-882; 1986.
10. Boyce, H.W. Palliation of advanced esophageal cancer. Semin. Oncol. 11:186-195; 1987.
11. Broadus, A.E.; Mangin, M.; Ikeda, K.; *et al.* Humoral hypercalcemia of cancer: identification of a novel parathyroid hormone-like peptide. New Engl. J. Med. 319:556-563; 1988.
12. Brown, A.E. Neutropenia, fever, and infection. In: Brown, A.E.; Armstrong, D. (eds). Infectious complications of neoplastic disease. Stoneham, MA: Yorke Medical Books; 1985:19-34.
13. Bruckman, J.E.; Bloomer, W.D. Management of spinal cord compression. Semin. Oncol. 5:135-140; 1978.
14. Brugieres, L.; Hartmann, O.; Travagli, J.P. Hemorrhagic cystitis following high-dose chemotherapy and bone marrow transplantation in children with malignancies. J. Clin. Oncol. 7:194-199; 1989.
15. Bunin, N.J.; Kunkel, K.; Callihan, T.R. Cytoreductive procedures in the early management of cases of leukemia and hyperleukocytosis in children. Med. Pediat. Oncol. 11:232-235; 1987.
16. Bunn, P.A.; Ridgway, E.C. Paraneoplastic syndromes. In: DeVita, V.T.; Hellman, S.; Rosenberg, S.A., (eds). Cancer: Principles and Practice of Oncology, 3rd ed. Philadelphia, PA: J.B. Lippincott Co.;1989:1896-1940.
17. Burtis, W.J.; Wu, T.L.; Insogna, K.L.; *et al.* Humoral hypercalcemia of malignancy. Ann. Intern. Med. 108:454-457; 1988.
17a. Byrne, T.N. Spinal cord compression from epidural metastases. N Engl J Med 327:614-618; 1992.
18. Crawford, J.B. Tumors. In: Vaughan, D.; Asbury, T. (eds). General ophthalmology. Los Altos, CA: Lange Medical Publications; 1986:325-335.
19. Culp, D.A. Palliative treatment of the patient with disseminated carcinoma of the bladder. Semin. Oncol. 6:249-253; 1979.
19a. Delaney, T.E.; Oldfield, E.H. Spinal cord compression. In: DeVita, V.T.; Hellman, S.; Rosenberg, S.A., (eds). Cancer: Principles and Practice of Oncology, 3rd ed. Philadelphia, PA: J.B. Lippincott Co.;1989:1978-1985.
20. DeMeester, T.R.; Barlow, A.P. Surgery and current management for cancer of the esophagus and Cardia. Curr. Probl. Cancer. 12:243-328; 1988.
21. Doolittle, G.C.; Wurster, M.W.; Rosenfeld, C.S.; *et al.* Malignancy-induced acidosis. South. Med. J. 81:533-536; 1988.
22. Fair, W.R. Urologic emergencies. In: DeVita, V.T.; Hellman, S.; Rosenberg, S.A., (eds). Cancer: Principles and Practice of Oncology, 3rd ed. Philadelphia, PA: J.B. Lippincott Co.;1989:2016-2028.
23. Feinstein, D.J. Diagnosis and management of disseminated intravascular coagulation: the role of heparin therapy. Blood 60:284-287; 1987.
24. Glover, D.J.; Glick, J.H. Metabolic oncologic emergencies. CA 37:302-320; 1987.
25. Glover, D.J.; Glick, J.H. Managing oncologic emergencies involving structural dysfunction. CA. 35:238-251; 1985.
26. Gostout, C.J. Acute gastrointestinal bleeding—a common problem revisited. Mayo Clin. Proc. 63:596-604; 1988.
27. Hathorn, J.W.; Rubin, M.; Pizzo, P.A. Empirical antibiotic therapy in the febrile neutropenic cancer patient: clinical efficacy and the impact of monotherapy. Antimicro. Agents Chemother. 31:971-977; 1987.
28. Hoyle, C.F.; Swirsky, D.M.; Fredman, L.; *et al.* Beneficial effect of heparin in the management of patients with acute promyelocytic leukemia. Br. J. Hematol. 68:283-289; 1988.
29. Jackson, D.P. Management of thrombocytopenia. In: Colman, R.W.; Hirsh, J.; Marder, V.J. (eds). Hemostasis and thrombosis: basic principles and clinical practice. Philadelphia, PA: J.B. Lippincott Co.; 1987:530-536.
30. Joshi, J.H.; Schimpff, S.C. Infection in patients with acute leuke-

mia. In: Mandell, G.L.; Douglas, R.G.; Bennett, J.E. (eds). Principles and practice of infectious diseases. New York, NY: John Wiley and Sons; 1985:1649-1654.

31. Kaplan, E.L.; Arganini, M.; Kang, S.J. Diagnosis and treatment of hypoglycemic disorders. Surg. Clin. N.Am. 67:395-410; 1987.

32. Lacy, J.H.; Wieman, T.J.; Shively, E.H. Management of malignant ascites. Surg. Gynecol. Obstet. 159:397-412; 1984.

33. Lichtman, M.A.; Rowe, J.M. Hyperleukocytic leukemias: rheological, clinical and therapeutic considerations. Blood 60:279-283; 1982.

34. List, A.F.; Hainsworth, J.D.; Davis, B.W.; et al. The syndrome of inappropriate secretion of antidiuretic hormone in small cell lung cancer. J. Clin. Oncol. 4:1191-1198; 1986.

35. Marder; V.J.; Martin, S.E.; Francis, C.W.; et al. Consumptive thrombohemorrhagic disorders. In: Colman, R.W.; Hirsh, J.; Marder, V.J.; Salzman, E.W. (eds). Hemostasis and thrombosis: basic principles and clinical practice. Philadelphia, PA: J.B. Lippincott, Co.; 1987:975-1015.

36. McKenna, R.J.; Khalil-Ali, M.; Ewer, M.J.; et al. Pleural and pericardial effusions in cancer patients. Curr. Probl. Cancer. 9:5-23; 1985.

37. Mundy, G.R.; Ibbotson, K.J.; D'Souza, S.M.; et al. The hypercalcemia of cancer: clinical implications and pathogenic mechanisms. New Engl. J. Med. 310:1718-1726; 1984.

38. Nussbaum, M.; Ghazi, A. Endoscopic applications of laser therapy. Surg. Annu. 18:225-241; 1986.

39. Perez-Soler, R.; McLaughlin, P.; Velasquez, W.S.; et al. Clinical features and results of management of superior vena cava syndrome secondary to lymphoma. J. Clin. Oncol. 2:260-266; 1984.

40. Peters, S.G.; Prakash, U.B.S. Pneumocystis carinii pneumonia. Am. J. Med. 82:73-77; 1987.

41. Peterson, B.A.; Levine, E.G. Uncommon subtypes of acute non-lymphocytic leukemia: clinical features and management of F.A.B. M5, M6, and M7. Semin. Oncol. 14:425-434; 1987.

42. Plum, F.; Posner, J.B. The diagnosis of stupor and coma, 3rd ed. Philadelphia, PA: F.A. Davis Co.; 1982.

43. Posner, J.B. Management of central nervous system metastases. Semin. Oncol. 4:81-91; 1977.

44. Posner, M.R.; Cohen, G.I.; Skarin, A.T. Pericardial disease in patients with cancer: the differentiation of malignant from idiopathic and radiation induced pericarditis. Am. J. Med. 71:407-413; 1986.

45. Potter, G.D.; Sellin, J.H. Lower gastrointestinal bleeding. Gastroent. Clin. N. Am. 17:341-356; 1988.

46. Ralston, S.H.; Gardner, M.D.; Dryburgh, F.J.; et al. Comparison of aminohydroxypropylidene diphosphonate, mithramycin and corticosteroids/calcitonin in treatment of cancer-associated hypercalcemia. Lancet 8461:907-909; 1985.

47. Raptopoulos, V. Computed tomography of the superior vena cava syndrome. C.R.C. Crit. Rev. Diag. Imag. 25:373-429; 1986.

48. Richter, M.P.; Coia, L.R. Palliative radiation therapy. Semin. Oncol. 12:375-383; 1987.

49. Rikkers, L.F. Variceal hemorrhage. Gastroent. Clin. N. Am. 17:289-302; 1988.

50. Ruckdeschel, J.C. Management of malignant pleural effusion: an overview. Semin. Oncol. 15(Suppl. 3):24-28; 1988.

51. Saral, R. Management of mucocutaneous herpes simplex virus infection in immunocompromised patients. Am. J. Med. 85(2A):59-60; 1988.

52. Saral, R. Acyclovir prophylaxis against herpes simplex virus infection in patients with leukemia. Ann. Intern. Med. 99:773-776; 1983.

53. Sculier, J.P.; Feld, R. Superior vena cava syndrome: recommendations for management. Cancer Treat. Rev. 12:209-218; 1985.

54. Shepherd, F.A.; Ginsberg, J.S.; Evans, W.K.; et al. Tetracycline sclerosis in the management of malignant pericardial effusion. J. Clin. Oncol. 3:1678-1682; 1985.

55. Thaler, M.; Pastakia, B.; Shawker, T.H. Hepatic candidiasis in cancer patients: the evolving picture of the syndrome. Ann. Intern. Med. 108:88-100; 1988.

56. Tsokos, G.C.; Balow, J.E.; Spiegel, R.J. Renal and metabolic complications of undifferentiated and lymphoblastic lymphomas. Medicine. 60:218-229; 1981.

57. Vanderspek, A.F.; Spargo, P.M.; Norton, M.L. The physics of lasers and implications for their use during airway surgery. Br. J. Anaesth. 60:709-729; 1988.

57a. Warrell, R.P., Bockman, R.S. Metabolic Emergencies. In: DeVita, V.T.; Hellman, S.; Rosenberg, S.A., (eds). Cancer: Principles and Practice of Oncology, 3rd ed. Philadelphia, PA: J.B. Lippincott Co.;1989:1986-2002.

57b. Warrell, RP; Murphy, WK; Schulman, P; O'Dwyer, PJ; Heller, G. A randomized double-blind study of gallium nitrate compared with etidronate for acute control of cancer-related hypercalcemia. J Clin Oncol. 9: 1467-1475; 1991.

58. Wilson, R.E. Surgical emergencies. In: DeVita, V.T.; Hellman, S.; Rosenberg, S.A., (eds). Cancer: Principles and Practice of Oncology, 3rd ed. Philadelphia, PA: J.B. Lippincott Co.;1989:2003-2015.

60. Wong, B. Parasitic diseases in immunocompromised hosts. Am. J. Med. 82:479-486; 1984.

61. Yahalom, J. Superior vena cava syndrome. In: DeVita, V.T.; Hellman, S.; Rosenberg, S.A., (eds). Cancer: Principles and Practice of Oncology, 3rd ed. Philadelphia, PA: J.B. Lippincott Co.;1989:1971-1977.

Michael H. Henrichs, Ph.D., Clinical Psychology

Chapter 14

PRINCIPLES OF PSYCHOSOCIAL ONCOLOGY

Greatness, after all, in spite of its name, appears to be not so much a certain size as a certain quality in human lives. It may be present in lives whose range is very small.

Phillips Brooks (15a)

PERSPECTIVE

The Psychosocial Interaction of Patients, Cancer, and Treaters

Cancer, in our society, in our schools and in our families, is still identified as a threatening, insidious and morbid process in the public's mind. Hardly a day goes by without reports (71) contributing to the impression that the potential for cancer is all about us—in the air we breathe, in the food we eat, the sexual relationships we pursue, and in the materials with which we work. In addition, statistics state that the disease, in its many forms, is the second most common cause of death in our society and that one out of four persons alive today will have cancer at some time in his or her lifetime. Is it any wonder that fear is generated by the latest agents announced as carcinogenic or, on the other hand, that hope springs from the latest announcement about a new anticancer agent or research finding? The long-awaited answer to the prevention or cure of this disease has yet to appear.

The physician and medical student must have an understanding of the emotional impact of the disease on the public at large and how it might influence the patient's behavior, work, and quality of life. However, physicians and other professionals are not immune from the emotional elements and the psychologically metastatic and malignant nature of cancer (37). On first impression, the pursuit of oncology and cancer treatment is not a glamorous profession (59).

This chapter addresses the principal psychosocial issues that arise in work with the cancer patient and traces the predominant psychosocial reactions and interactions of patients, families, and health care professionals, as the patient's cancer is diagnosed and treated, and the outcome is determined (Fig. 14-1). The prevalence of courage and hope among these patients, family members, and treaters is apparent as these topics are addressed.

Physicians are well aware of the impact that research has made on medical practice during the 20th century. These advances in the breadth and depth of medical information are staggering, and have led to the development of numerous specialties, including oncology. The concepts of General System Theory, such as Von Bertalanffy (73) introduced in 1950, help to cope with the proliferation of new knowledge and the theoretic and practical integration it requires. In this conceptual approach, an individual's internal as well external

environment can be understood as a hierarchy of open-ended systems, each having its own characteristics, self-regulating controls, and relationships with each other.

There have been many applications of these General System Theory concepts since the 1950s; however, for our purpose, a primary implication is to perceive and understand the cancer patient as an integrated and complex human being with biologic, psychologic, social, and cultural systems of levels or organization. A human is constantly functioning at many system levels and maintaining homeostasis internally, such as in cell growth, electrolyte balance, and thinking, and externally in such roles as that of parent, breadwinner, and teacher. Cancer, as any disease, tends to upset this homeostasis and such a disruption may reverberate through many systems.

The brain-mind system is the most integrated system functioning directly under the individual's control. Thus, the individual's awareness of how the body and bodily functions cope with cancer and its treatments may influence that person's thoughts, feelings, and actions. The brain-mind activities may in turn have specific effects on the functioning of the bodily systems. For example, a patient who has experienced vomiting in relation to receiving chemotherapy might become nauseated and vomit when thinking about the next treatment. However, this psychologic chain reaction may be successfully broken if it can be recognized as an interacting system. Patients and physicians will be better served if this systematic approach is kept in mind. It is a challenge for the attending physician to identify the several systems involved in the patient's disease. It is important, for example, for the physician to address the question, "How well are the patient, significant others, and the treatment-team members, including myself, functioning given this patient's cancer?"

This question and the concepts and processes that emerge comprise the essence of psychosocial oncology. Thus, medical and mental health professions of all disciplines and the general public are aggressively examining the process of how cancer affects people, not just physically, but emotionally and cognitively. Clinical, educational, and investigative projects on the psychosocial aspects of acquired immune deficiency

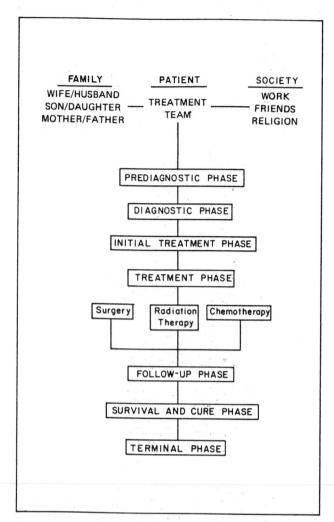

FAMILY	PATIENT	SOCIETY
WIFE/HUSBAND	TREATMENT	WORK
SON/DAUGHTER	TEAM	FRIENDS
MOTHER/FATHER		RELIGION

PREDIAGNOSTIC PHASE

DIAGNOSTIC PHASE

INITIAL TREATMENT PHASE

TREATMENT PHASE

Surgery   Radiation Therapy   Chemotherapy

FOLLOW-UP PHASE

SURVIVAL AND CURE PHASE

TERMINAL PHASE

Fig. 14-1. Schematic representation of a systematic approach used in identifying the several systems and groups involved in a cancer patient's movement through the stages of the disease. The interactions and relationships depicted here can be valuable to the physician and the student in attempts to give sound psychosocial help to the patient.

syndrome (AIDS), children with cancer, social support, children of adult cancer patients (35), siblings, quality of life (26) and bereavement (36) have begun to develop. Psychosocial oncology interests have focused less on predicting who will develop or survive cancer (20) and more on cancer prevention interventions for smoking cessation, AIDS education, and reducing harmful health practices. Likewise, the focus has included social systems, which involve the patient, family, work, friends, religion, schools, and community. Significantly, it has been recognized that the emotional impact of cancer reaches far beyond the patient alone. The needs and functioning of cancer survivors and bereaved family members of less fortunate patients who have died have begun to be addressed. It is noteworthy that professional journals in the health disciplines have published special series on psychosocial oncology during the past five years (1-3,5-7,9). Although the field is young, the movement has finally begun to be perceived as important for all patients, treaters, and society. These recent foci will become evident as we proceed in this discussion.

PATIENT AND FAMILY

An application of the General Systems Theory to oncology is to study the patient in the context of the family system. In this way, the behavior and experiences of any member of the family are recognized to have an effect and influence upon all the other members. For instance, the impact of a parent's cancer on the other family members can be either disastrous or manageable, depending upon the nature of the family and support that physicians, other professionals, and society at large provide (11). Although this idea of the influence of cancer on a family may appear to be a simple and common sense notion, all too often it is forgotten. Physicians and other treatment team members frequently assume that someone else is helping the family cope with the cancer. Furthermore, if family issues are not recognized and addressed, family members' behavior can interfere with the patient's treatment compliance.

What the physician can do to help the patient and the family will be discussed in the context of the phases of treatment. However, several general ideas are important whenever the patient or family are seen. Be aware of the possible impact of the cancer on the family and their anticipated or expressed reactions to the cancer diagnosis and its treatments (46). If one meets with the family, encourage open communication of thoughts and feelings about cancer (13). It is especially important to explain to children who have cancer and children whose parent has cancer what is happening to provide them with as much security and stability as possible and with enough information to allow them to know what to expect. And finally, it is important to remember that the self-esteem of the patient and other family members is frequently tied to the roles he or she has performed previous to the cancer. For example, the sexual relationship of patient and significant other may be affected by the disease and its treatment (78). These problems can and should be addressed as they emerge or even during inquiry (77). Education and support groups for children and parents as well as bereaved families have been recently developed. Such group interventions allow all family members to realize their experience and reactions are not abnormal, nor are they alone in their pain (35,36).

PATIENT AND SOCIETY

A cancer patient, like each of us, lives in a social system that extends beyond the family. The specific constellation of this system will vary in makeup and complexity according to the opportunity, interest, beliefs, and needs of the individual patient. The concepts of social support (23), networking, community and volunteer involvement, and communications have been activated into interventions for cancer patient families (17,25,43). In addition to family, the more common and significant elements of this network include work, friendships, and religion. These three areas frequently emerge as sources of both support and concern.

Work: A patient's self-image and sense of competence is often closely tied to career and daily work experiences. The life-threatening nature of cancer and treatment effects on everyday functioning can jeopardize the important avenue of satisfaction and livelihood that work provides for the patient. The cancer patient may assume that co-workers and supervisor do not want to work with someone who has or has had cancer. However, industry and life insurance companies are learning that cancer patients are good employees and have less absenteeism than the average, noncancer patient (76).

As might be expected, blue collar or manual labor employees have greater difficulty meeting the physical demands of their work than does the person with an office or desk job. Patients' perceptions of the interactions of their physical condition and their job will vary considerably, as is illustrated in these two brief descriptions. One middle-aged woman being treated for cancer described her bank teller job as a supportive endeavor that kept her mind focused on daily living and enabled her to continue important relationships with colleagues. In stark contrast, in his interview a middle-aged salesman revealed a serious concern that his company would find out he had cancer and proceed to replace him with a younger, healthier individual.

The physician should anticipate that the patient's employers will have questions and will display a reluctance to keep such a patient working, and a preference to avoid criticism by putting him on disability or sick leave. Although employer support is increasing (21), one should not assume that employers and co-workers will always be supportive of the patient. In this light, communication with the patient's employer, with the patient's consent, as well as the completion of health insurance forms, are responsibilities that the physician should think through carefully with the patient.

The phenomena of a patient returning to work and co-workers becoming aware that their colleague has cancer present a real challenge for all parties in the patient's and family's lives. It is not unusual for co-worker, friends, congregation members, children's classmates and teachers and spouse's acquaintances to suddenly change their normal, friendly, participatory behavior. Society as a whole and each of its members struggles with the dilemma of whether or not to initiate conversations and/or to continue relationships with the patient. In part this reluctance is due to the fear of upsetting or harming the patient or loved ones by bringing up a painful or seemingly morbid topic that might reduce the patient or loved one to tears. However, cancer in our midst reminds each of us of our own mortality and frailty, and thus it can be difficult to discuss (68). As a result of this nearly automatic isolating phenomenon, ironically it is often the patient or family member who must initiate communication or recontact with others. Thus, there is an additional burden of taking care of others who are afraid to address the patient's welfare and health with him or her on their own initiative.

Friends: The presence of friends in a patient's life can make a considerable difference in adjustment. It is not unusual to hear patients describe the sharing of their thoughts and feelings about their condition with a close friend whom they can trust and who will understand and accept them. On the other hand, caring for a friend can often provide an all-important focus for the cancer patient. We recall one elderly man who described how important it was for him and his wife to "check in on" and help a more elderly neighbor on a daily basis. Cancer patients often overcome the feelings of being ineffective, impotent, or helpless by discovering that *they* can continue to *help others.* This phenomenon is repeatedly demonstrated in education and support groups in which cancer patient families provide information and social support for each other (35).

Religion: Religious faith or beliefs enable some cancer patients to cope with their crisis and tolerate the consequences of their disease. The beliefs and affiliations provided by one's religion and philosophy of life can be a benefit as the patient copes with the initial crisis of cancer, as well as the long, tedious course of treatment and the illness itself.

However, a patient's religious beliefs are not necessarily a source of support. Some patients will harbor the belief that they deserve to have cancer because of a past wrongdoing. It should be readily apparent that such a belief of guilt or self-blame may consciously or unconsciously undermine treatment plans and the will to live (16,45). Or patients will ask, "Why me?" (30). They have lived a good life and have done what was expected of them. How could a just God allow this to happen to them? An awareness of a patient's religious beliefs and personal values will inform the treatment team members to better serve the holistic needs in the course of the illness (31,81).

TREATMENT TEAM

It is important for the physician to keep in mind that he or she is not alone in providing medical care and psychosocial support for the cancer patient and family. Other professionals, including nurses, social workers, psychologists, radiation technicians, receptionists, and aides, often spend more time with the patient than does the physician. Hence, these members can serve as supports as well as sources of information regarding the patient's and family's psychosocial problems and needs (70). These professionals will often look to the physician or to each other for guidance and support when problems arise (15).

In this context, treatment teams and cancer centers are fostering the use of support groups (67), group psychotherapy (33), educational groups (39,69), and dyadic peer support to accommodate the psychosocial needs of the patient. Professionals, paraprofessionals and volunteers from the community, including former or current patients, are demonstrating their willingness and effectiveness in helping patients and family members become better informed, more comfortable, and readier to comply with necessary treatment. In this manner, the truly collaborative nature of the multidisciplinary treatment *team* concept has emerged!

Treatment team members need to be aware of the signs and symptoms of cognitive and emotional difficulties that may develop in the course of the cancer and its very potent treatments. Two examples illustrate the purpose of this multidisciplinary awareness in cancer treatment. The radiation technician who had been treating a 55-year-old man on a daily basis noticed his emotional shift to a more depressive mood during the third week of radiation therapy. However, in an examination and interview with his primary physician during this same period, the man appeared to be as bright and cheerful as ever. Because of the close communication among the team members, the physician was alerted to this man's underlying depressed outlook by the technician. When the physician inquired about these feelings, the patient was able to set aside his need to protect the doctor from his problems. Patients often do not want to burden their physicians with personal problems. The patient—whose home was 150 miles away—was feeling sad and isolated from his wife (29). Having his wife join him for the remainder of his treatment greatly improved his outlook. Some severe emotional reactions of the patient or family members require special treatment, consultation, and future treatment planning. Such severe reactions may be first seen as a precipitant of the cancer or treatment or may be another regression in a pre-existing psychiatric disorder (27,38).

The second illustration relates to psychosocial effects brought about by shifts in the cognitive functioning of a patient. Research (64,82) has focused on the nervous system toxicity of chemotherapeutic agents and their effect on cognition, including memory, orientation, and judgment. It is not unusual for a family member to inform a patient's nurse that "He's been forgetting things lately," or "Her personality is different." Such information should be communicated to the physician so that its significance can be evaluated. Does it indicate evidence of a slight shift in the adjustment of an already limited elderly person, or is this a disease or treatment (iatrogenic) effect that requires an adjustment in treatment to maximize the patient's coping and quality of life (26)?

A final important consideration in discussing the treatment team is that the professionals might best consider the patient and the family as members of the treatment team, that is, as allies and collaborators in the struggle against cancer and in the decisions regarding and the support of the patient. Families report that when the physician and treatment team members share information, decision-making, and their emotional reactions with the patient and family trust and compliance is enhanced (37). One caution to consider is that the patient and the family members pay close attention to the words and the tone of delivery when treatment team members share information. Family members and patients report being influenced by the content and the affect of these communications which in some situations are felt to be helpful and in other circumstances unhelpful (70). Overall, however, family members appreciate being informed and included in these decisive conversations. The reader is encouraged to be mindful of these general psychosocial considerations as the various phases of cancer treatment are presented herein.

PREDIAGNOSTIC STAGE

The widespread concern and knowledge about the danger signs of cancer (71) create a number of psychologic reactions in those who think they might have the disease (44). Some of these individuals assume that any bodily symptom is an indication of the disease and seek repeated assurance from their physician that they do not have cancer. At the other extreme, there are individuals who either deny the presence of disease or delay seeking diagnosis because they fear the consequences of cancer. Such fear or fatalism may result from a prior unfavorable family experience with cancer, from advanced age with little interest in living longer, from anticipated prohibitive financial costs, or from other antecedent life or health problems that inhibit focusing on signs of the disease. These latter individuals either avoid the physician or try to conceal the symptoms or signs of cancer when they come for examinations such as their "reassuring" routine check-up or required insurance physical. Suffice it to say that the notion of contracting cancer is a very anxiety-provoking experience (44).

The physician might not perceive the full significance of the initial evidence of cancer or might minimize the possibility and therefore delay extensive testing. This is particularly possible when the patient complains constantly, exaggerates discomforts, or is a young and/or otherwise apparently healthy individual. The psychologically sensitive physician should be alert to, but not phobic about, the possibility of unconsciously conspiring with the patient to delay diagnosis.

If the patient is particularly concerned about the presence of cancer and the concern is unfounded, it is important for the physician to reassure the patient of the absence of the disease. Likewise, when the physician suspects a malignancy and refers the patient to a specialist for further study, the patient should be told the reasons for the referral and informed of the possible diagnosis. However, once the patient has been informed of the possibility of cancer, there should be as little delay as possible in either confirming or disproving the diagnosis.

DIAGNOSTIC PHASE

The initial reaction to being told, "you have a tumor, a mass or an unusual growth," is usually, "Does that mean I have cancer?" Most patients will ask and will want to know the diagnosis. They should be told the diagnosis and its consequences in terms that they are not only intellectually but emotionally prepared to understand (70). Even someone well-educated or of high intelligence might find it very difficult emotionally to tolerate or comprehend a detailed dissertation of the disease on first hearing the diagnosis. Patients will vary greatly in how much, how soon, and how often they want to discuss their diagnosis and its potential effects on the quality and strength of their life. This means that the physician should begin with a general statement. The amount of subsequent detail and the timing of the more specific ancillary statements should be related to the patient's responses (56). Thus, the physician should follow rather than lead the patient in exploring what the diagnosis may mean.

After being told their diagnosis, some patients will ask for the information again within hours or days, as if they had never been told. In such cases, one can assume that the patient wants to know, but that the meaning of the diagnosis is more than can be tolerated emotionally. Some patients will have specific requests regarding when and what members of their families are to be told. Some families will want the physician to discuss the diagnosis with the family first and to give them the option of telling the patient. This is especially true when the patient is a child (7,46). The emancipated youth or the elderly might insist that loved ones not be told. The physician must abide by the patient's wishes in regard to who is told; however, the physician may question and try to change the patient's decision. As mentioned earlier, children and other family members are often more secure knowing the truth than sensing something is amiss. At this initial phase of collaboration with the patient and family, the process of informed consent for sharing information, treatment regimen, and research protocols is essential (62). Therefore, it is also important that the spoken and written words are understood and readable for the patient (25).

The initial reaction to the diagnosis is predominantly one of disbelief. Feelings of shock and thoughts that it cannot be cancer may come and go or may persist for days (4). Because of this reaction, the physician should schedule a second visit within several days, after first telling the patient the diagnosis. This allows the patient time to collect herself or himself and to think through the various concerns. Such a diagnostic follow-up visit also gives the patient an opportunity to talk to others or to bring someone along to share in the more detailed discussion that ensues. Some physicians have tape recorded these patient-physician discussions and given the tape to the patient to listen to later when one can better focus on the information provided (11). If the final diagnosis is that of a benign tumor or some other noncancerous process, the patient and family might require repeated reassurance that a malignant disease is not present.

Once the need for treatment has been established, the significance of diagnosis is further confirmed by the physician's detailing the reasons for the specific treatment to be undertaken. Again, the patient should be given an opportunity to question and to discuss the facts as well as any fantasies and fears concerning the disease and treatment.

INITIAL TREATMENT PHASE

Initial cancer treatment is usually done by one or more specialists or clinics. This may mean that the primary physician will no longer be the treating physician. However, it is important for there to be someone who will continue to see the patient through and after any specialized treatment course. When possible, the primary physician should provide this continuity.

The first treatment course is anticipated with great anxiety, especially if it is surgical. When surgery is the treatment, the patient usually is told that the extent of the involvement of the cancer cannot be ascertained until the surgeon has a chance to observe directly and until further biopsies can be done. Whether the therapy is surgery, chemotherapy, or irradiation, there is great hope that the first treatment will be the only treatment and that cure will be the outcome. No matter how favorable the prognosis, some patients will view the outcome pessimistically. This group includes those who have a history of having anticipated the worst in other important situations. An attitude of pessimism protects them from being disappointed if the outcome is not favorable. If they do not understand the reason for it, such a negative attitude may anger those who are providing the treatment.

Surgery: Although it potentially causes the greatest amount of immediate discomfort and disability, surgery is tolerated best because most patients regard cutting and removing tissue as more permanent and complete than treatment by chemicals or irradiation. While the patient is occupied with the life-threatening possibilities of the cancer, the loss of sight, voice, sexual attractiveness (51), or reproductive potential is initially of secondary importance. The spouse, children, family, and close friends are frequently more immediately disturbed by the potential change in appearance or functioning than is the patient. These same individuals can be in the best position to support the patient (50). Exceptions to the above include individuals to whom physical appearance is important, either because of fantasies about their appearance, or the actual importance of such attributes in maintaining their valued relationships (68). These patients will often postpone surgery or try to find nonsurgical options. If acceptable alternatives are not available and surgery is performed, a postoperative depressive reaction may occur (60).

In addition, all losses of a body part (68) or bodily functioning, or a major change in body image will lead to a grief reaction. This is the "disembodied mind's" way of updating itself and adapting to the new reality. Such reactions are usually self-limited and require no specific psychologic intervention beyond an understanding, supportive attitude. At times, patients are reluctant to discuss their fears, anger, and feelings of hopelessness with the treating physician. Instead they tell a nurse, receptionist, medical student, or family member, explaining, "I know the doctor is busy." Hence, as discussed earlier, it is important to encourage staff and family members to keep the physician informed of the patient's concerns.

Radiation therapy: In its several therapeutic forms, radiation therapy is surrounded with the greatest mystery and fantasy because there is nothing to see, hear, or feel that indicates what is happening during the treatment. To help children who receive radiation therapy and children of adult patients address the mystery and the sometimes frightening nature of the machine, desensitizing demonstrations and tours of the radiation unit have been found most helpful. In most cases, radiation is given in small daily doses over an extended period of weeks. The patient and the treatment plan are examined weekly. The greatest psychologic distress usually is experienced at the beginning of the treatment course, during treatment when changes in therapy are required because of side reactions or extensions of disease, and at the end of treatment when the results of therapy are still unknown.

One of the most stressful aspects of radiation therapy is the waiting room experience. Here the patient faces other patients of varying ages, stages of disease, and degrees of disability. In general, the idea of having a separate waiting area for the sickest patients, and scheduling them at the beginning and end of the day when the facility is least congested, is desirable. The sensitivity of the nursing and administrative staff to the comfort and needs of waiting patients and family members is important to morale (58).

Chemotherapy: The waiting room experience also applies to the chemotherapy clinic setting. A wide array of drugs is involved in chemotherapy, some of which are given as the first treatment or at the initial stage of the disease. They may be used alone, in varying combinations, or with radiation therapy and/or surgery. Some of the drugs produce neurological (82) or gastrointestinal symptoms during or after administration. Occasionally, as a result of a symptom that has occurred as a side reaction to an earlier dose of medication, the patient will reexperience the symptom, such as nausea or vomiting, before the drug is given at a later time. This anticipation of discomfort may appear before the patient reaches the clinic or when the nurse starts to set up for treatment. Informing the patient of possible side reactions before the first treatment will be reassuring to most, although it will cause some to become anxious. If told briefly beforehand of the possible reactions to the drugs, and if assured that such reactions can be controlled, the likelihood of the patient becoming upset and the symptoms being created or magnified is minimized. Behavior and other therapeutic interventions have met with considerable success in helping the patient control nausea and vomiting (48). Such approaches contribute to better treatment compliance (57).

FOLLOW-UP PHASE

The patient might not have a primary physician to return to for general care or immediate follow-up at the end of the first treatment course. Indeed, the patient may never have had a primary physician or, after seeing one or more specialists over the course of the diagnostic work-up and treatment, might have to return to a physician seen only once before, or for a short period of time. Thus, it is important for the specialist—or whomever is responsible for the specific course of treatment—to ensure that the patient is to be followed by a physician who is interested in and knowledgeable about the patient's follow-up needs.

Previously, if a patient lived for 5 years without a recurrence, it was assumed that there was a cure. It is now recognized that a period of 8 to 10 years might be more realistic for predicting long-term survival or normal life expectancy. Thus, the waiting period has been extended. The follow-up physician, not necessarily an oncologist, must be interested and sensitive to physical changes and to the psychologic coping required during such an extended period.

The patient's physician also needs to know the possible long-term effects of cancer therapies the patient has received. The chance of a second cancer, the delayed accumulated effects of radiotherapy on the spinal cord, lung, blood vessels, bowel, and other systems, and the treatment effects of antimetabolites on growth centers, brain (64), and reproductive cells, are among the possible long-term complications. With many of the therapies used in combination— most of which are still experimental—it is important for the physician to keep abreast of the current literature on the long-term effects of the treatment.

RECURRENCE AND RETREATMENT PHASE

The importance of having a regular, scheduled time for a check-up is obvious. The first sign or symptom suggesting a recurrence may be difficult to perceive or, once so perceived, may be psychologically difficult for the patient to acknowledge and act upon. The possibility of a recurrence stirs up fantasies about physical or psychologic inadequacies, the relative importance of previous treatment and those providing the treatment, and the strength or virulence of the disease. Thus, for a number of reasons, there usually is a delay in returning for evaluation. Such a delay can be spotted or safeguarded against if the physician has a system of scheduling regular, periodic visits, and a follow-through system for all canceled or unkept appointments. Routine follow-up requirements of investigative treatment programs reduce the anxiety of the posttreatment visits. In these instances, the patient is informed of the follow-up requirements before committing to the treatment program.

The patient and family members may go through a series of reactions when evidence of a disease recurrence appears. Shock and disbelief might again be the initial reaction, and as with the initial treatment, might be followed by feelings of anger, guilt, or depression. These are usually phasic reactions related to the recognition, tolerance, and mastery of the realization that further treatment is necessary. The physician should be prepared for these reactions from the patient and family (75). If such are not voiced, the physician might indicate the possibility of experiencing these reactions. Reactions should be anticipated such as feeling inadequately treated and wondering if there is any treatment that will better protect them or if their bodies can resist or fight the new evidence of disease (8).

With disease recurrence, the inevitable thought is that cure is now less likely than once expected. This is a difficult time during which both physician and patient have to face reality together. Sometimes it is difficult to know or to predict what the immediate future may hold for the patient. This is a good time psychologically for a consultation. Such can be reassuring to patient, family, and physician and might increase the faith of all concerned in the new treatment plan. At this stage, patients and family members are understandably skeptical and hesitant to believe what they are told about therapy. This is also the time that patients and families are attracted to wild and far-out treatment claims made by charlatans hoping to capitalize on those who are looking for miracles. Here again, the physician should anticipate the attraction of claims that may be sought as treatment outside the usual medical channels. In a similar way, it is important for the physician to inform the patient of the risks and complications that may result from whatever treatment approaches or choices are offered as appropriate therapy.

Patients have to be repeatedly told the reasons for using a specific treatment plan, the expectations of the plan, and how these expectations are or are not being realistically fulfilled. For the physician to exaggerate the benefits or dangers of one therapy versus another, or to prematurely report the effects or lack of effect might facilitate the patient's continued cooperation at one point in time only to complicate the acceptance of or to make the patient mistrust and refuse the course of treatment at a later time.

After repeated courses of treatment with one or more periods of productive and comfortable living, the disease may progress to the stage where therapy is designed to slow progression of the disease while primarily keeping the patient as active and comfortable as possible. Most patients are psychologically aware of the irreversible and progressive nature of their disease when it reaches this stage, whether it has been discussed and explained to them or not. At this stage, the patient requires repeated assurance by word and deed that the physician and staff will be available when the patient needs them. Some physicians have difficulty caring for patients at this stage because of their feelings of sadness or defeat (4). The patient's primary need is to know that the physician is not going to abandon him or her. Often the patient's family has more difficulty than the patient in accepting the fact that the patient is not going to get better but is going to die as a result of the disease. This phase of care necessitates close communications between physician, staff, patient, and family. Because patient and family are sensitized to or denying the issue of death and when it might come, team members need to exercise caution in predicting the amount of time left. Accurate predictions are difficult to make and family members can be affected by misinformation.

TERMINAL-PALLIATIVE PHASE

When death seems to be near, one of the greatest challenges for physician and family is avoiding heroic and discomforting measures while keeping the patient comfortable and as aware of himself or herself and the surrounding environment as the patient desires (52). There should be little hesitation to use the amount or type of medication needed to keep the patient as comfortable as possible. The physician who is unwilling or unable to treat cancer pain, particularly for the dying patient, gives the impression of not caring and abandoning the patient when most in need (72).

Chronic pain and its treatment must be understood as being completely different from that of acute pain. The magnitude of chronic pain is primarily related to the learned and remembered response to prior pain and the peripheral somatic component(s) present are reinforced and exaggerated by these central psychologic components. To achieve and maintain adequate pain control the medication must be given in a more potent form or a dose higher than used previously and administered on an around-the-clock basis (47). This approach avoids the patient having to justify a request for pain relief and permits an accumulation of the analgesic at a level that will help to overcome any preoccupation with pain. After administering effective pain treatment schedule for 36 to 48 hours, it is possible to reduce the amount of some doses but not the frequency with which the medication is given. (It is important for the patient to know in advance that some doses will be reduced but not by how much and when. Liquid oral and injectable forms of analgesia are easiest to disguise.) The physician needs to be familiar with a range of different pain medications, potency, duration of action, and potentiation to treat chronic pain most effectively.

It is important for the patient to be kept as free from pain as possible without concern for habituation to the medication. Once preoccupation with pain is overcome by adequate analgesia and the patient is convinced that help is available, the amount of medication necessary to maintain comfort usually will lessen. The primary concern of most patients who recognize that their disease is progressing irreversibly is whether they will be able to tolerate whatever psychologic and physical discomfort dying may produce without losing their composure and dignity. It is important for the physician to accept the patient's awareness of dying and to relate to the patient on this basis (12,74). It is not easy to listen and respond to the patient's statement about readiness to die—especially for the young physician. Training in these interventions can be effective and reassuring (56). Relating to patients when they give up former neurotic patterns and defenses and involve themselves totally in the "here and now" may provide a unique experience for physicians. The use of groups and volunteers also can aid the patient's and family's adjustment (66). The family of the dying patient is particularly appreciative if the physician can help them be aware or can confirm their own but difficult-to-accept impression that death is near for the patient (52). Many patients and family members will have strong wishes regarding where the patient should die. Such wishes should be fulfilled, if possible. Unlike accidental or sudden deaths, a death by cancer may provide the family and patient time to address important issues and perhaps better prepare for the future (14,41).

BEREAVEMENT

After death has occurred, it is important to contact the family within a week or two to see if they have any final questions or concerns. The impact and long-range effects of death from cancer on surviving family members recently has received more attention (9,18). Frequently they will express a desire to come to the office for a more extensive discussion (79). Answering their questions and helping them to deal with the answers is extremely important. The physician should explore the family's thoughts and feelings about death (10) and the way the physician, the health professionals, and the

hospital discharged their responsibilities. Likewise, bereavement programs for treatment team members and staff are essential and are being developed within the hospital setting (49). The development of bereavement programs (36) for the children of adult cancer patients and the surviving parent is a positive movement in psychosocial oncology. Groups for bereaved family members can permit each individual to share information, support, and emotional reactions with people of similar ages in a confidential, comfortable, and supportive environment in which they can learn they are not alone in their grief. Likewise the typical reactions of guilt, anger, shame, sadness, and envy for others can be discovered to be common among peers and not abnormal as the child or adolescent might fear. In these group settings, the surviving parents are able to solve parenting problems, learn about children's reactions to grief, and other developmental information, and receive from and give support to other parents.

SURVIVAL AND CURE PHASE

The overall age-adjusted survival rate for all types of cancer is approaching 50%, while the results of treatment of some childhood tumors and leukemia, as well as adult lymphomas and testicular tumors are above 75%. These very encouraging, but recent, improvements have not yet been accepted psychologically by the patients, their families, or even the professionals (22). Perhaps the continued fear of cancer as a mysterious killer will be prominent until there is a better understanding of its etiology.

In general, although studies of long-term survivors are limited, the psychologic data available are consistent in their findings. Those who openly express their feelings—particularly negative feelings—and have a greater sense of self-esteem before treatment will be more likely to return to work (61) and survive longer. The long-term survivors (over 3- to 5-year remissions), including those cured of advanced cancer have a greater appreciation of time, life, people, and interpersonal reactions, and tend to live in the present rather than past or future (40). As might be expected, however, cancer survivors and parents of children with cancer are, in general, more sensitive to little aches and pains and worry about the possibility of recurrence, with little evidence of frank psychopathology resulting in later life (63). The quality of life of surviving cancer patients and their families requires more attention (26).

Data are needed on the adjustment of specific groups of cured patients. Questions remain about those with residual cosmetic defects, functional deficiencies (28), those who are unable to return to their previous jobs, or those who do not have family or social supports. Preliminary studies show that the cancer patient's long-term adjustment does not depend on, or in some case is inversely related to, the degree of physical disability experienced. It initially seems that those with the greatest residual reminders of the former cancer are the most appreciative of life, even though the quality of their lives by usual standards is compromised (24).

USE OF PSYCHOSOCIAL PROFESSIONALS

Within the past two decades, an increasing and widespread willingness to address mortality, and hence the dying patient's dilemma, has sparked research and literature on these problems. In step with the trend, the clinical applications of psychosocial principles and psychotropic medications to help with the specific needs of cancer patients and their families have also improved (65,70,80). The primary physician is most often in the optimal position to assess potential and ongoing psychosocial problems and to initiate the consultation and referral process to insure his or her patient's proper treatment.

The physician's experience and common sense will often serve him or her well in evaluating a patient and family for potential psychosocial problems. However, the physician should remember that patients will often use extraordinary coping skills and even massive defenses, such as denial, to adjust to the life-threatening impact of cancer. It is not unusual for the patient to become so caught up in his or her own defensive struggle so as to entice treaters into believing that everything (one's own feelings, family, and work) is fine. It often takes tactful courage to confront the patient gently and essentially give permission to accept professional help. The physician's attitude toward the patient's use of such help can often allow the patient to receive such support without feeling like he or she has failed the physician or family (53,70).

A number of modalities, including individual (32), group (35,54), family, peers (42), and telephone contact (55), have provided emotional support. A referral for psychologic consultation and/or psychologic testing should be made in the more acute situation in which a patient presents with delusional or psychotic functioning, suicidal ideation, or cognitive impairment. Most cases will be less acute and often will present with expressions of anxiety and/or depression by the patient and/or family. In these instances, a referral may result in a psychosocial professional working with the patient in individual or group counseling or psychotherapy, in parental counseling, in family meetings, or in cancer support groups (17,19,34). It is not unusual for volunteer self-help cancer support groups to provide beneficial information and support for a patient and his family (8).

SUMMARY

Continuity should be the watchword for the care of the cancer patient. Although often difficult to arrange, it is important to have a primary physician who will have an overview of the patient as an individual in a life setting, an intimate knowledge of the history of the disease, its meaning for patient and family, and most essentially, a primary relationship with the patient. Such a physician should follow the patient and maintain liaison with the specialists who may be involved in treatment. This follow-up during the different stages of the disease might extend over a period of years of the patient's life. The primary physician can help the specialists to understand the preoccupations, needs, and strengths of the patient and should be available to help explain the specialist's recommendations and actions to the patient. Working together, the primary physician and the oncologists, radiologists, and other specialists can provide the best care for the patient and the most appropriate therapies for the cancer. With this arrangement, the patient, the disease, and the significant others will never be treated as separate or only remotely related entities, but rather as interacting components in a life system. Likewise, should the patient die, the primary physician and other team members are best postured to help the surviving family members in the dying and bereavement process.

Recommended Reading

The reader's inquiry into the literature on psychosocial oncology would best be focused initially in three areas: the patient's experience of oneself and the disease; the experience and interaction of the patient with others, including physician and multidisciplinary team members; and the planning of psychosocial interventions. The references used in this chapter were chosen for their contribution to these three areas and for their succinct explications of the various related issues. Each reference should provide a unique contribution to the reader's knowledge.

Several references deserve special attention. Elizabeth Kubler Ross' earlier work, *On Death and Dying* (4), encompasses the phenomenology of dying patients and the struggles one encounters sharing their experiences was one of the first such works to capture the public's recognition. Weisman's book *On Death and Denying* (12) and Shanfield's article "On Surviving Cancer: Psychological Considerations" (63) on the experience of cancer are also very useful. In regard to the patient's social interactions, Von Bertalanffy's classic article "The Theory of Open Systems in Physics and Biology" (73) will help the reader gain a perspective of the disease, the patient, and the system that affects the processes of diagnosis and treatment. The knowledge of and planning for psychosocial interventions can be provided through journal articles (1-3,5,6) that contain updated, readily available and quite readable sources for the reader. Other practical interventions are thoroughly discussed in *Coping with Cancer* (8) and Rosenbaum's *A Comprehensive Guide for Cancer Patients and Their Families* (11).

REFERENCES

General References

1. Driscoll, C.E. (ed). Management of the Cancer Patient in Primary Care Clinics in Office Practice. Philadelphia, PA: W.B. Saunders Company; 1987:243-416.
2. Greer, S.; Watson, M. Towards a psychobiological model of cancer: Psychological considerations. Soc. Sci. Med. 20(8):773-777; 1985.
3. Hall, R.C.W. (ed). Psychiatric aspects of neoplastic disease: Cancer care issues for psychiatrists. In: Silverfarb, P. (Guest ed). Psychiatric Medicine. Longwood, FL: Ryandic Publishing, Inc.; 1987: 265-419.
4. Kubler-Ross, E. On Death and Dying. New York, NY: MacMillan Publishing; 1969.
5. McEwan, P.J.M. (ed). Cancer and the Mind. In: Social Science and Medicine. Elmsford, NY: Pergamon Press Inc.; 1985: 771-851.
6. McHugh, M.K. (ed). Psychosocial aspects of oncologic care. Topics in Clinical Nursing 7:1-86; 1985.
7. Michael, B.E.; Copeland, D.R. Psychosocial issues in childhood cancer. Am. J. Ped. Hem. Oncol. 9(1):73-83; 1987.
8. National Cancer Institute. Coping with cancer: An annotated bibliography prepared by Cancer Information Clearinghouse. Washington, DC: U.S. Dept. of Health, Education, and Welfare. National Institutes of Health. Publication No. 80-2129.
9. Osterweis, M.; Solomon, F.; Green, M. (eds). Bereavement: reactions, consequences, and care. Committee for the Study of Health Consequences of the Stress of Bereavement, Institute of Medicine, Washington, DC, National Academy Press; 1984.
10. Raphael, B. The anatomy of bereavement. New York, NY: Basic Books, Inc.; 1983.
11. Rosenbaum, E.H.; Rosenbaum, I. A Comprehensive Guide for Cancer Patients and Their Families. Palo Alto, CA: Bull Publishing Company; 1979.
12. Weisman, A.D. On Death and Denying. New York, NY: Behavioral Publication, Inc.: 1972.

Specific References

13. Abrams, R.D. The patient with cancer—his changing pattern of communication. N. Engl. J. Med. 274:317-322; 1966.
14. Adams-Greenly, M.; Moynihan, R.T. Helping the children of fatally ill parents. Am. J. Orthopsychiatry 53(2):219-229; 1983.
15. Artiss, K.L.; Levine, A.S. Doctor-patient relationship in severe illness. New Engl. J. Med. 288:1210-1214; 1973.
15a. Bartlett, J. Familiar Quotations. Boston, MA: Little, Brown and Co; 1955.
16. Bell, H.K. The spiritual cane component of palliative care. Seminars in Oncology 12(4):482-485; 1985.
17. Berger, J.M. Crisis intervention: A drop-in support group for cancer patients and their families. Social Work in Health Care 10(2):81-92; 1984.
18. Berman, H.; Cragg, C.E.; Kuenzig, L. Having a parent die of cancer: Adolescents' reactions. Oncology Nursing Forum 15(2):159-163; 1988.
18a. Billings, J.A. Specialized care of the terminally ill patient. In: DeVita, V.T., Hellman, S., Rosenberg, S.A. (eds). Cancer: Principles and Practice of Oncology. 3rd ed. Philadelphia, PA: JB Lippincott Co.; 1989:2237-2244.
19. Cain, E.N.; Kohorn, E.I.; Quinlan, D.M.; Latimer, K.; Schwartz, P.E. Psychosocial benefits of a cancer support group. Cancer 57:183-189; 1986.
20. Cassileth, B.R.; Walsh, W.P.; Lusk, E.J. Psychosical correlates of cancer survival: a subsequent report 3 to 8 years after cancer diagnosis. J. Clin. Oncol. 6(11):1753-1759; 1988.
21. Chamberlain, J.G.; Sparber, A.G. Are support groups meaningful in the workplace? AAOHN J 34(1):10-13; 1986.
22. Christ, G.H. Social consequences of the cancer experience. Am. J. Ped. Hem. Oncol. 9(1):84-88; 1987.
22a. Christ G.; Klein, L.L.; Loscalzo, M.; Weinstein, L.L. Community resources for cancer patients. In: DeVita, V.T., Hellman, S., Rosenberg, S.A. (eds). Cancer: Principles and Practice of Oncology. Philadelphia, PA: JB Lippincott Co; 1989:2225-2236.
23. Cohen, S.; Syme, S.L. (eds). Issues in the study and social application of social support. In: Social Support and Health. New York, NY: Academic Press; 1985; pp 3-22.
24. Craig, T.J.; Comstock, G.W.; Geiser, P.B. The quality of survival in breast cancer: A case controlled comparison. Cancer. 33:1451-1459; 1974.
25. Culver, C.M.; Gert, B. Ethical issues in oncology. Psychiatr. Med. 5(4):389-404; 1987.
26. deHaes, J.C.J.M.; van Knippenberg, F.C.E. The quality of life of cancer patients: a review of the literature. Soc. Sci. Med. 20(8):809-817; 1985.
27. Derogatis, L.; Morrow, G.; Fetting, J.; Penman, D.; Piasetsky, S.; Schmale, A.; Henrichs, M.; Caunrike, C. The prevalence of psychiatric disorders among cancer patients. J. Am. Med. Assoc. 249(6):751-757; 1983.
28. Dobkin, P.L.; Morrow, G.R. Long term side effects in patients who have been treated successfully for cancer. J. Psychosocial Oncology 3(4):23-52; 1985/86.
29. Goldberg, R.J.; Cullen, L.O. Factors important to psychosocial adjustment to cancer: A review of the evidence. Soc. Sci. Med. 20(8):803-807; 1985.
30. Gotay, C.C. Why me? Attributions and adjustment by cancer patients and their mates at two stages in the disease process. Soc. Sci. Med. 20(8):825-831; 1985.
31. Granstrom, S.L. Spiritual nursing care for oncology patients. Topics in Clinical Nursing 39-45; 1985.
32. Greer, S. Psychotherapy for the cancer patient. Psychiatr. Med. 5(4):267-279; 1987.
33. Harris, L.L.; Vogtsberger, K.; Mattox, D.E. Group psychotherapy for head and neck cancer patients. Laryngoscope 95:585-587; 1985.
34. Heinrich, R.L.; Schag, C.C. Stress and activity management: group treatment for cancer patients and spouses. J. Consult. and Clin. Psychol. 53:439-446; 1985.
35. Henrichs, M.; Bousha, D.; Sterling, S.; Thomassen, J. Preliminary evaluation of prevention project for children of cancer patients. Abstract. Proceeding of American Psychological Association, August 1987 and article in The Bulletin of the Rochester Psychiatric Center Medical Staff October, November, December 1987.
36. Henrichs, M.; Thomassen, J.; Bousha, D.; Sterling, S. The kids adjusting through support (K.A.T.S.) bereavement program: Preliminary look at a prevention program for bereaved families. Abstract. Proceedings of Action Research in the Community. Conference, May 1987 and article in The Bulletin of the Rochester Psychiatric Center Medical Staff April, May, June 1988.
37. Hermann, J.F. Psychosocial support: interventions for the physician. Seminars in Oncology 12(4):466-471; 1985.
38. Hyland, J.; Novotny, E.; Coyne, L.; Travis, J.; Area, H. The psychosocial team and the difficult-to-treat patient. J. Psychosocial Oncology 5(1):41-50; 1987.
39. Jacobs, C.; Ross, R.D.; Walker, I.M.; Stockdale, F.E. Behavior of cancer patients: a randomized study of the effects of education and peer support groups. Am. J. Clin. Oncol. 6:347-350; 1983.
40. Kennedy, J.; Tellegen, A.; Kennedy, S.; et al.: Psychological response to patients cured of advanced cancer. Cancer 38:2184-2191; 1976.
41. Koocher, G.P. Coping with a death from cancer. J. Consul. and Clin. Psychol. 54(5):623-631; 1986.
42. Lane, C.A.; Davis, A.W. Implementation: we can weekend in the rural setting. Cancer Nursing December 8(6):323-328; 1985.
42a. Lederberg, M.S.; Holland, J.C.; Massie, M.J. Psychologic aspects of patients with cancer. In: DeVita, V.T., Hellman, S., Rosenberg, S.A. (eds). Cancer: Principles and Practice of Oncology, 3rd ed. Philadelphia, PA: JB Lippincott Co; 1989:2191-2205.
43. Lev, E.L. Community support for oncology patient and family. Topics in Clin Nursing 71-78; 1985.
44. Levy, S. Behavior and Cancer: Life Style and Psychosocial Factors in the Initiation and Progression of Cancer. San Francisco, CA: Jossey-Bass; 1985.
45. Lynn, J. Legal and ethical issues in palliative health care. Seminars in Oncology 12(4):476-481; 1985.
46. Magni, G.; Silvestro, A.; Carli, M.; DeLeo, D. Social support and psychological distress of parents of children with acute lymphocytic leukaemia. Br. J. Med. Psychol. 59:383-385; 1986.
47. Marks, R.N.; Sachar, E.J. Undertreatment of medical inpatients with narcotic analgesics. Ann. Intern. Med. 78:173-181; 1973.
48. Morrow, G.; Dobkin, P.L. Behavioral approaches for the management of adversive side effects of cancer treatment. Psychiatr. Med. 5(4):299-314; 1987.
49. Moseley, J.R.; Logan, S.J.; Tolle, S.W.; Bentley, J.H. Developing a bereavement program in a university hospital setting. Oncology Nursing Forum 15(2):151-155; 1988.
50. Neuling, S.; Winefield, H. Social support and recovery after surgery for breast cancer: Frequency and correlates of supportive behaviours by family, friends and surgeon. Soc. Sci. Med. 27(4):385-392; 1988.
51. Northouse, L.L. Social support in patients' and husbands' adjustment to breast cancer. Nursing Research 1988; 37(2):91-95; 1988.
52. Patterson, G.W. Managing grief and bereavement. Primary Care 14(2):403-415; 1987.
53. Peterson, L. (ed). Biopsychosocial oncology: the role of psychology in the treatment of cancer. J. Consul. and Clin. Psychol. 54(5):591-632; 1986.
54. Plant, H.; Richardson, J.; Stubbs, L.; et al. Evaluation of a support group for cancer patients and their families. Br. J. Hosp. Med. 38(4): 317-320; 1987.
55. Rainey, L.C. Cancer counseling by telephone help-line: The UCLA psychosocial cancer counseling line. Public Health Reports 100(3):308-315; 1985.
56. Razavi, D.; Delvaux, N.; Farvacques, C.; Robaye, E. Immediate effectiveness of brief psychological training for health professionals dealing with terminally ill cancer patients: a controlled study. Soc Sci Med 27(4):369-375; 1988.
57. Richardson, J.L.; Marks, G.; Levine, A. The influence of symptoms of disease and side effects of treatment on compliance with cancer therapy. J. Clin. Oncol. 6(11):1746-1752; 1988.
57a. Rotman, M.; Torpie, R.J. Supportive care in radiation oncology. In: Perez, C.A., Brady, L.W. (eds). Principles and Practice of Radiation Oncology. Philadelphia, PA: JB Lippincott Co; 1992:1508-1516.
58. Sauer, R.; Seitz, M. Psychological and social support of cancer patients: Report on a program of the radiotherapy department, Erlanger. Recent Results in Cancer Research; 108:311-315; 1985.
59. Schmelkin, L.P.; Wachtel, A.B.; Hecht, D.; Schneiderman, B.E. Cancer opinionnaire: medical students' attitudes toward psychosocial cancer care. Cancer 58(3):801-806; 1986.

60. Schoenberg, N.; Carr, A.C. Loss of external organs: Limb amuptation, mastectomy, and disfigurement. In: Schoenberg, B.; Carr, A.C.; Peretz, D.; *et al.* (eds). Loss and Grief: Psychological Management in Medical Practice. New York, NY: Columbia University Press; 1970:119-131.

61. Schoenfeld, G. Psychological factors related to delayed return of an earlier lifestyle in successfully treated cancer patients. J. Psychosom. Res. 16:41-46; 1971.

61a. Schorer, L.R.; Schain, W.S.; Montague, D.K. Sexual problems of patients with cancer. In: DeVita, V.T., Hellman, S., Rosenberg, S.A. (eds). Cancer: Principles and Practice of Oncology, 3rd ed. Philadelphia, PA: JB Lippincott Co; 1989:2206-2224.

62. Senn, H.J.; Glaus, A.; Schmid, L. (eds). Supportive Care in Cancer Patients, Vol 108. Berlin, Germany: Springer-Verlag; 1988.

63. Shanfield, S.B. On surviving cancer: Psychological considerations. Compr. Psychiatry 21:128-134; 1980.

64. Silberfarb, P.M.; Ohilibert, D.; Levine, P.M. Psychosocial aspects of neoplastic disease. II. Affective and cognitive effects of chemotherapy in cancer patients. Am. J. Psychiatry 137:597-601; 1980.

65. Spiegel, D. Psychosocial Interventions with cancer patients. J. Psychosocial Oncology 3(4):83-95; 1987.

66. Spiegel, D.; Glafkides, M.C. Effects of group confrontation with death and dying. Int. J. Group Psychother. 33(4):433-447; 1983.

67. Taylor, S.E.; Talke, R.L.; Shoptaw, S.J.; Lichtman, R.R. Social support, support groups and the cancer patient. J. Consul. and Clin. Psychol. 54(5):608-615; 1986.

68. Tebbi, C.K.; Stern, M.; Boyle, M.; Mettlin, C.J.; Mindell, E.R. The role of social support systems in adolescent cancer amputees. Cancer 56(4):965-971; 1985.

69. Telch, C.F.; Telch, M.J. Group coping skills instruction and supportive group therapy for cancer patients: a comparison of strategies. J. Consul. and Clin. Psychol. 54(6):802-808; 1986.

70. Thorne, S.E. Helpful and unhelpful communications in cancer care: the patient perspective. Oncology Nursing Forum 15(2):167-172; 1988.

71. U.S. Public Health Service: The Health Consequences of Smoking: Cancer. A Report of the Surgeon General. Washington, DC: US Department of Health and Human Services, 1982.

72. Vachon, M.L.S. Bereavement programmes and interventions in palliative care. Progress in Clinical and Biological Research 1983: 451-461.

73. VonBertalanffy, L. The theory of open systems in physics and biology. Science 111:23-29; 1950.

74. Weisman, A.D. On Death and Denying. New York: Behavioral Publications, Inc.; 1972:192-211.

75. Weisman, A.D.; Worden, J.W. The emotional impact of recurrent cancer. J. Psychosocial Oncology 3(4):5-16; 1985/86.

76. Wheatley, G.M.; Cunnick, W.R.; Wright, B.P.; *et al.* The employment of persons with a history of treatment for cancer. Cancer 33:441-445; 1974.

77. Wise, T.N. Sexual problems in cancer patients and their management. Psychiatr. Med. 5(4):329-342; 1987.

78. Wolcott, D.L.; Fawzy, F.I.; Landserk, J.; McCombs, M. AIDS patients' needs for psychosocial services and their use of community service organizations. J. Psychosocial Oncology 4(1/2):135-146; 1986.

79. Worden, J.W. Bereavement. Seminars in Oncology 12(4):472-475; 1985.

80. Wortman, C.B. Social support and the cancer patient: conceptual and methodological issues. Cancer 53(suppl):2339-2362; 1984.

81. Wyszynski, A.A. The impact of spiritualism in the care of the cancer patient. J. Psychosocial Oncology 4(3):93-98.; 1986

82. Young, D.F.; Posner, J.B. Nervous system toxicity of the chemotherapeutic agents. In: Vinkin, P.J.; Bruyn, G.W. (eds). Handbook of Clinical Neurology 1980, vol. 39, part II. New York, NY: North-Holland Publishing Co.; 1980:91-129.

Philip Rubin, M.D., Radiation Oncology   Robert E. O'Mara, M.D., Radiology
David G. Bragg, M.D., Radiology

Chapter **15**

PRINCIPLES OF ONCOLOGIC IMAGING AND TUMOR IMAGING STRATEGIES

For the purposes of classification of extent of cancer and of comparability of the results of treatment, a basic requirement is that the data be measurable, verifiable by others, and codifiable.

A.R. Feinstein (20a)

PERSPECTIVE

The technical advances in tumor imaging have been as dramatic in radiologic diagnosis as multimodal advances have been in cancer treatment. In fact, they may be more so when we consider the innovations of the past two decades such computerized tomography (CT), ultrasound (US), magnetic resonance (MR) imaging, positron emission tomography (PET), and, potentially, labelled monoclonal antibodies (LMA). These newer modalities, coupled with electronic video displays controlled by computerization that enables quantification of images in static and dynamic modes, are revolutionary when compared to standard diagnostic roentgenographic procedures. Furthermore most standard radiologic procedures have improved. More accurate tumor visualization is due to better films with finer grains and higher resolution qualities as in mammography, better contrast media, selective catheterization for imaging of tumor vascularity, improved subtraction techniques such as digital angiography for viewing over bony sites, special procedure rooms, fluoroscopic control, and precise biopsies via skinny needles for pathologic confirmation of suspected malignant disease at primary sites, regional lymph nodes and/or remote visceral metastases, usually CT or US guided.

Currently, tumors can be diagnosed earlier and more precisely because of these advances. Those of us engaged in oncologic care and management realize that tumors are better and more accurately staged. An issue that is more debatable is the impact of tumor imaging on treatment and cancer curability. The caveat in this issue is the rising cost of medical care, particularly the high cost of tumor imaging by these newest techniques. To justify this type of investment of equipment, resources, and time, it would be highly desirable to show a definite correlation and a distinct contribution of improved tumor imaging and its impact on treatment and cancer curability at numerous disease sites. Such controlled studies are difficult to conduct but at some sites are underway and provide both suggestive and definite evidence of contributing to increasing survival rates and decreasing death rates.

For any radiologic imaging system, the quality of the images and their value in cancer detection can be characterized in terms of four fundamental properties, according to Hendee (25). These properties presented in Table 15-1, include spatial resolution, contrast discrimination, image noise, and the presence of distortion and artifacts. It is clear that no single procedure is best in all categories; contrast discrimination probably needs the most improvement. The emerging technologies important to oncologic diagnosis, are dependent upon the availability of computers and their sophisticated software packages for data handling and display. The concept of tumor threshold size is difficult to define. From an imaging standpoint, we can generally characterize the limits of resolution of the various imaging systems in use today. There are both objective and subjective limitations to these detection parameters of which we all must be aware. In part, they are related to equipment (spatial and contrast resolution), patient considerations, target organ considerations, and interobserver variations. Equipment design advances, new techniques and systems, as well as improvements in the educational process have reduced these limitations somewhat, but we have now reached some practical endpoints in lesion size resolution. Table 15-2 summarizes several common imaging techniques, broadly defines the advantages and limitations of each, and assigns an estimate of the tumor detection threshold for each system, by organ site. A number of assumptions have been made for the purposes of estimating rough approximations of tumor size "thresholds" visible by each technique to serve the purposes of comparison.

Decision Theory

Most oncologists understand the definitions of the terms sensitivity, specificity, true and false, positive and negative; however, this simple illustration will serve as a review (25).

Table 15-1. Imaging Characteristics of Selecteed Diagnostic Systems

Modality	Spatial Resolution	Contrast Resolution	Temporal Resolution	Signal-to-Noise Ratio	Distortion and Artifacts	Wide-Spread Application	Cost
Roentgenography	E	P	E	E	F	E	E
Fluoroscopy	F	P	E	F	F	F	F
Digital Subtraction Angiography	P	E	E	P	F	P	F
X-ray Computed Tomography	F	E	F	P	F	F	P
Ultrasonography	F	P	E	F	F	F	E
Positron Tomography	P	F	P	F	F	P	P
Nuclear Medicine	P	P	P	P	F	F	E
Magnetic Resonance	P	E	P	P	F	F	P

E = excellent; F = fair; P = poor.
*Reprinted from **Diagnostic Imaging**, May, 1983, with permission.*

Table 15-2. Imaging Detection Thresholds

Imaging Technique	Threshold (CM)							Comments
	Brain	Lung	Liver	Bone	Lymph Node	Pancreas	Kidney	
Plain films	NA	1.0	NA	2.0+	NA	NA	NA	Lung—low-contrast objects with obscure margine amplify problem Bone—must be large in medullary cavity or involve cortex
Film tomography	NA	0.5	NA	0.5	NA	NA	NA	Lung—improves detection efficiency Bone—allows matrix of tumor and soft tissue component to be seen
Ultrasound	NA	NA	1.5–2.0	NA	2.0+	1.5–2.0	1.0–2.5	Operator- and patient-dependent technology—"thresholds" variable and difficult to define
Computed tomography	1.0–1.5	0.2–0.5	1.0–1.5	0.5–1.0	1.0–2.0	1.5–2.-	1.0	Detection efficiency determined by anatomic location, size, and tumor tyupe
Lymphography	NA	NA	NA	NA	0.5	NA	NA	Able to define intrinsic node defects. Fails to opacify many node groups visible by CT
Angiography	1.5–2.0	limited application	1.0–1.5	variable	NA	1.5–2.0	1.0–1.5	Detection efficiency based on tumor vascularity
Digital techniques	2.0–3.0	?	0.5–1.0	NA	NA	1.5–2.5		Used as angio substitute. Will have reduced detection efficiency in return for less cost and morbidity. Digital imaging will allow contrast enhancement
Magnetic resonance imaging	1.0–1.5	0.5	1.0–1.5	NA	1.0–2.0	1.5–2.0	1.0	Assumes similar spatial resolution with CT with improved detection efficiency in base of brain, head and neck. Unknown with body imaging
Conventional nuclear imaging	1.5–2.0	Variable (67Ga)	2.0–2.5	0.5–1.0	variable (replaced nodes not visualized)	NA	NA	Brain—occasionally useful when CT not available or as adjunct Liver—cost-effective screen formats in appropriate setting Bone—essential for screening
Monoclonal antibody body imaging	?	?	?	?	?	?	?	Unknown impact—promises to define smaller tumor burdens in all body sites

NA = not applicable.

Any imaging procedure, or for that matter, any laboratory test will have an accuracy or predictive value based upon whether the result or time (positive or negative) correlates to the presence of disease.

	Disease Present	Disease Absent
Exam Positive	True Positive	False Positive
Exam Negative	False Negative	True Negative
	Sensitivity	Specificity

The *sensitivity* of a certain test or study is a function of the true positive rate compared to the sum of the true positives and false negatives.

$$\text{Sensitivity} = \frac{\text{true positives}}{\text{true positives + false negatives}}$$

The *specificity* of a test relates to the relationship of the true negative yield compared to the sum of the true negative plus false positive rate for the study.

$$\text{Specificity} = \frac{\text{true negatives}}{\text{true negatives + false positives}}$$

The *predictive value* of a study is a more important parameter of the potential usefulness of an examination in a certain disease state. The predictive value of a positive exam is determined by the true positive and false positive rate.

$$\text{Predictive value of a positive test} = \frac{\text{true positive}}{\text{true positive + false positive}}$$

$$\text{Predictive value of a negative test} = \frac{\text{true negative}}{\text{true negative + false negative}}$$

The accuracy rate of a procedure is the product of the sensivity and specificity.

$$\text{Accuracy} = \text{Sensitivity} \times \text{Specificity}$$

This brief review of some of the more common and useful terms involved in the decision process can be supplemented by consulting bibliographic reference 9. A tabulation of ten common imaging procedures most often applied to oncologic problems is described in Table 15-3 in terms of its limitations and applications and based upon its relative sensitivity and specificity.

Table 15-3. Specific Imaging Pprocedure: Limitations and Applications

Imaging Procedure	Relative Cost	Relative Sensitivity	Relative Specificity	Comments
Plain film radiography	low	varied	high	Plain films have excellent sensitivity and specificity in the soft tissues (mammography) and bones. In the chest, low-contrast tumor targets are a problem.
Xerography	low	high	moderate/high	Edge enhancement and wide exposure latitude allow soft tissue application (breast, neck, appendicular soft tissues, bone, and soft tissue tumor imaging).
Contrast GI studies moderate	high	high		Cancer screening applications can be justified for high-risk groups (esophagus, stomach, and colon).
Radionuclide liver scan	moderate	moderate	low	Displaced by CT/US as screening liver imaging modality of choice. ? still initial screen of choice.
Radionuclide bone scan	moderate	high	low	Procedure of choice in skeletal scanning. Abnormal sites must be verified by film radiography.
Radionuclide brain scan	moderate	moderate	low	CT has replaced radionuclide brain scanning except where CT access is limited.
Ultrasound abdominal scanning	moderate	high	moderate	Lack of radiation exposure, cost, and availability lend ultrasound to abdominal screening. Technique is operator dependent.
Computed tomography Brain	high	high	moderate	Procedure of choice for screening mass lesion suspect using contrast enhancement only.
Lung	high	high	low	
Abdomen	high	high	moderate	Highest sensitivity of all studies in detection of lung nodules. High false-positive rate.
Angiography	high	high	moderate	Cost, invasiveness, and time limit applications.
Magnetic resonance (MRI)	high	hith	high(?)	Resolution similar to CT. Elimination of bone artifacts makes CNS images better than CT. In chest, tumor and hilar node imaging improved over CT. Applications elsewhere—insufficient experience.

THE ONCOLOGIC DECISION PROCESS AND TUMOR IMAGING STRATEGIES

The first decision in cancer management most often determines whether the outcome will be successful. The most important factors in the decision are definition of the true anatomic extent or stage of the cancer and a multidisciplinary approach to treatment after the histiopathologic diagnosis of cancer is made. The oncologic decision process and imaging strategies need to be consistent and logical. There are several steps in the process (Table 15-4).

Accurate Diagnosis and Early Detection

To begin the oncologic decision process, the cancer needs to be detected and the diagnosis firmly established. Generally, this occurs in two populations — symptomatic or asymptomatic patients. The ability to detect a cancer depends upon the accuracy of the method and will be discussed later. The "gold standard" of diagnosis is the histopathologic verification of the cancer in the tissue in question. The essential element in establishing the validity of an imaging procedure is to demon- strate a high degree of correlation with histiopathologic findings (i.e., 90%). The use of an imaging technique for screening purposes is also contingent on the population, cost of the procedure, and potential curability of a cancer at the time of detection. Clearly, earlier detection of incurable cancers is of little value.

Precise Staging

At each major anatomic site it is essential to have a classification of cancer that is meaningful in terms of treatment and prognosis. A consistent cancer language and categorization allows the oncologist to develop treatment strategies in a multidisciplinary fashion. The Tumor, Node, Metastases (TNM) system as used by the American Joint Committee for Cancer Staging and End-Results Reporting (AJC) and the International Union Against Cancer (UICC), or other special classifications, are advocated. A dual classification that encompasses anatomic extent and histopathologic analysis is

the best form of oncotaxonomy. The challenge of oncologic imaging is complex and varies with each organ site and often, tumor type. To clarify the concept of tumor staging, decision flow diagrams are used—see example (Fig. 15-1). Obviously, the imaging process will often have to be tailored to suit the individual needs of the patient, the unique features of the tumor, and presenting characteristics of the disease.

Staging work-up is necessary at the time of diagnosis to define the true extent of the cancer in its three compartments (TNM) before the best treatment can be chosen. A distinction between clinical-radiographic versus surgical-pathologic staging is essential when reporting end results. Again, CT and MR are the critical non-invasive procedures to accurate clinical staging in most anatomic sites (Table 15-4).

Optimum Treatment — Clinical Trials

The treatment of choice is a function of those clinicians who make the choice and not solely of the cancer and its presentation. Optimal treatment today is based upon multidisciplinary decision-making in which all involved specialists participate and plan treatments using combined modalities rather than a single mode of therapy. The multimodal treatment selection is based upon staging as a first step and is most evident in clinical trial design. A carefully defined and similar target group of patients is the first step in protocol development. Such protocols are usually part of a cooperative group effort and usually test therapeutic options; however, they are

Table 15-4. Sequence of Imaging Process—Staging and Follow-up

Process	Problems Specific to Process
Detection and diagnosis ↓	Dictates staging workup
Staging workup (TNM) ↓	Dictated by tumor type, patient status, organ site, and procedural limitations
Definition of tumor response to treatment ↓	Imaging approach and sequence determined by therapeutic modality and tumor type
Follow-up ↓	Imaging approach and sequence determined by therapeutic modality and tumor type
Detection of relapse ↓	
Restage—before retreatment	Abbreviated restaging tailored to the tumor, patient status, and retreatment modality considered

Diagnostic Onco-Algorithm

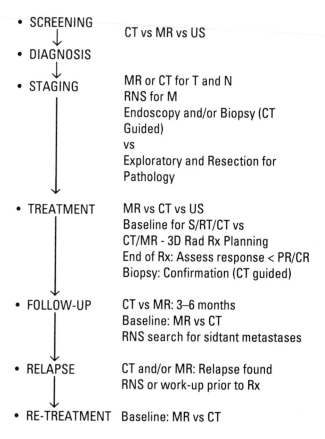

- SCREENING
  ↓   CT vs MR vs US
- DIAGNOSIS
  ↓
- STAGING   MR or CT for T and N
            RNS for M
            Endoscopy and/or Biopsy (CT Guided)
            vs
            Exploratory and Resection for Pathology

- TREATMENT   MR vs CT vs US
              Baseline for S/RT/CT vs
              CT/MR - 3D Rad Rx Planning
              End of Rx: Assess response < PR/CR
              Biopsy: Confirmation (CT guided)

- FOLLOW-UP   CT vs MR: 3–6 months
              Baseline: MR vs CT
              RNS search for sidtant metastases

- RELAPSE   CT and/or MR: Relapse found
              RNS or work-up prior to Rx

- RE-TREATMENT Baseline: MR vs CT

Fig. 15-1. Decision flow diagram.

equally effective in testing diagnostic procedures. Optimal protocols should allow complementary imaging techniques to evolve, as well as identify methods of triaging patients through a maze of alternate imaging modalities (25). There is a newly formed national cooperative group — The Radiologic Diagnostic Oncologic Group (RDOG) — assigned to design and assess competitive oncologic imaging procedures.

Better Follow-up

It is important to determine persistent cancer or early relapse as soon as possible so that salvage therapy or an alternate can be applied. The time of the first recurrence, a careful restaging work-up should document the precise failure pattern carefully. The patterns of failure allow us to determine whether the lack of success resulted from a local (T), nodal (N), or metastatic (M) failure, from complications of the treatment, or from unrelated disease. Once the reasons for failure are known, corrective measures can be taken and/or new therapeutic strategies in protocols can be developed for investigation. Clincial trials are based upon careful diagnostic criteria and staging to determine target groups for study and road maps of follow-up studies.

Relapse and Restaging

Whenever possible, we have recommended a strategy for the post treatment follow-up with similar assumptions and guidelines as were developed for the initial staging work-up prior to treatment. In no other instance is it more important for the radiologist to understand the treatment program than in the follow-up interval after treatment and the therapeutic approach will have a major influence on the selection and outcome of the imaging study. If tumor persistence or tumor progression is noted in the face of treatment, then a crossover to a new mode of therapy or new combination of agents are usually advised. Once a local-regional tumor relapse has been recognized, the staging process begins again, usually in a similar but modified form to be sure there is no metastatic disease. Restaging and biopsy proof is essential at the time of relapse or recurrence, before retreatment, with very few exceptions.

IMPACT OF TUMOR IMAGING STRATEGIES IN CANCER CURABILITY: FIVE HYPOTHESES

A number of hypotheses will be advanced to illustrate that improvements in tumor imaging may lead to the selection of optimal multimodal therapy and thereby improved outcome and survival.

1. Earlier diagnosis in symptomatic patients implies that smaller, more localized tumors without metastatic spread to nodes or viscera will be found, thereby increasing the potential for cure.
2. Improved screening procedures for occult tumors in asymptomatic patient cohorts which again implies the detection of smaller or minimal noninvasive cancers with a greater potential cure. The value of cancer screening has been questioned by many authors in recent years (21,41).
3. Precise staging or better tumor definition of the extensions of the primary, lymph node involvement and visceral metastases leads to more accurate staging and in turn more optimal treatment.

4. More precise outlining of the tumor volume three-dimensionally leads to better local regional treatment.
5. Evaluation of responses or detection of early relapses allows for the determination and application of another modality for salvage, hopefully leading to a better cure rate.

COMPARATIVE SURVEY OF MAJOR ORGAN SYSTEMS: THE "GOLD STANDARD" IN ONCO-IMAGING

In most areas of the body imaged, CT has become the standard against which other tumor imaging systems are measured. The applications of CT to mass lesion detection in the brain and staging in other body sites are now well established, particularly with contrast enhancement. Computerized tomography plays a dominant role in staging most anatomic areas with advantages in lesion detection and definition over conventional studies in a number of specific organ sites. Magnetic resonance imaging plays an increasingly important role in the staging process and at numerous anatomic sites challenges the superiority of CT. The ability of MR to provide 3D multiplanar views with great clarity lies in its T1 and T2 weighted images, spin echoes producing different signal intensities that can often discriminate normal tissue from tumors and provide an edge over CT. The cost is two to three times a CT exam and one needs to be certain of its value or complementarity to a CT exam. Its role in central nervous system (CNS) imaging is more easily understood and accepted than for other body sites. In a recent symposium (39) and seminar in cancer imaging (10), however, MR is in strong competition with CT for the "gold standard" at many major sites. The prospect for tumor versus normal tissue discrimination with MR as well as in vivo spectroscopy must await the trial of new, higher field strength magnets.

The "gold standard" in tumor imaging most accrately reflects the true pathologic state of the cancer being diagnosed or staged in the primary (T), nodal (N), or metastatic (M) compartment. Computerized tomography and MR are the most powerful tools available for noninvasive assessments of cancer invasion and dissemination, with US often directing interventional biopsy procedures. A brief overview of the comparison of CT/MR/US can be found in Table 15-5, with "gold standard" designations favoring the imaging procedure with highest predictive value. As can be gleaned from this table, both CT and MR contribute to staging, but when both are equal, CT is often used first due to availability and lower cost. Nevertheless, MR, with its sharp multiplanar imaging, has the edge in many organ sites and a concise summary follows in major organs.

NEW ADVANCES AND HORIZONS IN TUMOR IMAGING

Magnetic Resonance Spectroscopy (MRS) (17,39,42,49,50)

MRS coupled with MR imaging becomes perhaps the most powerful investigational tool to study tumor biology which is directly applicable to tumor diagnosis and management. Just as MR can generate high resolution anatomic images based on proton density maps and intensity signals based on the water proton content, MRS provides the information on regional biochemistry of several nucleii including ^{31}P, ^{1}H, ^{13}C, and ^{23}Na.

Table 15-5. "Gold Standard" in Oncologic Imaging

SITE	CT (CE)	MR (GE)	US
CNS	++	+++	0
HEAD & NECK	+++	+++	0
LUNG	+++	++	0
BREAST	+++	++	++
GIT			
Esopyagus	+++	+++	+
Gastric	+	+	0
Colon	+	+	0
Rectal	+	++	+
Pancreatic	+++	++	++
Liver	+++	+++(+)	++
GU			
Kidney	+++	+++	++
Bladder	++	+++	++
Prostate	++	+++	+++
MUSCULO-SKELETAL			
Osseous	+++	+++	0
STS	++	+++	+
LYMPHOID	+++	++	+

CE = contrast enhanced; GE = Gadolinium enhanced.

Plasma ^{1}H MRS: Perhaps the most exciting MRS discovery that proved to be disappointing was the initial report by Fossel *et al.* (21a) of the ability to detect the presence of a malignant tumor by using ^{1}H MRS of blood plasma. Eventually, a prospective randomized properly controlled study showed no difference between cancer patients, benign tumor patients, and normal patients.

Tumor characteristics "pathochemistry:" The search for a specific tumor signature has been thoroughly explored with T2 weighted MR images and US signals endlessly and elusively. However, if a suspicious lesion is found by MR and is suspected of being cancer, then MRS may be of value. Elevation of ^{31}P spectra, high concentrations of phosphomonoesteral (PME), inorganic phosphate (P$_i$), or phosphodieters (PDE), depressed nucleoside triphophates (NTP) in comparison to normal tissue would suggest malignancy. Alternately finding unique metabolite by MRS in a qualitative fashion has not yet been found.

Tumor pathophysiology: Tumor bioenergetics is characterized by ^{31}P MRS, which decreases with increasing tumor size and perfusion and is consistent with biochemical evidence that ATP levels are low in larger human cancers such as breast cancer. Metastatic potential has been associated with features of MRS proton spectra of cancer cells as in some rat mammary adenocarcinomas. Tumor metabolism through various catabolic and anabolic pathways could be studied for growth potential. That is, rapid growing tumors have a high metabolic rate that be correlated with enzyme kinetics such as the turnover of P$_i$ which tend to decline as tumors grow larger and slow down in proliferation. The observation that phosphorous MRS is sensitive to tumor hypoxia *in vivo* is now accepted and such can be used for determining sensitizing therapeutic strategies (14,42).

Drug sensitivity and resistance: MRS has the potential to offer a noninvasive means of monitoring tumor response to drugs by ^{31}P determinators *in vivo* in human tumor xenografts and some patient tumors. Study of different cell sublines — insensitive and resistant to a drug such as mitomycin or Adriamycin — show differences in ^{31}P MRS but this could reflect tumor killing mechanisms and growth delay. Pharmacokinetic studies may be possible *in vivo* using fluorinated compounds since ^{19}F is nearly as sensitive as ^{1}H (26). Drugs labelled with ^{19}F could be studied in specific tumors to determine then abiltiy to activate or detoxify chemotherapeutic agents.

Positron Emission Tomography

PET has been slow in its introduction to medicine and oncology due to its expense and complexity. A facility requires a cyclotron and a "hot" laboratory for producing short-lived positron emitting radioisotopes and a special twin headed PET scanners. Positrons decay by emitting two gammas at 180° angles so that their point of origin can be identified by time of detection by twin detections. With appropriate labelling of key compounds that can enter tumors through metabolic pathways, unique perfusion patterns or hypoxia in tumors can be diagnosed, monitored, and staged.

Applications of PET in oncology have been recently initiated for brain tumors. Although the resolution power of the equipment used and some of the theoretical models for quantitative studies of pathophysiological metabolism have limitations, the results obtained to date have provided important preliminary data indicating the usefulness of PET as a relatively non-invasive method for studying a variety of fundamental properties of tumors which could be very important for clinical management. Some of the areas that can be studied with PET include oxygen consumption and extraction efficiency, regional blood flow and volume, glucose consumption, pH, amino acid uptake/protein synthesis, metabolic effects of anti-tumor therapy, drug pharmacokinetics, and binding of agents to receptors.

Hypoxia in tumors (14,42): Tumors which contain hypoxic cells are resistant to radiation therapy and to many drugs. There is also reason to believe that hypoxia and the associated pathophysiological microenvironments that occur as tumors progress may be causally related to the developemnt of therapeutically resistant phenotypes. A major research effort has been directed at methods to overcome hypoxia-associated resistance and to predict which tumors may be hypoxic. This project involves measurement of ^{15}O$_2$ extraction ratio and tumor blood flow.

Tumor metabolism versus prognosis: There are indications that certain metabolic parameters measurable with PET may be related to tumor grade and patient survival. Glucose consumption is often high in brain tumors and has been correlated to grade.

Monitor effects of therapy: There is data for human tumors that suggest that PET may be used to monitor the effectiveness of therapy. Glucose consumption has been shown to remain decreased in tumors which are controlled and to increase again in recurrent tumors. In one study, radiation necrosis was distinguished from tumor recurrence by ^{18}FDG.

Tumor pharmacokinetics: The ability to take up drugs throughout the tumor is a critical determinant of therapeutic response. Drug uptake may be very heterogeneous within a large tumor or among different tumors of apparently similar pathology. In brain tumors, variability of integrity of the blood-brain barrier may cause significant variability in drug uptake. Published results with ^{11}C labelled BCNU indicate the potential of PET for such studies (50).

Assistance in staging tumors: Some reports suggest that PET sometimes defines tumor margins that extend beyond what is observed by the diagnostic methods such as CT scan. This may occur when the tumor cell population is metabolically heterogeneous and irregularly distributed morphologically in the tumor. Comparison of results with PET versus CT and MR imaging may provide important information for the therapist.

Binding to receptors: Antibodies with or without attached cytotoxins to tumor associated antigens or to growth factor receptors may be useful for diagnosis and therapy of malignancy. Positron emission tomography may be useful to monitor binding kinetics and to optimize development of reagents and their use in conjunction with other therapy modalities.

Radioautoimmunodetection (RAID) of Cancer (43)

Perhaps the most challenging and potentially wide reaching is the use of radiolabelled monoclonal antibodies (RMAB) to malignant tumor antigens for diagnostic and therapeutic purposes. Considerable advances have been made in the immunochemistry to improvement in antibody preparation and labelling coupled with improvements in instrumentation, especially single photon emission computed tomography (SPECT).

Radiolabelled monoclonal antibodies (RMAB) (19,40) are usualy cell surface antigens, commonly glycoproteins, commonly labelled with a diverse group of radioisotopes ^{131}I, ^{111}In, ^{123}I, and ^{99m}Tc. These are usually produced by murine hybridomas (fusion of a immunized donor lymphocyte with a mouse myeloma cell) which will elaborate the antibody. Two limiting factors are that less than 1% of RMAB usually enter the tumor so that signal to noise background obscures detection and toxicity caused by repeat study due to the prompt development of human antibodies to murine proteins.

Major immunodetection studies on clinical trials: A recent series of the literature by Hanson identified almost 2,000 patients studied in 61 trials, 52 of which were monoclonals. The tumors studied that show good targeting include such solid tumors as colorectal cancer, melanoma, breast, and ovarian cancer, lymphomas, i.e., cutaneous T cell lymphoma and neuroblastomas, human choriocarcinomas. The sensitivity varies form 39% to 90%. The results are variable and inconsistent and further investigation is currently recommended.

Single photon emission computed tomography: Most commonly used methods of *in vivo* detection of RMAB have been the planar gamma camera imaging with background subtraction techniques on sophisticated window techniques. Single photon emission computed tomography will allow detection of smaller lesions at depth (> 2.5 cm), but greater counting rates are required for RMAB than available from ^{131}I antibodies. With ^{123}I labelled antibodies, SPECT may yield much higher sensitivities close to 90%.

Interventional Ultrasonography (4)

Ultrasound is an established and effective technique and with the design of smaller probes which have allowed for the introduction into body cavities, this technique is increasingly used. Thus, transrectal US for prostate cancer and for determining rectal wall invasion, coupled with guided needle biopsy has increased the accuracy for diagnosis and staging. Other examples of endocavitary US applications are in esophageal cancer and for sampling tracheal and subcaronal nodes via transbronchial US detections. Intraoperative approaches at the time of craniotomy for brain tumors and laparotomy for liver nodules, with hepatobiliary techniques are undergoing extensive investigation.

CONCLUSION

As radiology continues to progress in its ability to increase resolution and gain information in noninvasive or minimally invasive forms, such changes must be assessed adequately to insure consistent effectiveness, true contribution to patient care, and the ability to replace or further enhance already existing diagnostic procedures in the oncological patient. Such information can usually only be ascertained through the means of well-controlled, multi-center type studies.

Recommended Reading

There are a recent number of important overviews of oncologic imaging modalities. First, "State of the Art in Oncologic Imaging" by Bragg (Dec. 1989) in *Seminars in Ultrasound, CT, and MR* (10) is a must. Then, the Second Conference on Radioimmunodetection and Radioimmunotherapy of Cancer (Feb. Suppl. 1990 Cancer Research) (4) provides the latest information and is an excellent review both for diagnosis and therapy. Thirdly recommended is a small volume by McGahan (editor) entitled *Interventional Ultrasound* (2).

REFERENCES

General References

1. Imaging in Cancer. American Cancer Society, Inc. New York, NY. 1987.
2. Interventional Ultrasound. John P. McGahan, ed. Baltimore, MD: Williams and Wilkins; 1990.
3. Seminars in Ultrasound, CT and MR. State of the Art Oncologic Imaging. Bragg, D.G. (Guest ed), H. Raymond, W. Zwiebel, H.R. Harnsberger, eds. Vol. 10, No. 6; Dec. 1989.
4. Supplement to Cancer Research. D.M. Goldenberg (ed). Second Conference on Radioimmunodetection and Radioimmunotherapy of Cancer. Vol. 50, No. 3, Feb. 1, 1990.

Specific References

5. Anderson, R.E.; Bragg, D.G.; Youker, J.E. Brain spinal cord neoplasms. In: Bragg, D.G.; Rubin, P.; Youker, J.E., eds. Oncologic imaging. New York: Pergamon Press, Inc.; 1985:23-46.
6. Balfe, D.M.; Heiken, J.P.; McClennan, B.L. Bladder cancer. In: Bragg, D.G.; Rubin, P.; Youker, J.E., eds. Oncologic imaging. New York: Pergamon Press, Inc.; 1985:389-404.
7. Balfe, D.M.; Heiken, J.P.; McClennan, B.L. Prostatic cancer. In: Bragg, D.G.; Rubin, P.; Youker, J.E., eds. Oncologic imaging. New York: Pergamon Press, Inc.; 1985:405-424.
8. Bragg, D.G. Imaging in primary-lung cancer: the roles of detection, staging, and follow-up. Semin. Ultrasound CT and MR 10:453-466; 1989.
9. Bragg, D.G. Imaging strategies for oncologic diagnosis and staging. In: Bragg, D.G.; Rubin, P.; Youker, J.E., eds. Oncologic imaging. New York: Pergamon Press, Inc.; 1985:13-22.
10. Bragg, D.G. State of the art oncological imaging. Semin. Ultrasound CT and MR 10:453-466; 1989.

11. Bragg, D.G.; Dodd, G.D. Imaging in cancer: state of the art. In: Bragg, D.G.; Dodd, G.D., eds. Imaging in cancer. New York: American Cancer Society, Inc.; 1987:3-4.

11a. Bragg, D.G.; Harnsberger, H.R; Thompson, W.M. Radiologic techniques in cancer. In: DeVita, V.T., Hellman, S., Rosenberg, S.A., eds. Principles and practice of oncology. Philadelphia, PA: J.B. Lippincott Co; 1989:440-463.

12. Bree, R.L. Prostate and other transrectally guided biopsies. In: McGahan, J.P., ed. Interventional ultrasound. Baltimore: Williams & Wilkins; 1990.

13. Bret, P.M. Pancreas. In: McGahan, J.P., ed. Interventional ultrasound. Baltimore: Williams & Wilkins; 1990.

14. Chaplin, D.J. Hydraliazine-induced tumor hypoxia: a potential target for cancer chemotherapy. J. Natl. Cancer Inst. 81:618-6232; 1989.

15. Chasen, M.H. Imaging primary lung cancers, pleural cancers, and metastatic disease. In: Bragg, D.G.; Dodd, G.D., eds. Imaging in cancer. New York: American Cancer Society, Inc.; 1987:58-74.

16. Cooperberg, P.; Coret, A.; Ajzen, S. Hepatobiliary techniques.In: McGahan, J.P., ed. Interventional ultrasound. Baltimore: Williams & Wilkins; 1990.

17. Daly, P.F.; Cohen, J.S. Magnetic resonance spectroscopy of tumors and potential *in vivo* clinical applications: a review. Cancer Res. 49:770-779.

18. Davidson, A.J.; Hartman, D.S. Imaging strategies for tumors of the kidney, adrenal gland, and retroperitoneum. In: Bragg, D.G.; Dodd, G.D., eds. Imaging in cancer. New York: American Cancer Society, Inc.; 1987:23-36.

19. Eckelman, W.C. Development of radiochemically pure antibodies. Cancer Res. 50(Suppl.):780s-782s; 1990.

20. Edeiken, J.; Karasick, D. Imaging in bone cancer. In: Bragg, D.G.; Dodd, G.D., eds. Imaging in cancer. New York: American Cancer Society, Inc.; 1987:103-109.

20a. Feinstein, A.R. Clinical Judgement. Huntington, NY. Robert E. Kreiger Publishing Co.; 1974.

21. Fornage, B.D. Interventional ultrasound of the breast. In: McGahan, J.P., ed. Interventional ultrasound. Baltimore: Williams & Wilkins; 1990.

21a. Fossel, E.T.; Carr, J.M.; Mcbonagh, J. Detection of malignant tumors: water suppressed proton nuclear magentic resonance spectroscopy of plasma. New Engl J Med. 315:1369-1376;1986.

22. Halvorsen, R.A. Jr.; Thompson, W.M. Gastrointestinal cancer: diagnosis, staging, and the follow-up role of imaging. Semin. Ultrasound CT and MR 10:467-480; 1989.

23. Harnsberger, H.R.; Dillon W.P. Imaging tumors of the central nervous system and extracranial head and neck. In: Bragg, D.G.; Dodd, G.D., eds. Imaging in cancer. New York: American Cancer Society, Inc.; 1987:89-102.

24. Harnsberger, H.R.; Dillon, W.P. The radiologic role in diagnosis, staging, and follow-up of neoplasia of the brain spine, and head and neck. Semin. Ultrasound CT and MR 10:431-452; 1989.

25. Hendee, W.R. The impact of future technology on oncologic diagnosis. In: Bragg, D.G.; Rubin, P.; Youker, J.E., eds. Oncologic imaging. New York: Pergamon Press, Inc.; 1985:629-644.

26. Joseph, A.; Davenport, C.; Kwock, L.; Furt, C.T.; London, R.E. Fluorine-19 NMR studies of tumor-bearing rats treated with difluoromethylornithine. Mag. Reson. Med. 4:137-143; 1987.

27. Kline, R.W.; Foley, W.D.; Gillin, M.T. Computed tomography and radiation therapy treatment planning. In: Bragg, D.G.; Rubin, P.; Youker, J.E., eds. Oncologic imaging. New York: Pergamon Press, Inc.; 1985:573-586.

28. Knop, R.H.; Carney, D.N.; Chen, C.W.; Cohen, J.S.; Minna, J.D. Levels of high energy phosphates in human lung cancer cell lines by 31P nuclear magnetic spectroscopy. Cancer Res. 47:3357-3359; 1987.

29. Larson, S.M. Clinical radioimmunodetection, 1978-1988: overview and suggestions for standardization of clinical trials. Cancer Res. 50(Suppl.):892s-898s; 1990.

30. Lawson, T.L.; Berland, L.L.; Foley, W.D. Malignant neoplasms of the pancreas, liver, and biliary tract. In: Bragg, D.G.; Rubin, P.; Youker, J.E., eds. Oncologic imaging. New York: Pergamon Press, Inc.; 1985:287-342.

31. Lindell, M.M. Jr.; Wallace, S. Soft tissue tumors of the appendicular skeleton. In: Bragg, D.G.; Rubin, P.; Youker, J.E., eds. Oncologic imaging. New York: Pergamon Press, Inc.; 1985:531-548.

32. Manaster, B.J.; Ensign, M.F. The role of imaging in musculoskeletal tumors. Semin. Ultrasound CT and MR 10:498-517; 1989.

33. Maris, J.M.; Evans, A.E.; McLaughlin, A.C.; D'Angio, G.J.; Bolinger, L.; Manos, H. Chance, B. 31P nuclear magnetic resonance spectroscopic investigation of human neuroblastoma *in situ*. New Engl. J. Med. 312:1500-1505; 1985.

34. McGahan, J.P. Gallbladder. In: McGahan, J.P., ed. Interventional ultrasound. Baltimore: Williams & Wilkins; 1990.

35. McGahan, J.P.; Montalvo, B.M.; Quencer, R.M.; Boggan, J.E. Intraoperative cranial and spinal sonography. In: McGahan, J.P., ed. Interventional ultrasound. Baltimore: Williams & Wilkins; 1990.

36. Milbrath, J.R.; Bragg, D.G.; Youker, J.E. Breast cancer. In: Bragg, D.G.; Rubin, P.; Youker, J.E., eds. Oncologic imaging. New York: Pergamon Press, Inc.; 1985:173-206.

37. Mountford, C.E.; Wright, L.C.; Holmes, K.T.; Mackinnon, W.B.; Gregory, P.; Fox, R.M. High-resolution proton nuclear magnetic resonance analysis of metastatic cancer cells. Science 226:1415-1417; 1984.

38. Mueller-Kleiser, W.; Walenta, S.; Paschen, W.; Kallinowski, F.; and Vaupel, P. Metabolic imaging in microregions of tumors and normal tissues with bioluminescence and photon counting. J. Natl. Cancer Instit. 80:842-848; 1988.

39. Okunieff, P.; Vaupel, P.; Neuringer, L.J. ATPase kinetics in malignant tumors measured by in vivo ^{31}P magnetic resonance spectroscopy. Abstract in Society of Magnetic Resonance in Medicine, San Francisco, CA, Vol. I: 413; 1988.

40. Order, S.E.; Sleeper, A.M.; Stillwagon, G.B.; Klein, J.L.; Leichner, P.K. Radiolabeled antibodies: results and potential in cancer therapy. Cancer Res. 50(Suppl.):1011s-1013s; 1990.

41. Paulus, D.D. Imaging in breast cancer. In: Bragg, D.G.; Dodd, G.D., eds. Imaging in cancer. New York: American Cancer Society, Inc.; 1987:5-22.

42. Rofstad, E.K.; DeMuth, P.; Fenton, B.M.; Sutherland, R.M. ^{31}P nuclear magnetic resonance spectroscopy studies of tumor energy metabolism and its relationship to intracapillary oxyhemoglobin saturation status and tumor hypoxia. Cancer Res. 48:5440-5446; 1988.

43. Sands, H. Experimental studies of radioimmunodetection of cancer: an overview. Cancer Res. 50(Suppl.):809s-813s; 1990.

44. Scheinberg, D.A.; Strand, M. Radioimmunotherapy in experimental animal models: principles derived from models. Cancer Res. 50(Suppl.):962s-963s; 1990.

45. Singer, J.; McClennan, B.L. The diagnosis, staging, and follow-up of carcinomas of the kidney, bladder, and prostate: the role of cross-sectional imaging. Semin. Ultrasound CT and MR 10:481-497; 1989.

46. Siu, A.; Teplitz, R.L. Fine needle aspiration/cytology for invasive ultrasound techniques. In: McGahan, J.P., ed. Interventional Ultrasound. Baltimore: Williams & Wilkins; 1990.

47. Smith, J.; Bragg, D.G. Tumors of the skeletal system. In: Bragg, D.G.; Rubin, P.; Youker, J.E., eds. Oncologic imaging. New York: Pergamon Press, Inc.; 1985:501-530.

48. Stark, P. Imaging mediastinal tumors. In: Bragg, D.G.; Dodd, G.D., eds. Imaging in cancer. New York: American Cancer Society, Inc.; 1987:75-88.

49. Steen, R.G. Response of solid tumors to chemotherapy monitored by in vivo ^{31}P nuclear magnetic resonance spectroscopy: a review. Cancer Res. 49:4075-4085; 1989.

50. Steen, R.G.; Tamargo, R.J.; McGovern, K.A.; Rajan, S.S.; Brem, H.; Wehrle, J.P.; Glickson, J.D. *In vivo* ^{31}P nuclear magnetic resonance spectroscopy of subcutaneous 9L gliosarcoma: effects of tumor growth and treatment with 1,3-bis(2-chloroethyl)-1-nitrosourea on tumor bioenergetics and histology. Cancer Res. 48:676-681; 1988.

51. Thompson, W.M. Esophageal cancer. In: Bragg, D.G.; Rubin, P.; Youker, J.E., eds. Oncologic imaging. New York: Pergamon Press, Inc.; 1985:207-242.

52. Thompson, W.M. Imaging strategies for tumors of the gastrointestinal system. In: Bragg, D.G.; Dodd, G.D., eds. Imaging in cancer. New York: American Cancer Society, Inc.; 1987:37-57.

53. Wallace, S.; Carrasco, C.H.; Charnsangavej, C.; Zornoza, J.; Chuang, V.P. Contributions of interventional radiology to diagnosis and management of the cancer patient. In: Bragg, D.G.; Rubin, P.; Youker, J.E., eds. Oncologic imaging. New York: Pergamon Press, Inc.; 1985:587-628.

54. Wong, W.S.; Goldberg, H.I. Gastric, small bowel, and colorectal cancer. In: Bragg, D.G.; Rubin, P.; Youker, J.E., eds. Oncologic imaging. New York: Pergamon Press, Inc.; 1985:243-286.

Lowell A. Goldsmith, M.D., Medical Oncology   Stephen E. Presser, M.D., Surgical Oncology
Elethea H. Caldwell, M.D., Surgical Oncology   Philip Rubin, M.D., Radiation Oncology

Chapter **16**

SKIN CANCER

On the window seat there stood a geranium diseased with yellow blotches, which had overspread all its leaves. Aylmer poured a small quantity of the liquid upon the soil in which it grew. In a little time, when the roots of the plant had taken up the moisture, the unsightly blotches began to be extinguished in a living verdure.

Nathaniel Hawthorne (25)

PERSPECTIVE

Skin tumors are visible to the naked eye of both patient and physician. Skin cancer is an excellent model for early diagnosis, prevention, and treatment of cancer. Sunlight, predominantly the UVB (290 to 320 nm) spectrum, is the major identified cause of skin cancer. Although there may be 300,000 to more than 600,000 skin cancers detected annually, the death rate from skin cancer is low—approximately 3,800 cases per year for nonmelanoma skin cancers. Most skin cancers can be treated on an outpatient basis and most are preventable. Malignant melanoma and lymphomas involving the skin, especially cutaneous T-cell lymphoma (mycosis fungoides) and malignant fibrous tumors of the skin are beyond the scope of this chapter.

EPIDEMIOLOGY AND ETIOLOGY

Epidemiology

1. Basal and squamous cell carcinomas (SCC) are the most common types of malignant skin disease. Basal cell carcinomas (BCC) is much more common than SCC.
2. Actinic keratoses (solar keratoses) are extremely common and only a tiny percent of them progress to frank neoplasia (35). Approximately 300,000 to 600,000 new BCC and SCC occur annually (4). Incidence rates in the United States are shown in Table 16-1 (27).
3. The annual death rate from skin cancer (nonmelanoma) is 3,800 cases (4).
4. Those of Celtic background, such as the Irish and Scottish, are highly prone to skin cancer. Individuals with type I skin (always burn; never tan) are a group at a very high risk for skin cancer. Nonmelanoma UV-related skin cancer is extremely rare in blacks; however, skin cancer in burn scars or atrophic skin lesions is as common in blacks as in whites.
5. The relative distributions of BCC and SCC according to site are shown in Fig. 16-1 (12).

Etiology

Sun Damage

This major cause of skin cancer has been known for some time. The UVB spectrum (290 to 320 nm) is the major carcinogenic wavelength both clinically and experimentally (58). There is an increase in sun-caused cancer, especially in BCC, as one approaches the latitudes of the equator. Sun-induced skin cancers are more prevalent on light-exposed areas of the body, for instance dorsal of the hands, and face, especially the nose. Occupations (e.g., farmers or sailors) with high sun exposure have an increased incidence of BCC and SCC. Depigmented areas of vitiligo have increased susceptibility to skin cancers, and genetic disorders of melanization, such as albinism, make one prone to skin cancers. Ozone absorbs UVB light from the sun. With destruction of the ozone layer through fluorinated hydrocarbons it is hypothesized that skin cancer may increase dramatically over the next several decades. In addition to direct carcinogenic effects, UVB affects local and systemic immune function in the skin and systemically (32).

Table 16-1. Histological Classification of Skin Tumors

Tumor Type	Incidence (%)
Basal cell carcinoma	
1. Superficial multicentric type	
2. Morphea type	75-90
3. Fibroepithelial	
Squamous cell carcinoma	
1. Adenoid squamous cell carcinoma	
2. Spindle-cell type	10-20
Metatypical	
Sweat gland tumors and related lesions	
Sebaceous gland tumors	
Tumors of hair follicle	
Paget's disease	
Undifferentiated carcinoma	<1
Cysts	
Tumor-like lesions	
Unclassified	

From World Health Organization (27) with permission.

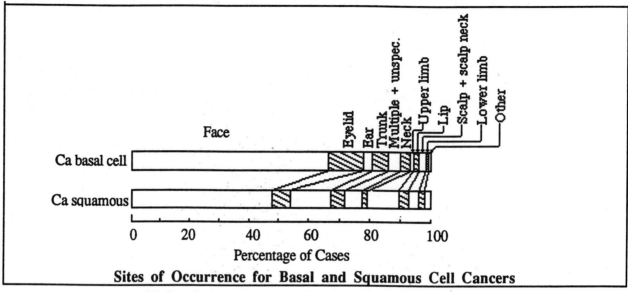

Fig. 16-1. Sites of occurrence for basal and squamous cell Skin cancers.

Genetics

Skin cancer is increased in a disorder of DNA repair, xeroderma pigmentosum (30). Basal cell nevus syndrome, another rare inherited disorder, has an increased incidence of BCC (30). Albinism has increased skin cancer risk due to decreased melanin.

Atrophic Skin Lesions

Skin diseases with chronic ulcerations and atrophic skin are situations in which skin cancer will arise (50). In burn scars, these malignancies are called Marjolin's ulcer. Skin diseases with atrophy, such as cutaneous tuberculosis, lupus erythematosus, and lichen planus, all may lead to SCC.

Chemical Carcinogenesis

Although not confirmed in animal research, arsenical exposure from pesticides or agricultural sprays and from increased arsenic in the drinking water is associated with increased skin cancers (57). Coal tar from industrial exposures (such as scrotal skin in chimney sweeps, first described by Percivall Pott in 1775) are situations where there are increased incidences of skin cancers (55).

Radiation Exposure

Radiation exposure is associated with increased incidence of skin cancers, including SCC, Bowen's disease (SCC in situ), and BCCs (51). Ionizing radiation, which was used previously to treat acne or tinea capitis, results in tumors about the head and neck; history of x-ray exposure should be sought.

Immunosuppression

Immunosuppression is associated with increased incidence of skin cancers (13). Immunosuppression may be the result of infection with human immunovirus; it is also commonly related to drugs used during transplantation. Multiple lesions and frequent local recurrence are common; most lesions are on sun-exposed areas. Papillomavirus may have a role in inducing skin cancers in these individuals.

Papillomavirus

Papillomavirus, especially in genital mucosa, is recognized as an etiologic agent in SCC (9), and has been found in skin malignancies (40).

DETECTION AND DIAGNOSIS

Clinical Detection

General examination of the skin. The patient should be completely disrobed and examined under good lighting so that all portions of the skin may be seen. Most skin cancers will occur on the trunk, head and neck, and arms. Skin examination should be preceded by a history, so that the presence of scars, burns, or previous irradiation have been considered. A five to ten times magnifying loop helps discern small, subtle skin lesions and aids in their characterization.

General Signs

These may be divided into early and subtle findings and later findings.

1. Early signs include:
   * small papule with telangiectasia
   * area of firmness and induration of the skin
   * small areas of irregular keratosis and scaling
2. Later signs include:
   * loss of skin markings
   * pinpoint or more diffuse changes in pigmentation, including hyperpigmentation
   * regular, heaped-up hyperkeratotic areas
3. Very late signs include:
   * lesions that ulcerate
   * persistent ulcerations with heaped-up border

In the nail bed there may be lesions that lead to destruction of the nail plate.

Premalignant Lesions

The borderline between malignancy and benignity is at times unclear both clinically and pathologically.

Actinic keratosis. A very common lesion is the actinic (solar) keratosis. These are usually multiple, red and rough ("grain of sand" quality) papules 1 to 3 mm in diameter and tend to be on sun-exposed areas, especially the dorsal of the hand, face, neck, and nose. It is debatable how frequently these lesions are truly premalignant (35), though the skin in which they occur is a common site for malignancy. The approach to these lesions, when they are actually atypical, may be treated as described below, but if there is any question of their malignancy or if they are extremely heaped up, a biopsy is required.

Arsenical keratoses. These are usually associated with a definite history of exposure to nonorganic arsenic which was present either in the drinking water or related to agricultural exposure (57). They are multiple, regular hyperkeratotic lesions on the palms and soles. These are accentuated on pressure areas. On the back, there may be irregular hyperpigmentation and hypopigmentation. They are associated with BCC and SCC.

Benign Lesions

Multiple benign lesions occur in the skin, many of which do not need a biopsy for diagnosis.

Seborrheic keratosis. These are flesh-colored to brownish lesions, well delineated from the surrounding skin, with a slightly irregular, nonshiny surface. The lesions may get irritated when caught or scratched. The lesion often appears to be stuck on to the skin. Biopsy is usually not necessary for diagnosis.

Warts. Warts are common lesions present at all ages. Small thrombosed capillaries can be seen and lesions may be hyperkeratotic or may have a filiform characteristic with multiple fronds being present; may have to be biopsied for definitive diagnosis.

Bowenoid papulosis. These are papillomavirus-induced lesions frequently in the genital area (9). They may be flesh-colored or somewhat brown.

Appendegeal lesions. A variety of epidermal appendages are associated with benign tumors. These include trichoepitheliomas from hair follicles and various sweat gland and vascular tumors. Biopsy is often needed for definitive diagnosis.

Malignant Skin Lesions (Table 16-1)

1. BCC is the most common skin malignancy (24,38,44,49). It starts as a painless, translucent, pearly nodule with telangiectasia on a sun-exposed area. It is clinically difficult, if not impossible, to diagnose accurately these tumors when they are less than 4 mm. As this tumor enlarges, it ulcerates and bleeds and has a rolled, shiny border. Since these are predominantly sun-induced, they commonly occur in photo-exposed areas such as the face. It is rare for these to metastasize. The morphea-like version may appear as a firm scar and not appear raised. The superficial type is plaque-like and could be mistaken for a persistent area of dermatitis.

2. SCC can be recognized as a red, irregular hyperkeratotic tumor (10,43). Later these tumors ulcerate and crust. Clinical diagnosis from a hyperplastic actinic keratosis can be challenging and requires biopsy confirmation. These occur in sun-exposed areas such as the head and neck and dorsal upper extremities. One to two percent of SCC can metastasize to local lymph nodes.

The prognosis is worse for SCC arising in chronically damaged skin (e.g., burn scars, lupus) or neglected, large, and/or recurrent lesions.

3. Keratoacanthoma is a hyperkeratotic tumor that clinically and histopathologically resembles SCC (46). The history, however, often is that of an abrupt (few weeks) onset instead of the chronic history of a SCC. Some authorities classify keratoacanthoma as a low-grade type of SCC, whereas others consider it a benign hair follicle derivative. Histopathology can help to differentiate a keratoacanthoma from a SCC although there are many debatable cases.

4. Bowen's disease usually appears as a single plaque with a definitive red and scaly border. The lesions are usually 1 to 3 cm and show no evidence of regression. There has been extensive discussion whether this lesion is associated with internal malignancy; most studies suggest that it is not. Biopsies are necessary for definitive diagnosis.

5. Paget's disease usually appears as a single plaque, usually on the nipple or in the genital area. The plaque may be red, slightly scaly and may be pigmented. This may be confused with eczematous dermatitis and biopsy is required for definitive diagnosis.

6. Verrucous carcinoma is a type of SCC that clinically appears wartlike, ulcerated, and fungating with sinus tracts (14). The soles are commonly affected. The history very often is that of a wart unresponsive to treatment that on biopsy shows marked atypia. Historically, depending on the location, this entity has been called epithelioma cuniculatum on the soles, condyloma acuminatum of Buschke-Lowenstein on the genitalia and laryngeal papillomatosis in the larynx.

7. Merkel's cell tumor starts as an asymptomatic nodule on the sun-exposed areas of the head and neck of an elderly individual (18,48). Definitive diagnosis is made by the electron microscopic demonstration of neurosecretory dense core granules or by immunohistochemical demonstration of neuron-specific enolase, a marker of amine precursor uptake and decarboxylation cells.

8. Skin metastases from primaries not in the skin can present as single to multiple bluish nodules and tumors. Histopathology, patient history, and tumor work-up are helpful in revealing the source of skin metastases.

Metastases from Skin Malignancies

The incidence of metastatic BCC is extremely low, reported as less than 0.1%. If metastasis occurs, it is usually to lymph nodes, lung, and bone. Lymphangiectatic and hematogenous spread occurs with equal frequency (54). Chemotherapy has been used. Distant metastases occur only when very advanced and favor the lung.

1. Regional lymph node metastases occur from SCC in 1% to 2% of patients. If the primary lesion occurs in the extremities, the prognosis is significantly poorer; there is a 5-year survival rate of 35% despite prompt node dissection (8,16). Squamous cell tumors in other areas such as scalp, ears, and nostril carry a high incidence of metastases (17,20,47). In a recent large series of 339

cases of skin cancer, Lovett *et al.* (34a) reported a 0.4% incidence of positive lymph nodes in BCC, a 15% incidence of positive lymph nodes for SCC, and a 39% incidence of recurrent SCC.

2. A lesion of special etiology, Marjolin's ulcer, also known as burn scar carcinoma, now includes SCCs arising in areas of previous trauma. The latent period from time of injury to onset of SCC varies with age. The younger the patient, the longer the latent period (34). The lesions are frequently slow-growing, but if recurrence occurs, they tend to metastasize rapidly. Wide local excision and regional node dissection is required. Burn scar carcinoma has shown a 34.8% incidence of nodal metastases (41). The aggressive nature of these tumors has led to consideration of a compromised immunologic barrier to these tumors (11).

Diagnostic Procedures

Excisional Biopsies

Excisional biopsy is undertaken in most cases with the goal of complete removal of the tumor with adequate surgical margins for cure. It is both a diagnostic and therapeutic procedure. The size of the lesion and the anatomic location of the lesion are important determinates in making the decision of whether a biopsy should be incisional for diagnosis only or excisional for both diagnosis and definitive treatment. If excisional biopsy is chosen, the issue of pathologic versus surgical margins should be considered. Abide *et al.* (6) address the question of adequate surgical margins and what is meant by the pathologist and surgeon when they refer to "close to the margin" or "all margins free of tumor." The authors postulate that the more completely a surgical margin is examined, the higher the correlation between presence or absence of tumor and subsequent cure. Abide *et al.* (6) recommend lateral margins of 5 mm when performing an excisional biopsy of a BCC.

Data regarding adequate margins for excisional biopsy of a SCC are less clear. It has been stated that as SCCs increase in size, high cure rates become more difficult to achieve because other margins become excessive (Cottel, WI, unpublished data, 1986).

Incisional Biopsies (56)

Incisional biopsy is performed with the goal of sampling only a part of the lesion. This may be done if:

1. The lesion is very large.
2. The lesion is benign and/or located in a cosmetically important place (e.g., nose).

The incisional biopsy may be:

1. Parallel incisional biopsy. A scalpel is used to incise in a horizontal plane. This is commonly done for BCC and SCC. It will not be useful in diagnosing a keratoacanthoma, as the "lips" of this lesion are needed for diagnosis.
2. Punch biopsy. A circular knife of 3 to 4 mm diameter may be used. A punch biopsy will not afford a certain diagnosis of a keratoacanthoma and if done for a BCC will make it difficult to adequately treat the BCC by curettage.

Special Diagnostic Techniques

Immunoperoxidase staining techniques can be helpful to diagnose certain tumors when standard (hemotoxylin and eosin) slides alone are not sufficient to make the diagnosis. Markers for keratin, CEA (carcinoembryonic antigen), and S-100 protein (of neural crest origin, such as melanoma) are available. This is most helpful for a histopathologically undifferentiated spindle cell tumor in which the diagnosis of a SCC or melanoma will dictate treatment and prognosis.

CLASSIFICATION AND STAGING

The anatomic staging for skin cancer is illustrated in Table 16-2 (12,28) and Fig. 16-2. This applies mainly to BCC and SCC of the skin. The current *American Joint Committee for Cancer Staging, 3rd ed.* (1a) and *International Union Against Cancer, 4th ed.* (28) of the classification of cancer are the same in context but differ from previous editions. The tumor (T) categories have been minimally modified and the node (N) categories are simply negative (N0) or positive (N1). However, differences exist as the stage grouping is largely based on clinical examination since this is a surface lesion. The T stage determines the group. T4 advanced and deeply invading cancer is equivalent to N1, which is equivalent to metastastic cancer.

PRINCIPLES OF TREATMENT

Multidisciplinary Decisions: Choice of Therapy (7)

The physician has a varied armamentarium to treat BCC and SCC and should not treat every skin cancer on every patient in the same way (Table 16-3). Treatment can be custom-tailored based on the following:

- size
- location
- aggressiveness of the tumor (based on histopathology)
- primary tumor versus recurrent or multiple recurrent tumor
- patient's life-style and preference
- patient's suitability for surgery

The treatment goals of BCC and SCC are to eradicate the local disease and to achieve the best functional and aesthetic results. In general, with well-trained physicians cure rates are in the 90% to 99% range using different treatment modalities. All these forms of treatment have their place; the variables of size, anatomic location, histologic character, and

Table 16-2. TNM Classification and Stage Grouping of Skin Carcinoma

TNM Classification		Stage Grouping			
T1	≤ 2 cm	Stage 0	Tis	N0	M0
T2	> 2 to 5 cm	Stage I	T1	N0	M0
T3	> 5 cm	Stage II	T2	N0	M0
T4	Deep extradermal structures		T3	N0	M0
	(cartilage, skeletal muscle,	Stage III	T4	N0	M0
	bone)		Any T	N1	M0
N1	Regional	Stage IV	Any T	Any N	M1

T = Tumor; N = node; M = metastasis.
From AJC/UICC (1a, 28), with permission.

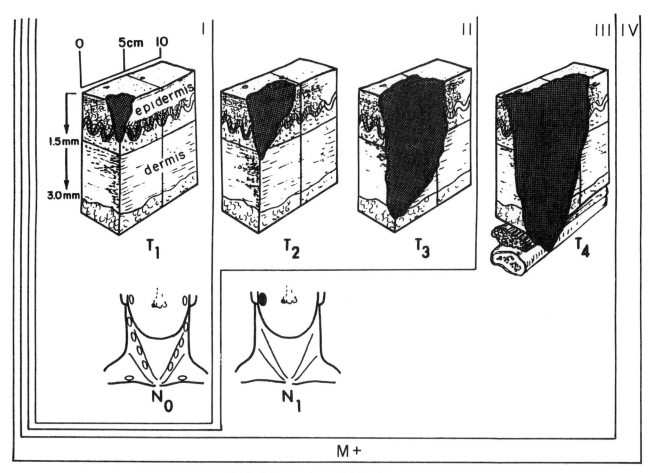

Fig. 16-2. Anatomic staging for skin cancer.

whether the lesions are primary or recurrent must be considered. However, practical considerations of patient convenience and the location of the lesion often affect treatment choice.

Surgery offers, in addition to a high cure rate, the opportunity of treating the patient with a single procedure in a short time. It provides good functional and aesthetic results and allows the opportunity to confirm histologically that adequate surgical margins have been obtained using excisional surgery. Curettage and discretion give good results but there is no histologic confirmation, as margins are usually not performed.

Small tumors (< 1 cm) in nonfacial locations and selected facial locations (excluding ears, nose, periorbital area) do well with curettage, excision with side-to-side closure, radiation therapy, or cryotherapy.

Radiotherapy offers similar advantages, but requires histologic confirmation before irradiation of the lesion is undertaken. It also requires multiple visits for the patient to complete treatment. If bone, cartilage, or tendon are involved at the time of initial treatment, most agree that radiotherapy should not be used for fear of radionecrosis. Radiation therapy is a good choice for elderly, nonsurgical candidates.

Mohs' surgery may be a lengthy procedure requiring special skills in preparing and interpreting the histologic sections. A second surgeon may be needed to carry out the reconstructive procedure after the tumor has been removed

Table 16-3. Multidisciplinary Treatment Decisions: Skin Cancer (3a,42a)

Stage	Surgery	Radiation Therapy	Chemotherapy
I $T_1N_0M_0$	Excision or Mohs' technique	CRT 3 Gy x 15 fx=45 Gy/3 wk	NR
II $T_2N_0M_0$	Mohs' technique	CRT 2.5 Gy x 20 fx=50 Gy/4 wk 2.0 Gy x 30 fx=60 Gy/6 wk	NR
III $T_3N_1M_0$	Mohs' technique	CRT 2.0 Gy x 30-35 fx=60-70 Gy/6-7 wk	NR
IV	Excision if possible	PRT if feasible	IC II

CRT = curative; IC II = investigational chemotherapy, phase I/II clinical trials; NR = not recommended; PRT = palliative; RT = radiation therapy. PDQ: NR

by the Mohs' surgeon. The Mohs' surgeon may allow the wound to heal by secondary intention.

Mohs' surgery is definitely indicated in the setting of recurrent BCC, large SCCs with ill-defined borders; in critical locations such as eyelids, where maximum preservation of uninvolved tissue is required; and sites such as periorbital, perinasal, and nasal, where recurrence rates are high. For recurrent or histologically aggressive malignancies (morpheaform, micronodular, or infiltrative BCC, perineural SCC or undifferentiated SCC), histologic margin control should be considered. Microscopically controlled Mohs' surgical excision should be considered when treating:

- recurrent cancers
- histologically aggressive cancers
- anatomic sites with potentially high recurrence rates (nose, ears, temples, periorbital area)
- anatomic sites where tissue preservation is most important (genitalia, nose, periorbital area)
- cancers with clinically ill-defined borders

Surgery

Excisional Surgery

After the limits of involvement of the lesion have been established, the limits of excision must be planned to include an adequate margin of normal tissue. In soft tissues, palpation of the surrounding tissue is helpful in assessing involvement. Immediate confirmation of marginal involvement can be obtained by frozen section examination. It is essential that the specimen be correctly oriented and clearly marked before being examined by the pathologist. Many pathologists prefer to examine the area of excision in the operating room for orientation prior to microscopic examination.

After the tumor is removed, repair must be planned. Some defects may be closed primarily, others will require complex reconstructive techniques to prevent or minimize disfiguring defects.

Timing of reconstruction in complex defects is influenced by the location of the defect and by whether the tumor is a primary or recurrent lesion. At present, most plastic surgeons feel that it is appropriate and in the patient's best interest to carry out repairs at the time of the ablative surgery. However, four categories of patients should be defined when discussing timing of repair:

- immediate repair mandatory
- immediate repair contraindicated
- immediate repair desirable
- secondary intention healing appropriate

Immediate repair is mandatory when vital structures are exposed. Such structures include brain, bone, cartilage, major vessels, or nerves. Primary closure, skin grafts, local flaps, and distant flaps may be used.

Immediate repair is contraindicated when adequacy of excision of margins cannot be determined with certainty or when technical difficulties place the patient at risk. The defect may be covered temporarily with a split-thickness skin graft or skin and mucosa may be closed primarily. Primary healing is used even if definitive repair is not possible.

Immediate repair is desirable if one is reasonably certain complete excision of the tumor has been achieved and if severe deformity or functional disturbance has resulted from the surgical resection. Other factors to be considered are age and

life expectancy of the patient, natural history of the tumor, physical and psychologic fitness of the patient, technical difficulties of primary repair, and the ability of the patient to cope with the deformity (21).

Curettage Surgery (29)

A curette (circular or oval cutting blade) is used to excise the tumor by an experienced clinician via a scraping technique. This method has been successfully used by dermatologists for more than 50 years. The curettage and electrodesiccation is performed three times at the same surgical session. The electrodesiccation itself, pressure, or chemical cautery is used for hemostasis. The surgical sites heal by secondary intention over 3 to 4 weeks without difficulty. There is usually scarring.

Mohs' Surgery (Microscopically Controlled Surgical Excision) (39,52)

Mohs' microscopically controlled surgery is named after general surgeon Frederick Mohs, who developed this technique more than 50 years ago. The tumor is excised with a scalpel and the margins are meticulously examined by the Mohs' surgeon, who serves both as pathologist and surgeon. Unlike standard histopathologic evaluation, the tumor is evaluated using multiple (many times over 50) horizontal microscopic sections. This is much more accurate than the traditional "bread loaf" technique which is subject to sampling error that results in false-negative margins. The Mohs' surgeon accurately maps out any positive deep and/or peripheral margins that require conservative re-excision. This re-excision results in continued meticulous microscopic evaluation and mapping until the margins are truly tumor-free. The minimum amount of normal tissue is excised using this method. The defect can then be sutured by an appropriate technique, or if not adjacent to an orifice (with a free margin), could heal by secondary intention. Secondary intention healing should be considered for large defects in the elderly, concave, level, or small convex defects, and in the fair-skinned patient. The technique described above, is the fresh tissue. The fixed-tissue technique (using zinc chloride) is rarely used today and is mainly of historic interest. Currently, there are about 200 Mohs' surgeons practicing in the United States.

Cryotherapy (23) and Lasers

Cryotherapy or cold therapy uses liquid nitrogen to create cold injury to the tumor and its periphery. The tumor is usually curetted for gross clinical margins prior to treatment with liquid nitrogen. An eschar forms and healing occurs by secondary intention. This form of therapy requires controlled freezing and specialized training. Liquid nitrogen therapy as used for warts, actinic keratosis, and seborrheic keratosis is inappropriate for the treatment of BCC or SCC. This technique is rarely favored and is confined to very small lesions and the elderly, debilitated patients (42a).

The carbon dioxide laser is a cutting tool with the advantage of producing hemostasis of small vessels while cutting. It has the advantage of keeping blood loss to a minimum.

Radiotherapy (12,26a,46)

Properly delivered, radiation treatment produces results comparable with those of surgery, with excellent cosmesis. It is essential to carefully palpate the margins of the lesion and provide a margin of 10 to 15 mm around the lesion for microspread, depending on the original size. All cancers should be treated in a customized fashion with special, cut-out, individualized lead shields and not with standard cones unless they perfectly fit the cancer outline plus a margin. If the excisional biopsy shows inadequate tumor margins, radiotherapy can be used. Radiation treatment might also be used in locations such as eyelids, ala and tip of the nose, and where surgical excision would involve extensive reconstructive surgery. Radiotherapy alone is usually contraindicated if the malignancy involves bone and cartilage; the hand, where preservation of fingers should be attempted, is the exception.

Radiation is often given in a highly fractionated schedule (e.g., a total dose of 4,500 cGy is given in 3 weeks in 300 cGy daily fractions with attention to shielding) (15), which is particularly the case in lesions overlying cartilage (ears and nose) and bone (in and about forehead and scalp). This long treatment process may be unacceptable to some patients. Shorter schedules in which equivalent doses are given in 1 to 2 weeks produce less satisfactory cosmesis, but may be used in elderly patients.

When bone and cartilage are deeply invaded, a combined approach of preoperative irradiation and surgery is often successful, particularly for extensive SCC about the ear and mastoid tip. Radiation therapy alone in this circumstance is rarely effective, and surgery is always preferable. The failure rate is usually high in deeply invading basal cell lesions, and although salvage by surgery is possible, recurrences may follow. Radiation therapy is contraindicated for patients with xeroderma pitmentosum, epidemodysplasia verruciformis, or the basal cell nevus syndrome because it may induce more tumors in the treatment area (42a).

Late radionecrosis with painful ulceration and failure of re-epithelialization can usually be avoided by proper fractionation during a course of radiation therapy.

Chemotherapy and Other Pharmaceuticals

Topical Fluouracil: 5-FU has been used for actinic keratoses with good success. By removing these lesions it may allow earlier detection of BCC and SCC in actinically damaged skin. It has an extremely limited role in the cure of Bowen's disease and superficial BCC. It should never be used to treat nodular BCC. It is used as a clinical diagnostic tool to define the clinical margins of an ill-defined skin cancer and has been injected to treat keratoacanthomas. Careful and prolonged follow-up is required, since deep follicular portions of the tumor may escape treatment and result in future tumor recurrence (3a).

Systemic Retinoids: Although several clinical trials have shown some efficacy for currently available systemic retinoids in both chemotherapy and chemoprevention, the long-term toxicity of these agents generally excludes them as treatment choices for most patients (34').

Alpha Interferon: Several early studies have shown variable responses of basal cell carcinoma to interlesional alpha interferon (23).

RESULTS AND PROGNOSIS

Local Control and Survival

The control of skin cancers by either surgery or chemotherapy is excellent if lesions are detected early and are small (i.e., <1 to 2 cm) (11a, 34a). Overall cancer control is 86%;

BCC is 91%, and SCC is 75%. For cancers less than 1 cm, 97% of BCC and 91% of SCC remain controlled. For larger lesions (1 to 5 cm), 87% of BCC and 76% of SCC are ablated. Excellent cosmesis is reflected in results: the complication rate was 5% overall and depended on tumor size (34a).

Primary Tumors

Most skin cancers are highly curable and both surgery and radiation therapy provide excellent cosmesis. Results are comparable with either modality (Table 16-4).

1. Surgery (Table 16-4): The 5-year cure rates are better than 90% for different techniques such as curettage, electrocoagulation, cold knife surgery, and chemosurgery (Mohs'). The latter two techniques have the advantage of histologic control of margins.
2. Radiation therapy (Table 16-4). The 5-year cure rates range from 92% to 100%. BCCs tend to be more curable than SCC.

Recurrences (33,37)

1. Recurrent skin cancer is more difficult to cure than primary skin cancer.
2. The recurrence rate for primary BCC is 5% to 10%. When BCCs are less than 1 cm, the recurrence rate approaches zero. Certain regions of the body, such as the nose and nasal labial folds, are more prone to recurrences, possibly related to their being at the sites of embryonic fusion planes. SCC has a recurrence rate of 20% to 25%.
3. Involved margins (19,42): The clinical management of positive residual margins for BCC remains controversial although many surgeons will re-excise. Data show that with follow-up for a 5-year period, one third of these tumors recur. If the following conditions exist, re-excision of BCC should be highly considered:
   - patient is not reliable
   - tumor is histopathologically aggressive or recurrent
   - tumor is near a vital structure (ear canal, eye)
   - positive margin is deep, rather than peripheral

   A 5-year probability of remaining relapse-free with incompletely excised basal cell cancers is approximately 90% if treated immediately, versus 61% if managed expectantly, according to Liu *et al.* (34'). Deep margins are of greatest concern since 33% fail versus 17% in lateral margins. Salvage is excellent in relapsed patients with 85% controlled by surgery or irradiation. Their 10-year outcomes are similar for each approach—more than 90% local control.
4. Positive margins of SCC: SCC with positive margins always should be re-excised because of the potential risk, albeit small, of metastasis. Skin cancer is best eradicated on the first treatment and the type of surgery and/or irradiation should be chosen with this in mind.

Cosmesis

Cosmesis is as important as local control since these cancers are highly curable. Depending on whether the lesion is primary or recurrent, and the size is 3 cm or less in diameter, cosmesis is good to excellent. Only large skin cancers (i.e., >3 cm and certainly > 5 cm) in diameter yield poor cosmesis (34a).

Table 16-4. Control of Malignant Skin Lesions with Radiation Therapy: Hahnemann University Experience, 1960–1980

From Crissey, JT: Curettage and electrodessication as a method of treatment for epitheliomas of the skin. J Surg Oncol 3:287, 1978. Copyright © 1978 J Surg Oncol. Reprinted by permission of Wiley-Liss, A Division of John Wiley and Sons, Inc.			(12) Control of Malignant Skin Lesions with Radiation Therapy: Hahnemann University Experience, 1960-1980	
Five-Year Cure Rate for Carcinomas of the Skin				
Method	Number of Lesions	Cure Rate (%)	Diagnosis	NED*, 4+ Years (%)
Curettage and electrocoagulation	1,400	92.6	Basal cell carcinoma	426/444 (95.9)
Cold knife surgery	4,628	95.5	Squamous cell carcinoma	144/156 (92.3)
Radiation therapy	3,228	94.7	Keratoacanthoma	12/12 (100)
Chemosurgery (Mohs') Overall rate	4,858	99.1		

* No evidence of disease

Retreatment

Irradiation failure always will be treated with a surgical approach (e.g., excision or Mohs). Surgical failures may be treated with irradiation.

Sun Protection

Instituting a sun-protection program in childhood and then maintaining it on a life-long basis could prevent all sun-induced skin cancer. Sun protection is still valuable when begun at any age.

CLINICAL INVESTIGATIONS

Photodynamic Therapy

The accessibility of skin tumors to the external environment has made them a focus for photodynamic therapy in which a porphyrin derivative, usually hematoporphyrin, is first given to the patient and the patient is exposed to high-intensity light which will be absorbed by the porphyrin (36). These therapies will be most useful in patients with basal cell nevus syndrome with malignant skin tumors.

Interferons

Interferons have been tried for local therapy in BCC (23). Injections with interferon over several weeks lead to a permanent regression of BCC. If therapy could be modified so that individuals responded to a limited number of intramuscular injections of interferon, this therapy could radically change the approach to skin cancers, since patients could be treated in an extremely early stage of progression.

Retinoids

Two systemic retinoids are approved by the Food and Drug Administration for other diseases. Accutane is approved for treatment of acne and Etretinate for treatment of psoriasis. Systemic retinoids are able to prevent or retard the appearance of skin cancers in those with genetic propensity to skin malignancy, basal cell nevus syndrome, or xeroderma pigmentosum (31). Trials using retinoids as a preventative at low doses are in progress to determine the effect of decreasing the recurrence of BCC in individuals with these diseases. As retinoids become a major therapeutic agent in medicine, this will be an extremely exciting area of research to follow.

Hyperthermia Combined with Radiation Therapy

Hyperthermia is a new modality (described in detail in Chapter 7, "Basic Concepts of Radiation Physics") in which tumors are heated to temperatures of 42° to 45°C, enhancing the response to irradiation and certain drugs, such as cisplatin. It has proven effective in controlling skin recurrences in breast cancer which mainly involve the chest wall. The investigation of combined approaches using hyperthermia is a promising field of research for extensive malignancies of the skin, either primary tumors, recurrences, or metastases.

Recommended Reading

An excellent introductory book on skin cancer that provides an understanding of the process of carcinogenesis and diagnosis is by Conti et al. (2a). The standard oncology textbooks have fine chapters devoted to skin cancers with thorough descriptions of surgical and radiotherapeutic techniques; these include "Skin", a chapter by Solan et al. (49a) in Perez and Brady's *Principles and Practice of Radiation Oncology* and Patterson's chapter in DeVita et al. (42').

REFERENCES

General References

1. Ackerman, L.V.; del Regato, J.A. Cancer: diagnosis, treatment, and prognosis. St. Louis, MO: C.V. Mosby, Co.; 1977.
1a. American Joint Committee on Cancer Staging and End Results Reporting. Manual for Staging of Cancer, 3rd ed. Philadelphia, PA : J.B. Lippincott, Co.; 1988.
2. Clark, R.L. Introduction to the 7th annual clinical conference. M.D. Anderson Hospital and Tumor Institute. In: Cumley, R.W.; McCay, J.; Aldridge, D.; et al., eds. Tumors of the skin. Chicago, Ill.; Year Book Medical Publishers; 1964:10.
2a. Conti, C.J.; Slaga, T.J.; Klein-Szanto, A.J.P. eds. Carcinogenesis: A comprehensive survey. Skin Tumors: Experimental and Clinical Aspects. New York, NY: Raven Press; 1989.
2b. del Regato, J.A.; Spjut, H.J.; Cox, J.D. (eds) Ackerman and del Regato's Cancer: Diagnosis, Treatment and Prognosis, 6th ed. St. Louis, MO: C.V. Mosby Co.; 1985.
3. MacComb, W.B.; Fletcher, G.H. Cancer of the head and neck. Baltimore, MD: Williams & Wilkins; 1967.
3a. Schwartz, R.A.: Skin Cancer: Recognition and Management. New York, NY: Springer-Verlag; 1988.
4. Silverberg E: Cancer statistics. Cancer 38:5022; 1988.
5. Symposium on Neoplasms of the Skin. M.D. Anderson Hospital. Chicago, Ill: Year Book Medical Publishers; 1962.

Specific References

6. Abide, J.M.; Nahai, F.; Bennett, R.G. The meaning of surgical margins. Plast. Reconstr. Surg. 73:492-496; 1984.

7. Albright, S.D. Treatment of skin cancer using multiple modalities. J. Am. Acad. Dermatol. 7:143-171; 1982.

8. Ames, F.C.; Hickey, R.C. Squamous cell carcinoma of the skin of the extremities. Intl. Adv. Surg. Oncol. 3:179-199; 1980.

9. Barrasso, R.; DeBrux, J.; Croissant, O.; Orth, G. High prevalence of papillomavirus-associated penile intraepithelial neoplasia in sexual partners of women with cervical intraepithelial neoplasia. New Engl. J. Med. 317:916-923; 1987.

10. Bernstein, G.; Forgaard, D.M.; Miller, J.E. Carcinoma *in situ* of the glands, penis and distal urethra. J. Dermatol. Surg. Oncol. 12:450-455; 1986.

11. Bostwick, J. III, Pendergrast, W.J. Jr., Vasconez, L.O. Marjolin's ulcer: an immunologically privileged tumor? Plast. Reconstr. Surg. 57:66-69; 1976.

11a. Brady, L.W. External irradiation of epithelial skin cancer. Int. J. Radiat. Oncol. Biol. Phys. 19:491-492; 1990.

12. Brady, L.W.; Binnick, S.A.; Fitzpatrick, P.J. Skin cancer. In: Perez, C.A.; Brady, L.W., eds. Principles and practice of radiation oncology. Philadelphia, PA: J.B. Lippincott Co.; 1987:377-394.

13. Cohen, E.B.; Komorowski, R.A.; Clowry, L.J. Cutaneous complications in renal transplant recipients. Am. J. Clin. Pathol. 88:32-37; 1987.

14. Coldiron, B.M.; Brown, F.C.; Freeman, R.G. Epithelial macuniculatum (carcinoma cuniculatum) of the thumb: a case report and literature review. J. Dermatol. Surg. Oncol. 12:1150-1155; 1986.

14a. Crissey, J.T. Curettage and electrodessication as a method of treatment for epitheliomas of the skin. J. Surg. Oncol. 3:287;1978.

15. Del Regato, J.A.; Vuksanovic, M. Radiotherapy of carcinomas of the skin overlying the cartilages of the nose and ear. Radiology 79:203-208; 1962.

16. Dzubow, L.M.; Rigel, D.S.; Robins, P. Risk factors for local recurrence of primary cutaneous squamous cell carcinomas. Treatment by microscopically controlled excision. Arch. Dermatol. 118:900-902, 1982.

17. Goepfert, H.; Guillamondegui, O.M.; Jesse, R.H.; Lindberg, R.D. Squamous cell carcinoma of the nasal vestibule. Archives of Otolaryngology — Head and Neck Surgery 100:8-10; 1974.

18. Goepfert, H.; Remmer, D.; Silva, E.; Wheeler, B. Merkel cells carcinoma (endocrine carcinoma of the skin) of the head and neck. Archives of Otolaryngology — Head and Neck Surgery. 110:707-712; 1984.

19. Gooding, C.A.; White, G.; Yatsuhashi, M. Significance of marginal extension in basal cell carcinoma. New Engl. J. Med. 273:923-924;1965.

20. Goodwin, W.J.; Jesse, R.H. Malignant neoplasms of the external auditory canal and temporal bone. Archives of Otolaryngology — Head and Neck Surgery. 106:675-679; 1980.

21. Grabb W.C. Smith. J.W., eds. Plastic surgery. Boston, MA: Little Brown and Co.; 1979:497-501.

22. Graham, G.F. Statistical data on malignant tumors in cryosurgery. J. Dermatol. Surg. Oncol. 9:238-239; 1983.

23. Greenway, H.T.; Cornell, R.C.; Tanner, D.J.; Peets, E.; Bordin, G.M. Treatment of basal cell carcinoma with intralesional interferon. J. Am. Acad. Derm. 15:437-443; 1989.

24. Grimwood, R.E.; Siegle, R.J.; Ferris, C.F.; Huff, J.C. The biology of basal cell carcinoma. J. Dermatol. Surg. Oncol. 12:805-808; 1986.

25. Hawthorne, N. The birthmark. In: The selected tales and sketches, 3rd ed. New York, NY: Holt, Rinehart, and Winston; 1970:264-281.

26. Haynes, H.A.; Mead, K.W.; Goldwyn, R.M. Cancers of the skin. In: Cancer: Principles and Practice of Oncology, 2nd Edition, V.T. DeVita, S. Hellman, S.A. Rosenberg, eds. Philadelphia, PA: J.B. Lippincott, Co., 1985:1343-1422.

27. International Histologic Classification of Tumors, Nos. 1-20. Geneva, Switzerland: World Health Organization; 1978.

28. International Union Against Cancer. TNM Classification of Malignant Tumors, 4th ed. New York, NY: Springer-Verlag; 1987:83-88.

29. Kopf, A.W.; Bart, R.S.; Schrager, D. Curettage and electrodessication treatment of basal cell carcinomas. Arch. Dermatol. 113:439-443; 1977.

30. Kraemer, K.H. Heritable diseases with increased sensitivity to cellular injury. In: Fitzpatrick, T.B.; Eisen, A.Z.; Wolff, K.; Freedberg, I.M.; Austen, K.F., eds. Dermatology in general medicine, 3rd ed. New York, NY: McGraw-Hill Book Co.; 1987:1791-1811.

31. Kraemer, K.H.; DiGiovanna, J.J.; Moshell, A.N.; Tarone, R.E.; Peck, G.L. Prevention of skin cancer in xeroderma pigmentosum with the use of oral isotretinoin. New Engl. J. Med. 318:1633-1637; 1988.

32. Kripke, M.L.; Applegate, L.A. Alterations in the immune response. In: Goldsmith, L.A., ed. Physiology, Biochemistry, and Molecular Biology of the Skin. 2nd ed. New York, NY: Oxford University Press, 1991:1222-1239.

33. Lang, P.G.; Maize, J.C. Histologic evolution of recurrent basal cell carcinoma and treatment implications. Arch. Dermatol. 14:186-196; 1986.

34. Lawrence, E.A. Carcinoma arising in the scars of thermal burns. Surg. Gynecol. Obstet. 95:579-588; 1952.

34'. Lippman, S.M., Shimm, D.S., Meyskens, F.L.: Nonsurgical treatments for skin cancer: Retinoids and alpha-interferon. J Derm Surg Oncol 14(8):862-869, 1988.

34a. Liu, F.F., Maki, E., Warde, P., Payne, D., Fitzpatrick, P. A management approach to incompletely excised basal cell carcinomas of skin. Int. J. Radiat. Oncol. Biol. Phys. 20:423-428, 1991.

34b. Lovett, R.D., Perez, C.A., Shapiro, S.J., Garcia, D.M. External irradiation of epithelial skin cancer. Int. J. Radiat. Oncol. Biol. Phys. 19:235-242, 1990.

35. Marks, R.M.; Rennie, G.; Selwood, T. The relationship to basal cell carcinomas and squamous cell carcinomas to solar keratoses. Arch. Dermatol. 124:1039-1042; 1988.

36. McCaughan, J.S. Jr.; Guy, J.T.; Hicks, W.; Laufman, L.; Nims, T.A. Photodynamic therapy for cutaneous and subcutaneous malignant neoplasms. Arch. Surg. 124:211-216; 1989.

37. Menn, H.; Robins, P.; Kopf, A.; Bart, R.S. The recurrent basal cell epithelioma: a study of 100 cases of recurrent retreated basal cell epitheliomas. Arch. Dermatol. 103:628-631; 1971.

38. Mikhail, G.R. Metastatic basal cell carcinoma. J. Dermatol. Surg. Oncol. 12:507-509; 1986.

39. Mohs, F.E. Chemosurgery for the microscopically controlled excision of cutaneous cancer. In: Epstein, E.; Epstein, Jr., eds. Skin surgery, 4th ed. Springfield, IL: Charles C. Thomas; 1977:526-541.

40. Moy, R.L.; Eliezri, Y.D.; Nuovo, G.J.; Zitelli, J.A.; Bennett, R.G.; Silverstein, S. Human papillomavirus type 16 DNA in periungual squamous cell carcinomas. J. Am. Med. Assoc. 261:2669-2673; 1989.

41. Novick, M.; Gard, D.A.; Hardy, S.B.; Spira, M. Burn scar carcinoma: a review and analysis of 46 cases. J. Trauma 17:809-817; 1977.

42. Pascal, R.R.; Hobby, L.W.; Lattes, R.; Crikelair, G.F. Prognosis of "incompletely excised" vs. "completely excised" basal cell carcinoma. Plast. Reconstr. Surg. 41:328-332; 1968.

42'. Patterson, J.A.K., Geronemus, R.G. Cancers of the skin. In: DeVita, V.T., Hellman, S., Rosenberg, S.A. (eds.). Cancer: Principles and Practice of Oncology, 3rd Edition. Philadelphia, PA: J.B. Lippincott, Co., 1989:1469-1498.

42a. Physicians's Data Query. Cancer of the Skin. Nat'l Cancer Inst., Bethesda, MD: January 1992.

43. Robins, P.; Dzubow, L.M.; Rigel, D.S. Squamous cell carcinoma treated by Mohs surgery: an experience with 414 cases in a period of 15 years. J. Dermatol. Surg. Oncol. 7:800-801; 1981.

44. Roenigk, R.K.; Ratz, J.L.; Bailin, P.L.; Wheeland, R.G. Trends in the presentation and treatment of basal cell carcinoma. J. Dermatol. Surg. Oncol. 12:860-865; 1986.

45. Rubin, P.; Cassarett, G. Skin and adnexae. In: Rubin, P.; Cassarett, G., eds. Clinical Radiation Pathology. Philadelphia, PA: W.B. Saunders Co.; 1968:62-119.

46. Shapiro, L.; Baraf, C.S. Subungual epidermoid carcinoma and keratoacanthoma. Cancer 25:141-152; 1970.

47. Shiffman, N.J. Squamous cell carcinomas of the skin of the pinna. Cancer J. Surg. 18:279-283; 1975.

48. Sibley, R.; Dehner, L.; Rosai, J. Primary neuro endocrine (Merkel cell) carcinoma of the skin. Am. J. Surg. Pathol. 9:95-108; 1985.

49. Siegle, R.J.; MacMillan, J.; Pollack, S.V. Infiltrative basal cell carcinoma: a non-sclerosing subtype. J. Dermatol. Surg. Oncol. 12:830-836; 1986.

49a. Solan, M.J., Brady, L.W., Binnick, S.A., Fitzpatrick, P.J. Skin. In: Perez, C.A., Brady, L.W. (eds.). Principles and Practice of Radiation Oncology, 2nd Edition. Philadelphia, PA: J.B. Lippincott, Co., 1992:479-495.

50. Stoll, H., Jr.; Schwartz, R.A. Squamous cell carcinoma. In: Fitzpatrick, T.B.; Eisen, A.Z.; Wolff, K.; Freedberg, I.M.; Austen, K.F., eds. Dermatology in General Medicine, 3rd ed. New York, NY: McGraw-Hill Book Co; 1987:746-758.

51. Traenkle, H.L. Late radiation injury and cutaneous neoplasia. In: Helm, F., ed. Cancer Dermatology. Philadelphia, PA: Lea & Febiger; 1979:31-37.

52. Tromovitch, T.A.; Stegman, S.J. Microscopic-controlled excision of cutaneous tumors. Cancer 41:653-658;1978.

53. Turk, L.L.; Winde, P.R. Carcinomas of the skin and their treatment. Semin. Oncol. 7:376-384; 1980.

54. Von Domarus, H.; Stevens, P.J. Metastatic basal cell carcinoma. Report of five cases and review of 170 cases in the literature. J. Am. Acad. Dermatol. 10:1043-1060; 1984.

55. Waldron, H.A. A brief history of scrotal cancer. British Journal of Industrial Medicine 40:390-401; 1983.

56. Winkelmann, R.D.K. Skin biopsy in skin surgery. In: Epstein, E.; Epstein, E. Jr., eds. Skin Surgery. Philadelphia, PA: W.B. Saunders Co; 1987:153-161.

57. Yeh, S. Skin cancer in chronic arsenicism. Human Pathol. 4:469-485; 1973.

58. Yuspa, S.; Dlugosz, A.A. Cutaneous carcinogeneis: natural and experimental. In: Goldsmith, L.A., ed. Physiology, Biochemistry, and Molecular Biology of the Skin. 2nd ed. New York, NY: Oxford University Press, 1991:1365-1402.

Virginia K. Langmuir, M.D., Surgical Oncology
Colin A. Poulter, M.D., Radiation Oncology

Raman Qazi, M.D., F.A.C.P., Medical Oncology
Edwin D. Savlov, M.D., Surgical Oncology

Chapter **17**

BREAST CANCER

Disease in man is never exactly the same as the same disease in an experimental animal, for in man the disease at once affects and is affected by what we call the emotional life.

Francis W. Peabody (14)

PERSPECTIVE

Breast cancer is the most common and a most dreaded malignancy in women. Its tremendous impact stems from many factors. Not only does it strike in the prime of life, and for no understood reason, but there is no known method of prevention. Because it affects a sexually important part of the body, its treatment may be physically and emotionally disfiguring. It has an unpredictable course and the risk of metastasis continues for 20 years or more. When it is fatal, it is often after a prolonged, painful, and disabling period of disease (156).

The past decade has seen considerable progress in our knowledge of the disease, the effectiveness of treatment, and the proper choice of treatment for individual patients. The equality of less radical surgery with traditional radical mastectomy has been demonstrated. In numerous studies, it has been shown that, for patients with localized, operable cancer, conservative surgery with breast preservation followed by full-dose radiation therapy results in excellent cosmesis, tumor control, and survival comparable with radical mastectomy.

Chemotherapeutic or hormonal agents, when used in the adjuvant setting, have been shown to delay recurrence and improve survival in certain patient subsets. They also have produced significant responses in patients with metastatic disease. Estrogen receptors (ER) and progesterone receptors (PR) have emerged as predictors of response to treatment and as prognostic indicators.

These advances are largely the result of carefully designed, randomized clinical trials, often carried out by multi-institutional cooperative study groups. Much of the hope for future progress rests with continued clinical research using the cooperative group mechanism. This chapter will summarize current knowledge and its application to patient care and point out promising investigational approaches for further improvements in the control of this disease.

EPIDEMIOLOGY AND ETIOLOGY

Epidemiology (12)

Breast cancer is slowly increasing in incidence and prevalence. For 1992, 186,000 new diagnoses were predicted (31). The prevalence of breast cancer is 100 per 100,000 females in any given year. Overall, breast cancer will strike one of every 10 females in the United States, accounting for 32% of all cancers in females. The mortality rate of 28 per 100,000 has remained essentially unchanged for 50 years. Breast cancer accounts for 19% of cancer deaths in females. The lack of change in the mortality rate may be because not all women take advantage of mammographic screening recommendations, and because many breast cancers still are quite advanced at initial diagnosis.

Breast cancer is more frequent in the left than the right breast, possibly because the left breast is usually larger than the right. It is more frequent in the upper outer quadrant of the breast. One percent of all breast cancer occurs in men. The major risk factors for the development of breast cancer are female sex and a personal or family (mother or sister) history of breast cancer. A history of benign proliferative breast disease is also associated with breast cancer. Table 17-1 (105) and Fig. 17-1 summarize breast cancer risk factors.

Natural History of Breast Cancer

It is always difficult to evaluate the natural history of any tumor because most patients receive some form of therapy. However, from analysis of old data on untreated patients and from extrapolations in treated patient populations, it is possible to gain some understanding of the natural history of this disease.

A British study (24), that analyzed 356 untreated breast tumors seen between 1902 and 1933, evaluated 250 of the cases that went to autopsy and had the diagnosis confirmed (Table 17-2) (24). In this group, the 5-year survival from onset of symptoms was 18% and the 10-year survival was 4%. Median survival was 2.7 years. These data are presumably biased toward the aggressive tumors, since the patients studied had been admitted to a cancer charity hospital and died and were autopsied while in the hospital. Seventy-four percent of these patients were admitted with stage IV disease. Survival data may appear worse in these patients because tumors were not reported until they had been present for a considerable period.

Fox (75) analyzed data from patients at the NCI. His analysis suggests that there is a subgroup of patients (60%) with less aggressive disease and a mortality rate of 2.5% per year. The remaining 40% have much more aggressive disease and die at a rate of 25% per year. However, other researchers

Table 17-1. Breast Cancer Risk Factors	Increased Risk*
FAMILY HISTORY	
Primary relative with cancer	1.2-3.0
Premenopausal	3.1
Premenopausal and bilateral	8.5-9.0
Postmenopausal	1.5
Postmenopausal and bilateral	4.0-5.4
MENSTRUAL HISTORY	
Age at menarche < 12 yr	1.3
Age at menopause > 55 yr with > 40 menstrual yrs	1.5-2.0
PREGNANCY	
First child after age 35 yr	2.0-3.0
Nulliparous	3.0
OTHER NEOPLASMS	
Contralateral breast cancer	5.0
Cancer of major salivary gland	4.0
Cancer of the uterus	2.0
BENIGN BREAST DISEASE	
Atypical lobular hyperplasia	4.0
Lobular carcinoma	7.2
PREVIOUS BIOPSY	1.86-2.13

* General population risk = 1.0

Courtesy of Love et al. (105). Reprinted by permission of the New England Journal of Medicine.

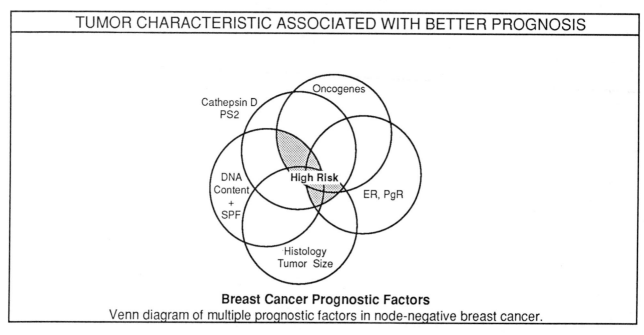

Breast Cancer Prognostic Factors
Venn diagram of multiple prognostic factors in node-negative breast cancer.

Fig. 17-1. High risk patients are T > 2cm, ER (-), PgR (-), undifferentiated tumor, poor nuclear grade, aneuploid, diploid with high S phase and less established are high levels of cathepsin D, amplification of HER-2/*neu* and/or *erb* B-2.

Table 17-2. Untreated and Treated Breast Cancer Survival According to Histologic Grade From Onset of Symptoms

Survival (yr)	Untreated* (1902–1933) (%)	Treated (1936–1949) (%)
Grade I		
5	5/23 (22)	264/321 (82)
10	2/23 (9)	107/190 (56)
15	0/23 (0)	31/83 (37)
Grade II		
5	7/32 (22)	299/563 (53)
10	1/32 (3)	93/308 (30)
15	0/23 (0)	29/136 (21)
Grade III		
5	0/31 (0)	120/362 (33)
10	0/31 (0)	44/216 (20)
15	0/31 (0)	8/84 (10)

* 86/250 cases with histological sections.

From Bloom et al. (24), with permission.

suggest a more realistic situation in which there is a continuum of patients with varying degrees of disease aggressiveness (148). A continued slow death rate extending out to 20 years or more has been demonstrated in several studies and suggests that, at least statistically, breast cancer cannot be cured. Certainly breast cancer is often a slow-growing tumor and recurrence may occur 20 to 30 years after initial therapy. But many patients are functionally cured in that they live out their normal life expectancy and die of other diseases.

The actual growth rate of breast cancer has been studied by measuring the diameter of metastatic nodules on serial chest x-rays. From this albeit inaccurate method, it has been suggested that it may take up to 8 years for a breast cancer to reach 1 cm in diameter. Obviously, an 8-year-old tumor is not an early tumor and it is not surprising that many of these patients with small primary tumors present with regional nodal involvement or eventually die of distant disease.

Etiology

There is no known single cause of breast cancer. However, genetic and/or hormonal factors may play a role in some patients.

1. Low-dose radiation exposure has been reported to cause carcinogenesis in the postpubertal breast and prior to menarche in: (a) patients being treated for mastitis with radiation therapy; (b) patients who have had repeated fluoroscopies for tuberculosis management; and (c) atom bomb survivors (101). Breast irradiation in adolescents or young adults has been shown to increase the risk of breast cancer (101).
2. Ingestion of dietary fat has been suggested as a risk factor for breast cancer because of marked international differences in rates of breast cancer and striking increases in incidence of breast cancer among populations migrating from low-to-high incidence areas. The relationship, however, remains controversial (154).
3. Unopposed estrogen stimulus has been postulated to increase risk, particularly in adolescent and premeno-

pausal females. Most current evidence as of now suggests that oral contraceptives do not increase the incidence of breast cancer (120).

DETECTION AND DIAGNOSIS

Clinical Detection

Because most breast cancers are found palpation by the patient or her physician, these tumors are usually 2 cm or more in diameter. As tumor size increases, the likelihood that distant metastasis has taken place rises and it has been suggested that, for each tumor, there is a critical volume before which distant metastasis does not occur (98). For this reason, screening patients for breast cancer before tumors are large enough to be palpable has been proposed as a way to decrease the risk of dying of the disease.

Any screening technique must fulfill a number of criteria to make it worthwhile. A high-risk population must be identifiable, since it is rarely cost-effective to screen large numbers of people for rare disorders. The technique must be rapid, relatively inexpensive, and easily learned by technicians performing it. False-positives and, especially, false-negatives must be low. The screened population must then benefit from the earlier diagnosis. Three main screening methods are available for the detection of breast cancer: self-breast examination (SBE), physical examination by a health care provider, and mammography. Other imaging techniques such as thermography and ultrasound have not been found to be effective screening methods.

Breast Examination

SBE should be performed monthly after the menstrual period by all women, beginning in their early twenties. With regular SBE, it is possible for a woman to "know" her breasts and potentially to detect lesions before her physician, particularly in cystic fibroid breast syndrome breasts that are difficult to examine. SBE has been estimated to have a sensitivity of only 20% to 30% (i.e., it only detects 20% to 30% of important lesions). Sensitivity can be improved with teaching, but the specificity then decreases (more false-positives). At present, there is no published evidence that SBE leads to improved survival from breast cancer (96,118). Physical examination is certainly important, particularly in patients who do not practice SBE. The most important fact to remember is that it is impossible to determine by palpation whether a lump is benign or malignant. A biopsy should be obtained for any discrete mass; lack of growth over time and a negative mammogram should not affect this decision.

Screening Mammography

The advantage of screening mammography is the potential to detect lesions before they are discernible by palpation. Mammographic findings that indicate malignancy include clustered microcalcifications; an irregular or spiculated mass; a solid nodule with ill-defined borders; architectural distortion; an enlarging, solid, well-circumscribed mass; a developing density indicated by comparison with previous films; and asymmetric density. The risk of developing breast cancer is quite low before the age of 35 years. It then increases with age continuously, with a small plateau between the ages of 45 and 55 years. Current recommendations by several groups for screening mammography are given in Table 17-3 (76). Patients at higher-than-average risk probably should be screened starting at an earlier age. In patients over age 50 years, it was found in one study that few cancers were found in the first 2 years after a negative mammogram. In 40- to 49-year-old patients, the number of cancers found in the first year after a negative mammogram was 40% of the number found in the unscreened controls, and this increased to 70% in the second year. For these reasons, an annual mammogram was recommended for the 40-to-49-year age group and every 2 years after age 50 (143).

Two mammographic techniques are currently in use: filmscreen mammography and xeroradiography (32). Both techniques have their particular advantages and disadvantages, but filmscreen mammography is used more widely. A major concern of the public has been the radiation dose from mammography. With present techniques, the mean glandular dose per view is 0.2 cGy or less. It has been estimated that if this dose were given to 100,000 45-year-old women, it would be equivalent to the risk of smoking eight cigarettes or driving 660 miles in a car (76).

One of the earliest studies of screening mammography, the New York City Hospital Insurance Plan study (137), revealed a mortality in the screened group that was 60% of the unscreened control group. Lead-time bias (diagnosing earlier but still dying at the same time) could not account for these differences. It is more difficult to determine whether length-time bias (selectively detecting the slowly growing, less aggressive cancers) is a factor in these studies. In a 14-year study by Frankel (76), 32% of patients with palpable lesions, 16% of those with nonpalpable infiltrating ductal carcinomas greater than 0.5 cm in diameter, and 2% with nonpalpable cancers 0.5 cm or less (infiltrating ductal, or lobular or ductal carcinoma in situ [CIS]) had died.

It is clear that screening mammography has the potential to reduce the mortality from breast cancer. Unfortunately, not all women are actually being screened, particularly in low income and minority groups. This is partially because some women never have a physical check-up, but there are many physicians who are not recommending mammography to their patients. Better education of physicians should help eliminate this barrier.

Diagnostic Procedures

Table 17-4 (3,121) summarizes current imaging modalities and their diagnostic capabilities.

Self Breast Examination

Although SBE, physical examination, and mammography can detect breast cancers, they are not 100% accurate and a tissue diagnosis is always necessary before proceeding to definitive therapy. Mammography always should be performed prior to definitive therapy of breast cancer because this procedure may detect other lesions in either breast; in addition, it is useful to have a baseline study for comparison with later films.

Fine Needle Aspiration (FNA) Cytology

Fine needle aspiration (FNA) cytology is used extensively in the diagnosis of both benign and malignant breast lesions (see Chapter 4, "Principles of Surgical Oncology"). With a skilled cytologist, false-positive results are almost nil and some surgeons will perform the definitive procedure on the basis of cytology alone. This approach is reasonable if lumpectomy is planned, but if total mastectomy is anticipated, it may be best to confirm the diagnosis with open biopsy. This confirmation will avoid the rare but devastating complication of removing a breast unnecessarily. It is often still advantageous to perform FNA in this setting because of the psychologic benefit to the patient of rapid diagnosis, since results can usually be obtained the same day. False-negatives do occur and a negative FNA should not dissuade the surgeon from biopsy if a discrete lump is present, particularly if there is a clinical suspicion of cancer.

Open-Breast Biopsy

Open-breast biopsy is the most common procedure for the diagnosis of breast cancer. Unless the lesion is very large, the whole mass should be excised with a margin of normal tissue. If there is any chance that lumpectomy may be the definitive procedure, the margins should be inked by the pathologist, since the original biopsy may be adequate therapy if the margins are clear. Open-breast biopsy can usually be performed as an outpatient procedure using local anesthesia. A portion of the tumor (≥ 0.5 cc) always should be submitted for measurement of ERs and PRs.

Table 17-3. Screening Mammography Guidelines

Patient Age (yrs)	Recommendations 8-5
35-40	Baseline mammogram (ACS, ACR)
35-50	Baseline mammogram (ACOG)
40-49	Annual or biennial mammogram (ACS, ACR) Frequency determined by physician
≥ 50	Annual mammogram (ACS, ACR, ACOG)

ACS = American Cancer Society; ACR = American College of Radiology;

ACOG = American College of Obstetrics and Gynecology.

From Frankel (76), with permission.

Table 17-4. Diagnositic Capabilities of Current Imaging Modalities in Breast Cancer

Method	Diagnosis and Staging Capability	Recommended For Use
Primary tumor and regional nodes		
Mammography	Visualizes approximately 90% of breast cancers	Film/screen and xeromammography have similar diagnostic accuracy
Ultrasound: dedicated	Limited to identification of cystic lesions and evaluation of dense breast	Dedicated units are expensive and not suitable for stand-alone screening
CT	Limited to evaluation of chest wall and internal mammary node involvement	Dedicated CT breast imaging system has been abandoned
MRI	Unproven	Experimental studies pending
Metastatic breast cancer: as required		
Chest x-ray film	Essential for all tumor types	
Radionuclide bone scan	Essential for baseline verification and evaluation of symptomatic patient	Abnormal bone scans require film
Liver imaging	Indicated with abnormal chemistries or symptoms	Initial imaging study radionuclide liver scan (requires validation of abnormal scan by ultrasound or CT)

CT = computed tomography; MRI = magnetic resonance imaging.

From Bragg et al. (3), with permission of McGraw-Hill, Inc.

Nonpalpable Lesions

It is becoming increasingly common for the surgeon to have to remove nonpalpable lesions detected by mammography. If the lesion contains microcalcifications, the likelihood of cancer is 20% to 30%. If there is only a mass lesion on the mammogram with no calcifications, the risk decreases to 14%. The result is that a large number of "unnecessary" biopsies are done. Improved predictive capabilities of the radiologist may be possible in the future if correlations can be made between mammographic appearance of these lesions and the final pathology. Specimen mammography with compression and magnification is important to correlate microcalcifications with the original mammogram and the pathologic specimen to determine whether the lesion has been completely excised. FNA cytology is now possible in these lesions at some centers because of the development of stereotaxic needle localization, which has an accuracy of plus or minus 1 mm.

In nonpalpable masses, a hooked wire is inserted into or adjacent to the lesion while the patient is in the radiology department. Methylene blue is usually injected also in case the wire should become dislodged. The patient is then taken to the operating room for excisional biopsy. The skin insertion site should be directly over the lesion, if possible. If there are microcalcifications in the lesion, the excised tissue should be x-rayed to confirm that the lesion was truly excised. If the lesion contained no microcalcifications, it is much harder to determine by specimen x-ray whether it was completely excised. All patients should have a mammogram within 2 months after biopsy to confirm that the abnormality is gone.

CLASSIFICATION AND STAGING

Histopathology

1. There are several histologic subtypes of adenocarcinoma of the breast. The classification used by the World Health Organization is widely accepted (158) (Table 17-5).

Table 17-5. Histologic Subtypes of Breast Cancer

Factors	Incidence (%)
Noninvasive	
Intraductal carcinoma (DCIS)	5 - 8
Lobular carcinoma in situ	
Invasive	
Invasive ductal carcinoma (invasive DC)	
Invasive DC with DCIS	70
Invasive lobular carcinoma	5-10
Mucinous carcinoma	3
Medullary carcinoma	5-7
Papillary carcinoma	1
Tubular carcinoma	1
Adenoid cystic carcinoma	
Secretory (juvenile) carcinoma	19
Apocrine carcinoma	
Others	
Paget's disease of the nipple	1-4

2. There are a number of histopathologic findings that correlate with prognosis. Tumor grade, as characterized by low nuclear grade, and the presence of tubule formation correlate with a good prognosis. Certain histologic types of breast cancer, such as pure tubular and mucinous carcinoma, are associated with a low incidence of distant metastases and thus a higher cure rate.

3. In the National Surgical Adjuvant Breast Project (NSABP), 36 pathologic and 6 clinical characteristics were documented in 581 patients. The single most important discriminant was positive axillary nodes; four or more positive nodes were worse than one to three. Multivariate analysis indicated that if nodes were negative, the presence of tumor necrosis, poor tumor differentiation (grade 3), and tumor size greater than 4 cm influenced treatment failure (58,69). In a more recent study of almost 1000 more favorable patients with stage I node N0 disease, 22 pathologic factors and 4 clinical features were analyzed. Three prognostically important features were identified: nuclear grade, histologic tumor type, and race. Tumor types with good prognosis are mucinous, tubular, and papillary tumors; poor prognosis types are atypical medullary and not otherwise specified. Blacks fared worse than whites.

Anatomic Staging

The current recognized anatomic staging system is reproduced in Table 17-6 (1) and Fig. 17-2. Stage assessment should be performed once at the clinical-diagnostic management phase and again at the postsurgical phase. Staging is a continuum that provides increasing accuracy in determining the organ involvement by the tumor. To indicate the chronology of the staging process, lower case "p" is inserted before the Tumor (T), Nodes (N), Metastasis (M) grade to indicate that pathologic examination has contributed to the stage. Reference (1) contains a detailed discussion of the classification system.

Primary Tumor

T staging is dependent on tumor size and the presence or absence of fixation to surrounding structures. Primary tumors should be described as precisely as possible with accurate measurement of diameters in centimeters and characterization of the shape, consistency, location, and involvement of skin, pectoral fascia, or ribs.

Regional Lymph Nodes

Clinically negative axillae associated with T1 or T2 breast tumors will contain histologically positive nodes in approximately 39% of cases, while clinically N1 axillae will be pathologically negative about 24% of the time (69). In gen-

Table 17-6. TNM Classification and Stage Grouping for Breast Tumors

TNM Classification			Stage Grouping			
Tis		In situ	Stage 0	Tis	N0	M0
T1		≤ 2 cm	Stage I	T1	N0	M0
	T1a	≤ 0.5 cm	Stage IIA	T0	N1	M0
	T1b	> 0.5 to 1 cm		T1	N1*	M0
	T1c	> 1 to 2 cm		T2	N0	M0
T2		> 2 to 5 cm	Stage IIB	T2	N1	M0
T3		> 5 cm		T3	N0	M0
T4		Chest wall/skin	Stage IIIA	T0	N2	M0
	T4a	Chest wall		T1	N2	M0
	T4b	Skin edema/ulceration, satellite skin nodules		T2	N2	M0
	T4c	Both 4a and 4b		T3	N1,N2	M0
	T4d	Inflammatory carcinoma	Stage IIIB	T4	Any N	M0
				Any T	N3	M0
N1	pN1	Movable axillary	Stage IV	Any T	Any N	M1
	pN1a	Micrometastasis only ≤ 0.2 cm				
	pN1b	Gross metastasis				
		i 1-3 nodes/> 0.2 to < 2 cm				
		ii ≥ 4 nodes/> 0.2 to < 2 cm				
		iii through capsule/< 2 cm				
		iv ≥ 2 cm				
N2	pN2	Fixed axillary				
N3	pN3	Internal axillary				
M1		Distant metastases (includes supraclav)				

* The prognosis of patients with pN1a is similar to that of patients with pN0.

T = tumor; N = node; M = metastasis; p = pathology.

From AJC (1), with permission.

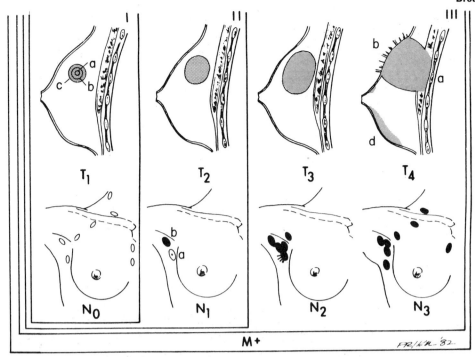

Fig. 17-2. Anatomic staging for breast cancer (see Table 17-6).

eral, larger tumors have more axillary nodal involvement (65,102) (Fig. 17-3). Internal mammary node involvement varies in frequency with the location of the primary breast cancer; it is more common with central and internal quadrant cancers and when there are axillary nodal metastases.

Staging Work-up

Staging work-up consists of selected procedures performed to determine the extent of local, regional, or distant cancer involvement. Careful mapping of the cancer on anatomic diagrams is recommended (Fig. 17-2). Pathologic evaluation

of any resected tissue not only establishes a diagnosis, but also provides staging (and, therefore, prognostic) information. Such information should include size of primary, adequacy of surgical margin, histologic subtype (Table 17-5), and number and extent of lymph node involvement (Tables 17-6 and 17-7).

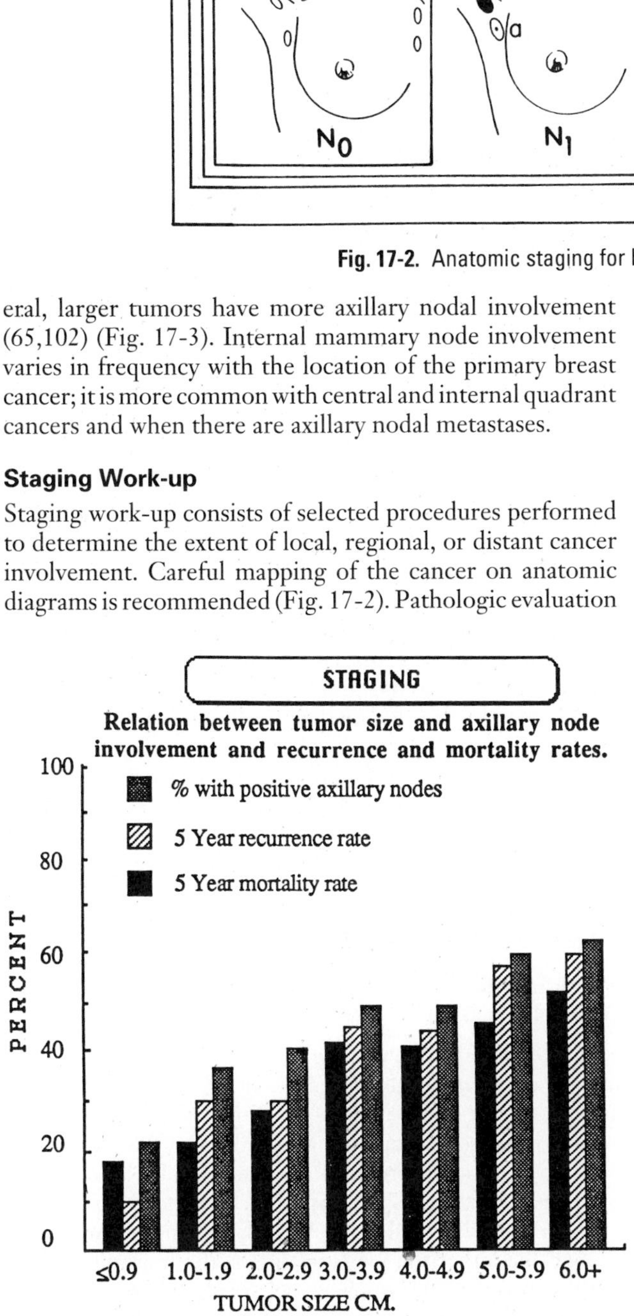

Recommended Procedures (Table 17-3)

1. *Physical examination* should include careful description of tumor size, location, fixation, and nodal status as described above. Histologic involvement of lymph nodes will occur in 35% to 40% of cases when no abnormal nodes can be felt.
2. *Mammograms* can be used to assess extent and size, multiple tumors, and invasion of the skin and chest wall.
3. *Excisional biopsy* (with or without mastectomy) and axillary nodal removal are advised for all but the most advanced (T4 or N3) lesions. This allows for complete pathologic staging.
4. *Routine studies* include chest x-ray, complete blood cell count, and liver function tests for all patients.
5. In the past, *metastatic work-up* included radioisotopic bone scan in all patients. However, less than 1% of stage I patients will have unsuspected bone metastases, and bone scan is therefore not recommended in these patients unless a baseline is required for participation in a clinical trial (10). Bone scan and targeted radiographs should be done if bone pain is present, because benign conditions such as osteoarthritis or spondylitis can produce "hot spots." Liver scans are usually not helpful unless abnormalities in the liver chemistries are found.
6. *ER and PR analysis* should be performed on any surgical specimen where there is sufficient tissue for both pathologic and receptor study. These receptors are cytoplasmic proteins that form complexes with the respective hormone. They are subsequently translocated to the cell nucleus to produce the final hormonal effect. ERs are found in approximately 60% of breast cancers in

STAGING

Relation between tumor size and axillary node involvement and recurrence and mortality rates.

- ▓ % with positive axillary nodes
- ▨ 5 Year recurrence rate
- ■ 5 Year mortality rate

(bar chart with PERCENT on y-axis from 0 to 100, TUMOR SIZE CM. on x-axis: ≤0.9, 1.0-1.9, 2.0-2.9, 3.0-3.9, 4.0-4.9, 5.0-5.9, 6.0+)

Fig. 17-3. Relation between tumor size and axillary node involvement and recurrence and mortality rates. Courtesy of Fisher *et al.* (65).

Table 17-7. Internal Mammary Node Involvement (%) In Breast Cancer

	PRIMARY SITE				
	UIQ	LIQ	CENTRAL	UOQ	LOQ
Total	27	33	32	14	13
Axilla					
Not involved	14	6	7	4	5
Involved	45	72	46	22	19

UIQ = upper inner quadrant; LIQ = lower inner quadrant; UOQ = upper outer quadrant;

LOQ = lower outer quadrant.

From Handley (83), with permission.

women under the age of 50 years, and in approximately 75% of those over the age of 50 years (11,67).

Optional and Investigative Procedures

1. Negative High-Risk Factors: In addition to negative ERs and PRs there are an increasing number of prognostic factors being identified to determine those patients at high risk for metastases, especially those who have negative axillary nodes. There is substantial evidence that estrogen receptor status, measures of proliferative capacity of the primary tumor (thymidine labeling index or flow cytometric measurements of S-phase and ploidy), and oncogene expression or amplification (c-erb-2) may have significant independent predictive value (138a).

   a. DNA Activity: The ability to quantitate the proliferative activity of breast cancer by flow cytometry and thymidine labelling index. In addition to histopathology and nuclear grade, ploidy and proliferative rates provide new predictive parameters for negative outcomes (50).
      - Aneuploid tumors *v* diploid tumors indicate a probability of 5-year disease-free survival (DFS) of 74% compared with 88%.
      - High S phase (>4-7%) *v* low S phase distinguishes the poor outcome for diploid tumors, i.e., 70% *v* 90% 5-year survival. Fortunately, only 13% of diploid tumors are in high S phase.

   b. Cathepsin D: a lyosomal enzyme that correlates with high percentages of positive nodes. Preliminary evidence in N0 patients correlates a decreased DFS interval with high levels of cathepsin D (144).

   c. Oncogenes: *HER-2/neu* and *erb* B-2 are increased and amplification correlates with positive-node tumor aggressiveness. Unfortunately, *HER-2-neu* does not correlate between amplification and negative outcome for N0 patients. A recent retrospective analysis suggested *HER-2/neu* can identify good risk N0 patients with a high probability of relapses. Analysis of *erb* B-2 also has been inconsistent (119a).

2. *Radiographic assessment* of lymph nodes with computed tomography (CT) or magnetic resonance imaging (MRI) is usually of little value and not recommended for routine staging. Arm lymphography also is not recommended.

3. *Radioisotopic examination* of internal mammary nodes using Technetium-99m colloid has been used for detection of metastases. This technique has not gained universal acceptance.

4. *Restaging before retreatment*: Recurrences of apparent solitary metastases require restaging to determine disease extent. A complete search for other metastases is especially important, and should include blood chemical, and radioisotopic evaluation of the major organs (liver, brain, lung, bone) commonly at risk for metastases, as well as radiographs and scans where lesions are suspected.

5. *Routine follow-up*: Following therapy of the primary tumor, in addition to a mammogram at least yearly, the breast cancer patient should have periodic physical examinations, at progressively longer intervals of 3- to 6-months, associated with serum alkaline phosphatase and transaminase determinations (as inexpensive screening tests for bone or liver metastases). Chest x-ray and bone scan should be done when clinically indicated. Positive areas on the bone scan should be examined radiographically for lytic lesions that might pose a threat of pathologic fracture. These lytic lesions might benefit from radiation therapy, usually with orthopedic bracing in long bones. Other tumor markers such as carcinoembryonic antigen, cystic disease fluid protein, and monoclonal antibody studies still are not widely accepted nor have their applicability been confirmed in the follow-up of breast cancer patients.

PRINCIPLES OF TREATMENT

Multidisciplinary Treatment Decisions (Table 17-8) (114)

Removal of the primary tumor by surgical excision is important for adequate local control. Removal of a portion of the axillary lymph nodes is done in clinically N0 patients for staging purposes, because it has been shown that pathologically positive nodes predict for an increased risk of distant metastases (as high as 75%). Systemic metastasis from breast cancer occurs independently from lymph node spread, although the larger the primary tumor, the more likely that both forms of metastasis have occurred. The treatment of breast cancer must therefore take these factors into account. Distant metastases occur most commonly in the bone, lungs,

Table 17-8. Multidisciplinary Treatment Decisions in Breast Cancer   (12a,109)

Stage	Surgery		Radiation Therapy		Chemotherapy
0 Tis	Lumpectomy to modified radical	and	CRT of breast		Adjuvant TAM and/or
I $T_1N_0M_0$	mastectomy	and	NR		MAC in subsets
	Nodal sampling				
					Adjuvant MAC and
II $T_{1,2}N_1M_0$	Lumpectomy to modified radical	and	CRT of breast and regional	and	TAM
	mastectomy		nodes		
	Nodal sampling				Adjuvant MAC and
IIIa $T_3N_0N_1$	Modified radical mastectomy	and	CRT of breast and regional	and	TAM
			nodes		
	Unresectable				MAC $\pm$ HT
IIIb $T_{1-3}N_3$			DRT of breast and regional	and	
T_4T_{any}			nodes		
	"Toilette" mastectomy				MAC $\pm$ HT
IV $T_{any}N_{any}M_1$	(optional)		PRT Optional		

RT = radiation therapy; CRT=curative; DRT = definitive; PRT=palliative; NR = not recommended; MAC = multiagent chemotherapy;
HT = hormonal therapy; TAM = tamoxifen.
PDQ: RCT - MAC = CMF, CAF, CA+II TAM, CMFF, CMFVP + other regimens.

liver, and brain. The use of adjuvant chemotherapy or hormonal therapy has led to decreased recurrence rates and increased survival in some patient subsets. Local recurrence also can occur after surgery, particularly after lumpectomy alone, and radiation therapy to the breast is indicated for these patients to reduce the risk of local recurrence (94). Table 17-7 provides a concise overview of the principles of multidisciplinary treatment.

Surgery

The purpose of surgery in the management of primary breast cancer is to remove the local and regional disease. If there has been no prior spread of tumor to distant sites, surgery may be curative. In the first 60 to 70 years of this century, it was believed that breast cancer underwent an orderly progression: from the primary site to the regional nodes and then on to distant sites. This concept inspired the Halsted radical mastectomy in which the breast, pectoralis muscles, and regional lymph nodes were removed *en bloc*. With the finding, however, that patients with negative lymph nodes were dying despite radical local therapy, it was suggested that distant metastasis could occur independent of lymph node metastasis. Some researchers were pessimistic enough to suggest that all breast cancers had metastasized by the time of diagnosis and that cure was impossible. Nevertheless, the enhanced survival in screened patients has made this possibility unlikely (88). This change in thinking led to the realization that, if radical surgery does not influence survival, it may be possible to use less aggressive local therapy (49).

Partial Mastectomy

Partial mastectomy usually has been subcategorized into lumpectomy, wide excision, or segmental mastectomy. However, probably there is no difference among them in local recurrence rates as long as the resection margins are free of

tumor (73,82). This operation is generally used in tumors less than 4 cm in diameter. The local recurrence rate at 8 years was reported by Fisher *et al.* (61) to be 39% after lumpectomy alone; however, if postoperative radiation therapy was given to the breast, this rate fell to 10%. Local recurrences usually occur near the previous excision site and are reduced if the initial resection margins are free of tumor (99,123). Other investigators have reported local recurrence rates between 4.9% and 13% for partial mastectomy plus irradiation. The presence of intralymphatic extension of tumor is also associated with an increased likelihood of local recurrence (126). Local recurrences usually can be managed with completion mastectomy with no apparent decrease in long-term survival (99).

Partial mastectomy has obvious psychologic advantages for the patient but must be performed correctly to avoid unacceptable distortion of the breast. The axillary dissection should be done through a separate incision and suction drains should be used only for the axillary dissection (Fig. 17-4). With present techniques, postoperative radiation therapy should not worsen the cosmetic result significantly.

Total Mastectomy

With total mastectomy, the whole breast, including the axillary tail, is removed, leaving the underlying pectoralis muscles intact. When axillary lymph node dissection is performed in continuity with the mastectomy, the operation is known as a modified radical mastectomy. Some surgeons will remove the pectoralis minor during this procedure. The rationale behind total mastectomy for breast cancer is the presumed multicentric nature of the disease. This determination generally has been made by histologic examination of mastectomy specimens, but it is unlikely that all histologic invasive and preinvasive cancers will develop into clinically significant cancers. Separate foci of cancer have been found

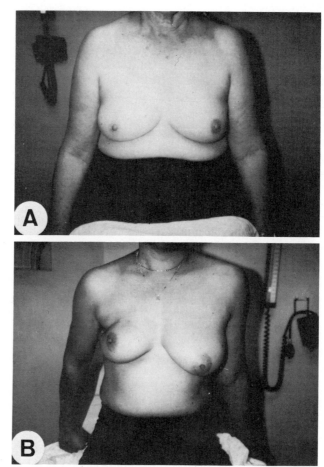

Fig. 17-4. (A) Post-operative appearance after segmental mastectomy and postoperative radiation therapy. Patient A had lumpectomy and axillary dissection done through separate incisions and (B) Patient B through the same incision. Note the distortion of the breast in B.

in 27% of patients when multiple histologic sections of the entire breast were examined. The rate was 18% in infiltrating cancers and 81% in intraductal cancers. However, 57% of these foci were within the same quadrant as the primary, suggesting spread rather than multicentricity.

Radical Mastectomy

This operation was developed by Halsted in the 1880's using the principles discussed above to treat women with extensive local disease. Fortunately, this advanced stage of disease rarely is encountered today. Radical mastectomy involved removal of the whole breast with its overlying skin, the pectoralis major and minor muscles, and all three levels of axillary lymph nodes (see below). Skin grafting was often necessary to close the defect. In some centers, the operation was extended to include excision of the internal mammary lymph nodes as well (113,150). This operation has been considered the gold standard for evaluation of all other operations for breast cancer (104).

There are several studies comparing radical mastectomy with total mastectomy or segmental mastectomy. The important conclusion drawn from these studies is that there is no significant difference in survival among these three treatment groups (21,60,109). Local recurrence rates are slightly lower after radical mastectomy than after total mastectomy (108). If irradiation of the remaining breast tissue is added to

segmental mastectomy, local recurrence rates are comparable with those for radical mastectomy (52,152).

Regional Lymph Nodes

The clinical assessment of axillary lymph node involvement is not especially accurate, in fact, false-positive and false-negative rates are reported to be between 25% and 30%. There is no evidence, however, that removal of clinically benign axillary nodes leads to improved survival. If clinically and pathologically positive nodes are removed, the regional recurrence rate is reduced (74).

For most patients, axillary node dissection is performed for staging purposes, as many patients may benefit from adjuvant chemotherapy or hormonal therapy (see below). There is some evidence that certain patient groups with pathologically negative nodes may also benefit from adjuvant therapy (53,57,106,110). If adjuvant therapy is planned for a patient, regardless of whether nodes are involved, axillary node dissection may become unnecessary other than for prognostic reasons.

The axillary lymph nodes have been divided into three groups. Level I nodes are inferior and lateral to the pectoralis minor muscle, level II nodes are beneath this muscle, and level III nodes are superior and medial. The development of lymphedema is a risk of axillary node dissection and increases in likelihood when levels II and III nodes are removed. The distribution of axillary node metastases was analyzed in 539 patients by Veronesi *et al.* (151). They found that, if level I nodes were negative, there was only a 1.5% chance that the higher levels would be involved. If both levels I and II were negative, level III was involved in only 0.4%. It is, therefore, safe to remove only level I or I and II nodes with little chance of concluding that a positive axilla is negative.

Reconstructive Surgery

Total mastectomy produces some degree of psychologic trauma in most patients. Breast reconstruction can alleviate this considerably. In the past, reconstruction was only done 6 to 12 months after all therapy, including adjuvant chemotherapy, had been completed. There was concern that an early local recurrence may be masked but, as the prosthesis is usually placed under the pectoralis major muscle, a recurrence still should be detected easily. Therefore, there is no reason to delay breast reconstruction for long periods and, in fact, immediate reconstruction at the time of mastectomy in selected patients is well tolerated, welcomed by patients, and does not compromise or delay the use of adjuvant chemotherapy (77) (Fig. 17-5).

Most breast reconstructions use a silicone implant filled with silicone gel or saline. When local tissues are inadequate, an expander that can gradually be filled with saline may be used, giving time for the tissues to stretch. When the local soft tissue is of poor quality because of previous radiotherapy, radical mastectomy, or skin grafting, it may be necessary to use a musculocutaneous flap using either the latissimus dorsi or rectus abdominis muscle to cover the prosthesis. It is also possible to reconstruct the breast in some patients without an implant by using autologous tissue from the lower abdominal wall (Fig. 17-5) (81).

Reconstruction of the nipple-areola complex should be delayed for a few months so that the reconstructed breast can attain its final contour. If the opposite breast requires reconstruction for symmetry, this should be done prior to nipple-areola reconstruction. Skin from the upper thigh is usually used for nipple-areola reconstruction, although the opposite areola and the vulva provide suitable tissue (85).

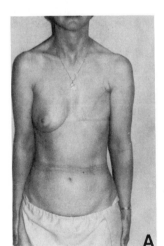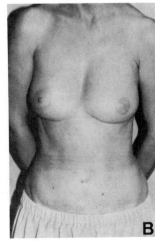

Fig. 17-5. (A) Surgical Reconstruction: Thirty-eight year old women after modified radical mastectomy. (B) Two years after reconstruction with transverse abdominal island flap. No alloplastic material was used in either breast. Courtesy of Hartrampf (85).

Radiation Therapy

Definitive Radiation Therapy

Due to the increasing use of SBE and clinical and mammographic screening, breast cancers are being discovered at an earlier stage when the tumor is smaller and axillary nodes clinically negative. Many patients in this stage are now suitable for breast-conserving treatment. Partial mastectomy followed by postoperative radiotherapy has been shown to have no adverse effect on long-term survival or local recurrence rates (52,152). Treatment choice in early breast cancer is a complex issue and many factors must be evaluated. The factors may be broken down into several categories.

Patient factors:

1. *Patient's wishes and feelings* regarding retaining the breast. Some patients are anxious about retaining a breast that may still harbor cancer and the risk of recurrence. However, with proper selection and treatment, this recurrence risk is no greater than that of chest wall recurrence after mastectomy, and salvage is still possible by mastectomy or further local excision if tumor recurs in the breast.

2. *Breast size:* A small breast may have a significant defect and poor cosmetic outcome if a relatively large amount of breast tissue must be removed to obtain clear margins. Larger breasts will have less deformity. Large and pendulous breasts, however, present technical difficulties for radiation therapy and the cosmetic outcome may be poorer. In addition, following mastectomy, patients with large breasts often have difficulty obtaining a comfortable prosthesis and are bothered by the uneven weight distribution. Also, breast reconstruction will require reduction mammoplasty of the opposite breast to obtain a good match (22).

Tumor factors:

1. *Size:* A large tumor may not give satisfactory cosmetic results. Partial mastectomy plus irradiation for tumors greater than 4 cm in diameter have not been studied in randomized, controlled clinical trials.

2. *Location:* Subareolar tumors present a problem of obtaining adequate margins without sacrifice of the nipple-areolar complex. However, this sacrifice may be acceptable to some patients. It may be difficult to obtain adequate margins with tumors at the periphery of the breast because of proximity to the skin and chest wall.

3. *Pathology:* Ductal CIS requires special consideration and is addressed later in this chapter. There is evidence that good results with breast preservation may be obtained (70).

4. *Multiple tumors:* The presence of two or more separate tumors clinically or mammographically usually will preclude breast preservation because of the extent of resection required (103).

5. *Extensive microcalcifications on mammography distant from the primary tumor:* These may indicate invasive, *in situ*, or benign disease, making mammographic follow-up difficult. Partial mastectomy is usually contraindicated in this situation.

Other considerations and comorbid conditions:

Breast-conserving treatment should be offered where access to surgery by someone familiar with the pathologic and radiotherapeutic procedures required is available. Careful cooperation of mammographer, surgeon, and pathologist is essential and must be planned before the procedure. Radiation therapy should be carried out in facilities with high-energy irradiation (4 to 6 MeV linear accelerator), which is preferable to cobalt-60, although the latter is adequate. High-energy electrons also are required for boost therapy. A treatment simulator is now considered highly desirable, and computerized treatment planning is essential. Access to state-of-the-art radiation therapy may require considerable travel, i.e., 5 days per week for 6 to 7 weeks. This may be a burden, especially for elderly patients. Most coexisting diseases are not serious contraindications for treatment. Serious pulmonary disease that might be further compromised by an otherwise trivial amount of lung irradiation is a consideration. Serious cardiac disease is a consideration in some tumors on the left side. Collagen vascular disease (71) and severe, uncontrolled diabetes are probable contraindications, because in such cases tissues tolerate irradiation poorly. The patient must be cooperative and able to lie still in the treatment position alone in the treatment room. Patients with serious psychiatric disorders and elderly demented patients usually are not suitable for this reason.

Partial mastectomy should be performed after consultation with the radiation therapist to rule out possible contraindications to radiotherapy and to give the patient a full understanding of this treatment modality. The incision should be directly over the tumor if possible or, if not, the tumor bed should be marked with clips to allow the radiation therapist to deliver a boost if it is required. Drains, if used, should be placed within the usual radiation portals. The assumption is that following surgery only a small volume of microscopic tumor will remain in the breast, which can be effectively sterilized by moderate doses of radiation in the range of 4,600 to 5,000 cGy and which will allow a good cosmetic outcome in regard to fibrosis, contraction, pigmentation, and telangiectasis. Several studies have shown that, even when margins appear clear of tumor, recurrence will occur in at least 25% of patients if postoperative radiotherapy is not given (52). Most recurrences are in the area of the primary tumor, indicating that despite the best pathologic technique, margins were not truly clear (134). Other studies on mastectomy specimens have demonstrated that other tumor is frequently present both close to the primary and in other quadrants of the breast.

Following local surgery, healing is usually adequate in 2 to 3 weeks to allow treatment to begin. The entire breast must be treated uniformly. The treatment field extends from the midline to the midaxillary line, and from 1.5 cm below the inframammary crease up to the level of the sternoclavicular joint. This is necessary because microscopic breast tissue extends beyond the obvious breast mound. Medial and lateral oblique portals are used and tissue compensation or wedge filters are essential for homogeneous dose. Careful field placement and simulation are required to avoid excessive underlying lung irradiation and to avoid the heart in tumors on the left side. The underlying chest wall, including muscle, ribs, and intercostal lymphatics, is included. Full discussion of the technique is beyond the scope of this chapter; however, it is one of the most demanding radiation therapy exercises requiring meticulous attention to detail and the best facilities and equipment, as well as excellent physics, dosimetry, and

technology staff. As previously stated, total doses of 4,600 to 5,000 cGy are required to sterilize microscopic disease. Fractions of 180 to 200 cGy/day should not be exceeded, since larger fractions decrease cosmetic outcome.

Boost therapy:

Many centers use a boost to raise the dose to 6,000 cGy in the immediate vicinity of the tumor. The boost includes the entire breast scar and the tumor bed. Therefore, it is important that the scar be located directly over the tumor or that the tumor bed be outlined with clips. Use of preoperative and postoperative mammograms is helpful to determine the site and depth of the tumor bed. The boost may be given most conveniently with electrons. Some centers use radioactive Iridium-192 seeds or wires in plastic afterloading catheters for the boost, but this technique is now used less frequently. Some groups carry out iridium implant boost at the time of local excision when the tumor bed is under direct vision, which avoids additional hospitalization. The NSABP B-06 trial used 5,000 cGy in 200 cGy fractions without boost and had an acceptable local recurrence rate, although some dosimetric details are lacking (52,61). The Milan trial used a boost with orthovoltage radiation (152). With tumors less than 1 cm and wide local excision with clear margins, a boost may not be necessary. Further long-term studies are required to determine the role of the boost.

Irradiation of nodal areas:

If the axillary nodes are histologically negative, irradiation to the axillary and supraclavicular areas is not required, significantly simplifying the radiation therapy. There is no consensus on the need for additional irradiation if the axilla is positive, but the following points should be considered. If there is only minimal microscopic involvement of a few (≤ 4) nodes and an adequate axillary dissection of levels 1 and 2 has been done, irradiation to the axilla may not be necessary. If there is gross axillary involvement or an inadequate dissection, postoperative irradiation will improve locoregional control of disease and should include the supraclavicular area. This treatment somewhat increases the incidence of edema, but such edema is often of minor degree and rarely cosmetically or functionally significant. The internal mammary nodes are at risk in centrally located subareolar and medial tumors, especially if the axilla is positive. A separate radiation portal may be used to treat these nodes, since trying to include this area in tangential portals exposes an unacceptable amount of lung and requires extension of the medial portal to the contralateral side of the midline. Electrons should be used for this area to minimize exposure of heart and lung.

The integration of chemotherapy and radiation therapy:

If chemotherapy is to be given, it is essential that it be started as soon after surgery as possible, while the systemic tumor burden is minimal. Concomitant radiation therapy and chemotherapy increase local tissue reaction and may worsen the cosmetic result. Doxorubicin should be especially avoided in this situation. If it is felt that the risk of residual disease in the breast and regional nodes is low, then irradiation may be delayed until chemotherapy is completed, provided the delay is not longer than 6 months. A compromise is to give 3 to 4 cycles of chemotherapy, suspend it during the radiation therapy and then resume and complete the chemotherapy for 3 or 4 more cycles. The actuarial 5-year breast failure rate was

4% when patients received radiotherapy before chemotherapy or 6-8% when given sequentially or concurrently before the completion of chemotherapy according to Recht *et al.* (125). However, the failure rate was 41% in patients who received all chemotherapy before radiotherapy. Results such as these suggest that delaying the initiation of radiotherapy may result in an increase or likelihood of local failure. Studies have shown that chemotherapy can be given in full dose after irradiation. As has always been true in breast cancer, many questions remain unanswered; however, earlier diagnosis provides an opportunity for breast preservation and abolition of the fear that a breast lump automatically means loss of the breast. This in itself should avoid the delay in therapy that so often occurred in the past. Breast preservation with acceptable cosmesis and low risk of recurrence or complications is now a reality for many women.

Time to initiate radiation therapy:

According to Harris *et al.*, there is an increase in breast failures (25-30%) in a small subset of early Stage I patients despite adjuvant chemotherapy if radiation therapy is delayed more than 16 weeks after surgical excision.

Postmastectomy Irradiation

This area remains controversial. Certain factors predict for a high risk of locoregional recurrence, and such gross recurrences can be difficult or impossible to control and lead to much suffering. It was hoped that the advent of multiagent, postoperative chemotherapy would prevent locoregional recurrence and improve disease-free and overall survival. It is now evident, however, that this has not occurred to the degree hoped for, probably because the remaining tumor burden was too great. It is unquestioned that postoperative radiation therapy properly delivered in adequate doses reduces locoregional failure. The challenge is to identify patients at significant risk, and to treat them adequately in conjunction with whatever systemic therapy they receive. It has been shown that there is no benefit from postoperative radiation therapy in patients with T1 or T2 tumors that have been treated with modified radical or radical mastectomy. Further studies on the use of adjuvant irradiation in patients with more advanced local disease are required to define treatment criteria (142).

Radiation Therapy in Locally Advanced Disease

When breast cancer presents at a stage at which surgery can no longer eradicate the disease, combination therapy is aimed at locoregional control. Because of the high risk of disseminated disease in this situation, systemic therapy is usually the initial approach, but primary radiotherapy has been suggested for locally advanced disease to avoid the difficult problems of recurrent local disease (38,138). If a good response is obtained, further consolidation may be achieved with surgery. The sequence depends on many factors and treatment is individualized. The aim is local control and cosmesis is sacrificed because full-dose irradiation must be used. Doses in excess of 6,000 cGy to the breast are given with external beam, sometimes supplemented with interstitial implantation. The regional nodes are also treated vigorously, but doses in excess of 5,000 cGy must be used cautiously because of the risk of brachial plexus injury.

Cosmesis

One of the major aims of radiation treatment is to provide excellent cosmesis after conservative surgery (22). If the surgical excision or lumpectomy is done carefully following the guidelines noted in Chapter 4, "Principles of Surgical Oncology," excellent cosmesis should result, presenting a normal appearing breast and nipple, free of distortion and disfigurement (Fig. 17-6). Hematomas in the breast and seroma after axillary node sampling increase the likelihood of persistent breast edema and lymphedema of the arm. Generally, good to excellent cosmesis is in the 80% to 90% range at 3, 5, and 7 years (44a,117) and patients tend to rate cosmesis as good to excellent more often than do physicians.

Chemotherapy and Hormonal Therapy

Adjuvant Chemohormonal Therapy: Occult Micrometastases

In the past decade, significant progress has been made in the systemic adjuvant treatment of breast cancer. The purpose of adjuvant therapy is to treat micrometastatic disease before it is clinically detectable in the hope that the smaller tumor burden will be easier to eliminate. Patients at high risk for developing metastatic disease are treated after their primary tumor is treated. Both chemotherapy and hormonal therapy have been used in the adjuvant therapy of breast cancer (132).

Adjuvant combination chemotherapy regimens used for breast cancer fall broadly into two groups: those consisting of CMF, and those containing doxorubicin. Recently, doxorubicin-containing regimens have been used for high-risk patients with more than four positive lymph nodes and negative ERs. Several prospective, randomized trials have demonstrated consistently that DFS of premenopausal women with breast cancer can be significantly prolonged by the use of adjuvant chemotherapy (27,127,157). In some of these trials, overall survival was increased as well. In one of the earlier adjuvant chemotherapy trials, 20% more of the patients treated with CMF were alive at the end of the ninth year compared with those treated with mastectomy alone (27). In

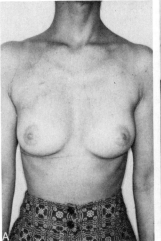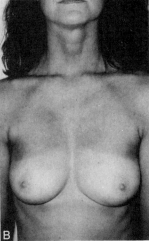

Fig. 17-6. Radiation Cosmesis: Excellent cosmesis results from the selective effect of irradiation. If breast surgery does not distort or disfigure the fine surgical result, ofen lumpectomy is maintained by radiation therapy.

postmenopausal women, on the other hand, most studies have shown improvement in DFS only. However, many of these trials have small sample sizes in which all but very large differences in survival are likely to be missed. To overcome the inadequate sample size of most trials, Early Breast Cancer Trialists' Collaborative Group conducted metaanalysis of 133 randomized trials involving 31,000 recurrences and 24,000 deaths among 75,000 women with early breast cancer worldwide (46a). This cooperative effort involves the largest evidence ever collected from randomized studies to assess the effect of cancer therapy on long-term outcome. The following is the summary of the important findings.

Tamoxifen produced highly significant reductions in the annual rates of both recurrence and of death in all women. Recurrence rate was reduced by 25% and mortality by 17% ($p < 0.00001$) (Fig. 17-7). In women older than 70 years, only tamoxifen was evaluated and recurrence was reduced by 28%; mortality by 21%. Recurrence was reduced in women younger than 50 years of age by 12% and mortality by 6%. Tamoxifen reduced overall tumor recurrence and mortality in estrogen receptor poor or negative patients as well, although the magnitude was significantly less than in estrogen receptor positive women. Interestingly, the risk of contralateral breast cancer was reduced by 39%. Long-term treatment (> 2 years) was also more effective.

Combination adjuvant chemotherapy reduced the annual recurrence rate by 28% and annual death rate by 16% in all women. However, the magnitude of reduction was greater in women younger than 50 years of age (Fig. 17-8). Long-term treatment (12 months) was no better than shorter regimens (6 months). Combination adjuvant chemotherapy was more effective than single agent chemotherapy (46a).

In women 50 years of age or younger, annual recurrence rate was reduced by 26% and annual death rate by 25% by ovarian ablation (46a).

Other conclusions include benefit of short term adjuvant chemotherapy continued during year 5 through 10 and cumulative differences in survival were greater at 10 years than at 5 years. Benefits for node-positive and node-negative women with use of tamoxifen and chemotherapy were similar, but absolute improvement in 10-year survival was about twice as great for node positive women. For women aged 50 to 69 years, direct comparisons show that chemotherapy plus tamoxifen is better than chemotherapy alone in terms of recurrence and mortality and better than tamoxifen alone in terms of recurrence (46a).

Whether to offer chemotherapy to large numbers of patients with node-negative breast cancer when there is, as of yet, no evidence of a survival advantage is a difficult decision for all physicians involved in the care of these patients. Determining subsets of patients with a poor prognosis within the node-negative group, rather than treating a large number of patients unnecessarily to benefit only a few, may prove useful because chemotherapy is not without side effects and there also may be some risk of secondary acute leukemia (42).

Guidelines for treatment of node-negative breast cancer patients are recommended based on standard and new prognosticators (80,111,112):

1. Minimal risk: Noninvasive tumors (ductal CIS and lobular CIS) or small invasive tumors at mammogra-

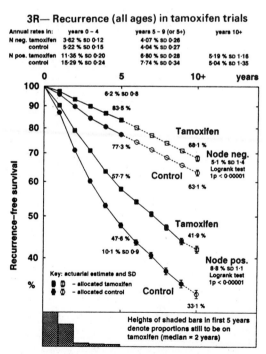

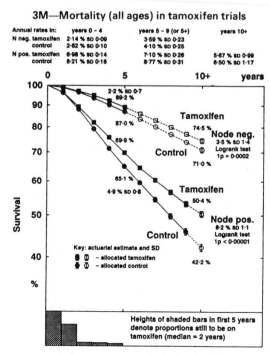

Fig. 17-7. Ten-year outcome in tamoxifen trials, subdivided by nodal status. The results are subdivided between "node-negative" (by dissection or by sampling) and "node-positive" (all other women, including the few with unrecorded nodal status). Among the node-negative women, the balanced totals were 761/6438 tamoxifen versus 917/6566 to causes other than breast cancer and 578 versus 715 (9.0% versus 10.9%) were other deaths, a proper overview of which indicated an odds reduction of 19% SD (3 7 standard deviations. 1p = 0.0001). Open symbols denote smoothed rates. From Early Breast Cancer Trialists' Collaborative Group (46a), with permission.

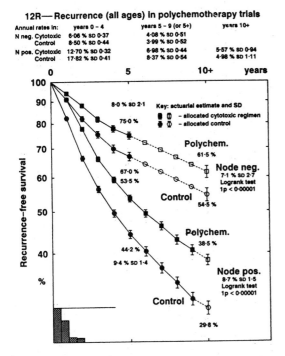

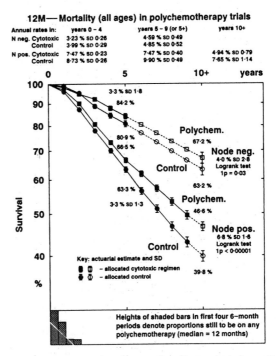

Fig. 17-8. Ten-year outcome in polychemotherapy trials, subdivided by nodal status. Among the node-negative women, the balanced totals were 273/1411 polychemotherapy versus 283/1360 control deaths (logrank O-E = -20.7, variance 121.2, 1p = 0.03), of which 18 versus 23 (1.3% versus 1.7%) were deaths before relapse attributed to causes other than breast cancer and 228 versus 260 (16.9% versus 19.1%) were other deaths, a proper overview of which yielded logrank O-E = -18.5, variance 111.9, odds reduction 15% SD9, 1p = 0.04. From Early Breast Cancer Trialists' Collaborative Group (46a), with permission.

phy, or at time of surgery for *in situ* benign disease—observation rather than adjuvant treatment.

2. Good risk: ER-positive, diploid, low S phase, T less than 2 cm, good nuclear grade, well-differentiated tumors, low level of cathepsin D—observation rather than adjuvant treatment.

3. Poor risk: ER-negative, aneuploid, diploid with high S phase, T greater than 2 cm, poor nuclear grade, poorly differentiated tumor, high levels of cathepsin D—adjuvant therapy, preferably in a mutual cooperative group protocol (postmenopausal: tamoxifen ± chemotherapy; premenopausal: chemotherapy).

Management of Metastatic Breast Cancer

Hormonal manipulation (Table 17-9) (90):

Totally unselected patients have a 30% probability of response to hormonal therapy. Ablative or additive hormonal treatment is useful in approximately 40% to 60% of the patients who have tumors that are ER positive and the response rates continue improving with increasing levels of the ER proteins (155). The presence of PRs is an even better predictor of response with response rates as high as 70 to 80% (155). Only 10% of patients who are receptor negative respond to hormonal manipulation. Often responses to hormonal manipulation are durable and the side effects are minimal. In postmenopausal women, hormonal treatment is the treatment of choice and should consist of tamoxifen followed by a progesterone. In patients with rapidly progressive tumors, however, cytotoxic chemotherapy is the treat-

ment of choice, as it is in patients with receptor-negative tumor or those who have had progression on hormonal therapy (44). Usually patients who have responded to one hormonal therapy also respond to another hormonal manipulation, although the duration for the second response is usually much shorter than the first. Postmenopausal status, osseous metastases, and durable disease-free interval usually predict a long response to hormones.

Oophorectomy: Previously, this procedure was the ablative treatment of choice in ER positive metastatic breast cancer in premenopausal women. As is true of other hormonal manipulations, metastatic disease in the liver and brain and lymphangitic lung metastases are less likely to respond. More recently, tamoxifen has been shown to be as effective as oophorectomy in premenopausal patients, although a small number of patients who had not responded to tamoxifen did respond to oophorectomy, and a lesser number of patients who initially did not respond to oophorectomy did respond to tamoxifen. In patients not suitable for surgical castration, ovarian ablation can be accomplished by irradiation with 1,500 to 2,000 cGy over 2 weeks.

Antiestrogen tamoxifen: Tamoxifen has become the treatment of choice in postmenopausal women who are ER positive and have metastatic disease likely to respond to hormones (126a). In a randomized study comparing tamoxifen with combination chemotherapy, the response rates, response duration, and survival were similar, although there was a marked difference in favor of tamoxifen in side effects and quality of life (146). In a similar comparison with dieth-

Table 17-9. Response (%) to Endocrine Therapy For Breast Cancer

Endocrine Therapy	Patient Group		
	Unselected	ERP+	ERP-
Tamoxifen*	32	54	9
Oophorectomy §	33	62	6
Progestins*	31	(35)	8
Aminoglutethimide	31	36	6
LHRH analogs §	42	-	-
Estrogens*	26	57	9
Androgens*	21	43	8
Adrenalectomy*	32	46	10
Hypophysectomy*	36	-	-

Response to Endocrine Therapy Correlated with Either ER Value or ER and PR Status				
ER Value (fmol/mg)	Response Rate (%)	Frequency PR Positive (%)	Combined ER/PR Status ER - / PR-	Response Rate (%)
<3	6	9		9
3-10		40	ER +/ PR-	
	46			32
10-100		70	ER +/ PR+	
>100	81	77		71

NOTE: Therapies listed in order of increasing toxicity.
* Primarily postmenopausal patients
§ Exclusively premenopausal patients
ERP = estrogen receptor protein; LHRH = luteinizing hormone-releasing factor; ER = estrogen receptor; PR = progesterone receptor.
Adapted from Henderson (90).

ylstilbestrol, tamoxifen was much better tolerated and has since replaced diethylstilbestrol as the initial treatment of choice for metastatic breast cancer in postmenopausal women. The usual dose is 10 mg orally twice daily. Side effects are infrequent and when they occur usually consist of nausea, vomiting, and hot flashes. A small percentage of patients might develop thrombocytopenia or hypercalcemia; the latter complication usually happens in the first few weeks after the tamoxifen initiation. During that period bone pains might also worsen, which is described as "flare phenomenon" and is not an indication for discontinuing treatment. Ten percent to 20% of patients who initially responded to tamoxifen and then progressed will again demonstrate a partial remission when tamoxifen is discontinued. Therefore, if the clinical condition permits before another treatment is started, the patient can be observed for several weeks to permit such a secondary response.

Progesterones: Approximately 30% of women with metastatic breast cancer who have previously responded to hormones will respond to progesterones. The most commonly used agent is megestrol acetate administered orally at a dosage of 40 to 300 mg/d. Side effects include weight gain, fluid retention, increased appetite, and thrombotic tendencies.

Medical adrenalectomy: Aminoglutethimide is an inhibitor of adrenal steroid biosynthesis and blocks the conversion of cholesterol to pregnenolone, and therefore reduces levels of adrenal androgens, which are a source of estrogens in both premenopausal and postmenopausal women. Although this inhibition may not be complete, the nonadrenal conversion of androstenedione to estrogens is also inhibited, thus effectively eliminating the source of estrogens. Aminoglutethimide

has produced an antitumor response in 50% or more of selected patients, most of whom have undergone prior therapy with either chemotherapy or hormonal manipulation. As is true of other hormonal responses, the highest response rates are observed in patients who are ER and/or PR positive.

A randomized comparison between surgical adrenalectomy and aminoglutethimide in women with advanced breast cancer has shown that the objective tumor regression is similar in the two treatments. The response does not differ significantly in frequency or duration either, so that aminoglutethimide has replaced surgical adrenalectomy and hyphosphysectomy.

Aminoglutethimide is administered as 250 mg tablets, starting with two tablets, and after 2 weeks increasing to four tablets, daily. To minimize the lethargy, dizziness, and skin rash that are often experienced by these patients, hydrocortisone should be administered concurrently (40 mg/d). Patients who develop postural hypotension need mineralocorticoid supplements as well. When aminoglutethimide is discontinued, adrenal function restores itself and slow tapering of hydrocortisone is not often required.

Androgens: The most commonly used androgen is fluoxymesterone administered orally 20 to 40 mg/d in divided doses. The side effects include virilization with increased facial hair, frontal balding, deepening of the voice, clitoral enlargement, and increased libido. Because of these side effects, androgens are poorly tolerated. They also cause unpleasant side effects such as cholestatic jaundice, hypercalcemia, and fluid retention. Responses to androgens are often not durable.

Adrenal corticosteroids: The adrenal corticosteroids often are used for supportive care of patients in the management of lymphangitic carcinomatosis, hypercalcemia, increasing intracranial pressure, bone pain, and anorexia. Objective responses are seen in 10% to 15% of cases.

Cytotoxic Chemotherapy

Metastatic breast cancer, unlike other solid tumors, is highly responsive to chemotherapy (Table 17-10) (89). With combination chemotherapy, response rates of 50% to 70% have been reported consistently, although there has not been a significant impact on long-term survival of these patients (6). As mentioned above, patients who have rapidly progressing disease, lack hormone receptors, have significant impairment of vital organs such as lung or liver by metastatic involvement, or whose disease has progressed on hormonal therapy should be treated with palliative combination chemotherapy. Metastatic disease to the brain does not respond to chemotherapy or hormonal manipulation and is best treated with radiation and steroids.

Single-agent chemotherapy rarely is used now in the treatment of these patients because combination chemotherapy gives superior, more durable response rates. Doxorubicin-containing regimens usually give higher response rates, but response duration and overall survival are not markedly improved. Since the median duration of response is only 8 to 18 months, attempts to improve results of current treatment are under way.

The toxicity of multiagent chemotherapy varies considerably, but, in general, nausea and fatigue are most common. Alopecia is frequent with cyclophosphamide- and doxorubicin-containing regimens. Doxorubicin is cardiotoxic as well, but this is usually not a problem below a total doxorubicin dose of 550 mg/m² BSA.

When resistance to chemotherapy is evident, change to a different combination of agents is indicated; however, response rates usually do not exceed 25%.

Currently, several newer investigational agents are being studied in patients with metastatic breast carcinoma. Use of alternating, non-cross-resistant chemotherapy regimens has not been particularly successful. The use of immunotherapy and high-dose chemotherapy, followed by autologous bone marrow transplant, is currently under investigation (19,47).

Radiation Therapy

Breast cancer may metastasize to any organ in the body: as mentioned, bone, lung, liver, and brain are frequent sites. Metastases usually are evident within a few years but notoriously for breast cancer, recurrence may occur, particularly in bone, many years later. Effective palliation and long-term survival often can be achieved by a variety of measures. The management plan for metastatic disease depends on many factors: age, menopausal status, hormone receptor status, if known, sites of metastases, and previous therapy. Systemic treatment is the mainstay but there are specific indications for irradiation and sometimes surgery. Planning and integration of therapy are essential by all involved. Radiation therapy is specifically indicated for relief of bone pain and prevention of fracture at critical sites. Orthopedic intervention may also be required. Metastases to the brain and choroid and the presence of spinal cord compression are indications for urgent radiation therapy. Because response to chemotherapy or hormonal treatment may be slow, radiation therapy that predictably affects palliation rapidly also may be indicated. It should be remembered that irradiation decreases or destroys bone marrow function, and will therefore decrease the patient's

Table 17-10. Response (%) to Combination Chemotherapy for Breast Cancer

| Regimen | Response Rate (%) | | Median Duration of | |
	PR + CR	CR	Response (mo)	Survival (mo)
CMFVP	46	11	9	12
CMFVP	59	18	8	14
CMFP	68	8	8	-
CMFP	53	5	6	16
CMF	53	11	11	17
CMF	53	15	6	12
CMF	37	10	7	14
CAF vs	47	-	6	-
CMF	41	-	6	-

| Study Design | Additional Benefit Observed with Doxorubicin Combination | | |
	Response (%) Rate	Duration (mo)	Survival (mo)
CMF vs CAF	+20	+3	+10
	+18	+4	+11
CMFP vs CAF	0	+5	+3
CMFVP vs CAFVP	+1	+2	-
	+31	+5	+3
CMFVP vs CAF	+31	+7	+6
	+15	0	+3

PR = partial response; CR = complete response; C = cyclophosphamide; M = methotrexate;; F = 5-fluorourcil; P = prednisone; V = vincrintine.
Adapted from Henderson, (89).

ability to tolerate chemotherapy. Careful integration of therapies and optimal sparing of bone marrow is therefore essential.

SPECIAL CONSIDERATIONS

Preinvasive Cancer

As more and more breast cancers are being detected at an early stage, preinvasive cancer, or CIS, is being diagnosed more often and now constitute 15-20%. Many of these lesions are nonpalpable and found on screening mammography. CIS can be divided into two categories, depending on where it arises. Ductal CIS arises in the ducts. Malignant epithelial cells are found within the ducts but there is no invasion through the basement membrane. Lobular CIS occurs in the lobules and may extend into the ducts in the same way that ductal CIS may extend into the lobules, resulting in occasional difficulty in distinguishing between the two.

Ductal CIS

Prior to screening mammography, most ductal CIS was detected by finding a mass in the breast due to extensive intraductal tumor. This presentation is now less common and often the lesion is detected by the presence of fine microcalcifications on mammography. Fifteen percent to 20% of breast cancers found by screening mammography are ductal CIS. It is believed that not all ductal CIS progress to invasive cancer. Those that do probably do so within 10 years.

Standard therapy has been total mastectomy. Breast conserving operations such as lumpectomy alone will yield high recurrence rate of 9-21% and half of these will reappear as invasive cancers (67a,110,138b). Recent data from an NSABP trial (69,70) of lumpectomy with or without radiotherapy revealed a small group of patients with ductal CIS that could be analyzed separately. The results suggested that lumpectomy with postoperative radiation therapy gave acceptable results and low local recurrence rates. Certainly, if we are treating invasive cancer with breast conserving surgery, it is reasonable to do so at an earlier disease stage. As with invasive cancer, as long as the resection margins are free of disease, this approach should be adequate (140).

A 2% rate of positive axillary nodes has been reported in ductal CIS, presumably because areas of invasion were not sampled by the examining pathologist. This is most likely to occur in patients with extensive ductal CIS; therefore, it may be wise to include axillary node dissection in this subgroup of patients. Because the risk of carcinoma in the opposite breast is not excessively high, careful follow-up by physical examination and mammography, rather than blind biopsy, is thought to be adequate.

Lobular CIS

Lobular CIS follows a different course than ductal CIS. It tends to be multicentric and may be bilateral. The risk of invasive cancer in the opposite as well as the ipsilateral breast is increased (128). Management of this tumor, at present, is controversial and has ranged from bilateral total mastectomy to complete excision with careful observation. The presence of lobular CIS is undoubtedly a risk factor for the development of invasive cancer but since the course can be indolent conservative surgery would appear to be the reasonable approach.

Inflammatory Carcinoma of the Breast

Locally advanced breast cancer includes patients with stages IIIA and B tumors and inflammatory carcinoma. Clinical features of the latter disease include erythema and edema of the breast with or without associated mass. Although originally at least one third of the breast had to be involved before making the diagnosis, recently it has been determined that lesser involvement has a similar prognosis. Dermal invasion of lymphatics is the histologic hallmark, but is not necessary, however, since the diagnosis is clinical. Virtually all inflammatory breast cancer patients have nodal involvement and incidence of systemic disease at presentation is high (93).

Because of the high incidence of systemic micrometastases and poor prognosis, radical mastectomy is contraindicated. Treatment with primary radiation therapy also has resulted in poor survival—less than 2 years.

To improve outcome by treating micrometastases present at diagnosis, systemic cytotoxic chemotherapy prior to local therapy with irradiation and/or surgery was introduced in early 1970. Several reports have been published documenting the salutary effect of maximum doses of doxorubicin-containing chemotherapy when combined with local radiation therapy (116,130,141).

Swain et al. (141) at the NCI treated 107 patients with locally advanced breast cancer; 45 of them had inflammatory breast cancer and received induction chemotherapy containing doxorubicin. After best response to induction chemotherapy, an open biopsy was repeated. If no tumor remained, the patient was treated with radiation therapy and chemotherapy. If tumor remained, local treatment consisted of mastectomy and radiation therapy. This was followed in either case by continued chemotherapy for 6 more months. The group reported 55% complete response and 43% partial response. Median survival of all patients was 50 months. The striking improvement is in chest wall failures: from 70% to 19% when combining all modalities. Current protocols with 2 to 3 cycles CAF, followed by surgery and postoperative irradiation (50 Gy) followed by maintenance chemotherapy have yielded a 37% DFS and 48% actuarial survival (15). Similarly, in a large study of 230 patients from France (130), there was significant improvement in DFS with a combined modality approach.

Though these survival rates represent improvement over single-modality treatment, newer treatments, including use of high-dose chemotherapy with autologous bone marrow transplantation (19,47) and use of colony-stimulating factors after high-dose chemotherapy, represent promising areas of research.

Paget's Disease

Paget's disease of the breast presents as an eczematoid, crusted lesion of the nipple and areola. Histologically, it is characterized by large cells with large nuclei and abundant cytoplasm in the epidermis. The origin of these cells is still controversial, but Paget's disease is almost always associated with an underlying noninvasive or invasive breast cancer. Treatment generally has been total mastectomy with axillary node dissection. Few studies of breast-conserving therapy have been reported.

Male Breast Cancer

Male breast cancer accounts for 1% of all breast cancers. It had been thought to carry a worse prognosis than breast cancer in women but this has not been confirmed by detailed studies (23). Total mastectomy is recommended with or without axillary node dissection. Skin grafting is often necessary to close the defect. Studies of adjuvant therapy in males have not been done because of the rarity of the disease but, as in women, positive axillary nodes predict a worse prognosis. Hormone receptor determinations should be done since ERs are positive in over 50% of patients and predict responsiveness to hormonal manipulation such as orchiectomy, tamoxifen, diethylstilbestrol, and aminoglutethimide.

Pregnancy and Lactation

Breast cancer during pregnancy and lactation does not appear to have a poorer prognosis than breast cancer detected at other times as long as therapy is not delayed. Mastectomy can be safely performed during pregnancy if particular care is taken with hemostasis. The urgent necessity for chemotherapy or radiation therapy because of rapid progression of disease may be an indication for therapeutic abortion but it is not recommended otherwise.

RESULTS AND PROGNOSIS

Staging Characteristics

Survival is shown relative to clinical and histologic stages using American Joint Committee on Cancer Staging and End Results (AJC) criteria and data from the NASBP and AJC (Table 17-11). Note that survival decreases with advancement of primary tumor and status of axillary lymph nodes (Table 17-12 and Figs. 17-3 and 17-9).

As noted, there are some major differences between the current and previous classifications that can result in stage migration or make results appear different when compared with previous classifications.

1. Axilla-negative patients are superior to axilla-positive in 5-year results, almost doubling overall survival outcome, i.e., overall survival 72% to 76% v 35% to 48%, respectively.

2. Axillary-positive one to three nodes prognosticates an outcome that is double in patients with greater than or equal to four nodes positive, i.e., overall survival 63% v 27%.

3. Ten-year survival can be projected accurately as a function of primary tumor size, axillary status, and level of involvement. There is a 20% decrease in survival with each 2 cm increase in tumor size and according to stage size, i.e., less than 2, 2 to 5, and greater than 5 cm (Fig. 17-3). Proximal level involvement is compatible with a high 5-year survival as contrasted to middle and distal levels, i.e., 65% v 31%.

Different Surgical Resections

There has been a trend to more conservative surgical resections without diminution of results: compare 91% 5-year survival for segmental mastectomy with 75% to 90% 5-year survival for radical mastectomy in Stage I breast cancer (Table 17-13).

Definitive Radiation Therapy for Localized Stages

Many studies now support the contention that simple excision of a tumor followed by radiation therapy is as effective as total mastectomy (Table 17-14). Several nonrandomized studies (17,34,38,43,85,87,116,124) as well as crucial randomized studies all support this conclusion. In the French studies (34,124), the primary tumor was often not completely excised. Despite this, their survival results were comparable with studies in which lumpectomy was performed in all patients. However, incomplete excision is associated with an increased local recurrence rate (123).

The results of the randomized studies can be summarized as follows (Table 17-13):

1. *The Italian Cancer Institute* study (152) showed no difference in survival between radical mastectomy and quadrantectomy plus breast irradiation (Fig. 17-10). This was independent of node status.

Table 17-11. Survival of Patients With Breast Cancer Relative To Clinical and Histologic Stage

Clinical Staging	Crude 5-year Survival (%)	Range of Survival (%)
Stage I	85	82-94
Stage II	66	47-74
Stage III	41	7-80
Stage IV	10	No data

(68)

Overall Survival (OS) and Disease-Free Survival (DFS) at 10 Years in Relation to Histologic Involvement of Axillary Lymph Nodes for Patients Treated by Radical Mastectomy

	DFS (%)	OS (%)
Histologically negative	72-76	72-76
Histologically positive	24-25	35-48
1-3 nodes	34-36	63
>4 nodes	14-16	27

Adapted from Henderson (91). Reprinted by permission of the New England Journal of Medicine.

Table 17-12. Ten-Year Survival Related to Primary Size and Level of Axillary Involvement In Breast Cancer

Axillary Status	<2cm (%)	2-5 cm (%)	>5cm (%)	TOTAL (%)
Negative	82	65	44	72
Positive, proximal only	73	74	39	65
Positive, middle or distal	*	28	37	31
Positive all	68	51	37	

* Insufficient data

Adapted from Schottenfeld et al. (135).

Table 17-13. Five-Year Survival In Breast Cancer — Surgical Results

	Clinical Stage I (%)	Clinical Stage II (%)
Segmental mastectomy	91	74
Segmental mastectomy plus radiotherapy	90-92	60-75
Simple mastectomy	75-82	66
Simple mastectomy plus radiotherapy	75-80	58-72
Modified radical mastectomy	89	
Radical mastectomy	75-90	50-60
Extended radical mastectomy	87-92	56-79

Adapted from Fisher et al. (52,58,60) and Versonesi et al. (149, 151).

Table 17-14. Treatment of Breast Cancer by Irradiation Only With a 5–10 Year Follow-up

Reference	Stage	Number of Patients	5-Year Survival (%)	Relapse-free Survival		Locoregional Recurrence (%)
Harris et al. (79)	I	62	94	No data		5
	II	122	73			7
Pierquin et al. (118)	T1	74	92	82		3
	T2	166	81	75	5-yr	6
	T3	22	70	54		15
Calle et al. (29)	T1 N0 N1a	559	No data	83		
	T2 N0 N1a	158		66		Some operated on
	T2 N1b	55		40	10-yr	(mastectomy)
	T3	125		29		
Amalric et al. (16a)	T1 N0	28	57	57		Some operated on
	T1 N1	20	80	80		(mastectomy)
	T2 N0	249	67	62		
	T2 N1	436	64	57		
	T3 N0	88	52	50		
	T3 N1	295	43	34		
Chu et al. (33)	I	146	75	-		8
	II		56	-		17
Clark et al. (35)	I, II	680	83	71	10-yr	8-12
Danoff et al. (36)	I	104	82 (~4 yr)	-		5
	II	80	70	-		
Hellman et al. (82)	I	176	96	-		5
	II		68	-		7
Montague (110)	I/ II	134/157	85/78	78/73	10-yr	6/5

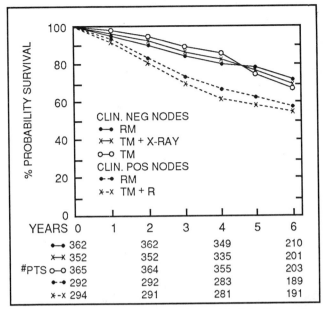

Fig. 17-9. Comparison of survival of patients with clinically negative nodes and patients with clinically positive nodes: National Surgical Adjuvant Breast Project information. RM = radical mastectomy; TM = total mastectomy; R = local/regional irradiation. Courtesy of Fisher and Redmond (60).

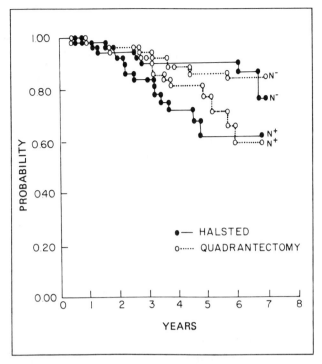

Fig. 17-10. Actuarial disease-free survival according to presence (N+) or absence (N-) of axillary node metastases (log-rank test, adjusted value, overall chi-square, 0.75 with 1 degree of freedom; p = 0.38). Courtesy of Veronesi et al. (151).

2. *The NSABP* conducted the most crucial studies establishing the role of definitive breast irradiation (Fig. 17-11) (61). The risk of recurrence in the breast was reduced substantially in all patients who received breast irradiation after lumpectomy (Fig. 17-11a). Overall survival and DFS after lumpectomy with or without irradiation was not significantly different from that for total mastectomy (Fig. 17-11b).

3. *The Stockholm* studies compared preoperative or postoperative irradiation to modified radical mastectomy alone (132). There was a definite improvement for both node-negative and node-positive patients with regard to a decrease in local recurrence and an increase in DFS for irradiated patients, but there was no impact on overall survival. Comparison of postoperative irradiation to chemotherapy and/or tamoxifen is noted in the following section.

4. *American series:*
   a. *Harvard series:* The long-term evaluation of complications in breast cancer comes from the follow-up of more than 1,000 patients over the past two decades at the Harvard Joint Center. Fortunately, the evolved radiation techniques and doses have lead to excellent outcomes with favorable therapeutic ratios. Pierce *et al.* (123a) (1,624 patients) report the likelihood of a late complication as less than 5% for severe effects such as brachial plexopathy, rib fracture, tissue necrosis and pericarditis. Chemotherapy as well as doses above 50 Gy add significantly though modestly to augmenting these undesirable events. The complications are low when using six new energies and limiting the dose to whole breast and axilla to 50 Gy or lower.
   b. *University of Pennsylvania series:* Fowble *et al.* (74a) report that in their series of 697 clinical Stage I and

II breast cancer patients treated over a decade by excision, axillary dissection, and definitive irradiation, the 10-year actuarial survival was 83% overall, 87% for Stage I, and 77% for Stage II patients. The important new finding is that the cumulative probability of isolate breast recurrence of 6% at 5 years rose to 16% at 10 years with or without distant metastases. Curiously, neither tumor size nor nodal status impacted on recurrence. The reason may be that the addition of adjuvant systemic chemotherapy significantly decreased the risk of isolated breast recurrence.

Adjuvant Chemotherapy and Hormonal Therapy

Localized Stage I/II Patients

For adjuvant chemotherapy, results have remained statistically significant for premenopausal women, whereas postmenopausal women have not shown consistently high responses (Table 17-15).

NSABP studies: Early efforts to improve DFS in postmastectomy patients by using cytotoxic chemotherapy include a study beginning in the late 1950s of the effects of triethylenethiophosphoramide injections around the time of surgery conducted by the NSABP (67). An improvement in survival lasting at least 10 years following treatment was found in a subset of premenopausal patients who had four or more nodes. No effect was seen in postmenopausal women.

Since 1972, the NSABP has carried out several large clinical trials. Two years of intermittent oral phenylalanine mustard demonstrated an improvement in both DFS and overall survival in mastectomized patients especially if they were premenopausal (54). Survival was also improved when patients both phenylalanine mustard and 5-FU, as compared

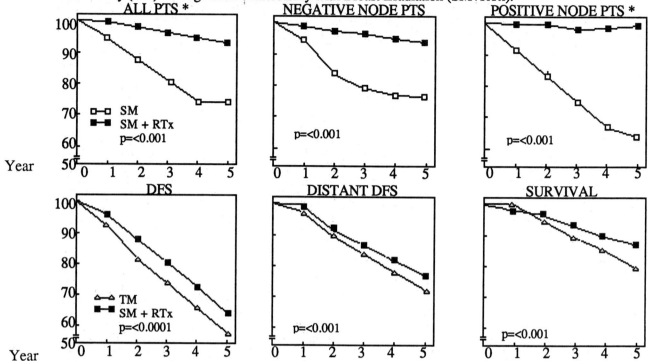

RESULTS

Life-Table Analysis Showing the percentage of Patients Remaining Free of Breast Tumor after Segmental Mastectomy (SM) or Segmental Mastectomy with Breast Irradiation (SM+RTx).

Fig. 17-11. Life-table (a) analysis showing the percentage of patients remaining free of breast tumor after lumpectomy (L) or with breast irradiation lumpectomy (L+XRT) and (b) rates of disease-free survival, distant disease-free survival, and overall survival of patients treated with total mastectomy (TM) of L+XRT. Courtesy of Fisher *et al.* (61).

with phenylalanine mustard alone (58). This survival improvement is especially significant in groups of premenopausal women with positive axillary nodes. The two-drug regimen also results in significantly improved survival in postmenopausal women with more than four involved lymph nodes. The addition of doxorubicin to phenylalanine mustard and 5-FU in ER negative patients has also been shown to increase DFS and overall survival (63).

Table 17-15. Ten-Year Results of NSABP and Milan Trials: Breast Cancer Patients with Histologically Involved Nodes Randomized to 1–2 Years of Adjuvant Chemotherapy or Mastectomy Alone

Patient Group	NSABP			Milan		
	Control	Melphalan	P	Control	CMF	P
Recurrence-free at 10 yrs (%)						
All patients	29	38	0.06	31	43	0.001
Premenopausal	29	46	0.02	31	48	0.0005
Postmenopausal	28	34	0.49	32	38	0.32
Premenopausal						
1-3 nodes	41	66	0.02	40	61	0.0002
> 3 nodes	17	22	0.42	15	26	0.03
Alive at 10 yrs (%)						
All patients	41	48	0.30	47	55	0.10
Premenopausal	37	61	0.02	45	59	<0.02
Postmenopausal	43	41	0.80	50	52	0.89
Premenopausal						
1-3 nodes	48	81	0.01	51	68	0.025
> 3 nodes	26	35	0.54	30	42	0.29

NSABP = National Surgical Adjuvant Breast Project; CMF = cyclophosphamide, methotrexate, 5-fluorouracil.

Adapted from Bonadonna et al. (25,29), Fisher et al. (54), and Henderson (89).

Milan Studies (25,26,28-30): The Milan study gave intensive monthly courses of CMF for 1 year following radical mastectomy (25).

- The results after 5 years showed that premenopausal women demonstrate significantly improved DFS after adjuvant combination chemotherapy. Postmenopausal women do not demonstrate such improved survival except for a subset that was able to tolerate over 85% of the full calculated dose of chemotherapy.
- The most recent report of a 10-year study shows an improved continued median survival that is largely attributable to the benefit in premenopausal women. No plateau has been shown (Table 17-15) (28). The relapse rate is greater in the untreated group in the first 2 years, and after that is the same as for the CMF-treated group (Fig. 17-12). There is a 3.5 year DFS benefit for CMF *v* control.
- Doxorubicin added before CMF for women with four or more positive nodes has improved DFS and overall survival compared with an alternating schedule of doxorubicin and CMF. Median follow-up time is 4.6 years (33).

The Stockholm Trials in adjuvant therapy of early breast cancer compared CMF adjuvant chemotherapy to postmastectomy radiation (132). There was a difference in DFS for these two groups after a mean follow-up of 6.5 years. However, postmenopausal patients treated with radiotherapy had fewer metastases and locoregional recurrences than those treated with CMF.

Peto and Early Breast Cancer Trialists' Collaborative Group: To overcome statistical heterogeneity among clinical trials on early breast cancer done worldwide, these investigators did meta-analysis of 133 randomized studies and showed a highly significant reduction in recurrence and death produced by tamoxifen (Fig. 17-7) (25% SD 2 recurrence and 17% SD 2 mortality: $2p$ = 0.00001), by ovarian ablation below age 50 (26% SD6 recurrence and 25% SD7 mortality $2p$ = 0.0004), and by polychemotherapy (Fig. 17-8) (28% SD 3 recurrence and 16% SD 3 mortality $2p$ < 0.00001). Cumulative differences in survival are larger at 10 than at 5 years.

Adjuvant Therapy in Other Patient Groups

1. Node-negative Patients: Adjuvant therapy is being explored in N0 patients with negative prognostic factors including negative ER status. Three clinical trials all showed a benefit in DFS, but not overall survival (57,92,110) (Table 17-16). Clinical trials are in active pursuit using chemical markers (ER, PR, cathepsin D, *HER-2/neu*, c-*erb* B-2) and flow cytometric analysis to select patients with pathologically negative nodes for chemotherapy or hormonal treatment (111).

2. Stage III (A+B) Locally Advanced Unresectable Cancers (T4 or N2): Response rates are high and combined modalities are able to render 80% to 90% of locally advanced cancer disease-free, but 5-year relapse and metastatic rates range from 50% to 70%. The DFS in a meta-analysis of a 9055 patient compilation of 33 studies of locally advanced breast cancer has a 33% 5-year survival. In a randomized study of 231 patients with non-metastatic Stage III breast cancer, Derman *et al.* (45) used adjuvant CMF chemotherapy in addition to primary local irradiation plus surgery. They failed to show a survival benefit. As with other studies, premenopausal subsets of patients showed improved DFS but overall survival did not increase. Local control was achieved in 90.9% of patients; this was attributed to irradiation and/or surgery. These findings suggest that the major effect of systemic treatment is to delay the onset of relapse rather than to eradicate clinically undetectable metastatic disease.

3. Inflammatory Cancers Without Metastases (M0): In a compilation of 865 patients, inflammatory cancers had a 5-year survival range of 10% to 70%, the average series was 40% to 60%. However, attrition occurs beyond 5 years and less than 25% are alive at 10 years. With aggressive multimodal treatment, the University of Texas M. D. Anderson Hospital Cancer Center report of Thoms *et al.* (147) notes a 27% overall 5-year survival. The positive note is for the 16% complete responders; their 5-year survival was 89%. Mastectomy made no difference in either locoregional control or distant metastatic rate, but mastectomy was recommended because cosmesis was poor with higher radiation doses when combined with multiagent chemotherapy, yielding a painful, "woody" breast.

4. High-Dose Combination Chemotherapy With Bone Marrow Transplants: High initial response rates (40% to 80%) and complete responses from 27% to 65% have been found after high-dose chemotherapy combinations. The early results indicate that 20% to 25% of patients in selected series are in unmaintained remission with a median 2-year follow-up (19).

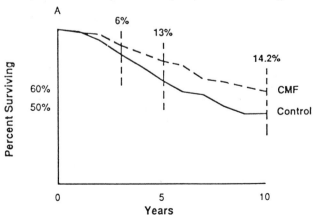
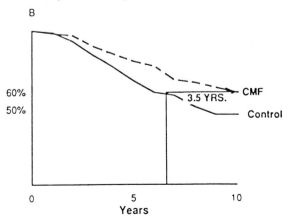

Fig. 17-12. Comparison of patients treated with CMF to control group. Note that there is a 3.5 yr DFS benefit for CMF vs control. Courtesy of Bonadonna *et al.* (29).

Table 17-16. Recent Adjuvant Chemotherapy Studies in Node-Negative Patients: Trial Characteristics and Summary of Results

Variable	Ludwig V [106]	NSABP B13 [57]	Intergroup [107]
No. patients	1275	679	406
ERP status	?*/neg/pos	Neg	Neg or pos
			T > 3 cm
Regimen	CMF	M′F	✦CMFP
Duration of therapy (mo)	1	13	6
Disease-free survival (yr)	4	4	3
Control	73%	71%	69%
Treated	77%	80%	84%
P	0.04	0.03	0.0001
Survival			
Control	86%	86%	88%
Treated	90%	87%	91%
P	0.24	0.8	0.3

NSABP = National Surgical Adjuvant Breast Project; ERP = estrogen receptor protein; CMF = cyclophosphamide, methotrexate, 5-fluorouracil; M′F = sequential methotrexate, 5-fluorouracil; CMFP = cyclophosphamide, methotrexate, 5-fluorouracil, prednisone.

* Patients were enrolled in the trial even if receptor status was unknown.

From Henderson et al. (92), with permission.

Prognostic Factors (119)

Size of Primary Tumor

The likelihood of distant metastasis increases as the primary tumor diameter increases. It has been estimated that there is a 50% probability of metastasis when a tumor reaches 3.6 cm in diameter. For each tumor, there may be a critical tumor volume below which metastasis does not occur.

Regional Lymph Node Status

Regional lymph node status has proved to be the most important prognostic factor in breast cancer management. Clinical evaluation of the axillary lymph nodes is not reliable and false-positive and false-negative rates are 25% to 30%. Therefore, pathologic examination of the nodes is necessary for accurate prognosis. Twenty-five percent of patients with pathologically negative axillary nodes will develop distant metastases. The percentage increases to 75% when the nodes are positive (67). The likelihood of positive nodes increases with increasing primary tumor size. The number of positive nodes also influences prognosis. Ten-year survival has been reported to be 38% if one to three nodes are positive, and 13% if four or more nodes are positive.

The internal mammary lymph nodes are more likely to be involved when the axillary nodes are positive, particularly in medial tumors. For this reason, extended radical mastectomy has been performed by some surgeons, including excision of the internal mammary nodes. This operation is extensive and there is little evidence to support its use. Tumor involvement of the internal mammary nodes predicts a high likelihood of distant metastases, and excision of the nodes would not be curative.

Distant Metastases

The presence of distant metastases indicates a dismal prognosis because cure is not possible. However, because breast cancer is often a slow-growing tumor, some patients can live for many years. Bone, lung, liver, and soft tissue are the most common sites for metastases and the prognosis for patients with bone or soft tissue metastases tends to be better than for those with visceral metastases.

DNA Analysis

Aneuploidy on flow cytometric analysis of dissociated primary breast cancers and a high labeling index correlate with a poor prognosis. It is now possible to estimate the growth fraction using a monoclonal antibody that reacts with a nuclear antigen associated with cell proliferation. This growth fraction has been shown to correlate to histologic grade and lymph node status (46,86).

Age (95)

It has been difficult to eliminate other important prognostic factors when analyzing the effect of age on survival from breast cancer (16). After corrections for stage, ER status, and lymph node status, the young (age < 30 years) and the elderly may do worse than other age groups (129). There is evidence that women age 35 to 49 may have the best prognosis. Elderly women (60 to 90 years) are often treated less aggressively. In one study, elderly women were denied irradiation after lumpectomy, leading to a worse outcome, i.e., more breast failures (70% to 90% depending upon decade) and life shortening (55% v 85% alive at 5 years).

In a large study of 1300 breast cancer patients stages I and II, patients aged less than 40 years had twice the local recurrence rate as those older than 40 years, i.e., 19% v 9%, but 15-year cancer-specific survival is identical. Salvage surgery was effective, with a 10-year survival of 64% if mastectomy was performed (100).

Hormone Receptors

The presence of ERs or PRs on breast cancer cells has been studied extensively, particularly because of the responsiveness of some tumors to hormonal manipulation. It has been found that recurrence and survival rates are worse for patients with ER negative tumors, independent of other prognostic factors (41,107). There is some evidence that the better prognosis in ER positive patients may not be sustained over time. This characteristic may be due to increased sensitivity of ER positive cells to therapy, resulting in eventual domination of ER negative cells. To support this, there is evidence that the clonogenic cells in breast cancer are not estrogen positive. The presence of positive PRs is also a favorable prognostic factor but it is unclear whether it adds any further prognostic information than ER status alone (37,59).

Histopathology

The importance of histologic subtypes and their impact on outcome is examined by Weiss et al. (153a). Seven subtypes are assessed with virtually no significant difference in 5-year actuarial survival, first failure, locoregional relapse despite significant differences in clinical T stage + pathologic node status, receptor negativity or positivity, and age. Tubular and celloid carcinomas are usually T1N0 and fare very well and invasive ductal carcinomas tend to have a higher rate of distant metastases only as first failure. All histologic subtypes can be effectively treated in early stages by lumpectomy and irradiation.

Other Prognostic Indicators

1. *Race:* Blacks appear to have a worse prognosis than whites when data are corrected for stage and ER status.
2. *Oncogenes:* The *HER-2/neu* or *c-erb* B-2 oncogene is amplified in some breast cancers. This gene amplification correlates with positive axillary nodes, reduced time to relapse, and decreased overall survival (145).
3. *Other markers:* Tumor levels of cathepsin D may also be of prognostic value, but results are not yet conclusive (144).

CLINICAL INVESTIGATIONS

Localized Cancers, Stages I and II

1. *Prevention.* NSABP is extending the use of tamoxifen to healthy women at high risk of breast cancer in a randomized comparison with placebo.

   The most compelling argument for extending the use of tamoxifen to this population is 38% reduction in contralateral breast malignancy in patients on adjuvant tamoxifen trials.
2. The evaluation of different surgical procedures in the treatment of operable breast cancer is being carried out in an NSABP study, evaluating more conservative treatment—total mastectomy *v* segmental mastectomy plus or minus radiation treatment. Axillary dissection is performed and if any positive axillary nodes are found, adjuvant chemotherapy in the form of melphalan and 5-FU is added. If tumor persists or recurs, a total mastectomy is performed for the tumor in the ipsilateral breast. This study will define the role of segmental mastectomies in the United States; they have become more standard forms of therapy in Europe, particularly in France, Scandinavia, and England, as well as in Canada. It will also answer the question raised by Clark (39,40) about the role of radiation therapy following segmental mastectomy; in his study a smaller, nonrandomized group of patients had an outcome comparable with segmental mastectomy and radiation therapy done by Peters (122).
3. The role of preoperative and postoperative radiation therapy is being defined in Scandinavian studies, particularly by investigators Wallgren et al. (153) at the Radiumhemmet. These studies have been completed and in time will establish the value of adjuvant radiation treatment in terms of both local recurrence, which is clearly reduced, and survival over the surgical radical mastectomy alone.
4. Other studies in some of the cooperative groups are exploring the combined use of radiation therapy and chemotherapy in the more locally advanced cancers. These stages II and III patients are being evaluated by a number of cooperative group protocols. Studies to date indicate that planned integration of radiation therapy does not increase the toxicity to bone marrow or decrease tolerance to drugs compared with the known hematologic toxicity of drugs themselves (79).

Advanced and Metastatic Cancer, Stages III and IV

Radiation therapy's role in the management of primary breast cancer as an alternative to radical mastectomy is an important question to be answered within the coming decade. It is being addressed by projected studies, including those of the NSABP. The combined use of irradiation and cytotoxic chemotherapy in the management of inoperable primary breast cancer is being studied by the Radiation Therapy Oncology Group in conjunction with the Eastern Cooperative Oncology Group.

Adjuvant therapy for primary breast cancer has been demonstrated to improve DFS in certain subgroups of patients, as discussed above. Current and future studies include modification of the drug combinations used in such treatment and the addition of hormonal agents to them and the use of hormonal agents alone, particularly for older women. Awaiting further clarification is the question of optimal combination and duration of adjuvant chemotherapy.

The improvement of cytotoxic chemotherapy will depend on the development of new agents identified in phase II trials, and their incorporation into combinations with standard drugs.

An important statement on hyperthermia and radiation therapy for locoregional recurrent breast cancer is presented by Kapp et al. (97a). This is a long-term assessment of what can and has been achieved by one of the dedicated working teams in actualizing hyperthermia clinically. In reviewing almost a decade of experience in approximately 90 patients, using hundreds of fields, the majority of which had extensive prior treatment with radiation therapy (68%) and chemotherapy (86%), intratumoral temperatures of average, maximal, and minimal levels were 42.4° C, 40.3° C, and 44.6° C. At 3 weeks following completion of radiation therapy (average dose 40 Gy) and hyperthermia (average of 3 therapies) there was a CR of 52%, a PR of 8%, with continuing regression in 22%, which led to a local control rate of 72%. As might be expected, this local control decays in time with an infield failure rate of 29% and a 31% complication rate (chest wall ulceration found often due to use of unbuffered xylocaine). Long-term local control as measured by patients and fields ranges from 30-40% at 1-3 years. A detailed analysis of prognostic factors is a valuable guide to expected outcome.

Recommended Reading

Writings on the detection, diagnosis, and treatment of breast cancer are voluminous—the student can best plunge into this sea of literature by addressing an aspect of a management problem based on patient contact to provide focus.

For general references, there are some excellent multi-authored texts that have been published recently providing the most up-to-date information. Two very active American university breast cancer clinical investigative groups that have compiled their multidisciplinary diagnostic and therapeutic approaches are Harris, Hellman, *et al.* (6a) at Harvard and Fowble and Goodman (4a) at the University of Pennsylvania. Another excellent general reference is the chapter on breast cancer by Henderson *et al.* in *Cancer: Principles and Practice of Oncology* (8).

For general historical reference, a starting point is Haagensen's monograph, *Diseases of the Breast* (5). This classic distills Haagensen's rich experience in breast cancer into the natural history of clinical and pathologic findings. Although his surgical treatment principles are being challenged, his criteria of inoperability remain with us today. For historical balance in this multidisciplinary era, it may be of interest to review different practices in breast cancer management of the 1970s in *Current Concepts in Cancer* series (13). For more recent references, see Haskell *et al.* in *Cancer Treatment* (7) and *Cancer of the Breast* by Donegan *et al.* (4).

There is no one standard approach in combining modalities, but there is more concordance than discordance, and the works by Bonadonna (25), Carbone (35,36), Ege (48), Fisher *et al.* (51,55,56,58,64,66,67), Fletcher *et al.* (72), Kaae and Johansen (97), McWirter (111), Peters (122), Rubin (131), Savlov *et al.* (133), all provide insights into the different aspects of diagnosis and treatment of this disease.

REFERENCES

General References

1. American Joint Committee for Cancer Staging and End Results. Manual for Staging of Cancer, 3rd ed. Philadelphia, PA: JB Lippincott Co; 1988.
2. Arseneau, J.C. Breast cancer. In: Rosenthal, S.M.; Bennett, J.M. (eds). Practical Cancer Chemotherapy. Garden City, NJ: Med Exam Publ Co; 175-198: 1981.
3. Bragg, D.G.; Rubin, P.; Youker, J.E. (eds). Oncologic Imaging. Elmsford, NY: Pergamon Press; 1985.
4. Donegan, W.L.; Spratt, J.S. (eds). Cancer of the Breast, 3rd ed. Philadelphia, PA: WB Saunders Co; 1988.
4a. Fowble, B.L.; Goodman, R.L.; Glick, J.H.; Rosato, E.F. (eds). Breast cancer treatment: A comprehensive guide to management. St. Louis, MO: Mosby-Yearbook, Inc.; 1991.
5. Haagensen, C.D. Diseases of the Breast, 2nd ed. Philadelphia, PA: WB Saunders Co; 1971.
6. Harris, J.R.; Hellman, S.; Henderson, I.C., Kinne, D.W. (eds). Breast Disease, 2nd ed. Philadelphia, PA: JB Lippincott Co.; 1991.
6a. Harris, J.R.; Lippmann, M.; Veronesi, U.; Willett, W. Breast cancer: A review in three parts. N Engl J Med 327:319-328; 473-479; 1992.
7. Haskell, C.M.; Sparkes, F.C. Thomson, R.W. Breast cancer. In: Haskell, C.M., ed. Cancer Treatment. Philadelphia, PA: W.B. Saunders Co; 159-196: 1980.
8. Henderson, I.C.; Harris, J.R.; Kinne, D.W., *et al.* Cancer of the breast. In: DeVita, V.T.; Hellman, S.; Rosenthal, S.A. (eds). Cancer: Principles and Practice of Oncology, 3rd ed. Philadelphia, PA: JB Lippincott Co.; 1197-1258: 1989.
9. Lewison, E.F.; Montague, A.C.W. (eds). Diagnosis and Treatment of Breast Cancer (International Clinical Forum). Baltimore, MD: Williams & Wilkins, Co; 1981.

10. Maisey, M.N. Imaging techniques in breast cancer. What is new? What is useful? — A review. Eur J Cancer Clin Oncol 24:61-68; 1988.
11. McGuire, W.L. Hormone receptors and the hormonal treatment of cancer. In: Carter, S.K.; Glatstein, E.; Livingston, R.B. (eds). Principles of Cancer Treatment. New York, NY: McGraw-Hill; 352-357: 1982.
12. Petrakis, N.L.; Ernster, V.L.; King, M.C. Breast. In: Schottenfeld, D.; Fraumeni, J.F. (eds). Cancer Epidemiology and Prevention. Philadelphia, PA: WB Saunders, Co; 855-870:1982.
12a. Physician's Data Query. Breast Cancer. Nat'l Cancer Inst., Bethesda, MD: January 1991.
12b. Robert, N.J. (ed). Breast Cancer. Semin Oncol 19(3):217-341; 1992.
13. Rubin, P., ed. Current Concepts in Cancer: Parts XXI-XXV, Carcinoma of the Breast. Chicago, IL: American Medical Association; 225-310: 1974.
14. Strauss, M.B. Familiar Medical Quotations. Boston, MA: Little, Brown & Co; 1968.

Specific References

15. Ackland, S.P.; Bitran, J.D.; Dowlatshahi, K. Management of locally advanced and inflammatory carcinoma of the breast. Surg Gynec Obstet 161:399-408; 1985.
16. Adami, H.O.; Malker, B.; Homberg, L., *et al.* The relation between survival and age at diagnosis in breast cancer. New Engl J Med 315:559-563; 1986.
17. Amalric, R.; Santamaria, F.; Robert, F., *et al.* Curative radiotherapy for operable breast cancer: 5 and 10 year results. In: Lewison, E.F., Montague, A.C.W. (eds). Diagnosis and Treatment of Breast Cancer (International Clinical Forum). Baltimore, MD: Williams & Wilkins, Co; 185-191: 1981.
18. Allred, D.; Clark, G.; Tandon, A., *et al.* HER-2/*neu* expression identified a group of node-negative breast cancer patients at high risk for recurrence. Proc Am Soc of Clin Oncol. 19:23;1990. Abstract.
19. Antman, K.; Gale, R.O.P. Advanced breast cancer: high-dose chemotherapy and bone marrow transplantation. Ann Intern Med 108:570-574; 1988.
20. Baker, J.A.; Bretsky, S.; Menendez-Botet, C; Kinne, D.W. Estrogen receptor protein of breast cancer as a predictor of recurrence. Cancer 55:1178-1181; 1985.
21. Baker, R.R.; Montague, A.C.; Childs, J.N. A comparison of modified radical mastectomy to radical mastectomy in the treatment of operable breast cancer. Ann Surg. 189:553-559; 1979.
22. Beadle, G.F.; Silver, B.; Botnick, L., *et al.* Cosmetic results following primary radiation therapy for early breast cancer. Cancer 54:2911-2918; 1984.
23. Bezwoda, W.R.; Hesdorffer, C.; Dansey, R., *et al.* Breast cancer in men: clinical features, hormone receptor status, and response to therapy. Cancer. 60:1337-1340; 1987.
24. Bloom, H.J.G.; Richardson, W.W.; Harries, E.J. Natural history of untreated breast cancer (1805-1933). Brit Med J 214:213-221; 1962.
25. Bonadonna, G. Present status of CMF adjuvant therapy in operable breast cancer. Int J Radiat Oncol Biol Phys 2:237-240; 1977.
26. Bonadonna, G.; Rossi, A.; Valagussa, P. Adjuvant CMF chemotherapy in operable breast cancer. Ten years later. World J Surg 9:707-713;1985.
27. Bonadonna, G.; Valagussa, P. Adjuvant systemic therapy for resectable breast cancer. J Clin Oncol 3:259-275; 1985.
28. Bonadonna, G.; Valagussa, P. Chemotherapy of breast cancer: current views and results. Int J Rad Oncol Biol Phys 19:279-297;1983.
29. Bonadonna, G.; Valagussa, P.; Rossi, A.; *et al.* Ten-year experience with CMF-based adjuvant chemotherapy in resectable breast cancer. Breast Cancer Res Treat 5:95-115; 1985.
30. Bonadonna, G.; Valagussa, P.; Zambetti, M., *et al.* Milan adjuvant trials for stage I - II breast cancet. In: Salmon, S.E. Adjuvant Therapy of Cancer V. 211-222, New York, NY: Grune & Stratton; 1987.
31. Boring, C.L.; Squires, T.S.; Tong, T. Cancer Statistics, 1992. CA-A Cancer Journal for Clinicians 42:19-38; 1992.
32. Bragg, D.G.; Harnsberger, H.R. Newer radiologic techniques. In: DeVita, V.T.; Hellman, S.; Rosenberg, S.A. (eds). Cancer: Principles and Practice of Oncology. Philadelphia, PA: JB Lippincott, Co; 388-405: 1985.

33. Buzzoni, R.; Bonadonna, G.; Valagussa, P., *et al.* Sequential vs alternating chemotherapy in the adjuvant treatment of breast cancer with more than 3 positive axillary nodes. Proc Am Soc of Clin Oncol. 9:19; 1990. Abstract.

34. Calle, R.; Viloq, J.R.; Schlienger, P. Radiation therapy for operable breast cancer with or without lumpectomy: 10-year results. In: Lewison, E.F., Montague, A.C.W. (eds). Diagnosis and Treatment of Breast Cancer (International Clinical Forum). Baltimore, MD: Williams & Wilkins, Co; 178-184: 1981.

35. Carbone, P.P. Chemotherapy in the treatment strategy of breast cancer. Cancer. 36:633-637; 1975.

36. Carbone, P.P. Progress in the systemic treatment of cancer. Cancer. 65:625-633;1990.

37. Chevallier, B.;Heintzmann, F.; Mosseri, V., *et al.* Prognostic value of estrogen and progesterone receptors in operable breast cancer. Cancer. 62:2517-2524; 1988.

38. Chu, A.M.; Cope, O.; Doucette, T., *et al.* Non-metastatic locally advanced cancer of the breast treated with radiation. Int J Rad Oncol Biol Phys 10:2299-2304; 1984.

39. Clark, R.M. Breast cancer — 20 years of conservative treatment. In: Lewison, E.F. Montague, A.C.W. (eds). Diagnosis and Treatment of Breast Cancer. (International Clinical Forum). Baltimore, MD: Williams & Wilkins, Co; 161-166: 1981.

40. Clark, R.M.; Wilkinson, R.H.; Mahoney, L.J.; Reid, J.G., *et al.* Breast cancer: a 21-year experience with conservative surgery and radiation. Int J Radiat Oncol Biol Phys 8:967-975; 1982.

41. Crowe, J.P.; Hubay, C.A.; Pearson, O.H., *et al.* Estrogen receptor status as a prognostic indicator for stage I breast cancer patients. Breast Cancer Res Treat 3:171-176;1982.

42. Curtis, R.E.; Boice, J.D., Jr.; Stoval, M.; *et al.* Risk of leukemia after chemotherapy and radiation treatment for breast cancer. N Engl J Med 326:1745-1751; 1992.

43. Danoff, B.F.; Pajak, T.F.; Solin, L. J., *et al.* Excisional biopsy, axillary node dissection and definitive radiotherapy for stages I and II breast cancer. Int J Radiat Oncol Biol Phys 11:479-483; 1985.

44. Davidson, N.E.; Lippman, M.E. Treatment of metastatic breast cancer. In: Lippman, M.E.; Lichter, A.S.; Danforth, D.N. (eds). Diagnosis and Management of Breast Cancer. Philadelphia, PA: WB Saunders Co; 375-406: 1988.

44a. de la Rochefordiere, A.; Abner, A.L.; Silver, B.; *et al.* Are cosmetic results following conservative surgery and radiation therapy for early breast cancer dependent on technique? Int J Radiat Oncol Biol Phys. 23(5):1992.

45. Derman, D.P.; Browde, S.; Kessel, I.L., *et al.* Adjuvant chemotherapy (CMF) for stage III breast cancer: A randomized trial. Int J Rad Oncol Biol Phys. 17:257-262;1989.

46. Dressler, L.G.; Seamer, L.C.; Owens, M.A., *et al.* DNA flow cytometry and prognostic factors in 1331 frozen breast cancer specimens. Cancer. 61:420-427; 1988.

46a. Early Breast Cancer Trialists' Collaborative Group. Systemic treatment of early breast cancer by hormonal, cytotoxic or immune therapy. Lancet 339:1-15, 17-85; 1992.

47. Eddy, D.M. High-dose chemotherapy with autologous bone marrow transplantation for the treatment of metastatic breast cancer. J Clin Oncol 10:517-519; 1992.

48. Ege, G.N. Internal mammary lymphoscintigraphy in breast cancer: a study of 1,072 patients. Int J Radiat Oncol Biol Phys. 7/8:755-762; 1977.

49. Epstein, A.H.; Connolly, J.L.; Gelman, R., *et al.* The predictors of distant relapse following conservative surgery and radiotherapy for early breast cancer are similar to those following mastectomy. Int J Radiat Oncol Biol Phys 17:755-760; 1989.

50. Fallenius, A.G.; Franzen, S.A.; Auer, G.U. Predictive value of nuclear DNA content in breast cancer in relation to clinical and morphologic factors. Cancer. 62:521-530; 1988.

51. Fisher, B. The surgical dilemma in the primary therapy in invasive breast cancer: a critical appraisal. Curr Probl Surg October:1-53; 1970.

52. Fisher, B.; Bauer, M.; Margolese, R., *et al.* Five-year results of a randomized clinical trial comparing total mastectomy and segmental mastectomy with or without radiation in the treatment of breast cancer. New Engl J Med 312:665-673; 1985.

53. Fisher, B.; Constantino, J.; Redmond, C., *et al.* A randomized clinical trial evaluating tamoxifen in the treatment of patients with node-negative breast cancer who have estrogen receptor-positive tumors. New Engl J Med 320:479-484; 1989.

54. Fisher, B.; Fisher, E.R.; Redmond, C. Ten year results from the NSABP clinical trial evaluating the use of L-phenylalanine mustard (L-PAM) in the management of primary breast cancer. J Clin Oncol 4: 929-941;1986.

55. Fisher, B.; Redmond, C. The surgical treatment of primary breast cancer — results of National Surgical Adjuvant Breast Project. In: Lewison, E.F.; Montague A.C.W. (eds). Diagnosis and Treatment of Breast Cancer. (International Clinical Forum). Baltimore, MD: Williams & Wilkins Co; 135-141: 1981.

56. Fisher, B.; Redmond, C.; Brown, A.; *et al.* Treatment of primary breast cancer with chemotherapy and tamoxifen. New Engl J Med 305:1-6; 1981.

57. Fisher, B.; Redmond, C.; Dimitrov, N.V., *et al.* A randomized clinical trial evaluating sequential methotrexate and fluorouracil in the treatment of patients with node-negative breast cancer who have estrogen-receptor-negative tumors. New Engl J Med 320:473-478;1989.

58. Fisher, B.; Redmond, C.; Fisher, E.R., *et al.* The contribution of recent NSABP clinical trials of primary breast cancer therapy to an understanding of tumor biology: an overview of findings. Cancer. 46:1009-1025; 1980.

59. Fisher, B.; Redmond, C.; Fisher, E.R., *et al.* Relative worth of estrogen or progesterone receptor and pathologic characteristics of differentiation as indicators of prognosis in node negative breast cancer patients: findings from National Surgical Adjuvant Breast and Bowel Project protocol B-06. J Clin Oncol 6:1076-1087;1988.

60. Fisher, B.; Redmond, C.; Fisher, E.R., *et al.* Ten-year results of a randomized clinical trial comparing radical mastectomy and total mastectomy with or without radiation. New Engl J Med 312:674-681; 1985.

61. Fisher, B.; Redmond, C.; Poisson, R., *et al.* Eight-year results of a randomized clinical trial comparing total mastectomy and lumpectomy with or without irradiation in the treatment of breast cancer. New Engl J Med 320:822-828; 1989.

62. Fisher, B.; Redmond, C.; Poisson, S., *et al.* Increased benefit from addition of Adriamycin and cyclophosophamide (AC) to tamoxifen (TAM, T) for positive-node, TAM-responsive postmenopausal breast cancer patients: results from NSABP B-16. Proc Am Soc Clin Oncol. 9:20;1990.Abstract.

63. Fisher, E.R.; Sass, R.; Fisher, B., *et al.* Pathologic findings from the National Surgical Adjuvant Breast Project (protocol 6) II. Relation of local breast recurrence to multicentricity. Cancer. 57:1717-1724; 1986.

64. Fisher, B.; Redmond, C.; Wolmark, N., *et al.* Disease-free survival at intervals during and following completion of adjuvant chemotherapy: the NSABP experience from 3 breast protocols. Cancer. 48:1273-1280; 1981.

65. Fisher, B.; Slack, N.H.; Bross, I.D., *et al.* Cancer of the breast: Size of neoplasm and prognosis. Cancer. 24:1071-1080;1969.

66. Fisher, B.; Slack, N.H.; Cavanaugh, P.J., *et al.* Postoperative radiotherapy in the treatment of breast cancer: results of the NSABP clinical trial. Ann. Surg. 172:711-732; 1970.

67. Fisher, B.; Slack, N.; Katrych, D., *et al.* Ten-year follow-up results of patients with carcinoma of the breast in a cooperative clinical trial evaluating surgical adjuvant chemotherapy. Surg Gynecol Obstet 140:528-534; 1975.

67a. Fisher, E.R.; Leeming, R.; Anderson, S.; *et al.* Conservative management of intraductal carcinoma (DCIS) of the breast. J Surg Oncol 47(3):139-147; 1991.

68. Fisher, E.R.; Redmond, C.; Fisher, B. Pathologic findings from the National Surgical Adjuvant Breast Project (protocol No. 4) VI. Discriminants for 5-year treatment failure. Cancer. 46:908-918; 1980.

69. Fisher, E.R.; Sass, R.; Fisher, B., *et al.* Pathologic findings from the National Surgical Adjuvant Breast Project (protocol 6) I. Intraductal carcinoma (DCIS). Cancer. 57:197-208; 1986.

69a. Fisher, E.R.; Sass, R.; Fisher, B., *et al.* Pathologic findings from the National Surgical Adjuvant Breast Project (protocol 6) II. Relation of local breast recurrence to multicentricity. Cancer. 57:1717-1724; 1986.

70. Fleck, R.; McNeese, M.D.; Ellerbroek, N.A., *et al.* Consequences of breast irradiation in patients with pre-existing collagen vascular disease. Int J Radiat Oncol Biol Phys 17:829-834; 1989.

71. Fletcher, G.H.; McNeese, M.D.; Oswald, M.J. Long-range results for breast cancer patients treated by radical mastectomy and postoperative radiation without adjuvant chemotherapy: an update. Int J Radiat Oncol Biol Phys 17:11-14;1989.

72. Fletcher, G.H.; Montague, E.; Nelson, E.A. Combination of conservative surgery and irradiation for cancer of the breast. AJR. 126:216-222; 1976.

73. Fourquet, A.; Campana, F.; Zafrani, B., *et al.* Prognostic factors of breast recurrence in the conservative management of early breast cancer: a 25-year follow-up. Int J Radiat Oncol Biol Phys 17:719-726; 1989.

74. Fowble, B.; Solin, L.J.; Schultz, D.J., *et al.* Frequency, sites of relapse, and outcome of regional node failures following conservative surgery and radiation for early breast cancer. Int J Radiat Oncol Biol Phys 17:703-710;1989.

74a. Fowble, B.L.; Solin, L.J.; Schultz, D.J.; Goodman, R.L. Ten-year results of conservative surgery and irradiation for stage I and II breast cancer. Int J Radiat Oncol Phys. 21:269-277; 1991.

75. Fox, M.S. On the diagnosis and treatment of breast cancer. JAMA. 241:489-494; 1979.

76. Frankel, G. The use of screening mammography. Cancer. 60:1979-1983; 1987.

77. Frazier, T.G.; Noone, R.B. An objective analysis of immediate simultaneous reconstruction in the treatment of primary carcinoma of the breast. Cancer. 55:1202-1205; 1985.

78. Glick, J. Meeting highlights: adjuvant therapy for breast cancer. JNCI. 80:471-475; 1988.

79. Glick, J.H.; Creech, R.H.; Torri, S.; *et al.* Tamoxifen plus sequential CMF chemotherapy versus tamoxifen alone in postmenopausal patients with advanced breast cancer: a randomized trial. Cancer. 45:735-741; 1980.

80. Glick, J.H.; Henderson, I.C. Adjuvant therapy for node-negative breast cancer: a. a proactive view. b. a cautious interepretation. In: Important Advances in Oncology 1990. DeVita, V.T., Hellman, S., Rosenberg, S.A. eds. Philadelphia, PA: JB Lippincott Co; 183-216: 1990.

81. Goldwyn, R.M. Breast reconstruction after mastectomy. N Engl J Med 317:1711-1714; 1987.

82. Haffty, B.G.; Goldberg, N.B.; Fischer, D., *et al.* Conservative surgery and radiation therapy in breast carcinoma: local recurrence and prognostic implications. Int J Radiat Oncol Biol Phys 17:727-732; 1989.

83. Handley, R.S. Carcinoma of the breast. Ann R Coll Surg Engl. 57:59-66; 1975.

84. Harris, J.R.; Levene, M.B.; Hellman, S. Primary radiation therapy for early breast cancer: the experience at the Joint Center for Radiation Therapy. In: Lewison, E.F.; Montague, A.C.W. (eds). Diagnosis and Treatment of Breast Cancer (International Clinical Forum). Baltimore, MD: Williams & Wilkins Co; 1981.

85. Hartrampf, C.R.; Bennett, G.K. Autogenous tissue reconstruction in the mastectomy patient. Ann Surg. 205:508-518; 1987.

86. Hatschek, T.; Fagerberg, G.; Stal, O., *et al.* Cytometric characterization and clinical course of breast cancer diagnosed in a population-based screening program. Cancer. 64:1074-1081;1989.

87. Hellman, S.; Harris, J.R.; Levene, M.B. Radiation therapy of early carcinoma of the breast without mastectomy. Cancer. 46:988-994; 1980.

88. Hellman, S.; Harris, J.R. The appropriate breast cancer paradigm. Cancer Res. 47:339-342;1987.

89. Henderson, I.C. Chemotherapy for advanced disease. In: Harris, J.R., Hellman, S., Henderson, I.C., *et al.* (eds). Breast Diseases. Philadelphia, PA: JB Lippincott Co; 428-479: 1987.

90. Henderson, I.C. Endocrine therapy in metastatic breast cancer. In: Harris, J.R., Hellman, S., Henderson, I.C., *et al.* (eds). Breast Diseases. Philadelphia, PA: JB Lippincott Co; 398-428:1987.

91. Henderson, I.C.; Canellos, G.P. Cancer of the breast: the past decade. New Engl J Med. 302:17-30; 1980.

92. Henderson, I.C.; Hayes, D.F.; Parker, L.M., *et al.* Adjuvant systemic therapy for patients with node-negative tumors. Cancer. 65:2132-2147; 1990.

93. Haagensen, C.D. Diseases of the Breast, 2nd ed. Philadelphia, PA: WB Saunders Co; 576-584: 1971.

94. Holmes, F.A.; Buzdar, A.U.; Kau, S.W., *et al.* 10-Year results of a combined modality approach for patients (PT) with isolated recurrences of breast cancer (IV-NED). Proc Am Soc Clin Oncol. 9:35;1990. Abstract.

95. Host, H.; Lund, E. Age as a prognostic factor in breast cancer. Cancer. 57:2217-2221; 1986.

96. Huguley, C.M.; Brown, R.L.; Greenberg, R.S., *et al.* Breast self-examination and survival from breast cancer. Cancer. 62:1389-1396; 1988.

97. Kaae, S.; Johansen, T. Breast cancer, 5-year results: 2 random series of simple mastectomy with postoperative irradiation versus extended radical matectomy. AJR. 87:82-88; 1962.

97a. Kapp, D.S.; Barnett, T.A.; Cox, R.S.; *et al.* Hyperthermia and radiation therapy of local-regional recurrent breast cancer: Prognostic factors for response and local control of diffuse or nodular tumors. Int J Radiat Oncol Biol Phys. 20:1147-1164; 1991.

98. Koscielny, S.; Tubiana, M.; Le, M.G.; *et al.* Breast cancer: relationship between the size of the primary tumour and the probability of metastatic dissemination. Br J Cancer. 49:709-715; 1984.

99. Kurtz, J.M.; Amalric, R.; Brandone, H., *et al.* Results of wide excision for mammary recurrence after breast-conserving therapy. Cancer. 61:1969-1972; 1988.

100. Kurtz, J.M.; Spitalier, J.-M.; Amalric, R., *et al.* Mammary recurrences in women younger than forty. Int J Radiat Oncol Biol Phys. 15: 271-276;1988.

101. Land, C.E. Low-dose radiation — a cause of breast cancer. Cancer. 46:868-873;1980.

102. Lelle, R.J.; Heidenreich, W.; Staunch, G., *et al.* The correlation of growth fractions with histologic grading and lymph node status in human mammary carcinoma. Cancer. 59:83-88; 1987.

103. Leopold, K.A.; Recht, A.; Schnitt, S.J., *et al.* Results of conservative surgery and radiation therapy for multiple synchronous cancers of one breast. Int J Radiat Oncol Biol Phys. 16:11-16;1989.

104. Levitt, S.H.; Potish, R. The gold standard and Pogo. Int J Radiat Oncol Biol Phys. 17: 235-236; 1989.

105. Love, S.M.; Gelman, R.S.; Silen, W. Fibrocystic "disease" of the breast — a nondisease? N Engl J Med. 307:1010-1014; 1982.

106. The Ludwig Breast Cancer Study Group. Prolonged disease-free survival after one course of perioperative adjuvant chemotherapy for node-negative breast cancer. N Engl J Med. 320:491-496; 1989.

107. McGuire, W.L. Hormone receptors: their role in predicting prognosis and response to endocrine therapy. Semin Oncol. 5:428-433; 1978.

108. McGuire, W.L.; Clark, G.M. Prognostic factors and treatment decisions in axillary-node-negative breast cancer. N Engl J Med 326:1756-1761; 1992.

109. McGuire, W.L.; Tandon, A.K.; Allred, D.C.; Chamness, G.C.; Clark, G.M. How to use prognostic factors in axillary node-negative breast cancer patients. J Nat'l Cancer Inst. 82:1006-1015; 1990.

110. McCormick, B.; Rosen, P.P.; Kinne, D.; *et al.* Duct carcinoma in situ of the breast: An analysis of local control after conservation surgery and radiotherapy. Int J Radiat Oncol Biol Phys. 21:289-292; 1991.

111. McWhirter, R. Should more radical treatment be attempted in breast cancer? Caldwell lecture, 1963. AJR. 92:3-13;1964.

112. Maddox, W.A.; Carpenter, J.T.; Laws, H.L., *et al.* A randomized prospective trial of radical (Halsted) mastectomy versus modified radical mastectomy in 311 breast cancer patients. Ann Surg. 198:207-212; 1983.

112a. Mansour, E.G.; Gray, R.; Shatila, A.H., *et al.* Efficacy of adjuvant chemotherapy in high-risk node-negative breast cancer. N Engl J Med. 320:485-490; 1989.

113. Meier, P.; Ferguson, D.J.; Karrison, T. A controlled trial of extended radical mastectomy. Cancer. 55:880-891; 1985.

114. Milbrath, J.R.; Bragg, D.G.; Youker, J.E. Breast cancer. In: Bragg, D.G.; Rubin, P.; Youker, J.E. (eds). Oncologic Imaging. Elmsford, NY: Pergamon Press; 173-206:1985.

115. Montague, E.D. Conservative surgery and radiation therapy in the treatment of operable breast cancer. Cancer. 53:700-704; 1984.

116. Noguchi, S.; Miyauchi, K., Nishizawa, Y., *et al.* Management of inflammatory carcinoma of the breast with combined modality therapy including intraarterial infusion chemotherapy as an induction therapy. Cancer. 61:1483-1491; 1988.

117. Olivotto, I.A.; Rose, M.A.; Osteen, R.T., *et al.* Late cosmetic outcome after conservative surgery and radiotherapy: analysis of causes of cosmetic failure. Int J Radiat Oncol Biol Phys. 17:747-754;1989.

118. O'Malley, M.S.; Fletcher, S.W. Screening for breast cancer with breast self-examination. JAMA. 257:2197-2203; 1987.

119. Osborne, C.K. Prognostic factors in breast cancer. PPO Uptakes. 4:3;1990.

119a. Paterson, M.C.; Dietrich, K.D.; Danyluk, J.; *et al.* Correlation between c-erbB-2 amplification and risk of recurrent disease in node-negative breast cancer. Canc Res. 51(2):556-567; 1991.

120. Paul, C.; Skegg, D.C.G.; Spears, G.F.S.; *et al.* Oral contraceptives and breast cancer: a national study. Br Med J. 293:723-726; 1986.

121. Paulus, D.D. Imaging in Breast Cancer. In: Holleb, A.I. (ed). Imaging in Cancer. New York, NY: American Cancer Society, Inc.; 1987:5-22.

122. Peters, M.V. The role of local excision and radiation in early breast cancer. In: Breast Cancer Early and Late. 13th Clinical Conference on Cancer, M.D. Anderson Hospital, 1968. Chicago, IL: Yearbook Medical Publishers; 1970.

123. Pexner, R.D.; Lipsett, J.A.; Desai, K.; *et al.* To boost or not to boost: Decreasing radiation therapy in conservative breast cancer treatment when "inked" tumor resection margins are pathologically free of cancer. Int J Radiat Oncol Biol Phys. 14:873-877; 1988.

123a. Pierce, S.M.; Recht, A.; Lingos, T.I.; *et al.* Long-term radiation complications following conservative surgery (CS) and radiation therapy (RT) in patients with early stage breast cancer. Int J Radiat Oncol Biol Phys. 23(5): 1992.

124. Pierquin, B.; LeBourgeois, P.; Brun, B.; *et al.* Radiotherapy and primary treatment of operable breast cancer. In: Lewison, E.F.; Montague, A.C.W. (eds). Diagnosis and Treatment of Breast Cancer (International Clinical Forum). Baltimore, MD: Williams & Wilkins Co;175-178: 1981.

125. Recht, A.R.; Come, S.E.; Gelman, R.S.; *et al.* Integration of conservative surgery, radiotherapy, and chemotherapy for the treatment of early-stage, node-positive breast cancer: Sequencing, timing and outcome. J Clin Oncol. 9:1662-1667; 1991.

126. Recht, A.; Schnitt, S.J.; Connolly, J.L., *et al.* Prognosis following local or regional recurrence after conservative surgery and radiotherapy for early stage breast carcinoma. Int J Radiat Oncol Biol Phys. 16:3-10; 1989.

126a. Rivkin, S.; Green, S.; Metch, K.B.; *et al.* Adjuvant combination chemotherapy (CMFVP) vs tamoxifen (TAM) vs CMFVP + TAM for postmenopausal women with ER + operable breast cancer and positive axillary lymph nodes: an Intergroup Study. Proc Am Soc Clin Oncol. 9:24; 1990. Abstract.

127. Rose, M.A.; Henderson, C.; Celman, R., *et al.* Premenopausal breast cancer patients treated with conservative surgery, radiotherapy and adjuvant chemotherapy have a low risk of local failure. Int J Radiat Oncol Biol Phys. 17:711-718; 1989.

128. Rosen, P.P.; Braun, D.W.; Lyngholm, B., *et al.* Lobular carcinoma in situ of the breast: preliminary results of treatment by ipsilateral mastectomy and contralateral biopsy. Cancer. 47:813-819; 1981.

129. Rosen, P.P.; Lesser, M.L.; Kinne, D.W., *et al.* Breast carcinoma in women 35 years of age or younger. Ann Surg. 199:133-142; 1984.

130. Rouesse, J.; Friedman, S.; Sarrazin, D.; *et al.* Primary chemotherapy in the treatment of inflammatory breast cancer: a study of 230 cases from the Institut Gustav-Roussy. J Clin Oncol. 4:1765-1771; 1986.

131. Rubin, P., ed. Introduction and comment: controlled clinical trials. JAMA. 199:732-746; 1967.

132. Rutqvist, L.E.; Cedermark, B.; Glas, U., *et al.* Radiotherapy, chemotherapy, and tamoxifen as adjuncts to surgery in early breast cancer: a summary of three randomized trials. Int J Radat Oncol Biol Phys. 16:629-640; 1989.

133. Savlov, E.; Witliff, J.L.; Hilf, R. Further studies of biochemical predictive tests in breast cancer. Cancer. 39:539-541; 1977.

134. Schmidt-Ullrich, R.; Wazer, D.E.; Tercilla, O., *et al.* Tumor margin assessment as a guide to optimal conservation surgery and irradiation in early stage breast carcinoma. Int J Radiat Oncol Biol Phys. 17:733-738; 1989.

135. Schottenfeld, D.; Nash, A.G.; Robbins, G.F., *et al.* Ten-year results of the treatment of primary operable breast carcinoma. Cancer. 38:1005; 1976.

136. Scottish Cancer Trials Office (MRC) Edinburgh: Adjuvant tamoxifen in the management of operable breast cancer: The Scottish trial. Lancet. ii:171-175; 1987.

137. Shapiro, S.; Venet, W.; Strax, P., *et al.* Ten- to fourteen-year effect of screening on breast cancer mortality. JNCI. 69:349-355; 1982.

138. Sheldon, T.; Hayes, D.F.; Cady, B., *et al.* Primary radiation therapy for locally advanced breast cancer. Cancer. 60:1219-1225; 1987.

138a. Sigurdsson, H.; Baldetorp, B.; Borg, A.; *et al.* Indicators of prognosis in node-negative breast cancer. N Engl J Med 322(15):1045-1053; 1990.

138b. Silverstein, M.J.; Waisman, J.R.; Bierson, E.D.; *et al.* Radiation therapy for intraductal carcinoma. Arch Surg 126:424-428; 1991.

139. Smalley, R.V.; Carpenter, J.; Barducci, A.; *et al.* A comparison of cyclophosphamide, adriamycin, 5-fluorouracil (CAF) and cyclophosphamide, methotrexate, 5-fluorouracil, vincristine, prednisone (CHFVPO) in various patients with metastatic breast cancer. Cancer. 40:625-632; 1977.

140. Stotter, A.T.; McNeese, M.; Oswald, M.J., *et al.* The role of limited surgery with irradiation in primary treatment of ductal in situ breast cancer. Int J Radiat Oncol Biol Phys. 18:283-288;1990.

141. Swain, S.M.; Sorace, R.A.; Bagley, C.A.; *et al.* Neoadjuvant chemotherapy in the combined modality approach of locally advanced breast cancer. Cancer Res. 47:3889-3894; 1987.

142. Sykes, H.F.; Sim, D.A.; Wong, C.J., *et al.* Local-regional recurrence in breast cancer after mastectomy and Adriamycin-based adjuvant chemotherapy: evaluation of the role of postoperative radiotherapy. Int J Radiat Oncol Biol Phys. 16: 641-648;1989.

143. Tabar, L.; Faberberg, G.; Day, N.E.; *et al.* What is the optimum interval between mammographic screening examinations? Br J Cancer. 55:547-551; 1987.

144. Tandon, A.K.; Clark, G.M.; Chamness, G.C., *et al.* Cathepsin D and prognosis in breast cancer. N Engl J Med. 322:297-302;1990.

145. Tandon, A.K.; Clark, G.M.; Chamness, G.C., *et al.* HER-2/*neu* oncogene protein and prognosis in breast cancer. J Clin Oncol. 7:1120-1128;1989.

146. Taylor, S.G.; Gelman, R.S.; Falkson, G., *et al.* Combination chemotherapy compared to tamoxifen as initial therapy for stage IV breast cancer in elderly women. Ann Intern Med. 104:455-461; 1986.

147. Thoms, W.W., Jr.; McNeese, M.D.; Fletcher, G.H., *et al.* Multimodal treatment for inflammatory breast cancer. Int J Radiat Oncol Biol Phys. 17:739-746; 1989.

148. Tubiana, M.; Koscielny, S. Cell kinetics, growth rate and the natural history of breast cancer. Eur J Cancer Clin Oncol. 24:9-14; 1988.

149. Valagussa, P.; Bignami, P.; Buzzoni, R.; *et al.* Are estrogen receptors alone a reliable prognostic factor in node negative breast cancer? In: Jones, S.E., Salmon, S.E. (eds). Adjuvant Therapy of Cancer IV. Orlando, FL: Grune & Stratton; 407-415: 1984.

150. Veronesi, U.; Valagussa, P. Inefficacy of internal mammary nodes dissection in breast cancer surgery. Cancer. 47:170-175; 1981.

151. Veronesi, U.; Rilke, F.; Luini, A., *et al.* Distribution of axillary node metastases by level of invasion. Cancer. 59:682-687; 1987.

152. Veronesi, U.; Saccozzi, R.; Del Vecchio, M., *et al.* Comparing radical mastectomy with quadrantectomy, axillary dissection, and radiotherapy in patients with small cancers of the breast. N Engl J Med. 305:6-11; 1981.

153. Wallgren, A.A.; Strender, L-E.; Arner, O., *et al.* Adjuvant pre- or postoperative radiotherapy in primary breast cancer. In: Lewison, E.S.; Montague, A.C.W. (eds). Diagnosis and Treatment of Breast Cancer (International Clinical Forum). Baltimore, MD: Williams & Wilkins Co; 209-211:1981.

153a. Weiss, M.C.; Fowble, B.L.; Solin, L.J.; *et al.* Outcome of conservative therapy for invasive breast cancer by histologic subtype. Int J Radiat Oncol Biol Phys. 23(5): 1992.

154. Willet, N.C.; Meir, M.J.; Colditz, G.A., *et al.* Dietary fat and the risk of breast cancer. N Engl J Med. 316:22-28; 1987.

155. Wittliff, J.L.; Day, T.G.; Dean, W.L., *et al.* Identification of endocrine responsive breast and endometrial carcinoma using steroid hormone receptors. In: Hall, T.C. (ed). Prediction of Response to Cancer Therapy. New York, NY: Alan R. Liss; 11-41:1988.

156. Woll, J.E. Breast cancer. In: Rosenthal, S.; Carignan, J.R.; Smith, B.D. (eds). Medical Care of the Cancer Patient. Philadelphia, PA: WB Saunders Co; 179-199:1987.

157. Wolmark, N.; Fisher, B. Adjuvant chemotherapy in stage II breast cancer: an overview of the NSABP clinical trials. Breast Cancer Res Treat. 3 Suppl:S19-26; 1983.

158. World Health Organization. The World Health Organization histological typing of breast tumors — 2nd ed. Am J Clin Pathol. 78:806-816; 1982.

Louis S. Constine III, M.D., Radiation Oncology   Raman Qazi, M.D., Medical Oncology
Philip Rubin, M.D., Radiation Oncology

Chapter 18

MALIGNANT LYMPHOMAS

This enlargement of the glands appeared to be a primitive affection of those bodies rather than the result of an irritation propagated to them from some ulcerated surface or other inflamed texture.

Thomas Hodgkin, 1832 (38)

PERSPECTIVE

Malignant lymphomas were first identified as a clinical entity in 1832, when Thomas Hodgkin described seven patients with enlarged lymph nodes not thought to result from inflammation (38). In 1845, Virchow distinguished lymphosarcoma from leukemia, but it was not until later in the 19th century that histologic criteria for the diagnosis of both Hodgkin's disease and "malignant lymphoma" were developed (58,107). The past 90 years have seen the continuing subclassification of this heterogeneous group of diseases of the lymphoreticular system by the contributions of Brill, Symmers, Gall, Mallory, Rappaport, Lukes, Burkitt, Dorfman, Berard, and others (53). The malignant lymphomas still present intriguing challenges to those seeking to clarify the etiology and pathogenesis of neoplastic disease. Progress in understanding the biology of the lymphomas has evolved with our greater understanding of the normal immune system. Moreover, investigations into the virologic and immunologic aspects of Hodgkin's disease and Burkitt's lymphoma have stimulated analogous investigations of many other malignancies. The current management of these diseases is a clear example of the advantages of multidisciplinary collaboration in staging and treating malignancy. The increasing capacity for curing lymphomas has inspired oncologists to approach less responsive neoplasms with more determination and optimism.

HODGKIN'S DISEASE

EPIDEMIOLOGY AND ETIOLOGY

Epidemiology (34)

1. Hodgkin's disease constitutes 40% of malignant lymphomas. The number of patients newly diagnosed each year in the United States has remained reasonably constant at about 7,400, with a male to female ratio of 1.3:1 (1).
2. A striking bimodal age peak is recognized in the incidence of Hodgkin's disease. Curiously, the age range for the first peak varies according to the economic development of the country, occurring prior to adolescence in underdeveloped countries, but in the mid to late 20s in industrialized countries. The second peak occurs in late adulthood (2). The disease is rare before the age of 5 years.
3. Although isolated clusters of this disease have been reported, conclusive evidence as to communicability is lacking (106).
4. Patients with a congenital immunodeficiency disease, such as ataxia telangiectasia, appear to have an increased risk for developing Hodgkin's disease (30). Similarly, it occurs more frequently in patients with iatrogenic or acquired immune deficiency syndromes, including AIDS (105).
5. Reports of Hodgkin's disease in first-degree relatives of affected patients, especially of the same gender, and in parent-child concordant pairs, are as yet unexplained (2). One possibility relates to an association with viruses. An increased incidence of Hodgkin's is seen in patients with elevated titers of various antibodies to the Epstein-Barr virus (EBV) (71), and such elevations recently have been shown to predate the diagnosis of Hodgkin's disease (69). Moreover, hybridization techniques have recently confirmed that a subset of patients with Hodgkin's disease have a clonal proliferation of EBV-infected cells, and that the EBV genomes are present in Reed-Sternberg (RS) cells (108).

Etiology

1. The pathogenesis of Hodgkin's disease remains an enigma, although recent investigations have provided a greater understanding of its nature. For example, it has been known that patients with untreated Hodgkin's disease have defective cellular but intact humoral immunity. Recent investigations suggest that this defect is secondary to an increased sensitivity of effector T cells to suppressor monocytes and T-suppressor cells (94). The abnormality may be a consequence of the neoplasm, or alternatively, an inherent genetic defect that disposes an individual to the development of Hodgkin's disease. Similar considerations relate to the association with the EBV. The expression of various antibodies (Immunoglobin (Ig)G or IgA against the capsid antigen, the E-B nuclear antigen, and early antigen D) is greater in a subset of individuals who develop Hodgkin's disease (108). It would appear that activation of the EBV

may dispose an individual for the induction of Hodgkin's disease by factors that to date are unidentified. However, an alternative explanation is that the observed pattern of EBV activity is simply a marker of the effect of a more fundamental factor (viral, environmental, genetic) that diminishes the immunologic control of latent infections in patients who develop Hodgkin's disease.

2. The evolution of this disease is well described. The process is likely to be unifocal in origin and, in 90% of patients, presents in a pattern of involvement that suggests contiguous lymphatic spread (53,68,98). Thus, clinical presentations fall in rather predictable patterns. Most patients present with supradiaphragmatic nodal disease, while vascular invasion with bone marrow involvement is relatively uncommon. However, if left unchecked, the tumor will grow, with direct extension into adjacent visceral organs or blood vessels. The para-aortic and left supraclavicular nodes are contiguous via the thoracic duct. The frequency of splenic involvement in situations not clearly explained by contiguous lymphatic spread suggests that it is a favored site for implantation and growth by Hodgkin's disease. Alternately, hypotheses relating its involvement to more convoluted patterns of contiguous spread can be offered. Although the evidence in support of this "continuity" theory is substantial, a "stochastic" theory has been proposed in which Hodgkin's disease is considered a multicentric systemic disorder, with its spread via the blood stream and a variable susceptibility of lymph nodes determining the pattern of distribution (95).

Biology

Another area of uncertainty relates to the cell that confers "malignancy" in Hodgkin's disease. The R S cell is the best candidate, yet its normal counterpart remains elusive. Arguments can be made that point to several possible cells, including B- and T-lymphocytes, monocytes or macrophages, interdigitating or dendritic reticulum cells, and progenitors of granulocytes. For example, using immunocytochemical techniques, T cell or B cell specific antigens can be detected on RS cells in 60% of patient materials, and the different pathologic subtypes are more closely associated with one of the two antigenic types (e.g., mixed cellularity Hodgkin's with T cells, lymphocyte predominant Hodgkin's with B cells) (5). Surface markers, such as the interleukin-2 receptor and human lympocyte antibody-DR antigens, can be demonstrated on the RS cell that are also found on activated T and B lymphocytes (45). In further support of a lymphocyte origin are recent demonstrations of clonal rearrangements of immunoglobulin heavy-chain or light-chain genes in tissue samples that contain large numbers of RS cells from patients with Hodgkin's disease (101). Since B cells are the usual host for the EBV, evidence invoking this virus in the causation of Hodgkin's disease suggests that this lymphocyte can be the relevant cell of origin for the malignancy. Other lines of evidence suggest that the interdigitating reticulum/dendritic cell is the normal counterpart of the RS cell. RS cells and their mononuclear variants have Fc and C3 receptors and Ia antigen, consistant with an origin from an antigen-presenting cell. The monocyte/macrophage is the other prominent antigen-presenting cell, but several characteristics of these cells are not shared with RS cells, diminishing the likelihood of an etiologic association. The continued difficulty in determining the lineage of the malignant Hodgkin's cell relates to the likelihood that there are few such cells compared with accompanying reactive cells, and they may become transformed at a primitive stage with an ability to partially differentiate.

DETECTION AND DIAGNOSIS

Clinical Detection (Fig. 18-1) (54a)

1. The typical presentation for patients with Hodgkin's disease is one of painless lymph node enlargement. Constitutional symptoms occur in one third of patients and most prominently include fever, sweating, or weight loss (53,68,98). Pruritis and malaise may also occur. Usually patients first notice lymphadenopathy above the diaphragm, involving cervical nodes in 60% to 80% of patients (53, 59,68,98). Axillary or mediastinal presentations are less common, and the latter may cause cough, dyspnea, or superior vena cava obstruction. Patients on occasion (3% to 10%) present with subdiaphragmatic involvement, usually with inguinal lymphadenopathy or an abdominal mass. Mesenteric nodes are rarely involved.

2. Contiguous growth of tumor into adjacent organs, and lymphatic spread or hematogenous dissemination to retroperitoneal nodes, spleen, liver, bone, or bone marrow will eventually occur if the disease is not treated.

DIAGNOSTIC PROCEDURES

1. Lymph node biopsy establishes the diagnosis. The largest, most central node in an enlarged group is most likely to be diagnostic (3,53). The biopsy of a cervical node is preferred because chronic inflammatory changes are more commonly present in inguinal or axillary nodes. Although lymph node aspiration may provide suitable material for a diagnosis (21), biopsy is preferred to provide material for full histopathologic, cytogenetic, and bacteriologic evaluation. The presence of RS

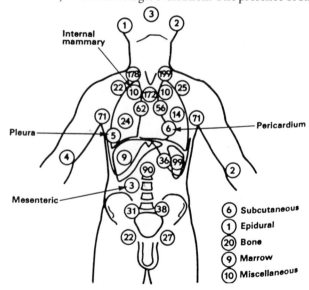

Fig. 18-1. Detection and diagnosis: Anatomical distribution of sites of involvement.

cells is essential for diagnosis, but these may be mimicked by cells of an infectious etiology (99). The classic RS cell is a large binucleate or polynucleate cell 25 to 30 μm in diameter, with an inclusion bodylike macronucleolus in each of the nuclei, prominent euchromatin, spider weblike heterochromatin, and prominent nuclear membrane with internal heterochromatin deposits. Phenytoin therapy may be associated with a Hodgkin's-like histology, but adenopathy due to this drug disappears after its cessation (8). Typical RS cells may be extremely rare in lymphocyte predominant-Hodgkin's disease.

2. A hematologic evaluation (including bone marrow) may reveal several abnormalities.

   a. Neutrophilic leukocytosis and mild normocytic, normochromic anemia are common. Eosinophilia may occur. Patients with extensive disease sometimes have lymphopenia (68).

   b. An idiopathic thrombocytopenic purpura-like picture may be seen rarely, with platelet-associated Ig demonstrable in some patients.

   c. Hemolytic anemia, usually Coomb's-test (antiglobulin) negative, may occur, usually in the setting of advanced disease (8).

   d. Bone marrow biopsy is advisable, but involvement with Hodgkin's disease is rare in patients with disease apparently confined to the supradiaphragmatic regions and without systemic symptoms (22,88).

   e. The erythrocyte sedimentation rate (ESR), hematocrit, and serum ferritin level should be obtained. When elevated, they may be associated with a worse prognosis (28,36,48).

   f. Elevated levels of leukocyte alkaline phosphatase and serum copper (as well as ESR) may be associated with exacerbations of disease and thus should be obtained at diagnosis and serially followed (68). An elevated alkaline phosphatase value may also reflect involvement of the liver, bone marrow, or bone with Hodgkin's disease.

   g. Hypergammaglobulinemia is common, while hypogammaglobulinemia may be seen in patients with advanced disease (68). A full immunologic evaluation of patients (response to intradermal recall antigens, phytohemogglutin (PHA) stimulation of lymphocytes) may show varying degrees of anergy, which can return to normal after successful therapy (103). However, abnormalities of cellular immunity (T cells) may persist for years (26).

3. Imaging studies play a prominent role in detection of disease and thus the evaluation for staging (Table 18-1) (see section on staging work-up).

CLASSIFICATION

Histopathology (4,11,61,64,65,70,85)

The first clinically useful subclassification of Hodgkin's disease was developed by Jackson and Parker (47) and included a large "granuloma" group. A subsequent scheme, developed by Lukes et al. (64), was later simplified into the Rye classification, which remains in use. Four subtypes of Hodgkin's disease are recognized in the most common application of this system (Table 18-2) (54).

1. *Nodular sclerosis Hodgkin's disease* constitutes about 75% of most recent series. Cellular nodules, containing plasma cells, neutrophils, and eosinophils, are surrounded by annular bands of polarizable collagen. RS cells are large (40 to 60 μm) and their abundant pale cytoplasm may retract during fixation, leaving lacunar spaces around the nuclei—thus the term lacunar cells. When these cells predominate and sclerosis is minimal, the term cellular phase is sometimes used.

2. *Lymphocyte predominance Hodgkin's disease* comprises about 5% of cases (90). The lymph node architecture may be completely or partially obliterated by a proliferation of benign-appearing lymphocytes with or without histiocytes. RS cells are few. Nodular and diffuse subtypes are recognized, with the former having a B-cell origin (5) and an indolent course with more frequent late relapses (83).

3. *Mixed cellularity Hodgkin's disease* Fifteen to twenty percent of patients have this subtype, in which a pleocellular infiltrate (plasma cells, neutrophils, eosinophils) and moderate numbers of RS cells are seen.

4. *Lymphocyte depletion Hodgkin's disease* is rare and characterized by a predominance of RS cells and few lymphocytes. This aggressive subtype must be carefully distinguished from nodular sclerosis Hodgkin's disease and non-Hodgkin's lymphoma. Some pathologists denote a less aggressive subtype, diffuse fibrosis, which is extremely hypocellular (85).

Anatomic Staging (Figs. 18-2 and 18-3) (54b)

The 1970 Ann Arbor Symposium on Staging in Hodgkin's disease (13) recommended a system using clinical and pathologic staging, and a modification of that system is accepted for staging classification (Figs. 18-2, 18-3, Table 18-3) (13). Of note is that B symptomatology is carefully defined. Unexplained weight loss of greater than 10% body weight must have occurred within 6 months of diagnosis, temperature elevation is greater than 38°C and recurrent during the previous month, and night sweats are drenching and recurrent during the previous month (13). Organ involvement is noted with letter symbols as follows: S = spleen, H = liver, L = lung, M = marrow, P = pleura, O = bone (osseous), and D = skin.

A relative weakness of the Ann Arbor system is its failure to consider disease bulk (including the number of involved sites), or specific patterns of involvement (96,97). For this reason subclassifications of the Ann Arbor staging system have been proposed, particularly for patients with stage IIIA disease. One proposal substages patients according to the location of involved abdominal sites. Patients with disease limited to the spleen, or splenic, celiac, or portal nodes are denoted anatomic substage III$_1$ and considered to have a more favorable prognosis than patients with involvement of para-aortic, iliac, or mesenteric nodes, denoted as III$_2$ (97). This system has not proven useful in some centers (42). Data from Stanford University, confirmed by others, indicate that the presence of five or more splenic nodules is an adverse prognostic factor; patients are thus designated as stage IIIAS+extensive or IIIAS+minimal (42).

Staging Work-up

Recommended procedures for a complete evaluation and classification are multiple.

Table 18-1. Imaging Modalities for Detection and Diagnosis of Hodgkin's Disease

Method	Diagnosis and Staging Capability	Recommended For Use
Primary tumor and regional nodes		
X-ray Chest	Intrathoracic disease is frequently adequately assessed	Always
CT Chest	Provides additional evidence of intrathoracic disease. CT is the preferred study when the following situations are being addressed: - Evaluation of a suspicious or equivocal mediastinum - Evaluation of the "normal" mediastinum (may contain enlarged lymph nodes demonstrable by CT) - Evaluation for chest wall involvement in the presence of bulky mediastinal disease - Evaluation for pulmonary parenchymal lesions - Evaluation for pleural or pericardial disease - Anatomic extent of disease for treatment planning	Yes
Abdominal and pelvic CT	Delineates extent of bulky lymph node disease. However, normal-sized lymph nodes that contain tumor deposits, at times readily demonstrable by lymphography, will not be detected by CT. Mesenteric lymphadenopathy is relatively reliably shown by CT in the non-Hodgkins lymphomas	Yes
MRI + gadolinium	Shows promise in delineating extent of disease. Pericardial involvement well demonstrated	Yes
Bipedal lymphography	Most accurate imaging test for evaluating retroperitoneal lymph nodes. Provides convenient means for follow-up regarding response to treatment or relapse	Yes
Ultrasonography	Exclusion of urinary tract obstruction with bulky lymphadenopathy	Selected
Gallium citrate radionuclide studies	Supradiaphragmatic disease. Proper technique is important for quality images	Selected

CT = computed tomography; MRI = magnetic resonance imaging.

Table 18-2. Interrelationships of Major Histopathology Classifications of Hodgkin's Disease

Jackson and Parker	Lukes, Butler, and Hicks	(Incidence %) Rye = Current	Distinctive Features
Paragranuloma	Lymphocytic histiocytic, diffuse; Lymphocytic histiocytic, nodular	Lymphocytic predominance (10-15) - (5)	Abundant stroma: mature lymphocytes and/or histiocytes; no necrosis: RS cells may be sparse
Granuloma	Nodular sclerosis	Nodular sclerosis (20-50) - (75)	Nodules of lymphoid tissue separated by bands of doubly refractile collagen; atypical "lacunar" Hodgkin's cells in clear spaces within the lymphoid nodules
	Mixed	Mixed cellularity (20-40) - (15-20)	Numerous RS cells and mononuclear Hodgkin's cells in pleomorphic stroma of eosinophils, plasma cells, fibroblasts, and necrotic foci
Sarcoma	Diffuse fibrosis; Reticular	Lymphocytic depletion (5-15) - (≤2)	RS cells usually abundant; marked paucity of lymphocytes; diffuse nonrefractile fibrosis and necrosis

RS = Reed-Sternberg.

Adapted from Kaplan (54).

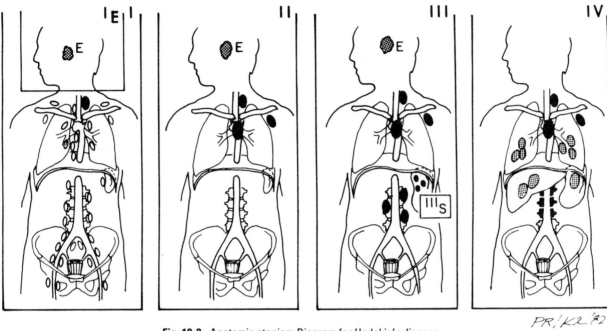

PR/KL '82.

Fig. 18-2. Anatomic staging: Diagram for Hodgkin's disease.

1. A detailed history records any systemic signs and symptoms, and evidence for cardiorespiratory compromise and organ dysfunction. The physical examination includes a careful determination of the location and size of all palpable lymph nodes. An evaluation of Waldeyer's ring, cardiorespiratory status, and organomegaly is vital.

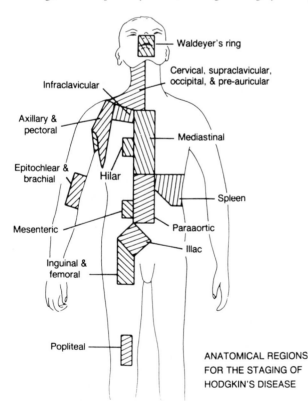

ANATOMICAL REGIONS FOR THE STAGING OF HODGKIN'S DISEASE

Fig. 18-3. Anatomic staging: Anatomic definition of separate lymph node regions.

2. Laboratory procedures include the following:
   a. A complete blood cell count with differential white blood cell count, reticulocyte count, and ESR.
   b. A direct Coomb's (antiglobulin) test in the setting of anemia.
   c. Blood chemistries, with particular attention to the serum alkaline phosphatase, liver, and renal function tests, and uric acid.
   d. Bone marrow biopsy in patients with B symptoms, clinical stage III or IV disease, or if there are blood cell count depressions, an elevated alkaline phosphatase, or bony abnormalties on imaging.
3. Imaging procedures are diverse in nature (Table 18-1):
   a. Chest x-ray and computerized tomography (CT) scan are obtained. The latter details the status of intrathoracic lymph node groups, lung parenchyma, pericardium, pleura, and the chest wall, and can alter eventual treatment in 10% of cases (16). Magnetic resonance imaging (MRI) of the chest offers the potential to better characterize the presence or absence of disease activity following therapy, and, accordingly, may be helpful as a baseline study (72).
   b. Bipedal lymphangiography (LAG) is important to guide the surgeon in subsequent laparotomy and to assist the radiation therapist in abdominal radiation field design. In a large series from Stanford University, the overall accuracy of LAGs in identifying involved nodes was 92%. There were no false-negatives, but the false-positive rate was 25% (15). Approximately 30% of clinical stage I and IIA patients (but only 14% of patients presenting only with cervical nodes), and more than 80% of clinical stage IIB patients will have abnormal retroperitoneal nodes on LAG, with the previous stated false-negative rate (89). Clinical stage IV patients should be spared the discomfort of LAG.

Table 18-3. Ann Arbor Stage/Substage Classification for Hodgkin's Disease

	Stage	Substage
Stage I	Single node region	I
	Single extralymphatic; Organ/site	I (E)
Stage II	Two or more node regions same side of diaphragm	II
	Single node region + localized single extralymphatic organ/site	II (E)
Stage III	Node regions both sides of diaphragm	III
	± localized single extralymphatic organ/site	III (E)
	Spleen, both	III (S)/(ES)
Stage IV	Diffuse involvement extralymphatic, organ/site ± node regions	IV
All stages divided	Without weight loss/fever/sweats	A
	With weight loss/fever/sweats	B

E = extralymphatic; S = spleen involved.

See Fig. 18-3 for sites.

Adapted from Carbone et al. (13).

c. Abdominal CT scanning is also effective in detecting abdominal and pelvic nodes. A node greater than 1 cm in diameter is considered suspicious, and one greater than 2 cm is considered abnormal (35). This technique cannot demonstrate the abnormal, "foamy" architecture of lymphomatous nodes as seen by LAG, or splenic involvement, but can suggest liver involvement and show enlarged mesenteric nodes, and upper para-aortic nodes (difficult to visualize by LAG).

4. Laparotomy and splenectomy should be undertaken only when they will influence therapeutic decisions (18,53,86,102). If the treatment policy is to use irradiation alone for patients with stages IA and IIA disease, then laparotomy is appropriate to exclude occult subdiaphragmatic involvement. Overall, 20% to 30% of patients with clinical stage I-II disease will be upstaged at laparotomy, and 90% of these patients will have splenic involvement (59). Select subgroups at low risk for upstaging include clinical stage I patients with mediastinal-only disease, clinical stage I women, and clincal stage I men with lymphocyte predominance Hodgkin's disease. Alternatively, laparotomy may also demonstrate the absence of disease thought to be present by imaging studies, and thereby downstage patients. Up to 50% of young patients (aged 40 years) with clinical stage III-IV disease will be down-staged. Subgroups with a low likelihood of downstaging include older patients with clinical stage IIIB-IVB mixed cellularity Hodgkin's disease/lymphocyte depletion Hodgkin's disease. In general, for patients who will be treated with chemotherapy alone or as an adjunct to irradiation, staging laparotomy cannot be recommended. Although treatment policies differ at major treatment centers, such patients are generally those with large mediastinal masses, with definite stage IIIB or IV disease, with multiple E sites, and perhaps with the previously defined III$_2$A disease (53,66,86,97).

When laparotomy is performed, all anatomic nodal stations should be sampled, with particular attention to nodes suspect on imaging studies; both lobes of the liver should be biopsied; clips should mark the location of the splenic pedicle and suspicious nodes, and oophoropexy should be performed if pelvic irradiation might be used. Complications include deaths (rare), wound infections and dehiscences, and small bowel obstructions. Young children undergoing splenectomy may be at an increased risk for serious infections by encapsulated bacteria.

5. Optional and investigative procedures:
   a. Gallium-67 scintigraphy may be useful as an adjunct imaging procedure. It has a 74%, true-positive rate, but also a high false-negative rate (43). It may be most useful in monitoring the response to therapy (46) for patients being assessed for the persistence of mediastinal disease (34a).
   b. Skeletal scintigrams are appropriate in the setting of bone pain or an elevated serum alkaline phosphatase value.
   c. Ultrasonograms, inferior cavography, or pyelograms occasionally will be indicated.

PRINCIPLES OF TREATMENT

Multidisciplinary Treatment Planning

The variety of possible therapeutic strategies for the treatment of patients with Hodgkin's disease, and the clear relationship of outcome to appropriate therapy, make it imperative that the surgeon, medical hematologist-oncologist, radiation oncologist, diagnostic radiologist, and pathologist jointly consider the characteristics of each patient in order to devise optimal therapy. Moreover, each participant must have expertise in the respective disciplines because of the complexity of each phase of evaluation and therapy. A concise overview of different treatment modalities is offered in Table 18-4 by stage of disease.

Surgery

1. The primary role of surgery is to obtain tissue diagnosis through biopsy (see section on diagnostic procedures). Abdominal exploration (laparotomy) with lymph node, bone marrow, and liver biopsies and splenectomy are performed in staging selected patients (see section on staging work-up). If definitive management of the patient should include laparotomy, but the patient's respiratory status is compromised by mediastinal adenopathy,

Table 18-4. Guidelines for Treatment in Hodgkin's Disease in Adults

Stage	Clinical Presentation	Treatment
IA or IIA	Supradiaphragmatic, absent or small mediastinal disease, laparotomy negative	Mantle + para-aortic-splenic pedicle RT (STNI) If hilar nodes clinically positive use partial transmission lung block (16.5 Gy) on involved side(s) If high cervical nodes, use preauricular field(s)
	As above but mediastinal adenopathy (LMA) (>1/3 intrathoracic diameter) or juxtapericardial tumor Laparotomy negative	STNI if LMA <1/3 intrathoracic diameter and selected patients with larger masses and no paracardiac disease, or MAC and mantle RT (or STNI)
	No laparotomy, but abdominal CT, lymphangiogram negative.	Combined MAC/RT as above (STNI or TLI alone are used in some centers)
	Subdiaphragmatic presentations with laparotomy staging	Inverted Y + mantle (RT) (TNI). If isolated pelvic disease, use inverted Y
IB or IIB	Night sweating ± either fevers or weight loss, and laparotomy staging	Treat as for IA and IIA above
	Fevers and weight loss	Combined MAC/RT
IIIA	Favorable: Absent or small mediastinal adenopathy, <5 splenic nodules, upper abdominal disease (IIIA1) Unfavorable: LMA, >5 splenic nodules, lower abdominal disease (IIIA2), no laparotomy	Mantle + para-aortic/splenic pedicle + pelvic RT (TNI) (partial hepatic RT if spleen involved), or combined MAC/RT Combined MAC/RT including pelvic RT if pelvic nodes positive or no laparotomy. Consider full course MAC Combined MAC/RT including pelvic RT if pelvic nodes positive or no laparotomy. Consider full course MAC followed by low-dose consolidation RT (20-30 Gy)
IIIB or IV	Limited disease extent (eg,two nodal regions or single focus of organ involvement)	Intensive MAC alone or combined MAC/RT including partial- or full-dose RT to involved organ. Consider RT to all sites of disease involvement
	Extensive disease	Intensive MAC. Consider RT to areas of bulky disease or to all involved sites
RECURRENT	If MAC alone was previously delivered, patient is young with recurrence >1 yr following MAC and isolated nodal recurrence	Total lymphoid RT or MAC followed by consolidation RT within tissue tolerance
	All others	MAC with consideration for consolidation RT within tissue tolerance, or bone marrow transplantation if remission is achieved. Consider RT to recurrent bulk disease.

MAC = multiagent chemotherapy; RCT = recommended chemotherapy; RT = radiation therapy; STNI = subtotal nodal irradiation; TNI = Total nodal irradiation; CT = computed tomography; LMA = large mediastinal adenopathy.
PDQ: RCT - MOPP/ABV hybrid, MOPP/ABVD alternating and other regimens.

then mantle irradiation should be considered prior to the administration of anesthesia to reduce the likelihood of related complications (77).

2. Radical excision of enlarged nodes is not justified in view of the efficacy of chemotherapy and radiotherapy.
3. Splenectomy for hypersplenism (persistent cytopenias with cellular bone marrow and reticulocytosis) may rarely be indicated in certain patients with advanced disease (93).

Radiation Therapy

The responsiveness of Hodgkin's disease to irradiation was first demonstrated by Pusey (80) in 1902. Gilbert (25) laid the foundations for the definitive radiotherapy treatment of Hodgkin's disease. Further definition of important principles was provided by Peters (74) in 1950. Systematic study

of the role of radiotherapy and use of supravoltage techniques was subsequently performed by Kaplan (54) at Stanford University.

Irradiation is the primary treatment modality for the majority of patients with early stages of Hodgkin's disease, including patients with stages I, II, and IIIA with microscopic splenic involvement or high abdominal nodal involvement, unassociated with other adverse prognostic factors such as massive mediastinal involvement or extensive juxtapericardial disease (53).

General techniques of radiation therapy:

1. The use of megavoltage irradiation (linear accelerators) and extended fields to include adjacent (contiguous) clinically uninvolved nodal sites is crucial in achieving high cure rates when radiotherapy alone is used to treat Hodgkin's disease (53,109). Segmental sequential

irradiation consists of treatment to major nodal stations on both sides of the diaphragm. Total nodal irradiation (TNI), also known as total lymphoid irradiation, sequentially irradiates a mantle field above the diaphragm, followed by irradiation of the para-aortic nodes and spleen (splenic pedicle) and the pelvis, separately or in one field (an inverted "Y"). Subtotal nodal irradiation (STNI) refers to a mantle followed by a para-aortic-splenic pedicle field and has become the arrangement most widely used in laparotomy-negative stages IA and IIA patients. Shielding and field shaping are used to protect lung, spinal cord, larynx, heart, humoral and femoral heads, kidneys, gonads, and iliac crest marrow. The subtotal nodal arrangement avoids all direct radiation dose to the pelvis and spares significant amounts of bone marrow with only minimal scattered irradiation to the gonads.

2. The dose required to eradicate Hodgkin's disease in demonstrably involved nodes is approximately 40-45 Gy (53), although recent data suggest that 30 to 40 Gy provide tumor control in most patients (56). This data notwithstanding, nodal sites on the same side of the diaphragm as the clinically apparent diseases are treated with 40 Gy with consideration for a 5 Gy boost to the involved nodal station(s) only (55a). Each treatment fraction delivers 1.5 to 2 Gy. A total dose of 35 Gy is adequate for nodal sites on the clinically uninvolved side of the diaphragm. Treatment to the para-aortic nodes and splenic pedicle area is recommended even in laparotomy-negative, supradiaphragmatic stages IA and IIA patients, since microscopic disease below the diaphragm cannot be dependably detected even at surgery. However, some clinicians treat with mantle irradiation only, reserving chemotherapy for those few patients whose disease recurs.

3. Consolidation irradiation is the term applied to relatively low-dose radiotherapy (15 to 25 Gy) delivered to sites of initial disease involvement in patients with advanced disease who achieve complete remission (CR) with chemotherapy (109). This technique remains investigational in terms of its efficacy. The concept of chemotherapy cytoreduction as induction for definitive radiotherapy, but in modified dose, was established by Bertino and Prosnitz who reported a better than 90% 5-year survival in chemoresponders. This approach allowed for modest half doses of irradiation to large portions of the anatomy. An Eastern Cooperative Oncology Group (ECOG) study did not confirm this finding on initial reporting, but if the radiation therapy was quality-controlled for both dose and volume, survival results were similiar for MOPP followed by ABVD consolidation or MOPP followed by consolidation low-dose 15 to 20 Gy irradiation. Prosnitz refers to his recent experience at Duke University with combined modality therapy, which was found to be more effective than chemotherapy in Stage IIB-IV Hodgkin's disease, where the 10-year actuarial survival (Hodgkin's death) was 93% for combined modality therapy versus 59% for chemotherapy patients (11a,78). Relapse occurred in a large number of chemotherapy-only patients, with 85% of these sites being initially involved at the time of diagnosis. To support the low-dose concept, Prosnitz

(78b) also refers to his earlier Yale experience, in which a less than 10% field failure and a high cure rate (>90%) occurred when patients responded to chemotherapy. Bonnadonna (9a) used larger doses (25 to 30 Gy) in combination with MOPP/ABVD with good-to-excellent results, i.e., 80% 5-year survival. The most recent experience confirms the role of irradiation to bulk disease in alternating or sequential schedules (107a).

4. Complications: Complications of radiotherapy include temporary bone marrow suppression in most patients. Less commonly, symptomatic radiation pneumonitis (5%) and pericarditis (5%) occur (53,56). Clinical hypothyroidism is rare (5% to 15%), but subclinical compensated chemical hypothyroidism is frequent (33% to 70%); it is detected by an elevation in thyroid-stimulating hormone and managed with thyroxin replacement (31). If the pelvis is irradiated, significant doses are received by the gonads even when appropriate shielding is used. Aspermia may occur with inguinal fields even with small doses of scattered irradiation when the total exceeds 1.5 to 2 Gy, but recovery is often seen at delayed time points of 2 to more than 5 years (73). Nevertheless, sperm banking prior to therapy is recommended. Menstrual dysfunction is common, but recovery usually takes place and pregnancies producing normal offspring occur (44). Second malignant tumors are common, particularly after combined modality therapy; the actuarial risk at 15 years is 17.6%, a fivefold excess compared with a nonpatient population (104).

Chemotherapy

Since it was demonstrated in the 1940s that nitrogen mustard had activity against Hodgkin's disease (33), great progress has been made in the treatment of generalized Hodgkin's disease with combinations of agents. The strategy, which has proven effective, entails the use of multiple non-cross-resistant agents with additive antitumor effects but without additive host toxicities (32) (see Chapter 8, "Basic Concepts of Cancer Chemotherapy"). A broad choice of agents exists with which to develop such combinations (Table 18-5). The timing of drug administration is designed to minimize acute toxicities, particularly gastrointestinal (GI) and hematologic, while delivering otherwise maximal tolerated doses. This intensive cyclic administration of drug combinations with periods of rest for normal tissue recovery may nevertheless be poorly tolerated by older patients. Such patients thus require close surveillance for infections and other intercurrent problems. The general approach of most chemotherapy programs has been to treat patients until they achieve a CR and then administer two additional cycles. The addition of maintenance chemotherapy has not proven beneficial.

1. Several three-to-five-drug programs have proven to be effective. The MOPP regimen (Table 18-5) was the first highly successful combination demonstrated. DeVita et al. at the National Cancer Institute reported CRs in 81% of 194 previously untreated patients with stage III or IV disease who were given the four-drug combination for 6 months or more (19,20). Once the efficacy of MOPP was shown, modifications were developed to decrease the acute toxicities of nausea, vomiting, peripheral neuropathy, constipation, and marrow suppression, and the chronic toxicities of sterility and

Table 18-5. Representative Results of Therapy in the Treatment of Hodgkin's Disease by Stage (5-7-10 YR Survival)

Stage	Patient No.	Treatment	RFS (%)	Survival (%)	Institution
IA, IIA	109	STNI or TNI	79*	96*	Stanford (87)
IA, IIA	315	STNI	82*	93*	JCRT (67)
IA, IIA	168	STNI	81*	96*	Yale (55)
IB, IIB	180	STNI, TNI	78+	87+	Stanford, JCRT (17)
		CMT (MOPP)	85+	91+	
IIIA	86	TNI	66#	86#	Stanford (42)
	85	CMT (MOPP)	86#	89#	
IIIA	21	TNI	65*	85*	St. Bartholomew (63)
	32	MVPP	85*	90*	
IIIB, IV	198	MOPP	52*	46*	NCI (20)
IIIB, IV	166	MOP/BAP	50#	70#	SWOG (51)
	125	MOPP/Bleomycin	40#	60#	
IIIB, IV	147	BCVPP	49#	67#	ECOG (6)
	146	MOPP	34#	61#	

\# = 5-year data; + = 7-year data; * = 10-year data.

RFS = relapse free survival; TNI = total nodal irradiation; STNI = subtotal nodal irradiation; CMT = combined modality therapy;

JCRT = Joint Center for Radiation Therapy; NCI = National Cancer Institute; SWOG = Southwest Oncology Group;

ECOG = Eastern Cooperative Oncology Group.

second maligancies. The BCVPP program was studied by ECOG (7) and the Southeastern Cancer Study Group (24) (Table 18-5). It proved to be at least as effective as MOPP. The PAVe regimen was developed at Stanford University (87) and is also effective. In the early 1970s, doxorubicin was developed and used in several regimens. The most prominent of these is the ABVD program (Table 18-5), which was carefully studied by Santoro *et al.* (91) and shown to provide a similar CR induction rate when compared with MOPP. It has been reported to be successful in salvaging patients who have recurrent disease after MOPP chemotherapy (92).

2. This lack of cross-resistance (ABVD following MOPP) was then used in the design of programs which alternated three or four drug combinations. Conceptually, this strategy appears to overcome the spontaneous development of multidrug resistant tumor cells. The Milan group (9,12) compared alternating cycles of MOPP and ABVD with MOPP treatment alone and showed the former to be superior, but other groups have not reproduced this apparent success. The most recent experience compares the use of alternating versus hybrid MOPP and ABVD in bulky stages I and IIA and advanced stages IIIB-IV. Results were similiar for both arms with regard to CR and survival; relapses were in major nodal sites of initial involvement (107a). Connors and Klimo (57) modifed the ABVD/MOPP regimen to omit dacarbazine and administer the other drugs within 14 days (MOPP/ABV). Radiation therapy is administered to sites of residual disease in selected patients. To date, the results have been excellent (90% disease-free survival (DFS) at more than 5 years) and toxicity has been modest. Nevertheless, the superiority of such alternating multidrug combinations over single multidrug regimens has not been unequivocally confirmed and is being investigated by several large coop-

erative group trials, particularly when low-dose consolidation radiotherapy is used with the latter type of regimen. The recent report of the Stanford experience by Ang *et al.* (5a) found PAVE + radiotherapy compares favorably with MOPP + radiotherapy and both multiple step therapies yield 5-year survival rates of 80% to 95% in unfavorable stages, with relapses mainly in sites of nodal bulk disease (79%) and extra nodal + nodes (21%).

Treatment Selection by Stage (Table 18-4)

A variety of different treatment strategies may be appropriate for any individual patient. Different programs may result in a similar likelihood of survival, but vary in the likelihood of freedom from first relapse. Moreover, the results vary in different institutions. Thus, variations in patient selection, staging evaluation, and definitions of response must be considered (39,53,62).

Stage I-II (A, B)

1. Most patients with stage I-II disease have supradiaphragmatic involvement (90%) and are appropriately treated with STNI. Although staging laparotomy is recommended, patients who are clinically staged should have irradiation to the entire spleen.
2. For patients with high cervical lymphadenopathy, the ipsilateral preauricular region is treated to 36 Gy (41).
3. Patients with lymphocyte-predominant disease limited to the high neck may be treated with mantle and preauricular irradiation alone, and the mediastinum can be shielded after 25 to 30 Gy (90).
4. For patients with pulmonary hilar lymph node involvement, the ipsilateral lung is treated with partial-transmission lung shielding to 16.5 Gy (41).
5. Patients with stage IIA or B disease with bulky mediastinal adenopathy may be treated with irradiation alone, or with combined irradiation and chemotherapy

(14,40,67). Patients treated with irradiation alone require careful planning using CT or magnetic resonance imaging (MRI), and irradiation techniques that include sequential field reductions and partial-transmission lung blocks. For patients with juxtapericardial disease, which would preclude cardiac blocking, and for patients with extensive mediastinal disease or other adverse prognostic factors (see section on prognostic factors), combined modality therapy is preferred. Two to three cycles of chemotherapy may be administered, followed by mantle irradiation and then completion of chemotherapy. Other strategies, such as initial chemotherapy followed by irradiation, are also used (29).

6. The optimal management of patients with B symptoms is still being defined. Subtotal nodal irradiation or TNI are effectively used. However, patients who have both fevers and weight loss have a worse prognosis than patients with other symptom constellations, and for these patients combined modality therapy or chemotherapy alone may prove to be superior (17).

Stage III A,B

The presence of multiple splenic nodules or lower abdominal involvement confers a worse prognosis for patients with IIIA disease. For patients with extensive infradiaphragmatic involvement, a large mediastinal mass, B symptoms, or clinical staging, combined modality therapy (using a technique that alternates cycles of chemotherapy with fields of irradiation) or chemotherapy alone is the treatment of choice (78a). TNI may be used effectively for patients with $IIIA_1$ disease and minimal splenic involvement, and a 50% transmission liver block with delivery of 20 to 22 Gy is frequently used. A further modification of this approach entails the use of STNI for patients with IIIA disease who have microscopic splenic involvement and no other abdominal disease.

Stage IV

Stage IV disease patients are treated with chemotherapy alone or combined modality therapy. Bone marrow involvements or multiple bone lesions are generally treated with such intensive chemotherapy that inclusion of irradiation may exceed normal tissue tolerances, although irradiation confined to regions of bulk disease should nevertheless be considered, particularly if a CR does not occur after chemotherapy.

Recurrent Disease

Relapse after initial therapy occurs most often within 4 years, but late relapse is not rare. Approximately 30% of patients with advanced Hodgkin's disease will not have CR with initial treatment or will relapse after a CR (63a). The choice of therapy for patients whose disease recurs after primary treatment is dependent on their disease characteristics at the time of relapse and the initial treatment. For patients who relapse less than 1 year after initial treatment with MOPP alone, alternative non-cross-resistant regimens such as ABVD have been used with variable success (8.5% to 22% 5-year DFS) (37,92). For young patients treated initially with chemotherapy alone and in whom relapse occurs more than one year after completing chemotherapy primarily in nodal sites and on one side of the diaphragm, wide field irradiation alone is effective, with or without additional chemotherapy. In this

setting 8-year freedom from relapse approaches 50% (27,84). Another treatment strategy for patients with chemotherapy-resistant Hodgkin's disease is the use of allogeneic or autologous bone marrow transplanation (BMT). In this subset of poor-prognosis patients, 20% to 25% have achieved long-term DFS (58a). However, this experience is based on patients with extremely poor disease characteristics who previously have had extensive therapy (49).

RESULTS AND PROGNOSIS

Survival Rates: Disease-Free Survival (DFS) and Overall Survival (Table 18-5)

In assessing the results of therapy in the treatment of Hodgkin's disease, consideration must be given to variations among different reports as to the following:

- definitions of DFS and overall survival
- characteristics of the patients reviewed in terms of staging evaluation and prognostic factors
- treatment regimens and techniques used
- morbidity of therapy

It is of special importance that attention is given to both DFS and overall survival when interpreting therapy results in early-stage disease, in view of the excellent potential of chemotherapy for salvaging patients treated initially with radiation therapy alone. Representative treatment results are presented in Table 18-5. As the therapy for Hodgkin's disease has become increasingly effective, the factors that influence outcome have declined in significance. Nevertheless, several factors continue to influence the success and certainly the choice of therapy.

1. The *stage or extent of disease* persists as the most important prognostic variable. Patients with stage IV disease have a 75% 5-year survival compared with 95% of patients with stages I and II disease (55,87). Within a given disease stage, other characteristics also influence the success of therapy.

   a. Large mediastinal adenopathy, defined as a mass exceeding one third the transverse diameter of the chest (intrathoracic width measured at the dome of the diaphragm) on a standard posterior-anterior chest radiograph, places a patient at a greater risk for disease recurrence. For patients with pathologic stage I-II disease treated with primary radiotherapy, DFS is inferior to that in patients treated with combined modality therapy, but overall survival remains high (80% to 90%), reflecting the effectiveness of chemotherapy as a salvage treatment. Nevertheless, patients without large mediastinal lymphadenopathy have a somewhat superior survival rate (67).

   b. Patients with extensive splenic involvement (five or more splenic nodules on cut section) have an inferior prognosis if treated with primary irradiation (42).

   c. Patients with stage IV disease who have multiple organ involvement fare worse than do patients with lesser amounts of disease (76).

   d. A large tumor burden, defined in terms of the tumor bulk and number of involved sites, has been reported to adversely influence outcome (96).

2. *B symptomatology* patients have a worse prognosis than

others, though the specific constellation of systemic symptoms appears to be relevant to this observation. That is, patients with night sweats only (at least among patients with pathologic stage I-II disease) appear to fare as well as pathologic stage I-IIA patients, while those with both fevers and weight loss have the worst prognosis (17).

3. *Age*: Among patients with advanced-stage disease, older age is an adverse prognostic variable (75), probably related to an inferior tolerance, and thus, the amount of therapy that can be administered.

4. *Laboratory studies* including the ESR, serum ferritin, and serum CD8 antigen levels have been reported to predict a worse outcome (28,36,48,79).

5. *Histologic subtype* appears to be more associated with patterns of disease involvement than with survival. For example, patients with pathologic stage I-II mixed cellularity Hodgkin's disease have an increased frequency of subdiaphragmatic relapse (67).

6. *Supradiaphragmatic versus Subdiaphragmatic*: Patients with isolated subdiaphragmatic Hodgkin's disease have a similar freedom from relapse and survival as do patients with equivalent stage supradiaphragmatic disease (60). Those with bulky splenic involvement fare the worst.

CLINICAL INVESTIGATIONS

Bone Marrow Transplantation

A variety of different treatment strategies have emerged for patients with advanced Hodgkin's disease who relapse or do not respond initially to treatment with chemotherapy regimens. BMT is an approach to circumvent the marrow toxicity resulting from the chemotherapy regimens. BMT is an approach to circumvent the marrow toxicity resulting from the use of high-dose chemotherapy with or without total body irradiation (107b).

   a. A recent update of autologous BMT literature provides information on 373 patients followed for 97 months. The median CR rate is 51%, of which 37% relapse, yielding a 32% 3-year survival rate. If a favorable and unfavorable cohort is identified, the CR rates are 63% versus 31% and 3-year survival is projected to be 77% and 18% of responders and nonresponders, respectively (55a).

   b. The most widely used chemotherapy program is cyclophosphamide, carmustine, and etoposide. Depending on whether patients are treated early and have recurrence with bulk disease (one or two chemotherapy regimens, < 10 cm in bulk nodes) or late (three or more chemotherapy regimens, > 10 cm in bulk disease), the 3-year DFS is 51% versus 22% and survival is 76% versus 38%, respectively (55a)

   c. The use of TNI and boost local radiation treatment for nodal involvement as well as aggressive chemotherapy produced a high CR rate, with 65% with no evidence of disease at 4 to 35 months (median, 20) (108a).

   d. Using more investigational approaches with radiolabelled Yttrium 90 bound to polyclonal antiferritin and radiolabeled monoclonal antibodies, in addition to TNI and aggressive chemotherapy, investigators project CR rates of 90% (107c,107d). Growth factors such as recombinant human granulocyte-macrophage colony stimulating factor reduce hematologic toxicity and allow for investigation of more aggressive forms and combinations of chemotherapy (137b).

PEDIATRIC HODGKIN'S DISEASE

The biology and natural history of Hodgkin's disease in children is similar to that in adults. However, when irradiation techniques and doses suitable for controlling disease in adults were translated to the pediatric setting, substantial morbidities (primarily musculoskeletal growth inhibition) were produced. It is within this context that new strategies for the treatment of pediatric Hodgkin's disease were developed. Historically, effected children were thought to have a worse prognosis than adults (53). It is now apparent that the converse is true. Not only do children (age <16 years) fare better than adults, but younger children (<10 years) fare better than adolescents. The explanation for this is not clear.

As initially stated, many characteristics of Hodgkin's disease in children are similar to that in adults. However, selected differences are noteworthy.

Epidemiology

1. A more striking male to female predominance is found among children, where the ratio is 4:1 for 3- to 7- year olds, 3:1 for 7- to 9- year olds, and more similar to adults (1.3:1) in older children (115).

2. Environmental factors, such as infection, may be associated with the risk for Hodgkin's. Supportive data include an increased risk in children from multiple-family homes, and a clustering of cases from a single school (112,113e,116).

Classification

A higher percentage of children have the lymphocyte-predominant subtype, and a lower percentage the lymphocyte-depleted subtype when compared with adults. The nodular sclerosing subtype is also somewhat less frequent in young children in contrast to adults (114).

DETECTION AND DIAGNOSIS

1. Most children (80%) present with cervical adenopathy (111).

2. While 60% of children have intrathoracic disease at diagnosis, mediastinal involvement is less frequent in 1- to 10- year olds (33%) as compared with adolescents (76%) (111).

3. The distinction of a normal or hyperplastic thymus from involvement with Hodgkin's disease is more problematic in children than in adults.

4. On staging laparotomy, reactive hyperplasia is more common in children aged 1 to 10 years (19%) as compared with older children (8%) (114).

5. As in adults, the decision to perform a staging laparotomy should depend on its value in influencing the therapeutic strategy. Because of the heightened desire to tailor therapy to disease extent in children in order to avoid potential morbidities of treatment, operative staging continues to be common.

PRINCIPLES OF TREATMENT AND RESULTS (Tables 18-6, 18-7, and 18-8)

Devising an optimal therapeutic approach for children with Hodgkin's disease is complicated by their increased risk for adverse effects from the treatments used for adults. In particular, standard radiotherapy doses and fields can cause profound musculoskeletal retardation (111). The successful use of chemotherapy in combination with lower doses of radiation therapy suggested new approaches for refining therapy to reduce morbidities (10,23,50,100). Investigators at Stanford University demonstrated the efficacy of six cycles of MOPP chemotherapy and low-dose involved field irradiation, achieving an 89% relapse-free survival at greater than 5 years (23) (Fig. 18-4). A recent report by Donaldson *et al.* compared results in early stage disease from Stanford (pathologic staging) extended-field radiation therapy alone or involved-field radiation therapy (plus chemotherapy) with those from St. Bartholomew's/Great Ormond Street (clinical staging, involved/regional-field radiation therapy). Overall survival from each institution was 91% at 10 years although more stage I patients at Barts/GOS relapse (23a). However, adverse sequelae of therapy include, most prominently, second malignancies and infertility. Consequently, other chemotherapeutic agents are under active investigation, both in the presence and absence of concomitant radiotherapy. Recommended approaches for therapy in children appear in Table 18-6. The data in Tables 18-7 and 18-8 present the results of trials in limited and advanced stage Hodgkin's disease, respectively, in which low-dose radiation therapy (15 to 25 Gy) is combined with chemotherapy, or high-dose (40 to 44 Gy) radiotherapy or chemotherapy alone is used.

Complications

1. Infection: Acute myelosuppression resulting from the chemotherapy incurs the risk for infection. The risk for serious bacterial infection at times distant from completion of therapy is well known. However, data from Stanford are persuasive in showing that the intensity of treatment, whether or not splenectomy has been performed, is most closely related to the occurrence of such infections (110). The use of prophylactic antibiotics appears to decrease this risk. Moreover, vaccines against pneumococci, Haemophilus influenzae, and meningococci may further decrease the frequency of serious infections.
2. The musculoskeletal morbidities of high-dose radiotherapy in young children include intraclavicular narrowing, shortened sitting height, decreased mandibular growth, and underdeveloped musculature.
3. Other long-term complications of therapy include injury to the lung, heart, and thyroid, as stated in the section on adults.

NON-HODGKIN'S LYMPHOMA

EPIDEMIOLOGY AND ETIOLOGY

Epidemiology (1)

1. Each year, approximately 31,700 patients in the United States are diagnosed as having non-Hodgkin's lymphoma (NHL), and about 16,500 patients die of this disease.
2. Peak incidence occurs after age 50 years, much later than that for Hodgkin's disease.
3. The incidence is slightly higher in males (1.4:1).

Table 18-6. Guidelines for Treatment Selection in Pediatric Hodgkin's Disease

Stage	Clinical Presentation	Recommendations
IA, IIA	Fully grown: Laparotomy negative, mediastinal mass not massive or juxtapericardial	Standard dose RT (STNI generally)
	Still growing: or Massive mediastinal mass or juxtapericardial	Low-dose RT (IF) + chemotherapy
IB, IIB	Night sweating without or with either fevers or weight loss, laparotomy negative	As for IA, IIA
	Fevers and weight loss	Low-dose RT (IF) + chemotherapy

IIIA1, IIIA1S+ minimal	Fully grown:
	  Mediastinal mass not massive or juxtapericardial
		Standard RT (STNI or TNI) or RT + chemotherapy
		  Hepatic RT if spleen involved

	Still growing: or Massive mediastinal or juxtapericardial	Low-dose RT (IF) + chemotherapy
IIIA1S+ extensive, IIIA2, IIIB, IVA, IVB		Chemotherapy ± low-dose RT(IF) (RT particularly recommended for large bulk disease)
Recurrent		Chemotherapy if none previously, otherwise consider BMT

Radiation therapy: Full-dose = 35-44 Gy, Low-dose = ≤ 25 Gy
RT = radiation therapy; STNI = subtotal nodal irradiation; IF = involved field; TNI = total nodal irradiation; BMT = bone marrow transplant.
Chemotherapy: 6 MOPP, 6 ABVD, 6-8 MOPP/ABVD, 6 OPPA/COP(P) or other experimental. Lesser amounts for early-stage disease experimental.

Table 18-7. Treatment Results in Children with Early-stage Hodgkin's Disease

Group/Institution	No. Patients		Stage and Treatment		% Survival		Follow-up interval	Reference
					Overall	Relapse-free		
Radiotherapy alone (full dose IF or EF)								
Children's Hospital of Philadelphia	31	PS	IA, IIA		83	64	10 yr	113c*
Joint Center/ Harvard	50	PS	I, IIA		98	82	5 yr	113d
St Bartholomew's/ Great Ormond Street	28	CS*	I, II		95.5	79	10 yr	111b*
Stanford University	48	PS **	I, II		86	82	10 yr	111b*
Intergroup Hodgkin's Study	39	PS	I, II	IF	95	41	5 yr	111f
	58			EF	96	67	5 yr	111f
	15	CS	I	IF†	93	82	10 yr	113b*
Full-dose RT + 3 or 6 courses of chemo								
Hospital of Saint-Louis	52	CS	I, II		94	88	10 yr	109a
Intergroup Hodgkin's Study	97	PS	I, II		90	95	5 yr	111f
St Bartholomew's Great Ormond Street	39	CS *	I, II		86	84	10 yr	111b*
Low-dose RT + 6 courses of chemo								
Stanford University	27	PS	I, II		100	96	10 yr	111a
Princess Margaret Hospital	27	CS	II, III		92	88	5 yr	113b
Children's Hospital of Philadelphia	30	CS	I, II		90	68	10 yr	113c*
Standord University	52	PS **	I, II		97	98	10 yr	111b*
Intergroup Hodgkin's Study	22	CS	II		93	89	10 yr	113b*
Chemotherapy alone								
Uganda	7	CS	I-II		100	100	5 yr	113e
South Africa	11	CS	I-II		91	100	5 yr	113a

*Some patients pathologically staged
** Some patients clinically staged
† Some received chemotherapy
CS = clinical stage; PS = pathologic stage; Full-dose radiotherapy = minimum dose to any nodal field ≥ 30 Gy; Low-dose radiotherapy = maximum dose to any nodal field ≤ 25.5 Gy; PA = para-aortic + spleen (pedicle); TNI = total nodal irradiation; IF = involved field; EF = extended field.

Etiology

1. A viral etiology for at least some lymphomas has been suggested by epidemiologic, cell culture, and immunologic investigations. These studies have implicated a herpes-like virus without proving a causal relationship. More recently, an association of NHL with certain lymphotrophic viral infections (human T-cell lymphocytic virus-I and human immunodeficiency virus) has been identified (138). This is highly compatible with a viral etiology or an induced immunologic defect permitting a malignant clone to proliferate (123,152,193).

An increased incidence of NHL in organ transplant patients with congenital immune deficiency syndromes also supports the above hypothesis (142,160,181).

2. Demonstration of the translocation of the c-myc oncogene into the immunoglobulin gene locus in Burkitt's lymphoma has provided a major breakthrough in the study of malignant transformation of lymphoid cells (156,187). (See Chapter 3, "Pathology of Cancer.")

3. An increased risk of NHL in persons exposed to agricultural herbicides, particularly of the phenoxyacetic acid group, has been reported (147).

Table 18-8. Treatment Results in Children with Advanced-stage Hodgkin's Disease

Group/Institution	No. Patients	Stage	Chemotherapy	Radiotherapy	% Survival Overall	Relapse-free	Follow-up interval	Reference
Stanford University	28	III/IV	6 MOPP	15-25 Gy IF	78	84	7.5 yr	111a
German (DAL)	50	IIIB/IV	2 OPPA/ 4 COP(P)	25-35 Gy IF	72	90	5 yr	114b
French (SFOP)	69	CS I-IIB, III, IV	3 MOPP/ 3 ABVD	20 Gy IF+PA	95	93	30 mo	111b**
Children's Hospital of Philadelphia	29	III/IV	6 COPP,ABVD, MOPP/ABVD	25-40 Gy EF	88	63	10 yr	113c*
Children's Cancer Study Group	64	III/IV	6 ABVD	21 Gy IF (region)	87	87 (IV = 54)	3 yr	111e
Pediatric Oncol. Group	62	IIB-IV	4 MOPP/ 4 ABVD	21 Gy TNI	91	77	3 yr	116a
Joint Center/ Harvard	15	III	6 MOPP	≥ 30 Gy	100	87	5 yr	113d
Intergroup Hodgkin's Study	20	CS III-IV	6 MOPP	20-30 Gy EF	60	65	10 yr	113b*
Joint Center/ Harvard	6	IV	6 MOPP	-	66	66	5 yr	113d
Australia/New Zealand	8	III/IV	6-12 MOPP	-	92	80	5 yr	111d

CS = clinical stage; IF = involved field; EF = extended field; PA = para-aortic + spleen (pedicle); TNI = total nodal irradiation.

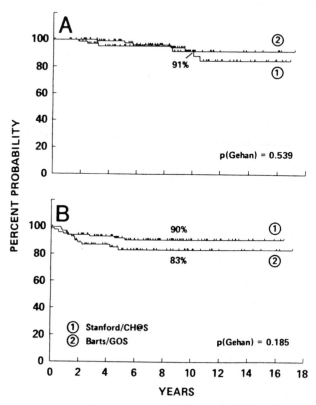

Fig. 18-4. Results: Actuarial survival and freedom from relapse. From Donaldson *et al.* (111b*), with permission.

Biology (Figs. 18-5 and 18-6) (130a,140b,165)

Advances in molecular genetics have provided new insights into the biology of the lymphoid malignancies. Integral components of these advances include:

1. Assays for markers of lymphoproliferative diseases based on the analysis of antigen receptor gene rearrangements.
2. Recognition of specific oncogenes relevant to the pathogenesis of various lymphoid malignancies (1).

NHLs are thought to arise from lymphocyte precursors in the bone marrow and thymus rather than immunocompetent lymphoid cells capable of participating in an immune response (123). These cells undergo specific and irreversible rearrangements of their immunoglobulin genes (B cells) or T-cell receptor genes (T cells) as they are committed to a specific lineage (152). These are clone-specific events that can be used to identify clonality, lineage, and degree of differentiation for the individual types. Thus, probes for the T-cell receptor and immunoglobulin subunits are used to assign each malignancy to a T- or B-cell group, though occasionally even these techniques prove to reveal less than straightforward information about the origin of specific lymphomas. Nevertheless, certain generalizations can be made.

1. B-cell types: Small, noncleaved lymphomas, which include Burkitt's and non-Burkitt's subtypes, and most large cell lymphomas are of B-cell phenotype. Surface immunoglobulins (usually of the IgM class) and B-cell

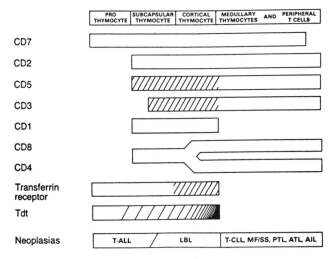

Fig. 18-5. Schematic diagram demonstrating molecular, genetic, and immunophenotypic correlates of normal B-cell differentiation.

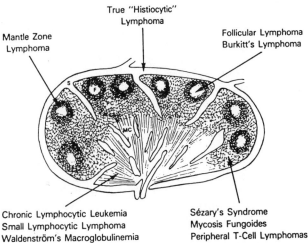

Fig. 18-6. Schematic diagram of normal lymph node illustrating anatomical and functional compartments of the immune system.

specific antigens (usually detected by the monoclonal antibodies B4 [CD19] and B1 [CD20] are expressed by these cells (138). Other types of B-cell lineage include the small lymphocytic well-differentiated lymphomas, the intermediate or small cleaved cell (mantle zone) lymphocytic lymphomas, and the follicular lymphomas.

   a. Approximately 10% of lymphoblastic lymphomas are considered to be of B-cell origin. They can more appropriately be considered to derive from stem cells that have an immature phenotype but are committed to B-cell differentiation pathways.

   b. The Burkitt's subtypes, which include equatorial African and North American forms, have differences in the precise locations of the chromosomal breakpoints associated with the specific translocations seen in these tumors (142,148a).

2. T-cell types: Lymphoblastic lymphomas are composed of immature lymphoid cells, which have the phenotype of early or common cortical thymocytes. They almost invariably have the enzyme terminal deoxynucleotidyl transferase (124a,193). Most lymphoblastic lymphomas (and some large cell lymphomas) also express T-cell markers (171a). All the other T-cell lymphomas apparently derive from cells with mature or postthymic phenotypes. Those that arise from mature cells bear the CD4 antigen and include adult T-cell leukemia/lymphoma, mycosis fungoides, Sezary's syndrome, angiocentric immunoproliferative lesions, and most of the peripheral T-cell lymphomas (152).

   a. The distinction between lymphoblastic lymphomas and leukemia is generally determined by the percentage of blast cells demonstrated in the bone marrow, with 25% the most commonly used cutoff point. The biologic correlate to this distinction is not unequivocally known, but appears to involve the degree of differentiation of the neoplastic cell. Malignancies with an immature thymocyte phentoype most frequently present as leukemia, whereas those with a more mature phenotype characteristically present with less marrow involvement but accumulations of cells in other areas (121,158).

3. The growth fractions of the lymphomas vary according to the subtype, and for some of the aggressive varieties may approach 100%. For these lymphomas the doubling times can be extremely short, from 12 hours to a few days (156). The B-cell tumors have the highest growth fractions, with up to 27% of the cells in S-phase (187).

4. Specific cytogenetic findings distinguish several of the different subtypes of NHL. Characteristic differences are found not only among different phenotypes, but even within an apparently homogeneous phenotype. Since particular genetic abnormalities may correlate with prognosis, such distinctions are important (181).

   a. Most follicular lymphomas carry the t(14;18) chromosomal translocation (200).

   b. Approximately one third of the diffuse large cell lymphomas also carry this translocation, suggesting a pathologic relationship with the follicular lymphoma (147). However, characteristic karyotypic abnormalities are not found for most of the large cell lymphomas, perhaps due to the phenotypically heterogeneous types in this category or because the genetic abnormalities do not involve karyotypic changes.

   c. In Burkitt's lymphoma the proto-oncogene c-myc is translocated from chromosome 8 to the heavy chain locus of chromosome 14 (180a,200a). The product of the c-myc oncogene is necessary for cellular proliferation and its abnormal expression may maintain the cell in an inappropriately proliferative state (120a,151).

DETECTION AND DIAGNOSIS

Clinical Detection

Symptoms and signs of NHL are similar to those in Hodgkin's disease except for the following generalizations.

1. Unlike Hodgkin's disease, noncontiguous spread is the rule in NHL, and the mediastinum is often spared. Unsuspected bone marrow involvement occurs much more frequently. Early involvement of oropharyngeal lymphoid tissue, skin, the GI tract, and bone is frequent (151).

2. In children, initial intra-abdominal manifestations are common, unlike Hodgkin's disease (168). (See Chapter 19, "Pediatric Tumors".)
3. Leukemic transformation with a high peripheral lymphocyte count occurs in about 13% of patients with lymphocytic lymphoma (151,184).
4. Autoimmune anemia with positive antiglobulin (Coombs) tests occurs in a significant minority of NHL patients (151).

Diagnostic Procedures

1. Surgical biopsy establishes the diagnosis.
   a. Although histology continues to be the primary decision-making criteria, immunophenotyping, and enzymatic and cytogenetic studies should supplement morphologic analysis.
   b. The most suspicious node should be selected for excisional biopsy. Frozen sections and needle biopsies are discouraged.
   c. Aspiration of bone marrow or effusions may provide the diagnosis and obviate the need for a lymph node biopsy.
2. The remainder of the required and suggested diagnostic procedures are listed under Classification: Staging Work-up and are similiar to Table 18-1 for Hodgkin's disease.

CLASSIFICATION

Histopathology

NHLs are a diverse group of diseases that differ with regard to histology, natural history, and response to therapy. This heterogeneity has led to several histopathologic classifications, which in turn have contributed to difficulty in interpreting study results (164,182,183,185).

In 1982, the National Cancer Institute appointed a panel of lymphoma pathologists to study the clinical applicability of six major histopathologic classification systems. The panel indicated that all six systems correlated well with clinical outcome and that none was superior to the others. A working formulation was introduced and recommended for the reporting of results (173). In 1985, this panel updated their report (172). In this classification, as in the Modified Rappaport System (185), architecture of the gland (follicular versus diffuse) and predominant cell type (small or large lymphocyte) are the two variables that best determine prognosis (Fig. 18-6). A follicular architecture and a small-sized lymphocyte characterize low-grade NHL and predict for an indolent course, while diffuse and large cell lymphomas are intermediate or high grade and are characterized by a more aggressive course (Table 18-9) (104).

As stated in the biology section, immunologic studies (immunofluorescence, erythrocyte rosettes, monoclonal antibodies, flow cytometry, immunoglobulin, and T-cell gene rearrangement) have begun to clarify these previously poorly understood lymphoproliferative disorders (118,189,199,200a, 200b). These studies have revealed that all NHLs of follicular type are of B-cell origin; the so-called histiocytic lymphoma is almost always a lymphocytic malignancy, usually of B-cell type, but occasionally of T-cell origin; mixed lymphomas are wholly of lymphocytic origin; Burkitt's lymphomas demonstrate a surface marker pattern; and immunoglobulin gene rearrangement is characteristic of B-cell origin (118,143,189).

Although the technology for determining the T-cell origin of lymphomas is less sophisticated, mycosis fungoides and Sezary syndrome are demonstrated to be of T-lymphocyte origin. Angioimmunoblastic lymphadenopathy, lymphomatoid papulosis, lymphomas arising in patients with celiac disease and sprue are also of T-cell origin (142a,199,200a). Lymphoblastic lymphomas are almost always of T-cell origin, while human T-cell leukemia/lymphoma virus-I associated lymphomas are exclusively T cell.

The distinction between malignant lymphoma and benign lymphadenopathy can sometimes be difficult. Monoclonality on immunophenotyping and gene rearrangement in such patients are the criteria used to diagnose a neoplastic process.

Anatomic Staging

Although the staging system is the same as that used for Hodgkin's disease, a report with long-term follow-up of 1,153 patients has shown that the stage of the disease is less predictive of outcome compared with Hodgkin's disease (190). Conversely, the histologic subtype of the NHL is the most important prognostic determinant (190), a finding not present in Hodgkin's disease.

Staging Work-up

Because of the noncontiguous spread of NHL, the majority of patients will manifest stage III or IV disease (119,190).

1. *Recommended procedures*: In addition to lymph node biopsy, the following procedures are recommended.
   a. Complete physical examination (including pelvic examination for women).
   b. Complete blood cell counts, including differential white blood cell and reticulocyte counts.
   c. Direct Coombs (antiglobulin) test. Autoimmune hemolytic anemia is significantly more frequent in NHL than in Hodgkin's disease.
   d. Blood chemistry analysis (including alkaline phosphatase, albumin, globulin, immunoglobulin, uric acid, creatinine).
   e. Bone marrow biopsy: The frequent presence of unsuspected bone marrow involvement in NHL has important implications for treatment planning (apparent stage I becomes stage IV). Therefore, bone marrow biopsy should be performed in virtually every case. Lymphocytic lymphomas have a high frequency (up to 50%) of bone marrow involvement, while large cell lymphomas have a much lower frequency.
   f. Chest x-ray (posteroanterior and lateral).
   g. CT is useful in detecting upper retroperitoneal and mesenteric nodes and liver involvement. This procedure has the advantage of being a noninvasive procedure and is applicable to all age groups. It is displacing the need for lymphangiography, since it can be useful for demonstrating many sites of lymphoid involvement, that is, mesentery, high abdominal lymph nodes, liver, spleen, and unusual deposits in retroperitoneal sites.
2. Procedures appropiate under selected circumstances:
   a. Additional radiographic procedures:
      1. Whole-chest tomography or MRI if any abnormality is noted or suspected on routine chest x-ray. In some institutions these studies are routinely obtained. MRI may prove useful as a follow-up study; a decrease in signal intensity is

Table 18-9. Working Formulation of Non-Hodgkin's Lymphoma for Clinical Use: Recommendations of an Expert International Panel: Comparisons to the Rappaport Scheme

Working Formulation	Rappaport Terminology
LOW GRADE	
Malignant lymphoma small lymphocytic	Diffuse well-differentiated lymphocytic
• consistent with chronic lymphocytic leukemia	
• plasmacytoid	
Malignant lymphoma, follicular,predominantly small cleaved cell	Nodular poorly differentiated lymphocytic
• diffuse areas	
• sclerosis	
Malignant lymphoma, follicular,mixed, small cleaved and large cell	Nodular mixed lymphocytic histiocytic
• diffuse areas	
• sclerosis	
INTERMEDIATE GRADE	
Malignant lymphoma, follicular predominantly large cell	Nodular histiocytic
• diffuse areas	
• sclerosis	
Malignant lymphoma, diffuse small cleaved cell	Diffuse poorly differentiated lymphocytic
Malignant lymphoma, diffuse mixed, small and large cell	Diffuse mixed lymphocytic-histiocytic
• sclerosis	
• epithelioid cell component	
Malignant lymphoma, diffuse large cell, cleaved cell, non-cleaved cell	Diffuse histiocytic
• sclerosis	
HIGH GRADE	
Malignant lymphoma large cell, immunoblastic	Diffuse histiocytic
• plasmacytoid	
• clear cell	
• polymorphous	
• epithelioid cell component	
Malignant lymphoma lymphoblastic	Diffuse lymphoblastic
• convoluted cell	
• non-convoluted cell	
Malignant lymphoma small noncleaved cell	Diffuse undifferentiated
• Burkitt's	
• follicular areas	

From Tucker et al. (104). Reprinted with permission from The New England Journal of Medicine, *318:76-81; 1988.*

likely to represent a CR, whereas a persistent increased signal may represent persistent disease or a CR (137a).

2. Bilateral lower-extremity lymphogram continues to be the optimal procedure for the evaluation of para-aortic lymph nodes, performed in institutions adept at this procedure.

3. Head or spinal CT or MRI for neurologic signs or symptoms.

4. Bone scan and plain bone radiographs for patients with symptomatic areas.

5. Gallium whole body scans and liver-spleen scans are at times appropriate.

b. Exploratory laparotomy and splenectomy should be considered if therapeutic decisions depend on the identitification of infradiaphragmatic involvement, such as for selected patients with stage I large cell lymphoma.

PRINCIPLES OF TREATMENT

Multidisciplinary Treatment Planning (Table 18-10) (118a,131b)

Because of the variety of potential staging and treatment options available to patients with NHL, an initial multidisciplinary planning conference is necessary for each patient as soon as the histologic diagnosis is made. The issues to be addressed include the need for pathologic staging and the optimal therapeutic strategy—primary or adjuvant chemotherapy or radiotherapy—and the sequence of multimodal therapy.

Surgery

1. The primary role of surgery is in establishing diagnosis.
2. Resection of extranodal GI primaries may rarely be curative, although additional treatment for microresidual or macroresidual disease is generally indicated.
3. Splenectomy may be rarely beneficial for hypersplenism.
4. Laparotomy may be rarely considered in carefully selected patients, especially in younger patients with apparently localized NHL, for whom radiation therapy is to encompass all disease with cure as the goal (126).

Radiation Therapy

The role of radiation therapy in the management of NHL has progressively decreased as chemotherapeutic regimens have become more effective. Yet it remains appropriate as either primary or adjuvant treatment in selected patients (144). Moreover, its role in these situations continues to be defined as chemotherapeutic approaches change. Once the overall treatment strategy has been determined, details of the administration of radiation therapy can be devised.

General Considerations

Important considerations in the administration of radiation therapy include timing and the volume, dose, and fraction size, each of which depends on whether chemotherapy is being used and the specific agents employed. The radiation therapy portals are designed with knowledge of the common routes of lymphatic spread and the chemotherapy and radiotherapy tolerances of the normal tissues in these regions. The dose and fraction size depend on the assessment of what is necessary for local disease control in light of the potential normal tissue morbidities.

Radiation therapy fields are customarily described according to the lymphoid regions being treated (127,173). Involved field irradiation denotes treatment limited to the involved nodal region(s), according to the Ann Arbor Staging System (See Table 18-3 and Fig. 18-3 in Hodgkin's section). Extended field irradiation involves treatment of both the involved lymphoid region(s) and those that are contiguous and presumed to be at a high risk for occult involvement. TNI entails the sequential treatment to all major lymphoid regions, usually in two or three segments. Total body irradiation (TBI) is treatment of the entire body in each treatment session. At times, the fields must be designed to treat specific extranodal sites or the whole abdomen when, for example, mesenteric nodes are involved with NHL. Partial transmission lead or cerrobend blocks are appropriate in situations where lower doses of irradiation are administered to organs concomitant with the treatment of nodal regions.

The dose of radiation necessary to achieve local control depends on the histologic type of the NHL and whether chemotherapy is also used. The low-grade and lymphocytic lymphomas may be locally controlled with doses of 30 to 40 Gy in 1.5 to 2 Gy fractions. Lymphomas with a large cell component require doses of 40 to 50 Gy (125). When TBI is used without BMT, daily doses of 0.10 to 0.15 Gy (weekly doses of 0.30 Gy) are administered to a total of only 1.2 to 1.5 Gy (146).

The complications of radiotherapy for NHL are similar to those that occur in the treatment of Hodgkin's disease (see section on radiotherapy in Hodgkin's disease section).

1. *Favorable histology or low-grade NHL* (nodular lymphocytic well-differentiated, nodular poorly-differentiated lymphocytic, nodular mixed, diffuse lymphocytic well-differentiated) (Table 18-9).

   a. *Stage I-II disease*: Following extensive staging, only 10% to 30% of patients with low-grade lymphoma will have localized disease, and most of these patients have follicular (nodular) subtypes. Radiation therapy is frequently effective for these patients, providing a 10-year DFS of 50% to 55% and survival of 60% to 65% (164,179,195). Patients with nonbulky disease (<10 cm) limited to two contiguous sites or less have a better prognosis, particularly if young (aged < 45 years) (170,179). There is no convincing evidence that extended radiation fields are superior to involved fields, and in particular, retrospective series show no advantage for the former in terms of overall survival (179). A small randomized trial performed at Stanford University showed no significant difference in either DFS or overall survival for TNI as compared with involved field irradiation (179). Yet some patients treated with involved field irradiation do relapse in contiguous unirradiated sites, and, thus, it seems appropriate to include the immediately adjacent clinically uninvolved nodal group(s). Adjuvant chemotherapy is of modest or no additional benefit for patients with early-stage low-grade lymphoma (175).

   b. *Stage III-IV low-grade lymphoma*: Patients with advanced-stage low-grade lymphomas are heterogeneous in their disease characteristics, and several possible treatment strategies can be considered (182a). Beyond this, controversy exists as to the optimal management for several of the subgroups. For patients with stage III disease and otherwise favorable characteristics (limited disease burden with fewer than five sites of nonbulky disease and no B symptoms), either TNI, combined modality therapy (e.g., BLEO-CHOP and involved field irradiation), or chemotherapy alone can afford durable responses (133,139,162,167,180). For other patients with stage III or IV disease, the prognosis is poorer, with DFS only 20% to 30% at 10 years despite initial CR rates of 60% to 80% (133,139,150,162). Overall survival is still 50% to 60% at 10 years, although those patients who relapse once can be expected to continue to relapse. As discussed in the section on chemotherapy, the spectrum of treatment approaches ranges from initial observation without therapy for asymptomatic patients, to aggressive primary chemotherapy programs. Primary radiotherapy pro-

Table 18-10. Guidelines For Treatment Selection in Non-Hodgkin's Lymphoma

Stage/Histology	Characteristics	Treatment
Favorable, low grade		
I	Nonbulky (<10 cm), age < 45 yr	RT (IF)
	All others	RT (IF) and consider adjuvant MAC
II	Two contiguous sites, nonbulky, young	RT (IF or EF) and consider adjuvant MAC
	All others	MAC and consider adjuvant RT (IF) if contiguous sites of disease
III	Limited disease burden (<5 sites of nonbulky disease), no B symptoms	MAC alone, combined MAC and RT (IF), or RT alone (TNI)
	All others (extensive disease)	Observation, no cytotoxic therapy for asymptomatic patients, or MAC alone
IV	Any	As for stage III, extensive disease burden
Unfavorable, intermediate & high grade		
I	Small disease burden (<2.5 cm), no B symptoms, age <60 yr	RT (IF/EF), consider adjuvant MAC
	All other	MAC and RT (IF)
	Any	MAC, consider adjuvant RT (IF), if contiguous sites of disease or bulk disease
II		MAC alone
III, IV	Any	
Recurrent	Any	Consider bone marrow transplantation after complete response with MAC. For bulk disease, consider boost RT.
Extranodal, IE or IIE		
Waldeyer's ring	Any	Regional RT (including cervical nodes), consider MAC for stage II, unfavorable histology
Other head & neck	Favorable histology	RT alone
	Unfavorable histology	Combined MAC and RT
	Parameningeal	include CNS therapy (intrathecal MAC + cranial RT)
Gastrointestinal	Complete resection, no nodes	Adjuvant RT or MAC
	Regional nodes involved	MAC; consider adjuvant RT
	Residual or unresected disease	Combined MAC and RT
Bone	Peripheral bones	RT. Consider adjuvant MAC
	Central bone	Combined MAC and RT
Thyroid	Localized to thyroid and adjacent nodes	RT. Consider adjuvant MAC
	Muscle invasion	Combined RT and MAC
Skin	Small disease extent (<2.5 cm) and no nodal involvement	RT. Strongly consider adjuvant MAC
	Extensive disease	MAC
Central nervous system	Any	RT. Consider MAC

RT = radiotherapy; IF = involved field; TNI = total nodal irradiation; EF = extended field; RCT = recommended chemotherapy; MAC = multiagent chemotherapy.
PDQ: RCT - PRO-MACE-MOPP, mBACOD, MACOP-B, PRO-MACE-CytaBOM CHOP, BACOP, COMLA, C(M)OPP
Modified from Armitage and Cheson (118a) and Devita et al. (131b).

grams have also been used and include TNI or, for stage IV patients, low-dose TBI as described previously (131,146). Although favorable short-term results are seen with TBI (90% CR for 2 to 3 years), hematologic toxicity can be profound and long-standing. For patients managed conservatively with initial observation only, local irradiation to sites of adenopathy that become problematic is appropriate.

Some patients who demonstrate rapid disease progression can be shown to have a histologic conversion of their low-grade lymphoma to one that is intermediate or high grade (117,148). The initial treatment does not seem to affect the likelihood of this occurrence. Subsequent response to therapy is probably similar to that for patients who initially present with the more aggressive histology, although patients who have previously received aggressive chemotherapy for their low-grade lymphoma can be expected to fare poorly (117,148).

2. *Unfavorable histology (intermediate- and high-grade) NHL* nodular histiocytic, diffuse histiocytic, diffuse lymphocytic poorly-differentiated, diffuse mixed, and including diffuse and large cell subtypes according to the working formulation (see Table 18-10)].

   a. *Stage I-II unfavorable NHL*: Following extensive staging, including laparotomy, 30% to 40% of patients will have stage I-II disease (126). About 25% of these patients will have an apparently extranodal origin for their disease, most commonly GI, Waldeyer's ring, thyroid, skin, bone, orbit, breast, or testis (136). The efficacy of radiotherapy alone for patients with early-stage large cell lymphoma appears to depend on selected prognostic factors, most importantly disease extent. Combined results from different series show a DFS of about 75% at 10 years for stage I patients, but only a 35% DFS at this interval for stage II patients (173,197). Younger patient age (< 60 years), the absence of B symptoms, limited disease extent (one involved region), and small disease bulk (less than 2.5 cm) identifies a particularly favorable group of patients in whom involved field or extended field irradiation is effective (194).

   The effectiveness of chemotherapy for stage II patients has been well demonstrated (see section below on chemotherapy). Most reports with large patient numbers have involved the use of adjuvant radiotherapy to sites of demonstrable disease, generally to doses of 30 to 36 Gy. In this setting, radiotherapy has generally followed the first half or completion of chemotherapy (124,130,176,183).

   b. *Stage III-IV unfavorable NHL*: Patients with advanced-stage disease are treated with chemotherapy (see section below on chemotherapy). Radiotherapy is generally inappropriate because of the systemic nature of the disease and the toxicity that would result from its administration to the several disease sites involved. Nevertheless, radiation therapy is a consideration for limited sites of residual disease after MAC. Radiotherapy is otherwise reserved for the treatment of emergencies (e.g., superior vena cava obstruction or spinal cord compression) or for palliation.

3. *Extranodal NHL*: Patients with extranodal NHL without associated nodal involvement, or with only regional involvement (stage IE or IIE) are generally treated similarly to other patients with early-stage NHL (178). However, selected extranodal sites require some individualization of therapy.

   a. *Waldeyer's ring*: When the lymphoid tissue of Waldeyer's ring is involved (stage IE), regional irradiation that includes the nasopharynx, tonsils, base of tongue, and cervical nodes down to the clavicles is delivered (145,198). A long-term survival rate of 50% to 70% can be expected. Adjuvant chemo-

therapy may be delivered, particularly for patients with stage II disease and unfavorable histology.

   b. *Other head and neck sites*: Patients with early-stage favorable histology NHL involving head and neck sites can be treated effectively with radiotherapy alone. Patients with unfavorable-histology NHL involving sinuses, base of tongue, and other sites are prone to relapse systemically unless adjuvant chemotherapy is also administered. Moreover, patients with parameningeal disease require an evaluation for disease involving the central nervous system (CNS) and should receive CNS therapy even if no direct involvement can be demonstrated (149).

   c. *GI tract*: This region is the most frequent site of extranodal NHL and most commonly involves the stomach (178). A complete resection of gastric lymphoma can cure only about one third of patients. Either adjuvant chemotherapy or radiotherapy improves the cure rate in this setting. If regional nodes are involved but resected, then the likelihood of systemic relapse is so high that chemotherapy is indicated. In the setting of known postsurgical residual disease, both modalities should be administered (140,169). For patients diagnosed with gastric lymphoma prior to gastrectomy, combined chemotherapy and radiotherapy alone have been reported to provide results similar to that involving gastrectomy while avoiding the morbidity of that procedure (180). Other reports, however, suggest that surgical resection and adjuvant chemotherapy are superior in terms of both DFS and overall survival (159,188).

   d. *Bone*: Resection of the involved bone does not improve survival compared with irradiation, which effectively provides local control for over 90% of patients (177). Patients with involvement of central bones, such as vertebral bodies, have a high likelihood of systemic relapse and should receive chemotherapy.

   e. *Thyroid*: Patients with disease localized to the thyroid or with involvement of immediately adjacent nodes are effectively treated with radiotherapy alone, which should include the cervical and upper mediastinal nodes as well as residual thyroid tissue. Although the importance and extent of the surgical procedure performed is not clearly known, it does identify those patients with more extensive involvement (e.g., tumor invading local muscle) who should receive adjuvant chemotherapy as well as irradiation (122,196).

   f. *Skin*: Patients who present with a single small (< 2.5 cm) lesion and no nodal involvement are effectively locally controlled with radiotherapy alone. Since one fourth of these patients will relapse systemically, adjuvant chemotherapy should be considered (132). Patients with more extensive involvement require chemotherapy.

   g. *CNS*: Patients who present with primary CNS lymphoma have a poor prognosis; their likelihood of local recurrence is high despite aggressive local radiotherapy, and some patients will systemically relapse. The frequency of cerebrospinal fluid involvement is low, and for patients with negative cerebrospinal fluid cytology, spinal axis irradiation does not appear to warrant its toxicity. Moreover, the increased use of adjuvant chemotherapy for patients with primary CNS lymphoma contraindicates the use of routine spinal axis irradiation because of associated bone marrow suppression (137,174).

Chemotherapy (Table 18-11) (118a,131b)

Chemotherapy is the mainstay of treatment for the majority of patients with NHL because only a minority of patients manifest truly localized disease. Patients with small lymphocytic lymphomas usually have disseminated or stage IV disease (81% in one large series) (190) mostly due to bone marrow involvement. The frequency of marrow involvement is lower in follicular lymphomas, but disseminated nodal disease is still common. Only 18% to 27% have disease confined to one side of the diaphragm (190). For unfavorable, more aggressive histology lymphomas like diffuse mixed, diffuse large cell, and immunoblastic subtypes, localized disease is more common and bone marrow involvement is less frequent. Yet the prognosis with radiation therapy alone is suboptimal except for selected stage I patients, and, therefore, chemotherapy alone or a combination of systemic chemotherapy and involved field irradiation is at present the preferred treatment (171,181a,186).

In addition to knowledge of the natural history as based on histology, age, and general health of the patient, the number of disease sites, tumor bulk, serum lactate dehydrogenase, and cytogenetic abnormalities are important prognostic determinants (120,118a,158).

1. *Low-grade or indolent stage III and IV* (See Table 18-9) (see section on radiation therapy for treatment of stage I-II disease): Treatment of patients with indolent NHL is controversial. Investigators at Stanford University

(152,186) believe that a significant percentage of these patients can be managed without therapy for prolonged periods, and some patients may even demonstrate spontaneous regression (155). Even when no immediate cytotoxic treatment is selected, these patients must be followed closely, because the majority will become symptomatic and require chemotherapy or radiotherapy.

Combination chemotherapy is advocated by others on the assumption that a CR may lead to an improved DFS and possible cure (133,139,162). CRs with various combinations have ranged from 50% to 79% (133,139,150,162), with higher CR rates with more intensive regimens. However, because of the indolent nature of these tumors, a long follow-up is necessary to document cure. Longo (162) reported a durable 57% CR with C-MOPP (Table 18-11). However, these results have not been confirmed in a large cooperative group trial (139). The treatment regimens used most frequently in low-grade lymphomas are listed in Table 18-11.

Recently, patients with low-grade lymphomas have been shown to have a 54% response rate to alpha-interferon, with an 8-month median duration of response (135). The mechanism of antitumor effect is presumably different from that resulting from conventional chemotherapy. (See Chapter 8, "Basic Concepts of Cancer Chemotherapy and Principles of Medical Oncology.") This clinical efficacy also has been documented in heavily pretreated patients. Virtually all patients experienced some degree of acute toxicity consisting of fever, malaise, muscular aches, fatigue, and anorexia, and a lowering of blood cell counts, and abnormalities of liver function are frequent. Combinations of chemotherapy and interferon are under investigation.

Table 18-11. Prospect for Long-Term Survival from More Recent Treatment Programs for Diffuse Aggressive Lymphoma

Regimen	CR (%)	RR (%)	Potential for Long-term Survival (CR) x (1-RR) (%)
ProMace/MOPP flexitherapy	80	35	52
m-BACOD	70	25	52
COP-BLAM	73	17	61
CAP-BOP	73	30	51
COP-BLAM III	84	9	76
BACOP-B	84	21	66
ProMACE-CytaBOM	84	25	63
	CR (%)	**% DFS**	**% Survival**
CHOP	67	70 (2 yr)	50 (22 mo)
	53	50 (7 yr)	30 (13.4 yr)
m-BACOD	72	80 (5 yr)	30 (5 yr)
	71	NA	50 (68 mo)
COMLA	55	50 (1.5 + yr)	68 (5 yr)
	44	50 (9 + yr)	50 (45 mo)
MACOP-B	84	88 (4 yr)	75 (4 yr)
	84	76 (5 yr)	69 (5 yr)

CR = complete remission; RR = relapse rate; DFS = disease-free survival.

Adapted from Armitage and Cheson (118a) and DeVita et al. (131b).

2. *Aggressive NHL, intermediate grade* (see Table 18-9 for definition): The curative potential of combination chemotherapy in aggressive intermediate-grade NHL has been demonstrated in the last 10 years (118a,129,134, 153,157,162). The recently reported regimens produce a CR rate and 5-year survival of 84% and 69%, respectively (118a,153). Because these tumors have a rapid growth rate, relapses are frequent within 2 years of diagnosis unless a CR has been achieved. CRs are generally durable, and in most patients tantamount to cure. Because of the tendency to early relapse and the potential for cure, prompt and intensive therapy for unfavorable lymphomas is indicated. Several effective regimens are described below.

   a. CHOP regimen. (See Table 18-11 for regimens) (150a).

   b. MACOP-B. This newer regimen was designed to emphasize frequent intensive myelosuppressive therapy alternating with weekly nonmyelosuppressive therapy, and unlike other regimens, the duration of treatment is only 12 weeks.

   In an effort to increase CR and cure rates obtained with CHOP, several other treatment programs have been introduced, including M-BACOD, ProMace-MOPP, ProMace-Cytabom, COP-BLAM, and MACOP-B (Table 18-11). At present, CR rates obtained with these intensive regimens exceed those reported with CHOP (Table 18-11) (161,188a). However, the follow-up period compared with the experience with CHOP has been brief, and initially reported dramatic results may have to be modified with longer follow-up (118a,129a,133a).

3. *Aggressive high-grade lymphomas* (see Table 18-9 for definition): These are relatively rare, with the exception of human T-cell leukemia/lymphoma virus-I associated NHL in adult patients. The therapies (listed above) that are effective in intermediate-grade lymphomas give uniformly poor long-term survival. Bone marrow and CNS involvement is frequent in these histologic subtypes. Mediastinal predilection in young male adults is an important clinical feature of lymphoblastic lymphoma. Recently, progress has been made in the treatment of high-grade lymphomas with the use of leukemia-like chemotherapy regimens and CNS prophylaxis. Coleman (127) reported 56% relapse-free survival at 3 years in 54 patients with lymphoblastic lymphoma. Because of the high relapse rate in high-grade lymphomas, some investigators are using high-dose chemotherapy, TBI, and BMT as initial therapy (Table 18-12). Follow-up on these studies is too short to make definitive conclusions. Treatment results for T-cell leukemia/lymphoma have been disappointing because of a high incidence of opportunistic infections during aggressive chemotherapy related to the underlying defect in T-cell function and immunosuppression from chemotherapy.

The above mentioned treatment regimens are complex, and have a great potential for toxicity. With MACOP-B, 21% of patients have profound life-threatening myelosuppression, and most have some degree of mucositis and neurologic dysfunction (153). These regimens should be administered only under the supervision of a physician experienced in the use of cancer chemotherapeutic agents. (See Chapter 8, "Basic Concepts of Cancer Chemotherapy and Principles of Medical Oncology.")

RESULTS AND PROGNOSIS

Results of Chemotherapy

1. *Indolent lymphomas*: Fig. 18-7 shows survival curves for low-grade and follicular large cell lymphomas. Heterogeneity among the four curves has borderline significance (P = .07). However, the survival for patients with the follicular large cell subtype is statistically significantly worse than the survival curve for those with the follicular small cleaved type (192a). Survival by stage is shown in Fig. 18-7 (190). Survival for stage I disease at 10 years is 83%. Survival curves for stages II, III, and IV disease do not differ significantly. Although a substantial proportion of patients with advanced stage are alive at 7 years, the majority of them are not disease free (190).

2. *Aggressive lymphomas*: A CR rate of 50%, and survival at 13 years of 30% with CHOP therapy (128) has raised hopes that the newer regimens noted above will produce higher cure rates (191). Early results (see Table 18-11) with several newer intensive regimens have been impressive, but because of a short follow-up (2-years) and variability in known prognostic factors, these results need confirmation by carefully designed, directly

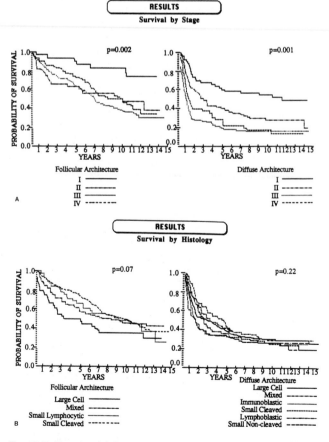

Fig. 18-7. Results: (a) Survival by stage. (b) Survival by histology. From Simon *et al.* (190), with permission.

Table 18-12. Autologous Bone Marrow Transplantation for NHL

Center	Patients (Number)	Preparative Regimen	Status of BMT	Projected Disease-Free Survival (%)
Dana Farber	100	Cy/TBI	All in CR or sensitive relapse	50
Center Leon, Bernard & others	100	Various	56% advanced relapse	19
Seattle	101	Cy/TBI, AraC/ TBI, others	73% advanced relapse	11
Hopkins	20	Cy/TBI	15% advanced relapse, others in second CR or sensitive relapse	50
Middlesex	50	Various, chemotherapy	Most advanced relapse	14
Tours/St. Antoine	46	Various	29% advanced relapse	60

Abbreviations: BMT = bone marrow transplant, Cy = cyclophosphamide, TBI = total body irradiation.
From Kurtzberg and Graham (155'), with permission.

comparative randomized studies, which are well-balanced for known prognostic factors (118a). Kwak *et al.* (155a) presents evidence for relative dose intensification of doxorubicin up to 75% of level as the single most important prognostic factor in survival following multivariate analysis of 115 patients with different regimens, i.e., 60% versus 40% 5-year survival (63a). The DFS for those receiving C-MOPP versus PROMACE/MOPP is shown in Fig. 18-7.

a. In stages I and II disease patients, Jones *et al.* (150a) report a 99% CR rate with a long-term survival of more than 80%, and a relapse rate of 20%. Longo (162) advocates PROMACE/MOPP and *IF radiation therapy* after the fourth cycle of chemotherapy, stating a 96% CR is possible, with virtually all CRs remaining with DFS at a median follow up of 4 years. A randomized study would be required to ascertain if additional toxicity is worth the gain in survival.

b. For stage II-IV (large cell lymphoma) treated by *M-BACOP* with a moderate dose of methotrexate versus standard high doses, CR rates are at the 76% level and 5-year DFS is 74% for those who achieve CR, giving a 56% overall survival. Prolonged follow-up indicates advanced-stage patients have a persistent failure rate of 7%/year for 2 to 5 years, but stage II patients have a relapse rate of 2.1%/year (188a,192).

CLINICAL INVESTIGATIONS

Currently a large number of intensive chemotherapy regimens are being tested against CHOP in an attempt to improve cure rates (129a,133a). Physicians should encourage their patients to participate in these trials so that questions concerning treatment intensity, frequency, and efficacy can be answered.

Presently, patients with unfavorable prognostic features or those who have failed front-line therapy are being treated with high-dose total body irradiation and chemotherapy followed by autologous BMT. In carefully selected series,

20% to 25% of patients have achieved long-term remission (Table 18-12) (140a,141,146a). However, older patients and previously heavily treated patients tolerate these demanding regimens poorly.

1. Depending on whether patients achieved a partial response or CR versus no response or disease progression after initial therapy, they are classified as "sensitive relapse" or "resistant relapse." Generally, there are better long-term responses in sensitive relapses as compared with resistant relapse, i.e., 36% versus 14% after autologous BMT. In a series of 100 patients in sensitive relapse treated by high-dose chemotherapy and anti—B cell monoclonal antibody, Freedman *et al.* (135a) report a 60% CR and an optimistic 50% DFS probability at 37.8 months. In another smaller series (140a), a CR rate of 60% was noted for high-dose chemotherapy + boost radiation therapy projecting to a long-term control rate of 25% with a sepsis rate of 21% proving fatal during BMT.

2. The role of TBI containing regimens in addition to high-dose chemotherapy needs to be determined in randomized studies and may favor certain subsets of lymphomas.

3. The role of bone marrow purging in autologous BMT needs to be better defined and has been shown to be of some benefit in Burkitt's tumor.

MULTIPLE MYELOMA

EPIDEMIOLOGY AND ETIOLOGY

Multiple myeloma (MM) is a neoplastic proliferation of plasma cells characterized by lytic bone lesions, anemia, and serum/urinary monoclonal globulin elevations. The resulting spectrum of clinical disease includes both localized and disseminated forms, which can behave in an indolent or aggressive manner.

Epidemiology

The incidence in 1991 is estimated to have been 12,300 new cases (6,200 males, 6,100 females). MM is the most common lymphoreticular neoplasm in nonwhites and the third most common in whites (202).

Etiology

Survivors of high-dose radiation exposure from atomic bombs in Hiroshima and Nagasaki show a 4.7 times greater incidence of MM than the general population. This did not become apparent until 20 years after exposure (205).

An increased incidence of MM in first degree relatives and in blacks strongly implicates a genetic susceptibility (205).

The demonstration of c-myc translocation to the immunoglobulin gene location has led to the speculation that this causes the increased B-cell proliferation (220).

Biology

Although MM has traditionally been considered a terminally differentiated B-cell malignancy, new evidence suggests that it is an early hematopoietic stem-cell disorder that becomes clinically evident at the mature stage of B-cell lineage (204). Data using cytogenetic and molecular biologic techniqes show DNA rearrangements similar to those seen in malignant lymphoma. The activation of oncogenes presumably occurs due to immunoglobulin gene rearrangement and resulting recombination errors. Chromosomal translocations may occasion these events (213).

DETECTION AND DIAGNOSIS

1. Bone pain accompanied by anemia often leads to the diagnosis. Pathologic fractures are common and may produce pleurisy-like or radicular pain.
2. Hypercalcemia and renal insufficiency develop in some patients. Hypercalcemia is primarily due to increased bone resorption. Myeloma cells in culture produce a number of osteoclast activating factors distinct from parathyroid hormone and vitamin D. Hypercalcemia and renal failure are more common in patients with Bence-Jones proteinuria (homogeneous free light chains of either the k or l type). Other causes of renal impairment include amyloid deposition, uric acid nephropathy, and pyelonephritis.
3. Patients with MM are at an increased risk for severe bacterial infection. Repeated pneumococcal pneumonias and life-threatening meningitis may precede other manifestations of disease. The decreased antibody response seems to result primarily from the activity of suppressor monocytes (211).
4. A tendency towards abnormal bleeding may result from interference with coagulation factors by markedly increased levels of circulating immunoglobulin or from thrombocytopenia.

Diagnostic Procedures (Table 18-1)

1. Diagnosis is based on the association of osteolytic lesions, elevated monoclonal serum or urine globulin, and marrow plasmacytosis.
2. Homogeneous (monoclonal) serum globulins can be detected by paper electrophoresis or immunoelectrophoresis. The latter will specifically identify mono-

clonal increases in IgG (54% of patients with MM), IgA (22%), IgD (less than 1%), and IgE (less than 1%). Serum ß-2-microglobulin can be used as a tumor marker (213a) . These abnormalities distinguish MM from conditions with increases in IgM.

3. Definitive diagnosis may be difficult because:
   a. Lytic bone lesions occur with other neoplasms (note that vertebral pedicles are rarely involved in myeloma, but commonly are in metastatic carcinoma).
   b. Plasmacytosis of the bone marrow may occur with drug sensitivity, collagen disease (e.g., rheumatoid arthritis), amyloidosis, cirrhosis, and occasionally with other disseminated neoplasms.
   c. Homogeneous serum globulins can occur in association with other neoplasms (e.g., of rectosigmoid, prostrate, and bile duct); although the significance of the association is unclear.

It is important to identify patients with monoclonal gammopathy of undetermined significance. These are elderly, asymptomatic patients with no bone lesions or marrow plasmacytosis and monoclonal immunoglobulin elevation of less than 2.0 g/dL. These patients remain clinically stable for many years although some may develop MM.

CLASSIFICATION (Table 18-13)

The clinical staging of multiple myeloma has evolved based on clinical correlations of outcome with tumor burden (measured with metabolic techniques) and renal function. Both direct and indirect reflections of the tumor burden include the character and number of bony lesions, hemoglobin and calcium levels, and M-component production rates. These criteria have thus been incorporated into the most widely used staging system for MM.

PRINCIPLES OF TREATMENT (Table 18-14)

Some patients with MM can have an indolent course. For this reason, evidence of progressive or symptomatic disease is usually required to initiate chemotherapy (201).

Chemotherapy (213a)

Without chemotherapy, median survival for patients with symptomatic disease is less than 1 year. With currently available treatments, survival can be extended to 3 to 4 years (222), although treatment strategies which include BMT over the potential to increase survival duration and rates.

Single Agent

1. Mephalan is the most commonly used alkylating agent. The addition of prednisone to melphalan doubles the response rate, but has little impact on survival. Melphalan is administered in 4-day high-dose intermittent courses every 4 to 6 weeks (10 mg/m²/d x 4). Prednisone is given concomitantly 40 to 100 mg/m²/d or 1 to 2 mg/kg/d x 4. It should be noted that oral melphalan is not consistently absorbed, so it should be given to the point of dose-limiting hematologic toxicity, which is defined as moderate leukopenia (white blood cell count 2,500 to 3,000/mm³). This combination produces a response in 50% to 60% of patients. Median survival of responders is about two to three times that of nonresponders (3 to 3.5 years versus 1 to 1.5 years) (219).

Table 18-13. Criteria for Staging Plasma Cell Myeloma

Stage REED	Criteria	Myeloma Cell mass (cells x 10^{12}/m^2)
I	All of the following:	
	Hemoglobin > 10 g/dL	
	• Normal serum calcium (< 12 mg/dL)	
	X-ray normal/solitary plasmacytoma	< 0.6
		(low)
	Low M-protein production rates:	
	IgG < 5.0 g/100 mL	
	IgA < 3.0 g/100 mL	
	Urine κ or λ < 4 g/24 h	
II	Fitting neither stage I nor III	0.6-1.2
		(intermediate)
III	One or more of the following:	
	• Hemoglobin < 8.5 g/dL	
	• Serum calcium > 12.0 mg/100 mL	
	• More than three lytic bone lesions	
	• High M-protein production rates	
	IgG > 7.0 g/100 mL	> 1.2
	IgA > 5.0 g/100 mL	(high)
	Urine κ or λ > 12 g/12 h	
	Subclassification	
A	Blood urea < 60 mg/100 mL, creatinine < 2.0 mg/100 mL	
B	Blood urea ≥ 60 mg/100 mL, creatinine ≥ 2.0 mg/100 mL	

Ig = immunoglobulin.

Table 18-14. Treatment Decisions for Multiple Myeloma

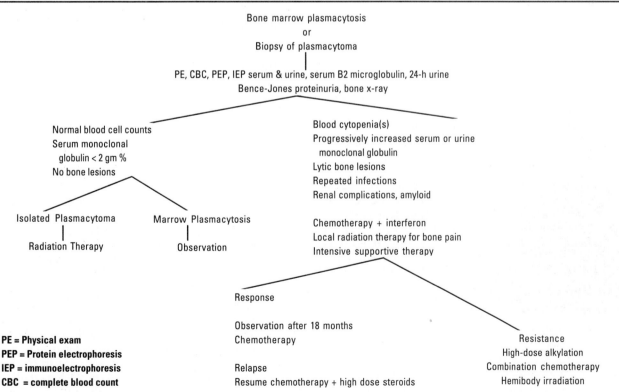

PE = Physical exam
PEP = Protein electrophoresis
IEP = immunoelectrophoresis
CBC = complete blood count

2. Cyclophosphamide may be adminstered orally or intravenously (IV) in intermittent courses. It may especially be of benefit to patients with thrombocytopenia. In such patients, 500 mg/m² IV every 2 weeks may be used initally along with prednisone.

Combination Therapy

1. Although the usefulness of combination chemotherapy in MM patients is still controversial, poor-risk patients with a high tumor load and elevated creatinine levels have been shown to have a survival advantage with a combination of IV alkylating agents.
   a. VBCMP (M2 regimen): vincristine 1.2 mg/m² IV day 1 (maximum dose 2.0 mg), carmustine 20 mg/m² IV d 1, cyclophosphamide 400 mg/m² IV day 1, melphalan 6 mg/m² orally days 1 through 4, prednisone 40 mg/m² PO days 1 through 7. This regimen (M2 protocol), developed at Memorial Sloan-Kettering Cancer Center, gave a response rate of 87% and a median survival of 50 months in a nonrandomized study (206).
2. Alternating combination chemotherapy was shown by the Southwest Oncology Group to improve remission rates and survival. A 53% remission rate with an alternating combination versus 32% with melphalan/prednisone (P = .002) was seen. Median survival was 43 months versus 23 months, P = .004 (221).
3. Maintenance therapy after initial induction of clinical remission has not been shown to prolong remission or survival duration. Chemotherapy reduces the myeloma cell burden by only one to two logs, and further chemotherapy has not resulted in a further decrease in myeloma cells.
4. VAD: For resistant myelomas, which are indicated by a failure to achieve more than 75% tumor cytoreduction, more than 50% serum myeloma protein, and/or more than 90% in Bence Jones proteinuria, VAD is an effective combination, resulting in responses in over 40% of patients with refractory MM, and a median survival of approximately 16 months (203,213a).

Interferon (IFN)- 2b (Interferon alpha 2)

Recently, IFN- 2b has shown significant activity in MM in patients who do not have a sustained response to chemotherapy. These IFN responses, unlike chemotherapy, take longer to develop and also appear to be more durable. The Eastern Cooperative Oncology Group used alpha IFN 2.5 MU/m2 subcutaneously three times per week in combination with chemotherapy; IFN was continued for 2 years (218). The 41% CR rate with VBMCP + IFN- 2b well exceeds results with chemotherapy alone. Neutropenia and a flu-like syndrome were more common in patients treated with the combination. A randomized comparison of VBMCP + IFN-2b versus VBMCP is planned by Eastern Cooperative Oncology Group.

Bone Marrow Transplantation

See section 5c below under "Radiation Therapy"

Radiation Therapy

Radiation therapy is a useful component of the overall management of patients with plasma cell tumors. Prior to the development of effective chemotherapy, radiation therapy was the primary therapeutic agent. It remains important in the following situations (215):

1. As primary therapy for patients with solitary plasmacytoma of bone or of isolated extramedullary sites.
2. As palliative therapy for painful lesions in patients with MM who are no longer responsive to chemotherapy.
3. As emergency therapy for patients with spinal cord or nerve root compression.
4. To prevent pathologic fractures in involved weight-bearing bones.
5. As TBI, particularly in the setting of BMT.

Techniques

1. Patients with solitary plasmacytoma of bone will frequently have disease extension into adjacent soft tissues. MRI is particularly useful for the demonstration and demarcation of this involvement. In the absence of such extension, the radiation portal generally includes the entire involved bone with a 2 to 3 cm soft tissue margin. When adjacent tissues are involved, the portal includes the disease with a more generous margin, depending on the neighboring normal tissue tolerances. The radiation dose required for sustained local control is 40 to 50 Gy administered over 4 to 5 weeks, although some patients will have recurring disease even with doses above this level (214,216). Evidence exists suggesting that treatment of solitary lesions will prevent subsequent disease dissemination in some patients, although most will nevertheless have widespread disease at some point (161).
2. Patients who have MM with painful bony involvement unresponsive to chemotherapy are treated with portals that involve the entire bone. In patients with vertebral body involvement, adjacent vertebral bodies are generally included. Although high radiation doses are necessary for durable local control, pain relief is accomplished with 10 to 20 Gy (in large fractions), which is generally appropriate for patients requiring palliation (216).
3. Patients with spinal cord compression are generally treated with 35 to 45 Gy to the involved vertebral body, one to two adjacent bodies above and below, and the soft tissue extension, with a margin.
4. Patients with impending pathologic fractures should be strongly considered for orthopedic intervention prior to radiation therapy.
5. *Large field radiotherapy:*
   a. TBI alone for patients with MM has been used with limited success (207,212). Its application is limited by the attendant marrow suppression that is common because of the previous chemotherapy most patients have received.
   b. Hemibody irradiation is currently being evaluated as an effective strategy for patients with multiple painful lesions. Several series suggest that subjective improvement occurs in 80% to 90% of patients treated with 8.5 to 9.5 Gy (212,223). Again, hematologic toxicity may occur. Some patients are able to tolerate administration to both the upper and lower hemibody given sequentially with a 4 to 6 week intervals between doses. Systemic radiation therapy following combination chemotherapy as primary treatment is under investigation.

c. Combined TBI and high-dose chemotherapy with either thiotepa or melphalan as a consolidation technigue in VAD-sensitive patients, followed by autologous BMT can lead to long-term survival in responders, i.e., 80% to 90% 2-year survival (213a).

SPECIAL CONSIDERATIONS OF TREATMENT

1. *Hypercalcemia* should be vigorously managed with saline hydration, diuretics, corticosteroids, calcitonin, and biphosphates. Plicamycin (mithramycin) can produce dramatic decreases in serum calcium (10 to 25 μg/kg by slow IV infusion), but pre-existing impairment of kidney function may preclude its use (217).
2. *Infection*: Infectious complications are frequent because of a variety of immune deficits described in patients with MM (211). Pneumoccal, meningococcal, and haemophilis B vaccines should be administered although their effectiveness in these patients has not been established. IV gammaglobulin in an uncontrolled study has been shown to be protective (209).
3. *Spinal cord compression*: If a patient with MM has persistent back pain, spinal cord impingement should be suspected until proven otherwise. Extradural compression from myelomatous involvement of a vertebral body is common. For diagnostic work-up and management, see Chapter 13, "Oncologic Emergencies."
4. An acute terminal phase, sometimes resembling acute myeloblastic or myelomonocytic leukemia, has been reported in up to one third of patients (205). These patients have been generally unresponsive to antileukemic regimens.

RESULTS AND PROGNOSIS

The use of intermittent prednisone and melphalan produces objective improvement with prolonged survival in at least half the patients treated (Table 18-15, Fig. 18-8) (206a,223a). The M2 protocol (see above) has been reported in an uncontrolled study to give the highest response rate (87%) with median survival of 50 months (206). Addition of IFN to combination chemotherapy has markedly increased the CR rate. Whether this translates into improved survival requires confirmation (218).

Staging (Table 18-13) reflects factors determining prognosis. Treatments of greater intensity are now considered for patients with stage III MM because of their worse prognosis (208).

DFS for solitary plasmacytoma of bone versus that of solitary soft-tissue disease is shown in Fig. 18-9 (208a).

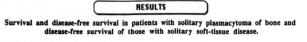

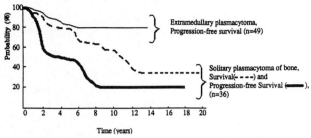

Fig. 18-8. Results: Survival and disease-free survival in patients with solitary plasmacytoma of bone and disease-free survival of those with solitary soft tissue disease. Adapted from Chak *et al.* (206a) and Wiltshaw (223a), with permission.

CLINICAL INVESTIGATIONS

Current chemotherapeutic regimens generally yield only partial remissions, and when relapse occurs a durable second remission is seldom obtained. Therefore, high-dose chemotherapy and TBI (207) followed by allogeneic or autologous BMT (210) are active areas of investigation.

Recommended Reading

For Hodgkin's disease, the writings of Kaplan (3a), in his classic book on the subject, is an excellent introduction to modern concepts of the pathogenesis of this disease, radiation therapy management, and combined modality clinical

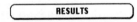

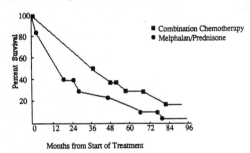

Fig. 18-9. Results: Long-term follow-up on a randomized trial comparing alternating combination chemotherapy to melphalan and prednisone in a Southwest oncology group study initiated in 1977. From Durie *et al.* (208a), with permission.

Table 18-15. Median Survival in Relation to Stage at Diagnosis for Multiple Myeloma

	Median Survival (mo)				
	Stage				
	I	**II**	**III**	**A**	**B**
Range	39 - >79	27 - 51	6 - 33	21 - >60	2 - 12
Total (1428 patients)	>60	41	23		

Adapted from Salmon and Cassady (220a).

trials. Hellman *et al.* (2a) and Hoppe *et al.* (2b) in *Cancer: Principles and Practice of Oncology* give excellent up-to-date overviews of Hodgkin's Disease. Other important author-investigators—pathogenesis: Rappaport (4); staging: Carbone *et al.* (13), DeVita *et al.* (20); combined modalities: Bonadonna (9), Kaplan and Rosenberg (54a,87).

For non-Hodgkin's lymphoma, to understand the pathologic criteria for classification subcategorizations and staging, read the National Cancer Institute's Non-Hodgkin's Classification Project Writing Committee report (172) and Rappaport's Armed Forces Institute of Pathology Atlas (185). In the management of non-Hodgkin's lymphoma, the benchmark reports from Rosenberg (186), DeVita (131b), and Tubiana (195) deserve review.

For multiple myeloma, chapters in the standard oncology texts and Salmon and Cassady (220a) and Wasserman (223') are recommended.

REFERENCES

General References

1. Cancer statistics. Boring, C.C., Squires, T.S., Tong, T. (eds). CA. 41:28; 1991.
2. Bennett, J.M., ed. Lymphomas I. Boston, MA: Martinus Nijhoff; 1981.
2a. Hellman, S.; Jaffe, E.S.; DeVita, V.T., Jr. Hodgkin's Disease. In: DeVita, V.T., Jr., Hellman, S., Rosenberg, S.A., (eds). Cancer: Principles and Practice of Oncology, 3rd ed. Philadelphia, PA: JB Lippincott Co.; 1989; 1696-1740.
2b. Hoppe, R.T.; Glatstein, E.; Wasserman, T. Hodgkin's Disease. In: Perez, C.A., Brady, L.W. (eds). Principles and Practice of Radiation Oncology, 2nd ed. Philadelphia, PA: JB Lippincott Co.; 1992:1307-1328.
3. Ioachim, H.L. Lymph node biopsy. Philadelphia, PA: JB Lippincott, Co; 1982.
3a. Kaplan, H.W. Hodgkin's Disease, 2nd ed. Cambridge, MA: Harvard University Press; 1980.
4. Rappaport, H. Tumors of the hematopoietic system. In: Atlas of Tumor Pathology, section III, fascicle I. Washington, DC: Armed Forces Institute of Pathology; 1966.

Specific References
Hodgkin's Disease

5. Agnarsson, B, Kadin, M. The immunophenotype of Reed-Sternberg cells: a study of 50 cases of Hodgkin's disease using fixed frozen tissues. Cancer. 63:2083-2087; 1989.
5a. Ang, P.T.; Horning, S.J.; Hoppe, R.T.; *et al.* Procarbazine, Alkeran and Velban (PAVe): efficacy in the combined modality therapy of unfavorable Hodgkin's disease (HD). Proc Am Soc Clin Oncol. 9: 254; 1990. Abstract.
6. Bakemeier, R.; Anderson, J.; Costello, W.; *et al.* BCVP chemotherapy for advanced Hodgkin's disease: evidence for a greater duration of complete remission, greater survival, and less toxicity than with a MOPP regimen: results of the Eastern Cooperative Oncology Group Study Ann Intern Med. 101:447-456; 1984.
7. Bakemeier, R.F.; Anderson, J.; Costello, W.; *et al.* BCVPP chemotherapy for advanced Hodgkin's disease: evidence for increased complete remission (CR) duration and less toxicity than with MOPP. Proc Am Soc Clin Oncol. (ASCO) 23:164; 1982. Abstract.
8. Bjorkholm, M.; Holm, G.; Merk, K. Cyclic autoimmune hemolytic anemia as a presenting manifestation of splenic Hodgkin's disease. Cancer. 49:1702-1704; 1982.
9. Bonadonna, G.; Valagussa, P.; Santoro, A. Alternating non-cross-resistant combination chemotherapy or MOPP in stage IV Hodgkin's disease. Ann Intern Med. 104:739-746; 1986.
9a. Bonadonna, G. Hodgkin's disease: The Milan Cancer Institute experience with MOPP and ABVD (Meeting abstract) Third International Conference on Malignant Lymphoma. June 10-13, 1987.
10. Botnick, L.; Goodman, R.; Jaffe, N.; *et al.* Stages I-III Hodgkin's disease in children: results of staging and treatment. Cancer. 39:599-603; 1977.
11. Braylan, R.C.; Jaffe, E.S.; Berard, C.W. Malignant lymphomas: currrent classification and new observations. In: Sommers, S.C. (ed). Pathology Annual. New York, NY: Appleton-Century-Crofts; 1975:213-270.
11a. Brizel, D.M.; Winer, E.P.; Prosnitz, L.R.; Scott, J.; Crawford, J.; Moore, J.O.; Gockerman, J.P. Improved survival in advanced Hodgkin's disease with the use of combined modality therapy. Int J Rad Oncol Biol Phys. 19: 535-542; 1990.
12. Canellos, G.; Propert, K.; Cooper, R.; *et al.* MOPP vs. ABVD alternating with ABVD in advanced Hodgkin's disease: a prospective randomized CALGB trial. Proc Am Soc Clin Oncol. 1988. Abstract.
13. Carbone, P.P.; Kaplan, H.S.; Mushoff, K.; *et al.* Report of the committee on Hodgkin's disease staging classification. Cancer Res. 31:1860-1861; 1971.
14. Carde, P.; Burgers, J.; Henry-Amar, M.; *et al.* Clinical stages I and II Hodgkin's disease: a specifically tailored therapy according to prognostic factors. J Clin Oncol. 6:239-252; 1988.
15. Castellino, R.; Billingham, M.; Dorfman, R. Lymphographic accuracy in Hodgkin's disease and malignant lymphoma with a note on the "reactive" lymph node as a cause of most false-positive lymphograms. Invest Radiol. 9:155; 1974.
16. Castellino, R.; Blank, N.; Hoppe, R.; Cho, C. Hodgkin disease: contributions of chest CT in the initial staging evaluation. Radiology. 160:603-605; 1986.
17. Crnkovich, M.; Leopold, K.; Hoppe, R.; Mauch, P. Stage I to IIB Hodgkin's disease: the combined experience at Stanford and the Joint Center for Radiation Therapy J Clin Oncol. 5:1041-1049; 1987.
18. DeLaney, T.; Glatstein, E. The role of the staging laparotomy in the management of Hodgkin's disease. In: DeVita, V.; Hellman, S.; Rosenberg, S. (eds). Updates, Cancer: Principles and Practice of Oncology, vol. 1. Philadelphia, PA: JB Lippincott Co.; 1987:1-14.
19. DeVita, V.T., Jr. The consequences of the chemotherapy of Hodgkin's disease. Cancer. 47:1-13; 1981.
20. DeVita, V.T., Jr.; Simon, R.M.; Hubbard, S.M.; *et al.* Curability of advanced Hodgkin's disease with chemotherapy. Long-term follow-up of MOPP-treated patients at the National Cancer Institute (NCI). Ann Intern Med. 92;587-595; 1980.
21. Dmitrovsky, E.; Martin, S.; Krudy, A.; *et al.* Lymph node aspiration in the management of Hodgkin's disease. J Clin Oncol. 4:306-310; 1986.
22. Doll, D.; Ringenberg, Q.; Anderson, S.; *et al.* Bone marrow biopsy in the initial staging of Hodgkin's disease. Med Pediatr Oncol. 17:1-5; 1989.
23. Donaldson, S.; Link, M. Combined modality treatment with low-dose radiation and MOPP chemotherapy for children with Hodgkin's disease. J Clin Oncol. 5:742-749; 1987.
23a. Donaldson, S.; Whitaker, S.; Plowman, N.; *et al.* Stage I-II pediatric Hodgkin's disease: Long-term follow-up demonstrates equivalent survival rates following different management schemes. J Clin Oncol. 8:1128-1137; 1990.
24. Durant, J.R.; Gams, R.A.; Velez-Garcia, E.; *et al.* BCNU, Velban, cyclophosphamide, procarbazine, and prednisone (BVCPP) in advanced Hodgkin's disease. Cancer. 42:2101-2110; 1978.
25. Gilbert, R. Radiotherapy in Hodgkin's disease (malignant granulomatosis): anatomic and clinical foundations: governing principles: results. AJR. 41:198-241; 1939.
26. Fisher, R. Implications of persistent T cell abnormalities for the etiology of Hodgkin's disease. Cancer Treat Rep. 66:681-687; 1982.
27. Fox, K.; Lippman, S.; Cassady, J.; *et al.* Radiation therapy slavage of Hodgkin's disease following chemotherapy failure. J Clin Oncol. 5:38-45; 1987.
28. Friedman, S.; Henry-Amar, M.; Cosset, J-M.; *et al.* Evolution of erythrocyte sedimentation rate as predictor of early relapse in post-therapy early-stage Hodgkin's disease. J Clin Oncol. 6:598-602; 1988.
29. Fuller, L.; Hagemeister, F.; North, L.; *et al.* The adjuvant fole of two cycles of MOPP and low-dose lung irradiation in stage IA through IIB Hodgkin's disease: preliminary results. Int J Radiat Oncol Biol Phys. 14:683-692; 1988.
30. Gatti, R.; Good R. Occurrence of malignancy in immunodefi-

ciency disease. A literature review. Cancer. 28:89-98; 1971.

31. Glatstein, E.; McHardy-Young, S.; Brast, N.; *et al.* Alterations in serum thyrotropin (TSH) and thyroid function following radiotherapy in patients with malignant lymphoma. J Clin Endocrinol Metab. 32:833-841; 1971.

32. Goldie, J.; Coldman, A.; Gudauskas, G. Rationale for the use of alternating non-cross-resistant chemotherapy. Cancer Treat Rep. 66:439; 1982.

33. Goodman, L.; Wintobe, M.; Daneshek, W.; *et al.* Nitrogen mustard therapy. JAMA. 132:126; 1946.

34. Grufferman, S.; Delzell, E. Epidemiology of Hodgkin's disease. Epidemiol Rev. 6:76-106; 1984.

34a. Hagenmerster, F.; Fesus, S.; Lamki, L.; Haynie. Role of Gallium scan in Hodgkin's disease. Cancer. 65:1090-1096; 1990.

35. Hamlin, D.J. Radiographic approach to the staging of lymphoma, including Hodgkin's disease. In: Bennett, J.M. Lymphomas I. Boston, MA: Martinus Nijhoff; 1981:177-233.

36. Hann, H.; Lange, B.; Stahlhut, M.; McGlynn, K. Serum ferritin and prognosis of childhood Hodgkin's disease. Proc Am Soc Clin Oncol. 6:A750; 1987. Abstract A750.

37. Harker, W.; Kushlan, P.; Rosenberg, S. Combination chemotherapy for advanced Hodgkin's disease after failure of MOPP: ABVD and B-CAVE. Ann Intern Med. 101:440-446; 1984.

38. Hodgkin, T. On some morbid appearances of the absorbent gland and spleen. Medico-Chirurgical Transactions 17:68-114; 1832.

39. Hoppe, R. The contemporary management of Hodgkin's disease. Radiology. 169:297-304; 1988.

40. Hoppe, R. The management of stage II Hodgkin's disease with a large mediastinal mass: a prospective program emphasizing irradiation. Int J Radiat Oncol Biol Phys. 11:349-355; 1985.

41. Hoppe, R. Treatment planning in the radiation therapy of Hodgkin's disease. Front Radiat Ther Oncol. 21:270-287; 1987.

42. Hoppe, R.T.; Rosenberg, S.A.; Kaplan, H.S.; *et al.* Prognostic factors in pathological stage IIIA Hodgkin's disease. Cancer. 46:1240-1246; 1980.

43. Horn, N.L.; Ray, G.R.; Kriss, J.P. Gallium-67 citrate scanning in Hodgkin's disease and non-Hodgkin's lymphoma. Cancer. 37:250-257; 1976.

44. Horning, W.; Hoppe, R.; Kaplan, H.; Rosenberg, S. Female reproductive potential after treatment for Hodgkin's disease. N Engl J Med. 304:1377-1382; 1982.

45. Hsu, S-M.; Yang, K.; Jaffe, E. Phenotypic expression of Hodgkin's and Reed-Sternberg cells in Hodgkin's disease. Blood. 70:96-103; 1987.

46. Israel, O.; Front, D.; Lam, M.; *et al.* Gallium 67 imaging in monitoring lymphoma response to treatment. Cancer. 61:2439-2443; 1988.

47. Jackson, H., Jr.; Parker, F., Jr. Hodgkin's Disease and Allied Disorders. New York, NY: Oxford University Press; 1947.

48. Jaffe, H.; Cadman, E.; Farber, L.; Bertino, J. Pretreatment hematocrit as an independent prognostic variable in Hodgkin's disease. Blood. 68:562-564; 1986.

49. Jagannath, S.; Armitage, J.; Dicke, K.; *et al.* Prognostic factors for response and survival after high-dose cyclophosphamide, carmustine, and etoposide with autologous bone marrow transplantation for relapse Hodgkin's disease. J Clin Oncol. 7:179-185; 1989.

50. Jereb, B.; Tan, C.; Bretsky, S.; *et al.* Involved field irradiation with or without chemotherapy in the management of children with Hodgkin's disease. Med Pediatr Oncol. 12:325-332; 1984.

51. Jones, S.; Haut, A.; Weick, J.; *et al.* Comparison of Adriamycin containing chemotherapy (MOP-BAP) with MOPP-bleomycin in the management of advanced Hodgkin's disease: a Southwest Oncology Group study. Cancer. 51:1339-1347; 1983.

52. Kadin, M. Possible origin of the Reed-Sternberg cell from an interdigitating reticulum cell. Cancer Treat Rep. 66:601-608; 1982.

53. Kaplan, H.S. Hodgkin's Disease. 2nd ed. Cambridge, MA: Harvard University Press; 1980.

54. Kaplan, H.S. Role of intensive radiotherapy in the management of Hodgkin's disease. Cancer. 19:356-367; 1966.

54a. Kaplan, H.S.; Dorfman, R.F.; Nelson, T.S.; *et al.* Staging laproatomy and splenectomy in Hodgkin's disease: Analysis of indications and patterns of involvement in 285 consecutive cases, unselected patients. NCI Monograph. 36: 291; 1973.

54b. Kaplan, H.S., Rosenberg, S.A: The treatment of Hodgkin's dis-

ease. Med Clin North Am. 50: 1591-1610;1966.

55. Kapp, D.; Prosnitz, L.; Farber, L.; *et al.* Patterns of failure in Hodgkin's disease: the Yale University experience. Cancer Treat. Symposia 2:145-156; 1983.

55a. Kessinger, A.; Nademanee, A.; Forman, S.J.; Armitage, J.O. Autologous bone marrow transplantation for Hodgkin's and non-Hodgkin's lymphoma. Hematol Oncol Clin North Am. 4:577-588; 1990.

56. Kinsella, T.; Fraass, B.; Glatstein, E. Late effects of radiation therapy in the treatment of Hodgkin's disease. Cancer Treat Rep. 66:991-1001; 1982.

57. Klimo, P.; Connors. MOPP/ABV hybrid program: combination chemotherapy based on early introduction of seven effective drugs for advanced Hodgkin's disease. J Clin Oncol. 3:1174-1182; 1985.

58. Kundrat, H. Uber Lympho-sarkomatosis. Wien Klin Wochenschr. 6:211-234; 1893.

58a. Lee, C.K.K.; Aeppli, D.M.; Bloomfield, C.D.; Levitt, S.H. Curative radiotherapy for laparotomy-staged IA,IIA, IIIA Hodgkin's disease: an evaluation of the gains achieved with radical radiotherapy. Int J Rad Oncol Biol Phys. 19: 547-560; 1990.

59. Leibenhaut, M.; Hoppe, R.; Efron, B.; Halpern, J.; Nelsen, T.; Rosenberg, S. Prognostic indicators of laparotomy findings in clinical stage I-II supradiaphragmatic Hodgkin's disease. J Clin Oncol. 7:81-91; 1989.

60. Leibenhaut, M.; Hoppe, R.; Varghese, A.; Rosenberg, S. Subdiaphragmatic Hodgkin's disease: laparotomy and treatment results in 49 patients. J Clin Oncol. 5:1050-1055; 1987.

61. Lennert, K.; Mohri, N.; Stein, H.; *et al.* The histopathology of malignant lymphomas. Br J Haematol. 31(Suppl):192-203; 1975.

62. Levitt, S.; Lee, C.; Aeppli, D.; Bloomfield, C. Radical treatment of Hodgkin's disease with radiation therapy: results of a 15-year clinical trial. Radiology. 162:623-630; 1987.

63. Lister, T.; Dorreen, M.; Faux, M.; J; *et al.* The treatment of stage IIIA Hodgkin's disease. J Clin Oncol. 1:745-749; 1983.

63a. Longo, D.L.; Young, R.C.; Wesley, M; *et al.* Twenty years of MOPP therapy for Hodgkin's Disease. J Clin Oncol. 4:1295-1306; 1986.

64. Lukes, R.J.; Butler, B.B.; Hicks, E.B. Natural history of Hodgkin's disease as related to its pathologic picture. Cancer. 19:317-344; 1966.

65. Mathe, G.; Rappaport, H.; O'Connor, G.T.; *et al.* Histological and cytological typing of neoplastic diseases of hematopoietic and lymphoid tissues. In: World Health Organization International Classification of Tumors, ed 14. Geneva, Switzerland: World Health Organzation; 1976.

66. Mauch, P.; Goodman, R.; Hellman, S. The significance of mediastinal involvement in early stage Hodgkin's disease. Cancer. 42:1039-1045; 1978.

67. Mauch, P.; Tarbell, N.; Weinstein, H.; *et al.* Stage IA and IIA supradiaphragmatic Hodgkin's disease: prognostic factors in surgically staged patients treated with mantle and para-aortic irradiation. J Clin Oncol. 6:1576-1583; 1988.

68. Moran, E.M.; Ultmann, J.E. Clinical features and course of Hodgkin's disease. Clin Haematol. 3:91-129; 1974.

69. Mueller, N.; Evans, A.; Harris, N.; *et al.* Hodgkin's disease and Epstein-Barr virus. Altered antibody pattern before diagnosis. N Engl J Med. 320:689-695; 1989.

70. The non-Hodgkin's Lymphoma Pathologic Classification Project. National Cancer Institute sponsored study of classifications of non-Hodgkin's lymphomas: summary and description of a working formulation for clinical usage. Cancer. 49:2112-2135; 1982.

71. Nonoyama, M.; Kawai, Y.; Huang, C.; *et al.* Epstein-Barr virus DNA in Hodgkin's disease, American Burkitt's lymphoma and other human tumors. Cancer Res. 34:1228-1231; 1974.

72. Nyman, R.; Rehn, S.; Glimelius, B.; *et al.* Residual mediastinal masses in Hodgkin disease: prediction of size with MR imaging. Radiology. 170:435-440; 1989.

73. Pedrick, T.; Hoppe, R. Recovery of spermatogenesis following pelvic irradiation for Hodgkin's disease. Int J Radiat Oncol Biol Phys. 12:117-121; 1986.

74. Peters, M. A study of survival in Hodgkin's disease treated radiologically. AJR. 63:299-311; 1950.

75. Peterson, B.; Pajak, T.; Cooper, M.; *et al.* Effect of age on therapeutic response and survival in advanced Hodgkin's disease. Cancer Treat Rep. 66:889-898; 1982.

76. Pillai, G.; Hagemeister, F.; Velasquez, W.; *et al.* Prognostic factors

for stage IV Hodgkin's disease treated with MOPP with or without bleomycin. Cancer. 55:691-697; 1985.

77. Prakash, U.; Abel, M.; Hubmayr, R. Mediastinal mass and tracheal obstruction during general anesthesia. Mayo Clin Proc. 63:1004-1011; 1988.

78. Prosnitz, L.R. Hodgkin's Disease: the right dose. Int J Rad Oncol Biol Phys. 19: 803-804; 1990.

78a. Prosnitz, L.; Cooper, D.; Cox, E.; Kapp, D.; Farber, L. Treatment selection for stage IIIA Hodgkin's disease patients. Int J Radiat Oncol Biol Phys. 11:1431-1437; 1985.

78b. Prosnitz, L.R.; Farber, L.R.; Scott, J.; et al. Combined modality therapy for advanced Hodgkin's disease: A 15-year follow-up data. J Clin Oncol. 6:603-612; 1988.

79. Pui, C-H; Ip, S.; Thompson, E.; et al. Increased serum CD8 antigen level in childhood Hodgkin's disease relates to advanced stage and poor treatment outcome. Blood. 73:209-213; 1989.

80. Pusey, W. Cases of sarcoma and of Hodgkin's disease treated by exposures to X rays: a preliminary report. JAMA. 38:166-170; 1902.

81. Rappaport, H.; Winter, W.J.; Hicks, E.B. Follicular lymphoma: A reevaluation of its position in the scheme of malignant lymphoma. Cancer. 9:792-821; 1956.

82. Raubitschek, A.; Glatstein, E. The never-ending controversies in Hodgkin's disease. Int J Radiat Oncol Biol Phys. 17:1115-1118; 1989.

83. Regula, D.; Hoppe, R.; Weiss, L. Nodular and diffuse types of lymphocyte predominance Hodgkin's disease. N Engl J Med. 318:214-219; 1988.

84. Roach, M.; Kapp, D.; Rosenberg, S.; Hoppe, R. Radiotherapy with curative intent: an option in selected patients relapsing after chemotherapy for advanced Hodgkin's disease. J Clin Oncol. 5: 550-555; 1987.

85. Rosen, P. Should we be subclassifying Hodgkin's disease? J Clin Oncol. 4:275-277; 1986.

86. Rosenberg, S. Exploratory laparotomy and splenectomy for Hodgkin's disease: a commentary. J Clin Oncol. 6:574-575; 1988.

87. Rosenberg, S.; Kaplan, H. The evolution and summary results of the Stanford randomized clinical trials of the management of Hodgkin's disease: 1962-1984. Int J Radiat Oncol Biol Phys. 11:5-22; 1985.

88. Rosenberg, S.A. Hodgkin's disease of the bone marrow. Cancer Res. 31:1733-1736; 1971.

89. Rubin, P.; Haluska, G.; Poulter, C.A. The basis for segmental sequential irradiation in Hodgkin's disease: clinical experience of patterns of recurrence. Am J Roentgenol Radium Ther Nucl Med. 105:814-817; 1969.

90. Russell, K.; Hope, R.; Colby, T.; et al. Lymphocyte predominant Hodgkin's disease: clinical presentation and results of treatment. Radiother Oncol. 1:197-205; 1984.

91. Santoro, A.; Bonadonna, G.; Bonfante, C.; et al. Alternating drug combination in the treatment of advanced Hodgkin's disease. N Engl J Med. 306:770-775; 1982.

92. Santoro, A.; Bonfante, V.; Bonadonna, G. Salvage chemotherapy with ABVD in MOPP-resistant Hodgkin's disease. Ann. Intern. Med. 96:139-143; 1982.

92a. Schewe, K.L.; Kun, L.E.; Cox, J.D. A step toward ending the controversies in Hodgkin's disease. Int J Radiat Oncol Biol Phys. 17:1123; 1989.

93. Schreiber, D.; Jacobs, C.; Rosenberg, S.; et al. The potential benefits of therapeutic splenectomy for patients with Hodgkin's disease and non-Hodgkin's lymphomas. Int J Radiat Oncol Biol Phys. 11:31-36; 1985.

93a. Shapiro, S.J.; Shapiro, S.D.; Mill, W.B.; Campbell, E.J. Prospective study of long-term pulmonary manifestations of mantle irradiation. Int J Rad Oncol Biol Phys. 19: 707-714; 1990.

94. Slivnick, D.; Nawrocki, J.; Fisher, R. Immunology and cellular biology of Hodgkin's disease. Hematol Oncol Clin North Am. 3(2):205-220; 1989.

95. Smithers, D. Modes of spread. In: Smithers, D.W. (ed). Hodgkin's Disease. Edinburgh and London, UK: Churchill-Livingstone; 1973:107-117.

96. Specht, L.; Nordentoft, A.; Cold, S.; et al. Tumor burden as the most important prognostic factor in early stage Hodgkin's disease. Cancer. 61:1719-1727; 1988.

97. Stein, R.; Golomb, M.; Werinik, P.; et al. Anatomic substages of stages IIIA Hodgkin's disease: follow-up of a collaborative study. Cancer Treat. Rep. 6:733-741; 1982.

98. Stein, R.S. Clinical features and clinical evaluation of Hodgkin's disease and the non-Hodgkin's disease. Cancer. 32:692-698; 1973.

99. Strum, S.B.; Park, J.K.; Rappaport, H. Observation of cells resembling Sternberg-Reed cells in conditions other than Hodgkin's disease. Cancer. 26:176-190; 1970.

100. Sullivan, M.; Fuller,. L.; Chen, T.; et al. Intergroup Hodgkin's disease in children study of stages I and I: a preliminary report. Cancer Treat Rep. 66:937-947; 1982.

101. Sundeen, J.; Lipford, E.; Uppenkamp, M.; et al. Rearranged antigen receptor genes in Hodgkin's disease. Blood. 70:96-103; 1987.

102. Sweet, D.L.; Kinnealey, A.; Ultmann, J.E. Hodgkin's disease: problems of staging. Cancer. 42:957-970; 1978.

103. Tan, C.; DeSousa, M.; Good, R. Distinguishing feature of the immunology of Hodgkin's disease in children. Cancer Treat Rep. 66:969-975; 1982.

104. Tucker, M.; Coleman, C.; Cox, R.; Varghese, A.; Rosenberg, S. Risk of second cancers after treatment for Hodgkin's disease. N Engl J Med. 318:76-81; 1988.

105. Unger, P.; Strauchen, J. Hodgkin's disease in AIDS complex patients. Report of four cases and tissue immunologic marker studies. Cancer. 58:821-825; 1986.

106. Vianna, N.; Polan, A. Epidemiologic evidence for transmission of Hodgkin's disease. N Engl J Med. 289:499; 1973.

107. Virchow, R. Weisses Blut. Neue notizen aus dem Gebiete der Natur und Heikunde (Froriep's neue notizen). 36:151-156; 1845.

107a. Viviani, S.; Bonadonna, G.; Santoro, A.; et al. Alternating vs Hybrid administration of MOPP-ABVD in Hodgkin's disease. Proc Am Soc Clin Oncol. 9:254; 1990. Abstract.

107b. Vose, J.M.; Bierman, P.J.; Weisenburger, D.D.; Armitage, J.O. The importance of early autologous bone marrow transplantation (ABMT) in the management of patients (Pts) with Hodgkin's disease. Proc Am Soc Clin Oncol. 9:256; 1990.

107c. Vriesendorp, H.M.; Blum, J.E.; Herpst, J.M.; et al. Refractory Hodgkin's disease: treatment with polyclonal Yttrium labeled antiferritin. Proc Am Soc Clin Oncol. 9:256; 1990. Abstract.

107d. Vriesendorp, H.M.; Order, S.E. Hodgkin's disease: new possibilities for clinical research. Int J Radiat Oncol Biol Phys. 17:1119-1122; 1989.

108. Weiss, L.; Movahed, L.; Warnke, R.; Sklar, J. Detection of Epstein-Barr viral genomes in Reed-Sternberg cells of Hodgkin's disease. N Engl J Med. 320:502-506; 1989.

108a. Yahalom, J.; Gulati, S.; Shank, B.; et al. Total lymphoid irradiation, high-dose chemotherapy and autologous bone marrow transplantation for chemotherapy-resistant Hodgkin's disease. Int J Radiat Oncol Biol Phys. 17:915-922; 1989.

109. Young, C.; Straus, D.; Myers, J.; et al. Multidisciplinary treatment of advanced Hodgkin's disease by an alternating chemotherapeutic regimen of MOPP/ABVD and low-dose radiation therapy restricted to originally bulky disease. Cancer Treat Rep. 66:907-914; 1982.

Pediatric Hodgkin's Disease

109a. Bayle-Weisgerber, C.; Lemercier, N.; Teillet, F.; et al. Hodgkin's disease in children: Results of therapy in a mixed group of 178 clinical and pathologically staged patients over 13 years. Cancer. 54:215-222; 1984.

109b. Cramer, P.; Andrieu, J.M. Hodgkin's disease in childhood and adolescence: results of chemotherapy-radiotherapy in clinical stages IA-IIB. J Clin Oncol. 3:1495-1502; 1985.

110. Donaldson, S. Glatstein, E.; Vasti, K. Bacterial infection in pediatric Hodgkin's disease. Relationship to radiotherapy, chemotherapy and splenectomy. Cancer. 41:1949-1958; 1978.

111. Donaldson, S.; Kaplan, H. A survey of pediatric Hodgkin's disease at Stanford University: Results of therapy and quality of survival. In: Rosenberg, S., Kaplan, H. (eds). Malignant Lymphomas. Etiology, Immunology, Pathology, Treatment. New York, NY: Academic Press; 1982.

111a. Donaldson, S.S.; Link, M.P. Combined modality treatment with low-dose radiation and MOPP chemotherapy for children with Hodgkin's disease. J Clin Oncol. 5:742-749; 1987.

111b. Donaldson, S.S.; Link, M.P.; McDougall, I.R.; et al. Clinical investigations of children with Hodgkin's disease at Stanford University Medical center: A preliminary overview using low dose irradiation and alternating ABVD/MOPP chemotherapy. In: Kamps, W.A., Poppema, S., Humphrey, B. (eds). In: Hodgkin's Disease in Children: Controversies and Current Practice. Boston, MA: Kluwer Academic Publishers; 1989:307-316.

111b*. Donaldson, S.; Whitaker, S.; Plowman, N. *et al*. Stage I-II pediatric Hodgkin's disease: long-term follow-up demonstrates equivalent survival rates following different management schemes. J Clin Oncol. 8:1128-1137; 1990.

111b**. Dionet, C.; Oberlin, O.; Habriand, J.L.; *et al*. Initial chemotherapy and low dose radiation in limited fields in childhood Hodgkin's disease: Results of a joint cooperative study by the French Society of Radiation Oncology (SFOP) and Hospital Saint-Louis, Paris. Int J Radiat Oncol Biol Phys. 15:341-346; 1988.

111c. Ekert, H.; Waters, K.D. Results of treatment of 18 children with Hodgkin's disease with MOPP chemotherapy as the only treatment modality. Med Pediatr Oncol. 11:322-326; 1983.

111d. Ekert, H.; Waters, K.D.; Smith, P.J.; Toogood, I.; Mauger, D. Treatment with MOPP or CHIVPP chemotherapy only for all stages of childhood Hodgkin's disease. J Clin Oncol. 6:1845-1850; 1988.

111e. Farah, R.; Weichselbaum, R. Substaging of stage III Hodgkin's disease. Hematol/Oncol Clin N Amer. 3:277-286; 1989.

111f. Gehan, E.A.; Sullivan, M.P.; Fuller, L.M.; *et al*. The Intergroup Hodgkin's disease in children. A study of stage I and II. Cancer. 65:1429-1437; 1990.

112. Gutensohn, N. Cole, P. Childhood social environment and Hodgkin's disease. N Engl J Med. 304:135; 1981.

113. Halperin, E.; Kun, L.; Constine, L.; Tarbell, N. Pediatric Radiation Oncology. Raven Press, New York, NY: 1989;434.

113a. Jacobs, P.; King, H.S.; Karabus, C.; *et al*. Hodgkin's disease in children: a ten-year experience in South Africa. Cancer. 53:210-213; 1984.

113b. Jenkin, D.; Chan, H.; Freedman, M.; *et al*. Hodgkin's disease in children: treatment results with MOPP and low-dose, extended-field irradiation. Cancer Treat Rep. 66:949-959; 1982.

113b*. Jenkin, D.; Doyle, J.; Berry, M.; *et al*. Hodgkin's disease in children: Treatment with MOPP and low-dose extended field irradiation without laparotomy late results and toxicity. Med. Pediat. Oncol. 18:265-272; 1990.

113c. Lange, B.; Littman. Management of Hodgkin's disease in children and adolescents. Cancer. 51:1371-1377; 1983.

113c*. Maity, A.; Goldwein, J.W.; Lange, B.; D'Angio, G.J. Comparison of high-dose and low-dose radiation with and without chemotherapy for children with Hodgkin's disease: An analysis of the experience at the Children's Hospital of Philadelphia and the Hospital of the University of Pennsylvania. J Clin Oncol. 10:929-936; 1992.

113d. Mauch, P.M.; Weinstein, H.; Botnick, L.; *et al*. An evaluation of long-term survival and treatment complications in children with Hodgkin's disease. Cancer. 51:925-932; 1988.

113e. Olweny, C.L.M.; Katongole-Mcbidde, E.; Kiire, C.; *et al*. Childhood Hodgkin's disease in Uganda — a ten-year experience. Cancer. 42:787-792; 1978.

114. Parker, B.; Castellino, R.; Kaplan, H. Pediatric Hodgkin's disease. I. Radiographic evaluation. Cancer. 37:2430; 1976.

114a. Pizzo, P.A.; Poplack, D.G. In: Principles and Practice of Pediatric Oncology. Philadelphia, PA: JB Lippincott Co; 1989.

114b. Schellong, G.; Bramswig, J.; Ludwig, R.; *et al*. Combined treatment-strategy in over 200 children with Hodgkin's disease: Graduated chemotherapy, involved field irradiation with low dose and selective splenectomy. Klin Pediatr. 198:137-146; 1986.

115. Smith, I.E.; Peckham, M.J.; McElwain, T.J.; *et al*. Hodgkin's disease in children. Br J Cancer 36:120; 1977.

115a. Tan, C.; Jereb, B.; Chan, K.W.; *et al*. Hodgkin's disease in children: results of management between 1970-1981. Cancer. 51:1720-1725; 1983.

116. Vianna, N.; Greenwald, P.; Davies, J. Extended epidemic of Hodgkin's disease in high school students. Lancet. 1:1209; 1971.

116a. Weiner, M.A.; Leventhal, B.G.l Marcus, R.; *et al*. Intensive chemotherapy and low-dose radiotherapy for the treatment of advanced-stage Hodgkin's disease in pediatric patients: A Pediatric Oncology Group Study. J Clin Oncol. 9:1591-1598; 1991.

Non-Hodgkin's Lymphoma

117. Acker, B.; Hoppe, R.; Colby, T.; *et al*. Histologic conversion in the non-Hodgkin's lymphoma. J Clin Oncol. 1:11-16; 1983.

118. Aisenberg, A.C.; Wilkes, B.M.; Jacobson, J.O.; Harris, N.L. Immunoglobulin gene rearrangement in adult non-Hodgkin's lymphoma. Am J Med. 83:738-744; 1987.

118a. Armitage, J.O.; Cheson, B.D. Chemotherapy for patients with diffuse large cell lymphoma. J Clin Oncol. 6:1335-1347; 1988.

119. Anderson, T.; Chabner, B.A.; Young, R.C.; *et al*. Malignant lymphoma: I. The histology and staging of 473 patients at the National Cancer Institute. Cancer. 50:2699-2707; 1982.

120. Anderson, T.; DeVita, V.T., Jr.; Simon, R.M.; *et al*. Malignant lymphoma: II. Prognostic factors and response to treatment of 473 patients at the National Cancer Institute. Cancer. 50:2708-2721; 1983.

120a. Armelin, H.; Armelin, M.; Kelly, K.; *et al*. Functional role for c-myc in mitogenic response to platelet-derived growth factor. Nature. 310:655-660; 1984.

121. Bernard, A.; Boumsell, L.; Reinherz, E. *et al*. Cell surface characterization of malignant T cells from lymphoblastic lymphoma using monoclonal antibodies. Evidence for a phenotypic difference between malignant T cells from patients with acute lymphoblastic leukemia and lymphoblastic lymphoma. Blood. 57:1105; 1981.

122. Blair, T.; Evans, R.; Buskirk, S.; *et al*. Radiotherapeutic management of primary thyroid lymphoma. Intl J Radiat Oncol Biol Phys. 11:365-370; 1985.

123. Blayney, D.W.; Jaffe, E.S.; Blattner, U.A.; *et al*. The human T cell leukaemia/lymphoma virus associated with American adult T cell leukaemia/lymphoma. Blood. 62:401-405; 1983.

124. Bonadonna, G. Chemotherapy of malignant lymphomas. Semin Oncol. 12:1-14; 1985.

124a. Braziel, R.; Keneklis, T.; Donlon, J. *et al*. Terminal deoxynucleotidyl transferase in non-Hodgkin's lymphoma. Am J Clin Pathol. 80:655-659; 1983.

125. Bush, R.; Gospodarowicz, M.; Sturgeon, J.; *et al*. Radiation therapy of localized non-Hodgkin's lymphoma. Cancer Treat Rep. 61:1129-1136; 1977.

126. Chabner, B.A.; Fisher, R.I.; Young, R.C.; *et al*. Staging of non-Hodgkin's lymphoma. Semin Oncol. 7:285-291; 1980.

127. Coleman, C.N.; Picossi, V.J.; Cos, R.S.; *et al*. Treatment of lymphoblastic lymphoma in adults. J Clin Oncol. 4:1628-1637; 1986.

128. Coleman, M. Chemotherapy for large cell lymphoma: optimism and caution. Ann Intern Med. 103:140-142; 1985.

129. Coltman, C.A.; Dahlberg, S.; Jones, S.E.; *et al*. CHOP is curative in thirty percent of patients with large cell lymphoma. A twelve-year Southwest Oncology Group study follow-up. In: Advances in chemotherapy: Update on Treatment for Diffuse Large Cell Lymphoma. New York, NY: Urley; 1986:71-77.

129a. Connors, J.M. The clinician's decision of whether CHOP chemotherapy should be standard therapy for treatment of patients with diffuse histiocytic lymphoma. In: Important Advances in Oncology 1990. DeVita, V.T., Hellman, S., Rosenberg, S.A. (eds). Philadelphia, PA: JB Lippincott Co; 1990:227-233.

130. Connors, J.M.; Klimo, P.; Fairey, R.N.; *et al*. Brief chemotherapy and involved field radiation therapy for limited stage histiologically aggressive lymphoma. Ann Intern Med. 107:596-602; 1985.

130a. Cossman, J.; Chused, T.M.; Fisher, R.I.; Magrath, I. Diversity of immunologic phenotypes of lymphoblastic lymphomas. Cancer Res. 43:4486; 1983.

131. Cox, J.D.; Komaki, R.K.; Kun, L.; *et al*. Stage III nodular lymphoreticular tumors (non-Hodgkin's lymphoma): results of central lymphatic irradiation. Cancer. 47:2247-2252; 1981.

131a. Desch, C.E.; Lasala, M.R.; Smith, T.; Hillner, B.E. The timing of autologous bone marrow transplantation (ABMT) in Hodgkin's disease patients following a chemotherapy relapse. Proc Am Soc Clin Oncol. 9:272; 1990.

131b. DeVita, V.; Jaffe, E.; Mauch, P.; Longo, D. Lymphocytic lymphomas, In: DeVita, V., Hellman, S., Rosenberg, S. (eds). Cancer Principles and Practice of Oncology. JB Lippincott Co., 3rd ed, 1989:1741-1798.

132. Esche, B.; Fitzpatrick, P. Cutaneous malignant lymphoma. Int J Radiat Oncol Biol. 12:2111-2115; 1986.

133. Ezdinli, E.Z.; Anderson, J.R.; Melvin, F.; *et al*. Moderate versus aggressive chemotherpay of nodular lymphocytic poorly differentiated lymphoma. J Cli. Oncol. 3:769-775; 1985.

133a. Fisher, R.I. CHOP Chemotherapy as standard therapy for treatment of patients with diffuse histiocytic lymphoma. In: Important Advances in Oncology 1990. DeVita, V.T., Hellman, S., Rosenberg, S.A., (eds). Philadelphia, PA: JB Lippincott Co; 1990:217-225.

134. Fisher, R.I.; Miller, T.P.; Daun, B.W.; *et al*. Southwest Oncology Group clinical trials of intermediate and high grade non-Hodgkin's lymphoma. Semin Hematol. 24(suppl 1):21-25; 1987.

135. Foon, K.A.; Roth, M.S.; Bunn, P.A. Interferon therapy of non-Hodgkin's lymphoma. Cancer. 59:601-604; 1987.

135a. Freedman, A.S.; Takvorian, T.; Anderson, K.C.; *et al.* Autologous bone marrow transplantation in B-Cell non-Hodgkin's lymphoma: very low treatment-related mortality in 100 patients in sensitive relapse. J Clin Oncol. 8:784-791; 1990.

136. Freeman, C.; Berg, J.W.; Cutler, S.J. Occurrence and prognosis of extranodal lymphomas. Cancer. 29:252-260; 1972.

137. Freeman, C.; Shustik, C.; Brisson, M.; *et al.* Primary malignant lymphoma of the central nervous system. Cancer. 58:1106-1111; 1986.

137a. Fultz, P.; Rubens, D.; Carigrian, J.; *et al.* MR Imaging of Hodgkin's and non-Hodgkin's lymphoma. Radiology. 165(P):201; 1987.

137b. Gianni, A.M.; Bregni, M.; Siena, S.; *et al.* Recombinant human granulocyte-macrophage colony-stimulating factor reduces hematologic toxicity and widens clinical applicability of high-dose Cyclophosphamide treatment in breast cancer and non-hodgkin's lymphoma. J Clin Oncol. 8:768-778; 1990.

138. Gibbs, W.N.; Wycliffe, S.; Lofters, M.B.; *et al.* Non-Hodgkin's lymphoma in Jamaica and its relation to adult T cell leukaemia-lymphoma. Ann Intern Med. 106:361-368; 1987.

139. Glick, J.H.; Barnes, J.M.; Ezdinli, E.Z.; *et al.* Nodular mixed lymphoma: results of a randomized trial failing to confirm prolonged disease-free survival with COPP chemotherapy. Blood. 58:920-925; 1981.

140. Gospodarowicz, M.; Bush, R.; Brown, T.; *et al.* Curability of gastrointestinal lymphoma with combined surgery and radiation . Int J Radiat Oncol Biol Phys. 9:3-9; 1983.

140a. Gribben, J.G.; Goldstone, A.H.; Linch, D.C.; *et al.* Effectiveness of high-dose combination chemotherapy and autologous bone marrow transplantation for patients with non-Hodgkin's lymphomas who are Still responsive to conventional-dose therapy. J Clin Oncol. 7:1621-1629; 1989.

140b. Grignani, F.; Dalla-Favera, R. Molecular biology of lymphoid malignancies. Current Opinion in Oncology. 1:4-9; 1989.

141. Gulati, S.C.; Shank, B.; Black, P.; *et al.* Autologous bone marrow transplantation for patients with poor-prognosis lymphoma. J Clin Oncol. 6:1303-1313; 1988.

142. Hanto, D.W.; Frizzera, G.; Gajl-Pecazlska, K.J.; Simmons, R.L. Epstein-Barr virus, immunodeficiency and B cell lympho-proliferation. Transplantation. 39:461-472; 1985.

142a. Haynes, B. Human T lymphocyte antigens as defined by monoclonal antibodies. Immunol Rev. 57:127-261; 1981.

143. Hoppe, R. The non-Hodgkin's lymphomas: pathology, staging, treatment. Curr Prob Cancer. 11(6):363-447; 1987.

144. Hoppe, R. The role of radiation therapy in the management of the non-Hodgkin's lymphomas. Cancer. 55:2176-2183; 1985.

145. Hoppe, R.; Burke, J.; Glatstein, E.; *et al.* Non-Hodgkin's lymphoma. Involvement of Waldeyer's ring. Cancer. 42:1096-1104; 1978.

146. Hoppe, R.; Kushlan, P.; Kaplan, H.; *et al.* The treatment of advanced stage favorable histology non-Hodgkin's lymphoma: a preliminary report of a randomized trial comparing single agent chemotherapy, combination chemotherapy, and whole body irradiation. Blood. 58:592-598; 1981.

146a. Horning, S.J.; Nademanee, A.P.; Chao, N.J.; *et al.* Regimen-related toxicity and early post-transplant survival in patients undergoing autologous bone marrow transplantation (ABMT) for lymphoma: Combined experience of Stanford University and the City of Hope National Medical Center. Proc Am Soc Clin Oncol. 9:271; 1990. Abstract.

147. Hours, S.; Blave, A.; Holmes, F.F.; *et al.* Agricultural herbicide use and risk of lymphoma and soft tissue sarcoma. JAMA. 256:1141-1147; 1986.

148. Hubbard, S.; Chabner, B.; DeVita, V.; *et al.* Histologic progression in non-Hodgkin's lymphoma. Blood 59:258-264; 1982.

148a. Iverson, U.; Iverson, O.; Ziegler, J.; *et al.* Cell kinetics of African cases of Burkitt's lymphoma. A preliminary report. Eur J Cancer. 8:305-310; 1972.

149. Jacobs, C.; Hoppe, R. Non-Hodgkin's lymphomas of head and neck extranodal sites. Int J Radiat Oncol Biol Phys. 11:357-364; 1985.

150. Jones, S.E.; Grozea, P.N.; Miller, T.P.; *et al.* Chemotherapy with cyclophosphamide, doxorubicin, vincristine and prednisone alone or with levamisole plus BCG for malignant lymphoma: a Southwest Oncology Group study. J Clin Oncol. 1:1318-1324; 1985.

150a. Jones, S.E.; Miller, T.P.; Connors, J.M. Long-term follow-up and analysis for prognostic factors for patients with limited-stage diffuse large-cell lymphoma treated with initial chemotherapy with or without adjuvant radiotherapy. J Clin Oncol. 7:1186-1191; 1990.

151. Jones, S.E.; Rosenberg, S.A.; Kaplan, H.S.; *et al.* Non-Hodgkin's lymphoma. IV. Clinicopathologic correlation in 405 cases. Cancer. 31:806-823; 1973.

152. Kalyanaraman, V.S.; Sarngadharan, M.G.; Nakao, Y.; *et al.* Natural antibodies to the structural core protein (p 24) of the human T cell leukaemia (lymphoma) retrovirus found in sera of leukaemia patients in Japan. Proc Natl Acad Sci. U.S.A. 79:1653-1657; 1982.

153. Klimo, P.; Connors, J.M. MACOP-B chemotherapy for the treatment of diffuse large cell lymphoma. Ann Intern Med. 102:596-602; 1985.

154. Knowles, D.M.; Chamulak, G.A.; Subar, M.; *et al.* Lymphoid neoplasia associated with acquired immunodeficiency syndrome (AIDS). Ann Intern Med. 108:744-753; 1988.

155. Krikorian, J.G.; Portlock, C.S.; Cooney, D.P.; *et al.* Spontaneous regression of non-Hodgkin's lymphoma: a report on nine cases. Cancer. 46:2093-2099; 1980.

155 . Kurtzberg, J.; Graham, M.L. Non-Hodgkin's lymphoma: Biologic classification and implication of therapy. Ped Clin N Am. 38(2):443-456; 1991.

155a. Kwak, L.W.; Halpern, J.; Olshen, R.A.; Horning, S.J. Prognostic significance of actual dose intensity in diffuse large-cell lymphoma: results of a tree-structured survival analysis. J Clin Oncol. 8:963-977; 1990.

156. Leder, P.; Battey, J.; Lenovi, G.; *et al.* Translocations among antibody genes in human cancer. Science. 222:765-771; 1983.

157. Lee, R.; Cabanillas, F.; Bodey, G.P.; Fredreich, E.J. A ten-year update of CHOP-bleo in the treatment of diffuse large cell lymphoma. J Clin Oncol. 4:1455-1461; 1986.

158. Levine, E.G.; Arthur, D.C.; Frissera, G.; *et al.* Cytogenetic abnormalities predict clinical outcome in non-Hodgkin's lymphoma. Ann. Intern. Med. 108:14-20; 1988.

159. List, A.; Greer, J.; Cousar, J.; *et al.* Non-Hodgkin's lymphoma of the gastrointestinal tract: an analysis of clinical and pathologic features affecting outcome. J Cin Oncol. 6:1125-1133; 1988.

160. List, A.F.; Greco, A.; Vogler, B. Lymphoproliferative diseases in immunocompromised hosts: the role of Epstein-Barr virus. J Clin Oncol. 5:1673-1689; 1987.

161. Longo, D.L. Chemotherapy for advanced aggressive lymphoma: more is better...isn't it? J Clin Oncol. 8:952-955; 1990.

162. Longo, D.L.; Young, R.C.; Hubbard, S.M.; *et al.* Prolonged initial remission in patients with nodular mixed lymphomas. Ann Intern Med. 100:651-656; 1984.

163. Lopez, T.M.; Hagemeister, F.B.; McLaughlin, P.; *et al.* Small noncleaved cell lymphoma in adults: superior results for stages I-III disease. J Clin Oncol. 8:615-622; 1990.

164. Lukes, R.J.; Collins, R.D. Immunologic characterization of human malignant lymphoma. Cancer. 34:1488-1503; 1974.

165. Mann, R.B.; Jaffe, E.S.; Berard, C.W. Malignant lymphomas: a conceptual understanding of morphologic diversity. Am J Pathol. 94:1-3; 1979.

166. McLaughlin, P.; Fuller, L.; Velasquez, W.; *et al.* Stage I-II follicular lymphoma: treatment results for 76 patients. Cancer. 58:1596-1602; 1986.

167. McLaughlin, P.; Fuller, L.; Velasquez, W.; *et al.* Stage III follicualr lymphoma: durable remissions with a combined chemotheray-radiotherapy regimen. J Clin Oncol. 5:867-874; 1987.

168. Magrath, I. Malignant non-Hodgkin's lymphomas. In: Pizzo, P., Poplack, D. (eds). Principles and Practice of Pediatric Oncology. JB Lippincott Co., Philadelphia, PA: 1988:415-455.

169. Maor, M.; Maddux, B.; Osborne, B.; *et al.* Stages IE and IIE non-Hodgkin's lymphomas of the stomach: comparison of treatment modalities. Cancer. 54:2330-2337; 1984.

170. Mauch, P.; Leonard, R.; Skarin, A.; *et al.* Improved survival following combined radiation therapy and chemotherapy for unfavorable prognosis stage I and II, non-Hodgkin's lymphoma. J Clin Oncol. 3:1301-1308; 1985.

171. Miller, T.P.; Jones, S.E. Initial chemotherapy for clinically localized lymphomas of unfavorable histology. Blood. 62:413-418; 1983.

171a. Murphy, S.; Melvin, S.; Mauer, A. *et al.* Correlation of tumor cell kinetic studies with surface marker results in childhood non-Hodgkin's lymphoma. Cancer Res. 39:1534-1538; 1979.

172. National Cancer Institute Non-Hodgkin's Classification Project

Writing Committee. Classification of non-Hodgkin's lymphomas: reproducibility of major classification systems. Cancer. 55:91-95; 1985.

173. National Cancer Institute sponsored study of classifications of non-Hodgkin's lymphomas. Cancer. 49:2112-2135; 1982.

174. Neuwelt, E.; Frenkel, E.; Gumerlock, M.; et al. Developments in the diagnosis and treatment of primary CNS lymphoma. Cancer. 58:1609-1620; 1986.

175. Nissen, N.I.; Ersboll, J.; Hansen, H.S.; et al. A randomized study of radiotherapy versus radiotherapy plus chemotherapy in stage I and II non-Hodgkin's lymphoma. Cancer. 52:1-7; 1983.

176. O'Connell, M.; Harrington, D.; Earle, J.; et al. Chemotherapy followed by consolidation radiation therapy for the treatment of clinical stage II aggressive histologic type non-Hodgkin's lymphoma. Cancer. 61:1754-1758; 1988.

177. Ostrowski, M.; Unni, K.; Banks, P.; et al. Malignant lymphoma of bone. Cancer. 58:2646-2655; 1986.

178. Paryani, S.; Hoppe, R.; Burke, J.; et al. Extralymphatic involvement in diffuse non-Hodgkin's lymphoma. J Clin Oncol. 1:682-688; 1983.

179. Paryani, S.; Hoppe, R.; Cox, R.; et al. Analysis of non-Hodgkin's lymphomas with nodular and favorable histologies, stages I and II. Cancer. 52:2300-2307; 1983.

180. Paryani, S.; Hoppe, R.; Cox, R.; et al. The role of radiation theray in the management of stage III follicular lymphomas. J Clin Oncol. 2:841-848; 1984.

180a. Pellici, P-G.; Knowles, D.; Macgrath, I. et al. Chromosomal breakpoints and structural alterations of the c-myc locus differ in endemic sporadic forms of Burkitt lymphoma. Proc Natl Acad Sci USA. 83:2984; 1986.

181. Penn, I. Tumors of the immunocompromised patients. Ann Rev Med. 39:63-73; 1988.

181a. Peterson, B.A.; Anderson, J.R.; Frizzera, G.; et al. Combination chemotherapy prolongs survival in follicular mixed lymphoma (FML). Proc Am Soc Clin Oncol. 9:259; 1990. Abstract.

182. Portlock, C.S. Non-Hodgkin's lymphomas. Advances in diagnosis, staging and management. Cancer. 65(suppl):718-722; 1990.

182a. Portlock, C.S.; Rosenberg, S.A. No initial therapy for stage III and IV non-Hodgkin's lymphomas of favorable histologic types. Ann Intern Med. 90:10-13; 1979.

183. Prestidge, B.; Horning, S.; Hoppe, R. Combined modality therapy for stage I-II large cell lymphoma. Int J Radiat Biol Phys. 15:633-639; 1988.

184. Proceedings of the Conference on non-Hodgkin's Lymphoma. Cancer Treat Rep. 61; 1977.

185. Rappaport, H. Tumors of the hematopoietic system. In: Atlas of tumor pathology, section III, fascicle VIII. Washington, DC: Armed Forces Institute of Pathology; 1966.

186. Rosenberg, S.A. Current concepts in cancer. Non-Hodgkin's lymphoma—selection of treatment on the basis of histologic type. N Engl J Med. 301:924-928; 1979.

187. Rowley, J.D. The biological implications of consistent chromosome rearrangements. Cancer Res. 44:3159-3169; 1984.

187a. Sandlund, J.; Kiwanuka, J.; Marti, G.; et al. Characterization of Burkitt's lymphoma cell lines with monoclonal antibodies using an ELISA technique. In: Reinherz, E., Hayes, B., Nadler, L., Berstein, I. (eds). Leukocyte Typing. vol. 2. Proceedings of the 2nd International Congress of Human Leukocyte Antigens, New York, NY: Springer-Verlag; 1986:403-410.

188. Shepherd, F.; Evans, W.; Kutas, G.; et al. Chemotherapy following surgery for stages IE and IIE non-Hodgkin's lymphoma of the gastrointesinal tract. J Clin Oncol. 6:253-260; 1988.

188a. Shipp, M.A.; Yeap, B.Y.; Harrington, D.P.; et al. The m-BACOD combination chemotherapy regimen in large-cell lymphoma: analysis of the completed trial and comparison with the M-BACOD regimen. J Clin Oncol. 8:84-93; 1990.

189. Siminovitch, K.A.; Jensen, J.P.; Epstein, A.L.; Korsmeyer, S.J. Immunoglobulin gene rearrangements and expression in diffuse histiocytic lymphomas reveal cellular lineage, molecular defects and sites of chromosomal translocation. Blood. 67:391-397; 1986.

190. Simon, R.; Durreleman, S.; Hoppe, R.T.; et al. The non-Hodgkin's Lymphoma Pathologic Classification Project. Long-term follow-up of 1,153 patients with non-Hodgkin's lymphoma. Ann Intern Med. 109:939-943; 1988.

191. Skarin, A.T. Diffuse aggressive lymphomas: a curable subset of non-Hodgkin's lymphomas. Semin Oncol. 13(suppl. 5):10-25; 1986.

192. Skipp, N.A.; Harrington, D.P.; Klar, M.M.; et al. Identification of major prognostic subgroups of patients with large cell lymphoma treated with M-BACOD or M-BACOD. Ann Intern Med. 104:757-765; 1986.

192a. Soubeyran, P.; Eghbali, H.; Bonichon, F.; et al. Follicular lymphomas. Prognostic and survival in a retrospective series of 281 patients. Proc Am Soc Clin Oncol. 9:263; 1990.

193. Sullivan, J.L.; Medveczky, P.; Forman, S.J.; et al. Epstein-Barr virus induced lymphoproliferation, implication for antiviral chemotherapy. N Engl J Med. 311:1163-1167; 1984.

194. Sutcliffe, S.; Gospodarowicz, M.; Bush, R.; et al. Role of radiation therapy in localized non-Hodgkin's lymphoma. Radiother Oncol. 4:211-223; 1985.

195. Tubiana, M.; Carde, P.; Burgers, J.; et al. Progostic factors in non-Hodgkin's lymphoma. Int J Radiat Oncol Biol Phys. 12:503-514; 1986.

196. Tupchong, L.; Hughes, F.; Harmer, C. Primary lymphoma of the thyroid: clinical features, prognostic factors, and results of treatment. Int J Radiat Oncol Biol Phys. 12:1813-1821; 1986.

197. Vokes, E.; Ultmann, J.; Golomb, H.; et al. Long-term survival of patients with localized diffuse histiocytic lymphoma. J Clin Oncol. 3:1309-1317; 1985.

198. Wang, D.S.; Fuller, L.M.; Butler, J.J.; et al. Extranodal non-Hodgkin's lymphomas of the head and neck. Am J Roentgenol. 123:471-481; 1975.

198a. Wasserman, T.H.; Glatstein, E. Non-Hodgkin's lymphomas. In: Perez, C.A., Brady, L.W. (eds). Principles and Practice of Radiation Oncology, 2nd ed. Philadelphia, PA: JB Lippincott Co; 1992:1329-1344.

199. Weiss, J.W.; Winter, M.W.; Phylikly, R.L.; Banks, P.M. Peripheral T cell lymphomas: histologic, immunohistologic and clonical characterization. Mayo Clin Proc. 61:411-426; 1986.

200. Weiss, L.; Warnke, R.; Sklar, J.; et al. Molecular analysis of the t(14;18) chromosomal translocation in malignant lymphomas. N Engl J Med. 317:1185; 1987.

200a. Weiss, L.M.; Strickler, J.G.; Dorfman, R.F.; et al. Clonal T cell populations in angioimmunoblastic lymphadenopathy and angio-immunoblastic lymphadenopathy-like lymphoma. Am J Pathol. 122:392-397; 1986.

200b. Yunis, J.; Oken, M.; Kaplan, M. et al. Distinctive chromosomal abnormalities in histologic subtypes of non-Hodgkin's lymphoma. N Engl J Med. 307:1231; 1982.

Multiple Myeloma

201. Alexanian, R.; Hart, A.; Khan, A.V.; et al. Treatment for multiple myeloma. JAMA. 208:2680-1685; 1969.

202. American Cancer Society. Cancer statistics. CA. 41:28; 1991.

203. Barlogie, B.; Alexanian, R.; Dicke, K.; et al. High-dose chemotheray and autologous bone marrow transplantation for resistant multiple myeloma. Blood. 70:869-873; 1987.

204. Barlogie, B.; Epstein, J.; Selvanayagam, P.; Alexanian, R. Plasma cell myeloma-new biological insights and advances in therapy. Blood. 73:865-879; 1989.

205. Bergsagel, D.E.; Rider, W.D. Plasma cell neoplasm. In: DeVita, V.T.; Hellman, S.; Rosenberg, S.A., (eds). Cancer: Principles and Practices of Oncology. Philadelphia, PA: JB Lippincott Co; 1985:1753-1786.

206. Case, D.C.; Lee, B.J.; Clarkson, B.D. Improved survival times in multiple myeloma treated with melphalan, prednisone, cyclophosphamide, vincristine and BCNU: M2 protocol. Am J Med. 63:897-903; 1977.

206a. Chak, L.Y.; Cox, S.; Bostwick, D.G. Hoppe, R.T. Solitary plasmacytoma of bone: treatment, progression, and survival. J Clin Oncol. 5: 1811-1815; 1987.

207. Coleman, M.; Saletan, S.; Wolf, D.; et al. Whole bone marrow irradiation for the treatment of multiple myeloma. Cancer. 49:1328; 1982.

208. Durie, B.M. Staging and kinetics of multiple myeloma. Semin Oncol. 13:300-309; 1986.

208a. Durie, B.G.M.; Dixon, B.; Carter, S.; et al. Improved survival duration with combination chemotherapy induction for multiple myeloma: A Southwest Oncology Group study. J Clin Oncol. 4:1127-1237; 1986.

209. Forden, D.S. Phase I study of intravenous gammaglobulin in multiple myeloma. Am J Med. 76:111-116; 1984.

210. Gahrton, G.; Tura, S.; Flesch, M.; et al. Bone marrow transplan-

tation in multple myeloma: report from the European Cooperation Group for bone marrow transplantation. Blood. 69:1262-1264; 1987.

211. Jacobson, D.R.; Zolla-Pazner, S. Immunosuppression and infection in multiple myeloma. Semin Oncol. 13:282-290; 1986.

212. Jaffe, J.P.; Bosch, A.; Raich, P.C. Sequential hemi-body radiotherapy in advanced multiple myeloma. Cancer. 43:124-128; 1979.

213. Klein, G.; Klein, E. Mye/1g juxtaposition by chromosomal translocation: Some new insights, puzzles, and paradoxes. Immunol Today. 6:208; 1985.

213a. Kyle, R.A. Multiple myeloma: therapeutic approaches in 1990. Am Soc Clin Oncol Educational Booklet. 1990:167-188.

214. Mendenhall, C.; Thar, T.; Million, R. Solitary plamacytoma of bone and soft tissue. Int J Radiat Oncol Biol Phys. 6:1497; 1980.

215. Mill, W.; Wasserman, T. Multiple myeloma and plasmacytomas. In: Perez, C.; Brady, L., (eds). Principles and Practice of Radiation Oncology. Philadelphia, PA: JB Lippincott Co; 1987:1086-1100.

216. Mill, W.; Griffith, R. The role of radiation therapy in the management of plasma cell tumors. Cancer. 45:647-652; 1980.

217. Mundy, G.R.; Bertoline, D.R. Bone destruction and hypercalcemia in plasma cell myeloma. Semin Oncol. 13:291-299; 1986.

218. Okrn, M.M.; Kyle, R.A.; Griepp, P.R.; et al. Alteranting cycles of VBMCO with interferon (INF 2) in treatment of multiple myeloma Proc Am Soc Clin Oncol. 7:225; 1988.Abstract.

219. Olson, J.P. Multiple myeloma and related disorders. In: Rosenthal, S.; Carignan, J.; Smith, B.D., (eds). Medical care of the cancer patient. Philadelphia, PA: WB Saunders Co; 1987:163-173.

220. Potter, M. Plasmacytomas in mice. Semin Oncol. 13:275-281; 1986.

220a. Salmon, S.E.; Cassady, R.J. Plasma Cell Neoplasms. In: DeVita, V.T., Jr, Hellman, S., Rosenberg, S.A. (eds). Cancer Principles and Practice of Oncology. Philadephia, PA: JB Lippincott Co.; 1989.

221. Salmon, S.E.; Hart, A.; Bonnet, J.D.; et al. Alternating combination chemotherapy and levamisole improves survival in multiple myeloma. A Southwest Oncology Group study. J Clin Oncol. 1:453-461; 1983.

222. Sporn, V.; McIntyre, O.R. Chemotherapy of previously untreated multiple myeloma patients. An analysis of recent treatment results. Semin Oncol. 13:318-325; 1986.

223. Tomas, R.; Daban, A.; Bontoux, D. Double hemibody irradiation in chemotherapy resistant multiple myeloma. Cancer Treat Rep. 68:1173; 1984.

223'. Wasserman, T.H. Multiple myeloma and plasmacytomas. In: Perez, C.A., Brady, L.W. (eds). Principles and Practice of Radiation Oncology, 2nd ed. Philadelphia, PA: JB Lippincott Co.; 1992:1345-1355.

223a. Wiltshaw, E. The natural history of extramedullary plasmacytoma and its relation to solitary myeloma of bone and myelomatosis. Medicine. 55:217-238; 1976.

Cindy L. Schwartz, M.D., Pediatric Oncology   Louis S. Constine III, M.D., Radiation Oncology
Thomas C. Putnam, M.D., Pediatric Surgery   Harvey J. Cohen, M.D., Pediatric Oncology

Chapter 19

PEDIATRIC SOLID TUMORS

We can say with some assurance that although children may be the victims of fate, they will not be the victims of our neglect.

John F. Kennedy (7a)

PERSPECTIVE

The study of childhood cancer has resulted in both a greater understanding of the neoplastic process and a paradigm for the therapy of responsive cancers. Investigations into the biology of childhood cancer have resulted in the identification of certain genes associated with malignant processes and others that are associated with prognosis and stage. In addition, we have learned that certain chromosomal abnormalities can predispose an individual to specific forms of cancer. The treatment of childhood solid tumors has progressed over the past 20 years so as to better use the modalities of surgery, radiation therapy, and chemotherapy, intertwined for maximum efficacy and minimum toxicity (Fig. 19-1). The appropriate use of these modalities has resulted in an improved outlook for a child diagnosed with a solid tumor, so that approximately two-thirds of such children will survive their disease (Table 19-1) (7,8). The current issues facing pediatric oncology include identifying the high-risk patients, optimizing therapeutic:toxic ratios of the modalities we use, and investigating and minimizing the long-term effects of the diseases and their therapies.

General Introduction to Pediatric Tumors

Epidemiologic Characteristics

Neoplastic diseases are second only to accidents as a cause of death in children. The relative incidence of childhood malignancies is noted in Table 19-1. Over half of all childhood malignancies are of the solid tumor variety (2).

Biology

Advances in the field of genetics and molecular biology have dramatically increased our understanding of malignancy, particularly of childhood tumors. Knudson hypothesized that certain pediatric tumors (retinoblastoma, Wilms') could develop only if two independent mutations occurred in a single cell (3b). This "two hit" theory suggested that germinal mutations predispose to hereditable tumors since only the "second hit" is necessary for tumor development. Specific chromosomal loci that predispose to these tumors have been defined (13q14 for retinoblastoma and 11p13 for Wilms'). The nonhereditable tumors require two post-zygotic mutations and hence are less likely to be bilateral. The theory of Knudson paved the way for the concept of multiple step mutagenesis that explains common adult forms of carcinoma (e.g., colon carcinoma).

The recognition that cancer is related to genetic abnormalities and the current ability to study genetic material at the molecular level has led to the determination of genetic rearrangements that play a role in oncogenesis. Rearrangements may result in oncogene activation or loss of tumor suppression genes. Specific genetic alterations have been recognized as noted in Table 19-2b. Other genetic markers have been found (e.g., amplification of n-myc in neuroblastoma) that predict for a poor prognosis. Resistance to drug therapy has been found to be related to the expression of the mdr-1 oncogene in pediatric malignancies (1a). Understanding of such genetic alterations in cancer cells may lead to the development of therapeutic modalities that will facilitate cure by directly affecting the genetic abnormality.

Etiology

Dramatic advanced in the understanding of childhood tumors has resulted from progress in cellular biology, particularly recombinant DNA technology (4) (Table 19-2a [3a]). These include the elucidation of genetic events, e.g., the location of oncogenes near structural genetic rearrangements, mechanisms by which proto-oncogenes might be activated, and specific chromosomal (recessive) alterations in some pediatric malignancies, such as 13q14 for retinoblastoma and osteogenic sarcomas, and 11p13 for Wilm's tumor. (Tables 19-2b [3a]).

Therapeutic Advances: Optimization of Multimodal Treatment

Initial advances in the treatment of childhood malignancies were due to the addition of one modality to another sequentially. Radical surgery was followed by regional radiation treatment of the tumor bed and nodes and the use of cyclic chemotherapy in multi-drug combinations for occult disseminated disease. The efficacy of the cytotoxic therapies allowed for the use of more conservative surgical procedures. A steady reduction in radiation field size and dose has become standard practice in Hodgkin's disease and childhood solid tumors. For some drug sensitive tumors (e.g., non-Hodgkin's lymphomas, neuroblastoma, germ cell tumors), it became possible to rely on chemotherapy for the treatment of residual disease. In some settings, the duration of chemotherapy can be reduced (e.g., stage I Wilms' tumor can be treated in only 24 weeks). For those tumors in which long-

251

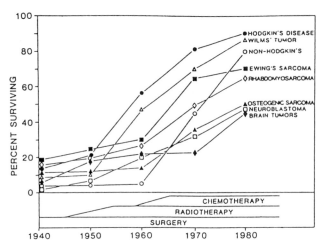

Fig. 19-1. Improvement in 2-year survival rates of the principle tumors of children.

term survival can be achieved in the majority of patients, protocol investigations can attempt to minimize toxicity (23,24).

In the past decade, cure rates have continued to increase as a result of the survival of patients with more advanced or aggressive disease. In some instances this is a result of newer chemotherapeutic agents (cisplatin, etoposide), but more often it is a result of more accurate staging of disease and the use of dose intensive regimens (including bone marrow transplantation). Advances in other disciplines (particularly radiology, infectious disease, blood banking and surgery) have helped make this possible.

Essential Advances in Other Disciplines

Radiology

The revolution in imaging procedures has allowed for greater accuracy in clinical staging and improved correlations with surgical pathologic evaluations. The impact of noninvasive methods preceding and directing the surgical and radiotherapeutic attack is critical to the design of clinical trials. Ultrasound, a nonionizing mode of imaging, is readily available and is particularly effective in detecting abdominal or soft tissue masses. Computed tomography (CT) and magnetic resonance imaging (MRI) allow for more accurate determination of tumor extent. These modalities have the advantage of three-dimensional plain displays. In the future, MR spectroscopy may add biochemical information that could be helpful.

Supportive Care

In the past 15 years, the ability to use chemotherapy and radiation in a dose-intensive manner have depended on being able to support the patient through periods of marrow aplasia. The development and empiric use of broad spectrum antibiotics has facilitated the delivery of cytotoxic agents in ways that would not have been conceivable two decades ago (bone marrow transplantation, dose-intensive regimens).

Hematopoietic colony-stimulating factors that decrease the duration of myelosuppression after chemotherapy are now being incorporated in treatment regimens. A new era is beginning in which the maximal tolerated doses for many myelosuppressive agents will rise, hopefully increasing the cure rates.

Advances in transfusion medicine have also been essential in this era of intensive chemotherapeutic regimens. Blood

Table 19-1. Pediatric Malignancies: Magnitude of the Problem

Type	1985 Estimated			Trends in Survival for children under 15 Relative 5-Year Survival Rates (%)				
				Year of Diagnosis				
	New Cases	Deaths	New Cases (%) Distribution	1960-63 [1]	1970-73 [1]	1974-76 [2]	1977-79 [2]	1980-85 [2]
All Sites	6550	2175	21	28	45	55.0	61.2	65.2 *
Acute lymphocytic leukemia	2000	850	6	4	34	53.0	68.6	70.7 *
Acute myeloid leukemia				3	5	16.1	24.5 †	23.2 †
Wilms' tumor	410	75	6	33	70	74.1	80.1	80.9
Brain and nervous system	1230	550	19	35	45	54.5	55.5	57.0
Neuroblastoma	525	250	8	25	40	48.4	49.7	55.4
Bone	320	85	5	20	30	51.9 †	47.3 †	50.8 †
Hodgkin's disease			6	52	80	80.4	84.5	89.3 *
Non-Hodgkin's lymphomas	780	160	8	18	26	42.3	49.6	64.2 *

[1] Rates are based on Surveillance, Epidemiology and End Results (SEER) data from a series of hospital registries and one population-based registry.

[2] Rates are from the SEER program. They are based on data from population-based registries in Conn, New Mexico, Utah, Iowa, Hawaii, Atlanta, Detroit, Seattle-Puget Sound, and San Francisco-Oakland. Rates are based on follow-up of patients through 1986.

* The difference in rates between 1974-1976 and 1980-1985 is statistically significant ($P<0.05$).

† The standard error of the survival is between 5 and 10 percentage points.

Adapted from Silverberg (7) and Young (8).

Table 19-2. Genetics of Pediatric Malignancies

a. Oncogenes Located near Structural Genetic Rearrangements in Selected Pediatric Malignancies

Oncogene	Genetic Rearrangement	Tumor
c-myc	t(8;14) (q24;q32)	Burkitt's lymphoma
abl, bcr	t(9;22) (q34;q11)	Chronic myelogenous leukemia
N-myc	DMs, HSRs	Neuroblastoma
rel	t(2;11) (q37;q14)	Rhabdomyosarcoma
ets	t(11;22) (q24;q12)	Ewing's sarcoma, Neuroepitheliomas

b. Pediatric Malignancies with Recognized Recessive Genetic Alterations

Tumor	Chromosomal Alterations
Retinoblastoma	13q14
Osteosarcoma	13q14
Wilms' tumor	11p13
Embryonal tumors of Beckwith-Wiedemann syndrome	11p
Acoustic neuroma and meningioma	22
Meningioma	22

Adapted from Israel (3a).

products are now relatively free from infections (e.g., hepatitis A and B, cytomegalovirus, HIV). Platelet products are available virtually on demand and can be HLA matched in instances of alloimmunization. Neutrophils may be lifesaving in the setting of sepsis that is unresponsive to antibiotics.

The administration of multiple chemotherapeutic agents, antibiotics, transfusions, and nutritional support is possible only now that venous access can be assured with the use of tunnelled central venous catheters.

Late Effects and Toxicities Following Multimodal Treatment (Tables 19-3 and 19-4)

Multimodality therapy results in significant toxicity, both acute and long term. Toxicities of radiation therapy may be intensified by the use of chemotherapy and vice versa. The addition of chemotherapy may lead to heightened reactions within the radiation field, referred to as a recall phenomenon, but which actually represents independent but additive injury to normal tissue cells. For example, actinomycin D can cause a skin reaction that outlines the original radiation field months and even years later (23). A hypothesis on pediatric radiosensitivity and chemosensitivity of normal tissue and organs has been proposed by Rubin *et al.* (6). The successful use of multimodality therapy has resulted in a large contingent of long-term survivors. They need to be followed closely for late effects (Tables 19-3 and 19-4).

*Radiation therapy :*The chronic sequelae of radiation include retardation of bone and cartilage growth, intellectual impairments, myelosuppression, nephropathy, hepatopathy, and pneumonitis Table 19-4).

Chemotherapy may cause such late effects as infertility and late cardiac decompensation after anthracyclines. Late effects in other organs such as lung (after bleomycin) and kidney (after cisplatinum) are being actively studied (Table 19-3).

Combined-modality therapy has resulted in enhancement of many of the above complications, particularly encephalopathies, pneumonitis, pulmonary fibrosis, cardiomyopathies, hepatopathies, and myelosuppression.

Table 19-3. Long-Term Side Effects of Chemotherapy

Drugs	Potential Organ Damage
Antracyclines Doxorubicin	Cardiac — myocardial damage congestive failure arrhythmias
Bleomycin	Lungs — fibrosis, impaired diffusion capacity, exacerbated by increased O_2 (e.g., anesthesia)
Cyclophosphamide, Isofosphamide	Gonadal Damage — infertility, sterility, early menopause Bladder — hemorrhagic cystitis, bladder cancer Marrow — secondary AML
CCNU/BCNU	Gonadal, lungs
Cisplatinum	Kidney — decreased glomerular filtration rate Ears — hearing loss (high frequency)
Methotrexate	Liver dysfunction CNS — learning impairment (high dose IV)
6-Mercaptopurine 6-Thioguanine Actinomycin-D	Liver dysfunction
Steroids	obesity, cataracts, osteoporosis
Epidophyllotoxins	peripheral neuropathy, secondary leukemia

Table 19-4. Long-Term Effects of Radiation

Irradiated Area	Risks
Cranium and Nasopharynx	Cataracts Growth — impaired Central Nervous System — learning impairment Dentition — abnormal formation High dose (> 2500) Hypothalamic dysfunction (decreased growth hormone) (decreased gonadotropins, thyroid stimulating hormones, hyperprolactinemia) Hearing (especially w/cisplatinum)
Neck and Mandible	Hypoplasia of bone/soft tissues Dentition — abnormal formation — abnormal salivary function Thyroid — overt or compensated hypothyroidism
Thorax	Hypoplasia (includes impaired chest wall growth) Lungs — fibrosis, decreased capacity Cardiac — pericardial and valvular thickening Breasts — impaired growth, ? increased malignancy
Abdomen/Pelvis	Hypoplasia (including scoliosis) Liver (if in field) Kidneys (if in field) Gonads (if in field) Gastrointestinal tract
Extremities	Hypoplasia

Second malignancies, including leukemias and sarcomas, are of great concern and may be more often attributable to combined modality therapy than to chemotherapy or radiotherapy in isolation. Genetic predispositions for malignancy are relevant in some instances.

Psychosocial Aspects

Psychosocial aspects critical to pediatric oncology include impact of the disease, and treatments and their sequelae, not only on the child, but on the entire family. Since the majority of children will be cured, an emphasis on maintaining appropriate school achievement, discipline, behavior, and socialization should be stressed. Parental concerns regarding their role in the occurrence of cancer should be allayed in most instances, since childhood cancers are not related to parenting styles (ie diet, environment). Families with potentially inherited malignancies should receive genetic counselling. The ethical rights of the child patient (3) and the impact of cancer on the family, particularly siblings, need special attention (14).

NEUROBLASTOMA

Neuroblastoma (NB) originates from the neural crest cells that normally give rise to the sympathetic nervous system. It is a tumor that has given us insights into the biologic processes of malignancy. Patients older than 1 year of age with disseminated disease are rarely cured with aggressive use of known active agents, while infants sometimes experience spontaneous tumor regression. The tumor may also spontaneously mature to a benign ganglioneuroma. If we could learn the mechanisms by which regression and maturation occur in malignancies, we might be better able to treat most cancer.

EPIDEMIOLOGY AND ETIOLOGY

Epidemiology

Neuroblastoma is the most common malignancy of infants, accounting for half of infantile cancer (23). Two-thirds of patients with NB are under 5 years of age. Overall, NB occurs in approximately 8.7 white children and 7.4 black children per million in the United States each year (7% of all children with cancer) (59). Fifteen percent of childhood cancer mortality is due to NB.

Etiology

The high incidence of NB in early infancy suggests that its development may be related to abnormal maturation of fetal neural crest cells. Of interest is the finding of microscopic nodules of adrenal NB in infants less than 3 months of age who have died of nontumor related causes (11).

Genetics

Rarely, families have been reported in which NB has occurred in multiple siblings, or occasionally in multiple generations of a family. In one family, four of five siblings had NB. Their mother had a mediastinal mass and an elevated catecholamine level (17). In another family, the parents of a child with NB each had had a child with NB in a previous marriage. In addition, the father's grandchild (of an unaffected son) was found to have NB (34,48). Knudson and Strong (41) have proposed that 2% to 25% of NB arises in patients with a prezygotic germinal mutation similar to the mechanism described for familial retinoblastoma.

Neuroblastoma has been reported to occur with an increased incidence in patients with fetal hydantoin syndrome, von Recklinghausen's disease, Beckwith-Wiedemann syndrome, and Hirschsprung's disease.

Molecular Biology

Cytogenetic abnormalities have been demonstrated in the tumor cells of many patients with NB (15). A deletion or rearrangement of the short arm of chromosome 1 is found most commonly, but is not specific for NB.

Homogeneous staining regions are long nonbanding regions of metaphase chromosomes that stain homogeneously with trypsin-Giemsa. Double minute chromosomes are small paired chromatin bodies of varying size and number. Either may be seen in NB cells and cell lines. It is thought that double minute chromosomes result from the breakdown of homogeneous staining regions. Both forms of chromatin contain regions of amplified chromosomal DNA. Cell line studies have revealed that HSR contain amplified N-myc sequences. Amplified N-myc oncogene occurs more commonly in patients with advanced stage disease. The degree of amplification appears to be an intrinsic biologic property of a given NB, which is consistent from the time of diagnosis through periods of progressive disease (14).

The DNA content of NB tumor cells appears to be of prognostic importance. Flow cytometry has been used to determine whether NB cells are pseudodiploid, diploid, or hyperdiploid. For patients with disseminated disease, pseudodiploidy and diploidy have been associated with N-myc amplification and poor response to cyclophosphamide and doxorubicin therapy (39,45). Hyperdiploidy has been associated with early stage disease and good prognosis (24,44).

To date, molecular biology has been a research tool, used to better understand the factors associated with the biologic behavior of these tumors. In the near future, studies of the molecular biology of a given tumor may play an important role in the therapy chosen.

Biological Markers

Eighty-five percent to 90% of patients with NB excrete abnormally high levels of catecholamines (25,44,57). Vanillylmandelic acid (VMA) and homovanillic acid (HVA) are commonly measured. While their absolute values are not of prognostic significance, a higher VMA:HVA ratio suggests a better prognosis for patients with disseminated disease. Although a 24-hour urine collection for catecholamines is most accurate, a single urine collection can be evaluated by comparing the ratio of catecholamine:creatinine present in a sample (38). Rapid tests for VMA have been used to follow patients with VMA-secreting tumors (25,44). Urinary levels of cystathionine are elevated in 50% to 80% of patients and may correlate with poor prognosis (24,27). Serum dopamine levels are also elevated in approximately 90% of patients (9).

An elevated serum level of neuron specific enolase (> 100 mg/mL) has been associated with poor prognosis (38,60). Elevated ferritin levels have been noted in approximately half of patients with advanced-stage NB and have also been associated with poor prognosis (28).

G_{D2} ganglioside is present on the surface of NB cells and is shed into the circulation. This ganglioside is being investigated to determine whether serum levels have prognostic significance. In addition, monoclonal antibodies to this ganglioside may be used for diagnostic scanning (18,58).

Maturation/Immunology

Neuroblastoma has an amazing ability to spontaneously regress and mature. Spontaneous regression is noted most commonly in infants under 1 year of age. Microscopic residual tumor in these patients rarely results in recurrence. Malignant tumors may spontaneously mature into benign ganglioneuromas. Immunologic mechanisms and maturational processes have been hypothesized to explain these findings. Cell-and antibody-mediated cytotoxicity against NB cells has been demonstrated in patients and in their mothers (35). Neuroblasts may also differentiate and mature. In vitro, a variety of substances such as 5-trifluoromethyl-2-deoxyuridine and papaverine (both which increase cyclic adenosine monophosphate), retinoic acid, and bromodeoxyuridine induce maturation. The level of N-myc expression in NB tumor cells decreases following in vitro differentiation (37). N-myc may thus play an important role in regulating the differentiation of NB cells.

DETECTION AND DIAGNOSIS

Infants with localized NB often appear well, with a mass being the major presenting feature. Older children, however, often have metastatic disease, and may present with nonspecific complaints of fever, weight loss, general malaise, and fatigue. A reasonable rule is that a child older than 2 years of age with an abdominal mass who appears well is likely to have Wilms' tumor, while one who appears chronically ill is more likely to have NB.

Clinical Detection

1. The clinical presenting features of NB are dependent on the location of tumor. Neuroblastoma may arise anywhere along the sympathetic nervous system chain. The most common primary site of involvement is in an adrenal gland (40%).
2. Other sites of occurrence are in the paraspinal regions of the abdomen (25%), the thorax (15%), the neck (5%), and the pelvis at the organ of Zuckerkandl (5%).
3. An abdominal mass is frequently the first presenting sign of disease. Such a mass may be large, firm, irregular, and may cross the midline.
4. Thoracic masses may be detected by chest x-ray of a child with a persistent cough or respiratory distress. Cervical masses are often initially diagnosed as lymphadenitis. However, if Horner's syndrome or heterochromia iridis is noted, NB should be suspected.
5. Pelvic masses may cause disturbances of bowel or bladder function due to compression.
6. In some patients, the presenting symptoms are related to secretory products of the tumor. Intractable diarrhea due to secretion of a hormone called vasoactive intestinal polypeptide has been found in 7% to 9% of children with neural crest tumors, most frequently ganglioneuromas or ganglioneuroblastomas (51).
7. The syndrome of opsoclonus-myoclonus is an unusual presenting feature of NB. Patients have acute cerebellar ataxia and rapid, dancing, eye movements. Although these patients often have localized disease, they have a tendency for residual neurologic dysfunction, including recurrence of ataxia, mental retardation, and extrapyramidal deficits (12). The etiology of this syndrome is unclear, although an autoimmune factor, perhaps an antibody directed against NB, which cross-reacts with a cerebellar cell antigen, may cause this damage.
8. Neuroblastomas that arise in paravertebral ganglion have a tendency to grow into intervertebral foramena, forming a dumbbell-shaped mass. The intraspinal component may cause spinal cord compression, with paralysis, extremity weakness, or incontinence. Such a situation is an oncologic emergency that has often been treated by surgical decompression or radiation therapy, or more recently, by rapid institution of chemotherapy. Permanent paraplegia may result if this complication is not recognized early.
9. Many children with NB have metastatic disease at the time of diagnosis. In these children, the presenting features are commonly related to the metastatic tumor, rather than to the primary tumor.
   a. Infants may present with bluish skin nodules of NB. This has been reported to occur in 32% of neonatal patients (52). Catecholamines may be released when these nodules are palpated. This results initially in an erythematous flush that lasts for 2 to 3 minutes, followed by blanching due to vasoconstriction (29).
   b. The liver is a common site for metastatic NB in infancy. Rapid hepatic enlargement may result in marked abdominal distention, followed by respiratory compromise.
   c. Neuroblastoma may infiltrate the marrow cavity, causing pancytopenia and resulting complications, e.g., fevers, infection, pallor, lethargy, and bleeding.

d. Bone involvement may produce pain with or without palpable bone masses. Skeletal metastases are usually lytic and are often seen in the skull, orbit, and proximal long bones. Those patients with bone lesions of the orbit may present with a raccoon-like appearance secondary to proptosis and ecchymoses of the upper and lower eyelids.

e. Intracranial metastatic disease is usually meningeal (42). Intracerebral lesions are extremely rare. In infants, meningeal involvement may be manifested by separation of the cranial sutures.

Diagnosis

1. Evaluation of NB requires an examination of the area of primary disease as well as those areas to which NB is known to spread. In all instances of suspected NB, a 24-hour urine collection should be obtained if possible to assess catecholamine (VMA, HVA) secretion. If this is not feasible, as may be the case in infants, a urine collection may be analyzed for VMA:Cr and HVA:Cr ratios.

2. In addition to the chest x-ray, a CT scan of the abdomen, pelvis, and chest should be performed. Those patients with cervical masses should also have a CT scan of this area.

3. Paravertebral lesions have a propensity to extend into the intervertebral foramena, which may cause spinal cord compression. Therefore, any patient with a paravertebral lesion that appears to be approaching the spinal cord should be further evaluated for possible spinal cord compression. Myelogram has been commonly used, although MRI can also detect such lesions.

4. A skeletal survey and bone scan should be performed in all patients to detect bony lesions. Small lytic lesions at the end of long bones may be demonstrable on radiographic scan but not by bone scan (40). However, the bone scan may be more sensitive in finding lesions of the skull and tubular bones (36,55). In addition, a bone scan will reveal the primary tumor in as many as 60% of patients (54). It may be useful in this regard for those patients in whom the primary tumor is not easily localizable by CT scan.

5. Since the bone marrow is a common site of metastatic involvement, a bone marrow aspirate and biopsy should be performed in all patients with NB. Marrow involvement can, at times, be found when monoclonal antibodies to NB are used to detect tumor cells. The prognostic implications of finding marrow tumor cells in this way have not been studied in a prospective manner.

6. The liver should be examined by contrast CT scan or by a liver-spleen scan. The Pediatric Oncology Group is currently recommending a liver biopsy for those patients with abdominal disease.

CLASSIFICATION AND STAGING

Histopathology

Sympathoblasts are the neural crest cells from which NB arises and thus give rise to the sympathetic nervous system. These cells may also differentiate into paraganglionic cells from which pheochromocytomas and paragangliomas are derived. Neuroblastoma is composed of small round cells with scant cytoplasm and must be differentiated from similar cell tumors of childhood, such as rhabdomyosarcoma, lymphoma, leukemia, Ewings' sarcoma, and retinoblastoma.

Neuron specific enolase may be helpful in differentiating NB from other small round cell tumors which are not of neuroectodermal origin. Periodic acid-Schiff staining is usually positive in Ewing's sarcoma and rhabdomyosarcoma, but negative in NB. Lymphoid markers can be used to rule out a lymphoma. Neuroblastoma cells may be densely packed, separated by thin fibrils or bundles, and necrosis and calcification can be seen. The small round cells often form clusters surrounded by pink neurofibrillary material. These "rosettes" are characteristic of NB. With increasing maturation, more fibrillary material is apparent and ganglionic differentiation may be seen. Electron microscopy may be helpful, particularly if the neurofibrillary material is not distinct. Cytoplasmic structures, consisting of neurofilaments, neurotubules, and neurosecretory granules, which contain catecholamines, may be noted (46).

Histologic grading systems have attempted to evaluate the cellular maturation of NB. Correlation of prognosis with degree of tumor maturation has not been successful (26,47). A histologic grading system based on the cellularity and the number of mitotic-karyorrhectic cells in the tumor has been proposed by Shimada (53). Although it has been reported to be predictive of prognosis (53), the system is complicated and has not been assessed by a large number of pathologists to date. A new age-linked prognostic categorization based on a new histologic grading system has been presented by POG to compare and test with that proposed by Shimada (38a).

Staging

The classic staging system of NB is that of Evans et al. (21), based on the presurgical extent of disease. An alternative staging system used by the Pediatric Oncology Group, derived from the St. Jude Children's Research Hospital, is based on the degree of the resectability of the primary tumor as well as metastatic spread (19,30,33,,35). The Pediatric Oncology Group staging system was an attempt to improve the prognostic value of the staging system. In particular, lymph node involvement is used as a major criterion in this system, because 83% of patients with Evans stage II and III tumors without nodal disease survive, compared with 31% of those with nodal disease (13).

The Evans staging system also includes a group called stage IVS NB, which consists of patients who would otherwise be stage IV but have remote disease confined to special selected sites such as liver, skin, or bone marrow. Most often, these are children younger than 1 year of age. Overall their prognosis is considerably better than others with stage IV disease (20).

Other factors that have been associated with prognosis include serum factors such as lactate dehydrogenase, ferritin, and serum neuron specific enolase, as well as the histologic grading of the tumor, the urinary VMA:HVA ratio, and tumor cell ploidy by flow cytometry (39,44,45,49,53). The association of the N-myc oncogene amplification and expression with the likelihood of progressive NB is very exciting from a biologic perspective (14).

Anatomic staging according to the pathologic American Joint Committee for Cancer Staging and End Results Reporting/International Union Against Cancer tumor, node, metastasis classification is correlated with the Evans and D'Angio and POG systems (Table 19-5 [3]).

Table 19-5. Neuroblastoma Staging Systems

Evans & D'Angio	Pediatric Oncology Group	International Staging System for Neuroblastoma
Stage I Tumor confined to the organ or structure of origin. **Stage II** Tumor extending in continuity beyond the organ or structure of origin but not crossing the midline. Regional lymph nodes on the ipsilateral side may be involved. **Stage III** Tumor extending in continuity beyond the midline. Regional lymph nodes may be involved bilaterally. **Stage IV** Remote disease involving the skeleton, bone marrow, soft tissue, and distant lymph node groups, etc. (see stage IV-S). **Stage IV-S** Patients who would otherwise be stage I or II, but who have remote disease confined to liver, skin, or bone marrow (without radiographic evidence of bone metastases on complete skeletal survey).	**Stage A** Complete gross resection of primary tumor, with or without microscopic residual. Intracavitary lymph nodes, not adhered to and removed with primary (nodes adhered to or within tumor resection may be positive for tumor without upstaging patient to stage C), histologically free of tumor. If primary in abdomen or pelvis, liver histologically free of tumor. **Stage B** Grossly unresected primary tumor. Nodes and liver same as stage A. **Stage C** Complete or incomplete resection of primary. Intracavitary nodes not adhered to primary histologically positive for tumor. Liver as in stage A. **Stage D** Any dissemination of disease beyond intracavitary nodes, i.e., extracavitary nodes, liver, skin, bone marrow, bone.	**Stage 1** Localized tumor confined to the area of origin; complete gross excision, with or without microscopic residual disease; identifiable ipsilateral and contralateral lymph nodes negative microscopically. **Stage 2A** Unilateral tumor with incomplete gross excision; identifiable ipsilateral and contralateral lymph nodes negative microscopically. **Stage 2B** Unilateral tumor with complete or incomplete gross excision; with positive ipsilateral regional lymph nodes; identifiable contralateral lymph nodes negative microscopically. **Stage 3** Tumor infiltrating across the midline with or without regional lymph node involvement; or, unilateral tumor with contralateral regional lymph node involvement; or, midline tumor with bilateral regional lymph node involvement. **Stage 4** Dissemination of tumor to distant lymph nodes, bone, bone marrow, liver, and/or other organs (except as defined in 4S). **Stage 4S** Localized primary tumor as defined for stage 1 or 2 with dissemination limited to liver, skin.

PRINCIPLES OF TREATMENT

Neuroblastoma is a chemotherapy-and radiation therapy-sensitive tumor. However, for those patients with localized disease, surgical therapy alone is frequently sufficient. Although those children with disseminated disease will respond to chemotherapy and radiation therapy, permanent disease control is infrequently achieved. It is only with intensive regimens, including bone marrow transplantation (BMT), that the cure rate of those patients with advance-stage disease may be increasing. The multidisciplinary approach is summarized in Table 19-6.

Surgery

For those patients with localized disease, complete removal of tumor offers the best chance of cure, although residual tumor in patients with stages I and II disease may regress spontaneously.

Patients with advanced disease have tumors that cannot be completely resected either due to the extent of bulky disease or to metastases. In these instances, a diagnostic biopsy is often the only recommended surgical procedure. In patients with stage IV disease and bone marrow involvement, a bone marrow aspirate demonstrating pseudorosettes, together with the presence of elevated urinary catecholamines, is sufficient to make the diagnosis. Since tumor recurrence in patients with advance-stage disease is often at the primary site of tumor, surgical reduction of this primary tumor mass after initial cytoreductive therapy, may affect the likelihood of cure.

Radiotherapy

Neuroblastoma is a radiosensitive tumor. Radiation therapy is often used for emergency situations, particularly at the time of diagnosis, when a large mediastinal mass may produce respiratory symptoms or a dumbbell lesion protruding into the intervertebral foramen may cause cord compression. Patients with early-stage disease can often be treated with surgery alone, or surgery plus a small amount of chemotherapy; thus, the use of radiation therapy in localized disease has been decreasing. Patients with advanced disease often receive radiation therapy after initial chemotherapy in an attempt to make residual disease either surgically resectable or less likely to recur. Radiation therapy is a component of the preparative regimen prior to autologous or allogenic BMT, which is being used in the treatment of stage IV NB. Radiation therapy may also play an important role in the palliative treatment of patients in terminal-stage of NB for whom bone pain or compression of organs such as the trachea, bowel, or urinary tract are causing significant symptoms.

When radiation therapy is used in the initial treatment of NB, megavoltage equipment and careful attention to sparing normal tissue are necessary. Doses range from 1,500 to 3,500 cGy. No clear dose response curve has been demonstrated.

Chemotherapy

Chemotherapy is the major modality for most patients with NB. The following agents have been found to produce responses (CR and partial) when used as single agents: cyclo-

Table 19-6. Multidisciplinary Treatment Decisions in Neuroblastoma

Pediatric Oncology Group

Stage/(Evans-Stage)	Surgery	Radiotherapy	Chemotherapy
A (I, node negative II-III)	Complete resection	None	None
B (II, III)*	Incomplete resection	None **	CY/DOX
C-D in infants	Complete resection/incomplete resection	None **	CY/DOX/VP-16/CDDP intense therapy/reserved for infants with poor prognostic factors
C in children (usually III)	Complete resection/incomplete resection	None **	CY/DOX/VP-16/CDDP
D in children† (IV)	Biopsy for diagnosis	TBI in the setting of BMT/Radiotherapy for palliation	CY/DOX/VP-16/CDDP (ifosfamide)
(IV- S††) —	Complete resection of primary	Radiotherapy sometimes for hepatomegally or primary	CY/DOX sometimes used

* If complete excision at second surgery, no radiotherapy

** Unless poor response to chemotherapy and surgery

† Optimal therapy, MAC vs BMT is being tested

†† Observation alone for some patients

TBI = total body irradiation; BMT = bone marrow transplant; CY = cyclophosphamide; DOX = doxorubicin; VP-16 = etoposide; CDDP = cisplatin.

phosphamide (59%), doxorubicin (41%), cisplatin (46%), epidophyllotoxin (30%), vincristine (24%), and actinomycin-D (14%) (16). Ifosfamide and carboplatin are also active agents.

For patients with localized disease, cyclophosphamide or vincristine have been used as single agents or in combination. A current regimen uses cyclophosphamide (100 mg/m^2/d) for 7 days, followed by doxorubicin 35 mg/m^2 on day 8 has been effective in low stage patients (32). Epidophyllotoxin and cisplatin have been found to be effective in low-stage patients who do not respond to cyclophosphamide and doxorubicin, as well as in advanced-stage patients (31).

More recently, these four agents as well as ifosfamide and carboplatin have been used concurrently for patients with advanced disease. It is not yet clear whether this approach will increase the cure rate in these patients.

The impact of using four drugs in subsets of infants with aggressive disease was analyzed by Bowman et al. (11a) and found to be an independent variable in improving survival.

SPECIAL CONSIDERATIONS

Bone Marrow Transplantation

Although most patients with NB respond to chemotherapy and irradiation, the cure rate of patients with disseminated disease is extremely low. Intensive regimens currently used are at the limits of bone marrow tolerance. In an attempt to increase the likelihood of long-term survival, higher doses of chemotherapy and total body irradiation (TBI) have been used. Because the amount of therapy necessary to eradicate disease would produce irreversible bone marrow damage, BMT is used to restore hematopoiesis.

Allogenous BMT is usually limited to those with human lymphocyte antigen matched donors and carries with it the risk of graft-versus-host disease. Autologous BMT has been used, particularly when marrow specimens can be purged of NB tumor cells. Bone marrow may be incubated with magnetic beads coated with anti-NB antibodies and passed over a magnet to remove tumor cells (56). Using these and other transplantation techniques, a number of long-term survivors of stage IV NB have been reported (10). Recent analysis of two POG studies by Shuster et al. (53a) found no significant prognostic benefit in bone marrow transplantation (BMT) versus surgery plus chemotherapy for patients in remission and, therefore, urges a large randomized trial of autologous BMT be undertaken to establish its value. However, in smaller studies, progression-free survival at 2 years is 40% compared to 10% in historical controls ($p < .05$) (53b).

RESULTS AND PROGNOSIS

Results (Table 19-7 [3], Fig. 19-2 [33])

1. Age and stage of disease at diagnosis are predictors of outcome as reflected in the classic survival curves shown in Fig. 19-2c (33).
2. Older studies report 2-year survivals of 80%, 60%, 13%, 7%, and 75% for patients with stages I, II, III, IV, and IVS, respectively (21). Although it is commonly quoted that multi-agent chemotherapy has not significantly improved cure rates, a review of patients treated with intensive approaches from 1970 through 1980 at

Table 19-7. Disease-Free Survival in Localized Neuroblastoma

	No. Patients	Relapse-free Survival (% Range)	Average Survival (%)
Node-negative (POG stage A), treated with surgery alone, 7 series	130	85-100	94
Node-negative and/or Evans-D'Angio stage II, not irradiated, 6 Series	83	80-100	90
Node-negative and/or Evans-D'Angio stage II, irradiated, 8 series	96	60-100	80
Node-positive and/or Evans-D'Angio stage III, not irradiated, 3 series	51	11-73	42
Node-positive and/or Evans-D'Angio stage III, irradiated, 7 series	86	64-86	75

POG = Pediatric Oncology Group.
Adapted from Halperin et al. (3).

the Dana Farber Cancer Institute indicates survival of 100%, 93%, 81%, 23%, and 90% (Fig. 19-2a) for Evans stage I, II, III, IV, and IVS, respectively (51). These patients were 2 to 12 years from the time of therapy, with a mean follow-up of 46 months for all patients (66 months for surviving patients). The St. Jude experience (11a) shows a similar improvement in survival rate with the addition of more agents (Fig. 19-2b).

3. Nodal invasion is a powerful prognosticator of treatment outcome. The Pediatric Oncology Staging System takes this into account, resulting in a remarkable ability to predict survival by consideration of stage (A/B vs C/D - Fig. 19-2c).

CLINICAL INVESTIGATIONS

1. Oncogenes: A better understanding of the genetic events that result in disease progression may be helpful for future studies. For example, it has been noted that agents that mature NB cells, particularly retinoic acid, decrease the expression of N-myc RNA. Such maturational agents may be incorporated into intensive regimens to decrease the likelihood of tumor recurrence in advanced-stage disease. Combined analysis of DNA ploidy and N-*myc* genomic content could predict clinical outcome in Stage IVS neuroblastoma and could predict patients for more aggressive chemotherapy (11').

2. Intensive Therapy and BMT: Increasingly intensive regimens using BMT may improve disease-free survival (DFS) in the near future. Using biologic parameters to determine therapy may permit us to know who will need such intensive therapies.

3. New Screening Techniques: Alternatively, because NB is usually more advanced in older children, the newly established techniques for screening populations of young infants may enable us to diagnose and treat infants when the disease is still localized (50). A recent consensus statement has not found screening at 6 months of age to reduce the mortality associated with NB (47a).

Recommended Reading

The current treatment of children with neuroblastoma is reviewed in the articles by Hayes (33) and Finklestein (22).

WILMS' TUMOR (NEPHROBLASTOMA)

Wilms' tumor (nephroblastoma), the second most common abdominal tumor in children, is an ideal model for the successful treatment of cancer in childhood. Two major factors are responsible for this success: (1) a multidisciplinary approach to treatment (surgery, radiotherapy, and chemotherapy) has proven far superior to any one therapy alone; (2) development of national cooperative study groups such as The National Wilms' Tumor Study (NWTS) has made possible the collection and analysis of data not available at individual institutions. A sequence of protocols has yielded valuable information including:

1. the prognostic significance of tumor histology
2. a refinement of the staging system that improves the ability to predict outcome and select therapy
3. the benefits of multiple agent chemotherapy
4. the identification of patients who do not need radiation

In addition, the development of newer imaging modalities, such as ultrasound, CT, and MRI, has made possible better delineation of the tumor, vascular spread, and metastatic disease. This has provided valuable information for planning the surgical approach, more accurate staging, and detection of local tumor regrowth or the detection of metastases. The remarkable improvement over the past 30 years in the outcome for patients with Wilms' tumor is illustrated in Fig. 19-1.

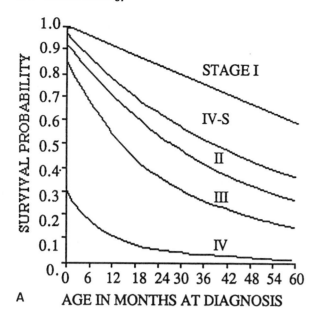

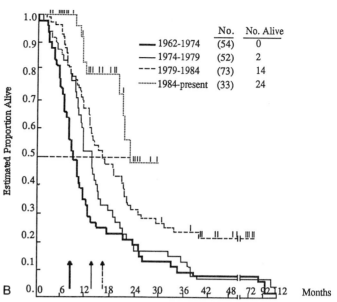

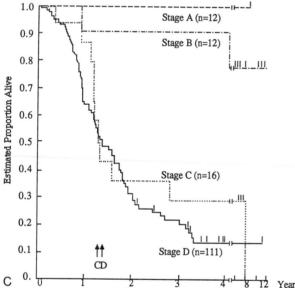

Fig. 19-2. Results: (A) Survival by stage and age. From Breslow and McCann (13), with permission. (B) Survival of children older than 1 year of age. (C) Survival of children older than 1 year of age with POG staged diseases. From Hayes and Smith (33), with permission.

EPIDEMIOLOGY AND ETIOLOGY

Epidemiology

Incidence

Wilms' tumor is the second most common solid abdominal tumor in childhood (sixth overall), occurring in 7.6 per million children in the U.S. (63,74) (Table 19-1). Only neuroblastoma exceeds it in incidence. It is a highly malignant tumor that almost always arises from the kidney. It rarely develops in extrarenal sites (96).

Age and Sex

The tumor occurs most frequently between the ages of 2 and 5 years. The mean age at presentation is 3 to 3.5 years (74,82). The sex ratio is close to 1:1, although some series report a slight male predominance (62,116).

Wilms' tumor in the infant is rare (88,114). Renal tumors in the newborn are most likely to be congenital mesoblastic nephroma or pathologic variants of that tumor. Wilms' tumor may also occur in teenagers and adults (90).

Bilateral Wilms' Tumor

This occurs in 4% to 8% of patients whose mean age is younger than those with unilateral Wilms' tumor (66,95).

Etiology

The tumor may arise in three renal tissue elements: embryonic kidney blastema, epithelium, and stroma (64). Not all tumors contain all three elements.

Biology

1. Genetics: Wilms' tumor is considered to be of genetic origin in up to 40% of children with the lesion, but epidemiologic data from NWTS suggests a lower incidence (70,91). D'Angio (74) has stated that as few as 1% of patients with Wilms' tumor have other family members with the disease.

2. Proto-oncogenes are important genes for cell proliferation. However, when these genes are altered or mutated, they may permit the development of a malignant tumor. These oncogenes are dominant and therefore can permit malignancy in the heterozygous state. Another classification of gene is termed a tumor suppressor gene. These genes are important in cellular development and seem required for cell differentiation. When they are mutated, development of a malignant tumor becomes possible. Anti-oncogenes are recessive and therefore tumor expression occurs in the homozygous state (91).

a. Most patients with Wilms' tumor have normal constitutional chromosomes. Patients with Wilms' tumor and congenital aniridia frequently have a constitutional deletion of band 13 on the short arm of chromosome 11 (11 p13) (Table 19-2). This deletion has also been noted in Wilms' tumor patients with otherwise normal constitutional chromosomes. This suggests that an abnormal allele may play a role in Wilms' tumorigenesis (91).

b. Familial forms of Wilms' tumor are inherited in an autosomal dominant fashion, with a penetrance of about 50%. Carriers constitutionally lack one allele for the "tumor gene." If the existing allele is lost or altered, malignancy can develop. The gene is a tumor suppressor gene or an anti-oncogene and functions even though it is a recessive gene. There is at present no evidence that the familial Wilms' tumor gene is located at 11p13 (91).

c. Knudson and Strong (92) have proposed a "two-hit hypothesis" for carcinogenesis due to genetic mutation. The first event may be either constitutional or acquired. For the tumor to develop, a second event (hit) is required to alter the gene and permit the development of a malignant cell (92).

3. Associated congenital anomalies: Certain congenital anomalies occur frequently in children diagnosed with Wilms' tumor and are noted more often in patients with bilateral disease (68). There is an increased risk of Wilms' tumor in Beckwith-Wiedemann syndrome and in patients with hemihypertrophy or aniridia (111).

a. Aniridia may be either familial or sporadic. One third of patients with aniridia have the sporadic form. Wilms' tumor is associated only with the sporadic form and will develop in one third of those individuals. Aniridia occurs in one of 73 patients with Wilms ' tumor compared with 1 of 50,000 in the general population (99). The constellation of aniridia, Wilms' tumor, mental retardation, and ambiguous genitalia has been associated with the deletion of band 13-14 in the short arm of chromosome 11 p13-14) (117).

b. Nephroblastomatosis (residual renal blastema) has been associated with the deletion of the 11 p band on the short arm of chromosome 11 and Wilms' tumor (86).

c. WAGR syndrome is the association of Wilms' tumor, aniridia, gonadoblastoma, and mental retardation (100).

d. Drash syndrome represents the association of Wilms' tumor with male pseudohermaphroditism and diffuse glomerular disease. The latter presents as the nephrotic syndrome and is responsible for the mortality in Drash syndrome (77,78,79).

e. Rare patients with Wilms' may develop acquired von Willebrand's disease with significant bruising and bleeding (103,108).

DETECTION AND DIAGNOSIS

1. Evaluation begins with an accurate history and physical examination.

2. A family history may reveal other members with Wilms' tumor. In addition, attention is paid to congenital anomalies known to be associated with Wilms' tumor.

3. An abdominal mass is the most common presenting sign and is noted in more than 80% of patients (83). Abdominal pain and vomiting have been noted in 50% (61).

4. A smooth, large abdominal mass filling one side of the abdomen is typical in this disorder. An enlarged liver suggests hepatic metastases.

5. Microscopic hematuria occurs in 20% to 30% (74,82).

6. Hypertension may be present at diagnosis as a result of increased renin production (80,113).

7. Laboratory studies: Laboratory evaluation of a child with a suspected Wilms' tumor should include a complete blood cell count, urinalysis, and liver and renal function blood studies. Hypercalcemia in an infant with an abdominal mass suggests a rhabdoid tumor or a congenital mesoblastic nephroma rather than a true Wilms' tumor (89,110,115). An elevated hemoglobin may indicate a rare erythropoietin-secreting Wilms' tumor (109). Clotting abnormalities may exist due to acquired von Willebrand's disease.

8. Imaging studies

a. A plain radiograph of the abdomen and chest is the initial assessment. Coarse calcifications may occur in a Wilms' tumor but fine stipple calcifications are noted more frequently in neuroblastoma.

b. A chest x-ray may reveal pulmonary metastases, the most common site of metastatic spread (93) Abdominal CT with contrast or intravenous pyelography (IVP) will reveal an intrarenal mass displacing and distorting the collecting system of the involved kidney. The opposite kidney is scrutinized for bilateral involvement. Occasionally, Wilms' tumor is misdiagnosed on IVP when the lesion is actually a neuroblastoma that has distorted the renal collecting system (105).

c. Ultrasonography is especially useful in complementing the IVP, but is essential to look for tumor growth into the renal vein, vena cava, and right side of the heart. Liver metastases may also be demonstrated by ultrasound.

d. CT of abdominal areas are commonly performed to determine exact dimensions and extension of renal mass.

e. CT of the chest is a more sensitive method than a plain film for diagnosing small pulmonary metastases.

f. Bone scans are indicated in patients with the clear cell sarcoma variant of Wilms' tumor. Angiography is rarely indicated.

CLASSIFICATION AND STAGING

Histopathology: Pathologic Behavior

Wilms' tumor frequently infiltrates through the kidney capsule into adjacent structures. There may be direct extension into the pelvis and ureter or the renal vein and vena cava. Hilar and peri-aortic lymph node involvement is relatively common. The lung represents the most common site of distant metastases.

Grossly, the tumor is generally solid and confined by the renal capsule. The tumor may contain necrotic or cystic areas. Gross tumor may extend into the pelvis and ureter or into the renal vein and vena cava. Microscopically, the tumor may contain varying amounts of three tissue elements: blastema, epithelia, and stroma.

An important contribution by the first NWTS was the recognition that tumor histopathology affected prognosis. Certain pathologic categories were defined. Anaplasia and sarcomatous changes were noted in a small group of patients, 49 out of 427 tumors studied. Twenty-eight (57%) died, as compared with 26 deaths in the remaining 376 patients (6.9%). Anaplasia and sarcomatous changes are termed unfavorable histology (65). Anaplasia is rarely found in children under age 2 years. Succeeding NWTS data have confirmed the poor prognosis of tumors with unfavorable histology with several exceptions. Stage I anaplastic Wilms' tumors behave clinically like stage I, with favorable histology. Clear cell sarcomas respond to a three-drug regimen of doxorubicin/ vincristine/ dactinomycin (94). In addition, rhabdoid tumor has been dropped from the Wilms' tumor classification because it is probably of neuroectodermal origin (84).

There are two other pathologic entities associated with Wilms' tumor: congenital mesoblastic nephroma and nephroblastomatosis. The former is a benign mesenchymal tumor of renal origin, distinct from Wilms' tumor seen during the first 3 months of life (67,87,106). Cellular variations of this tumor with less benign behavior have recently been described in infants (66,112). The persistence of embryonic renal blastema beyond 36 weeks' gestation is termed nephroblastomatosis. This has been noted in one-fourth to one-third of Wilms' tumors (64,69).

Staging

Staging likewise affects prognosis. The official AJC and UICC TNM staging systems are not widely used, but their pathologic stage groupings, as illustrated in Fig. 19-3 correspond with the NWTS staging system (see Table 19-8), which has been modified over the past decade (NWTS I/II versus III and IV).

Positive prognostic factors are lower-stage disease and a favorable histology. Negative prognostic factors are unfavorable histology, lymph node involvement, tumor thrombus in the inferior vena cava, and tumor rupture before or during surgery. An exception is that patients with stage I disease with unfavorable histology do as well as those with favorable histology. Stage IV and unfavorable histology have similar relapse-free survival. Two-year survival for patients with negative lymph nodes is 54% with unfavorable histology and 90% with favorable histology (76).

Independent information reveals that patients with stages III and IV disease are at a high risk of relapse if they have a DNA tetraploid pattern (104).

PRINCIPLES OF TREATMENT

The principles of treatment have evolved from NWTS clinical trials. With the evolution of these clinical trials, the control arm of each succeeding protocol is the better outcome of the earlier trial. A summary of NWTS clinical trials provides a concise overview of the multidisciplinary approach that has been so successful (Table 19-9) (3).

Table 19-8. Clinicopathologic Staging* of WILMS' TUMOR

Group	(NWTS I,II)	Stage*	(NWTS III, IV)
I	Limited to kidney, completely resected Capsule intact, not ruptured. No residuum beyond margins of resection	I	Limited to kidney, completely excised. Capsule intact. Not ruptured before or during removal. No residuum
II	Extends beyond kidney, completely resected Local extension of tumor (i.e., penetration beyond pseudocapsule into perirenal soft tissues, or periaortic lymph node involvement). Renal vessel outside kidney substance infiltrated or contains tumor thrombus. No residuum	II	Extends beyond kidney, completely excised. Regional extension (i.e., penetration through outer surface of capsule into perirenal soft tissues). Vessels outside kidney infiltrated or contain tumor thrombus. May have been biopsied or local spillage confined to flank. No residuum
III	Residual nonhematogenous tumor confined to abdomen. Any of following: Ruptured before or during surgery, or biopsy performed Implants found on peritoneal surfaces Lymph nodes involved beyond abdominal periaortic chains Not completely resectable because of local infiltration into vital structures	III	Residual nonhematogenous tumor confined to abdomen. Any of following: Lymph nodes on biopsy found to be involved in hilus, periaortic chains, or beyond Diffuse peritoneal contamination, e.g., spillage beyond flank or penetration through peritoneal surface Implants found on peritoneal surfaces Extends beyond surgical margins either microscopically or grossly Not completely resectable because of local infiltration into vital structures
IV	Hematogenous metastases. Deposits beyond group III (e.g., lung, liver, bone, brain)	IV	Hematogenous. Deposits beyond stage III (e.g., lung, liver, bone, brain)
V	Bilateral renal involvement either initially or subsequently	V	Bilateral renal involvement at diagnosis. An attempt should be made to stage each side according to above criteria based on disease extent prior to biopsy

* Clinical stage decided by surgeon in operating room, confirmed by pathologist who also evaluates the histology. Staging is the same for tumors with favorable and with unfavorable histologic features. Statement of both criteria (e.g., stage II/favorable histology or stage II/unfavorable histology) necessary.

NWTS = National Wilms' Tumor Study.

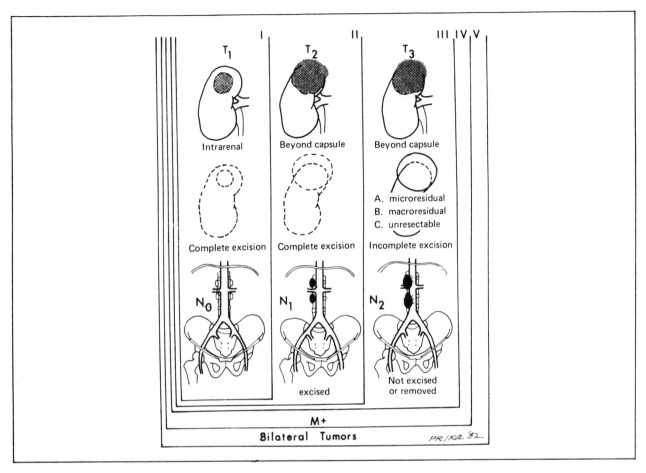

Fig. 19-3. Anatomic staging for Wilms' tumor.

Surgery

The importance is stressed of careful and gentle surgical technique to prevent rupture of the tumor during its removal. A large transabdominal incision is required to facilitate exploration and excision. Sometimes a combined thoracicoabdominal incision is required. An attempt is made to ligate the renal vessels early in the resection to reduce tumor emboli, but early ligation is abandoned if it increases the risk of tumor rupture. The entire ureter, which may have tumor extension, is excised with the specimen. This also reduces the incidence of subsequent urinary tract infections caused by stasis in a retained portion of ureter.

Hilar and peri-aortic lymph nodes are sampled for prognostic determination. Thorough inspection of the abdominal cavity is made for extension or metastatic disease. Suspicious sites are biopsied. To prevent tumor spillage, involved contiguous tissue is taken in continuity with the tumor.

Gerota's fascia of the contralateral kidney is opened and the kidney is inspected both anteriorly and posteriorly. Surgical treatment for bilateral Wilms' tumors has varied from nephrectomy with tumor excision on the more involved side and partial nephrectomy on the opposite side, to bilateral nephrectomy and renal transplantation. A recent study of 145 patients with synchronous bilateral Wilms' tumor registered in NWTS II and III revealed 94 who underwent initial surgery followed by chemotherapy with or without irradiation with a 3-year survival of 82%. The recommended treatment for bilateral Wilms' tumor (stage V) is bilateral biopsy, chemotherapy for the most advanced stage, followed by excision of tumor, avoiding bilateral nephrectomy (66).

Should preoperative ultrasound reveal tumor in the vena cava or right atrium, planning surgical excision may involve cardiopulmonary bypass with or without hypothermia (71,102). Alternately, preoperative chemotherapy may be used to facilitate removal of tumor. Aggressive surgical excision is indicated for metastatic disease in certain situations: isolated pulmonary lesions at diagnosis or metastatic disease not responding to chemotherapy and irradiation.

Radiation Therapy

Radiation therapy is integrated with surgery and chemotherapy. Its goal is to prevent local and regional recurrences. For patients with unfavorable histology or the clear cell variant, and for all patients with stages III and IV disease, irradiation is necessary. Megavoltage apparatus and beam shaping devices are used to tailor therapy to the patient, carefully excluding normal tissues beyond the target volume. Daily doses are 1.5 to 1.8 Gy to large and small volumes, respectively. Current total doses and volumes are based on experience gained from NWTS I, II, and III.

Timing: Radiation therapy is initiated within 10 days following surgery (if possible) because of the increased risk of abdominal recurrence when it is delayed (113a). It should be

Table 19-9. Multidisciplinary Treatment Decisions in Wilms' Tumor: NWTS Trials 1-4

Group/Stage[1] Study Number	I	II	III	IV
1 ('69-'74)	S+AD (15)* •RT + •RT -	S+RT (18-40 Gy) •AD (15)* •V (15)* •AD/V (15)*	As II	S+RT+AD/V •V pre-S •without
2 ('74-'79)	S+AD/V •(6)*	S+RT(18-40 Gy) •AD/V (15)* •AD/V/A (15)*	As II	As II
3 ('79-'86)	FH:S+AD/V •(2.5)*	FH:S±RT(20 Gy) •AD/V (15)* •AD/V/A(15)*	FH:S+RT (10 vs 20 Gy) •AD/V (15)* •AD/V/A(15)*	•AD/V/A (15)* •VAC (15)*
4 ('86--)	FH: S+AD/V Ana •(2.5 - P/I ***) •(6)*	FH:S+AD/V •(6)* •(15)* •(6-P/I) •(15-P/I) Ana:S+RT(12.6-37.8 Gy) •AD/V/A (15)* •AD/V/A/C (15)*	FH:S+RT(10.8GY)[2] + AD/V/A CCSK (I-IV):As FH III,IV Ana: As II	•(6)* •(15)* •(6-P/I) •(15-P/I) Ana: As II

[1] Group/Stage: NWTS group for studies 1,2; NWTS stage for studies 3,4

* (duration in months)   ***___(P/I = pulsed, intensive drug schedule S = surgery, RT = radiation therapy; (dose)** with range age-dependent for NWTS--1,2; 4-anaplastic AD = actinomycin-D; V = vincristine; A = adriamycin; C = cyclophosphamide; FH = favorable histology; UH = unfavorable histology; Ana = anaplastic; CCSK = clear cell sarcoma of kidney; RT (NWTS-4): dose plus additional "boost" of 10.8 Gy permitted for residual disease > 3cm diameter

[2] NWTS = National Wilms' Tumor Study

Adapted from Halperin et al. (3).

noted, however, that the relapses that were related to this delay occurred primarily in patients with unfavorable histology.

For stage III disease with favorable histology without gross residual disease, radiation therapy is delivered to the tumor bed defined as the involved kidney and areas of associated disease as imaged preoperatively or defined surgically. The radiation therapy portal always includes the entire width of adjacent vertebrae to avoid scoliosis. The whole abdomen is treated (10 to 12 Gy fractionated for favorable histologies) in patients who have peritoneal seeding or tumor rupture prior to or during surgery. Boost doses are administered to sites of residual gross disease (3 cm).

For stage IV (favorable histology) disease, the primary lesion is treated according to the stage it would be in the absence of metastases. If the lung is involved, by X-ray the entire thorax is treated (10-12 Gy fractionated for favorable histologies). Recent studies show that small pulmonary lesions, recognized only on CT scan, may be successfully treated with chemotherapy alone (76a). Patients with stage II and IV (unfavorable-histology) disease are treated as outlined for stage III disease but with doses based on patient age. An additional boost is given to sites of known residual disease (12 to 38 Gy).

Chemotherapy

In 1966, Farber (77a) reported the utility of dactinomycin as adjuvant chemotherapy for the treatment of Wilms' tumor. Vincristine was noted to be effective shortly thereafter. The NWTS I revealed that radiation therapy and either dactinomycin or vincristine would provide approximately 55% relapse-free survival (RFS) in groups II and III patients, but when the two drugs were used in combination, RFS was 81%. The two drugs have since been the mainstay of therapy for Wilms' tumor. Current chemotherapy is stage dependent. Low-stage disease can be adequately treated with dactinomycin and vincristine without irradiation. Doxorubicin is added to dactinomycin and vincristine in higher-stage disease. It is unclear if the addition of cyclophosphamide to the above three-drug regimen increases survival in children with unfavorable histology. Radiation therapy is not necessary for any patient with stage I disease or stage II disease with favorable histology. Less radiation therapy is required when doxorubicin is added to vincristine and dactinomycin in stage III disease. Six months of drug therapy for 6 months provides good results in stage I disease (93% 2-year DFS). The drug dosage must be reduced in children under 1 year of age to reduce serious toxicity from 49% to 13% and drug-related death from 6% to 0% (101). This can be performed without compromise in therapeutic effectiveness. Improved survival for anaplastic Wilms' tumor histology treated with VAC and abdominal radiation therapy resulted in good disease-free survival and overall 5-year survival of 87.5% that was not significantly different from favorable histology. Sarcomatous histology responded poorly (71a).

The new NWTS IV continues the previous approach of trying to improve overall survival while limiting therapeutic toxicities. Dose-intensified regimens are compared with standard intensity therapies, and the possibility of decreasing the therapy duration is also being examined (75).

RESULTS (Tables 19-10 and 19-11) (4)

Two-year RFS or 5-year survival from nephrectomy is considered a cure in Wilms' tumor (97). There are isolated reports of recurrences beyond 5 years. These may represent

true bilateral Wilms' tumors or nephroblastomatosis. The 4-year RFS for stage I disease (FH) is 89%, 88% for stage II (FH), 78% for stage III (FH), and 75% for stage IV (FH). For stages I-III (UF) 4-year RFS is 66%, and for stage IV (UF) is 55%. Seventy-five percent of relapses occur within 1 year and fewer than 3% occur after 2 years from onset of therapy. Some patients with low-stage disease who develop metastases can be cured with intensive chemotherapy and radiation therapy (82a). Unfortunately, patients who develop local abdominal recurrences are rarely cured of their disease.

The successive NWTS trials provided increasingly efficacious therapy while decreasing its morbidity for patients with favorable prognoses. In the first NWTS, group I patients younger than 2 years were found to be highly curable with chemotherapy alone, whereas the older children required local radiotherapy. In NWTS-2, more intensive chemotherapy (actinomycin-D plus vincristine) obviated the need

Table 19-10. NWTS Outcomes in Group I Patients*

Age	RT	NWTS-1			NWTS-2		
		N	RFS(%)	OS(%)	N	RFS(%)	OS(%)
<2 yr	Yes	38	90	97	–	–	–
	No	36	88	94	117	86	95
≥2 yr	Yes	39	77	97	–	–	–
	No	41	58	91	77	89	97

* RT = postoperative radiotherapy; N = number patients; RFS = 2-year relapse-free survival; OS = overall survival; NWTS = National Wilms' Tumor Study.

Adapted from Pizzo et al. (4).

Table 19-11. Results in Randomized NWT = 3 Patients*

Stage/Histology	Regimen	N	2-Year Survival (%)	
			Relapse Free	Overall
I/FH	AD+V, 10 wk v. 6 mo	469	90 v. 93	98
II/FH	15 mo. AD + V v. AD+V+A* (±RT)	262	91 v. 90	99 v. 93
II/FH	AD+V ± A No RT v. 2000 cGy*	262	90 v. 91	95 v. 96
III/FH	AD+V v. AD+V+A* (15 mo; +RT)	264	77 v. 88	88 v. 95
III/FH	AD+V+A 1000 v. 2000 cGY*	264	82 v. 83	92 v. 91
Any IV, Any UH	AD+V+A vs. AD+V+A+C (15 mo; + RT)	291	63 v. 69	78 v. 80

* Collapsed regimens from the factorial design; persistent disease at last follow-up in stage IV was scored as relapse. Data indicate that, in general, FH stages II and III patients can be treated successfully with the less intensive regimens and that better treatment is needed for patients with UH and/or metastases, especially those with rhabdoid tumors. Stage I/FH children present particular problems for analysis. These results show the less intensive 10-week regimen to be no worse than 6 months, but other analyses suggest that 6 months of treatment may be better. Of the four possible treatment combinations for stage III/FH, AD+V+1000 cGy appears to produce inferior results when both relapse-free survival and infradiaphragmatic relapse are considered.

FH = favorable histology; UH = unfavorable histology; AD = Actinomycin-D; V = vincristine; A = doxorubicin; C = cyclophosphamide; RT = radiation therapy.

Adapted from Pizzo et al. (4).

for radiotherapy in any group I patient. The third NWTS has demonstrated that intensive chemotherapy can effectively treat stage II patients without radiotherapy and that the three-drug regimen of actinomycin-D, vincristine, and doxorubicin was not superior to intensively administered actinomycin-D and vincristine for these patients. Patients with stage III-IV disease receive intensive drug regimens and radiotherapy. The current NWTS-4 primarily is testing the duration and optimal method of drug administration. Results from these trials are given in Tables 19-10 and 19-11.

Long-term follow-up is essential for all patients (77'). Irradiation affects growing cartilage and bone as well as soft tissues. This can result in scoliosis, shortened height, and slipped epiphyses. Second malignancies are known to develop in patients treated for Wilms' tumor (98). A median of 10 years has been noted for the development of a second tumor in the irradiated field and a median of 5 years for those to whom no irradiation was given (97). Both solid tumors and leukemias have developed (107). Some investigators believe that genetic influences are the prime factors determining the development of secondary malignancies (85).

CLINICAL INVESTIGATIONS

1. Oncogenes: Exciting new work in the relationship of genetic material to oncogenesis is ongoing.
2. New chemotherapeutic agents: Etoposide, cisplatinum, and ifosfamide are new chemotherapeutic agents that have been effective in recurrent Wilms' tumor. Their role in improving the prognosis in children with high-stage disease needs to be evaluated.
3. Optimization of treatment often means less rather than more treatment. Variations in dosages and duration of drug and radiation treatment are being studied to reduce toxicity without compromising results in children with favorable histology and to improve survival in those with unfavorable histology.

Recommended Reading

The best current articles giving an overview of Wilms' tumor, its biologic behavior and how treatment has evolved through coordinated studies are those of D'Angio (72), Gannick (81), and Green (82).

NON-HODGKIN'S LYMPHOMA

Childhood non-Hodgkin's lymphomas (NHL) are a heterogeneous group of malignancies that arise from T cells, B cells, and their precursors in the lymphoid system. The variability in their presentation and patterns of spread, and their systemic nature, reflect their origin from a lineage of cells that migrate throughout the body (144). Similarly, progress in their treatment mirrors the recognition of their systemic nature and underlying biology. This has led to the development of effective chemotherapeutic regimens tailored to characteristics of the cancer. In this regard, prognosis and response to therapy depend on the underlying cell type, primary site, and the extent of disease. In the past, local therapy resulted in an overall survival of 10% to 30% (121,131,163). Current aggressive multiagent protocols result in overall survivals of 50% to 80% (118,154,166). Child-

hood NHL is distinguished from adult NHL by differing frequencies of immunohistopathologic types, and the relative infrequency of nodal as compared with extranodal presentations. There is a greater propensity for NHL in children to disseminate noncontiguously, evolve into leukemia, and to involve the central nervous system (157).

EPIDEMIOLOGY AND ETIOLOGY

Epidemiology

1. Lymphomas comprise 10% of all pediatric cancers. Sixty percent are NHL and 40% are Hodgkin's disease (170).
2. NHL is uncommon under the age of 5 years and increases in frequency steadily with age throughout life (133).
3. The male to female ratio is 2 or 3:1 (133).
4. The frequency of NHL varies markedly in various geographic regions. In equatorial Africa, approximately 50% of childhood cancers are lymphomas, primarily Burkitt's (145). In this setting, an association with Epstein-Barr virus (EBV) (172) and specific chromosomal breakpoints (resulting in a characteristic 8:14 chromosomal translocation) are seen (145).
5. The incidence of NHL is increased in patients with disorders associated with an abnormal regulation of the immune system.
   a. Immunodeficiency states, usually inherited but also acquired (such as the acquired immune deficiency syndrome [AIDS]), are associated with the development of lymphomas. These are histologically predominantly large cell or immunoblastic, and generally of B-cell origin (129). A defect in T-cell regulation that permits the expansion of EBV-infective clones of B cells may explain this association. The X-linked lymphoproliferative syndrome, ataxia telangiectasia, Wiscott-Aldrich syndrome, and common variable immune deficiency disease, are all examples of underlying disorders that place patients at risk for the development of NHL (129).
   b. Children who receive renal, cardiac, or bone marrow allografts are also at a substantially increased risk because of their immunosuppressive therapy (150).
   c. NHL is also an uncommon second malignant neoplasm in patients treated for their primary cancer with combined chemotherapy and radiotherapy (126).

Biology

1. Most childhood NHLs are thought to arise from lymphocyte precursors in the bone marrow and thymus rather than from immunocompetent lymphoid cells capable of participating in an immune response (123).
   a. Small noncleaved lymphomas, which include Burkitt's and non-Burkitt's subtypes, and most large cell lymphomas are of B-cell phenotype (136,152). Surface immunoglobulins (Ig) (usually of the IgM class) and B-cell specific antigens (usually detected by the monoclonal antibodies B4 [CD19] and [B1CD20]) are expressed by these cells (164). The Burkitt's subtype, which includes equatorial African and North American forms, have differences in the precise locations of the chromosomal breakpoints

these tumors (162).

b. Lymphoblastic lymphomas are composed of immature lymphoid cells that almost invariably have the enzyme TdT (124). Most lymphoblastic lymphomas (and some large cell lymphomas) also express T-cell markers. The distinction between lymphoblastic lymphoma and leukemia is generally determined by the percentage of blast cells demonstrated in the bone marrow, with 25% the most commonly used cutoff point. The biologic correlate to this distinction is not unequivocally known, but appears to involve the degree of differentiation of the neoplastic cell. Malignancies with an immature thymocyte phenotype most frequently present as leukemia, whereas those with a more mature phenotype characteristically present with less marrow involvement but accumulations of cells in other areas (135).

2. Childhood lymphomas generally grow rapidly due to high growth fractions (approaching 100% in some cases) and short doubling times (12 hours to a few days) (137). B-cell tumors have the highest growth fractions, with up to 27% of the cells in S phase (156).

3. Specific cytogenetic findings distinguish several of the different subtypes of childhood NHL (140). Characteristic differences are found not only among different phenotypes, but even within an apparently homogeneous phenotype. Since particular genetic abnormalities may correlate with prognosis, such distinctions are important (145).

a. In Burkitt's lymphoma, the proto-oncogene c-myc is translocated from chromosome 8 to the heavy chain locus of chromosome 14 (128). The product of the c-myc oncogene is necessary for cellular proliferation, and its abnormal expression may maintain the cell in an inappropriately proliferative state (120).

b. In lymphoblastic lymphoma, specific nonrandom chromosomal abnormalities have not been established but several translocations have been described (141).

c. Characteristic karyotypic abnormalities also have not yet been shown for large cell lymphomas. This may be due to the phenotypically heterogeneous tumors in this category or it may be because the genetic abnormalities do not involve karyotypic changes.

DETECTION AND DIAGNOSIS

Clinical Detection

In general, patients present with a limited number of syndromes that correspond to the cell type. Symptoms are usually of short duration prior to diagnosis.

1. Thirty percent to 40% of patients present with supradiaphragmatic adenopathy (157), which may include a mediastinal mass (especially in males) or involvement of Waldeyer's ring, among other locations. Typical presentation in patients with mediastinal mass is malaise and cough progressing to dyspnea. Supradiaphragmatic disease frequently disseminates to involve bone marrow (80% to 90%), CNS or gonads (30%) (141,157,159). It is usually of lymphoblastic histology.

2. Thirty percent to 40% of patients present with an abdominal mass associated with ascites, an acute abdomen, or intussusception, or a malnutrition syndrome with colitis symptoms (157). The disease involves the ileocecal region, mesentery, ovaries, or retroperitoneum. The abdominal disease frequently spreads to the CNS (171). It is usually of undifferentiated histology.

3. A variety of primary extranodal sites (e.g., tonsils, lung, bone, testicles, soft tissue) cause presentations referable to the involved region (139,169).

a. At the time of diagnosis, the likelihood of bone morrow involvement depends on the histologic subtype. In small noncleaved lymphomas, the bone marrow is involved in 20% of patients (146,148), and evidence from cytogenetic studies of microscopically uninvolved marrow shows involvement in another 20% (122).

b. The CNS is not commonly involved at diagnosis except in patients with marrow involvement.

Diagnostic Procedures

1. Surgical biopsy establishes the diagnosis. Although histology remains as the primary decision-making criterion, immunophenotyping, enzymatic, and cytogenetic studies should supplement morphologic analysis.

a. The most suspicious node should be selected for excisional biopsy. Frozen sections and needle biopsies are discouraged.

b. Staging laparotomy is unnecessary because it does not influence treatment or prognosis (158).

2. Aspiration of bone marrow or effusions may provide the diagnosis and obviate the need for a lymph node biopsy.

3. Laboratory evaluation should include complete blood cell count with differential, platelets, and reticulocytes. Electrolytes, uric acid, calcium, phosphorus, renal ,and liver function tests should also be obtained. Other studies, such as catecholamines, may be useful in excluding the diagnosis of other tumors.

4. Lumbar puncture with cytocentrifugation of cerebrospinal fluid (CSF) should be performed.

5. Imaging studies include chest x-ray, CT, or MRI of the chest and abdomen (as well as areas of obvious involvement), bone scan, and plain radiographs as indicated.

CLASSIFICATION AND STAGING

Histopathology

Essentially all pediatric NHL are diffuse lymphomas of intermediate or high grade, according to the International Working Formulation. Table 19-12 lists the various histopathologic subtypes according to the Rappaport Classification System as modified by the International Working Formulation. The correlation with immune markers and approximate frequency are also noted.

Staging

The Ann Arbor Staging System for Hodgkin's disease is not appropriate for pediatric NHL because of noncontiguous patterns of involvement and frequency of extranodal disease. Several systems are used for staging (145), based in some manner on the burden of tumor present at diagnosis, since this correlates to survival. The system used at the National

Table 19-12. Distribution of Histopathologic Types of non-Hodgkin's Lymphoma With Corresponding Immunophenotypes

Histology	Phenotype	Frequency (%)
Nodular (follicular)		Extremely rare
Diffuse		
Large cell (histiocytic)		15-20
Cleaved	Mostly B-cell and non-B,	
Noncleaved	non-T neoplasms	
Immunoblastic	Rarely T cell	
Lymphoblastic		30-50
Convoluted	Virtually all T cell	
Nonconvoluted	Few non-T, non-B	
	neoplasms ("common ALL	
	phenotype")	
	Few pre-B cell	
Undifferentiated (small non-cleaved)		20-30
Burkitt's	B cell (surface IgM)	
Non-Burkitt's (pleomorphic)		

Cancer Institute was originally devised for Burkitt's lymphoma and should not be applied to patients with lymphoblastic lymphoma. It differs from the St. Jude scheme by excluding the diaphragm as a determinant of disseminated disease. This exclusion is appropriate for NHL in contrast to Hodgkin's disease. It also reflects the advantage of complete surgical resection of abdominal disease.

PRINCIPLES OF TREATMENT

Local treatment with surgery or radiation therapy produced long-term survivors in only 10% to 30% of children with NHL (121,131,163). These children had localized disease and favorable presentations. Since the vast majority of patients have occult disseminated disease at diagnosis, intensive multiagent chemotherapeutic protocols were developed. Moreover, advances in clinical staging methods and immunohistologic identification of tumor subtypes have been coupled with the development and appropriate application of effective agents. Optimal initial therapy is essential, since patients who recur are rarely salvaged.

Surgery

1. Routine staging laparotomy, is not indicated. It is unlikely to alter systemic therapy and may delay it (157).
2. In patients with abdominal presentations, laparotomy may be indicated for treatment of an acute abdomen or to establish the diagnosis. If disease is limited to the gastrointestinal (GI) tract, complete resection should be considered (160). In patients with Burkitt's lymphoma, one should consider debulking if greater than 90% of the tumor can be removed with minimal morbidity (149).

Radiation Therapy

1. The role of radiotherapy in the management of NHL in children has progressively decreased as chemotherapeutic regimens have become more effective. It retains an important role in selected situations, but in general

does not improve DFS and may add unnecessary morbidity. Recent reports from the Pediatric Oncology Group (142) and St. Jude Children's Research Hospital (155) demonstrate successful local and systemic control with chemotherapy alone for children with Murphy/St. Jude stages I and II disease regardless of histology. The addition of localized radiation therapy to chemotherapy has also shown no benefit for patients with advanced-stage disease (125,155).

2. Situations in which radiotherapy is appropriate include:
   a. Emergency, x-ray radiotherapy is used in the setting of acute airway compromise or spinal cord compression. A hyperfractionated regimen should be considered.
   b. Some form of presymptomatic treatment of the CNS is warranted in the majority of cases, because 30% to 35% of children will develop CNS lymphoma in its absence. However, intrathecal chemotherapy alone is effectively used in most settings without the added morbidity of cranial irradiation. Specific indications for cranial x-ray radiotherapy include the following: overt leptomeningeal lymphoma at diagnosis, and evidence for leukemic transformation (bone marrow involvement with greater than 25% blasts) at diagnosis (153).
   c. The role of x-ray radiotherapy for primary NHL of bone in children is unknown. Excellent local control is afforded by its use, and data that demonstrate similar results when x-ray radiotherapy is omitted are not yet available (at least for large cell, nonlymphoblastic histologies). Radiotherapy is thus appropriately administered in this setting. Unfortunately, the frequency of second malignancies may be increased following its use (143).
   d. Radiotherapy is given to selected patients who do not achieve a CR following initial chemotherapy with or without surgery.
   e. Radiotherapy is used to palliate pain associated with uncontrolled disease.

f. Radiotherapy may be administered for consolidation prior to BMT in patients with recurrent disease.

3. Patients with CNS involvement, especially those with cranial nerve palsies or spinal cord compression, are treated with radiation therapy and intrathecal chemotherapy on an urgent basis to prevent permanent neurologic sequelae.

Chemotherapy

Even children with apparently localized NHL have a high likelihood of having micrometastatic disseminated disease. For this reason, all children, regardless of stage or histology, are treated with chemotherapy (161). All childhood NHL responds to a wide range of agents, but different combinations and schedules are optimal for particular histologies and stages.

1. For children with NHL, the most effective regimens include cyclophosphamide, vincristine, prednisone, methotrexate, and doxorubicin (COMP, ACOP, APO (119,130,138).

2. For children with lymphoblastic NHL, the LSA2-L2 regimen has proven effectiveness; it includes the abovementioned agents as well as thioguanine, asparaginase, carmustine, cytarabine, and hydroxyurea with methotrexate given both intravenously and intrathecally (139).

SPECIAL CONSIDERATIONS

1. Treatment of children with NHL can be complicated by a tumor lysis syndrome that has severe metabolic consequences or renal failure. Hyperuricemia, hyperkalemia, hyperphosphatemia, and hypocalcemia are associated with this syndrome, which most commonly complicates therapy for Burkitt's lymphoma. Careful management is demanded and the temporary use of dialysis may be required. In a recent study from St. Jude Children's Research Hospital, renal failure could not be attributed to hyperuricemia or hyperphosphatemia in the majority of patients. Renal failure was more closely correlated with oliguria in the 12 hours preceding and 24 hours following initiation of chemotherapy, suggesting the importance of careful fluid management (165).

2. Children with recurrent NHL should be considered for BMT (132).

RESULTS AND PROGNOSIS

Results of Therapy (Fig. 19-4) (155) (TK)

Prior to 1975, when therapy was primarily directed to the identifiable gross tumor, few children survived this disease (131). Those children who did well had favorable presentations, including limited resectable abdominal disease, or involvement of a single nodal region or of a single bone. With current intensive multiagent regimens, survival is excellent for all patients except those with grossly disseminated disease. Most recurrences in NHL occur within 12 months of diagnosis and are uncommon beyond 2 years (151,158). Histology is no longer of great prognostic significance for outcome. It is, however, the basis for choosing the therapeutic regimen.

1. Children with stage I-II disease have an 85% to 97% 2-year DFS (139,156). Patients with nonlymphoblastic histologies may fare somewhat better than those with lymphoblastic disease.

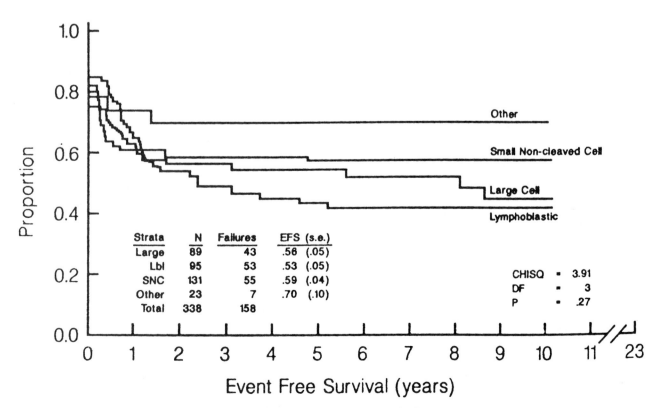

Fig. 19-4. EFS for childhood NHL. From Murphy *et al.* (155), with permission.

2. Children with stage III disease have a 60% to 80% 2-year DFS, with follow-up in most studies substantially longer than 2 years (155).
3. Children with stage IV non-lymphoblastic NHL have a much poorer prognosis with a 35% to 55% likelihood of remaining in remission for more than 2 years (156). Those with stage IV lymphoblastic lymphoma (T-cell ALL) have 60-80% event-free survival.

Prognostic Factors

1. The tumor burden at presentation is the most prominent determinant of treatment outcome (147,155). The clinical stage assigned to the patient, which is determined by the tumor burden and by disease extent, also predicts outcome.
2. The serum levels of several substances also appear to correlate to prognosis. It is likely that they also reflect tumor bulk, although other biologic explanations are possible. The most predictive substances include lactic dehydrogenase (127) and the interleukin-2 receptor (167).
3. Bone marrow or CNS involvement at diagnosis has been associated with a poor prognosis (119). However, newer intensive therapies appear to have overcome this association, at least for bone marrow involvement (134,161).
4. Although histology is no longer prognostically significant for outcome, it is extremely important in that it determines the specific therapy used (119,155).

CLINICAL INVESTIGATIONS

New approaches to diagnosis and therapy are under way that may improve the ability to cure children with NHL.

1. A more refined identification of prognostic factors based on biochemistry and molecular genetics may allow a more tailored approach to therapy.
2. For patients with particularly poor prognostic factors, such as those with undifferentiated (small noncleaved cell) NHL involving the CNS or bone marrow, more intensive therapies, perhaps coupled with BMT, are under investigation.
3. New chemotherapeutic agents and monoclonal-antibody-targeted immunotoxins are being developed, and biologic response modifiers such as alpha-2 interferon are being tested for their ability to enhance therapy.
4. Substances to protect or overcome the adverse effects of therapy may improve the therapeutic ratio by allowing more drug administration. Examples include mesna to protect the bladder and hematopoietic growth factors to ameliorate myelosuppression.
5. Advances in delineating the nature (e.g., chromosomal translocations, c-myc gene activity) of the neoplastic proliferation may permit therapy that is targeted toward these abnormalities.

Recommended Reading

An historical perspective of NHL in childhood is offered by Rosenberg *et al.* (163). Magrath (145) provides an updated review on the treatment of NHL in childhood. The article by Zigler *et al.* (172) reviews the role of EBV and human malignancy.

RHABDOMYOSARCOMA

Rhabdomysarcoma (RMS) is an aggressive tumor that arises from embryonal mesenchyme with the potential for differentiating into skeletal muscle (199). Since Stout's (217) landmark series in 1946, progress in the understanding and treatment of this complex neoplasm has been rapid. It can arise almost anywhere in the body, is locally invasive, and readily disseminates early in its course. In the past, the only cures were accomplished with radical surgery and these were only possible in the few children without metastases. Significant disfigurement and loss of function were common sequelae. High-dose radiation therapy increased the potential for local control but caused a different set of morbidities. As chemotherapy has become increasingly effective in both eliminating micrometastatic disease and assisting in local control, the need for aggressive surgery and large-volume irradiation has diminished (186,203,208,210,221). Overall survival rates have concomitantly increased from less than ~20% in the 1960s to as high as 70%. A paramount role in this progress has been played by investigators comprising the Intergroup Rhabdomyosarcoma Studies (IRS), which is now in its fourth generation of protocols (202).

EPIDEMIOLOGY AND ETIOLOGY

Epidemiology

1. Rhabdomyosarcoma accounts for 4% to 8% of childhood malignancies and 5% to 15% of childhood solid tumors, and is the most common pediatric soft tissue sarcoma (174,228).
2. Annual incidence in the United States is 4.5 per million in whites and 1.3 per million in blacks, a ratio of 3:1 (174,228).
3. Thirty-eight percent of RMS occur in children under 5 years of age, 47% in those 5 to 14 years old, and 15% in those 15 years and older (202).
4. Rhabdomyosarcoma can arise in any site where striated muscle is located as well as in mesenchymal tissue in other areas (190).

Etiology

1. The etiology of RMS is unknown, although reports of tumors in children with neurofibromatosis, and in families with multiple tumors, have genetic implications (198,199). An increased frequency of congenital anomalies CNS, GI, genitourinary, cardiac among children with RMS has been noted (215). An increased relative risk for RMS has also been associated with paternal cigarette smoking and exposure to chemicals (187).
2. A variety of karyotypic abnormalities have been found, and a greater frequency of DNA-aneuploidy appears to be present as compared with other childhood sarcomas (225). The most consistent anomaly is a homozygosity for a mutant allele on chromosome 11, a finding similar to that for Wilms' tumor and hepatoblastoma (195). This phenomenon in these three embryonal tumors suggests a common pathogenetic mechanism.

DETECTION AND DIAGNOSIS

Clinical Detection

Rhabdomyosarcoma commonly presents as an asymptomatic mass with poorly defined margins. Specific presentations relate to the primary disease site (178).

Orbit: Swelling, proptosis, discoloration, limitation of extraocular motion.

Other head and neck sites: Hoarseness, polyps, obstruction, dysphagia, decreased hearing, persistent otitis, sinusitis or parotitis, and cranial nerve palsies (particularly the facial nerve). Penetration into the brain can occur with parameningeal sites and mimic an intracranial mass, with headache, vomiting, and diplopia.

Retroperitoneum: GI discomfort or other mass-related symptoms.

Genitourinary tract: Urethal, vaginal or other perineal masses, hematuria, urinary frequency or retention. Paratesticular RMS can appear as a hydrocele, incarcerated hernia, testicular torsion, or mass.

Extremity: Painful or asymptomatic mass.

Trunk: Mass simulating a hernia or hematoma, or causing a classic superior vena cava syndrome.

Diagnostic Procedures

1. *Laboratory tests*, including complete blood cell count with differential, liver and renal function tests, and urinalysis.
2. *Radiographs*, CT, and MRI of the involved area and adjacent structures as indicated (225). Specific examinations may include the following:
   a. Head and neck: Skull or dental films, middle ear tomography, lumbar puncture with CSF cytology.
   b. Retroperitoneum: IVP.
   c. Genitourinary tract: Barium enema, IVP, voiding cystourethrogram, ultrasound, cystoscopy, and pelvic examination under anesthesia.
   d. An arteriogram or inferior venacavagram may assist in determining operability.
   e. Evaluation for metastases with bone marrow biopsy, chest CT, bone scan, and liver scan abdominal scan.
   f. Myelogram or spinal MRI if spinal cord-related symptoms are present.
   g. Biopsy of the lesion establishes the diagnosis and should be performed before extensive surgery.

CLASSIFICATION AND STAGING

Histopathology

Most RMS subtypes are soft, fleshy tumors with variation in the extent of invasion and necrosis. The exception is the botryoides subtype, which has a grapelike myxoid polypoid appearance (177,190). Cross-striations and periodic acid-Schiff positivity (from cytoplasmic glycogenic) may be seen by light microscopy. Intracytoplasmic filaments and Z-band material may be identified by electron microscopy. Table 19-13 (33) (202) shows the relative frequency of the four classically described histologic types, which are described as follows (182).

1. *Embryonal*: Primitive spindle-shaped small cells with elliptical nuclei. Botryoides is a subtype of embryonal. The embryonal histology is usually found in head and neck, genitourinary, and retroperitoneal sites.
2. *Alveolar*: Alveolar microarchitecture, sometimes with multinucleated giant cells. This subtype is usually found in older children with extremity lesions (212a).
3. *Pleomorphic*: Large, sometimes multinucleated cells with extensive pleomorphism, mixed with spindle and strap cells. This uncommon subtype is usually found in trunk and extremity lesions.
4. *Other*: Includes undifferentiated mesenchymal sarcoma and other special types, usually found in extremity and head and neck sites.

Despite previous publications to the contrary, recent correlations of the outcome of patients with tumors classified according to the above conventional schema have shown a lack of prognostic significance (210). Consequently Palmer and Foulkes (206), in connection with the IRS, have proposed a cytologic-based (i.e., cell nucleus) based classification scheme as follows.

1. *Monomorphous*: Cells with uniform size. Five percent of patients have this subtype and their prognosis is poor.
2. *Anaplastic*: Enlarged and bizarre mitotic figures are frequent. Again, 5% of patients have this subtype and their prognosis is poor.
3. *Mixed*: Includes all other tumors and is associated with a more favorable prognosis.

Because of additional classification systems and a lack of either acceptance or efficacy of any one, an international workshop is attempting to construct a single acceptable system (175,210).

Table 19-13. Conventional Pathologic Subtypes and Sites of Rhabdomyosarcoma and Undifferentiated Sarcoma

Pathologic Type	Predominant Primary Sites	Relative Frequency (%)	Usual Age Range (yr)
Embryonal RMS	Head and neck, genitourinary tract	57	3-12
Botryoides RMS	Bladder, vagina; nasopharynx	6	0-3;4-8
Alveolar RMS	Extremities, trunk	19	6-21
UDS	Extremities, trunk	10	6-21
Other	Extremities, trunk	8	6-21

Adapted from Hayes and Smith (33).

Staging

The IRS classification system is most widely used and is based on disease extent, including status of regional nodes, and tumor resectability (Fig. 19-5, Table 19-14) (196). Patient outcome is highly predictable using this system. Drawbacks relate to the emphasis on surgical reduction of tumor bulk implicit in this system. This may lead surgeons to perform unnecessarily, morbid surgery at inappropriate times. In addition, the surgical approach is not uniformly applied and this may obfuscate interpretation of the results. Consequently, other systems have been proposed based on tumor extent, lymph node involvement, the presence of metastases, and tumor histology (179,184,196) (Table 19-13). Evaluations of these systems are currently in progress.

PRINCIPLES OF TREATMENT

With the exception of patients with orbital or genitourinary primary sites, aggressive surgery and radiation therapy alone has been curative less than 25% of the time (192,193,219). Substantial functional and cosmetic morbidity may result from this approach to therapy. Recognition that combination chemotherapy can eradicate micrometastatic disease and reduce the extent of local disease, and that radiation therapy can control local disease has led to a decrease in aggressive surgery except in selected situations (181,186,191,194). The optimal sequencing and intensity of the three modalities are continually evolving (Table 19-15).

Surgery

1. Initial surgery should be an incisional biopsy for diagnosis.
2. Wide resection of the primary tumor, including surrounding normal tissue, offers a good chance for local control.
3. The extent and timing of surgical excision depends on the site of tumor. The overall treatment strategy is related to the prospects for survival without excessive morbidity.
4. Reoperation for microscopic residual disease following an initial excision, or when the first operation was carried out without knowledge of the type of neoplasm involved, may be indicated prior to further management. This is site-dependent (see section on special considerations). Reoperation following chemotherapy and radiotherapy as a salvage procedure, sometimes necessitating an exenterative procedure, is sometimes appropriate (210).
5. Elective en bloc lymph node dissection is rarely indicated, although staging biopsy for enlarged regional nodes should be done (197,203).

Radiation Therapy

1. Rhabdomyosarcoma may infiltrate tissues extensively and radiation portals must encompass the entire extent of the tumor volume. Margins are based on the confidence with which this volume can be identified and on

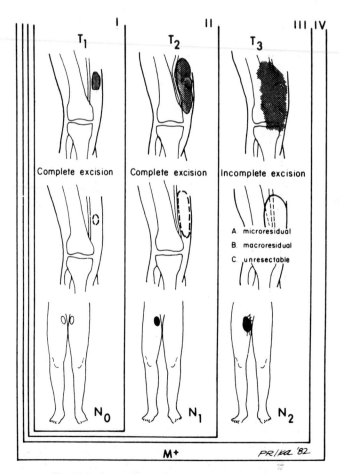

Fig. 19-5. Anatomic staging for rhabdomyosarcoma.

Table 19-14. Intergroup Rhabdomyosarcoma Study Clinical Grouping System

Clinical Group	Definition
I A	Localized, completely resected, confined to site of origin
I B	Localized, completely resected, infiltrated beyond site of origin
II A	Localized, grossly resected microscopic residual
II B	Regional disease, involved lymph nodes, completely resected
II C	Regional disease, involved lymph nodes, grossly resected with microscopic residual
III A	Local or regional grossly visible disease after biopsy only
III B	Grossly visible disease after >50% resection of primary tumor
IV	Distant metastases present at diagnosis

the location of critical normal tissues that should be excluded. In the setting of surgical reduction of gross disease and multiagent chemotherapy, a 2 to 5 cm margin is generally appropriate.

2. Aggressive radiation therapy to doses of 50 to 65 Gy can provide local control of gross residual or microscopic disease in 90% of patients; however, the higher dose may result in substantial late morbidity (180,220). With the concomitant use of chemotherapy in the first IRS trial, local control rates were generally high, but did depend on the radiation dose, with an increased recurrence rate found at lower doses (200a,202). A recent report from Memorial Sloan-Kettering by Mandell *et al.* (200a) found 40Gy with chemotherapy was effective for microscopic residuum. Larger tumor volumes (greater than 5 cm) were also associated with higher recurrence rates. The implication of the above is that higher radiation doses are necessary, yet they are known to be associated with substantial long-term morbidity. To deal with this dilemma, trials of new strategies using multiple fractions of irradiation are under way (200). Until such studies are complete, dose

ranges will remain at 40 to 45 Gy for microscopic disease (199a) and 50 to 55 Gy for gross disease. Children less than 6 years of age will generally receive 5 Gy less.

3. Interstitial radiation therapy will occasionally be advantageous for selected sites and circumstances (201).

4. Radiation therapy must be carefully coordinated with other therapies so as not to impair surgical healing or drug administration. Major considerations include the primary site (see special considerations section), the suppression of bone marrow, and the interaction of radiation therapy with chemotherapeutic agents.

Chemotherapy

Since the widespread adoption of chemotherapy as part of the therapy of RMS, progressive refinements have occurred. IRS-I tested whether VAC (vincristine, actinomycin-D, cyclophosphamide) was superior to VA in group II disease and whether pulse VAC plus doxorubicin was superior to pulse VAC alone in groups II and III disease. No benefit was found for cyclophosphamide in group II disease nor to the addition

Table 19-15. Rhabdomyosarcoma (Intergroup Rhabdomyosarcoma Studies-III Guidelines)

Group	Surgery	Radiotherapy (Gy)	Chemotherapy
I Non alveolar	CR	None	MAC
I Alveolar	CR	41.4	MAC
II	GR	41.4	MAC
III + IV (except special pelvic)	IR*	41.4 (< 6 yr, < 5 cm)	MAC
		45 (< 6 yr, ≥ 5 cm ≥ 6 yr, < 5 cm)	MAC
		50.4 (≥ 6 yr, ≥ 5 cm)	MAC
III Special pelvic: (bladder, prostate vagina, uterus)	Incisional or cytoscopic biopsy only	Same as III-IV†	MAC

New IRS-IV protocols include hyperfraction radiotherapy for group III patients, and radiotherapy for all patients with pelvic presentation.

*For group IV, excise if possible.
†Some patients with second surgery, complete resection may avoid radiotherapy.
IR = incomplete resection; MAC = multiagent chemotherapy; CR = complete resection; GR = gross resection.

of doxorubicin in groups III and IV (202). In IRS-II, no benefit was found for "pulse" VAC as compared to VA for group II. In groups III and IV, pulse VAC was better than a VAC plus doxorubicin-containing combination, but statistical significance was lacking. IRS-IV is comparing VAC, VAI (vincristine, actinomycin, ifosfamide) and VIE (vincristine ifosfamide, etoposide) for stage I-III. Newer agents are being piloted for stage IV.

SPECIAL CONSIDERATIONS

Specific Sites

Bladder: Bladder RMS usually arises in the submucosa and subsequently invades the bladder wall. The morbidity of excision, when necessitating partial or total pelvic exenteration, is inappropriate in light of the efficacy of radiation therapy and chemotherapy in providing local disease control (185,207). Several IRS trials have attempted to define the situations where surgical excision is appropriate or when radiation therapy is necessary. In general, primary bladder dome tumors that can be completely excised with bladder preservation might be properly managed without radiation therapy. This approach, however, is less efficacious for trigone or bladder neck lesions (209a). IRS-III guidelines for patients with residual gross disease after initial surgery entail initial chemotherapy alone. If a CR or partial response occurs, then surgery is performed and radiation therapy is avoided. If tumor remains after surgery, then radiation therapy is given. Surgery is then performed to document a CR or to excise residual disease, if present. Radiation therapy should be designed with consideration for shielding the femoral epiphyseal plates and proximal femurs.

Prostate: Because prostate RMS tends to be locally invasive and disseminates early, radical surgery is rarely possible or indicated (185,207). The current therapeutic approach is to start with vigorous chemotherapy in an attempt render the tumor resectable and avoid radiation therapy. If a complete surgical excision is not possible, radiation therapy is given at that time and surgery is used to document the response or remove residual disease. Chemotherapy is then continued.

Paratesticular: The spermatic cord is generally the site of origin although the epididymis or tunics may also be the primary. An orchiectomy is performed through an inguinal incision with a high ligation of the spermatic cord. Although controversy exists as to the need for retroperitoneal lymph node dissection, this practice is recommended until additional data are available (212). An ipsilateral dissection alone is less morbid and probably appropriate in view of the rarity of cross-over nodal metastasis. Radiation therapy is administered postoperatively to both the lymph nodes (again, until data obviating this practice are available) and to any violated scrotal tissues.

Orbit: The effectiveness of radiation therapy for controlling local disease while preserving vision has reduced the need for enucleation (226).

Other head and neck sites: Superficial lesions may be completely resected with satisfactory cosmesis and function, but deeper lesions routinely require irradiation (180,227). Portals are carefully constructed to avoid uninvolved normal tissues.

Children with parameningeal head and neck disease present a major therapeutic problem in that complete surgical extirpation is essentially impossible and both local and CNS failures are common without optimal therapy (211,218). When intracranial extension is present at diagnosis, radiation therapy is given at the beginning of the course of therapy. In other instances chemotherapy is given first. In the absence of intracranial extension (negative CSF cytology, no nerve palsies, and no erosion of the base of the skull) the primary lesion is irradiated with a margin including the adjacent meninges. If intracranial extension is present but CSF cytology is negative, then prophylactic whole brain irradiation is also administered. If CSF is also positive, craniospinal irradiation is necessary. Intrathecal chemotherapy is routine.

Extremity: Disease extent and nodal status should be assessed, including the sampling of adjacent lymph nodes. As in other sites, radical surgical procedures, particularly amputation, are excessive (189). However, if substantial morbidity can be avoided, gross excision of the tumor remains superior to biopsy alone. The radiation therapy volume is generous, although generally does not include the entire muscle compartment. A strip of the extemity is spared to avoid lymphedema.

Vagina: The botryoides form of RMS, is frequent in this location. Chemotherapy with or without surgery is frequently used. When radiation therapy is used in order to avoid excessive surgical morbidity or because of residual disease, interstitial radiation therapy or contact brachytherapy may be appropriate (181a,188).

Uterus: Difficulty sometimes exists in distinguishing uterine from vaginal RMS. In IRSIII, chemotherapy was administered followed by surgery in group III and radiotherapy when necessary (173).

Retroperitoneum: Rhabdomyosarcoma in this site is frequently of large bulk at diagnosis. Complete resection is generally not feasible. Unfortunately, radiation therapy is limited by normal tissue tolerances. New strategies such as intraoperative radiation therapy are under investigation.

Paraspinal. Paraspinal tumors may require extended field radiation therapy and more intensive chemotherapy because of high local regional failure and to achieve systemic control (205a).

RESULTS AND PROGNOSIS

Results of Therapy

The overall survival for RMS, according to histology, site, and stage are depicted in Fig. 19-6 (205).

1. By stage: Groups I and II are clearly superior with more localized and resectable disease. At best, 50% to 90% survival is probable if metastatic disease is in its occult stage. Patients with metastasis (stage IV) do not fare well (20% survival) (Fig. 19-6a) (202).
2. By histopathology: Sarcoma botryoides is the most favorable type, with a 90% survival at 10 years, followed by embryonal 65% ; alveolar is the worst, at 45% (Fig. 19-6b) (202).
3. By site: Orbital tumors are the most favorable with a 90% survival, followed by those with genitourinary origins (75%). In the more common head and neck and extremity locations survival is 50%, whereas larger truncal and retroperitoneal tumors have 30% survival (Fig. 19-6c) (205).

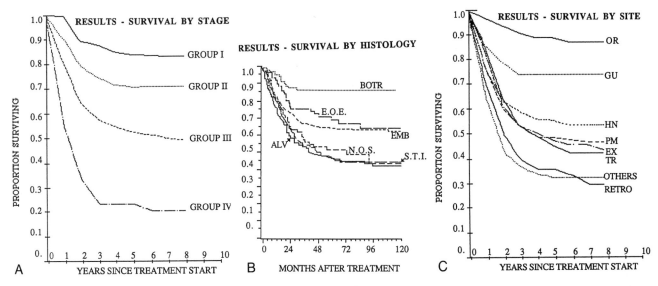

Fig. 19-6. Results. (A) Survival by stage. From Mauer *et al.* (202), with permission. (B) Survival by histology. From Mauer *et al.* (202), with permission. (C) Survival by site. From Newton *et al.* (205), with permission.

Patterns of Relapse

Time to Relapse

Eighty percent of recurrences occur in the first 2 years following completion of localized therapy for patients who recur after having achieved a CR. If disease recurs while the patient is undergoing primary therapy, the median survival is 20 weeks, with long-term survival currently unobtainable. For patients whose disease recurs after having achieved CR and completed therapy, 20% can be successfully salvaged, depending on certain pretreatment characteristics (209).

Sites of Relapse

Rhabdomyosarcoma is a systemic disease and essentially all patients are presumed have at least micrometastatic disease. Twenty percent have demonstrable metastases. Rhabdomyosarcoma spreads via blood and lymphatics. Relapse is most frequent locally. Distant spread occurs, in order of decreasing frequency in the lungs, CNS, lymph nodes, bone, liver, bone marrow, and soft tissues (182, 203).

Prognostic Factors

The most important determinant to date is the clinical group of the patient, that is, disease extent at the time chemotherapy is initiated (176, 183, 196, 202, 204,212a,213a,214).

Metastatic disease is present in 20% of patients at diagnosis, and their long-term survival remains poor (a 7% probability with bone marrow involvement, 23% with other sites) (216).

Lymph node involvement is identified in 10% to 14%, of patients without distant metastases at diagnosis (26). The percentage is highest for prostatic (41%), paratesticular (26%), and genitourinary (24%) sites. Sites with a small percentage of proven involvement were the orbit (0%), trunk (3%), nonorbital head and neck (7%), and extremities (12%). Patients with lymph node involvement had a 3-year survival estimate of 54%, compared with 78% for patients without lymph node involvement.

The primary site of disease is of prognostic importance (183, 196). The tumor location determines the presenting signs and symptoms, which may be associated with the rapidity of diagnosis. The propensity for lymphatic spread depends on the location. The location of the lesion influences the ability to use aggressive surgery or radiotherapy.

CLINICAL INVESTIGATIONS

IRS-IV was recently implemented. New drug combinations, radiation strategies, and sequencing with surgery are under investigation. BMT continues to be tested in selected patients with metastatic or recurrent disease.

Recommended Reading

A brief but comprehensive overview of childhood rhabdomyosarcoma is provided by Raney *et al.* (210). For further detailed discussions, please see Hays *et al.* (188), Maurer *et al.* (203), Raney *et al.* (211, 212), and Tefft *et al.* (223). An overview of the pathologic differential diagnosis of childhood sarcomas can be found in Dehner (177) and a classic article by Horn and Enterline (190). Schema and complications of therapy are discussed in articles by Tefft *et al.* (221, 222).

GERM CELL TUMORS AND TERATOMA

Germ cell tumors (GCT) are benign or malignant growths that arise from the primordial germ cells. Germs cells first appear in the yolk sac endoderm and migrate around the hindgut to the genital ridge of the embryo on the posterior abdominal wall, where they congregate and subsequently become part of the developing gonad (290). Tumors of the gonads often arise from these cell (239).

It has been postulated that a slightly aberrant path of migration may account for the occurrence of extragonadal germ cell tumors along the dorsal wall of the embryo in midline sites, primarily the sacrococcygeal, retroperitoneal, mediastinal, and pineal regions (231). An alternative theory suggests that totipotential cells that develop from Hensen's node (primitive knot) escape organizing forces and become independent neoplasms, resulting in the midline and paraxial distribution of these tumors (285). The high incidence of sacrococcygeal tumors can be accounted for by the fact that the primitive knot migrates through a caudal area to the region of the coccyx.

Independent of mechanism of origin, the type of tumor that results is determined by the subsequent development of the germ cell (280). Those cells that undergo gonadal differentiation become the germinomas, also known as seminomas or dysgerminomas. Those that maintain their totipotentiality may become embryonal carcinomas. The development of extraembryonic structures results in endodermal sinus tumors (yolk sac tumors) or choriocarcinomas (placental tumors). Embryonic differentiation into ectoderm, mesoderm, and endoderm results in teratomas (274) (Fig. 19-7) (3).

EPIDEMIOLOGY AND ETIOLOGY

Epidemiology

The most common GCT is the sacrococcygeal teratoma, from the Greek "teras," or monster. This tumor occurs in 1 of 35,000 live births and is two to four times more frequent in girls than in boys. Eighty percent of these tumors are benign. Approximately 40% of childhood GCT originate in the sacrococcygeal area. The remainder of GCT arise in other locations, including the gonads, mediastinum, neck, intracranial region, and retroperitoneum. Four malignant GCTs occur per million children under the age of 15 years, accounting for 3% of tumors in children (291).

Children with sacrococcygeal teratomas have a 12% to 18% incidence of associated anomalies, most often of the anorectal region (e.g., imperforate anus, rectal stenosis) (249). The frequent association of a family history of twinning with the occurrence of sacrococcygeal teratomas, resulted in early theories suggesting that teratomas were abortive attempts at the development of twins. It is of interest to note that the common sites of teratomas — the brain, mediastinum, abdomen, and sacrococcygeal regions — are all sites of conjoined twin attachments.

ETIOLOGY

Genetics

Although most GCT occur in otherwise normal individuals, a genetic tendency for abnormal germ cell development may exist in some families. Instances of malignant GCT have been reported in siblings, twins, and up to three generations of individuals in families (252,262,281). Gonadal dysgenesis (particularly in phenotypic females with 46XY karyotypes) has been associated with gonadoblastoma or dysgerminoma (250). In one family, a phenotypically normal brother of two such females was diagnosed with a testicular choriocarcinoma containing elements of embryonal carcinoma and seminoma (257). These findings suggest that abnormal germ cell development may play a role in the ultimate appearance of GCT.

In testicular and ovarian tumors, an isochromosome marker of the short arm of chromosome 12 (ipl2) has been noted (232,253). More recent studies using flow cytometry, have shown variations in the ploidy of various teratoma and germinoma specimens (270). Aneuploidy may be associated with an unfavorable prognosis. The proliferative activity of disseminated GCT, determined by flow cytometric study of cells obtained from paraffin imbedded tissue, correlated with duration of survival (278). Such studies may be clinically useful in the future.

Markers

Malignant GCT, with evidence of extraembryonic differentiation, often produce proteins commonly elaborated by the corresponding normal extraembryonic structure. These markers have use in the detection, diagnosis, and subsequent monitoring of patients with these tumors (277).

Alpha-fetoprotein (AFP) is present in the serum of human fetuses, particularly at 12 to 15 weeks' gestation. The fetal liver and the yolk sac both produce this protein. AFP has been found in GCT specimens that have endodermal sinus tumor histology (yolk sac origin). Serum levels of AFP are elevated in these patients' sera as well as in the serum of patients with malignant teratomas without detected yolk sac tumor elements. The latter finding suggests that yolk sac tumor elements are present and that more aggressive therapy may be necessary. When evaluating AFP levels, it is important to recognize that the child must reach 9 months of age before the high levels present at birth have fallen to adult levels (282). The *in vivo* half-life of AFP is 4 to 5 days. The rate of disappearance of serum AFP following resection of an AFP-producing tumor correlates with the adequacy of tumor removal. Radiolabelled antibodies to AFP have been developed and may be useful for *in vivo* detection and localization of these neoplasms.

Beta human chorionic gonadatropin (beta-HCG) is a glycoprotein normally produced by specialized placental cells to enable the fertilized egg to remain implanted in the uterine wall. Germ cell tumors with trophoblastic elements (choriocarcinomas), hydatidiform moles, and pregnancy all produce beta-HCG. The finding of an elevated serum beta-HCG level in a patient whose teratoma does not have histologically recognizable chorionic elements, suggests that such elements are nonetheless present within the tumor.

PRESENTATION AND EVALUATION

The presentation and evaluation of a patient depends on the location of the GCT.

Sacrococcygeal (230,288): This tumor arises from the anterior portion of the coccyx and generally presents as an external mass between the anus and coccyx. The appearance

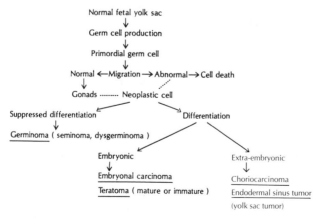

Fig. 19-7. Classification of germ cell tumors. From Halperin *et al.* (3), with permission.

varies from a small mass with a dimple to a large pendulous lesion. The overlying skin may be normal or roughened, shiny, hairy, tense, wrinkled, or ulcerated. An intrapelvic component may cause the patient to experience urinary or rectal obstruction. This may occur in association with an external mass or in the absence of any external tumor. Intradural tumor extension is found in 3% to 5% of the lesions. Maternal polyhydramnios has been associated with sacrococcygeal teratoma in infants (275).

Evaluation of the patient includes a physical examination, with particular attention to the abdominal and rectal examination. Intrapelvic or abdominal extensions of an external mass should be sought with a barium enema, ultrasound, and IVP or an abdominal and pelvic CT scan. AFP and beta-HCG levels should be determined preoperatively. The most frequent alternative diagnosis is meningocele.

Ovarian (235,240,259,265,269,272): In infants, ovarian tumors almost always present as an abdominal mass. Older girls present with symptoms of abdominal pain (most common), nausea, vomiting, constipation or urinary tract obstruction. Only half have palpable masses. Acute abdominal pain may be caused by torsion of the tumor on its pedical or hemorrhage within the tumor. About 5% of children will have bilateral tumors.

Evaluation consists of a physical examination searching for an abdominal mass. An abdominal x-ray will reveal calcification in approximately half of the children, most of which will be benign. Ultrasound of a teratoma will show both cystic and solid components. Mature elements such as bone or teeth may be noted. CT scans may be useful in evaluating larger lesions. Preoperative values of AFP and beta-HCG should be obtained.

Testicular (246,260,287): Testicular tumors present as an asymptomatic scrotal mass. Coexisting hydroceles may be present in 15% to 25% of the patients. There is no preponderance of one side over the other. Occasionally, bilateral tumors are noted. Torsion of tumors in undescended testes may present as acute abdominal pain. Malignancy of the testis is 20 to 40 times higher in patients with undescended testes. However, the incidence of cancer is increased not only in undescended testis of these patients, but also in the contralateral testis, suggesting that testicular cancer may result from an intrinsic testicular defect (267).

Evaluation consists of a scrotal examination, a CT scan of the chest and abdomen for pulmonary metastases and retroperitoneal adenopathy, a bone scan, and preoperative measurements of AFP and beta-HCG serum levels. The differential diagnosis for an intrascrotal mass includes testicular torsion, epididymitis, and testicular infarction. Abdominal, pelvic, and scrotal ultrasounds may prove helpful in following patients during treatment.

Mediastinal tumors (258,268): Patients with anterior mediastinal masses often have cough, wheezing, dyspnea, and chest pain. Newborns may require immediate intubation for respiratory distress. Intrapericardial tumors may cause congestive heart failure and cardiac tamponade.

Evaluation should include chest x-ray and a CT scan of the chest. Mediastinal teratomas are calcified in approximately 35% of cases. Echocardiography is useful for the delineation of intrapericardial tumors. For these tumors, cardiac catheterization is necessary to determine whether other cardiac anomalies exist and to evaluate the course of the great blood vessels as well as the blood supply to the tumor. Serum AFP and beta-HCG values should be obtained preoperatively.

Abdominal (244,271): Most abdominal GCT are located in the retroperitoneum, although gastric and hepatic tumors have been reported. Retroperitoneal teratomas in children under aged 2 years usually present as asymptomatic abdominal masses. Older children with retroperitoneal GCT may have anorexia, vomiting, and abdominal pain. Rarely, intradural extensions may develop, resulting in neurologic disorders of the lower extremities. Gastric tumors commonly cause abdominal distention and masses. Vomiting and hematemesis may occur.

Evaluation includes abdominal and chest x-rays. Teratomas will often contain calcifications. A CT scan of the abdomen defines the relationship of the tumor mass to adjacent structures. An upper GI series may be necessary, particularly for gastric tumors. A 24-hour urine sample is collected for catecholamines to distinguish this tumor from the more common neuroblastoma. Serum samples for AFP and beta-HCG are obtained.

Head and neck germ cell tumors (254): Germ cell tumors of the head and neck occur most commonly in infants. Cervical teratomas in the newborn present as an obvious neck mass, frequently causing respiratory obstruction. Maternal polyhydramnios has been observed in 22% of patients and is believed to be due to the inability of the fetus to swallow. Oropharyngeal teratomas usually present as large masses protruding from the mouth, frequently causing respiratory distress and cyanosis.

Management of these tumors consists of endotracheal intubation for respiratory distress and an x-ray of the neck. Patients with oropharyngeal teratomas should also have skull films obtained to detect calcifications and bony abnormalities. Calcifications suggest a teratoma. Ultrasound will reveal mixed, cystic, or solid tissues. A CT scan can reveal the extent of cervical teratomas. Preoperative thyroid function studies are required for appropriate evaluation. Serum samples are obtained preoperatively for the measurement of AFP and beta-HCG.

Intracranial tumors (273,286): The pineal region is the most common site of an intracranial GCT, although 20% are located in suprasellar or infrasellar regions. Infants present with hydrocephalus and symptoms of increased cranial pressure. In teenagers, headaches are common presenting features. In addition, there may be lethargy, vomiting, visual disturbance, diabetes insipidus, and seizures associated with this tumor.

Skull films in the newborn with a teratoma frequently demonstrate calcification, almost always in a supratentorial location. A CT scan may reveal the extent of a tumor and the associated ventricular enlargement. Arteriorography may be helpful to demonstrate the effect on blood supply and aid in planning the surgical approach. Measurements are made of AFP and beta-HCG in the serum and CSF.

Vaginal (233,292): Girls with vaginal GCT are usually less than 3 years of age and often present with a bloody vaginal discharge. Vaginal examination in such a young child should be performed under anesthesia. Chest x-ray, CT scan of the chest, abdomen, and pelvis and a bone scan will be necessary in addition to serum AFP and beta-HCG. The tumor must be differentiated from a rhabdomyosarcoma of the vagina (sarcoma botyroides).

CLASSIFICATION

Histopathology

GCT arise from pluripotential germ cells that may remain in an undifferentiated state (embryonal carcinoma), may differentiate along a pathway of gonadal differentiation (germinoma), or may differentiate into either embryonic (teratoma) or extraembryonic (endodermal sinus tumor or a choriocarcinoma) structures (274,280) (Fig. 19-7) (3). Germ cell tumors are thus a diverse group of tumors with pathologic and clinical characteristics specific to the type of cells involved.

Teratoma (248): Teratomas are unusual tumors in that they are composed of all three germ layers: the ectoderm, mesoderm, and endoderm. They present as a mixture of both cystic and solid elements. Although all types of germ layer tissues are seen, neural tissues often predominate. Mature structures may be found: hair, teeth, bone. Malignancy from any of these tissues may arise, the most common being adenocarcinoma and rhabdomyosarcoma. Extraembryonic tissues may result in endodermal sinus tumor or choriocarcinoma. Histologically, teratomas have been classified into three main types: mature, immature, and teratoma with malignant components (264). Mature teratomas with well-differentiated tissues present are benign. Immature teratomas have embryonic-appearing neuroglial or neuroepithelial elements in addition to mature elements. Mature and immature teratomas are most commonly found in infants. Although malignant evolution is more likely to occur in immature teratomas than in mature teratomas, malignancy has occurred years after removal of an apparently benign tumor (279). This occurs most commonly in the sacrococcygeal area. Whether this represents a recurrence or a second primary is unclear. The sacrococcygeal region is also the most common site for a teratoma with malignant components — usually endodermal sinus tumors and embryonal carcinoma. Teratomas display positive staining for AFP or beta-HCG only when malignant elements are present.

Endodermal sinus tumor: This is the most common malignant germ cell tumor in the pediatric age group. Grossly, the endodermal sinus tumors are pale, tan-yellow, with foci of necrosis and small cystic areas. They are soft and fall apart easily. Microscopically, the cells are pale and resemble those of the yolk sac, with reticular, pseudopapillary, polyvesicular, vitelline or solid patterns, or mixtures of the above. Perivascular cuffs of tumor cells, called Schiller-Duval bodies, are characteristic of this type of tumor.

Embryonal carcinoma: Microscopically these tumors consist of undifferentiated cells, usually densely packed. Embryonal, glandular, papillary, or clear cell adenocarcinomatous patterns are characteristic. Embryonal carcinoma is rarely a pure histologic pattern in infants and children. It is commonly seen in association with teratomas and endodermal sinus tumors.

Choriocarcinoma: Choriocarcinoma has two distinct forms, gestational and nongestational. The former arises within the placenta, and the latter from extraplacental tissue of a nonpregnant person. Histologic features are the same for both types, with cells resembling the chorionic layer. The two main components are cytotrophoblasts (large round cells with clear cytoplasm) and syncytiotrophoblasts (syncytia-forming large cells with abundant homogeneous, vacuolated cytoplasm, and dark irregular nuclei). Levels of beta-HCG are elevated in patients with choriocarcinoma.

Germinoma (seminoma, dysgerminoma): These tumors are composed of uniform polyhedral cells with fibrous tissue and infiltrates of lymphocytes. AFP and beta-HCG are negative if no other malignant germ cell elements are present. However, germinomas are most often found in combination with other GCT.

Staging

Because of the diverse location of these tumors, no satisfactory method of staging appropriate for all tumors has been developed. A variety of staging systems are available for testicular and ovarian tumors (283,284).

PRINCIPLES OF TREATMENT

If at all possible, teratomas should be completely removed surgically. Although most are benign, malignancy has been observed to develop in children years after the removal of an apparently benign tumor. Therefore, careful follow-up is necessary for all patients who have had teratomas excised. In the past, malignant teratomas, embryonal carcinoma, endodermal sinus tumor, and choriocarcinoma were almost informally fatal, even with apparently complete surgical resection. The one exception was embryonal carcinoma of the infant testis in which radical orchiectomy was sometimes curative. In the 1960s, Li *et al.* (261a) demonstrated the efficacy of chemotherapy for gestational choriocarcinomas and testicular germ cell tumors. Subsequently, major advances have been made in the treatment of germ cell tumors (242,247,256,266).

Surgery

For all localized GCT, complete surgical excision should be attempted. Surgical excision alone is the recommended treatment for benign germ cell tumors. Complete excision of the coccyx is recommended by some for the surgical treatment of the sacrococcygeal lesions. Since surgical complications of sacrococcygeal lesions usually involve hemorrhage, control of the tumor vasculature is important. In malignant lesions, extension along tissue planes may preclude complete removal. Second-look surgery may be of benefit after chemotherapy to completely excise tumor.

Radiation Therapy

In the past, radiation therapy to the tumor bed was coupled with chemotherapy for malignant GCT. In many instances, little effect by radiation therapy was noted. Radiation therapy may be beneficial for some patients who do not completely respond to chemotherapy and surgery (255).

Chemotherapy

For malignant GCT and some immature teratomas, particularly those with increased numbers of neuroglial cells, chemotherapy plays a major role. Responsiveness to chemotherapy was first noted for gestational choriocarcinoma (261). When treated with methotrexate, a 47% CR rate was observed. However, nongestational choriocarcinoma was not responsive. Responses to chemotherapy were noted in the 1960s for ovarian tumors, most commonly with drugs such as vincristine, actinomycin-D, cyclophosphamide (VAC) (236,289).

In the 1970s additional drugs (e.g., vinblastine, cisplatin) were found to have significant single-agent response rates in testicular GCT of young men (234,251,276). Einhorn and Donohue (241) used PVB to produce a 70% CR rate and a 55% long-term DFS for all patients with testicular carcinoma. Although maintenance therapy was initially used after a period of more intensive therapy, subsequent studies revealed that intensive therapy alone was effective (244).

PVB was shown to be more effective than VAC for patients with ovarian GCT (236), particularly for those with pure endodermal sinus tumors. Patients with GCT whose disease recurs after PVB may often be salvaged using other agents, including ifosfamide, etoposide, and doxorubicin (243,263).

Results of Therapy

The regimens described above, which were first used in adults, have been found to be effective in children as well. The Children's Cancer Study Group reported the results of treating 79 children with malignant germ cell tumors (39% of whom had widely disseminated metastases at diagnosis) with vinblastine, bleomycin, cisplatinum, actinomycin D, cyclophosphamide and doxorubicin. CRs were seen in 69%. Four years from diagnosis, 45% percent remained free of disease (229).

Prognostic Factors

The prognosis for patients with teratomas is dependent primarily on the degree of maturity — the prognosis for mature teratomas being better than that for immature teratomas. Malignant teratomas or other forms of malignant GCT are difficult to treat. Prognosis is also affected by the degree of disease spread.

For teratomas, age can be of prognostic significance. Sacrococcygeal teratomas are almost always benign in children under 2 months of age, but the likelihood of malignant evolution increases rapidly after this early period. It is thought that later diagnosis explains the increased incidence of malignancy in patients whose teratomas arise within the pelvis or abdomen compared with those with externally visible primaries. Mediastinal teratomas behave in a benign manner in children and young teenagers, but are more aggressive and often fatal in older patients (238). Cervical teratomas and intracranial teratomas in infants are usually benign, while those presenting in the teenage years or in adult life are frequently malignant.

Future Investigations

Studies involving the use of multiple chemotherapeutic agents continue. The roles of ifosfamide, etoposide, and high-dose cisplatin (200 mg/m²) are being explored. These previously fatal tumors are now curable in a high percentage of patients. With better use of the available agents, it is hoped that the percentage of cured patients will continue to increase.

Recommended Reading

The report of Grosfeld et al. (249) is recommended because it reports a series of teratomas with reference to location, age, and incidence of malignancy. The article by Tapper and Lack (279) is similarly helpful. Ovarian tumors in children and adolescents are reviewed by Ehren et al. (240). Testicular cancer in children has been reviewed by Exelby (345).

LANGERHANS CELL HISTIOCYTOSIS (HISTIOCYTOSIS X)

The Langerhans' cell histiocytoses (LCH) are a spectrum of diseases often referred to as histiocytosis X (301) that include eosinophilic granuloma, Hand-Schuller-Christian disease, and Letterer-Siwe disease. Unlike neoplasms, which are characterized by a clonal population of tumor cells, the lesions of LCH contain heterogeneous populations of morphologically normal reactive cells. The predominant cell is the macrophage or histiocyte, hence the grouping of clinically diverse syndromes under one subtitle. Langerhans' cell histiocytoses are characterized by frequent spontaneous remissions and exacerbations, with a 30% to 40% survival in untreated patients (296). Although the traditional therapeutic modalities are those used for malignant disorders, the approach to therapy is vastly different. The goal of therapy is to maintain control over the proliferating cells rather than to completely eradicate an abnormal clone. Since the approach to treatment differs, malignant proliferations of macrophage lineage such as monocytic leukemias, histiocytic lymphomas, and malignant histiocytoses must be distinguished from the LCH. Also to be distinguished are other nonmalignant histiocytoses, in which the involved histiocyte is of a phagocytic type. Disorders of this type include infection associated hemophagocytic syndrome, familioerythrophagocytic lymphohistiocytosis, and sinus histiocytosis.

EPIDEMIOLOGY AND ETIOLOGY

Epidemiology

The incidence of LCH is not well known, although it has been estimated to occur in 1 of 200,000 children. The disseminated form of the disease is more common in younger children (296).

Etiology

Langerhans' cell histiocytoses have been attributed to infection, autoimmune phenomena, hypersensitivity reactions, and neoplasia. Although speculations abound, the etiology of LCH is unknown. The various clinical presentations may represent a spectrum of one disease or distinct diseases of different etiologies grouped together by virtue of the associated histiocytic proliferation.

Biology

The Langerhans' cell of apparent monocyte-macrophage lineage that proliferates in the LCH appears to be related to the dermal macrophage. Both cell types are characterized by Birbeck's granules, the lymphocyte differentiation antigen CD-1 and presence of the S-100 antigen (303). In the skin, the dermal macrophage is an antigen-processing cell, suggesting that the LCH might be an immunologic proliferative response to an unknown antigen (298).

It has also been postulated that the Langerhans cell is responding to an abnormal signal from another part of the immune system. The findings of pathologic changes in the thymus gland and a deficiency of suppressor T cells have been cited as suggestive of an abnormality of T lymphocytes (3e).

Further investigation of this Langerhans' cell, and the factors that affect its proliferation and differentiation, may improve our understanding of these diseases.

DETECTION AND DIAGNOSIS

Clinical Detection

The clinical presentation of LCH varies, depending on the involved organs. Lytic bone lesions are present in the majority of cases. Skin, lung, liver, spleen, and bone marrow may also be affected, and may lose function as a result of cellular infiltration. Three classic presentations have been described (Table 19-16).

1. *Eosinophilic granuloma* is characterized by localized lesions confined to the bone. This form of disease occurs predominantly in older children or young adults.
2. *Hand-Schuller-Christian disease* has multiple-site involvement and often includes the classic triad of skull defects, diabetes insipidus, and exophthalmus. This form occurs primarily in children aged 2 to 5 years. The triad of symptoms may not arise concurrently. In particular, diabetes insipidus may appear long after other symptoms are in remission (294). Chronic otitis media and loss of teeth due to gum infiltration and the radiographic picture of "floating teeth" may occur. The flat bones of the skull, ribs, pelvis, and scapula are most commonly involved, although the long bones and lumbosacral vertebrae may be affected (307).
3. *Letterer-Siwe disease*, disseminated form of the disease, occurs primarily in infants and children younger than 2 years of age. Visceral lesions involve the skin, liver, lungs, lymph nodes, spleen, and other reticuloendothelial organs. In contrast to older children with LCH, these infants may be quite ill, with failure to thrive, hepatosplenomegaly, anemia, liver dysfunction, and significant pulmonary symptoms. Draining ears are often mistaken for otitis media, and the skin rash may be confused with infantile seborrhea or eczema.

Diagnosis

If a patient's physical examination and history are suggestive of histiocytosis X, a surgical biopsy must be performed for pathologic confirmation. Accessible soft tissue sites, such as skin or mucosal nodules, should be used when possible. Radiographic studies that should be performed include a chest x-ray, a skeletal survey including skull films, a bone scan, and an abdominal ultrasound to assess the size of the liver and spleen. Laboratory evaluations include a complete blood cell count and liver function tests that include total protein, albumin, transaminases, and prothrombin time/partial prothrombin time.

CLASSIFICATION AND STAGING

Histopathology

The Langerhans' cells are large histiocytic cells with pale nuclei that are often indented or folded, and contain up to three nucleoli (295). In addition to these cells, variable numbers of plasma cells, lymphocytes, and eosinophils are seen in biopsy specimens. Occasionally granulomas are found. The finding of Birbeck's granules by electron microscopy is considered pathognomonic of this disease. CD-1 is expressed and S-100 is positive.

Staging

A clinical staging system based on the prognostic factors of Lahey (302), in which stage is determined by the age of presentation (< 2 years versus > 2 years), the number of organs involved (< four organs or ≥ four organs), and the presence of organ dysfunction (302). Organs evaluated include the skin, bone, liver, lungs, spleen, pituitary, or hematopoietic system. More recently, it has been shown that the degree of dysfunction of certain organs (liver, lungs, and hematopoietic system) is of greater prognostic importance. A more complex system for staging has been devised by Greenberger *et al.* (297).

Each of these staging systems attempts to correlate with prognosis. An adolescent or an adult who presents with a solitary bone eosinophilic granuloma has the best prognosis, while an infant with multiple affected organs (Letterer-Siwe disease) has the worst. Skin involvement, liver dysfunction (demonstrated by hypoproteinemia or hyperbilirubinemia), pulmonary involvement (demonstrated by tachypnea, dyspnea, cyanosis, cough, pneumothorax, or pleural effusions), or hematopoietic dysfunction (demonstrated by anemia or thrombocytopenia) are particularly poor prognostic signs (300). Skel-

Table 19-16. Diagnostic Criteria For "Histiocytosis X" Syndromes

	Letter-Siwe Disease	Hand-Schüller-Christian Disease	Eosinophilic Granuloma of Bone
Age	**<2 years**	**>2 years**	**Older children**
Symptoms	Seborrheic or purpuric rash, anorexia, failure to thrive, lymphadenopathy, oraganomegaly	Exophthalmos, skeletal defects, diabetes insipidus, chronic otitis media, dental problems	Solitary or multiple bony lesions
Physical examination	Hepatosplenomegaly, lymphadenopathy, hemorrhages	Bone tenderness and swelling over lesions, exophthalmos	Bone tenderness and swelling over lesions
Biopsy	Diffuse proliferation of histiocytes, some eosinophils, and occasional granuloma	Diffuse proliferation of histiocytes, some eosinophils, and occasional granuloma	Diffuse proliferation of histiocytes, some eosinophils, and occasional granuloma
Course	Death may occur from pancytopenia, infection, or organ failure	Chronic, fluctuating	May be recurrent

etal involvement and diabetes insipidus are not associated with an unfavorable outcome (296). The natural history of histiocytosis is that a CR may be followed by relapse and death after months or years (304).

PRINCIPLES OF TREATMENT

As a disorder of excessive cellular proliferation, LCH responds to treatment modalities used for cancer therapy, including surgery, radiation, and chemotherapy (299). The goal, however, is to maintain control over the abnormal proliferation rather than to eradicate all cells. The side effects of therapy should not be greater than those related to the disease itself.

Surgery

Patients with single-site eosinophilic granulomas may be treated by surgical curettage. Extensive surgical procedures should be avoided.

Radiation Therapy

The lesions of histiocytosis X are exquisitely radiation-sensitive and usually regress with small doses, in the range of 450 to 900 cGy (Fig. 19-8) (296). Higher doses apparently do not provide increased local control. No dose response curve has been established. Care should be taken to avoid radiating potentially sensitive normal structures, such as the lens of the eye, thyroid, and kidney if at all possible. Except for patients who are at risk for skeletal deformity, visual loss secondary to exophthalmus, pathologic fractures, vertebral collapse, diabetes insipidus, or those suffering from severe pain, chemotherapy is the treatment of choice if multiple lesions exist (305).

Chemotherapy

The basic principle of systemic chemotherapy is to begin with the most benign treatment and then to add increasingly toxic agents if necessary, never making the treatment worse than the disease. The ultimate goal is to try to prevent permanent disability. Combination chemotherapy may be used initially in the most severely ill patients. Once a response is obtained, the doses and frequency of drug administration are reduced to find an effective regimen with the least amount of toxicity. Response to chemotherapy varies from 30% to 80% (306). Corticosteroids with or without vincristine or vinblastine are the preferred agents for initial therapy. If these agents fail, methotrexate and 6-mercaptopurine are often used. Other agents frequently used include cyclophosphamide, chlorambucil, and nitrogen mustard (297). More recently, etoposide at a dose of 200 mg/m^2 for 3 days was shown to induce a response in 15 of 18 patients (83% response rate) (293). Disease recurred in one of the 12 children who achieved a CR (301).

Immunotherapy

In vitro studies of lymphocyte activity have demonstrated that patients with LCH have abnormal, autoreactive lymphocytes. Incubation of their lymphocytes with thymic extracts prevents this autocytotoxicity (304). Recent investigations have explored the use of thymic extracts as therapy for children with LCH (304). Initial clinical studies showed a 51% response rate for 37 patients treated with thymic hormones. Further studies of this form of therapy are ongoing.

RESULTS AND PROGNOSIS

The outcome of LCH is extremely variable (Table 19-17). In most instances, the disease resolves with time, if the immediate complications of the disease are kept under control. This is particularly true for those patients with eosinophilic granuloma and Hand-Schuller-Christian disease. The time course for the disease may be quite prolonged. Those infants with disseminated Letterer-Siwe disease are at greater risk of succumbing to their disease. Greenberger *et al.* (296) analyzed 127 children with LCH according to his staging system. Approximately 80% of patients with stages I and II disease survived, compared with 60% of patients with stage III disease. All patients with stage IV disease were dead by 2 years of age. Although some of these stage IV patients may now be treated adequately, the prognosis for this group of patients remains poor.

When choosing a therapeutic regimen, both the immediate and long-term effects must be considered. Radiation therapy may have local effects on the growth of normal tissue in the irradiated area. Of the 127 patients reviewed by Greenberger *et al.* (296), 84 received chemotherapy, five of whom developed a late malignancy. All five of these patients received chlorambucil. Four patients received radiation therapy as well, and two of these four patients also received nitrogen mustard. Three of these patients developed acute leukemia, one developed thyroid carcinoma, and one developed hepatocellular carcinoma. An additional patient who was treated with radiation therapy alone developed thyroid carcinoma. Alkylating agents, particularly chlorambucil, should be avoided in patients with LCH unless it is absolutely essential to control active disease.

CLINICAL INVESTIGATIONS

Current therapies for this disease are aimed at controlling the proliferative response to the histiocytic cells. If the etiology

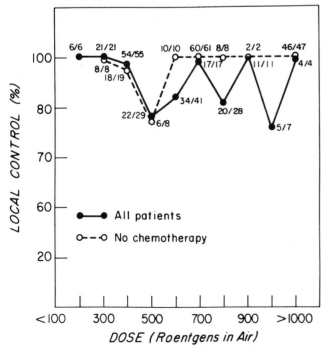

Fig. 19-8. Bone lesion radiotherapy in histiocytosis (127 Pts). From Greenberger *et al.* (296), with permission.

Table 19-17. Clinical, Prognostic, and Therapeutic Aspects of the Major Childhood Histiocytoses

Class I (LHC)	Class I (IAHS)	Class II (FEL)	Class III
Prognosis			
Variable, but a self-resolving disease process in most cases	Excellent, provided underlying infection is controlled and immunosuppression can be reversed	Extemely poor; uniformly rapidly fatal	Poor for acute monocytic leukemia. Improving for MH and NHL; up to 75% survival at 40 months reported with appropriate therapy
Recommended			
None to mild irradiation or chemotherapy (vinblastine and steroids) for certain lesions	Avoidance of all immunosuppressive therapy	Experimental	Doxorubicin in a combination chemotherapy regimen for MH and NHL; appropriate treatment for acute monocytic leukemia

MH = malignant histiocytosis; NHL = non-hodgkins lymphoma.
Adapted from Ladisch and Jaffe (299).

or etiologies of these disorders were better understood, it might be possible to use therapies which directly affect the primary cause. Until such knowledge is available, evaluation of standard cytotoxic therapies will continue.

Recommended Reading

Ladisen *et al.* (298) provide a comprehensive review of the histiocytoses both in terms of the biology, clinical presentation, and treatment. The article by Lahey (300) provides a review of prognostic factors. Greenberger *et al.* (296) review the results of treating patients with systemic histiocytosis.

PEDIATRIC OSTEOGENIC SARCOMA

PERSPECTIVE

Osteogenic sarcoma is a relatively rare tumor, although it is the most frequently encountered malignant primary tumor of bone (321). The hallmark of this disease is osteoid or immature bone produced by a malignant proliferating spindle cell stroma. In spite of its rarity, the history of this tumor's treatment provides an education in the methodology of clinical cancer research.

EPIDEMIOLOGY AND ETIOLOGY

Epidemiology

Osteogenic sarcoma is the most common bone tumor encountered in the first three decades of life; there are approximately 2,000-3,000 newly diagnosed patients per year in the United States (312). The incidence of osteogenic sarcoma is seven per million teenagers annually, with a male to female ratio of approximately 1.5:1. The peak incidence occurs at age $13\frac{1}{2}$ for girls and $14\frac{1}{2}$ for boys, corresponding to their respective growth spurts. Taller people appear to be at increased risk, as are individuals with Paget's disease (317).

Etiology

Osteogenic sarcoma is a rapidly proliferating tumor, the etiology of which is unknown. The relatively high incidence of this tumor in adolescents undergoing rapid skeletal growth

and in individuals with Paget's disease of the bone suggests that increased bone activity may play a role in the induction of this malignancy (319). The molecular basis for the phenomena is unknown. Viral induction of osteogenic sarcoma has been noted in animals, but no evidence currently exists in humans for a viral etiology (316,337,342). Many patients will have had a history of trauma prior to the diagnosis. It is likely that this observation is due to the fact that injuries allow recognition of the already proliferating tumor.

The incidence of osteogenic sarcoma is increased in bones which have previously been irradiated. For this reason X rays have been implicated as potentially causative. It must be kept in mind that these patients have usually been treated for a malignancy. Patients with one tumor may also be at a higher than normal risk of developing a spontaneous second primary malignancy. Patients with hereditary retinoblastoma who have a constitutive deletion in chromosome 13 (13q14) have an increased incidence of osteogenic sarcoma, only half of which occurs within the radiation field. Thus the abnormality in chromosome 13 may predispose to osteogenic sarcoma. Two prepubertal American Indian sisters, with a constitutional translocation between chromosome 13 and 14, who developed osteogenic sarcoma have been described (318).

Recently, the DNA content of osteogenic sarcoma has been examined. In one study, 92 of 96 high grade osteogenic sarcomas were found to have a hyperdiploid DNA content, whereas low grade periosteal sarcomas and benign bone tumors had diploid DNA content (308). Using flow cytometry, a correlation between the DNA index and outcome after surgery and chemotherapy has also been noted in patients with high grade osteogenic sarcoma (327). The development of pulmonary metastasis occurs more frequently in patients with hyperdiploid tumor cells than those with near diploid cells.

DETECTION AND DIAGNOSIS

Clinical Detection

1. Pain is by far the most common presenting symptom of osteogenic sarcoma occurring in virtually all patients.
2. Palpable masses, swelling, and limitation of motion are common.

3. Systemic symptoms such as anorexia and weight loss are rarely seen. If they are present, one should suspect overt metastatic disease.

4. Patients infrequently present with fractures. Those with pulmonary metastases may have symptoms such as cough, chest pain or dyspnea.

5. Osteogenic sarcomas usually arise in the metaphyses of the bones. The lower extremities are involved more frequently. Approximately 60% of tumors occur about the knee (40% distal femur and 20% proximal tibia), with 76% occurring in the bones of the upper and lower extremities (346). Lesions of the sacrum, jaw, and phalanges are much less common.

6. The disease rarely occurs in bones of the skull, and when it does, it is usually a complication of Paget's disease of the bone in adults or a secondary complication of radiation therapy.

7. The diagnosis is initially suspected by the presenting symptoms and the X ray. X rays of the involved bone characteristically show bone destruction and periosteal new bone formation. When tumor erupts through the cortex, the formation of new bone produces a "sunburst" appearance and soft tissue swelling is noted.

8. The diagnosis of osteogenic sarcoma, as with any malignant lesion rests on an adequate biopsy and histologic examination. To be conclusive, the biopsy must show the presence of osteoid within a sarcomatous tumor.

9. Other tests may further define the extent of the primary lesion. Computed tomography or MRI scanning of the involved region is recommended. Arteriography may be necessary in patients being considered for limb salvage procedures where the vascular and neurologic integrity of the limb must be assured.

10. The lung must be examined by chest X ray and CT scan in order to detect metastatic disease.

11. Since radionuclides are incorporated into new bone, bone scans can outline the primary tumor, multifocal primary lesions, and metastatic lesions.

CLASSIFICATION AND STAGING

Osteogenic sarcomas have been classified in a number of different ways. Radiologically, they have been classified on the basis of having an osteolytic, sclerosing, or telangiectatic appearance. The latter is considered to be a poor prognostic sign.

Histopathology

Osteogenic sarcomas have also been classified by their primary site of origin. Classic osteogenic sarcomas arise from the medullary cavity. A less aggressive form of osteogenic sarcoma arises in the periosteal area of the bone. It tends to spread along the shaft of the bone but does not invade the cortex and is associated with a low incidence of metastasis (325). Periosteal, intracortical, and extraskeletal osteogenic sarcomas have also been described.

Histologically, most osteogenic sarcomas in children are the classic osteoblastic form, with osteoblasts demonstrating pleomorphism and bizarre mitoses. Necrosis, fibrosis, and calcification may also be noted. Chondroblastic, fibroblastic, telangiectatic, and small cell types have also been described but are considerably less common in children.

Osteogenic sarcoma in the child or adolescent is almost always high grade osteoblastic osteogenic sarcoma. Prognostic factors are related to the site of the tumor (patients with distal tumors do better than those with proximal or central axis tumors) and age (prognosis improves with age). Biologic response to therapy has been used to predict eventual outcome of therapy with a given therapeutic regimen. A recent study using flow cytometry has suggested that a DNA index suggestive of diploidy predicts for better survival than does an increased DNA index suggestive of hyperdiploidy (327).

Patients who present with obvious metastatic disease in the lungs have a significantly worse prognosis than patients with apparent localized disease. With modern chemotherapeutic approaches and aggressive resection of pulmonary nodules, even the former group of patients are potentially curable (340). Patients with multifocal osteogenic sarcoma continue to have an exceedingly poor prognosis (336).

PRINCIPLES OF TREATMENT

Multidisciplinary Treatment Decisions

The natural history of surgically resected (amputation) osteogenic sarcoma is notable for a rapid appearance of pulmonary metastases 6 to 12 months after diagnosis (328). Five years from the time of diagnosis, only 15-20% of patients are alive (312,328). The results with high dose radiotherapy alone are worse (343). Chemotherapy offered little hope until the early 1970s when both high dose methotrexate with leucovorin rescue and doxorubicin were found to be effective agents (310,322). Early single arm studies of adjuvant chemotherapy after amputation showed markedly improved survivals (40-50%), compared to historical controls treated only with amputation (311,323). The Mayo Clinic then reported 50% survival after surgery alone, raising the possibility that improved outcomes reported in the 1970s were due to improved surgical techniques rather than adjuvant chemotherapy (344). As a result, effective adjuvant chemotherapy was not universally made available to patients until the 1980s, when controlled randomized studies showed that adjuvant chemotherapy improves the disease-free survival of patients with osteogenic sarcoma (313,326). Studies have now shown the importance of chemotherapy dose intensity for this aggressive tumor. The possibility of evaluating biologic response to therapy has been pioneered in the treatment of osteogenic sarcoma (see below).

Surgery

The mainstay of treatment of osteogenic sarcoma is the attainment of local control. Because the tumor is relatively chemosensitive but radioresistant, the management of the primary tumor is surgical removal of all gross and microscopic tumor. When possible, this is achieved most easily by amputation with a wide margin of normal tissue. Instances in which the tumor recurred in the stump was attributed to "skip lesions" of tumor in the affected bone, separated from the primary tumor by several centimeters of normal bone (315). To prevent this, disarticulations were previously used. In the current era of adjuvant chemotherapy and improved CT/MRI scanning, it is no longer felt necessary to remove entire bones unless dictated by the location and extent of tumor.

With improvement in the survival of patients with osteogenic sarcoma, subamputative, or limb-sparing, surgery has been used in the hope of reducing the functional and psychological morbidity of amputation (329). The portion of bone involved with tumor is removed and replaced by an artificial prosthesis or a bone graft. This procedure can be performed only if the vascular and neurologic integrity of the limb is not compromised. In many instances, pre-operative chemotherapy may reduce the size of the mass sufficiently to make limb-sparing surgery possible. The disease-free survival of those patients who have had limb-sparing surgery appears similar to that of those who have had an amputation (314,329). This procedure is limited to those patients with lower extremity tumors who have already undergone most of their growth. For patients with lesions of the humerus, any preservation of function in the hand can significantly improve long-term functional results.

Although pulmonary lesions of osteogenic sarcoma may occur in patients who have received adjuvant chemotherapy, fewer nodules may be present at the time of recurrence than in those who have not received chemotherapy (314,324). In many such instances, the number of nodules is sufficiently low that they can be surgically removed. Long-term survival has been documented in patients after undergoing such procedures (332,333,345).

Radiation Therapy

Osteogenic sarcoma is a relatively radioresistant tumor. The doses required for clinical response often result in severe tissue damage and subsequent amputation. For this reason, radiation therapy is not used when surgical resection is possible. Radiation therapy has been administered to patients those primary tumor has not been amenable to surgical resection. Cure with this approach is unusual. Radiation therapy has also been used to prevent and control pulmonary metastases, but again is of limited value in this setting. Palliative radiation for pain or temporary control of metastases can be beneficial.

Chemotherapy

Prior to 1972, chemotherapy for osteogenic sarcoma was ineffective. In 1972, it was shown almost simultaneously that doxorubicin or high doses of metbotrexate followed by leucovorin could produce objective tumor regression in 42% of patients (310,322). Since then, these two agents have been the basis for adjuvant chemotherapy. The early studies showed the importance of treatment with full dose doxorubricin (309). Cisplatin has also been shown to be an active agent in this tumor (334,335).

Although 80% of patients appear to be free of metastases at diagnosis, the rapid onset of pulmonary metastases within a year of diagnosis despite adequate local control suggests that micrometastases are present at the time of diagnosis and surgery. The ideal time for initiating chemotherapy in this disease is unclear. One could rationalize either immediate surgery to remove the tumor burden or immediate chemotherapy to control micrometastasis. Rosen et al. use chemotherapy before complete excision of tumor (341). In addition to treating micrometastatic disease early, this approach allows assessment of the degree of necrosis in the surgical specimen as a measure of the tumor response to chemotherapy. Shrinkage of a large tumor may allow limb salvage

procedures to become feasible. In his T-10 study, Rosen found that patients whose tumors did not optimally respond to bleomycin, cytoxan, actinomycin-D (BCD), and methotrexate could be better treated by deleting subsequent courses of methotrexate and using, instead, doxorubicin, cisplatinum and BCD (339). Other investigators prefer nontailored regimens, with or without pre-operative chemotherapy, followed by chemotherapeutic regimens using known active agents (326,347).

Immunotherapy

In past years, in conjunction with surgical resection and in some instances, chemotherapy, several centers have treated patients with osteogenic sarcoma with various forms of immunotherapy. Attempts to increase or enhance immunologic response to the presence of a tumor have included the use of the bacillus Calmette-Guerin (BOG) vaccine, transfer factor, and more recently, interferon (312). To date, none of these methods have demonstrated a clear improvement over surgically treated controls. In one study, warfarin, an anticoagulant, was found to decrease the incidence of pulmonary metastasis. However, this was an extremely small study and has never been confirmed (320).

RESULTS AND PROGNOSIS

The role of adjuvant chemotherapy in significantly improving the long-term disease-free survival of patients with nonmetastatic osteogenic sarcoma has been confirmed in two randomized studies (313,326). Approximately 65-70% overall disease-free survival can be obtained in patients with nonmetastatic disease at diagnosis (339) who receive adjuvant chemotherapy while patients treated with surgery alone have only a 20% relapse-free survival rate, unchanged from historical controls (313,326). Rosen et al. have reported 2-3 year survivals of approximately 80-90% in all patients treated with pre-operative chemotherapy followed by a tailored regimen. However, similar results were not found by the Children's Cancer Study Group who continued to show only a 40% long-term disease-free survival in those patients with poor initial responses to therapy (338). It is not yet clear that tailoring of therapy is better than extremely aggressive early chemotherapy for all patients with osteogenic sarcoma. The role of pre-operative chemotherapy versus immediate surgical excision is also unclear. Certainly, pre-operative chemotherapy allows for the possibility of limb salvage in a number of patients for whom prosthesis need to be made and for whom some shrinkage of the tumor will make the surgical procedure possible. The effects of possible delays in therapy due to complicated surgical procedures such as limb salvage is unknown.

CLINICAL INVESTIGATIONS

The optimal treatment approach for osteogenic sarcoma remains unclear. Areas to be explored include the importance of pre-operative chemotherapy versus immediate resection, the effects of limb salvage procedure and subsequent surgical delays, and the appropriateness of tailoring the therapy versus an aggressive approach for all patients with this disease. There is hope that further biologic studies, such as those of the DNA index, will allow classification of patients prognostically by virtue of the tumor biology itself rather than entirely based on response to therapies. This type of analysis may allow us to determine which patients will need the extremely aggressive approach using all known agents versus those for whom less toxic therapies may be adequate. New approaches are needed for those patients with metastatic disease at diagnosis as well as those who relapse after chemotherapeutic regimens. New agents, such as ifosfamide, may prove helpful for these patients (330). There are anecdotal reports of prolonged survival in patients with metastatic disease at diagnosis when complete resection of pulmonary lesions can be accomplished.

Complete excision of gross disease continues to be an absolute necessity for the achievement of cure in osteogenic sarcoma. One would hope that sometime in the future, we might be able to treat this disease with less disabling interventions. Limb salvage is a step along this pathway, but it too, is a complicated and traumatic procedure that often results in continual disability for the patients. Investigators have tested, in small numbers of patients, the possibility of using chemotherapy alone or radiation sensitizers that might allow for successful treatment without complete surgical excision (331). To date, these studies are in their infancy and do not offer patients their best chance at long-term survival. Surgery and chemotherapy remain the mainstay of treatment for this disorder.

Recommended Reading

The articles by Marcove (328) and Dahlin (312) provide an excellent source for understanding the natural history and epidemiology of osteogenic sarcoma. The effect of adjuvant chemotherapy is provided in the article by Link (326). Rosen (339) explores the use of preoperative chemotherapy. Alterations in the pattern of disease, in the era of adjuvant chemotherapy, are described by Jaffe (324).

PEDIATRIC EWING'S SARCOMA

PERSPECTIVE

Ewing's sarcoma is a highly malignant nonosseous tumor that usually arises in bone, but occasionally occurs in soft tissues (351). It is the most common bone tumor in children under 10 years of age, and second only to osteogenic sarcoma in the second decade of life (382). In 1921 James Ewing described this tumor as one which arose in the shaft of long bones but was not associated with bone production. It did, however, diffusely alter bone structure, and was, unlike osteogenic sarcoma, radiosensitive (355).

Ewing's sarcoma is one of the small round cell tumors of childhood and is similar to the others in its propensity to metastasize and in its responsiveness to chemotherapy. Treatment with surgery, radiotherapy and chemotherapy has dramatically changed the outlook for patients with nonmetastatic disease, achieving local control of the tumor in 75-85% of patients, and producing 5-year disease-free survival of 50-55% (348,349,360,361,369,373,374,377). Most deaths occur within 2 years of diagnosis, but late recurrences after 10-12 years have been reported (372,374).

EPIDEMIOLOGY AND ETIOLOGY

Epidemiology

1. Ewing's sarcoma accounts for 3% of childhood cancers, with an incidence of 200 per year in the United States (382).
2. The age range is 5 months to 60 years with the peak incidence between 11 and 17 years (350). Ninety percent of patients are diagnosed before the age of 30 years. The tumor is rare, however, in children under the age of 5 years.
3. The disease is rare in Blacks and Chinese (362,382).

Etiology

1. The cell of origin for Ewing's sarcoma has not been unequivocally established. Certain characteristics suggest that Ewing's sarcoma cells are derived from primitive mesenchymal cells that are not yet committed to differentiation (352). Cytogenetically, Ewing's sarcoma cells have a distinctive reciprocal translocation of chromosome 22 at the q12 locus, a feature shared with peripheral neuroepithelioma, which has a neural phenotype. This would suggest the possibility of a neural origin for Ewing's sarcoma (381).
2. In contrast to retinoblastoma and Wilms' tumor which may result from deletion of an antioncogene, the lack of a constitutional karyotypic abnormality in patients with Ewing's sarcoma suggests that it is associated with a dominantly expressed oncogene (367).
3. The immunochemical and cytogenetic features of Ewing's sarcoma are similar to a spectrum of other neoplasms referred to as primary "blastomas," which demonstrate a variable expression of mesenchymal, epithelial, and neuronal markers. Extraosseous Ewing's sarcoma is included within this group (368). Ewing's sarcoma has not been associated with known congenital syndromes, and there is no known evidence for hereditary transmission.
4. Children with Ewing's sarcoma have a higher than expected frequency of osteosarcoma developing in irradiated areas, further supporting a cytogenetic abnormality in this tumor (375).

DETECTION AND DIAGNOSIS

Clinical Detection

Pain is the most common presenting symptom in patients with Ewing's sarcoma, noted in 80% of individuals (371) Tenderness and swelling are also common.

Symptoms are frequently present for several months before diagnosis. A mass is palpable in up to 60% of patients, demonstrating the propensity for the tumor to break through the cortex and involve surrounding tissue.

The sites of presentation, as well as the age distribution of affected patients, is shown in Fig. 19-9, taken from a series by Dahlin *et al.* (351). Overall, the primary lesion occurs in the extremities in 59%, of patients (femur 22%, fibula or tibia 21%, humerus 11%), in the pelvis in 22% (ilium 14%), in the ribs in 5%, and elsewhere in 14% (usually in the vertebral bodies).

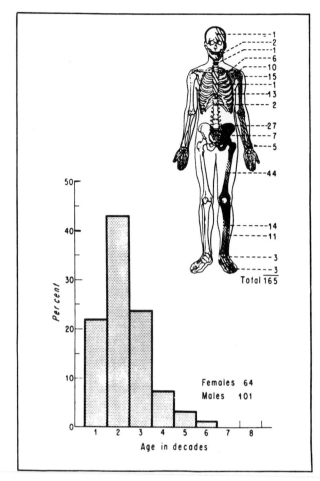

Fig. 19-9. Distribution according to age and sex, and skeletal distribution of 165 Ewing's sarcomatas seen at the Mayo Clinic prior to January 1, 1960. The regions of predilection are indicated by the density of the cross-hatching. From Dahlin, D.C.; Coventry, M.P.; Scanlon, P.W. Ewing's sarcoma: a critical analysis of 165 cases. J. Bone Joint Surg. 43A:185-192; 1961; with permission.

Systemic symptoms such as weight loss, fatigue, and fever are frequent. The association of leukocytosis and an elevated erythrocyte sedimentation rate in this setting may erroneously suggest the diagnosis of osteomyelitis.

Neurologic abnormalities occur in 15% of patients, either as spinal cord or peripheral nerve compression.

Demonstrable metastatic lesions are present at diagnosis in 14-35%, of patients. The lesions occur in the lungs, bones, lymph nodes, and bone marrow and less frequently in the central nervous system (378).

Diagnostic Evaluation

1. Radiographs of an involved bone typically demonstrate an expanding destructive lesion in the diaphysis (353). Periosteal reaction in the form of periosteal elevation and subperiosteal new bone formation may occur as tumor extends through the cortex, producing the "onion skin" appearances. This picture, as well as a "sunburst" pattern resulting from radiating spicules may occur in both osteogenic and Ewing's sarcoma. Other radiographic findings in Ewing's sarcoma include mottled rarefaction resulting from bone destruction, sclerosis, and cystic loculation. It is notable that the observed size of the lesion may underestimate extensive bone marrow space involvement.

2. An associated soft tissue mass is typical, occurring in over 50% of long bone presentations. Computerized Tomography scanning and, more recently, MRI have been useful in the determination of disease extent.

3. *Radioculide bone scan* may reveal metastatic lesions, although this technique may exaggerate the linear tumor extent of the primary lesion.

4. *Chest X ray and CT scan* are obtained to determine if pulmonary metastases are present.

5. *Laboratory evaluation* includes complete blood count with differential, ESR, renal and liver function tests, including lactate dehydrogenase. Urine vanillylmandelic acid and monovanillic acid can aid in excluding neuroblastoma from consideration.

6. *Bone marrow aspiration* and biopsy are performed to determine if there is marrow involvement.

7. *Lumbar puncture with cytopathology* is obtained in the setting of parameningeal presentations or if neurologic abnormalities are present.

8. *Biopsy of the lesion* establishes the diagnosis and is therefore important. Diagnostics tissue should be obtained from soft tissue and not cortical bone, if possible. This reduces the potential for pathologic fracture. The scar should be small, easily encompassed by the radiation portal (vertical along the limb), and in a region with a reasonable underlying connective tissue bed, thus reducing the propensity for soft tissue necrosis secondary to irradiation (380).

CLASSIFICATION AND STAGING

Histopathology

The histologic pattern of Ewing's sarcoma is one of monomorphic sheets of small round cells with hyperchromatic nuclei and relatively little cytoplasm. The amount of associated stroma is small, but it can produce a compartmental effect. Tremendous cellularity may be present, with a solidly packed, highly undifferentiated and, at times, dimorphic pattern with large as well as the previously noted small cells present. Glycogen in granules with periodic acid-Schiff's positivity can usually be demonstrated, but is not diagnostic (359,365). Primitive neural features have been described with less frequency and maturation than in peripheral primitive neuroectodemal tumors. Recent histochemical studies indicate that Ewing's sarcoma tumor cells are uniformly vimentin positive and frequently cytokeratin positive, indicating origin from epithelial and neuronal elements (368). The other small round cell tumors of childhood, neuroblastoma, non-Hodgkin's lymphoma, and rhabdomyosarcoma, must be excluded.

Staging

No standard staging system for Ewing's sarcoma is accepted. Tumors are classified as localized or disseminated.

PRINCIPLES OF TREATMENT

Most patients with Ewing's sarcoma present with what appears to be localized disease, but surgery or radiotherapy alone is unlikely to be curative due to the presence of micrometastases. Chemotherapy has become increasingly effective in eliminating these cells, as well as assisting in obtaining local control. This has permitted strategies to reduce the need for radical surgery or high dose, large volume irradiation. The goal of therapy is to eradicate all tumor while preserving as much function as possible, and the optimal integration of the three modalities of therapy in terms of their aggressiveness remains to be determined. Fifteen to 35% of patients have demonstrable metastatic disease at diagnosis, and for most of these patients long-term survival is unobtainable, even with aggressive treatment including transplantation.

Surgery

1. Biopsy using optimal techniques (see section on "Evaluation") establishes the diagnosis.
2. The nature of the surgery used on the primary tumor is determined by its location and extent, and on the presence or absence of known metastases. Although surgeons vary in terms of their approaches, the data available suggest that selective interventions are most appropriate. Aggressive surgery including amputation or, if possible, a limb-sparing procedure should be used when a severe pathologic fracture is present, or when there is a potential for substantial growth impairment as a consequence of radiotherapy. Surgical resection of expendable bones can achieve local control without an undue functional deficit (372). For patients with bulky (greater than 8 cm) tumors, radical surgery is performed by some surgeons but morbidity may be great. In this setting more limited surgery with little normal tissue margin or microscopically positive margins followed by radiation therapy is at least as efficacious in achieving local control. Another strategy is pre-surgical chemotherapy, with the definitive surgical procedure followed by radiotherapy if necessary. In the setting of favorable distal extremity lesions, either surgery or radiation therapy can be successful, and the expected resulting morbidity should guide the choice.

Radiation Therapy

1. The potential for radiation therapy, to achieve local control is dependent on the location and extent of the tumor. In general, radiation therapy is successful, together with combination chemotherapy, in greater than 90% of patients with distal extremity lesions, 75% with proximal extremity lesions, but only 65% with central lesions (376). Thus the use of radiotherapy is considered in light of the surgical procedure deemed appropriate and the morbidities of each alone or in combination. Radiation therapy is appropriate for distal extremity lesions in nonexpendable bones and in the setting of subtotal or marginal resection of a bulky tumor.
2. For patients with metastatic Ewing's sarcoma, irradiation to the lungs and sites of osseous metastases have been of some value in overall disease control.
3. Improvements in chemotherapy and imaging techniques and information regarding the characteristics of local tumor recurrence have allowed for refinements in the administration of radiotherapy. The traditional volume included a generous margin around the soft tissue component and the entire bone, with successive field reductions to doses of 55-60 Gy. Recent data supports the exclusion of one epiphyseal center at the opposite end of the bone from an eccentrically located lesion (360,369) with peak doses of 50-60 Gy depending on the tumor bulk and surgical procedure. Moreover,

clinical trials are in process that further tailor the treatment volume. Important radiotherapy considerations include treating the surgical scar and shaping fields to maintain lymphatic drainage.

Chemotherapy

1. Ewing's sarcoma is an extremely chemotherapy sensitive tumor with a significant response rate to a number of single agents. These include high dose melphalan, cyclophosphamide, doxorubicin, vincristine, 5-fluorouracil, BCNU, ifosfamide, etoposide and actinomycin-D. Multi-agent chemotherapy has a role both in terms of improved systemic and local control, translating into improved overall survival. A number of regimens have been evaluated with the most successful generally including cyclophosphamide, doxorubicin, vincristine and actinomycin D. High dose-intensity use of the more active agents, cyclophnsphamide and doxorubicin, has played a particular role in improving disease free survival (373).
2. Although chemotherapy typically follows surgery and is administered in part prior to radiotherapy, in selected situations chemotherapy may also precede surgery as well (361).

SPECIAL CONSIDERATIONS

1. *Central nervous system prophylaxis*: Prophylactic treatment of the CNS with whole brain irradiation or intrathecal methotrexate has been recommended (364,371). However, extension of tumor or metastatic involvement of the CNS is rare, and the need for such therapy is questionable except in the instance of direct intracranial extension or parameningeal involvement
2. *Bone marrow transplantation*: Recent results using autologous bone marrow transplantation for patients with metastases at diagnosis or other prognostically poor presentations are promising (359,363).

RESULTS AND PROGNOSIS

Results

1. Prior to the use of multiagent chemotherapy, few children with Ewing's sarcoma survived, with 85% dying within 2 years of diagnosis (356) Currently, the overall 5-year disease-free survival is 50-55% (361,369,370,374, 378) with some institutions reporting superior results (359,363,373).
2. The extent and location of the patient's disease affects the likelihood of survival, with 75-85% of patients with limited volume distal extremity Ewing's sarcoma surviving, in contrast to 25-35% of patients with large central lesions (348,354,361,374,378).

Prognostic Factors

The extent of disease at diagnosis is the most important prognostic factor. Several variables directly or indirectly relate to this factor, making it difficult to determine the independent significance of any one.

1. The presence of grossly metastatic disease at diagnosis is associated with a generally poor outcome. In earlier studies, patients with bone or bone marrow involvement fared worse than patients with limited pulmonary

involvement (349,351,369,373). Progress in treating patients with metastatic disease has occurred (359).

2. Patients with an extensive soft tissue component of the primary have a less favorable prognosis than patients with limited or no soft tissue involvement (365).
3. The size of the primary as it involves the bone (greater or less than 8 cm) may influence the likelihood of a successful outcome (354,360).
4. High serum levels of lactic dehydrogenase are associated with a poorer outcome, possibly because they reflect the burden or activity of tumor (357,373).
5. The site of involvement is relevant to the likelihood of the success of therapy. Involvement of the pelvis or sacrum is associated with a worse prognosis than is involvement of the proximal extremities (humerus, femur) or central sites such as the rib or vertebrae. These sites are less favorable than involvement of a distal extremity site. Local recurrence in the primary site occurs in 15% of children with extremity lesions, 47% with rib primaries, and 69% with pelvic tumors (348).
6. A high leukocyte count may also be associated with an increased risk of tumor recurrence (360,370).

CLINICAL INVESTIGATIONS

1. A further understanding of the molecular pathology and pathologic diversity of Ewing's sarcoma will improve the ability to subclassify this tumor and may provide important prognostic information.
2. The histologic response of the unresected tumor to chemotherapy may prove useful in tailoring subsequent therapy (360,370).
3. New radiotherapy techniques such as hyperfractionation may enhance the likelihood of local control without increasing local morbidity.
4. Additional chemotherapeutic agents (etoposide, ifosfamide) (366) are being studied in an attempt to improve disease-free survival.

Recommended Reading

Early studies that provide a perspective on the natural history of Ewing's sarcoma prior to modern therapeutic techniques include those by Wang and Schulz (380), Dahlin et al. (350,351), and Falk (356). Modern approaches to Ewing's sarcoma are reviewed in articles by Hayes (359,360), Jurgens (361), Rosen (373), Tepper (376) and Thomas (377). An overall review of the tumor, its biology, presenting features, and appropriate therapy is available in the report by Miser (367).

MALIGNANT HEPATIC TUMORS

PERSPECTIVE

Primary liver tumors in infancy and childhood are frequently malignant. The most common malignant tumors are hepatoblastoma (HBA) and hepatocellular carcinoma (HCC). They comprise the third most common type of intra-abdominal malignant tumor, exceeded only by neuroblastoma and Wilms' tumor. Only total surgical excision has resulted in long-term survival. Recent data, however, appear to indicate that chemotherapy can make a previously inoperable tumor operable. In addition, chemotherapy has made possible long-term survival even when pulmonary metastases are present.

EPIDEMIOLOGY AND ETIOLOGY

Epidemiology

1. Childhood liver tumors occur at a rate of 1.9 per million per year (405). The incidence of malignancy in hepatic tumors varies from one-half to two-thirds in affected patients (387,397).
2. Hepatoblastoma is the most frequently noted malignant liver tumor accounting for 50-60% of all such tumors. Hepatocellular carcinoma occurs with the next greatest frequency, 20-30% (387,388,394,395). Other less frequently occurring malignant tumors include rhabdomyosarcoma, leiomyosarcoma, mesenchymoma, and undifferentiated sarcoma.
3. HBA usually occurs in the very young with a mean age of 17 months (394). There is a male predominance, 1.5:1 to 2:1(390,394,397). Hepatocellular carcinoma usually occurs in the older child, mean age 9.7 years (395). There is also increased incidence in the male, 1.7:1 (390,394,397).

ETIOLOGY

Both HBA and HCC arise in hepatocytes. Hepatoblastoma is more frequently isolated to one lobe of the liver with the right lobe predominating. Hepatocellular carcinoma is more likely to occur in both lobes or to be multicentric (387,394,395). Vascular invasion occurs frequently and the lung is the most common organ for metastases. Metastases are often identified at the time of initial diagnosis. Lymphatic invasion and regional lymph node metastases occur less frequently (390,394,395).

Isosexual precocity has been noted in tumors secreting human chorionic gonadotropin (HCG) and regresses with extirpation of the tumor (390,394,397,399).

The incidence of coexisting anomalies in HBA is difficult to assess accurately. Hemihypertrophy has been noted as has Beckwith-Wiedemann syndrome. Hepatoblastoma has occurred in families with familial polyposis coli (388,393,394, 396,397). There is a high association between HCC and macronodular cirrhosis, and also hepatitis B surface antigen (384,389,391,395,402). Hepatitis B viral DNA has been found in the host genome of both HCC and noncancerous liver tissue and suggests an oncogenic etiology.

Hepatic malignancy has been reported in patients with biliary atresia or neonatal hepatitis (383,395). Hepatomas have also been associated with the chronic form of hereditary tyrosinemia (390,395).

DETECTION AND DIAGNOSIS

Detection

The average duration of signs and symptoms for HBA and HCC is short, 2.2 and 1.5 months, respectively (394,395). Greater than 90% of patients present with an abdominal mass. Less frequently occurring signs and symptoms are abdominal pain, fever, weight loss, and icterus. Occasionally isosexual precocity may be the presenting sign.

Diagnosis

Evaluation consists of an abdominal and chest X ray to look for intrahepatic calcifications and metastatic disease. An ultrasound will note the lesion in the liver and evaluate the hepatic veins and inferior vena cava for tumor extension. A CT scan of the abdomen will give additional information regarding size, location, and multiplicity of the tumor. Angiographic studies of the hepatic and tumor vasculature is essential to determine resectability and aid in planning the surgical approach (388,390,394). In addition, a routine CBC is obtained. Anemia with a hemoglobin less than 10 gm is frequently noted (390). Liver function tests including studies of clotting factors are obtained. These values are usually normal unless jaundice is present. Finally, serum measurements are made of alpha-fetoprotein (AFP) and HCG. When elevated (AFP in two-thirds of HBA and one-half of HCC) they are excellent tumor markers to follow the results of therapy and to detect recurrent disease (388,390,400). Serum cholesterol levels may be of prognostic value. In a series of patients with HBA, the five with elevated serum cholesterol levels had a poor outcome (397,398).

CLASSIFICATION

Pathology

The histologic classification of HBA is based on the work of Willis (403) modified by Ishak and Glunz (392). The most frequently noted tumor type is of conventional histology and is separated into several categories. Epithelial histology is predominantly of either fetal or embryonal tissue. Less frequently noted is mixed epithelial and mesenchymal histology. A small number noted are of an indeterminate type. The other and least frequently noted tumor type is of anaplastic histology. These tumors are much more cellular and consist of poorly differentiated small to medium-sized cells. The histologic patter for HCC is usually a microtrabecular pattern with neoplastic hepatocytes grouped in clusters. Occasionally multinucleated giant cells are noted. A less frequently noted pattern is fibrolamellar type. Those tumors are characterized by hyaline bands of collagen often laminated and interspersed between clumps of plump polygonal neoplastic cells.

Staging

The Children's Cancer Study Group Hepatoma Study uses the following system of surgical-pathologic classification.
- Group I: Complete tumor excision.
- Group II: Tumor excision with microscopic residual disease.
- Group III: Gross residual disease, unresectable, or tumor spillage.
- Group IV: Metastatic disease.

PRINCIPLES OF TREATMENT

Total excision of the primary tumor is still the major goal of therapy. More than half of hepatoblastomas are resectable (388,394,397). Evidence is mounting that preoperative chemotherapy may convert a previously unresectable tumor to a surgically excisable tumor, and postoperative chemotherapy will improve survival in patients who have had complete surgical excision (388,397). There are also reports of survival with chemotherapy in patients with pulmonary metastases (388,397).

Surgery

A generous bilateral subcostal incision is made for the celiotomy. Occasionally the chest must be entered for inferior vena cava control superior to the liver. The liver is inspected and any invasion of tumor into adjacent viscera is noted. Suspicious lymph nodes in the hepatoduodenal ligament are biopsied. The liver and tumor are evaluated along with the angiogram for resectability. Lobectomy or extended lobectomy are the surgical procedures required for complete tumor excision. Occasionally deep hypothermia and cardiac arrest have been used for successful tumor excision (385). Biopsy of the tumor is reserved only for those tumors deemed unresectable. Uncontrolled blood loss is the most common cause of operative mortality and may reach 20% (387,397).

Radiation

Radiation has not been shown to affect prognosis but has been used in combination with chemotherapy in long-term survivors.

Chemotherapy

Various chemotherapeutic regimens have been used that improve survival. These include doxorubicin and cis-platinium (388,397,401). In addition, vincristine and cyclophosphamide have been added. In small series, the preoperative use of chemotherapy shrank the tumors and lowered the levels of AFP. This is now used routinely (388). Continued chemotherapy postoperatively has resulted in survival of 18 in a series of 29 patients (388). Fourteen survived without recurrence of metastases from 2-11 years after therapy. Four more survived with normal AFP levels and no evidence of recurrence from six months to two years.

RESULTS

Long-term survival has increased from 25-70% through the addition of chemotherapy to complete surgical excision. In addition, pre-operative chemotherapy can render a previously inoperable lesion operable.

PROGNOSTIC FACTORS

Hepatoblastoma has a more favorable prognosis than HCC, with a 25-40% versus 0-9% long-term survival (394,395). The fibrolamellar variant of HCC has a better prognosis with long term survivors noted in up to 75% in small series (390,395,404). The average survival in patients with fibrolamellar disease is 28.5 months as compared to 4.2 months in other forms of HCC. Those with the anaplastic type of HBC rarely survive.

The prognosis has been poor if the primary tumor cannot be completely excised, with greater than 95% dying of the disease. The symptom complex of pallor, weight loss, fatigue, and loss of appetite usually indicates a fatal outcome.

Recommended Reading

Exelby's article (387) is recommended for further reading on malignant liver tumors. An article by Mahour et al. (397) reports the improved survival in children with malignant tumors in the modern era.

REFERENCES

General References

1. Bragg, D.G.; Rubin, P.; Youker, J.E., eds. Oncologic Imaging. Elmsford, NY: Pergamon Press; 1985.

1a. Chan, H.; Thormer, P.; Hadad, G.; Ling, V. Immunohistochemical analysis of P-glycoprotein: Prognostic correlation in soft tissue sarcoma of childhood. J Clin Oncol 8:689-704;1990.

2. Green, D. Long-term complications of therapy for cancer in childhood and adolescence. The Johns Hopkins University Press; 1989:171.

3. Halperin, E.C.; Kun, L.E.; Constine, L.S.; Tarbell, N.J. Pediatric Radiation Oncology. New York, NY: Raven Press; 1989.

3a. Israel, M.A. Molecular and cellular biology of pediatric malignancies. In: P.A. Pizzo, D.G. Poplack (eds). Principles of Pediatric Oncology. Philadelphia, PA: JB Lippincott Co; 1989.

3b. Knudson, A.G. Mutation and cancer: Statistical study of retinoblastoma. Proc Natl Acad Sci USA 68:620-623;1971.

3c. Pizzo, P.A.; Horowitz, M.A.; Poplack, D.G.; Hays, D.M.; Kun, L.E. Solid tumors in childhood. In: DeVita, V.T., Hellman, S., Rosenberg, S.A., eds. Cancer: Principles and Practice of Oncology. 3rd ed. Philadelphia, PA: JB Lippincott Co.; 1989:1612-1670.

4. Pizzo, P.A.; Poplack, D.G., eds. Principles of Pediatric Oncology. Philadelphia, PA: J.B. Lippincott Co.; 1989.

4a. Poplack, D.G.; Kun, L.E.; Cassady, J.R.; Pizzo, P.A. Leukemias and lymphomas of childhood. In: DeVita, V.T., Hellman, S., Rosenberg, S.A., eds. Cancer: Principles and Practice of Oncology. 3rd ed. Philadelphia, PA: JB Lippincott Co.; 1989:1671-1695.

5. Rubin, P.; Constine III, L. Nelson, D. Complications of cancer treatment. In: Perez, C.; Brady, L.W., eds. Principles and Practice of Radiation Oncology. 2nd ed. Philadelphia, PA: JB Lippincott Co.; 1992.

6. Rubin, P.; Van Houtte, P.; Constine, L. Radiation sensitivity and organ tolerance in pediatric oncology: a new hypothesis. Front Radiat Ther Oncol 16:62-82; 1982.

7. Silverberg, E. Cancer Statistics. CA. 40:9-19; 1990.

7a. Strauss, M.B. Familiar Medical Quotations. Boston, MA: Little, Brown and Co; 1968.

8. Young, J.L. Jr.; Ries, L.F.; Silverberg, E. et al. Cancer incidence, survival, and mortality for children younger than age 15 years. Cancer. 58:598-602; 1986.

Specific References

Neuroblastoma

9. Alvarado, C.; Faraj, B.; Kim, T.; Camp, V.; Bain, R.; Ragab, A. Plasma dopa and catecholamines in the diagnosis and follow-up of children with neuroblastoma. Am. J. Pediatr. Hematol Oncol. 7:221-227; 1985.

10. August, C.S.; Serota, F.T.; Koch, P.A.; Burkey, E; et al. Treatment of advanced neuroblastoma with supralethal chemotheray, radiation and allogeneic or autologous marrow reconstitution. J. Clin. Oncol. 2(6):609-616; 1984.

11. Beckwith, J.B.; Perrin, E.V. In situ neuroblastoma: a contribution to the natural history of neural crest tumors. Am. J. Pathol. 43:1089-1104; 1963.

11a. Bowman, L.C.; Hancock, M.L.; Santana, V.M. et al. Impact of intensified therapy on clinical outcome in infants and children with neuroblastoma: The St. Jude Children's Research Hospital experience 1962 to1988. J Clin Oncol. 9:1599-1608;1991.

11'. Bourhis, J.; Dominici, C.; McDowell, H.; et al. N-myc genomic content and DNA ploidy in stage IVS neuroblastoma. J. Clin. Oncol. 9(8):1371-1375; 1991.

12. Bray, P.F.; Ziter, F.A.; Lahey, M.E.; et al. The coincidence of neuroblastoma and acute cerebellar encephalopathy. J. Pediatr. 76:983-990; 1969.

13. Breslow, N.; McCann, B. Statistical estimation of prognosis for children with neuroblastoma. Cancer Res. 31:2098-2103; 1971.

14. Brodeur, G.; Gayes, F.A.; Green, A.; Casper, J.; Lee, H.; Seeger, R. Consistent N-myc copy number in simultaneous or consecutive neuroblastoma samples from a given patient's tumor. Proc. Am. Soc. Clin. Oncol. 5:13; 1986. Abstract.

15. Brodeur, G.M.; Sekhon, G.S.; Goldstein, M.N. Chromosomal aberrations in human neuroblastomas. Cancer. 40:2256-2263; 1977.

16. Carli, M.; Green, A.; Hayes, F.A.; Pratt, C. Therapeutic efficacy of single drugs for childhood neuroblastoma: a review. In: Raybaud, C.; Clement, R.; LeBreuil, G.; Bernard, J., eds. Pediatric Oncology Excerpt Media. Amsterdam, The Netherlands; 1982:141-150.

17. Chatten, J.; Voorhees, M.L. Familial neuroblastoma. New Engl. J. Med. 277:1230-1236; 1967.

18. Cheung, N.K.; Saarinen, U.; Neely, J.; Landmeier, B.; Donovan, D.; Coccia, P. Monoclonal antibodies to a glycolipid antigen on human neuroblastoma cells. Cancer Res. 45:2642-2649; 1985.

19. Evans, A.E.; D'Angio, G.J.; Sather, N.; et al. A comparison of four staging systems for localized and regional neuroblastoma: a report from the Children's Cancer Study Group. J Clin Oncol. 8(4):678-688; 1990.

20. Evans, A.E.; D'Angio, G.J.; Propert, K.; Anderson, J.; Hann, H.W.L. Prognostic factors in neuroblastoma. Cancer. 59:1853-1859; 1987.

21. Evans, A.E.; D'Angio, G.J.; Randolph, J. A proposed staging for children with neuroblastoma. Cancer. 27:374-378; 1971.

22. Finklestein, J.Z. Neuroblastoma: the challenge and frustration. Hematol. Oncol. Clin. North Am 1: 675-694; 1987.

23. Gale, G.; D'Angio, G.; Uri, A.; Chatten, J.; Koop, C.E. Cancer in neonates: the experience at the Children's Hospital of Philadelphia, PA: Pediatrics. 70:409-413; 1982.

24. Geiser, C.F.; Edron, M.L. Cystathioninuria in patients with neuroblastoma or ganglioneuroblastoma. Cancer.22:856-860; 1968.

25. Gitlow, S.E.; Bertani, L.M.; Rausen, A.; Gribetz, D.; Dziedzic, S.W. Diagnosis of neuroblastoma by qualitative and quantitative determination of catecholamine metabolites in urine. Cancer. 25:1377-1383; 1970.

26. Gitlow, S.E.; Dziedzic, L.B.; Strauss, L.; et al. Biochemical and histologic determinants in the prognosis of neuroblastoma. Cancer. 32:898-905; 1973.

27. Gjeissing, L.R. Cystathioninuria in neuroblastoma. Biochem. J. 89:42-43; 1963.

28. Hann, H.; Evans, A.; Siegel, S.; Wong, K.; Sather, H.; Dalton, A.; Hammond, D.; Seeger, R. Prognostic importance of serum ferritin in patients with stage III and IV neuroblastoma: the CCSG experience. Cancer Res. 45:2843-2848; 1985.

29. Hawthorne, H.C.; Nelson, J.S.; Witzleben, C.L.; et al. Blanching subcutaneous nodules in neonatal neuroblastoma. J. Pediatr. 77:297-300; 1970.

30. Hayes, F.A.; Green, A.; Hustu, H.O.; Kumar, M. Surgicopathologic staging of neuroblastoma: prognostic significance of regional lymph node metastases. J. Pediatr. 102:59-62; 1983.

31. Hayes, F.A.; Green, A.A.; Casper, J.; Cornet, J.; Evans, W.E. Clinical evaluation of sequentially scheduled cisplatin and VM26 in neuroblastoma: response and toxicity. Cancer. 48:1715-1718; 1981.

32. Hayes, F.A.; Green, A.A.; Mauer, A.M. Correlation of cell kinetic and clinical response to chemotherapy in disseminated neuroblastoma. Cancer Res. 37:3766-3770; 1977.

33. Hayes, F.A.; Smith, E.I. Neuroblastoma. In: Pizzo, P.A.; Poplack, D.G., eds. Principles and Practice of Pediatric Oncology. Philadelphia, PA: J.B. Lippincott Co; 1989:614.

34. Hecht, F.; Kaiserhecht, B.; Northtrup, S.C.; et al. Genetics of familial neuroblastoma: long-range studies. Cancer Genet. Cytogenet. 7:227-230; 1982.

35. Hellstrom, K.E.; Hellstrom, I.E.; Bill, A.H.; Pierce, G.E.; Yang, J.P.S. Studies on cellular immunity to human neuroblastoma cells. Intl J Cancer. 6:172-188; 1970.

36. Howman-Giles, R.B.; Gilday, D.L.; Ash, J.M. Radionuclide skeletal survey in neuroblastoma. Radiology. 131:497-502; 1979.

37. Ihiele, C.J.; Reynolds, C.P.; Israel, M.A. Decreased expression of N-myc precedes retinoic acid induced morphological differentiation of human neuroblastoma. Nature. 313:404-406; 1985.

38. Ishiguro, Y.; Kato, K.; Ito, T.; et al. Nervous system-specific enolase in serum as a marker for neuroblastoma. Pediatrics. 72:696-700; 1983.

38a. Joshi, V.V.; Cantor, A.B.; Altshuler, G.; et al. Age-linked prognostic categorization based on a new histologic grading system of neuroblastomas. Cancer 69(8):2197-2211; 1992.

39. Kaneko, Y.; Danda, N.; Maseki, N.; Sakurai, M.; Tsuchida, Y.; Takida, T.; Okabe, I.; Sakurai, M. Different karyotypic patterns in early and advanced stage neuroblastoma. Cancer Res. 47:311-318; 1987.

40. Kauffman, R.A.; Thrall, J.H.; Keyes, J.W.; et al. False negative

bone scans in neuroblastoma metastatic to the ends of long bones. AJR. 130:131-135; 1978.

41. Knudson, A.G.; Strong, L.C. Mutations and cancer. Neuroblastoma and pheochromocytoma. Am. J. Hum Genet. 24:514-532; 1972.

42. Koizumi, J.H.; Dal Canto, M.C. Retroperitoneal neuroblastoma metastatic to brain, report of a case and review of the literature. Child's Brain. 7:267-279; 1980.

43. LaBrosse, E.H. Biochemical diagnosis of neuroblastoma: use of a urine spot test. Proc. Am. Assoc. Cancer Res. 9:39; 1968.

44. Laug, W.; Siegel, S.; Shaw, K.; Landing, B.; Baptista, J.; Gutenstein, M. Initial urinary catecholamine metabolite concentrations and prognosis in neuroblastoma. Pediatrics. 62:77-83; 1978.

45. Look, A.T.; Hayes, F.A.; Nitschke, R.; McWilliams, N.B.; Green, A.A. Cellular DNA content as a predictor of response to chemotherapy in infants with unresectable neuroblastoma. N Engl J Med. 311:231-135; 1984.

46. Mackay, B.; Masse, S.R.; King, O.Y.; et al. Diagnosis of neuroblastoma by electron microscopy of bone marrow aspirates. Pediatrics. 56:1045-1049;1975.

47. Makinen, J. Microscopic patterns as a guide to prognosis of neuroblastoma in childhood. Cancer. 29:1637-1646; 1972.

47a. Murphy, S.; Cohn, S.; Craft, A.W. et al. Consensus statement from the ACS Workshop on Neuroblastoma Screening. CA-A Cancer J for Clinicians 41:227-230;1991.

48. Pegelow, G.H.; Ebbin, A.J.; Powars, D.; et al. Familial neuroblastoma. J. Pediatr. 87:763-765; 1975.

49. Rosen, E.M.; Cassady, R.; Frantz, C.N.; Kretschmar, C.; Levey R.; Salla, S.E. Neuroblastoma: the Joint Center for Radiation Therapy/Dana-Farber Cancer Institute/Children's Hospital experience. J Clin Oncol. 2:719-731; 1984.

50. Sawada, T.; Nakata, T.; Takasugi, N.; et al. Mass screening for neuroblastoma in infants in Japan. Lancet . ii:271-273; 1984.

51. Scheibel, E.; Rechnitzer, C.; Fahrenkrug, J.; et al. Vasoactive intestinal polypeptide (VIP) in children with neural crest tumors. Acta Paediatr. Scand. 71:721-725; 1982.

52. Schneider, K.M.; Becher, J.M.; Drasna, I.H. Neonatal neuroblastoma. Pediatrics. 36:359-365; 1965.

53. Shimada, H.; Chatten, J.; Newton, J.; Sachs, W.; Hamoudi, N.; Chiba, T.; Marsden, H.; Misugi, K. Histopathologic prognostic factors in neuroblastic tumors: definition of subtypes of ganglioneuroblastoma and an age-linked classification of neuroblastomas. JNCI. 73:405-416; 1984.

53a. Shuster, J.J.; Cantor, A.B.; McWilliams, N.; et al. The prognostic significance of autologous bone marrow transplant in advanced neuroblastoma. J. Clin. Oncol. 9(6):1045-1049; 1991.

54. Smith, F.W.; Gilday, D.L.; Eng, G.; et al. Primary neuroblastoma uptake of ^{99m}technetium methylene diphospohnate. Radiology. 137:501-504; 1980.

55. Sty, J.R.; Kun, L.E.; Casper, J.T. Bone imaging as a diagnostic aid in evaluating neuroblastoma. Am J Pediatr Hematol Oncol. 2:115-118; 1980.

55a. Thomas, P.R.M. Neuroblastoma. In: Perez, C.; Brady, L.W., eds. Principles and Practice of Radiation Oncology. 2nd ed. Philadelphia, PA: JB Lippincott Co.; 1992:1449-1455.

56. Treleaven, J.G.; Ugelstad, J.; Philip, T. Removal of neuroblastoma cells from bone marrow with monoclonal antibodies conjugated to magnetic microspheres. Lancet i:70-73; 1984.

57. von Studnitz, W.; Kaser, H.; Sjoersdma, A. Spectrum of catecholamine biochemistry in patients with neuroblastoma. N Engl J Med. 209:232-235; 1983.

58. Wu, Z.L.; Schwartz, E.; Seeger, R.; Ladisch, S. Expression of G_{D2} ganglioside by untreated primary human neuroblastomas. Cancer Res. 46:440-443; 1986.

59. Young, J.L.; Ries, L.G.; Silverberg, et al. Cancer incidence, survival and mortality for children younger than age 15 years. Cancer. 58:598-603; 1986.

60. Zeltzer, P.M.; Parma, A.M.; Dalton, A.; et al. Raised neuron-specific enolase in serum of children with metastatic neuroblastoma. Lancet. ii:361-363; 1983.

Wilms' Tumor (Nephroblastoma)

61. Aron, B.S. Wilms' tumor: clinical study of 81 patients. Cancer. 33:637-646; 1974.

62. Arthur, D.C. Genetics and cytogenetics of pediatric cancer. Cancer. 58:535-540; 1986.

63. Austin, D.F.; Nelson, V.E.; Johnson, L.F. Epidemiologic characteristics of childhood cancer. In: Vaeth, J.M., ed. Childhood Cancer: Triumph Over Tragedy. Frontiers of Radiation Therapy and Oncology. vol 16. Basel, Germany: S. Karger; 1982:9-17.

64. Beckwith, J.B. Wilms' tumor and other renal tumors of childhood. Hum. Pathol. 14:481-192; 1983.

65. Beckwith, J.B.; Palmer, N.F. Histopathology and prognosis of Wilms' tumor. Cancer. 41:1937-1948; 1978.

66. Blute, M.L.; Kelalis, P.P.; Offord, K.P.; Breslow, N.E.; Beckwith, J.B.; D'Angio, G.J. Bilateral Wilms' tumor. J. Urol. 138:968-973; 1987.

67. Bolande, R.P.; Brough, A.J.; Izant, R.J. Congenital mesoblastic nephroma of infancy. Pediatrics. 40:272-278; 1967.

68. Bond, J.V. Bilateral Wilms' tumor, age at diagnosis, associated congenital anaomalies and possible patterns for inheritance. Lancet . ii:482-484; 1975.

69. Bove, K.E.; McAdams, A.J. The nephroblastomatosis complex and its relationship to Wilms' tumor: a clinicopathologic treatise. Perspect. Pediatr. Pathol. 1:185-223; 1973.

70. Breslow, N.E.; Beckwith, J.B. Epidemiologic lectures of Wilms' tumor: results of the National Wilms' Tumor Study. JNCI. 68:429-436; 1982.

71. Chang, J.H.; Janik, J.S.; Burrington, J.D.; Clark, D.R.; Campbell, D.N.; Pappas, G. Extensive tumor resection under deep hypothermia and circulatory arrest. J. Pediatr. Surg. 23:254-258; 1988.

71a. Corey, S.J.; Anderson, J.W.; Vawter, G.F.; et al. Improved survival for children with anaplastic Wilms' tumor. Cancer 68:970-974; 1991.

72. D'Angio, G.J. Oncology seen through the prism of Wilms' tumor. Med. Pediatr. Oncol. 13:53-58; 1985.

73. D'Angio, G.J.; Thomas, P.R.M. The optimization of radiation therapy and chemotherapy: the price of success. Int J Radiat Oncol Biol Phys. 19:1097-1098;1990.

74. D'Angio, G.J. Wilms' tumor and neuroblastoma in children. Pediatr. Rev. 6:16-19; 1984.

75. D'Angio, G.J.; Breslow, N.E.; Beckwith,J.B.; et al. Treatment of Wilms' Tumor: results of the third national Wilms' tumor study. Cancer 64:349-360; 1989.

76. D'Angio, G.J.; Evans, A.E.; Breslow, N.; et al. The treatment of Wilms' tumor: results of the second national Wilms' tumor study. Cancer. 47:2302-2311; 1981.

76a. deKraker, J.; Lemerle, J.; Voute, P.A.; et al. Wilms' tumor with pulmonary metastases at diagnosis. The significance of primary chemotherapy. J Clin Oncol. 8:1187-1190;1990.

77. Drash, A.; Sherman, F.; Hartmann, W.I.T.; et al. A syndrome of pseudohermaphrodism, Wilms' tumor, hypertension, and degenerative renal disease. J. Pediatr. 76:585-593; 1970.

77a. Farber, S. Chemotherapy un the treatment of leukemia and Wilms'tumor. JAMA. 198:826-838;1966.

77'. Evans, A.E.; Norkool, P.; Evans, I.; et al. Late effects of treatment for Wilms' tumor. Cancer 67:331-336; 1991.

78. Friedman, A.L.; Finlay, J.L. The Drash syndrome revisited: diagnosis and follow-up. Am. J. Med. Genet. 3:293-296; 1987.

79. Gallo, G.E.; Chemes, H.E. The association of Wilms' tumor, male pseudohermaphroditism and diffuse glomerular disease (Drash syndrome): report of eight cases with clinical and morphologic findings and review of the literature. Pediatr. Pathol. 7:175-189; 1987.

80. Ganguly, A.; Gribble, J.; Tune, B.; et al. Renin-secreting Wilms' tumor with wevere hypertension. Ann. Intern. Med. 79:835-837; 1973.

81. Ganick, D.J.; Wilms' tumor. Hematol Oncol. Clin. North Am. 1:698; 1987.

82. Green, D.M. The diagnosis and management of Wilms' tumor. Pediatr. Clin. North. Am. 32:735-754; 1985.

82a. Green, D.M.; Fernbach, D.J.; Norkool, P.; et al. The treatment of Wilms' tumor patients with pulmonary metastases detected only with computed tomography: A report from the National Wilms' Tumor Study. J. Clin. Oncol. 9(10):1776-1781; 1991.

83. Green, D.M.; Jaffe, N. Wilms' tumor: model of a curable pediatric malignant solid tumor. Cancer Treat. Rev. 5:143-172; 1978.

84. Haas, J.; Palmer, N.F.; Weinberg, A.G.; et al. Ultrastructure of malignant rhaboid tumor of the kidney. Hum. Pathol. 12:646-657; 1981.

85. Haselow, R.E.; Nesbit, M.; Dehner, L.P.; et al. Second neoplasms following megavoltage radiation in a pediatric population. Cancer. 42:1185-1191; 1978.

86. Heideman, R.L.; McGravran, L.; Waldstein, G. Nephroblastomatosis and deletion 11p. Am. J. Pediatr. Hematol. Oncol. 8:231-234; 1986.

87. Howell, C.G.; Othersen, H.B.; Kiriat, N.E.; *et al.* Therapy and outcome in 51 children with mesoblastic nephroma: a report of the national Wilms' tumor study. J. Pediatr. Surg. 17:826-831; 1982.

88. Hrabovsky, E.E.; Othersen, H.B.; deLorimier, A.; *et al.* Wilms' tumor in the neonate: a report from the national Wilms' tumor study. J. Pediatr. Surg. 21:385-387; 1986.

89. Jayabose, S.; Iqbal, K.; Newman, L.; San Filippo, J.A.; Davidian, M.M.; Noto, R.; Sagel, I. Hypercalcemia in childhood renal tumors. Cancer. 61:788-791; 1988.

90. Kilton, L.; Matthews, M.J.; Cohen, M.T. Adult Wilms' tumor: a report of prolonged survival and review of the literature. J. Urol. 124:1-5; 1980.

91. Knudson, A.G. Hereditary cancer, oncogenes, antioncogenes. Cancer Res. 45:1437-1443; 1985.

92. Knudson, A.G.; Strong, L.C. Mutation and cancer: a model for Wilms' tumor of the kidney. JNCI. 48:313-324; 1972.

93. Kraker, J. de; Lemerle, J.; Voute, P.A.; *et al.* Wilms' tumor with pulmonary metastases at diagnosis: the significance of primary chemotherapy. J Clin Oncol. 8(7):1187-1190; 1990.

94. Kumar, A.P.M.; Pratt, C.B.; Coburn, T.P.; *et al.* Treatment strategy for nodular renal blastoma and nephroblastomatosis associated with Wilms' tumor. J. Pediatr. Surg. 13:281-185; 1978.

95. Laberge, J.M.; Nguyen, L.T.; Homsy, Y.L.; Doody, D.P. Bilateral Wilms' tumor: changing concepts in management. J. Pediatr. Surg. 22:730-735; 1987.

96. Lai, H.S.; Hung, W.T.; Hou, S.W. Extrarenal Wilms' tumor — a case report. J. Pediatr. Surg. 23:454-456; 1988.

97. Lemerle, J.; Voute, P.A.; Tournade, M.F.; *et al.* Effectiveness of pre-operative chemotherapy in Wilms' tumor: results of an International Society of Paediatric Oncology (SIOP) clinical trial. J. Clin. Oncol. 1:604-609; 1983.

98. Meadows, A.T.; Baum, E.; Fossati-Bellani, F.; *et al.* Second malignant neoplasms in children: an update from the Late Effects Study Group. J. Clin. Oncol. 3:532-538; 1985.

99. Miller, R.W.; Fraumeni, J.R.; Manning, M.D. Association of Wilms' tumor with aniridia, hemihypertrophy and other congenital malformations. N Engl J Med. 270:922-927; 1964.

100. Mochon, M.C.; Blanc, J.F.; Plauchu, H.; Philip, T. WAGR syndrome, Wilms' tumor aniridia, gonadoblastoma, mental retardation: a review apropos of 2 cases. Pediatrics. 42:249-252; 1987.

101. Morgan, E.; Baum, E.; Breslow, N.; Takashima, J.; D'Angio, G. Chemotherapy-related toxicity in infants treated according to the second national Wilms' tumor study. J. Clin. Oncol. 6:51-55; 1988.

102. Nakayama, D.K.; Norkool, P.; deLorimier, A.A.; O'Neill, J.A., Jr.; D'Angio, G.J. Intracardiac extension of Wilms' tumor. A report of the national Wilms' tumor study. Ann. Surg. 204:693-697; 1986.

102a. National Wilms' Tumor Study Committee. Wilms' tumor: Status report, 1990. J. Clin. Oncol. 9(5):877-887; 1991.

103. Noronha, P.A.; Hruby, M.A.; Maurer, H.S. Acquired von Willebrand disease in a patient with Wilms' tumor. J. Pediatr. 95:997-999; 1979.

104. Rainwater, L.M.; Hosaka, Y.; Farrow, G.M.; Kramer, S.A.; Kelalis, P.P.; Lieber, M.M. Wilms' tumors: relationship of nuclear acoxyribonucleic acid ploidy to patient survival. J. Urol. 138:974-977; 1987.

105. Rosenfield, N.S.; Leonidas, J.C.; Barwick, K.W. Aggressive neuroblastoma simulating Wilms' tumor. Radiology. 166:165-167; 1988.

106. Sandstedt, B.; Delemarre, J.F.M.; Krul, E.J.; *et al.* Mesoblastic nephromas: a study of 29 tumors from the SIOP nephroblastoma file. Histopathology. 9:741-750; 1985.

107. Schwartz, A.D.; Lee, H.; Baum, E.S. Leukemia in children with Wilms' tumor. J. Pediatr. 87:374-376; 1975.

108. Scott, J.P.; Montgomery, R.R.; Tubergen, D.G.; *et al.* Acquired von Willebrand's disease in association with Wilms' tumor, regression following treatment. Blood. 58:665-669; 1981.

109. Shalet, M.F.; Holder, R.M.; Walters, T.R. Erythropoietin-producing Wilms' tumor. J. Pediatr. 70:615-617; 1967.

110. Shanbhogue, L.B.; Gray, E.; Miller, S.S. Congenital mesoblastic nephroma of infancy associated with hypercalcemia. J. Urol. 135:771-772; 1986.

111. Sotelo-Avila, C.; Gonzales-Crussi, F.; Fowler, J.W. Complete and incomplete forms of Beckwith-Wiedemann syndrome. Pediatrics 96:47-50; 1980.

112. Steinfeld, A.D.; Crowley, C.A.; O'Shea, P.A.; *et al.* Recurrent and metastatic mesoblastic nephroma in infancy. J. Clin. Oncol. 2:956-960; 1984.

113. Stine, K.C.; Goertz, K.K.; Poisner, A.M.; *et al.* Congestive heart failure, hypertension, hyperreninemia in bilateral Wilms' tumor: successful medical management. Med. Pediatr. Oncol. 14:63-66; 1986.

113a. Thomas, P.R.M.; Tefft, M.; Compaan, P.J.; *et al.* Results of two radiation therapy randomizations in the Third National Wilms' Tumor Study. Cancer 68:1703-1707; 1991.

114. Ugate, N.; Gonzales-Crussi, F.; Hsueh, W. Wilms' tumor: its morphology in patients under one year of age. Cancer. 48:346-353; 1981.

115. Vido, L.; Cacli, M.; Rizzoni, G. Congenital mesoblastic nephroma with hypercalcemia. Am. J. Pediatr. Hematol. Oncol. 8:149-152; 1986.

116. Young, J.L.; Miller, R.W. Incidence of malignant tumors in U.S. children. J. Pediatr. 86:254-258; 1975.

117. Yunis, J.J.; Ramsey, N.K.C. Familial occurrence of aniridia Wilms' tumor syndrome with deletion 11 p13-14, 1. J. Pediatr. 96:1027-1030; 1980.

Non-Hodgkin's Lymphoma

118. Anderson, J.; Jenkin, R. Treatment of childhood non-Hodgkin's lymphoma. N Engl J Med. 309:311; 1983. Letter to Editor.

119. Anderson, J.; Wilson, J.; Jenkin, R.; *et al.* Childhood non-Hodgkin's lymphoma: the results of a randomized therapeutic trial comparing a 4-drug regimen (COMP) with a 10-drug regimen (LSA-L). N Engl J Med. 308:559-565; 1983.

120. Armelin, H.; Armelin M.; Kelly, K.; *et al.* Functional role for c-myc in mitogenic response to platelet-derived growth factor. Nature. 310:655-660; 1984.

121. Bailey, R.J.; Burgert, E.O.; Dahlin, D.C. Malignant lymphoma in children. Pediatrics. 28:985-992; 1961.

122. Benjamin, D.; Magrath, I.; Douglass, E.; Corash, L. Derivation of lymphoma cell lines from microscopically normal bone marrow in patients with undifferentiated lymphomas: evidence of occult bone marrow involvement. Blood. 61:1017-1019; 1983.

123. Bernard, A.; Boumsell, L.; Reinherz, E.; *et al.* Cell surface characterization of malignant T cells from lymphoblastic lymphoma using monoclonal antibodies. Evidence for a phenotypic difference between malignant lymphoma. Blood. 57:1105; 1981.

125. Braziel, R.; Keneklis, T.; Donlon, J.; *et al.* Terminal deoxynucleotydyl transferase in non-Hodgkin's lymphoma. Am. J. Clin. Pathol. 80:655-659; 1983.

125. Camitta, B.; Lauer, S.; Casper, J.; *et al.* Effectiveness of a six-drug regimen (APO) without local irradiation for treatment of mediastinal lymphoblastic lymphoma in children. Cancer. 56:738-741; 1985.

126. Coleman, C. Adverse effects of cancer therapy: risk of second neoplasms. Am. J. Pediatr. Hematol. Oncol. 4:103-111; 1982.

127. Csako, G.; Magrath, I.; Elin, R. Serum total and isoenzyme lactate dehydrogenase activity in American Burkitt's lymphoma. Am. J. Clin. Pathol. 78:712-717; 1982.

128. Dalla-Favera, R.; Bregini, M.; Erikson, J.; *et al.* Human c-myc onc gene is located on the region of chromosome 8 that is translocated in Burkitt lymphoma cells. Proc. Natl. Acad. Sci. USA. 79:7824; 1982.

129. Filipovitch, A.; Zerbe, D.; Spector, B.; *et al.* Lymphomas in persons with naturally occurring immunodeficiency disorders. In: Magrath, I.; O'Connor, G.; Ramot, B., eds. Pathogenesis of Leukemias and Lymphomas: Environmental Influences. New York, NY: Raven Press; 1984:225-234.

130. Finlay, J.; Trigg, M.; Link, M.; Frierdich, S. Poor-risk non-lymphoblastic lymphoma of childhood: results of an intensive pilot study. Med. Pediatr Oncol. 17:29; 1989.

131. Glatstein, E.; Kim, H.; Donaldson, S.S.; *et al.* Non-Hodkin's lymphomas. VI. Results of treatment in childhood. Cancer. 34:204-211; 1974.

132. Gribben, J.; Hudson, B.; Linch, D. The potential value of very intensive therapy with autologous bone marrow rescue in the treatment of malignant lymphomas. Hematol Oncol. 5:281-293; 1987.

133. Grundy, G.W.; Greagan, E.T.; Fraumeni, J.F.; *et al.* Non-

Hodgkin's lymphoma in childhood: epidemiologic features. JNCI. 51:767-776; 1973.

134. Haddy, T.; Keenan, A.; Jaffe, E.; Magrath, I. Bone Involvement in young patients with non-Hodgkin's lymphoma: efficacy of chemotherapy without local radiotherapy. Blood. 72:1141; 1988.

135. Haynes, B. Human T lymphocyte antigens as defined by monoclonal antibodies. Immunol. Rev. 57:127-161; 1981.

136. Hutchison, R.; Murphy, S.; Fairclough, D. et al. Diffuse small noncleaved cell lymphoma children, Burkitt's versus non-Burkitt's types. Cancer. 64:23; 1989.

137. Iverson, U.; Iverson, O.; Ziegler, J.; et al. Cell kinetics of African cases of Burkitt's lymphoma. A preliminary report. Eur. J. Cancer. 8:305-310; 1972.

138. Jenkin, R.; Anderson, J.; Chilcote, R.; et al. The treatment of localized non-Hodgkin's lymphoma in children: a report from the Children's Cancer Study Group. J. Clin. Oncol. 2:88-97; 1984.

139. Kellie, S.; Pui, D.; Murphy, S. Childhood non-Hodgkin's lymphoma involving the testit: clinical features and treatment outcome. J Clin Oncol .7:106; 1989.

140. Kristoffersson, U.; Heim, S.; Heldrup, J. Cytogenetic studies of childhood non-Hodgkin lymphomas. Hereditas. 3:77; 1985.

141. Lemerle, M.; Gerrard-Marchant, R.; Sancho, H.; et al. Natural history of non-Hodgkin's lymphoma in children. Br. J. Cancer. 31(suppl 2):324-331; 1975.

142. Link, M.; Donaldson, S.; Berard, C.; Shuster, J.; Murphy, S. High cure rate with reduced therapy in localized non-Hodgkin's lymphoma (NHL) of childhood. Proc Am Soc Clin Oncol.. 6:190; 1987.

143. Loeffler, J.; Tarbell, N.; Kozakewich, H.; Cassady, J.; Weinstein, H. Primary lymphoma of bone in children: analysis of treatment results with Adriamycin, prednisone, Oncovin (APO), and local radiation therapy. J. Clin. Oncol. 4:496-501; 1986.

144. Magrath, I. Lymphocyte differentiation pathways — an essential basis for the comprehension of lymphoid neoplasia. JNCI. 67:501; 1981.

145. Magrath, I. Malignant non-Hodgkin's lymphomas. In: Pizzo, P.; Poplack, D., eds. Principles and Practice of Pediatric Oncology. Philadelphia, PA: JB Lippincott Co.; 1988:415-455.

146. Magrath, I.; Shiramizu, B. Biology and treatment of small non-cleaved cell lymphoma. Oncology. 3:41; 1989.

147. Magrath, I.; Lee, Y.; Anderson, T.; et al. Prognostic factors in Burkitt's lymphoma: importance of total tumor burden. Cancer. 45:1507-1515; 1980.

148. Magrath, I.; Ziegler, J. Bone marrow involvement in Burkitt's lymphoma and its relationship to acute B-cell leukemia. Leuk. Res. 4:33-59; 1980.

149. Magrath, I.T.; Lwanga, S.; Carswell, W.; et al. Surgical reduction of tumor bulk in management of abdominal Burkitt's lymphoma. Br. Med. J. 2:308-312; 1974.

150. Matas, A.; Hertel, B.; Rosai, J. Post-transplant malignant lymphoma, distinctive morphologic features. Am. J. Med. 61:716-720; 1976.

151. Meadows, A.; Sposto, R.; Jenkin, R.; et al. Similar efficacy of 6 and 18 months of therapy with four drugs (COMP) for localized non-Hodgkin's lymphoma of children: a report from the Children's Cancer Study Group. J. Clin. Oncol. 7:92-99; 1989.

152. Muller-Weihrich, S.; Ludwig, R.; Reiter, A.; et al. B-type non-Hodgkin's lymphomas and leukemia: the BFM study group experience. In: Cavalli, F.; Bonnadonna, G.; Rosencweig, M., eds. Proceedings of the Third International Conference on Malignant Lymphoma; Lugano, Switzerland; June 10-13, 1987.

153. Murphy, S.; Bleyer, W. Cranial irradiation is not necessary for central-nervous-system prophylaxis in pediatric non-Hodgkin's lymphoma. Intl. J. Radiat. Oncol. Biol. Phys. 13:467-468; 1987.

154. Murphy, S.; Bowman, W.; Abromowitch, M.; et al. Results of treatment of advanced stage Burkitt's lymphoma and B-cell (Sig+) acute lymphoblastic leukemia with high-dose fractionated cyclophosphamide and coordinated high-dose methotrexate and cytarabine. J. Clin. Oncol. 4:1732; 1986.

155. Murphy, S.; Fairclough, D.; Hutchison, R.; Berard C. Non-Hodgkin's lymphomas of childhood: an analysis of the histology, staging, and response to treatment of 338 cases at a single institution. J. Clin. Oncol. 7:186-193; 1989.

156. Murphy, S.; Melvin, S.; Mauer, A.; et al. Correlation of tumor cell kinetic studies with surface marker results in childhood non-Hodgkin's lymphoma. Cancer Res. 39:1534-1538; 1979.

157. Murphy, S.B. Classification, staging, and end results of treatment of childhood non-Hodgkin's lymphomas: dissimilarities from lymphomas in adults. Semin. Oncol. 1:332-339; 1980.

158. Murphy, S.B.; Husto, H.O. A randomized trial of combined modality therapy of childhood non-Hodgkin's lymphoma. Cancer. 45:630-637; 1980.

159. Nathwani, B.; Kim, H.; Rappaport, H. Malignant lymphoma, lymphoblastic. Cancer. 38:964-983; 1976.

160. Nelson, D.F.; Cassady, J.R.; Traggis, D.; et al. The role of radiation therapy in localized resectable intestinal non-Hodgkin's lymphoma in children. Cancer. 39:89-97; 1977.

161. Patte, C.; Philip, T.; Rodary, C.; et al. Improved survival rate in children with stage II and IVB cell non-Hodgkin's lymphoma and leukemia using multi-agent chemotherapy: results of a study of 114 children from the French Pediatric Oncology Society. J. Clin. Oncol. 4:1219-1226; 1986.

162. Pellici, P-G.; Knowles, D.; Magrath, I.; et al. Chromosomal breakpoints and structural alterations of the c-myc locus differ in endemic sporadic forms of Burkitt lymphoma. Proc. Natl. Acad. Sci. USA. 83:2984; 1986.

163. Rosenberg, S.A.; Diamond, H.D.; Dargeon, H.W.; et al. Lymphosarcoma in childhood. New Engl. J. Med. 259:505-512; 1958.

164. Sandlund, J.; Kiwanuka, J.; Marti, G.; Goldschmidts, G.; Magrath, I. Characterization of Burkitt's lymphoma cell lines with monoclonal antibodies using an ELISA technique. In: Reinherz, E.; Hayes, B.; Nadler, L.; Bernstein, I., eds. Leukocyte Typing. vol. 2. Proceedings of the 2nd International Congress of Human Leukocyte Antigens. New York, NY: Springer-Verlag; 1986:403-410.

165. Stapleton, F.; Strother, D.; Roy, S.; Wyatt, R.; McKay, C.; Murphy, S. Acute renal failure at onset of therapy for advanced stage Burkitt lymphoma and B cell acute lymphoblastic lymphoma. Pediatrics. 82:863-868; 1988.

166. Sullivan, M.; Boyett, J.; Pullen, J. Pediatric Oncology Group experience with modified LSA-L therapy in 107 children with non-Hodgkin's lymphoma (Burkitt's lymphoma excluded). Cancer. 5:323-336; 1985.

166a. Thomas, P.R.M. Lymphomas in children. In: Perez, C.; Brady, L.W., eds. Principles and Practice of Radiation Oncology. 2nd ed. Philadelphia, PA: JB Lippincott Co.; 1992:1470-1475.

167. Wagner, D.; Kiwanuka, J.; Edwards, B.; et al. Soluble interleukin II receptor levels in patients with undifferentiated and lymphoblastic lymphomas. J. Clin. Oncol. 5:1262-1274; 1987.

168. Wollner, N.; Burchenal, J.H.; Lieberman, P.H.; et al. A comparative study of 2 modalities of therapy. Cancer 37:123-134; 1976.

169. Wollner, N.; Mandell, L.; Filippa, D.; et al. Primary nasal-paranasal oropharyngeal lymphoma in the pediatric age group. Cancer. 65:1438; 1990.

170. Young, J.L.; Miller, R.W. Incidence of malignant tumors in US children. J. Pediatr. 87:254-258; 1975.

171. Ziegler, J.L.; Bluming, A.Z.; Morrow, R.H.; et al. Central nervous system involvement in Burkitt's lymphoma. Blood. 36:718-728; 1970.

172. Ziegler, J.L.; Magrath, I.T.; Gerber, P.; et al. Epstein-Barr virus and human malignancy. Ann. Intern. Med. 86:323-336; 1977.

Rhabdomyosarcoma

173. Brand, E.; Berek, J.; Nieberg, R.; Hacker, N. RMS of the uterine cervix, sarcoma botryoides. Cancer. 60:1552-1560; 1987.

174. Breslow, N.; Langholz, B. Childhood cancer incidence: geographical and temporal variations. Intl. J. Cancer 32:703-716; 1983.

175. Caillaud, J.M.; Marchant, R.G.; Marsden, H.B. Histopathology classification of childhood rhabdomyosarcoma: a report from the International Society of Pediatric Oncology pathology panel. Med Pediatr Oncol. 17:391-400; 1989.

176. Crist, W.; Garnsey, L.; Beltangady, M. Prognosis in children with rhabdomyosarcoma: a report of the intergroup rhabdomyosarcoma studies I and II. J. Clin. Oncol. 8:443-452; 1990.

177. Dehner, L.P. Soft tissue sarcomas of childhood: the differential diagnostic dilemma of the small blue cell. NCI Monogr. 56:43-59; 1981.

177a. Donaldson, S.S. Rhabdomyosarcoma. In: Perez, C.; Brady, L.W., eds. Principles and Practice of Radiation Oncology. 2nd ed. Philadelphia, PA: JB Lippincott Co.; 1992:1456-1466.

178. Donaldson, S. In: Carter, S.; Glatstein, E.; Livingston, R.B., eds. Principles of Cancer Treatment. New York, NY: McGraw-Hill; 1982:852-862

179. Donaldson, S.; Belli, J. A rational clinical staging system for childhood RMS. J. Clin. Oncol. 2:135-139; 1984.

180. Donaldson, S.; Castro, J.; Wilbur, J.; Jesse, R. RMS of the head and neck in children: combination treatment by surgery, irradiation and chemotherapy. Cancer. 31:16-35; 1973.

181. Dritschilo, A.; Weichselbaum, R.; Cassidy, J.R.; et al. The role of radiation therapy in the treatment of soft tissue sarcomas of childhood. Cancer. 42:1192-1203; 1978.

181a. Flamant, F.; Gerbaulet, A.; Nihoul-Fekete, C.; et al. Long-term sequelae of conservative treatment by surgery, brachytherapy, and chemotherapy for vulval and vaginal rhabdomyosarcoma in children. J. Clin. Oncol. 8(11):1847-1853; 1990.

182. Gaiger, A.M.; Soule, E.H.; Newton, W.A. Pathology of rhabdomyosarcoma, experience of the Intergroup Rhabdomyosarcoma Study, 1972-1978. NCI Monogr. 56:19-27; 1981.

183. Gehan, E.A.; Gover, N.; Marer, H.M. Prognostic factors in children with rhabdomyosarcoma. NCI Monogr. 56:83-92; 1981.

184. Ghavimi, F.; Exelby, P.R.; D'Angio, G.J.; et al. Multidisciplinary treatment of embryonal rhabdomyosarcoma in children. Cancer. 35:677-686; 1975.

185. Ghavimi, F.; Herr, H.; Jereb, B.; Exelby, P. Treatment of genitourinary RMS in children. J. Urol. 132:313-319; 1984.

186. Green, D.; Jaffe, N. Progress and controversy in the treatment of childhood rhabdomyosarcoma. Cancer Treat. Rev. 5:7-27; 1978.

187. Grufferman, S.; Wang, H.; DeLong, E.; Kimm, S.; Delzell, E.; Falletta, J. Environmental factors in the etiology of RMS in childhood. JNCI. 68:107-113; 1982.

188. Hays, D.M.; Shimada, H.; Raney, B.; et al. Clinical staging and treatment results in RMS of the female genital tract among children and adolescents. Cancer. 61:1893-1903; 1988.

189. Hays, D.M.; Sutow, W.W.; Lawrence, W.; et al. Rhabdomyosarcoma: surgical therapy in extremity lesions in children. Orthop. Clin. North Am. 8:883-902; 1977.

190. Horn, R.C.; Enterline, H.T. Rhabdomyosarcoma: a clinicopathological study and classification of 39 cases. Cancer. 11:181-199; 1958.

191. Jereb, B.; Cham, W.; Lattin, P.; et al. Local control of embryonal rhabdomyosarcoma in children by radiation therapy when combined with concomitant chemotherapy. Intl. J. Radiat. Oncol. Biol. Phys. 1:217-225; 1976.

192. Johnson, D.G. Trends in surgery for childhood rhabdomyosarcoma. Cancer. 35:916-920; 1975.

193. Jones, I.S.; Reese, A.B.; Kraut, J. Orbital rhabdomyosaroma: an analysis of 65 cases. Trans. Am. Ophthalmol. Soc. 63:223-225; 1965.

194. Kilman, J.W.; Clatworthy, H.W.; Newton, W.A.; et al. Reasonable surgery for rhabdomyosarcoma: a study of 69 cases. Ann. Surg. 178:346-351; 1973.

195. Koufos, A.; Hansen, M.; Copeland, N.; et al. Loss of heterozygosity in three embryonal tumors suggests a common pathogenetic mechanism. Nature. 316:330-334; 1985.

196. Lawrence, W.; Gehan, E.; Hays, D.; Beltangady, M.; Mauer, H. Prognostic significance of staging factors of the UICC staging system in childhood RMS: a report from the Intergroup Rhabdomyosarcoma Study (IRS-II). J. Clin. Oncol. 5:46-54; 1987.

197. Lawrence, W.; Hays, D.; Heyn, R.; et al. Lymphatic metastases with childhood RMS: a report from the Intergroup Rhabdomyosarcoma Study. Cancer. 60:910-915; 1987.

198. Li, F.; Fraumeni, J. Prospective study of a family cancer syndrome. JAMA. 247:2692-2696; 1982.

199. McKeen, E.; Bodurtha, J.; Meadows, A.; Douglass, E.; Mulvihill, J. RMS complicating multiple neurofibromatosis. J. Pediatr. 93:992-993; 1978.

199a. Mandell, L.; Ghavimi, F.; Peretz, T.; et al. Radiocurability of microscopic disease in childhood rhadomyosarcoma with radiation doses less than 4,000 Gy. J. Clin. Oncol. 8(9):1536-1542; 1990.

200. Mandell, L.; Ghavimi, F.; Exelby, P.; Ruks, Z. Preliminary results of alternating combination chemotherapy (CT) and hyperfractionated radiotherapy (HART) in advanced rhabdomyosarcoma (RMS). Intl. J. Radiat. Oncol. Biol. Phys. 15:197-203; 1988.

200a. Mandell, L.; Ghavimi, F.; LaQuaglia, M.; Exelby, P. Prognostic significance of regional lymph node involvement in childhood extremity rhabdomyosarcoma. Med. Pediatr. Oncol. 18:466-471; 1990.

201. Martinez, A.; Goffinet, D.R.; Donaldson, S.S.; et al. The use of interstitial therapy in pediatric malignancies. Front. Radiat. Ther. Oncol. 23:91-100; 1978.

202. Maurer, H.M.; Beltangady, M.; Gehan, E.A. The Intergroup Rhabdomyosarcoma Study-1: a final report. Cancer. 61:209-220; 1988.

203. Maurer, H.M; Donaldson, M.; Gehan, E.; et al. Rhabdomyosarcoma in childhood and adolescence. Curr. Probl. Cancer. 2:3-36; 1977.

204. Maurer, H.M.; Donaldson, M.; Gehan, E.A.; et al. The Intergroup Rhabdomyosarcoma Study. Update, November 1978. NCI Monogr. 56:61-68; 1981.

205. Newton, W.A. Jr.; Soule, E.H.; Hamoudi, A.B.; Reiman, H.M.; et al. Histopathology of childhood sarcomas, Intergroup Rhabdomyosarcoma Studies I and II: clinicopathologic correlation. J. Clin. Oncol. 6:67-75;1988.

205a. Ortega, J.A.; Wharam, M.; Gehan, E.A.; et al. Clinical features and results of therapy for children with paraspinal soft tissue sarcoma: A report of the Intergroup Rhadbomyosarcoma Study. J. Clin. Oncol. 9(5):796-801; 1991.

206. Palmer, N.; Foulkes, M. Histopathology and prognosis in the second Intergroup Rhabdomyosarcoma Study (IRS-II). Proc. Am. Soc. Clin. Oncol. 2:229; 1983. Abstract C-897.

207. Plowman, P. Radiotherapy of pediatric genitourinary tumors. In: Broecker, B.; Klein, F., eds. Pediatric Tumors of the Genitrourinary Tract. New York, NY: Alan R. Liss, Inc.; 1988:263-281.

208. Pratt, C.; Huster, H.; Fleming, I.; et al. Coordinated treatment of rhabdomyosarcoma with surgery, radiotherapy, and combination chemotherapy. Cancer Res. 32:606-610; 1972.

209. Randy, R.; Crist, W.; Maurer, H.; Foulkes, M. Prognosis of children with soft tissue sarcoma who relapse after achieving a complete response. A report from the Intergroup Rhabdomyosarcoma Study I. Cancer. 52:44-50; 1983.

209a. Raney, R.B.; Gehan, E.A.; Hays, D.M.; et al. Primary chemotherapy with or without radiation therapy and/or surgery for children with localized sarcoma of the bladder, prostate, vagina, uterus, and cervix. A comparison of the results in Intergroup Rhabdomyosarcoma studies I and II. Cancer 66:2072-2081; 1990.

210. Raney, R.; Hays, D.; Tefft, M.; Triche, T. Rhabdomyosarcoma and the undifferentiated sarcomas. In: Pizzo, P.; Poplack, D., eds. Principles and Practice of Pediatric Oncology. Philadelphia, PA: JB Lippincott Co.; 1988:635-658.

211. Raney, R.; Tefft, M.; Newtron, W.; et al. Improved prognosis with intensive treatment of children with cranial soft tissue sarcomas arising in nonorbital parameningeal sites: a report from the Intergroup Rhabdomyosarcoma Study. Cancer. 59:147-155; 1987.

212. Raney, R.; Tefft, M.; Lawrence, W.; et al. Paratesticular sarcoma in childhood and adolescence. A report from the Intergroup Rhabdomyosarcoma Studies I and II, 1973-1983. Cancer. 60:2337-2343; 1987.

212a. Reboul-Marty, J.; Quintana, E.; Mosseri, V.; et al. Prognostic factors of alveolar rhabdomyosarcoma in childhood. Cancer 68:493-498; 1991.

213. Rodary, C.; Flamant, F.; Donaldson, S.S. for the SIOP-IRS Committee. An attempt to use a common staging system in rhabdomyosarcoma: a report of an international workshop initiated by the International Society of Pediatric Oncology (SIOP). Med Pediatr Oncol. 17:210-215; 1989.

213a. Rodary, C.; Gehan, E.A.; Flamant, F.; et al. Prognostic factors in 951 nonmetastatic rhabdomyosarcoma in children: A report from the International Rhabdomyosarcoma Workshop. Med. Pediatr. Oncol. 19:89-95; 1991.

214. Rodary, C.; Rey, A.; Olive, D.; et al. Prognostic factors in 281 children with nonmetastatic rhabdomyosarcoma (RMS) at diagnosis. Med. Pediatr. Oncol. 16:71-77; 1988.

215. Ruymann, F.; Maddux, H.; Ragab, A.; et al. Congenital anomalies associated with RMS: an autopsy study of 115 cases. A report from the Intergroup Rhabdomyosarcoma Study Committee. Med. Pediatr. Oncol. 16:33-39; 1988.

216. Ruymann, F.; Newton, W.; Ragab, A.; Donaldson, M.; Foulkes, M. Bone marrow metastases at diagnosis in children and adolescents with RMS, a report from the Intergroup Rhabdomyosarcoma Study. Cancer. 53:368-373; 1984.

217. Stout, A. Rhabdomyosarcoma of the skeletal muscle. Ann. Surg. 123:447-472; 1946.
218. Tefft, M.; Fernandez, C.; Donaldson, M.H.; et al. Incidence of meningeal involvement by rhabdomyosarcoma of the head and neck in children: a report of the Intergroup Rhabdomyosarcoma Study (IRS). Cancer. 42:253-258; 1978.
219. Tefft, M.; Jaffe, N. Sarcoma of the bladder and prostate in children: rationale for the role of radiation therapy based on a review of the literature and a report of 14 additional patients. Cancer. 32:1161-1177; 1973.
220. Tefft, M.; Lattin, P.; Jereb, B.; et al. Acute and late effects on normal tissues following chemo- and radiotherapy for childhood RMS and Ewing's sarcoma. Cancer. 37:1201-1217; 1986.
221. Tefft, M.; Lattin, P.; Jereb, B.; et al. Treatment of rhabdomyosarcoma and Ewing's sarcoma of childhood: acute and late effects on normal tissues following combined chemo- and radiotherapy for childhood rhabdomyosarcoma and Ewing's sarcoma. Cancer. 37:1202-1213; 1973.
222. Tefft, M.; Lindberg, R.D.; Gehan, E.A. Radiation therapy combined with systemic chemotherapy of rhabdomyosarcoma in children: local control in patients enrolled in the Intergroup Rhabdomyosarcoma Study. NCI Monogr. 56:75-81; 1981.
223. Tefft, M.; Wharam, M.; Gehan, E. Local and regional control of RMS by radiation in IRS II. Intl. J. Radiat. Oncol. Biol. Phys. 15(suppl 1):159; 1988.
224. Trent, J.; Casper, J.; Meltzer, P.; Thompson, F.; Fagh, J. Nonrandom chromosome alterations in rhabdomyosarcoma. Cancer Genet. Cytogenet. 16:189-197; 1985.
225. Trotty, W.; Murphy, W.; Lee, J. Soft-tissue tumors: MR imaging. Radiology. 160:135-141; 1986.
226. Weichselbaum, R.R.; Cassady, J.R.; Albert, D.M.; et al. Multimodality management of orbital rhabdomyosarcoma. Intl. Ophthalmol. Clin. 20:247-259; 1980.
227. Wharam, M.; Foulkes, M.; Lawrence, W.; et al. Soft-tissue sarcoma of the head and neck in childhood. Non-orbital and non-parameningeal sites. a report of the Intergroup Rhabdomyosarcoma Study I. Cancer. 53:1016-1019; 1984.
228. Young, J.; Miller, R. Incidence of malignant tumors in U.S. children. J. Pediatr. 86:254-258; 1975.

Germ Cell Tumors and Teratomas

229. Ablin, A.R.; Krailo, M.; Ramsay, N.; et al. Malignant germ cell tumors in childhood: an outcome analysis. Proc. Am. Soc. Clin. Oncol. 5:213; 1986.Abstract.
230. Altman, R.P.; Randolph, J.G.; Lilly, J.R. Sacrococcygeal teratoma: American Academy of Pediatrics surgical section survey, 1973. J. Pediatr. Surg. 9:389-398; 1974.
231. Ashley, D.J.B.; Path, F.R.C. Origin of teratomas. Cancer. 32:390-394; 1973.
232. Atkin, N.B.; Baker, M.C. i (12p): specific chromosomal marker in seminoma and malignant teratoma of the testis. Cancer Genet. Cytogenet. 10:199-204; 1983.
233. Beller, F.K.; Nienhaus, H.; Schmundt, V.; et al. Endodermal germ cell carcinoma (endodermal sinus tumor) of the vagina in infant girls. J. Cancer Res. Clin. Oncol. 94:295-306; 1979.
234. Blum, R.H.; Careter, S.S.; Agre, K. A clinical review of bleomycin — a new antineoplastic agent. Cancer. 31:903; 1973
235. Breen, J.L.; Maxson, W.S. Ovarian tumors in children and adolescents. Clin. Obstet. Gynecol. 20:607-623; 1977.
236. Cangir, A.L.; Smith, J.; van Eys, J. Improved prognosis in children with ovarian cancers following modified VAC (vincristine sulfate, dactinomycin and cyclophosphamide) chemotherapy. Cancer. 42:1234-1238; 1978.
237. Carlson, R.W.; Sikic, B.I.; Turbow, M.M.; et al. Combination cisplatinum, vinblastine, and bleomycin chemotherapy (PVB) for malignant germ-cell tumors of the ovary. J. Clin. Oncol. 10:645-651; 1983.
238. Carter, D.; Bibro, M.C.; Touloukian, R.J. Benign clinical behavior of immature mediastinal teratoma in infancy and childhood: report of two cases and review of literature. Cancer. 49:398-402; 1982.
239. Dehner, L.P. Gonadal and estragonadal germ cell neoplasms-teratomas in childhood. In: Finegold, M.; Benington, J.L., eds. Pathology of Neoplasia in Children and Adolescents. Major Problems in Pathology. vol. 18. Philadelphia, PA: WB Saunders Co; 1986:282-312.
240. Ehren, I.M.; Mahour, G.H.; Isaacs, H., Jr. Benign and malignant ovarian tumors in children and adolescents: a review of 63 cases. Am. J. Surg. 147:339-344; 1984.
241. Einhorn, L.H.; Donohue, J.P. Cis-diaminodichloroplatinum, vinblastine, and bleomycin combination chemotherapy in disseminated testicular cancer. Ann. Intern. Med. 87:293; 1977.
242. Einhorn, L.H.; Donahue, J.P. Combination chemotherapy in disseminated testicular cancer. Semin. Oncol. 6:87-93; 1979.
243. Einhorn, L.H.; Williams, S.D. Chemotherapy of disseminated testicular cancer: a random prospective study. Cancer. 46:1339-1344; 1980.
244. Einhorn, L.H.; Williams, S.D.; Troner, M.; et al. The role of maintenance therapy in disseminated testicular cancer. N. Engl. J. Med. 305:727; 1981.
245. Engel, R.; Eakins, R.; Fletcher, B. Retroperitoneal teratoma: review of the literature and presentation of an unusual case. Cancer. 22:1068; 1968.
246. Exelby, P.R. Testicular cancer in children. Cancer. 45:1803-1809; 1980.
247. Golbey, R.B.; Reynolds, T.F.; Vugrin, D. Chemotherapy of metastatic germ cell tumors. Semin. Oncol. 6:82-86; 1979.
248. Gonzalez-Crussi, F. Extragonadal teratomas. Atlas of Tumor Pathology. 2nd series, fascicle 18. Washington, D.C: Armed Forces Institute of Pathology; 1982.
249. Grosfeld, J.L.; Ballantine, T.V.N.; Lowe, D.; et al. Benign and malignant teratomas in children: analysis of 85 patients. Surgery. 80:297-305; 1976.
250. Hart, W.R.; Burkons, D.M. Germ cell neoplasms arising in gonadoblastomas. Cancer. 43:669-678; 1979.
251. Higby, D.J.; Wallace, H.J.; Albert, D.; et al. Diaminodichloro-platinum in chemotherapy of testicular tumors. J. Urol. 112:100; 1974.
252. Jackson, S.M. Ovarian dysgerminoma in three generations. J. Med. Genet. 4:112-113; 1967.
253. Jenkyn, D.J.; McCartney, A.J. A chromosome study of three ovarian tumors. Cancer Genet. Cytogenet. 26(2):327-337; 1987.
254. Jordan, R.B.; Gauderer, M.W. Cervical teratomas: an analysis. literaure review and proposed classification. J. Pediatr. Surg. 23(6):583-591; 1988.
255. Kersh, C.R.; Constable, W.C.; Hahn, S.S.; et al. Primary malignant extragonadal germ cell tumors: an analysis of the effect of radiotherapy. Cancer. 65:2681-2685; 1990.
256. Kiffer, J.D.; Sandeman, T.F. Primary malignant mediastinal germ cell tumors: a study of eleven cases and a review of the literature. Intl. J .Radiat. Oncol. Biol. Phys. 17:835-841; 1989.
257. Kingsbury, A.C.; Frost, F.; Cookson, C.M. Dysgerminoma, gonadoblastoma and testicular germ cell neoplasia in phenotypically female and male siblings with 46XY genotype. Cancer. 59:288-291; 1987.
258. Lack, E.E.; Weinstein, J.H.; Welch, K.J. Mediastinal germ cell tumors in childhood. A clinical and pathologic study of 21 cases. J. Thorac. Cardiovasc. Surg. 89:826-835; 1985.
259. Lawson, A.P.; Adler, G.F. Radiotherapy in the treatment of ovarian dysgerminomas. Intl. J. Radiat. Oncol. Biol. Phys. 14:431-434; 1988.
260. Li, F.P.; Fraumeni, J.F. Jr. Testicular cancers in children. JNCI. 44:1575-1582; 1972.
261. Li, M.C.; Hertz, R.; Spencer, D.B. Effect of methotrexate on choriocarcinoma and chorioadenoma. Proc. Soc. Exp. Biol. Med. 96:361; 1956.
261a. Li, M.C.; Whitmore, W.R.; Golbey, R.B.; et al. Effects of combined drug therapy in metastatic cancer of the testis. JAMA. 174:1291-1299; 1960.
262. Liber, A.F. Ovarian cancer in mother and 5 daughters. Arch. Pathol. 42:280-290; 1950.
263. Loehrer, P.J.; Einhorn, L.H.; Williams, S.D. VP-16 plus ifosfamide plus cisplatin as salvage therapy in refractory germ cell cancer. J. Clin. Oncol. 4:528-536; 1986.
264. Mahour, G.H.; Landing, B.H.; Wooley, M.M. Teratomas in children: clinicopathologic studies in 133 patients. Z. Kinderchir. 23:365-380; 1978.
265. Mahour, G.H.; Woolley, G.H.; Landing, B.H. Ovarian tumors in children: a 33 year experience. Am. J. Surg. 63:367-370; 1976.
266. Mann, J.R.; Pearson, D. Barrett, A.; et al. Results of the United Kingdom Children's Cancer Study Group's malignant germ cell tumor studies. Cancer. 63:1657-1667; 1989.

267. Martin, D.C. Malignancy in the cryptorchid testis. Urol. Clin. North Am. 9:371-376; 1982.

268. Norohna, P.A.; Noronha, R.; Rao, D.S. Primary anterior mediastinal endodermal sinus tumor in childhood. Am. J. Pediatr. Hematol. Oncol. 7:312-316; 1985.

269. Norris, H.J.; Zirkin, H.J.; Benson, W.L. Immature (malignant) teratoma of the ovary: a clinical and pathologic study of 58 cases. Cancer. 37:2359-2372; 1976.

270. Oosterhuis, J.W.; Castedo, S.M.; deJong, B.; Cornelisse, C.J.; Dam, A. Ploidy of primary germ cell tumors of the testis. Pathogenetic and clinical relevance. Lab. Invest. 60(1):14-21; 1989.

271. Oronez, N.G.; Manning, J.T., Jr.; Alyala, A.G. Teratoma of the omentum, abdominal wall and peritoneum. Cancer. 51:955-958; 1983.

272. Orr, P.S.; Gibson, A.; Young, O.S. Ovarian tumours in children: a 27 year review. Br. J. Surg. 63:367-370;1976.

273. Packer, R.J.; Sutton, L.M.; Rosenstock, J.G.; et al. Pineal region tumors of childhood. Pediatrics 74:97; 1984.

274. Reamen, G.H.; Cohen, L.F. Less frequently encountered malignant neoplasms. In: Levine, A.S., ed. Cancer in the Young. New York, NY: Masson Publishers; 1982:707-727.

275. Rosenfeld, C.R.; Coln, C.D.; Duenhoelter, J.H. Fetal cervical teratoma as a cause of polyhydramnios. Pediatrics. 64(2):176-179; 1979.

276. Samuels, M.L.; Howe, C.D. Vinblastine in the management of testicular cancer. Cancer. 25:1009; 1970.

277. Scardino, P.T.; Cox, H.D.; Waldmann, T.A.; et al. The value of serum tumor markers in the staging and prognosis of germ cell tumors of the testis. J. Urol. 118:994-999; 1977.

278. Sledge, G.W.,Jr.; Eble,J.N.; Roth, B.J.; Wuhrman, B.P.; Fineberg, N.; Einhorn, L.H. Relation of proliferative activity to survival in patients with advanced germ cell cancer. Cancer Res. 48(13):3864-3868; 1988.

279. Tapper, D.; Lack, E.E. Teratomas in infancy and childhood. A 54 year experience at the Children's Hospital Medical Center. Ann. Surg. 198:398; 1983.

280. Teilum, G. Special Tumors of Ovary and Testis and Related Extragonadal Lesions. 2nd ed. Philadelphia, PA: JB Lippincott Co; 1977.

281. Trentini, G.P.; Palmieri, B. An unusual case of gonadic germinal tumor in a brother and sister. Cancer. 33:250-255; 1974.

282. Tsuchida, Y.; Endo, Y.; Saito, S.; Kaneko, M.; Shiraki, K.; Ohmi, K. Evaluation of alpha-fetoprotein in early infancy. J. Pediatr. Surg. 13(2):155-156; 1978.

283. Tsuji, L.; Nakajima, F.; Nishida, T.; et al. Testicular tumors in children. J. Urol. 110:127-129; 1973.

284. Ulfelder, H. Staging system for cancer at gynecologic sites. In: American Joint Committee. Manual for Staging of Cancer. Philadelphia, PA: JB Lippincott Co; 1978:94-97.

285. Waldhausen, J.A.; Kilman, J.W.; Vellios, F.; Battersby, J.S. Sacrococcygeal teratoma. Ped. Surg. 54(6):933-949; 1963.

286. Wara, W.M.; Jenkin, D.T.; Evans, A.; et al. Tumors of the pineal and suprasellar region: Children's Cancer Study Group treatment results 1960-1975. Cancer. 43:698-701; 1979.

287. Weissbach,J.; Altwein,J.E.; Stiens, R. Germinal testicular tumors in childhood. Eur. Urol. 10:73-85; 1984.

288. Whalen, T.; Mahour, G.; Landing, B.; Woolley, M.M. Sacrococcygeal teratomas in infants and children. Am. J. Surg. 150:373; 1985.

289. Wider, F.A.; Marshall, J.R.; Basridin, C.A.E.; et al. Sustained remissions after chemotherapy for primary ovarian cancer containing choriocarcinoma. N. Engl. J. Med. 280:1439-1442; 1969.

290. Witshi, E. Migration of the germ cells of human embryos from the yolk sac to the primitive gonadal fold. Contrib. Embryol. 32:69; 1988.

291. Young, J.L.,Jr.; Ries, L.G.; Silverberg, E.; et al. Cancer incidence survival and mortality for children younger than age 15 years. Cancer. 58:598-602; 1986.

292. Young, R.H.; Scully, R.E. Endodermal sinus tumor of the vagina: a report of nine cases and review of the literature. Gynecol. Oncol. 18:380-392; 1984.

Langerhans' Cell Histiocytosis (Histiocytosis X)

293. Ceci, A.; de Terlizzi, M.; Colella, R.; Balducci, D.; Roma, M.G.; Zurlo, M.G.; Macchia, P.; Mancini, A.; Indolfi, P.; Locurto, M.; et

al. Etoposide in recurrent childhood Langerhans' cell histiocytosis: an Italian cooperative study. Cancer. 62:2528-2531; 1988.

294. Dunger, D.B.; Broadbent, V.; Yeoman, E.; et al. The frequency and natural history of diabetes insipidus in children with Langerhans-cell histiocytosis. N. Engl. J. Med. 321:1157-1162; 1989.

295. Favara, B.E. The pathology of "histiocytosis." Am. J. Pediatr. Hematol. Oncol. 3:45-56; 1981.

296. Greenberger,J.S.; Cassady,J.R.: Jaffe, N. et al. Radiation therapy in patients with histiocytosis: management of diabetes insipidus and bone lesions. Int. J. Radiat. Oncol. Biol. Phys. 5:1749-1755;1979.

297. Greenberger, J.S.; Crocker, A.C.; Vawter, G.; et al. Results of treatment of 127 patients with systemic histiocytosis (Letter-Siwe syndrome, Schuller-Christian syndrome and multifocal eosinophilic granuloma). Medicine. 60:311; 1981.

298. Ladisch, S.; Jaffe, E.S. The histiocytoses. In: Pizzo, P.A.; Poplack, D.G. eds. Principles and Practice of Pediatric Oncology. Philadelphia, PA: JB Lippincott Co.;1980.

299. Ladisch, S.; Jaffe, E.S. The histiocytoses. In: Pizzo,P.A.; Poplack, D.G. eds. Principles of Pediatric Oncology. Philadelphia,PA: JB Lippincott Co; 1989:491-504.

300. Lahey, M.E. Histiocytosis X: an analysis of prognostic factors. J. Pediatr. 87:184-189; 1975.

301. Lichtenstein, L. Histiocytosis X: integration of eosinophilic granuloma of bone, "Letterer-Siwe disease," and "Schuller-Christian disease" as related manifestations of a single nosologic entity. Arch. Pathol. 56:84-102;1953.

302. Lahey, M.E. Prognosis in reticuloendotheliosis in children. J. Pediatr. 60:664-671; 1962.

303. Mierau, G.W.; Favara, B.E. S-100 protein immunohistochemistry and electron microscopy in the diagnosis of Langerhans cell proliferative disorders: a comparative assessment. Ultrastruct. Pathol. 10:303-309; 1986.

304. Osband, M.E.; Lipton, J.M.; Lavin, P.; et al. Histiocytosis X: demonstration of abnormal immunity, T-cell histamine receptor deficiency, and successful treatment with thymic extract. N. Engl. J. Med. 304:146-153; 1981.

305. Selch, M.T.; Parker, R.G. Radiation therapy in the management of Langerhans cell histiocytosis. Med. Pediatr. Oncol. 18:97-102; 1990.

306. Starling, K.A.; Donaldson, M.H.; Haggard, M.E.; et al. Therapy of histiocytosis X with vincristine, vinblastine, and cyclophosphamide. Am. J. Dis. Child. 123:105-110; 1972.

307. Vogel, J.M.; Vogel, P. Idiopathic histiocytosis: a discussion of eosinophilic granuloma, the Hand-Schuller-Christian syndrome, and the Letterer-Siwe syndrome. Semin. Hematol. 9:349; 1972.

Osteogenic Sarcoma

308. Bauer, H.; Kreicbergs, A.; Silfversward, C..; Tribukait, B. DNA analysis in the differential diagnosis of osteosarcoma. Cancer 61:2532-2540; 1988.

309. Cortes, E.P.; Holland, J.F.; Glidewell, O. Adjuvant therapy of operable primary osteosarcoma-cancer and leukemia group B experience. Cancer Res. 68:16-24; 1979.

310. Cortes, E.P.; Holland, J.F.; Wang, J.J.; et al. Doxorubicin in disseminated osteosarcoma. J. Am. Med. Assoc. 221:1132-1138; 1972.

311. Cortes, E.P.; Holland,J.F.; Wang,J.J.; Sinks, L.F.; Blom,J.; Senn, H.; Bank, A.; Glidewell, O. Amputation and Adriamycin in primary osteosarcoma. New Engl. J. Med. 291:998-1000; 1974.

312. Dahlin, C.D.; Coventry, M.B. Osteogenic sarcoma: a study of 600 cases. J. Bone Joint Surg. (Am.) 49:101-110; 1967.

313. Eilber, F.; Giuliano, A.; Eckardt, J.; Patterson, K.; Moseley, S.; Goodnight, J. Adjuvant chemotherapy for osteosarcoma: a randomized prospective trial. J. Clin. Oncol. 5:21-26; 1987.

314. Eilber, F.R.; Morton, D.L.; Eckardt,J.; Grant, T.; Weisenburger, T. Limb salvage for skeletal and soft tissue sarcomas. Cancer 53:2579-2584; 1984.

315. Enneking, W.F.; Kagan, A. Transepiphysieal extension of osteosarcoma: incidence, mechanisms, and implications. Cancer 41:1526-1527; 1978.

316. Finkle, M.P.; Biskis, B.O.; Jinkins, P.B. Virus induction of osteosarcomas in mice. Science 151:698-700; 1966.

317. Frauman, J.F. Stature and malignant tumors of bone in childhood and adolescence. Cancer 20:967-973; 1967.

318. Gillman, P.A.; Wang, N.; Fan, S.F.; Reede, J.; Khan, A.; Levanthal,

B.G. Familial Osteosarcoma associated with 13;14 chromosomal rearrangement. Cancer Genet. Cytogenet. 17:123-132; 1985.

319. Hems, G. Aetiology of bone cancer, and some other cancers, in the young. Br. J. Cancer 24:208-214; 1970.

320. Hoover, H.C.; Ketcham, A.S.; Millar, R.C.; et al. Osteosarcoma: improved survival with anticoagulation and amputation. Cancer 41:2475-2480; 1978.

321. Jaffe, N. Malignant bone tumors. Pediatr. Ann. 4:10-32; 1975.

322. Jaffe, N. Recent advance in the chemotherapy of metastatic osteogenic sarcoma. Cancer 30:1627-1631; 1972.

323. Jaffe, N.; Frei, E.; Traggis, D.; Bishop, Y. Adjuvant methotrexate and citrovorum-factor treatment of osteogenic sarcoma. New Engl. J. Med. 291:994-997; 1974.

324. Jaffe, N.; Smith, E.; Abelson, H.T.; Frei, E. Osteogenic sarcoma: alterations in the pattern of pulmonary metastases with adjuvant chemotherapy. J. Clin. Oncol. 1:251-254; 1983.

325. Johnson, R.J. Parosteal osteosarcoma. Clin. Orthop. 68:78-83; 1970.

326. Link, M.P.; Goorin, A.M.; Miser, A.W.; Green, A.A.; Pratt C.B.; Belasco, J.B.; Pritchard, J.; Malpas, J.S.; Baker, A.R.; Kirkpatrick, J.A.; Ayala, A.G.; Shuster, J.J.; Abelson, H.T.; Simone, J.V.; Vietti, T.J. The effect of adjuvant chemotherapy on relapse-free survival in patients with osteosarcoma of the extremity. New Engl. J. Med. 314:1600-1606; 1986.

327. Look, T.A.; Douglass, E.C.; Meyer, W.H. Clinical importance of near-diploid tumor stem lines in patients with osteosarcoma of an extremity. New Engl. J. Med. 318:1567-1572; 1988.

328. Marcove, R.C.; Mike, V.; Hajek, J.V.; Levin, A.G.; Hutter, R. Osteogenic sarcoma in childhood. New York State J. Med. 71:855-859; 1970.

329. Marcove, R.C.; Rosen, G. En bloc resections for osteogenic sarcoma. Cancer 45:3040-3044; 1980.

330. Marti, C.; Kroner, T.; Remogen, W.; et al. High-dose ifosfamide in advanced osteosarcoma. Cancer Treat. Rep. 69:115-117; 198?.

331. Martinez, A.; Goffinet, D.R.; Donaldson, S.S.; Bagshaw, M.A.; Kaplan, H.S. Intra-arterial infusion of radiosensitizer (BUdR) combined with hypofractionated irradiation and chemotherapy for primary treatment of osteogenic sarcoma. Intl. J. Radiat. Oncol. Biol. Phys. 2:123-128; 1984.

332. Martini, N.; Huvos, A.G.; Mike, V.; Marcove, R.C.; Beattie, E.J. Multiple pulmonary resections in the treatment of osteogenic sarcoma. Ann. Thorac. Surg. 12:271-280; 1971.

333. Meyer, W.H.; Schell, M.J.; Kumar, A.P.; Rao, B.N.; Green, A.A.; Champion, J.; Pratt, C.B. Thoracotomy for pulmonary metastatic osteosarcoma. Cancer 59:374-379; 1987.

334. Nitschke, R.; Starling, K.A.; Vats, T.; Bryan, H.H. Cis-diamminedichloroplatinum (NSC-119875) in childhood malignancies: a southwest oncology group study. Med. Pediatr. Oncol. 4:127-132; 1978.

335. Ochs, J.J.; Freeman, A.L.; Douglass, H.O.; Higby, D.S.; mindell, E.R.; Sinks, L.F. Cis-dichlorodiammineplatinum (II) in advanced osteosarcoma. Cancer Treat. Rep. 62:239-245; 1978.

336. Parham, D.M.; Pratt, C.B.; Parvey, L.S.; Webber, B.L.; Champion, J. Childhood multifocal osteosarcoma. Cancer 55:2653-2658; 1985.

337. Pritchard, D.J.; Reilly, C.A.; Finkle, M.P. Evidence for a human osteosarcoma virus. Nature (New Biol.) 234:126-127; 1971.

338. Provisor, A.; Nachman, J.; Krailo, M.; Ettinger, L.; Hammond, D. Treatment of non-metastatic osteogenic sarcoma of the extremities with pre- and post-operative chemotherapy. ASCO Proc. 6:217; 1987.

339. Rosen, G.; Caparros, B.; Huvos, A.G.; Kosloff, C.; Nirenberg, A.; Cacavio, A.; Marcove, R.C.; Lane, J.M.; Mehta, B.; Urban, C. Preoperative chemotherapy for osteogenic sarcoma. Cancer 49:1221-1230; 1982.

340. Rosen, G.; Huvas, A.G.; Mosendo, C.; et al. Chemotherapy and thoracotomy for metastatic osteogenic sarcoma: a model for adjuvant chemotherapy and the rationale for the timing of thoracic surgery. Cancer 41:841-849; 1978.

341. Rosen, G.; Marcove, R.C.; Caparros, B.; Nirenberg, A.; Kosloff, C.; Juvos, A.G. Primary osteogenic sarcoma. Cancer 43:2163-2177; 1979.

342. Rous, P.; Murphy, J.B.; Nirenberg, A.; et al. Osteogenic sarcoma: selection of adjuvant chemotherapy based upon the resonse of the primary tumor to preoperative chemotherapy based upon the response of the primary tumor to preoperative chemotherapy,

abstract C-378. In: Proceedings of the 17th annual ASCO meeting, Washington, D.C., April 1981:429.

343. Sweetnam, R.; Knowelden, J.; Jedden, H. Bone sarcoma: treatment by irradiation, amputation, or a combination of the two. Br. Med. J. 2:363-367; 1971.

344. Taylor, W.F.; Ivins, J.C.; Dahlin, D.C.; Edmonson, J.H.; Pritchard, D.J. Trends and variability in survival from osteosarcoma. Mayo Clin. Proc. 53:695-700; 1978.

345. Telander, R.L.; Pairolero, P.C.; Pritchard, D.J.; et al. Resection of pulmonary metastatic osteogenic sarcoma in children. Surgery 84:335-341; 1978.

346. Uribe-Botero, G.; Russell, W.O.; Sutow, W.W.; Martin, R.G. Primary osteosarcoma of bone. A clinicopathologic investigation of 243 cases with necropsy studies in 54. Am. J. Clin. Pathol. 67:427-435; 1977.

347. Weiner, M.A.; Harris, M.B.; Lewis, M.; Jones, R.; Sherry, H.; Feurer, E.J.; Johnson, J.; Lahman, E. Neoadjuvant high-dose methotrexate, cisplatin, and doxorubicin for the management of patients with nonmetastatic osteosarcoma. Cancer Treat. Rep. 70:1431-1432; 1986.

Ewing's Sarcoma

348. Brown, A.; Fixsen, J.; Plowman, P. Local control of Ewing's sarcoma: an analysis of 67 patients. Br. J. Radiol. 60:261-268; 1987.

349. Chan, R.C.; Suton, W.W.; Lindberg, R.D.; et al. Management and results of localized Ewing's sarcoma. Cancer 43:1001-1006; 1979.

350. Dahlin, D.C. Bone tumors: general aspects and data on 6,221 cases. Springfield, IL: C.C. Thomas; 1978.

351. Dahlin, D.C.; Coventry, M.P.; Scanlon, P.W. Ewing's sarcoma: a critical analysis of 165 cases. J. Bone Joint Surg. 43A:185-192; 1961.

352. Dickman, P.; Liotta, L.; Triche, T. Ewing's sarcoma: characterization in established cultures and evidence of its histogenesis. Lab. Invest. 47:375-382; 1982.

353. Edeiken, J.; Hodes, P.J. Roentgen diagnoses of bone, 2nd ed. Baltimore: Williams & Wilkins; 1973.

354. Evans, R.; Nesbit, M.; Askin, F.; et al. Local recurrence, rate and sites of metastases, and time to relapse as a function of treatment regimen, m size of primary and surgical history in 62 patients presenting with non-metastatic Ewing's sarcoma of the pelvic bones. Intl. J. Radiat. Oncol. Biol. Phys. 11:129-136; 1985.

355. Ewing, J. Diffuse endothelioma of bone. Proc. N.Y. Pathol. Soc. 21:17-24; 1921.

356. Falk, S.; Albert, M. Five-year survival of patients with Ewing's sarcoma. Surg. Gynecol. Obstet. 124:319-324; 1967.

357. Farley, F.; Healey, J.; Caparros-Sisson, B.; Godbold, J.; Lane, J.; Glasser, D. Lactase dehydrogenase as a tumor marker for recurrent disease in Ewing's sarcoma. Cancer 59:1245-1248; 1987.

358. Frankel, R.S.; Jones, A.E.; Cohen, J.A.; et al. Clinical correlations of gallium-67 and skeletal whole body radionuclide studies with radiography in Ewing's sarcoma. Radiology 110:597-603; 1974.

359. Hayes, F.; Thompson, E.; Parvey, L.; et al. Metastatic Ewing's sarcoma: remission induction and survival. J. Clin. Oncol. 5:1199-1204;

360. Hayes, F.; Thompson, W.; Meyer, W.; et al. Therapy for localized Ewing's sarcoma of bone. J. Clin. Oncol. 7:208-213; 1989.

361. Jurgens, H.; Exner, U.; Gadner, H.; et al. Multidisciplinary treatment of primary Ewing's sarcoma of bone. A 6-year experience of a European Cooperative trial. Cancer 61:23-32; 1988.

362. Li, F.; Tu, J.; Liu, F.; et al. Rarity of Ewing's sarcoma in China. Lancet 1:1255; 1980.

363. Marcus, R.; Graham-Pole, J.; Springfield, D.; et al. High-risk Ewing's sarcoma: end-intensification using autologous bone marrow transplantation. Intl. J. Radiat. Oncol. Biol. Phys. 15:53-59; 1988.

364. Mehta, Y.; Hendrickson, F.R. CNS involvement in Ewing's sarcoma. Cancer 33:859-862; 1974.

365. Mendenhall, C.; Marcus, R.; Enneking, W.; et al. The prognostic significance of soft tissue extension in Ewing's sarcoma. Cancer 51:913-917; 1983.

366. Miser, J.; Kinsella, T.; Triche, T.; et al. Ifosfamide with mesna uroprotection and etoposide: and effective regimen in the treatment of recurrent sarcomas and other thumors of children and young adults. J. Clin. Oncol. 5:1191-1198; 1987.

367. Miser, J.; Triche, T.; Pritchard, D.; Kinsella, T. Ewing's sarcoma and the nonrhabdomyosarcoma soft tissue sarcomas of childhood. In: Pizzo, P.; Poplack, D., eds. Principles and practice of pediatric oncology. Philadelphia: J.B. Lippincott Co.; 1989:659-688.

368. Moll, R.; Lee, I.; Gould, V.; Berndt, R.; Roessner, A.; Franke, W. Immunocytochemical analysis of Ewing's tumors. Am. J. Pathol. 127:288-304; 1987.

369. Perez, C.A.; Tefft, M.; Nesbit, M.E.; et al. Radiation therapy in the multimodal management of Ewing's sarcoma of bone: report of the intergroup Ewing's study. Natl. Cancer Inst. Monogr. 56:255-262; 1981.

370. Pomeroy, T.; Johnson, R. Prognostic factors for survival in Ewing's sarcoma. Am. J. Roentgenol. 123:598-606; 1975.

371. Pomeroy, T.C.; Johnson, R.E. Combined modality therapy of Ewing's sarcoma. Cancer 35:36-47; 1975.

372. Pritchard, D.; Dahlin, D.C.; Dauphine, R.T.; et al. Ewing's sarcoma: a clinicopathological and statistical analysis of patients surviving 5 years of longer. J. Bone Joint Surg. 57A:10-16; 1975.

373. Rosen, G.; Caparros, B.; Nirenberg, A.; et al. Ewing's sarcoma ten year experience with adjuvant chemotherapy. Cancer 47:2204-2213; 1981.

374. Sailer, S.; Harmon, D.; Mankin, H.; Truman, J.; Suit, H.; Phil, D. Ewing's sarcoma: surgical resection as a prognostic factor. Intl. J. Radiat. Oncol. Biol. Phys. 15:43-52; 1988.

375. Strong, L.; Herson, J.; Osborne, B.; et al. Rish of radiation-related subsequent malignant tumors in survivors of Ewing's sarcoma. J. Natl. Cancer Inst. 62:1401-1406; 1979.

376. Tepper, J.; Glaubiger, D.; Lichter, A.; Wackenhut, J.; Glatstein, E. Local control of Ewing's sarcoma of bone with radiotherapy and combination chemotherapy. Cancer 46:1969-1973; 1983.

377. Thomas, P.; Perez, C.; Neff, J.; Nesbit, M.; Evans, R. The management of Ewing's sarcoma: role of radiotherapy in local tumor control. Cancer Treat. Rep.. 68:703-710; 1984.

378. Trigg, M.; Glaubiger, D.; Nesbit, M. The frequency of isolated CNS involvement in Ewing's sarcoma. Cancer 49:2404-2409; 1982.

379. Vietti, T.J.; Gehan, E.A.; Nesbit, M.E.; et al. Multimodal therapy in metastatic Ewing's sarcoma: an intergroup study. Natl. Cancer Inst. Monogr. 56:279-284; 1981.

380. Wang, C.C.; Schulz, M.D. Ewing's sarcoma. New Engl. J. Med. 248:571-576; 1953.

381. Whang-Peng, J.; Triche, T.; Knutsen, T.; et al. Chromosome translocation in peripheral neuroepithelioma. New Engl. J. Med. 311:584-585; 1984.

382. Young, J.L.; Miller, R.W. Incidence of malignant tumors in U.S. children. J. Pediatr. 86:254-258; 1975.

Malignant Hepatic Tumors

383. Altman, ; Schwartz, . Malignant diseases of infancy, childnood and adolescence. Philadelphia: W.B. Saunders; 1983:524.

384. Blumberg, B.S.; London, W.T. Hepatitis B virus: pathogenesis and prevention of primary cancer of theliver. Cancer 50:2657-2665; 1982.

385. Chang, J.H.; Janik, J.S.; Burrington, J.D.; Clark, D.R.; Campbell, D.N.; Pappas, G. Extensive tumor resection under deep hypothermia and circulatory arrest. J. Pediatr. Surg. 23:254-258; 1988.

386. Chen, W.J.; Lee, J.C.; Hung, W.T. Primary malignant tumor of liverin infants and children in Taiwan. J. Pediatr. Surg. 23:457-461; 1988.

387. Exelby, P.R.; Filler, R.M.; Grosfeld, J.L. Liver tumors in chidlren in the particular reference to hepatoblastoma and hepatocellular carcinoma. American Academy of Pediatrics Surgical Section Survey. J. Pediatr. Surg. 10:329-337; 1975.

388. Gauthier, F.; Valayer, J.; Thai, B.L.; Sinico, M.; Kalifa, C. Hepatoblastoma and hepatocarcinoma in children: analysis of a series of 29 cases. J. Pediatr. Surg. 21:424-429; 1986.

389. Giacchino, R.; Pontisso, P.; Navone, C.; Alberti, A.; Dini, G.; Facco, F.; Ciraregna, B. Hepatitis B virus (HBV)-DNA-positive hepatocellular carcinoma following hepatitis B virus infection in child. J. Med. Virol. 23:151-155; 1987.

390. Giacomantonio, M.; Ein, S.H.; Mancer, K.; Stephens, C.A. Thirty years of experience with pediatric primary malignant liver tumors. J. Pediatr. Surg. 19:523-526; 1984.

391. Hsu, H.C.; Wu, M.Z.; Chang, M.H.; Su, I.J.; Chen, D.S. Child-hood hepatocellular carcinoma develops exclusively in hepatitis B surface antigen carriers in three decades in Taiwan. Report of 51 cases strongly associated with rapid development of liver cirrhosis. J. Hepatol. 5:260-267; 1987.

392. Ishak, K.G.; Glunz, P.R. Hepatoblastoma and hepatocellular carcinoma in infancy and childhood. Report of 47 cases. Cancer 20:396-422; 1967.

393. Kingston, J.E.; Herbert, A.; Draper, G.J.; Mann, J.R. Association between hepatoblastoma and polyposis coli. Arch. Dis. Child 58:959-962; 1983.

394. Lack, E.E.; Neare, C.; Vawter, G.F. Hepatoblastoma: a clinical and pathologic study of 54 cases. Am. J. Surg. Pathol. 6:693-705; 1982.

395. Lack, E.E.; Neave, C.; Vawter, G.F. Hepatocellular carcinoma. Review of 32 cases in childhood and adolescence. Cancer 52:1510-1515; 1983.

396. Li, F.P.; Thurber, W.A.; Seddon, J.; Holmes, G.E. Hepatoblastoma in families with polyposis coli. J. Am. Med. Assoc. 257:2475-2477; 1987.

397. Mahour, G.H.; Wogu, G.U.; Siegel, S.E.; Isaacs, H. Improved survival in infants and children with primary malighant liver tumros. Am. J. Surg. 146:236-240; 1983.

398. Muraji, T.; Woolley, M.M.; Sinatra, F.; Siegel, S.M.; Isaacs, H. The prognostic implication of hypercholesterolemia in infants and children with hepatoblastoma. J. Pediatr. Surg. 20:228-230; 1985.

399. Navarro, C.; Corredeger, J.M.; Sancho, A.; Rovira, J.; Morales, L. Paraneoplastic precocious puberty. Report of a new case with hepatoblastoma and review of the literature. Cancer 56:1725-1729; 1985.

400. Pritchard, J.; daCunha, A.; Cornbleet, M.A.; Carter, C.J. Alpha-fetoprotein (alpha FP) monitoring of response to Adriamycin in hepatoblastoma. J. Pediatr. Surg. 17:429-430; 1982.

401. Quinn, J.J.; Altman, A.J.; Robinson, H.T.; Cooke, R.W.; Hight, D.W.; Foster, J.H. Adriamycin and cisplatin for hepatoblastoma. Cancer 56:1926-1929; 1985.

402. Sun, T.T.; Chu, Y.R.; Ni, Z.Q.; Lu, J.H.; Huang, F.; Ni, Z.P.; Pei, X.F.; Yu, Z.I.; Liu, G.T. A pilot study on universal immunization of newborn infants in an area of hepatitis B virus and primary hepatocellular carcinoma prevalence with a low dose of hepatitis B vaccine. J. Cell. Physiol. (Suppl.) 4:83-90; 1986.

403. Willis, R.A. The pathology of the tumours of children. In: Cameron, R.; Wright, G.P., eds. Pathological monographs. London: Oliver and Boyd, Ltd.; 1962:57-61.

404. Wood, W.J.; Rawlings, M.; Evans, H.; Lim, C.N. Hepatocellular carcinoma: importance of histologic classification as a prognostic factor. Am. J. Surg. 155:663-666; 1988.

405. Young, J.L.; Miller, R.W. Incidence of malignant tumors in U.S. children. J. Pediatr. 86:254-258; 1975.

Steven S. Searl, M.D., Ophthalmology
Henry S. Metz, M.D., Ophthalmology

Louis S. Constine III, M.D., Radiation Oncology
Philip Rubin, M.D., Radiation Oncology

Chapter **20**

TUMORS OF THE EYE

The eye altering alters all.

William Blake (16)

PERSPECTIVE

Although loss of an eye is well worth the long-term survival resulting from eradication of a malignant tumor, with multimodal approaches there is an effort to preserve, if possible, the globe and vision. With modern irradiation techniques, melanomas of the eye have become radiocurable, with preservation of the eye. Similar techniques have been developed and often applied to the remaining eye and retinoblastoma. Soft tissue sarcomas of the head and neck area, particularly of the orbit, respond especially well to chemotherapy and irradiation and preservation of the eye is possible.

There is a large variety of neoplasms of the eye, affecting all age groups. Although this is a highly specialized area of treatment, some of these eye tumors offer a unique insight and a challenge to understanding malignant disease in its broadest sense. It is essential that the student and physician be aware of the common malignancies and their signs. In Table 20-1 (13), the most common tumors of the eye are listed by anatomic site and histology.

Retinoblastoma is a unique tumor. Its fascination relates to hereditary patterns. It is the first human cancer in which the causative gene has been identified. Clinical methods are being developed to detect high-risk offspring and siblings of affected individuals (93,95,98,117,118). Although it is a tumor of childhood, it is not as common as embryonal rhabdomyosarcoma, a mass lesion that can present in the orbit and has proven to be highly curable. Hemangiomas about the eyelids are common at birth and most often require no specific therapy because their natural history is to regress spontaneously.

The most common adult tumors differ from those found most often in children (Table 20-1). Among primary intraocular tumors, melanoma of the choroid is most frequent. However, metastasis, usually from breast or lung, is the most common intraocular malignancy. An orbital mass is usually metastatic from another cancer, or is part of the dissemination process of lymphomas or leukemias. Eyelid neoplasms include the familiar skin cancers, particularly of the basal cell variety, but sebaceous cell cancer, the third most common, is almost unique to eyelids.

The team approach is best to obtain optimal results. The ophthalmologist, ophthalmic echographer, and diagnostic radiologist need to diagnose precisely and localize the tumor, often through noninvasive imaging techniques to avoid losing the eye by direct biopsy of the tumor. With the introduc-tion of computed tomography (CT) and magnetic resonance imaging (MRI), a surgeon and radiation oncologist are more able to plan their treatment techniques (Table 20-2) (14). The desire for eye preservation has led to the development of highly refined radiation therapy techniques, such as precisely shaped megavoltage photon and electron beams, careful immobilization procedures, surgically controlled placement of cobalt discs, and, most recently, high-energy beams with well-defined Bragg peaks. The use of chemotherapy reflects the general developments in tumor response; it is highly effective in pediatric tumors such as rhabdomyosarcoma, it is lesser valuable in treating the common adult tumors.

TUMORS OF THE EYELID AND ADNEXAE (6,12,22): EPIDEMIOLOGY AND ETIOLOGY

Epidemiology

Benign eyelid tumors, such as papillomas, nevi, hemangiomas, and xanthomas, occur with great frequency. Carcinoma (epithelioma) of the eyelids is the most common malignant tumor in ophthalmology. Basal cell carcinomas (BCC) in the eyelids outnumber squamous cell carcinomas (SCC) 40 to one. In the conjunctiva, (SCC) occurs ten times more often than (BCC) (13). The general behavior of both these tumors is similar to that of skin carcinomas of other sizes. They show a predilection for the junction of skin and conjunctiva at the margin of the eyelid. (BCC) is often locally invasive, but does not metastasize. SCCs, like those elsewhere, metastasize.

Pigmented tumors of the lids, and especially of the conjunctiva, are rare. They are often difficult to manage because the onset or degree of malignancy is not always apparent on clinical examination (5). Primary acquired melanosis can be particularly difficult to manage because of its widespread involvement of the conjunctiva and eyelids. Since histopathologic examination of involved tissue can differentiate melanosis from low malignant potential, repeat biopsy of suspicious areas is indicated. In some cases, because of extensive involvement of the ocular surface, surgical excision is impractical. In these cases, controlled cryotherapy of the involved epithelial surfaces is effective in eradicating malignant cells with minimal destruction of ocular tissues (26).

A special type of cancer involving the eyelids or caruncle is sebaceous carcinoma; it is one of the "great masqueraders" and can resemble chronic inflammation or a benign mass

Table 20-1. The Most Common Tumors of the Eye

	ADULTS			CHILDREN		
Site	Tumor Type	Sign	Visual Loss	Tumor Type	Sign	Visual Loss
Lid	Basal cell carcinoma	Scabbing ulcer	None	Hemangioma	Red strawberry mass	Closed eyelid
Conjunctiva	Squamous cell carcinoma	Fleshy lesion	None	Leukemia	Raised, inflected mass	None
Intraocular	Melanoma	Black to brownish elevated area in choroid	Scotoma	Retinoblastoma	White reflex	Blindness
Intraorbital	Lymphoma	Mass, displacement of globe	Diplopia	Embryonal rhabdomyosarcoma	Mass, displacement of globe	Diplopia
Metastatic	Breast (lung)	Raised area in retina	Scotoma	Neuroblastoma	Proptosis, ecchymosis, pain	Diplopia

Adapted from Sagerman (13).

Table 20-2. Imaging Modalities Eye and Orbit

METHOD	DIAGNOSIS AND STAGING CAPABILITY	RECOMMENDED FOR USE
CT	Provides excellent anatomic detail of globe, orbital content and bony orbit. Can distinguish smooth, round cysts from infiltrative tumors vs. pseudotumors and detect bone destruction and sinus invasion.	Yes
Primary tumor ultrasonography and fine needle aspiration biopsy	A scan and B scan can be used to screen intraocular and orbital tumors and cysts, especially melanomas	No
MRI	Provides excellent 3D view, orbital fat hyperintense and vitreous hypointense in tumor (T1) and reverse in T2. Can detect tumors vs. pseudotumors and cysts. May be superior for diagnosis of vascular lesions, demyelinating disease	Yes
Endoscopy	Orbital endoscopy with fiber optic light is used in conjunction with CT and/or MRI for obtaining core biopsy	Yes, when indicated
Standard orbital view	Useful for assessing optic nerve foramen and supraorbital fissure, but supplanted by CT; can detect intraocular calcification	No
Orbital phlebography	Venography particulary useful for detecting orbital varices, but is less efficient and more invasive than CT	No
Carotid angiography	Useful in diagnosis of vascularized tumors and aneurysms, but replaced by CT/MRI	No
Fluourescein angiography	Sometimes used in diagnosis of ocular melanoma	No
Biopsy	Usually an incisional or excisional biopsy is indicated to confirm malignant vs. pseudotumors. Directed stereotactically by CT/MRI. Contraindicated for melanomas due to high risk of seeding	Yes, if indicated

CT = computed tomography; MRI = magnetic resonance imaging.
Adapted from Shields (14).

lesion known as chalazion (33). Pterygium is a common benign condition characterized by abnormal vascularity of the cornea.

Etiology

Etiologic agents for carcinomas of the eyelid and conjunctiva are similar to skin cancer and usually relate to exposure to actinic rays (sun), wind, and weather and other environmental factors. Hemangiomas of the eyelids are mostly found at birth or shortly after (61% at birth and 25% during the first month after birth) (13).

DETECTION AND DIAGNOSIS

Clinical Detection (Table 20-1)

1. Typical presentation is a sore that fails to heal or a persistent warty growth.
2. SCC shows a predilection for the upper eyelid, from

which lymphatics drain into the preauricular nodes. In the conjunctiva, the limbus is the most common site of origin and the lesion is commonly preceded by leukoplakia (13).

3. BCC occurs most frequently in the lower eyelid: 54% in the lower eyelid, 28% in the inner canthus; 13% in the upper eyelid; and 5% in the outer canthus (28).

4. Carcinomas in the region of the medial canthus are common and must be recognized and treated promptly. Invasion of the orbit by tumors in this location tends to occur early.

Diagnostic Procedures

1. External inspection with palpation occasionally is useful. Inspection must include everting the eyelids for examination of the conjunctival surfaces.

2. Evidence of bony invasion can be detected by x-ray.

3. Confirmation by histopathologic study of incisional or excisional biopsy is mandatory.

CLASSIFICATION

Histopathology

1. Tumors of the eyelids:
   - benign lesions: Nevus, papilloma, molluscum contagiosum, xanthelasma, hemangioma, senile keratosis, inverted follicular keratosis, and keratoacanthoma
   - precancerous lesions: Senile keratosis, carcinoma in situ, radiation dermatosis, xeroderma pigmentosum, and melanosis
   - malignant lesions: BCC and SCC, adenoacanthoma, sweat gland and hair follicle carcinomas, sebaceous or Meibomian gland carcinomas, malignant melanoma, and Merkel's tactile cell tumor

2. Conjunctival tumors:
   - benign lesions: Nevus, papilloma, desmoid, dermolipoma, and angioma

   - precancerous lesions: Squamous dysplasia, carcinoma in situ (conjunctival intraepithelial neoplasia), acquired melanosis
   - malignant lesions: SCC, mucoepidermoid carcinoma, melanoma, lymphoma

ANATOMIC STAGING (1)

The staging system is similar to that used for skin cancers (Fig. 20-1).

Staging Work-up

1. Extent of primary is determined by inspection, palpation, and by radiographs, if bone invasion is suspected.

2. Palpation of preauricular area to identify enlarged nodes.

3. Metastatic work-up is required for melanoma, sebaceous cell carcinoma, lymphoma, and Merkel's cell tumor.

PRINCIPLES OF TREATMENT

A multidisciplinary approach is essential for best results. Treatment options for each entity are summarized in Table 20-3.

Surgery

1. Most benign tumors of the lids and conjunctiva are excised easily for cosmetic purposes and there are generally no complications or recurrences. However, large keratoacanthomas, though technically benign, may cause extensive tissue destruction and resultant functional disability, mandating aggressive surgical treatment (18).

2. Cauterization can remove some papillomas involving the lid margins.

3. Biopsy is essential because inspection is some times misleading concerning the benign or malignant nature of a tumor of the eyelid. Most lid lesions receive excisional biopsy. For a large lesion of suspected malignancy,

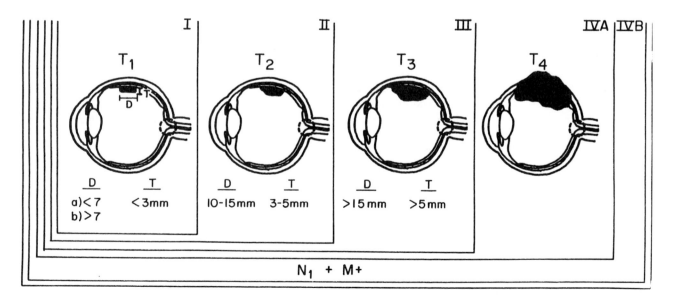

Fig. 20-1. Anatomic staging and classification for choroid melanoma (see Table 20-4). T = tumor; D = diameter; N = node; M = metastasis.

Table 20-3. Treatment Decisions for External Eye and Adnexae Tumors (10,11a,12a)

TUMOR	SURGERY	RADIATION THERAPY	CHEMOTHERAPY
Eyelid basal cell **Small < 0.5 cm**	Excision with no reconstruction	Inner canthus lesion for punctum and nasolacrimal duct preservation	-
Intermediate **>0.5 cm - > 1.0 cm**	Excision or requires reconstruction	CRT to avoid large reconstruction 45-50 Gy, 2.5 Gy fractionated, protect lens	-
Massive	Enucleation with globe and orbital content	CRT if globe and vision can be preserved 55-60 Gy, 2.0 Gy fractionated	-
Conjunctival carcinoma **Squamous cell carcinoma**	Excision if small, with margin control	CRT 50-60 Gy. Protect lens	-
Conjunctival lymphoma	-	CRT 24-36 Gy Lens protection rarely possible	If regional lymph nodes positive or orbit invaded
Conjunctival melanoma **Superficial <0.75 mm**	Excision with margin control	CRT - Special radioisotope applicator 20 Gy to 100-140 Gy	If metastatic, IC II
Massive	Enucleation	-	IC II
Hemangiomas	-	CRT - Observe but if no vision or giant with thrombocytopenia. 50-100 Gy to 2.5-3 Gy	-
Lacrimal gland	Excision	PRT - Postop 60-65 Gy Shield lens	-

RT = radiation therapy; CRT = curative; PRT = palliative; IC II = investigational chemotherapy, phase I/II clinical trials.
PDQ: NR

diagnostic biopsy should precede any major lid reconstruction procedure.

4. Surgery is used for most skin cancers of the eyelids because the ophthalmologist can perform it without great difficulty and with reasonably good cosmetic results.
   a. There are specific limitations to surgery that are indications for primary (definitive) radiation therapy, including a lesion so strategically located that excision would carry significant morbidity (e.g., lesion of the medial canthus where excision may require removal of the lacrimal duct, resulting in a continuous and permanent flow of tears to the patient's cheek).
   b. Patients may also be referred for radiation therapy when there have been one or several postsurgical recurrences, and when pathologic examination determines tumor remains in the resection margins.
5. Wide excision, including the eye and indicated portions of the eyelids and orbital contents, may be required for carcinomas and melanomas of the lid and conjunctiva. Complete exenteration of the orbit may also be indicated.

Radiotherapy

1. Diagnostic biopsy should always precede radiation therapy.
2. Radiation therapy can play an important role in the management of tumors of the eyelid and conjunctiva. The key to success, as with tumors elsewhere in the body, rests on an early diagnosis.

3. *Irradiation techniques:*
   a. There are many techniques to accomplish adequate irradiation for skin cancers in the eyelids. These tumors are usually localized to the free margin of the lower lid or surface of the upper lid with an insignificant incidence of direct extension to deeper or vital structures or to lymph nodes.
   b. At the University of Rochester, the preferred schedule is 4,500 cGy in 3 weeks with 250 cGy fractions, using superficial irradiation (150 kv 1.0 to 3.0 mm Al).
   c. Alternate schedules: Rapid schedules delivering 2,000 cGy in a single exposure are acceptable for small, superficial lesions (i.e., ≤ 1 mm^2) (37). Five thousand cGy in 3 weeks with six equal fractions can be delivered without undue reaction and with good cosmetic results (13). Equally effective for larger tumors are more protracted regimens such as 6,000 cGy in 30 fractions, five fractions per week with more penetrating beams (i.e., 250 kv 1.0 mm^2 Cu or electron beams).
   d. One may treat benign lesions of the cornea, such as recurrent pterygium, with a ß-applicator such as the strontium-90 disc (13,21,38), which comes in various sizes and shapes and performs different functions. The irradiation is confined to the area directly beneath the applicator so that specific corneal shielding is not required.
   e. Irradiation cataractogenesis: Irradiation has the disadvantage of endangering the ocular lens. There-

fore, when indicated, careful shielding is required to prevent cataracts. Normally, cells from the anterior lens epithelium at the pre-equatorial region actively proliferate and progressively migrate and elongate, becoming clear as they pass to the posterior pole of the lens. Irradiation interferes with the orderly progression of these cells, which fail to differentiate and which degenerate, so that debris accumulates. Because the lens has little cell loss, the cell damage from irradiation appears as an opaque zone in the posterior pole (13,19,35). The irradiation-induced cataract may be stationary if the dose is low or administration is protracted. However, it can become progressive and obscure vision if radiation doses greater than 1,200 cGy are delivered to the lens (30,31,34). Lead eyeshields to protect the lens are essential. Tolerance to the cornea is rarely exceeded, since the cornea is fairly radioresistant; however, for conjunctival lesions, this precaution becomes critical. Irradiation delivered in the region of the inner canthus can destroy the epithelium of the lacrimal puncta and canaliculi; this can result in permanent and troublesome epiphora unless careful fractionation schemes are used.

Cryotherapy

Some lid and conjunctival tumors respond well to cryotherapy. Papillomata have been shown to shrink, disappear, and not recur following repeated freeze-thaw cycles (24). Good results have been reported in the treatment of widespread conjunctival melanosis (25).

Special Considerations of Treatment

1. SCC of the conjunctiva: This invasive malignancy represents one end of a continuous spectrum from mild intraepithelial dysplasia, to severe dysplasia, carcinoma in situ, and finally, invasive carcinoma. The vast majority of these lesions can be definitively treated by surgical excision with histopathologic evaluation of margins (32,75). Enucleation and exenteration is seldom necessary except in the case of mucoepidermoid carcinoma, which follows a more aggressively malignant course. Early and accurate histopathologic diagnosis is crucial in this situation (37). Radiation therapy is feasible for larger lesions, with preservation of globe function and vision. Depending on tumor size, 50 to 60 Gy would be used, with 2.0 Gy fractions.

2. Leukemia: Acute leukemic infiltrates of the conjunctiva and orbit are exquisitely radiosensitive. Straight-on radiation fields delivering 100 cGy daily for 5 days of orthovoltage irradiation to an anterior field that includes the entire orbit is usually effective (13).

3. Hemangiomas: Over 90% of these lesions regress — 16% before 6 months of age; 65% between 6 and 12 months; and the remaining 19% between aged 1 and 5 years (9,12). Therefore, it is advisable to do absolutely nothing until later in life, except where deprivation amblyopia is of concern. In a small percentage of cases (7% to 10%), persistence is seen beyond 7 years of age. In such instances, Reese (12) recommends cryotherapy and sclerosing solutions. However, excellent involution can be obtained by small doses of superficial irradiation delivering 50 to 100 cGy per fraction to a total dose of 250 to 500 cGy (13). A direct beam is avoided to decrease the possibility of inducing cataracts.

4. Conjunctival melanomas: These tumors have a course different from melanomas elsewhere in the eye. Prognosis is based on tumor thickness. In most cases of discrete melanoma, (< 0.75 mm in thickness) excision with adequate margins is curative. In conjunctival melanomas greater than 1.5 to 2.0 mm in thickness, prognosis is poor, regardless of treatment modality. Lederman (27) has achieved successful control with preservation of vision in the majority of patients using the strontium-90 applicator (single doses of 2,000 cGy weekly to 10,000 to 14,000 cGy total), radon seeds (Gamma-irradiation in tantalum wire), and/or external orthovoltage irradiation (5,000 to 6,000 cGy in 10 to 14 days).

5. Merkel's cell tumors and sebaceous cell tumors: These more aggressive malignancies must be treated by excision and histologic confirmation of clear margins (33,36).

6. Conjunctival lymphomas are often confined and treatment with irradiation provides excellent local control. Specially designed lens shields can reduce possibility of inducing radiation cataracts (i.e., <10%) and preserve vision. Doses of 24 to 30 Gy in 8 to 16 fractions in 9 to 20 days is highly successful, with no local failures up to 10 years. There is a small incidence of systemic failures, often less than 10%. (22)

RESULTS AND PROGNOSIS

Results for BCC are excellent and similar to those for other skin cancer, that is, 95% cure without recurrences. Large radiation therapy series have shown a control rate of 95% (23,28). Malignant epibulbar melanoma of the eye has been treated successfully by Lederman (27) utilizing local excision and a variety of radiation techniques. The results, 84% (30/37) 3-year survival and more than 50% 5-year survival, attest to the effectiveness of this approach.

INTRAOCULAR TUMORS (6,12)

Benign intraocular tumors occur relatively infrequently. There are several types.

A nevus of the uveal tract may occur in the iris, ciliary body, or choroid. It can be recognized by its clinical appearance and course. The principle concern about a nevus of the eye is that it be distinguished from a melanoma. This usually is possible because of its unchanging size, the absence of much elevation, and the fact that it interferes little with the function of the overlying retina when it occurs in the choroid. However, differentiation of a large nevus from a small, dormant melanoma can be virtually impossible. In this case, routine, continued observation is mandatory.

Hemangiomas of the uveal tract can be more troublesome and can show some signs of growth over a period of many years. It is usually possible to identify these tumors by use of intravenous fluorescein combined with examination of the fundus with cobalt blue light. Under these circumstances, hemangiomas fluoresce brightly.

An angioma of the retina is a rare, benign, intraocular tumor that may be associated with angiomatous malformations in other organs, especially the brain. This association comprises the Von Hippel-Lindau disease. Although it is benign as a tumor, an untreated retinal angioma can destroy the eye. Transscleral cryopexy can result in complete destruction and scarring of the hemangioma and prevent secondary, effusive retinal detachment.

The lesions of tuberous sclerosis and neurofibromatosis occasionally are seen in the fundus of the eye. Neurilemoma in the ciliary body and astrocytoma of the retina rarely occur.

Choroidal osteoma may resemble a metastatic tumor or an amelanotic melanoma. Ultrasound and CT scanning are the two most useful diagnostic tests in identifying this benign tumor. The heavy density of the osteoma's bony matrix helps confirm the diagnosis (41).

Metastatic tumor to the eye is the most common form of intraocular tumor. The diagnosis may be difficult preoperatively or prior to autopsy, especially if no primary site of malignancy has been identified. The most common primary sites are breast, lung, kidney, and the gastrointestinal tract (89).

There are two principal malignant intraocular tumors: melanoma of the uveal tract and retinoblastoma. Each of these tumors is of special interest and of great importance. A vast amount of information has been accumulated on both.

MELANOMA OF THE CHOROID: EPIDEMIOLOGY AND ETIOLOGY

Epidemiology

1. Intraocular malignant melanoma is estimated to occur in about 0.05% of the eye-patient population. It is a tumor of adults; the average age is 50 years. It is rare in blacks (7).
2. Intraocular melanoma is the most common primary intraocular malignancy in Caucasian countries with mainly white populations. Metastatic disease is the most common intraocular malignancy. In Africa and Asia, retinoblastoma is the most common primary intraocular malignancy.
3. There is no difference in distribution between the sexes; nor is there any significant genetic relation except for the tumor's predilection for whites. It is rarely associated with other melanomas, such as those of the skin. Conversely, cutaneous malignant melanomas do not commonly metastasize to the eye; however, ten such cases were collected by Font *et al.* (55).

Etiology

The derivation of melanomas of the uvea has been the subject of a great deal of study and theory. It is possible that the stromal melanocytes of the uvea are the precursors of malignant melanoma. The pigment epithelium of the retina, or of other neural-crest-derived cells, is also implicated by some observers. Another hypothesis is that most melanomas arise in pre-existing nevi.

DETECTION AND DIAGNOSIS

Clinical Detection (Table 20-1)

Typical presentation depends on ophthalmoscopic examination. However, the term intraocular melanoma may refer to a tumor appearing in any part of the uveal tract; this may include the iris, in which case the tumor may be visible on direct inspection. Iris melanomas may be diffuse rather than discrete nodules, presenting as heterochromia, or darkening of the iris. Acquired heterochromia in the presence of increased intraocular pressure is particularly piceious (49).

When it occurs in the choroid, the tumor most characteristically appears in an equatorial position within the eye. It is possible for the tumor to reach a relatively large size before it produces symptoms, such as loss of side vision or a sensation of floating spots. Therefore, the investigation of minor visual symptoms may be important. Tumor growth produces deterioration of vision as the retina overlying the tumor loses its function. The tumor frequently produces secondary changes within the eye, such as the induction of cataract, secondary glaucoma, iridocyclitis, and retinal detachment.

Of 626 melanomas reported by Reese (12,76), 78% occurred in the choroid, 12% in the iris, and 10% in the ciliary body. The most common patterns of spread are intraocular via the choroid and through the sclera extraocularly into the orbit (13). Distant metastatic spread is blood borne and can involve any organ, most commonly the liver. Lymphatic spread can occur, but is less common (13).

Diagnostic Procedures

Since biopsy is not acceptable, it is essential to rely on noninvasive imaging studies to establish the diagnosis (Table 20-2).

1. Diagnostic procedures principally consist of ophthalmoscopic examination. The tumor can be recognized with a high degree of clinical accuracy, although there are a few conditions that sometimes make differential diagnosis difficult.
2. CT and magnetic resonance imagery (MRI) scans, are the most accurate means of tumor delineation for orbital tumors (45,47,65).
3. Fluorescein angiography sometimes is useful in the diagnosis of intraocular melanoma (72).
4. Radioactive uptake study with radioactive phosphorus-32 has been claimed to be useful in distinguishing benign from malignant tumors. Phosphorus-32 is concentrated in rapidly growing tumor cells during DNA replication. Currently, with the accuracy of ultrasonography, CT scanning, and MRI scanning, phosphorus-32 uptake studies are seldom used.
5. Ultrasonic A or B scan can be significant diagnostically in the study of intraocular melanoma, especially when visualization is not possible. Ultrasound is particularly helpful in measuring tumor height.
6. X-ray examination is of little value except in advanced lesions with bone destruction.
7. Biopsy of melanomas of the choroid is not acceptable because of a high incidence of consequent orbital spread. Melanomas of the iris, and less often, of the anterior portions of the ciliary body can sometimes be excised and the eye preserved.

The former accuracy of clinical diagnosis was only fair; false-positives occurred in 10% to 20% of cases (12). Ferry (55) studied 744 cases of enucleated eyes with a diagnosis of probable malignant melanoma. He observed that this diagnosis was mistaken in 100 of 744 instances. Hemorrhage, retinal detachment, retinal cysts, parasites, other tumors, and inflammatory conditions were responsible for the mistakes in clinical diagnosis. Since the use of diagnostic ultrasound has become widespread, there has been a significant improvement in diagnostic accuracy. In a classic study, unsuspected melanomas were found in 4% of eyes with opaque media submitted to ophthalmic pathology laboratories. The use of ophthalmic diagnostic ultrasound and CT scanning has greatly reduced the number of unsuspected melanomas, but cases are still occasionally missed, particularly in eyes undergoing phthisis bulbi or histologic disorganization of the eye. As a general rule, blind eyes with opaque media in whites should be examined by ophthalmic diagnostic ultrasound, particularly if pain or bleeding in otherwise quiet eyes occurs.

CLASSIFICATION

Histopathology

1. *Callender's classification:*
   a. Small, spindle-shaped cells with small condensed nuclei, referred to as spindle A are the most benign type. The 5-year mortality rate is less than 5% (7).
   b. The spindle B type of melanoma is characterized by larger, more loosely packed spindle cells with prominent nucleoli. It is also relatively benign and has a 14% 5-year mortality rate (7).
   c. The pure epithelioid cell type occurs least frequently. This type is large and polygonal and has round nuclei, prominent cytoplasm, and resembles epithelial tumors. The mortality rate is 69% (7).
2. Half of the melanomas of the eye have a mixture of cell types. The dangerous epithelioid cell types exhibit a 51% 5-year mortality rate (7).
3. Necrosis is rare in melanomas and occurs in only 7% of tumors (7). When it occurs, it may create severe inflammatory signs and secondary glaucoma.
4. Pigmentation of the tumor varies from intense to amelanotic. The degree of pigmentation correlates only slightly with the degree of malignancy. Reticulin fibers are frequent and heavy in some tumors, and light in others. Reticulin content is only slightly correlated with prognosis.
5. Newer prognostic parameters include number of mitotic figures per high-power field, and inverse standard deviation of tumor cell nucleolar area (78).

Anatomic Staging

The classification is the same as that published in the previous editions of the American Joint Committee (AJC) and International Union Against Cancer (UICC) and is detailed in Table 20-4 (8) and Fig 20-1.

Staging Work-up

The most important goal is to exclude metastases. In melanoma, the most frequent target is the liver (52).

PRINCIPLES OF TREATMENT

Different approaches to the treatment of ocular melanomas are summarized in Table 20-5 (145).

Surgery

1. Treatment of intraocular melanoma consists of removal of the affected eye. An exception is melanoma of the iris. This can be excised from the eye if observation indicates that it is growing. In the unusual instance when extraocular extension into the orbit has occurred, exenteration of the orbit can be performed. However, the value of the procedure is questionable in melanoma because distant metastases are almost certain by this time.
2. It has been suggested that enucleation may have an adverse rather than a beneficial effect for many patients with respect to the development of metastatic disease (81). The mortality rate before enucleation is low (1% per year) (81). Mortality rises abruptly after enucleation. Some investigators feel that approximately two thirds of fatalities could be attributed to the dissemination of tumor emboli at the time of enucleation (81). Others disagree (69), feeling that the fatalities seen within 2 years after enucleation are only exceptionally secondary to dissemination of tumor cells, as the growth rate of uveal melanomas is generally very slow and tends to be non-metastatic.
3. A "no-touch" technique has been described to prevent tumor spread from occurring secondary to ocular manipulation during enucleation (57).

Table 20-4. TNM Classification and Stage Grouping for Choroid Melanoma

	TNM Classification		Stage Grouping			
T1		≤ 10 mm greatest dimension, ≤ 3mm elevation	Stage IA	T1a	N0	M0
	T1A	≤ 7 mm greatest dimension, ≤ 2mm elevation	Stage IB	T1b	N0	M0
	T1B	> 7 to 10 mm greatest dimension, > 2 to 3 mm elevation	Stage II	T2	N0	M0
T2		> 10 to 15 mm greatest dimension, > 3 to 5 mm elevation	Stage III	T3	N0	M0
T3		> 15 mm greatest dimension or > 5 mm elevation	Stage IVA	T4	N0	M0
T4		Extraocular extension	Stage IVB	Any T	N1	M0
				Any T	Any N	M1
		All sites				
N 1		Regional				

T = tumor; N = node; M = metastases.
From UICC (8).

Table 20-5. Treatment Decisions for Intraocular and Orbital Tumors (10,11a,12a)

TUMOR	SURGERY	RADIATION THERAPY	CHEMOTHERAPY
Intraocular			
Choroid melanoma	Resection of tumor or more often enucleation of globe	CRT - Proton beam (70 Gy) Helium ion beam Co^{60} or I^{125} plaques 30-50 Gy minimum dose, 150-200 Gy maximum dose	For metastatic disease IC II (see Chapter 33)
Retinoblastoma	Enucleation, especially if vision cannot be preserved and unilateral	CRT - For eye preservation especially with bilateral and contralateral tumors. 35-50 Gy (4-6 MV) photons or electrons	IC II of extraocular extension or if metastases ITMTX + CSF
Orbital			
Embroyonal rhabdomyosarcoma	Tumor excision with eye preservation	CRT - Radioresponsive 40-50 Gy, with dose fractionation for eye preservation	RCT: VACA*
Histiocytosis-X	Tumor excision	CRT - Radiosensitive 10 Gy (5-20 Gy)	MAC (see Chapter 19)
Lymphoma		CRT - Radiosensitive 20-40 Gy	MAC:CHOP (see Chapter 18)
Metastatic neuroblastoma		PRT - Radiosensitive 30 Gy	MAC (see Chapter 19)
Adult lung or breast		PRT - Radiosensitive 30-50 Gy	MAC (see Chapter 33)

RT = radiation therapy; CRT = curative; PRT = palliative; MAC = multiagent chemotherapy; RCT = recommended chemotherapy; IC II = investigational chemotherapy, phase I clinical trials; ITMTX = intrathecal methotrexate; CSF = cerebral spinal fluid.

PDQ: RCT - *VACA = vincristine, doxorubicin, cytoxin; CHOP = cyclophosphamide, doxorubicin, vincristine, prednisone.

4. Isolated melanomas of the anterior chamber angle and ciliary body may be treated with iridocyclectomy (56).
5. Full-thickness eye wall resections have also been attempted by Peyman and Raichand (74), but this approach presently must be considered experimental.
6. Pre-enucleation radiation may improve survival (43).

Radiation Therapy (Fig. 20-2)

Melanomas are generally radioresistant, but high tumor doses can be focally and precisely delivered to eradicate small tumors. Radiation therapy can be considered for a tumor in the patient's remaining eye. Some refined techniques have been developed to spare the lens of the eye and deliver the high doses required to obliterate these tumors (63). However, some investigators feel radiation therapy is not appropriate treatment for uveal melanomas (54,66).

1. Proton beam: Uveal melanomas are highly curable by proton beam irradiation. This method avoids cataract production, saving the eye and its vision. Results are as high as 90% tumor control (58,59,77).
2. A cobalt-60 disc (113) technique makes it possible to deliver 3,000 to 4,000 cGy minimum and 15,000 to 20,000 cGy maximum to the tumor base (7). If external irradiation is contemplated, large daily doses of 500 to 600 cGy to a tolerable maximum have been yielding better results than conventional fractionation schemes (Fig. 20-2). This treatment may produce significant morbidity. Rapid regression suggests a poor prognosis (116).
3. Radon seeds: Some arrests of tumor growth are reported with radon seeds sewn temporarily to the sclera (97). This procedure is no longer recommended.
4. Iodine-125 or ruthenium Ru-106 plaques: Irradiation of choroidal melanomas with iodine-125 ophthalmic

plaques has been performed. Tumors were found to be sterilized; the eyes suffered less irradiation damage than did eyes treated with cobalt-60 (73,74).
5. Helium ions: Helium ion-charged particle therapy allows uniform dosage to be delivered to the entire tumor. There was no evidence of postirradiation enlargement, and no metastases or tumor-related deaths in one series (48). The incidence of radiation retinopathy may be reduced.

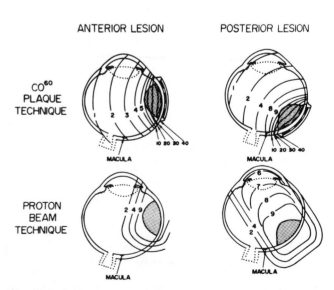

Fig. 20-2. Comparison of proton beam and cobalt-60 irradiation techniques for anterior Isodose curves are drawn, labeled with doses of thousands of cGy (cobalt cGy equivalents for protons). From Gragoudas et al. (60). Published courtesy of Ophthalmology (1980; 87:571-81).

Chemotherapy

Treatment with chemotherapy alone is not yet significant. In widespread metastatic disease — metastatic melanomas of the skin — cytotoxic agents are used (68).

Photocoagulation

Photocoagulation of small melanomas is under investigation and may become a generally accepted treatment modality for small, favorably located accessible tumors.

Cryotherapy

Some melanomas may be destroyed by transscleral cryopexy (40). This technique may be better for small tumors.

Thermal/Ultrasound

Early work has been reported on the histopathologic effects of ultrasonically induced hyperthermia in uveal melanomas. It is speculated that this technique may enhance the effect of radiotherapy (50).

RESULTS AND PROGNOSIS

1. Local control for uveal melanomas is excellent, either with enucleation or radiation therapy. Surgery means loss of the eye. Eye preservation is possible by proton beam therapy; in 1,006 cases Munzenrider et al. (71) reported a 2.3% failure and 96.3% local control (Fig. 20-3a) (71). Lindstadt et al. (62) used helium ion beam in 307 patients to achieve a 96.8% local control rate with 81% survival and 83% eye retention. Approximately two thirds of patients have useful vision (62) (Fig. 20-3b).

2. The size of a melanoma of the choroid has bearing on the prognosis; large tumors are associated with higher mortality. The results of surgical treatment, that is, removal of the eye with a melanoma, are good if the tumor is small and has not exhibited extraocular extension. The ability to eradicate tumor varies with size (Fig. 20-3a) is also related to vision preservation (Fig. 20-3b) (62,71).

3. Anatomic extensions along the ciliary vessels and the nerves penetrating the sclera or extraocular extension under the conjunctiva make the prognosis worse. Distant metastases are frequent if extraocular extension is present, or if the eye harbors a relatively large tumor.

4. Histopathology: There are a variety of histopathologic types with spindle cell A and B and fascicular types (i.e., >70% survival) having favorable prognosis in contrast to the necrotic, mixed and especially epithelioid types, particularly the latter, which is highly metastatic (Table 20-6) (145).

5. Melanomas of the iris and anterior portions of the ciliary body are equally radiosensitive melanomas of the choroid. Such tumors are being excised in increasing numbers, successfully preserving both life and vision. Decker et al. (51) found, despite a 5-year local control rate of 98% for ciliary body melanomas, there was only a 59% 5-year disease-specific survival with a higher degree of salvage enucleation (26%) than with uveal tumors.

6. The time lapse between surgical removal of the diseased eye and appearance of symptomatic metastases is not as significant as with many other tumors. The incidence rate of symptomatic metastases 5 to 10 years after enucleation is only a little higher than in the 10- to 15-year period (see Fig. 20-4 [46] or a comparison of survival between cobalt-60 treatment and enucleation). Evidently metastases may lie dormant for many years. What may excite the growth of temporarily stationary metastases is unknown.

7. The age of the patient affects the prognosis; it is worse for elderly adults.

8. The reported incidence of primary malignant melanoma of the skin metastatic to the eye has been relatively low (80).

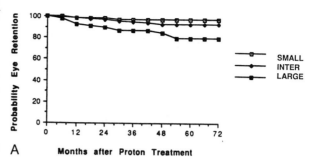

Eye Retention in 1006 Patients

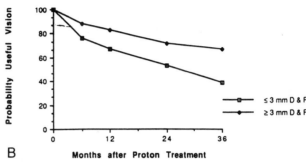

Useful Vision in Eyes 20/200 or Better

Fig. 20-3. (A) Kaplan-Meier plot of eye retention probability after proton therapy in 1,006 patients with small (<3 mm height and <10 mm diameter), intermediate (3.1 to 8 mm height and/or 10.1 to 16 mm diameter), and large (>8 mm height and >16 mm diameter) uveal melanomas; (B) Kaplan-Meier plot of the probability of retaining useful vision in patients with tumors, 3 mm from the optic disc (D) and fovea (F) and >3 mm from the optic disc and/or fovea in 562 eyes with initial visual acuity 20/200 (6/60) or better. From Munzenrider (69), with permission.

CLINICAL INVESTIGATIONS

The National Eye Institute is currently conducting a Collaborative Ocular Melanoma study investigating the role of radiation therapy in the treatment of ocular melanoma (79). To date, many individual studies, using a variety of radiotherapeutic techniques, suggest that radiotherapy offers little advantage over enucleation in terms of mortality, but does provide preservation of vision for a variable length of time (41,42,44,60,61,63,64,67).

Table 20-6. Results of Enucleation of CHOROID MELANOMA

	5-Year		10-Year	
	Number of Patients	Survival (%)	Number of Patients	Survival (%)
Spindle A	63	89	31	81
Spindle B	337	77	159	64
Fascicular	52	71	25	56
Necrotic	83	46	48	29
Mixed	502	37	320	22
Epithelioid	27	33	15	0
Total	1,064	55	598	38

From Wilder and Paul (145), with permission.

RETINOBLASTOMA: EPIDEMIOLOGY AND ETIOLOGY

Epidemiology

1. Retinoblastoma occurs in approximately one of 20,000 live births (12). This makes it about as common as hemophilia (94).
2. There is no known difference in the incidence between whites and blacks, males and females, or in children in various parts of the world (99).
3. Thirty percent of retinoblastomas are bilateral and all bilateral tumors are germinal. Forty percent of all retinoblastomas are germinal (i.e., 25% of all unilateral tumors are germinal). In these cases there is a 100% chance of an autosomal dominant pattern of hereditary transmission to the next generation as well as a lifelong significant risk of development of a second nonocular malignancy (85).
4. More than 90% of retinoblastoma cases are diagnosed before aged 5 years. The median age of diagnosis is 14 months for bilateral cases and 23 months for unilateral tumors.

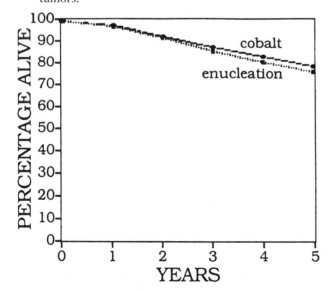

Fig. 20-4. Statistically adjusted comparison of survival in patients with uveal melanoma treated with cobalt-60 plaque therapy and with enucleation. From Brady *et al.* (46), with permission.

5. There is a 5% association with other congenital defects of which mental retardation is the most common (102). In the syndrome designated Dq-, one half of the patients have retinoblastoma, as well as a high incidence of other defects including psychomotor retardation, skeletal abnormalities, congenital heart disease, and other eye defects (112,115,138).
6. Spontaneous regression occurs in 1% of all retinoblastoma patients (106). This has been attributed to the tumor's outgrowing its vascular supply and becoming necrotic, thus releasing toxic products that ultimately may eliminate the lesion (12).

Etiology

Retinoblastoma has been documented to result from a genetic mutation (Fig. 20-5) (95).

1. Retinoblastoma behaves like an autosomal dominant syndrome with higher than 90% penetrance (12), but the abnormal tumor-producing mutant allele is recessive.
2. Seventy percent of retinoblastomas present as unilateral tumors. In all the bilateral and in 25% of the unilateral presentations, a germinal mutation affecting all cells in the body has occurred (99).
3. Despite the high occurrence rate of germinal mutations (40% of cases), only 12% of patients have a positive family history; the other 88% representing the first germinal mutation in the family (83).
4. Retinoblastoma conforms to the two-hit Knudson's hypothesis (104) in which two chromosomal mutational events are necessary to cause cancer. In the hereditary form, the mutational event affects a germ cell and thus all cells in the body, whereas in nongerminal cell cases, a single retinal cell is affected.
5. The normal allele at the retinoblastoma locus is currently thought to act as a controller gene or suppressor of the malignant retinoblastoma growth (95). Thus, both alleles must be lost before malignant growth can ensue. In the hereditary cases, all cells have lost one normal allele, and the chance of several retinal cells losing the second allele is quite high, resulting in bilateral or multicentric tumor growth at an earlier age (14 months). In the nonhereditary or somatic form, one retinal cell has lost one allele and must lose the second

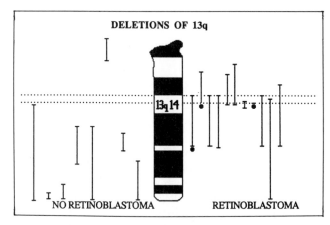

DELETIONS OF 13q

NO RETINOBLASTOMA   RETINOBLASTOMA

Fig. 20-5. Schematic representation of chromosome 13 showing reported deletions with and without associated retinoblastoma. The dotted band represents the Q14 band of the chromosome. On the left of the chromosome are shown reported deletions that do not include the Q14 band. These deletions do not cause retinoblastoma. To the right are shown reported deletions that do include all or part of the Q14 band, and that result in retinoblastoma. For more specific information on the reports of deletions, see Weichselbaum *et al.* (118).

before a unicentric, unilateral tumor arises, usually at a later age (23 months). Thus, in nongerminal cases, the chance of bilateral mutations (two hits) on two separate retinal cells is low, and the chance that a bilateral tumor would be nongerminal or somata is equally low (101).

6. Since 50% of offspring of germinal retinoblastoma patients will be affected, prenatal or presymptomatic diagnosis is crucial (5). A few laboratories have developed diagnostic tests to identify the retinoblastoma gene in this group of patients. Detection of the gene in the 15% of patients with unilateral disease that have the germinal mutation is also important because they carry a lifelong risk of secondary malignancies (92,95,98,101).

7. Healthy parents who have a single affected child can expect an attack rate of 6% among their other offspring (12).

8. An unaffected sibling of a child with sporadic retinoblastoma, like one of his parents, may be a carrier; the risk is extremely low (< 1%) (103).

9. If retinoblastoma occurs more than once in a given pedigree, there is a 40% to 48% chance that the affected members of this pedigree will have offspring with retinoblastoma. The unaffected members have a chance of only 5% to 20% (108).

DETECTION AND DIAGNOSIS:

Clinical Detection (Table 20-1)

1. Typical presentation usually occurs when the tumor fills the eye to the point that the pupil is whitened by the underlying tumor, or when a secondary strabismus, an inflammatory reaction, or secondary glaucoma produces signs and symptoms (12,90).

2. The differential diagnosis of retinoblastoma includes Coat's disease, nematode endophthalmitis, persistent hyperplastic primary vitreous, retrolental fibroplasia, uveal coloboma, retinal dysplasia, and congenital or early-onset cataract.

3. Early detection for high-risk individuals, such as those with a history of familial retinoblastoma, indicates repeated funduscopic studies in infancy and in childhood.

DIAGNOSTIC PROCEDURES (TABLE 20-2)

1. Examination by external inspection, ophthalmoscopy, slit-lamp microscopy, and transillumination is necessary. Since the tumor is bilateral in 30% of cases, detailed examination of the second eye is essential. This usually must be done under general anesthesia with a widely dilated pupil using direct and indirect ophthalmoscopy with depression of the anterior sclera to bring all parts of the vitreous cavity into the range of view of the ophthalmoscope.

2. Echograms with ultrasonic devices have been investigated to delineate the tumor, especially when the view of the tumor may be clouded by cataract, intraocular hemorrhage, calcification, etc.

3. CT scans are accurate in delineating the tumor and its extensions. CT is sensitive in detecting calcifications and can show nerve involvement and intracranial extension in advanced lesions (82).

4. MRI can show retinoblastomas as an intense signal, and with gadolinium, can show optic nerve and intracranial extensions more accurately than can CT. Coronal and sagittal reconstructions are helpful for treatment planning.

5. Radioactive uptake study with radioactive phosphorous has been claimed to be useful in distinguishing benign from malignant tumors. However, this technique is confined to adults because it involves an exposure to an amount of irradiation that is considered hazardous to children.

6. Biopsy of intraocular tumors is not practical and has led to dangerous spread and orbital involvement.

7. Elevated aqueous tumor levels of the enzyme lactic dehydrogenase may be a helpful indicator of an eye that harbors a retinoblastoma (84). This test is more accurate when the sample is fresh, not frozen, and free of blood cells.

CLASSIFICATION

Histopathology

1. Retinoblastoma usually arises from the posterior portion of the retina and consists of small, closely packed, round or polygonal cells with dark staining nucleus and scanty cytoplasm. In many cases, the tumor cells are arranged in rosettes, but their absence does not necessarily exclude this diagnosis (7).

2. Histopathologic classification of retinoblastoma permits a certain amount of separation between more differentiated and less differentiated tumor varieties. The more differentiated tumors show small rosettes that are thought to represent differentiated spongioblasts (neuroepitheliomas).

3. The tumor often outgrows its blood supply. Areas of necrosis are common and are responsible for the formation of calcium deposits. Rarely, the tumor may become so necrotic as to destroy itself entirely, giving rise to the rare instance of spontaneous regression. The necrotizing tendency of the tumor is one of the factors responsible

for the occasional intense ocular inflammation that may be highly misleading clinically.

4. The tumor spreads readily within the eye. It can seed itself throughout the interior of the eye and include the iris and anterior chamber. Distant spread of retinoblastoma commonly occurs along the optic nerve. Here the tumor can spread readily along the meningeal spaces of the optic sheath and soon reach the cranial cavity. Distant spread can also occur through the blood stream, most commonly to bone, lungs, and liver.

5. The causes of death in this tumor are interesting. More than 90% of the patients have intracranial involvement; in almost 50% of all deaths, disease is confined to the head and spinal cord; the remaining half have distant metastases. Distant metastasis occurs with equal incidence (≈ 50%) of spread to lymph nodes, skull bones, distant bones, and viscera (105).

6. Trilateral retinoblastoma occurs when both eyes are involved and pineoblastoma occurs in the pineal gland. This rare but interesting combination illustrates that the pineal or third eye shares the same developmental anlage as the retina. This diagnosis must be considered in a patient with bilateral retinoblastoma who subsequently develops headache or lethargy (107).

ANATOMIC STAGING

There are a number of different classification and staging schemas (Table 20-7 [1,82] and Fig. 20-6).

The AJC/UICC categories are made equivalent to the Reese and St. Jude systems that are more widely used.

Staging Work-up

It is most important to exclude metastases, the most common site being the central nervous system. The recommended work-up includes (46):

- CT scan for detailing potential involvement of eye bilaterality and extensions into orbit, optic nerve, and base of the brain.
- MRI scanning (6,11).
- Lumbar puncture for colony tumor cells seeding the colony stimulation factor.

- For patients with advanced disease, a radioisotopic oncologic survey including brain, bone, and liver.
- Complete blood cell count and sequential multiple analysis.

PRINCIPLES OF TREATMENT

A multidisciplinary decision is essential for best outcome and survival as illustrated in Table 20-5.

Surgery

The treatment of retinoblastoma is usually removal of the affected eye. Because biopsy is associated with an unacceptable risk, accurate clinical diagnosis is essential. When the tumor grows in an endophytic fashion into the vitreous cavity, direct observation with indirect ophthalmoscopy is possible with high diagnostic accuracy. However, when tumor growth is exophytic into the subretinal space, alternative imaging techniques such as echography, CT or MRI scanning must be used to make the correct diagnosis.

In the surgical removal of the eye, it is important that as much of the optic nerve as possible, 10 to 15 mm, be removed along with the eye. The cut end of the nerve must be examined histopathologically.

Photocoagulation

Photocoagulation of retinoblastoma, is rarely undertaken, but is generally not indicated and may increase the likelihood of extraocular extension or metastasis.

Radiotherapy

1. Unilateral tumor: Experience is being accumulated in radiation treatment of small, unilateral tumors, such as might be found in genetically determined high-risk patients. The response to radiation therapy can be monitored by observation with the ophthalmoscope (89).

2. Residual tumor: If tumor is present at the cut end of the optic nerve, elective radiation therapy to the intracranial portion of the optic nerve, including the chiasm, is recommended. Spread to the meningeal spaces can be evaluated by spinal fluid cytology (89).

Table 20-7.   STAGING: TNM Classification Summary for Retinoblastoma

Reese	AJC			St. Jude
Group I	T1/pT1	≤ 25% of retina		IA
Group II	T2/pT2	> 25% to 50% of retina		IB
	T3/pT3	> 50% of retina and/or intraocular beyond retina		IC
Group III	T3a/pT3a	> 50% of retina and/or cells in vitreous		IIA > IID
	T3b	Optic disc	pT3b	Optic nerve up to lamina cribrosa	IIB
Group IV				
	T3c	Anterior chamber and/or uvea	pT3c	Anterior chamber and/or uvea and/or intrascleral	IIC
Group V	T4/pT4	Extraocular		III
	T4a	Optic nerve	pT4a	Beyond lamina cribrosa not at resection line	IIIA
					> C
					IIIB
	T4b	Other extraocular	pT4b	Other extraocular and/or at resection line	
	N1/pN1	Regional		IIID
	M1	Distant metastases		IV

T = tumor; N = node; M = metastasis.
Adapted from AJC/UICC (1,8).

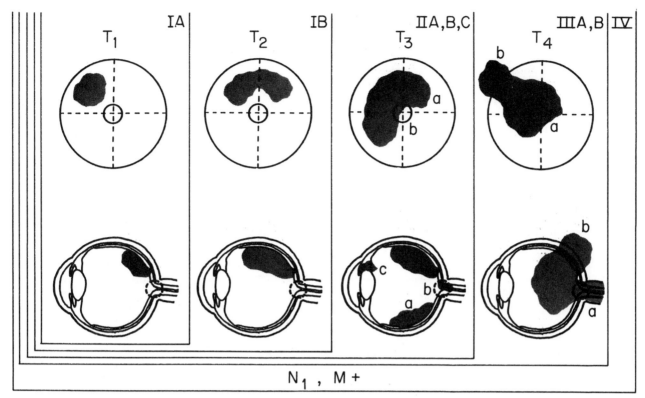

Fig. 20-6. Anatomic staging for retinoblastoma (see Table 20-7). T = tumor; N = node; M = metastasis.

3. Bilateral or contralateral involvement: If the affected eye has been removed and tumor is found in a small or localized area in the second eye, it can be eradicated by carefully directed irradiation combined with chemotherapy. The tumor can be observed directly with the ophthalmoscope; thus, the results of treatment can be closely monitored. If treatment is obviously not succeeding, the eye can be removed without unreasonably endangering the patient by the delay.

4. Techniques (88, 89, 90,91, 97,100, 102, 108, 113, 114, 116, 119)
   a. Retinoblastoma is sensitive to relatively moderate doses of irradiation, which the normal retina can withstand. A few retinoblastomas may be well differentiated and thus somewhat more radioresistant. Because of the multifocal behavior of this neoplasm, the entire retina is at risk (100,116).
   b. The usual technique of irradiation is to deliver 3,500 to 4,500 cGy by either high energy electrons (4 to 6 MeV) or megavoltage irradiation. Lateral (temporal) portals are preferred and the time of delivery is from 3.5 to 4.5 weeks. Recently, Weiss *et al.* (116) have found that use of a single lateral field results in multiple recurrences in the anterior portion of the retina; and therefore, they have added an anterior port (with lens protection) to the conventional temporal field.
   c. Stallard (113) has developed a technique using radioactive cobalt discs sewn to the globe localized over small tumors (group 1); these replace radon seeds (97). The minimum dose is 3,500 cGy in 7 days at the apex of the treated volume and 19,000 cGy at its base. Results in Stallard's series are outstanding (91% for

small tumors) and similar to those from external-beam therapy (84%) (113).
   d. Delivery of radiation therapy for retinoblastoma should be precise. The patient can be sedated but an immobilizing cast is preferred because treatment lasts usually 1 month. The eye lens is quite sensitive to radiation damage and despite many attempts at shielding with precise direction of x- rays, a radiation cataract is often the price of cure of the tumor. Such a cataract can be successfully removed.
   e. In infants, an important complication of radiation treatment in the ocular area is the growth-retarding effect of irradiation on the bones of the orbital region. This can produce considerable facial asymmetry if the patient is under 2 years of age at treatment time. Radiation therapy for retinoblastoma also has been responsible for the late appearance of orbital osteogenic sarcoma and rhabdomyosarcoma. This risk is much reduced by smaller, but still adequate, treatment dosage.

Chemotherapy

1. Treatment with chemotherapy alone is not yet significant. In recent years, the use of chemotherapy in metastatic retinoblastoma has revealed the effectiveness of certain drugs, among which are nitrogen mustard, triethylenemelamine (TEM), actinomycin D, 5-FU, cyclophosphamide, vincristine, and doxorubicin. Uracil mustard, melphalan, and hydroxyurea are ineffective (12).
2. In the past, cytotoxic agents were given for this disease by intra-arterial infusion into the carotid arteries. The procedure is difficult and risky and, at present, reserved for drastic circumstances.

3. Combination chemotherapy (i.e., vincristine/cyclophosphamide/intrathecal methotrexate; or vincristine/cyclophosphamide/doxorubicin) is being used for the treatment of extraocular extension of the tumor with widespread metastatic disease (12). The St. Jude Children's Research Hospital uses combination chemotherapy as an adjuvant to irradiation and surgery (109). The combination of TEM (12) or cyclophosphamide (111), with irradiation has also been used.

Cryotherapy

Encouraging results have been reported with cryotherapy (96). The applications can be controlled ophthalmoscopically. The technique is ideal for lesions anterior to the equator. Bruch's membrane as well as the internal limiting membrane of the retina are preserved with no specific complications. Very large lesions — greater than 7 disc diameters (87) — are not destroyed by cryotherapy.

RESULTS AND PROGNOSIS

1. Prognosis and results of treatment for vision and for survival depend heavily on the stage at which the tumor is first observed. Untreated, retinoblastoma is almost invariably fatal. With treatment, the mortality rate is about 20%, but is highly dependent on the size and location of the tumor when treatment is started (12). The tumor can be extensive in one eye before the patient exhibits any signs or seeks examination. This is mainly responsible for the 20% mortality rate associated with the tumor (12).
2. Occasionally one has to decide between risking the patient's life by retaining the second eye harboring tumor and treating it with nonsurgical alternatives, or removing the second eye and thereby protecting life at the expense of vision.
3. Approximately 50% (12) of all retinoblastomas subjected to radiation therapy are controlled. (Table 20-8). Radiation failures can be reirradiated or the eyes can be enucleated as salvage procedures (114). Long-term survivors of irradiation have a 1.5% chance of developing second primaries; the most common is osteosarcoma. Nonradiogenic neoplasms also have been reported (102).
4. There is a high incidence of multiple retinal tumors in patients with retinoblastoma. These other tumors may

be treated with light photocoagulation and/or cryotherapy in an attempt to maintain vision (110).
5. The prognosis for patients with metastatic retinoblastoma is poor.

CLINICAL INVESTIGATIONS

Research on retinoblastoma has recently shifted and currently stands at the frontier of understanding genetic influences in human malignancy. Current studies are directed towards earlier detection of the germinal carrier in retroblastoma and development of techniques to further explore genetic factors in other neoplasias (86).

TUMORS OF THE ORBIT (6,12)

Perspective

Tumors of the orbit are any tumors that might be expected within or on the anatomic structures the orbit encloses, or that might reach the orbit by either extension from adjacent areas or metastatic routes. There is, therefore, no tumor that is peculiar to the orbit. The uniqueness of orbital tumors is the large range of diagnostic possibilities which calls for extensive use of various diagnostic techniques. The differential diagnosis of an orbital tumor can present a difficult and stimulating problem.

Epidemiology and Etiology

There is no specific information on this subject because of the variety of tumors.

Detection and Diagnosis

Clinical Detection (Table 20-1)

Typical presentations:
1. Unilateral exophthalmos or changes in the contour of the eyelids are the most common presenting signs. These signs, however, are not pathognomonic of tumors because they may result from inflammatory and metabolic diseases.
2. The second most common sign associated with orbital tumor is double vision. This is produced by mechanical or neurologic involvement of the extraocular muscles.
3. Less common in most orbital tumors is involvement of visual acuity or loss of visual field.
4. Eyelid swelling, ptosis, and orbital pain also are seen.

Table 20-8. Results of Control of Retinoblastoma by Irradiation

Group	Cassady et al. Control Rate	Cassady et al. Control (%)	Thompson et al. Control Rate	Thompson et al. Control (%)	Total Control Rate	Total Control (%)
I	36/43	84	12/17	71	48/60	80
II	30/45	67	1/3	33	31/48	65
III	22/32	69	3/5	60	25/37	68
IV	11/37	30	1/4	25	12/41	29
V	10/66	15	3/5	60	13/71	18
Total	109/223	49	20/34	59	129/257	50

Adapted from Cassady et al. (91) and Thompson et al. (114).

Diagnostic Procedures (Table 20-2)

1. External inspection and careful examination are essential and should include evaluation of exophthalmos, including any displacement of the globe up, down, or to the side. For example, lacrimal gland tumors arising in the upper outer quadrant of the orbit frequently displace the eye not only forward, but down and in as well.
   a. An orbital tumor can sometimes be palpated in the space between the orbital rim and the eyeball.
   b. Visual acuity and visual field studies might be necessary. Optic nerve tumors, for example, can produce vision loss before producing exophthalmos.
2. CT scans and MRI scanning can be helpful diagnostic tools in delineating intraorbital tumors, bone orbital erosions, and/or intracranial extension (126).
3. Ultrasonography is being applied to the study of orbital masses and intraocular lesions with success.
4. Differential diagnosis of other malignancies: In the investigation of orbital tumors, the possibility of invasion from neighboring areas, particularly the nasal sinuses, must be considered. The primary site of tumors metastatic to the orbit, such as breast, lung, prostate, or adrenals, must be determined by procedures such as physical examination (55) and x-ray. Peripheral blood tests and sometimes bone marrow biopsy also must be done to determine the presence of leukemia or lymphosarcoma. There is a limited differential diagnosis in children when orbital metastases are suspected; neuroblastoma is the most common, but histiocytosis X demands careful consideration.
   a. Separation of the sutures with increased intracranial pressure in young children with histiocytosis X may show irregular defects in the skull. When associated with proptosis and diabetes insipidus, this constitutes the triad of Hand-Schuller-Christian disease.
   b. In neuroblastoma, skull x-rays may show diffuse lytic defects associated with sutural separation (13).
5. Differential diagnosis of hyperthyroidism: Unilateral exophthalmos is commonly associated with suppressed overt hyperthyroidism. Unexplained unilateral proptosis might deserve surgical exploration and biopsy of suspicious tissue. Other causes of unilateral exophthalmos can be orbital rhabdomyosarcoma, histiocytosis X, ethmoid carcinoma, lymphomas, metastatic neuroblastoma, retinoblastoma, angiofibromatosis, pseudolymphoma, and premature closure of the coronal sutures (13).
   Bilateral and symmetrical exophthalmos are most often produced by hyperthyroidism, leukemia, and cavernous sinus thrombosis (13).
6. Carcinoembryonic antigen (CEA) can be helpful in the work-up. Serum CEA has been found to be elevated in various malignancies, while it is low in benign lesions (124).

Classification

Histopathology

Grade (G)$_1$ (well-differentiated), G$_2$ (moderately well-differentiated), G$_3$ (undifferentiated) (142).

Orbital tumors are usually classified as primary benign, primary malignant, and metastatic tumors. An extremely wide range of tumor types in the orbit has been described. Most of these are remarkably rare, and only the more common are listed below.

1. Primary benign tumors:
   a. Hemangioma is the most common orbital tumor. Other vascular tumors include telangiectases, aneurysms, fibroangiomas, and hemangiopericytoma (144).
   b. Lymphangiomas can resemble hemangiomas.
   c. An infrequent orbital tumor is congenital dermoid tumor, characteristically occurring in the superior temporal portion during childhood.
   d. Benign lacrimal gland tumors occur.
2. Primary malignant tumors:
   a. Embryonal rhabdomyosarcoma is the most common childhood primary malignant tumor.
   b. Malignant orbital tumors of the lacrimal gland include adenoidcysticsarcoma (adenocarcinoma), malignant mixed tumors, and rarely, mucoepidermoid carcinomas.
   c. Rarely, other sarcomas appear as primary in the orbit, such as lymphosarcoma or reticulum cell sarcoma.
3. *Metastatic tumors* (55):
   a. Metastatic tumors to the orbit include neuroblastoma of childhood, carcinoma of the breast, and, occasionally, carcinoma of the lung.
   b. Invasion of the orbit by carcinoma of the nasal sinuses or from the skin epitheliomas, particularly in the region of the nasal canthus, sometimes occurs.

Anatomic Staging

Because of the diversity and the rarity of orbital tumors, no effort at classification has been made for the majority of them. The exception is rhabdomyosarcoma, for which a staging system exists based on size of the tumor (T), involvement of lymph nodes (N), presence of distant metastases (M), and histologic grade (G) (20). The grading system is an innovation (see Chapter 19, "Pediatric Solid Tumors").

Staging Work-up

A careful search is necessary to exclude metastases or to find the primary if the lesion is metastatic. Radioisotopic oncologic survey of the skeleton is important for both primary and metastatic orbit tumors.

Metastatic tumors to the eye occur in 70% of cases from breast primaries, 15% from lung, 7% from alimentary tract, and 8% from other tumors, including neuroblastoma and leukemia (13,121,122). Breast and lung are the most common primary sites in adults; neuroblastoma is the most common condition in children (34). Tumor emboli are usually to the choroid; the favored locus is the posterior pole of the globe. Retinal detachment and bilateral lesions are known to occur. The incidence of bilateral lesions is as high as 25% to 30% (13,66,67). Conjunctival lymphosarcomas may be limited to the conjunctiva or may represent a focus of widespread disease; it is vital to exclude metastasis elsewhere and/or to search for the primary.

Principles of Treatment

Occasionally orbital tumors are sufficiently anterior that biopsy can be done simply and tissue diagnosis can be obtained before definitive surgery. Usually orbital tumors are not readily accessible to simple biopsy; a major procedure exposing orbital tissues is required. Deeper orbital tumors are generally biopsied only by total excision. Exploration of the orbital contents and removal of an orbital tumor carries considerable risk to function of the extraocular muscles and to the integrity of the optic nerve, which receives nourishment from several small vessels in the orbit. Again, a multidisciplinary approach to management is important for optimal outcomes (Table 20-5).

Surgery

1. Anterior approach is either through the skin or through the conjunctiva between the eye and the bony orbit. In most cases, however, there is sufficient space between the eye and the bony orbit to permit adequate exploration of the orbital contents.
2. Lateral approach through the bony wall of the orbit permits exploration of the anterior and middle third of the orbit. If the tumor is in a nasal quadrant, temporal decompression of the bony orbit can permit the eye to be retracted, giving better nasal access.
3. Superior approach with retraction of the frontal lobe of the brain and uproofing of the orbit exposes the posterior orbit. This approach is advantageous because extension of a tumor from the posterior third of the orbit into the cranial cavity can be determined and perhaps treated at the time of surgery.

Radiotherapy (120-123,125,127,128,130,131-143)

1. Primary and metastatic orbital tumors behave essentially as they do in other areas, and are subject to the same treatment modalities.
2. Radiotherapy is used for treatment of lymphosarcoma of the orbit and of metastatic orbital tumors such as neuroblastoma and breast and lung cancers. Pseudolymphomas of the orbit are very responsive to irradiation and are eradicated with 2,000 cGy doses given in regular daily doses of 200 cGy (129).
3. In treating orbital rhabdomyosarcoma with radiation therapy, the "poor man's wedge" technique yields the best results. This technique consists of delivering 200 cGy daily to an anterior field until 500 cGy have been absorbed at 4 cm depth. Then a lateral booster field is applied to raise the dose at the posterior orbit to 5,500 to 6,000 cGy, usually in four increments, moving the field posteriorly 1 cm each day (140,141).
4. Operative removal is usually the treatment of choice for lacrimal gland carcinoma; radiation therapy is preferred for lymphomas. Exenteration may be necessary if tumor extends posteriorly. If complete excision cannot be accomplished, or if there is concern about residual disease, postoperative irradiation is indicated. A wedge-field arrangement is angulated to miss the contralateral eye. Tumor doses range between 5,000 and 6,000 cGy in 5 to 6 weeks. A supplementary boost of 1,000 to 2,000 cGy can be delivered with intracavitary radium (or substitute) using a specially loaded prosthesis. A similar arrangement can be used for local recurrences at any time after surgery (13). A special circumstance occurs with lymphosarcomas of the lacrimal gland; these are radiosensitive and 2,000 cGy (200 cGy x 10) give excellent results (13).
5. The treatment of histiocytosis X in the orbit consists of a small retro-orbital field including bony defects; doses necessary to control the lesion vary from 500 to 2,000 cGy (13), but doses less than 1,000 cGy currently are considered sufficient (130).
6. The treatment for neuroblastoma metastatic to the orbit is the same as for histiocytosis X, although levels of 3,000 cGy should be used if response is slow. With metastatic orbital neuroblastoma, in contrast to histiocytosis X, death is almost universal and special protection of the lens and cornea is rarely indicated (13).
7. The treatment of metastatic eye tumors is mainly palliative. Enucleation is rarely justified unless secondary glaucoma or severe unremitting pain occurs. Once the diagnosis is established, radiotherapy, properly applied, can allow for restoration of vision. Although orthovoltage irradiation at doses of 2,500 to 3,000 cGy in 3 weeks has been advocated, a single lateral megavoltage field delivering 4,000 to 5,000 cGy is preferred for a solitary focus, particularly if the primary is under control and there is a chance to protect the anterior chamber of the eye to avoid cataracts (13).

Chemotherapy

1. Cytotoxic agents definitely play a role in the treatment of metastatic orbital tumors that have metastasized elsewhere (i.e., melanoma, neuroblastoma, and lymphoma).
2. The use of chemotherapy prospectively in tumors with a high propensity for dissemination, such as embryonal rhabdomyosarcoma occurring primarily in the orbit, has proven highly effective when combined with surgery and/or irradiation (128).

Hormonal Therapy

Hormonal therapy can be used to treat metastatic breast carcinoma. The estrogen receptor assay measures the hormonal sensitivity of metastatic breast carcinoma and predicts the beneficial effect of hormonal manipulation (adrenalectomy, oophorectomy, hypophysectomy) (78).

Results and Prognosis

1. Lymphosarcomas of the orbit have an excellent prognosis. Schultz (143) has reported survival rates of 60% to 70%.
2. In rhabdomyosarcomas of the head and neck in children, combination chemotherapy (vincristine, actinomycin D, and cyclophosphamide) and radiation therapy recently have yielded a 2-year survival of 74% and local control of 89% (128). Sagerman et al. (141) have treated orbital rhabdomyosarcoma in children primarily with radiation therapy yielding tumor control in 100% of patients (15 of 15) from 2 to 7 years of age. In their experience, five children died of metastatic disease, but with local control in the orbit (141). Such results indicating the radiocurability of localized rhabdomyosarcoma have prompted some to advocate radiation therapy following biopsy as the primary treatment (127).

Clinical Investigations

There are many studies on metastatic tumors (particularly melanoma), which include orbital location. There are also many studies on advanced sarcomas (particularly rhabdomyosarcoma). An especially important protocol is that of the

Children's Cancer Study Group (CCSG-212), which studies the effect of postoperative irradiation with actinomycin D, vincristine, cyclophosphamide, and doxorubicin on childhood rhabdomyosarcoma. A similar protocol for rhabdomyosarcoma exists in the CCSG-A 614.

Recommended Reading

General study on the subject of eye tumors should begin with appropriate chapters in Spenser's *Ophthalmic Pathology* (15). Other important works include Shields' *Diagnosis and Management of Intraocular Tumors* (14), Ferry's *Ocular and Adnexal Tumors* (5), and Yanoff and Fine's *Ocular Pathology—A Text and Atlas* (17). Reese's monograph, *Tumors of the Eye* (12) beautifully illustrates and correlates clinical and pathology aspects of tumor of the eye and remains a classic. The multivolume work, *System of Ophthalmology* , especially volumes 7 (3), 9 (4a), and 10 (4) are excellent, although somewhat dated, references. Duane's *Clinical Ophthalmology* (2) is a multivolume, loose-leaf format that is updated annually. For point of view more specifically directed towards eye tumors in children, see Nicholson and Green's chapter in *Pediatric Ophthalmology* (10) and *Diseases of the Orbit* (12a).

Some of the classic sources for Radiation Oncology may be sought in specific case circumstances and include for Late Effects: Merriam and Focht(31), Rubin and Casarret (35); for Conjunctival Melanomas: Lederman (27); for Choroidal Melanomas: Munzenrider *et al.* (71), Markoe, Brady *et al.* (67a); for Retinoblastoma: Bagshaw *et al.* (89), Cassady *et al.* (91); for Orbital Rhabdomyosarcoma: Donaldson *et al.* (129); and for Histocytosis X: Greenberger *et al.* (130).

REFERENCES

General References

1. American Joint Committee on Staging and End-Results Reporting. Manual for Staging of Cancer. 3rd ed. Chicago, IL: AJC; 1987.
2. Duane, T.D., ed. Clinical Ophthalmology. Philadelphia, PA: Harper & Row; 1989.
3. Duke-Elder, W.S.; Ashton N.; Smith R.J.H.; *et al.* The foundations of ophthalmology, vol. In: Duke-Elder, W.S., ed. System of ophthalmology. vol.7. London: Henry Kimpton; 1962.
4. Duke-Elder, W.S.; Dobree, J.H. Diseases of the retina, In: Duke-Elder, W.S., ed. System of Ophthalmology. vol 10. London, UK: Henry Kimpton; 1967.
4a. Duke-Elder, W.S.; Perkins E.S. Diseases of the uveal tract. In: Duke-Elder, W.S., ed. System of ophthalmology. vol. 9. London, UK: Henry Kimpton; 1966.
5. Ferry, A.P., ed. Ocular and Adnexal Tumors, vol. 12. International Ophthalmology Clinics. Boston, MA: Little Brown and Co; 1972.
6. Hammerschlag, S. B.; Hesselink, J.R.; Weber, A.L. Computed Tomography of the Eye and Orbit. Norwalk,CT: Appleton-Century-Crofts; 1983.
7. Hogan, M.; Zimmerman, L. Ophthalmic Pathology, An Atlas and Textbook. 3rd ed. Philadelphia, PA: WB Saunders Co; 1985-86.
8. International Union Against Cancer. TNM Classification of Malignant Tumors. 4th ed. Berlin, Germany: Springer-Verlag; 1987.
9. Jakobiec, F.A., ed. Ocular and Adnexal Tumors. Birmingham, UK: Aesculapius Press; 1978.
9a. Markoe, A.M.; Brady, L.W.; Karlsson, U.L.; Shields, J.A.; Augsburger, J.J.: Eye. In: Perez, C.A., Brady, L.W. (eds). Principles and Practice of Radiation Oncology. 2nd ed. Philadelphia, PA: JB Lippincott Co., 1992:595-609.
10. Nicholson, D.H.; Green, W.R. Ocular tumors in children. In: Nelson, L.B., Calhoun, J.H., Harley, R.D. (eds). Pediatric Oph-

thalmology, 3rd ed. Philadelphia, PA: WB Saunders Co; 1991:382-426.
11. Peyster, R.G.; Hoover, E.D. Computerized Tomography in Orbital Disease and Neuro-Ophthalmology. Chicago, IL: Year Book Medical Publishers; 1984.
11a. Physician's Data Query. Tumors of the Eye. Nat'l Cancer Inst., Bethesda, MD; January, 1992.
12. Reese, A.B. Tumors of the Eye. New York, NY: Harper and Row; 1976.
12a. Rootman, J. Diseases of the Orbit. Philadelphia, PA.: JB Lippincott Co.; 1988.
13. Sagerman, R.H. Moments of Decision in Cancer of the Eye. Chicago, IL: American College of Radiology; 1972.
14. Shields, J.A. Diagnosis and Management of Intraocular Tumors. St. Louis, MO: C V Mosby Co; 1983.
15. Spenser, W.H., ed. Ophthalmic Pathology. 3rd ed. Philadelphia, PA: WB Saunders Co.; 1986.
16. Strauss, M.B. Familiar medical quotations. Boston, MA: Little Brown and Co; 1968.
17. Yanoff, M.; Fine, B.S. Ocular Pathology — A Text and Atlas. 3rd ed. New York, NY: Harper and Row; 1989.

Specific References

Eyelid and Adnexae

18. Boynton, J.R.; Searl, S.S.; Caldwell, E.H. Large periocular keratoacanthoma: the case for definitive treatment. Ophthalmic Surg. 17:565-569; 1986.
19. Cogan, D.B.; Donaldson, D.D. Experimental radiation cataracts. Arch. Ophthalmol. 45:508-522; 1951.
20. Donaldson, D.D. Orbit, lacrimal apparatus, eyelids and conjunctiva. In: Donaldson, D.D., ed. Atlas of External Diseases of the Eye. vol II. St. Louis, MO: CV Mosby Co; 1963.
21. Duggan, H.E. Results using the strontium-90 ß-ray applicator on eye lesions. J. Can. Assoc. Radiol. 17:132-137; 1966.
22. Dunbar, S.F.; Linggood, R.M.; Doppke, K.P.; *et al.* Conjunctival lymphoma: results and treatment with a single anterior electron field. A lens sparing approach. Int. J. Rad. Oncol. Biol. Phys. 19(2):249-257; 1990.
23. Fitzpatrick, P.J.; Jamieson, D.M.; Thompson, G.A.; Allt, W.E. Tumors of the eyelids and their treatment by radiotherapy. Radiology. 104:661-665; 1972.
24. Harkey, M.; Metz, H.S. Cryotherapy of conjunctival papillomata. Am. J. Ophthalmol. 66:872-874; 1968.
25. Jakobiec, F.A.; Brownstein, S.; Wilkinson, R.D.; Khalil, M.; Cooper, W.C.; Shibata, H.R. Combined surgery and cryotherapy for diffuse malignant melanoma of the conjunctiva. Arch. Ophthalmol. 98:1390-1396; 1980.
26. Jakobiec, F.A.; Folberg, R.; Iwamoto, T. Clinicopathologic characteristics of premalignant and malignant melanocytic lesions of the conjunctiva. Ophthalmology. 96:147-166; 1989.
27. Lederman, M. Radiotherapy of malignant melanomata of the eye. Br. J. Radiol. 34:21-42; 1961.
28. Martin, M.E. Cancer of the eyelids. Arch. Ophthalmol. 22:1-20; 1939.
29. Martin, O.L. Long-term survivals of patients with cancer of the eye and surrounding structures treated with radiation therapy. Am. J. Roentgenol. 105:566-578; 1969.
30. Merriam, G.R., Jr.; Focht, E.F. A clinical study of radiation cataracts and the relationship to dose. AJR. 77:759-785; 1957.
31. Merriam, G.R., Jr.; Focht, E.F. Radiation dose to the lens in the treatment of tumors of the eye and adjacent structures. AJR. 71:357-369; 1958.
32. Ni, C.; Searl, S.S.; Kriegstein, H.J.; Wu, B.F. Epibulbar carcinoma. In: Ni, C.; Albert, D.M.; ed. Ocular Tumors and Other Ocular Pathology. Intl. Ophthalmol. Clin. 22(3):1-33; 1982.
33. Ni, C.; Searl, S.S.; Kuo, P.K.; Chu, F.R.; Chong, C.S.; Albert, D.M. Sebaceous cell carcinomas of the ocular adnexae. In: Ni, C.; Albert, D.M., eds. Tumors of the Eyelid and Orbit. Intl. Ophthalmol. Clin. 22(1):23-61; 1982.
34. Parker, R.G.; Burnett, L.L.; Wootton, P.; McIntyre, D.J. Radiation cataract in clinical therapeutic radiology. Radiology. 82:794-798; 1964.
35. Rubin, P.; Casarett, G.W. Organs of special sense: the eye and the ear. In: Rubin, P.; Casarett, G.W., eds. Clinical Radiation Pathology. Philadelphia, PA: W B Saunders Co; 1968:622-720.

36. Searl, S.S.; Boynton, J.R.; Markowitch, W.; diSant'Agnese, P.A. Malignant Merkel cell neoplasm of the eyelid. Arch. Ophthalmol. 102:907-911; 1984.

37. Searl, S.S.; Kriegstein, H.J.; Albert, D.M.; Grove, A.S., Jr. Invasive squamous cell carcinoma with intraocular mucoepidermoid features: conjunctival carcinoma with intraocular invasion and diphasic morphology. Arch. Ophthalmol. 100:109-111; 1982.

38. van der Brenk, H.A.S. Results of prophylactic postoperative irradiation in 1,300 cases of pterygium. Am. J. Roentgenol. 103:723-733; 1968.

Intraocular Tumors

39. Baum, M.D.; Pikerton, A.R.; Berler, D.K.; Kramer, K.K. Choroidal osteoma. Ann. Ophthalmol. 11:1849-1851; 1979.

Choroid Melanoma

40. Abramson, D.H.; Lisman, R.D. Cryopexy of a choroidal melanoma. Ann. Ophthalmol. 11:1418-1421; 1979.

41. Adams, K.S.; Abramson, D.H.; Ellsworth, R.M.; Haik, B.G.; Bedford, M.; Packer, S.; Seddon, J.; Albert, D.; Polivogianis, L. Cobalt plaque versus enucleation for uveal melanoma: comparison of survival rates. Br. J. Ophthalmol. 72:494-497; 1988.

41a. Albert, D.M.; Earle, J.D.; Sahel, J.A. Intraocular melanomas. In: DeVita, V.T., Jr., Hellman, S., Rosenberg, S.A. (eds). Cancer: Principles and Practice of Oncology. 3rd ed. Philadelphia, PA: JB Lippincott Co; 1989:1543-1556.

42. Ammar, F.; Robertson, A.G.; Dudgeon, J. Radiotherapy of choroidal malignant melanomas. Clinical Radiol. 38:21-23; 1987.

43. Augsburger, J.J.; Eagle, R.C.; Chiu, M.; Shields, J.A. The effects of pre-enucleation radiotherapy on mitotic activity of choroidal and ciliary body melanomas. Ophthalmology. 94:1627-1630; 1987.

44. Augsburger, J.J.; McNeary, B.T.; von Below, H.; Gamel, J.W.; Shields, J.A.; Brady, L.W.; Markoe, A.M.; Day, J.L. Regression of posterior uveal malignant melanomas after cobalt plaque radiotherapy. Graefes Arch. Clin. Exp. Ophthalmol. 224:397-400; 1986.

45. Augsburger, J.J.; Peyster, R.G.; Markoe, A.M.; Guillet, E.G.; Shields, J.A.; Haskin, M.E. Computed tomography of posterior uveal melanomas. Arch. Ophthalmol. 105:1512-1516; 1987.

46. Brady, L.W.; Markoe, A.M.; Amendola, B.E.; Karlsson, U.L.; Micaily, B.; Sheilds, J.A.; Augsburger, J.J. Tumors of the eye and orbit. In: Wilson, J.F., ed. Syllabus: A Categorical Course in Radiation Therapy: Cure with Preservation of Function and Aesthetics. Oak Brook, IL: Radiological Society of North America, Inc.; 1988:7-11.

47. Chambers, R.B.; Davidorf, F.H.; McAdoo, J.F.; Chakeres, D.W. Magnetic resonance imaging of uveal melanomas. Arch. Ophthalmol. 105:917-921; 1987.

48. Char, D.H.; Castro, J.R.; Quivey, J.M.; Chen, G.T.; Lyman, J.T.; Stone, R.D.; Irvine, A.R.; Barricks, M.; Crawford, J.B.; Hilton, G.F.; Lonn, L.I.; Schwartz, A. Helium ion charged particle therapy for choroidal melanoma. Ophthalmology 87:565-570; 1980.

49. Char, D.H.; Crawford, J.B.; Gonzales, J.; Millu, T. Iris melanoma with increased intraocular pressure. Differentiation of focal solitary tumors from diffuse or multiple tumors. Arch. Ophthalmol. 107:543-51; 1989.

50. Coleman, D.J.; Silverman, R.H.; Iwamoto, T.; Lizzi, F.L.; Rondeau, M.J.; Driller, J.; Rosado, A.; Abramson, D.H.; Ellsworth, R.M. Histopathologic effects of ultrasonically induced hyperthermia in intraocular malignant melanoma. Ophthalmology. 95:970-981; 1988.

51. Decker, M.; Castro, J.R.; Linstadt, D.E.; Char, D.; Petti, P.L.; Quivey, J.M.; Ahn, D. Ciliary body melanoma treated with helium particle irradiation. Int. J. Rad. Oncol. Biol. Phys. 19(2):243-247; 1990.

52. Einhorn, L.H.; Burgess, M.A.; Gottlieb, J.A. Metastatic patterns of choroidal melanoma. Cancer 37:1001-1004; 1974.

53. Ferry, A.P. Lesions mistaken for malignant melanoma of the posterior uvea. Arch. Ophthalmol. 72:463-469; 1964.

54. Fine, S.L.; Straatma, B.R.; Earle, J.D.; Hawkins, B.S.; McLaughlin, J.A. Failure of preenucleation radiation to decrease uveal melanoma mortality. The Collaborative Ocular Melanoma Study Staging Committee. Am. J. Ophthalmol. 107:440-442; 1989.

55. Font, R.L.; Naumann, G.; Zimmerman, L.E. Primary malignant melanomas of the skin metastatic to the eye and orbit. Am. J. Ophthalmol. 63:738-754; 1967.

56. Forrest, A.W.; Keyser, R.B.; Spencer, W.H. Iridocyclectomy for melanomas of the ciliary body. Ophthalmology. 85:1237-1249; 1978.

57. Fraunfelder, F.T.; Boozman, F.W., III; Wilson, R.S.; Thomas, A.H. No-touch technique for intraocular malignant melanomas. Arch. Ophthalmol. 95:1616-1620; 1977.

58. Gragoudas, E.S.; Goitein, M.; Verhey, L.; Munzenrider, J.; Suit, H.D.; Koehler, A. Proton beam irradiation: an alternative to enucleation for intraocular melanomas. Ophthalmology. 87:571-581; 1980.

59. Gragoudas, E.S.; Seddon, J.M.; Egan, K.; Glynn, R.; Munzenrider, J.; Austin-Seymour, M.; Goitein, M.; Verhey, L.; Urie, M.; Koehler, A. Magnetic resonance imaging in the evaluation and differentiation of uveal melanoma. Ophthalmology. 94:349-353; 1987.

60. Gragoudas, E.S.; Seddon, J.H.; Egan, K; Glynn, R.J.; Goitein, M.; Munzenrider, J.; Verhey, L.; Urie, M.; Koehler, A. Metastasis from uveal melanoma after proton beam irradiation. Ophthalmology. 95:992-999; 1988.

61. Kinkaid, M.D.; Folberg, R.; Torczynski, E.; et al. Complications after proton beam therapy for uveal malignant melanoma. Ophthalmology. 95:982-991; 1988.

62. Linstadt, D.; Castro, J.; Char, D.; Decker, M; Ahn, D.; Petti, P.; Nowakowski, V.; Quivey, J.; Phillips, T.L. Long-term results of helium ion irradiation of uveal melanoms. Int. J. Rad. Oncol. Biol. Phys. 19(3):613-618; 1990.

63. Lommatzsch, P.K. Results after ß-irradiation (^{106}Ru/^{106}Rh) of chroidal melanomas. Am. J. Clin. Oncol. 10(2):146-151; 1987.

64. Lommatzsch, P.K.; Kirsch, J.H. ^{106}Ru/^{106}Rh plaque radiotherapy for malignant melanomas of the choroid. Documeta Ophthalmologica 68:225-238; 1988.

65. Mafee, M.F.; Peyman, G.A.; Peace, J.H.; Cohen, S.B.; Mitchell, M.W. Magnetic resonance imaging in the evaluation and differentiation of uveal melanoma. Ophthalmology. 94:341-348; 1987.

66. Manschot, W.A.; Van Strik, R. Is irradiation a justifiable treatment of choroidal melanoma? Br. J. Ophthalmol. 71:348-352; 1987.

67. Manschot, W.A.; von Peperzell, H.A. Choroidal melanoma. Arch. Ophthalmol. 98:71-77; 1980.

68. Moon, J.H.; Gailani, S.; Cooper, M.R.; Hayes, D.M.; Rege, V.B.; Blom, J.; Falkson, G.; Maurice, P.; Brunner, K.; Glidewell, O.; Holland, J.F. Comparison of the combination of 1,3 bis (2-chloroethyl)-1-nitrosourea (BCNU) and vincristine with 2 dose schedules of 5-(3,3-dimethyl-1-triazeno) imidazole 4-carboxamide (DTIC) in the treatment of dissemination malignant melanoma. Cancer. 35:368-371; 1975.

69. Munzenrider, J.E. Particle treatment of the eye. Presented at the 31st Annual Scientific Meeting at the American Society for Therapeutic Radiology and Oncology. Refresher Course No. 107. Monday, October 2, 1989.

70. Munzenrider, J.E.; Gragoudas, E.S.; Seddon, J.M.; Sisterson, J.; McNulty, P.; Birnbaum, S.; Johnson, K.; Austin-Seymour, M.; Slater, J.; Goitein, M.; Verhey, L.; Urie, M.; Ruotolo, D.; Egan, K.; Osuna, F. Conservative treatment of uveal melanoms: Probability of eye retention after proton treatment. Int. J. Rad. Oncol. Biol. Phys. 15:553-558;1988.

71. Munzenrider, J.E.; Verhey, L.J.; Gragoudas, E.S.; Seddon, J.M.; Urie, M.; Gentry, R.; Birnbaum, S.; Ruotolo, D.M.; Crowell, C.; McManus, P.; Finn, S.; Sisterson, J.; Johnson, K.; Egan, K.; Lento, D.; Bassin, P. Conservative treatment of uveal melanoma: local recuurence after proton beam therapy. Int. J. Rad. Oncol. Biol. Phys. 17:493-498;1990.

72. Norton, E.W.D.; Smith, J.L.; Curtin, V.T.; et al. Fluorescein fundus photography: an aid in the differential diagnosis of posterior ocular lesions. Trans. Am. Acad. Ophthalmol. Otolaryngol. 68:755-765; 1964.

73. Packer, S. Iodine-125 radiation of posterior uveal melanoma. Ophthalmology. 94:1621-1626; 1987.

74. Packer, S.; Rotman, M.; Fairchild, R.G.; Albet, D.M.; Atkins, H.L.; Chan, B. Irradiation of choroidal melanoma with iodine-125 ophthalmic plaque. Arch. Ophthalmol. 98:1453-1457; 1980.

75. Peyman, G.A.; Raichand, M. Full thickness eye wall resection of choroidal neoplasms Ophthalmology. 86:1024-1036; 1979.

76. Reese, A.B. Precancerous and cancerous melanosis. Am. J. Ophthalmol. 61:1272-1277; 1966.

77. Seddon, J.M.; Gragoudas, E.S.; Egan, K.M.; et al. Uveal melanomas near the optic disc or fovea. Ophthalmology. 94:354-361; 1987.

78. Seddon, J.M.; Polivogianis, L.; Hsieh, C.C.; Albert, D.M.; Gamel,

J.W.; Gragoudas, E.S. Death from uveal melanoma. Arch. Ophthalmol. 105:801-806; 1987.

79. Straatsma, B.R.; Fine, S.L.; Earle, J.D.; Hawkins, B.S.; Diener-West, M.; McLaughlin, J.A. Enucleation versus plaque irradiation for choroidal melanoma. Ophthalmology. 95:1000-1004; 1988.

80. Vida, L.O.; Binder, P.S. Simultaneous metastasis of skin melanoma to the eye and orbit. Ann. Ophthalmol. 10:431-433; 1978.

81. Zimmerman, L.E.; McLean, I.W.; Foster, W.D. Does enucleation of the eye containing a malignant melanoma prevent or accelerate the dissemination of tumor cells? Br. J. Ophthalmol. 62:420-425; 1978.

Retinoblastoma

82. Abramson, D.H.; Ellsworth, R.M. Ancillary tests for the diagnosis of retinoblastoma. Bull NY Acad. Med. 56:221-231; 1980.

83. Abramson, D.H.; Ellsworth, R.M.; Grumbach N.; Kitchin, F.D. Retinoblastoma: survival, age at detection and comparison 1914-1958; 1958-1983. J. Pediat Ophthalmol. Strabismus. 22:246-250; 1985.

84. Abramson, D.H.; Piro, P.A.; Ellsworth, R.M.; Kitchin, F.D.; McDonald, M. Lactate dehydrogenase levels and isoenzyme patterns: measurements in the aqueous humor and serum of retinoblastoma patients. Arch. Ophthalmol. 97:870-871; 1979.

85. Abramson, D.H.; Ellsworth, R.M.; Kitchin, F.D.; Jung, G. Second nonocular tumors in retinoblastoma survivors: are they radiation-induced? Ophthalmology. 91:1351-1355; 1984.

86. Albert, D.M. Historic review of retinoblastoma. Ophthalmology. 94:654-662; 1987.

87. Albert, D.M.; Dryja, T.P. Recent studies of the retinoblastoma gene. Arch. Ophthalmol. 106:181-182; 1988.

88. Armstrong, D.I. The use of 4-6 MeV electrons for the conservative treatment of retinoblastoma. Br. J. Radiol. 47:326-331; 1974.

89. Bagshaw, M.A.; Kaplan, H.S. Retinoblastoma, megavoltage therapy, and unilateral disease. Trans. Am. Acad. Ophthalmol. Otolaryngol. 70:944-950; 1966.

90. Bettman, J.W.; Bagshaw, M.A.; Kaplan, H.S.; et al. The therapy of retinoblastomas: a critical appraisal with special emphasis on the linear accelerator. Trans. Pac. Coast Otoophthal. Soc. 32:257-272; 1958.

91. Cassady, J.R.; Sagerman, R.H.; Tretter, P.; Ellsworth, R.M. Radiation therapy in retinoblastoma: an analysis of 230 cases. Radiology. 93:405-409; 1969.

92. Cavenee, W.K.; Murphree, A.L.; Shull, M.M.; Benedict, W.F.; Sparkes, R.S.; Kock, E.; Nordenskjold, M. Prediction of familial predisposition to retinoblastoma. New Engl. J. Med. 314:1201-1207; 1986.

93. Cowell, J.K.; Hungerford, J.; Jay, M.; et al. Retinoblastoma: clinical and genetic aspects: a review. Journal of the Royal Society of Medicine. 8l(4):220-223;1988.

94. Devesa, S.S. The incidence of retinoblastoma. Am. J. Ophthalmol. 80:263-265; 1975.

95. Dryja, T.P.; Rappaport, J.M.; Joyce, J.M.; Peterson, R.A. Molecular detection of deletions involving band q14 of chromosome 13 in retinoblastomas. Proc. Natl. Acad. Sc. USA 83:7391-7394; 1986.

96. Faris, B.M.; Tarkji, M.S.; Baghdasserian, S.A.; To'mey, K.F. The role of cryotherapy in the management of early lesions of retinoblastoma. Ann. Ophthalmol. 10:1005-1008; 1978.

97. Fingerhut, A.G.; Collins, V.P. Local treatment of retinal tumors with radon. Radiology. 81:1003-1007; 1963.

98. Friend, S.H.; Bernards, R.; Rogelj, S.; Weinberg, R.A.; Rapaport, J.M.; Albert, D.M.; Dryja, T.P. A human DNA segment with properties of the gene that predisposes to retinoblastoma and osteosarcoma. Nature. 323:643-646; 1986.

99. Grabowski, E.F.; Abramson, D.H. Intraocular and extraocular retinoblastoma. Hematol Oncol Clin North Am. 1:721-735; 1987.

100. Hill, D.R.; Margolis, L.W. Radiation therapy management of retinoblastoma. Radiol. Clin. Biol. 41:139-144; 1972.

101. Horsthemke, B.; Barnert, H.J.; Greger, V.; Passarge, E; Hopping, W. Early diagnosis in hereditary retinoblastoma by detection of molecular deletions at gene locus. Lancet. 288:511-512; 1987.

102. Jensen, R.D.; Miller, R.W. Retinoblastoma: epidemiologic characteristics. New Engl. J. Med. 285:307-311; 1971.

103. Kitchin, F.D. Genetics of retinoblastoma. In: Reese, A.B., ed. Tumors of the Eye. New York, NY: Harper and Row; 1976:125-131.

104. Knudson, A. Mutation and cancer: statistical study of retinoblastoma. Proc. Natl. Acad. Sci. USA. 68:820; 1971.

105. Merriam, G.R. Jr. Retinoblastoma, analysis of 17 autopsies. Arch. Ophthalmol. 44:71-108; 1950.

106. Parks, M.N.; Zimmerman, L.E. Retinoblastoma. Clin. Proc. Child. Hosp. (Dist. Columbia) 16:77-84; 1960.

107. Pesin, S.R.; Shields, J.A. Seven cases of trilateral retinoblastoma. Am. J. Ophthalmol. 107:121-126;1989.

108. Pieromi, D.; Lashmet, M.H.; Helveston, E.M. Retinoblastoma. J. Pediatr. Ophthalmol. Strabismus. 6:182-185; 1969.

109. St. Jude Children's Research Hospital; Pratt, C.; Mayer, D.; Hustu, H.D.; et al. (principal investigators) Protocol for the treatment of childhood retinoblastoma with surgery, radiotherapy, and chemotherapy. Oct 1970.

110. Salmonsen, P.C.; Ellsworth, R.M.; Kitchin, F.D. The occurrence of new retinoblastomas after treatment. Ophthalmology. 86:837-840; 1979.

111. Skeggs, B.L.; Williams, I.G. The treatment of advanced retinoblastoma by means of external irradiation combined with chemotherapy. Clin. Radiol. 23:169-172; 1966.

112. Sparkes, R.S.; Muller, H.; Klisak, I. Retinoblastoma with 13q-chromosomal deletion associated with maternal paracentric inversion of 13q. Science. 203:1027-1029; 1979.

113. Stallard, H.B. The treatment of retinoblastoma. Ophthalmologica. 151:214-230; 1966.

114. Thompson, R.W.; Small, R.C.; Stein, J.J. Treatment of retinoblastoma. AJR. 114:16-23; 1972.

115. Weichselbaum, R.R.; Zakov, Z.N.; Albert, D.M.; Friedman, A.H.; Nove, J.; Little, J.B. New findings in the chromosome 13 long-arm deletion syndrome and retinoblastoma. Ophthalmology. 86:1191-1198; 1979.

116. Weiss, D.R.; Cassady, J.R.; Peterson, R. Retinoblastoma: a modification in radiation therapy technique. Radiology. 114:705-708; 1975.

117. Wiggs, J.L.; Dryja, T.P. Predicting the role of hereditary retinoblastoma. Am. J. Ophthalmol. 106:346-352; 1988.

118. Wiggs, J.L.; Nordenskjold, M.; Yandell, D.; Rapaport, J.; Grondin, V.; Janson, M.; Werelius, B.; Petersen, R.; Craft, A.; Riedel, K.; Liberfarb, R.; Walton, D.; Wilson, W.; Dryja, T.P. Prediction of the risks of hereditary retinoblastoma, using DNA polymorphisms within the retinoblastoma gene. New Eng. J. Med. 318:151-157; 1988.

119. Williams, I.G. The treatment of advanced retinoblastoma by means of external irradiation combined with chemotherapy. Clin. Radiol. 17:169-172; 1966.

Tumors of the Orbit

120. Abramson, D.H.; Ellsworth, R.M.; Tretter, P.; Wolff, J.A.; Kitchin, F.O. The treatment of orbital rhabdomyosarcoma with irradiation and chemotherapy. Ophthalmology. 86:1330-1335; 1979.

121. Albert, D.M.; Rubinstein, R.A.; Scheie, H.G. Tumor metastases of the eye. Am. J. Ophthalmol. 63:4-12; 1967.

122. Arnott, E.J.; Greaves, D.P. Metastases in the orbit. Br. J. Ophthalmol. 49:43-48; 1965.

123. Ashton, N.; Morgan, S. Embryonal sarcoma and embryonal rhabdomyosarcoma of the orbit. J. Clin. Pathol. 18:699-714; 1965.

124. Bullock, J.D.; Yanes, B. Metastatic tumors of the orbit. Ann. Ophthalmol 12:1392-1394; 1980.

125. Byers, R.M.; Berkeley, R.G.; Luna, H.; Jesse, R.H. Combined therapeutic approach to malignant lacrimal gland tumors. Am. J. Ophthalmol. 79:53-55; 1975.

126. Byrd, S.E.; Harwood-Nash, D.C.; Fitz, C.R.; Barry, J.F.; Rogovitz, D.M. Computed tomography of intraorbital optic nerve gliomas in children. Radiology. 129:73-78; 1978.

127. Cassady, J.R.; Sagerman, R.H.; Tretter, P.; Ellsworth, R.M. Radiation therapy for rhabdomyosarcoma. Radiology 91:116-120; 1968.

128. Donaldson, S.S.; Castro, J.R.; Wilbur, J.R.; Jesse, R.H. Rhabdomyosarcoma of the head and neck in children. Combination treatment by surgery, irradiation, and chemotherapy. Cancer. 31:26-34; 1973.

129. Donaldson, S.S.; McDougall, I.R.; Egbert, P.R.; Enzmann, D.R., Kriss, J.P. Treatment of orbital pseudo-tumor (idiopathic orbital inflammation) by radiation therapy. Int. J. Radiat. Oncol. Biol. Phys. 6:79-86; 1980.

130. Greenberger, J.S.; Cassady, J.R.; Jaffe, N.; Vawter, G.; Crocker, A.C. Radiation therapy in patients with histiocytosis: management of diabetes insipidus and bone lesions. Int. J. Radiat. Oncol. Biol. Phys. 5:1749-1755; 1979.

131. Hood, C.I.; Font, R.L.; Zimmerman, L.E. Metastatic mammary carcinoma of the eyelid with histiocytoid appearance. Cancer. 31:793-800; 1973.

132. Johnston, S.S.; Ware, C.F. Iris involvement in leukemia. Br. J. Ophthalmol. 57:320-324; 1973.

133. Jones, I.S.; Reese, A.B.; Kront, J. Orbital rhabdomyosarcoma: an analysis of 62 cases. Trans. Am. Ophthalmol.Soc. 57:320-324; 1973.

134. Lewis, R.A.; Clark, R.B. Infiltrative retinopathy in systemic leukemia. Am. J. Ophthalmol. 79:48-52; 1975.

135. Mortada, A. Nature of lymphoid tumors of the orbit, conjunctiva, eyelids, lacrimal gland. Am. J. Ophthalmol. 57:821-826; 1964.

136. Orestein, M.M.; Anderson, D.P.; Stein, J.J. Choroid metastasis. Cancer. 23:1101-1108; 1972.

137. Porterfield, J.F.; Zimmerman, L.E. Rhabdomyosarcoma of the orbit: a clinico-pathologic Study of 55 cases. Arch. Pathol. Anat. 335:329-344; 1962.

138. Rubin, P.; Green, J. Solitary setastasis. Springfield, MA: CC Thomas Co; 1968.

139. Russell, W.O. Staging of soft tissue sarcomas. In: American Joint Committee for Cancer Staging and End-Results Reporting. Classification and Staging of Cancer by Site — a Preliminary Handbook. Chicago, IL: AJC; 1976:261-266.

140. Sagerman, R.H.; Cassady, J.R.; Tretter, P. Radiation therapy for rhabdomyosarcoma of the orbit. Trans. Am. Acad. Ophthalmol. Otolaryngol. 72:849-853; 1968.

141. Sagerman, R.H.; Tretter, P.; Ellsworth, R.M. The treatment of orbital rhabdomyosarcoma of children with primary radiation therapy. AJR. 114:31-34; 1972.

142. Schenk, N.L.; Ogura, J.H.; Pratt, L.L. Cancer of the lacrimal sac — presentation of 5 cases and review of the literature. Ann. Otol. Rhinol. Laryngol. 82:153-161; 1973.

143. Schultz, M.D. Radiation therapy of lesion of the orbit and ocular adnexae. Trans. Am. Acad. Ophthalmol. Otolaryngol. 63:449-454; 1959.

144. Searl, S.S.; Ni, C. Hemangiopericytoma. In: Ni, C.; Albert, D.M., eds. Tumors of the Eyelid and Orbit. Intl. Ophthalmol. Clin. 22:141-162; 1982.

145. Wilder, H.C.; Paul, E.V. Malignant melanoma of choroid and ciliary body: a study of 2,535 cases. Milit. Surg. 109:370-378; 1951.

Gunar K. Zagars, M.D., Radiation Oncology   Julia L. Smith, M.D., Medical Oncology
John D. Norante, M.D., Surgical Oncology   Sandra McDonald, M.B., Ch.B., Radiation Oncology

Chapter **21**

TUMORS OF THE HEAD AND NECK

Reduce the deformity, maintain the reduction, restore the function.

Russell John Howard (33)

PERSPECTIVE

Although head and neck cancers constitute a small proportion (5%) (1b) of all malignancies, pronounced functional deficits and cosmetic deformities associated with these diseases heighten their relative importance. Functionally, the aerodigestive tract is complicated by the curious arrangement of respiratory and digestive tracts wherein the airway crosses the alimentary path. A variety of complex adaptations in the tongue, palate, pharynx, and larynx have evolved to protect the trachea from inundation by food and to assure smooth swallowing (22,32,100). Malignant disease of one part of this complex functional unit may indirectly have far-reaching influence on other regions. Functionally, too, the head and neck region is the sole location of several sensory functions (vision, hearing, balance, taste, smell), the loss of which, either by disease or by treatment, produces significant morbidity.

From a cosmetic standpoint, it is crucial to remember that facial-oral-laryngeal structures are key mediators of social interaction and that treatment as well as disease can be deforming and debilitating. A cured but mutilated and socially inhibited human being is not the goal of treatment. Rehabilitation, plastic surgical reconstruction, and prosthesis construction may be as important as resection (9a). Eradication of the tumor by irradiation optimally should allow for preservation of normal tissue resulting in maintenance of function and cosmesis. Survival cannot be measured simply in terms of mortality.

The multifaceted problems presented by head and neck cancer dictate a multidisciplinary approach involving the primary care physician, otolaryngologic surgeon, radiation oncologist, plastic surgeon, chemotherapist, pathologist, diagnostic radiologist, dental surgeon, nutritionist, oncology nurse, and social worker. The patient, family, friends, and employer are also intimately involved in the management process. Cooperative joint consultations prior to treatment and posttherapy follow-up clinics are essential in the optimal treatment of these diseases.

To the student, the management of head and neck cancers can be perplexing. With a shift of a few centimeters in location, a histologically identical carcinoma can have a different natural history and can pose distinct therapeutic problems. Many of these variations will be discussed, but considerable experience is required to detect the subtleties of a particular circumstance that dictate a unique nuance in the management approach. Although general principles of management will be presented, individualization of each case is necessary.

EPIDEMIOLOGY AND ETIOLOGY

Epidemiology

1. Head and neck cancers account for 5% of all malignancies and rank as the fourth most common cancer in males (approximately 30,000 new cases yearly in the United States) (2).
2. The larynx is the most common site, followed by oral cavity, pharynx, and salivary glands (2,10,15,35).
3. Mortality rates are at 2.4% of all cancer deaths. Rates are higher for males (3%) than for females (1%) (32d).
4. In certain regions of the world, such as India (buccal mucosa) and China (nasopharynx), particular head and neck subsites are especially common and provide clues to possible etiologic factors (10,35).

Etiology

1. In the majority of patients, there is not a clear-cut etiology.
2. Smoking and high alcohol intake (particularly in combination) are strikingly common in head and neck cancer patients and are implicated as etiologic factors (35).
3. Poor oral hygiene is another important factor.
4. Carcinoma of the nasopharynx is especially common among southern Chinese and seems to be related to environmental rather than genetic factors (159,171).
5. Epstein-Barr virus (EBV) is associated with nasopharyngeal carcinoma (NPC) in all races (152,157,158).
6. There is a higher frequency of premalignant and malignant oral lesions in young Americans because of the increasing use of smokeless tobacco (32f).
7. Carcinoma of the buccal mucosa is common in India and is associated with betel nut chewing (35).
8. Carcinomas of the nasal cavity have shown increased incidence in furniture workers and are somehow related to wooddust inhalation (179).
9. Chronic iron deficiency (Plummer-Vinson syndrome) is an etiologic factor in tongue and postcricoid carcinomas in females (35).

319

10. In the preantibiotic era, tertiary syphilis was implicated in tongue carcinoma (35).
11. Papillomavirus: The availability of the various human papilloma virus (HPV) DNA probes has permitted extensive screening of a variety of human carcinomas for HPV sequences. Based on the animal models, it would seem that carcinomas of any squamous epithelium, or any epithelium that may undergo squamous metaplasia, would be potential candidates for being associated with a papillomavirus. HPV DNA has been found in oral papillomas (18a,22c), in leukoplakia lesions (22c) and in oral carcinomas (22c). A recent study has demonstrated HPV-16 sequences in a verrucous carcinoma of the larynx (8b). The role of HPV in the etiology of squamous cell carcinoma (SCC) is, however, not clear.

Biology

Patients with squamous cell carcinoma of the head and neck (SCCHN) in comparable stages have diverse clinical courses and responses to similar treatment. Biologic parameters that may have prognostic importance in the natural history and treatment sensitivity have been investigated.

1. *DNA flow cytometry:* A number of studies using flow cytometry to assess DNA content have suggested an association of abnormal or aneuploid DNA histograms to tumor stage and patient prognosis (15a,15b,18b,35a). A recent study (20a) demonstrated that patients with aneuploid SCC had significantly decreased relapse-free and overall survival rates compared with patients with diploid SCC, independent of all clinicopathologic features examined.
2. *Epithelial cell surface antigens:* The A, B, and H antigens, normally present at epithelial cell surfaces, have been reported as reduced or lost in neoplastic epithelium, and this loss may provide a marker for malignant change. These antigens have been evaluated in the oral mucosa and results suggest that loss of the H antigen may be a marker for primary SCC (9e,10d,32c).
3. *Involucrin:* Involucrin is an important structural component of the insoluble protein envelope of mature, stratified squamous epithelial cells, and diminished expression has been found in dysplastic, carcinoma *in situ*, and invasive malignant lesions in the oral cavity (10b).

DETECTION AND DIAGNOSIS (Table 21-1) (8)

Clinical Detection

1. Most cancers of the head and neck grow and present as malignant *ulcerations* of a surface mucosa with raised, indurated edges and underlying infiltration-induration. These infiltrative, *endophytic* growths are more aggressive and difficult to control than the less common fungating, elevated, *exophytic* growths. Palpation may sometimes disclose an endophytic growth that otherwise is hard to detect.
2. Symptoms and signs depend on location.
   a. *Oral cavity:* Swelling or ulcer that fails to heal. Local pain is not always present. Ipsilateral referred otalgia is not uncommon. Inspection and palpation reveal an indurated ulcer.
   b. *Oropharynx:* Silent (symptoms delayed) area. Dysphagia, local pain, pain on swallowing, and referred otalgia are common symptoms. Inspection, including a mirror exam, should be supplemented with palpation. Topical anesthesia is often helpful.
   c. *Hypopharynx:* Silent area. Dysphagia, odynophagia, referred otalgia, or neck mass (node) are common presentations. Examination is the same as for the oropharynx.
   d. *Larynx:* Persistent hoarseness, pain, referred otalgia, dyspnea, and stridor. Indirect mirror examination (laryngoscopy) is essential.
   e. *Nasopharynx:* Bloody nasal discharge, obstructed nostril, conductive deafness (Eustachian obstruction), and neurologic problems (atypical facial pain, diplopia, hoarseness, Horner's syndrome) due to cranial nerve involvement. An otherwise asymptomatic neck mass is also a common problem. Examination involves indirect nasopharyngoscopy and cranial nerve assessment.
   f. *Nose and sinuses:* Bloody nasal discharge, nasal obstruction, facial pain, facial swelling, and diplopia

Table 21-1. Imaging

SITE	MODALITY	DIAGNOSIS & STAGING CAPABILITY	RECOMMENDED ROUTINE STAGING PROCEDURE
ALL Head and Neck	**Primary tumor and nodes**		
	CT	Extent of primary tumor and nodal involvement	Yes
	MRI	Offers 3-D views of primary site and nodes	Yes
	Metastatic Chest x-ray	Look for metastases/second primary tumor	Yes
	Radionuclide studies	Look for metastases if suspected	Yes

CT = computed tomography; MRI = magnetic resonance imaging.
From Bragg et al. (8), with permission.

(direct orbital extension). Examination includes anterior rhinoscopy, palpation of orbital margin, and inspection and palpation of roof of mouth and gingivobuccal sulcus.

   g. *Parotid and submandibular glands:* Painless local swelling, hemifacial paralysis due to facial nerve involvement.

3. A *metastatic cervical node* may be part of the clinical presentation of any of the above tumors. The most common enlarged node is the *jugulodigastric node,* which is just behind the angle of the mandible. Occasionally a neck mass is the sole presenting complaint. Any enlarged cervical node in an adult that persists for more than 1 week is regarded as malignant (Figs. 21-1a and 21-1b).

Diagnostic Procedures

1. Careful *inspection,* directly and via mirror of oral cavity, nasopharynx, oropharynx, larynx, and hypopharynx is necessary. Fiber-optic aerodigestive endoscopy is often valuable.

2. Careful *palpation* often allows one to detect more than by visual examination. A routine for systematic palpation of cervical lymphatics must be followed. Normal cervical nodes are soft, flat, mobile, and less than 1 cm in size. Metastatic cervical nodes become hard, oval, or round, and are readily detected once they grow beyond 1 cm in diameter.

3. *Biopsy* of all suspicious lesions is necessary. If clinical suspicion is high but the first report is negative, then repeat the biopsy. Verrucous carcinomas may be easier to diagnose clinically than microscopically.

4. *Radiographic studies* (Table 21-1) (8) selected according to needs are essential in the staging work-up.

   a. *Plain films:* Skull, sinuses, base of skull, and lateral soft tissue view of neck.

   b. *Computerized tomography (CT) scans* and *magnetic resonance imaging (MRI):* Increasingly useful in staging (24,36), especially for nasopharynx, oropharynx, larynx, and paranasal sinuses.

   c. *Orthopantomogram of mandible:* Useful to evaluate floor of mouth and gingival lesions, as well as bone erosion.

   d. *Barium swallow:* Standard and cinefluorograph, especially for pyriform sinus and hypopharynx.

   e. *Laryngogram:* For larynx and hypopharynx.

   f. *Chest x-ray:* For detection of metastasis or second primary.

   g. *Bone scan:* For bony metastases in symptomatic patients.

   h. *Arteriogram:* For diagnosis of chemodectomas.

   i. *Anti-EBV antibody titers:* Immunoglobulin G and immunoglobulin A are fairly specific for nasopharyngeal carcinoma and may aid in the diagnosis of cervical node cancer with unknown primary.

CLASSIFICATION

Histopathology (15) (Table 21-2)

More than 80% of cancers arising from the epithelial lining of the aerodigestive tract are SCCs and can be graded as well-differentiated, moderately well-differentiated, or poorly differentiated. Grading has been correlated with prognosis (4). A variety of SCCs are recognized (Table 21-2). Adenocarcinoma may arise from minor salivary glands in the mucosal lining of the aerodigestive tract, or from major salivary glands. A wide variety of nonepithelial malignancies can arise in the head and neck region, including lymphoma, plasmacytoma, melanoma, and soft tissue sarcoma. These are the subjects of separate chapters.

Anatomic Staging (3) (Table 21-3) (3,17b)

More than 80% of head and neck cancers arise from the epithelium of the mucosa lining the aerodigestive tract (15,35). The tumor (T) classifications for the primary tumor are similar for all aerodigestive sites but differ in some detail for different sites, as shown in Table 21-3. The node (N) classification for cervical lymph node metastases is uniform for all head and neck sites (Fig. 21-2). The staging systems presented in this chapter are all clinical-diagnostic stages, based on the best possible estimate of the extent of disease before treatment. Although surgical-pathologic classifications are possible, they are of less practical importance in the management of these tumors. However, when surgical treatment is carried out, cancer of the head and neck can be staged during these periods of management, using all information available. Such surgical-pathologic staging information may be crucial in deciding the need for and type of adjuvant treatment. It is important to note that staging systems for cancer have changed over the years. The current American Joint Committee for Cancer Staging and End Results Reporting (AJC) 3rd ed (3) and International Union Against Cancer (UICC) 4th ed (17b) editions of the classification of cancer are the same in context but differ from previous editions.

Staging Similarities

Most tumor (T) and node (N) definitions remain the same for most sites. As noted, the AJC and the UICC have agreed so there are no differences in the T or N categories. The head

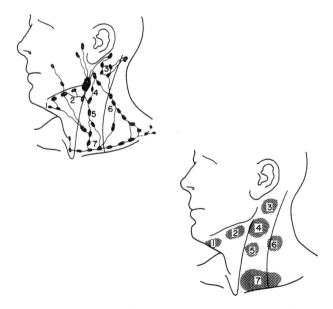

Fig. 21-1. Cervical node anatomy. 1: submental; 2: submandibular; 3: high posterior cervical; 4: jugulo-digastric; 5: mid-cervical; 6: mid-posterior triangle; 7: supraclavicular.

Table 21-2. Histopathology Classification: Common Cancers of Aerodigestive Tract

| Squamous Cell Carcinoma | | Adenocarcinoma |
Macroscopic Variants	Microscopic Variants	(Major or Minor Salivary Gland
Carcinoma in leukoplakia	Keratinizing well-differentiated; moderately well-differentiated; poorly differentiated	Malignant mixed salivary tumor
Carcinoma in erythroplasia	Nonkeratininzing; anaplastic squamous carcinoma	Adenoid cystic Mucoepidermoid (low or high grade)
Infiltrative carcinoma	Lymphoepithelioma	Acinic cell
Exophytic carcinoma	Transitional cell carcinoma	Poorly differentiated adenocarcinoma
Verrucous carcinoma	Spindle cell squamous carcinoma	

Table 21-3. TNM Classification and Stage Grouping of the Oral Cavity and Pharynx

"Largest Dimension" T Staging (oral cavity, oropharynx)	"Number of Subsites" T Staging (nasopharynx, hypopharynx, larynx)
TX Tumor cannot be assessed	TX Tumor cannot be assessed
T0 No evidence of primary tumor	T0 No evidence of primary tumor
Tis Carcinoma in situ	Tis Carcinoma in situ
T1 Greatest dimension ≤ 2 cm	T1 Tumor confined to one site
T2 Greatest dimension > 2 cm and ≤ 4 cm	T2 Involving more than one site in region of origin
T3 Greatest dimension > 4 cm	T3 Extension beyond region (nasopharynx to nose; larynx to pyriform sinus) or fixation of vocal cord if laryngeal or hypopharyngeal wall
T4 Massive tumor >4 cm with deep invasion of muscle, or invasion of bone, cartilage, or skin	T4 Massive tumor involving bone, cartilage, deep muscle, or skin

Nodal Involvement	Stage Grouping			
NX Regional nodes cannot be assessed	Stage 0	Tis	N0	M0
N0 No regional lymph node metastases	Stage I	T1	N0	M0
N1 Single, ipsilateral involved node < 3 cm	Stage II	T2	N0	M0
N2 Single or multiple ipsilateral, contralateral, or bilateral involved nodes, none > 6 cm	Stage III	T3	N0	M0
		T1, T2 or T3	N1	M0
N2a Single ipsilateral node > 3 cm but < 6 cm	Stage IV	T4	N0 or N1	M0
N2b Multiple ipsilateral nodes none > 6 cm		Any T	N2 or N3	M0
N2c Bilateral or contralateral nodes none > 6 cm		Any T	Any N	M1
N3 Involved node > 6 cm				

T = tumor; N = node; M = metastases.
From AJC/UICC (3,17b), with permission.

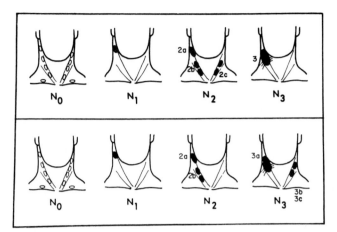

Fig. 21-2. Anatomic staging for cervical nodes (N categories). Upper panel shows the current staging system (AJCC, 1988) and lower panel is the old system. In the new system the number, size and laterality relative to the primary tumor are factors in staging nodes. The diameters <3 cm, 3–6 cm, >6 cm (N1, N2, N3) were chosen because these are determined more objectively than fixation.

and neck sites are carefully defined anatomically as are regional nodes. Approximately half the sites are predominantly determined by size of primary and half are determined by anatomic subsites. The size-oriented classifications include lip, oral cavity, oropharynx, salivary gland, and thyroid. In all sites 2 to 4 cm are used as the divisions between T1 (<2 cm) versus T2 (2 to 4 cm) versus T3 (>4 cm). The exception is thyroid, which uses 1 to 4 cm criteria. The subsite-oriented classification includes nasopharynx, hypopharynx, larynx, and maxillary antrum. Extensions into adjacent subsites escalate stage so that T1 versus T2 is one or two sites. With extension into surrounding tissues, depth of invasion usually becomes T3 with T4 being massive extensions beyond site as defined.

The N definitions are based primarily on size: 3 to 6 cm, with N1 (<3 cm) versus N2 (3 to 6 cm) versus N3 (>3 cm) being so determined. The major shift is in location of nodes, with contralateral and bilateral nodes no longer being considered a poor prognostic sign and downstaged from N3 to N2. The same N designations exist for all sites but thyroid.

Equivalence of TNM (tumor, node, metastases) categories is important to note. The T extent that is the same as N1 is either T3 and T4, depending on sites, and N2, N3 are considered to be the same as metastatic disease.

Staging Differences

Oral Cavity

The definition of T4 has been made more specific for lip and oral cavity. The definitions for N2 and N3 have been modified so that bilateral (b) and contralateral (c) nodes are considered N2b and N2c instead of N3b and N3c, respectively.

Oropharynx and Nasopharynx

The T definitions remain the same. The N definitions for N2 and N3 have been modified as noted above.

Larynx and Hypopharynx

The T definitions remain the same. The N definitions for N2 and N3 have been modified as noted.

Maxillary Sinus

The T definitions have changed from the number of extensions to emphasis on location and surrounding site invasions. That is, infrastructure is T2 versus surprastructure origin for T3. Massive involvement beyond paranasal sinuses is T4. Neck nodes are compatible with new definitions.

Salivary Gland

The T definitions have changed in that size, which was the predominant characteristic, is modified by extension so that all categories are a and b with or without local extension into skin, soft tissue, bone, and nerve. The change only applies to macroscopic, not microscopic extension.

Patterns of Spread

The (TNM) classification is a summary statement about the extent of any cancer, but of itself is not adequate to formulate the best treatment approaches for any given case. Careful attention to particular routes of local spread, of nodal involvement, and of metastatic disease in any given patient is necessary for optimal individualization of treatment. Spread patterns will be described in the sections dealing with specific tumor sites.

Staging Work-Up

The AJC rules for staging classification allow different types of evaluative evidence for classifying the extent of disease at different sites and at different times in a patient's history:

1. *Clinical-diagnostic staging (clinical TNM)* includes the standard clinical and radiologicl procedures short of surgery. This staging is fundamental and most important.

2. *Surgical-pathologic staging (pathologic TNM)* includes surgical exploratory procedures (staging surgery) and consists of biopsy samples of tissue or complete resection of primary and/or nodes with careful histopathologic study of extent of disease.

3. *Retreatment staging (retreatment TNM)* is used for evaluation of recurrent disease or for re-evaluation when additional treatment is necessary.

Recommended Staging Procedures

1. Careful *clinical evaluation* of primary site and cervical lymphatics as outlined herein in the section on clinical detection is recommended. Re-emphasized are visual inspection, mirror examination, and palpation. The T criteria for each site must be carefully documented and measurements (preferably three-dimensional) are recommended for all sites.

2. Careful *palpation, mapping, and measurement* of cervical nodes are important. Any enlarged, firm cervical node (> 1 cm) in an adult is regarded as malignant until disproved. Clinically false-positive cervical nodes in head and neck cancer patients are not common (15%) (238). The number of palpable nodes is an important prognostic factor. Mobility is often subjectively evaluated. Reduced mobility is taken to imply escape of the tumor from the confines of the node into tissue planes. Reduced mobility alone does not adversely influence prognosis. Complete fixation (complete immobility of node) means invasion of prevertebral muscle, base of skull, or cervical spine and is an objective finding carrying poor prognosis (238). Size is regarded as a more

objective measure than mobility, and studies have shown that nodes greater than 6 cm in diameter are most often unresectable.

3. *Examination under anesthesia* permitting direct inspection of relatively inaccessible sites such as nasopharynx, hypopharynx, and larynx is an important component of evaluation and should only rarely be omitted. Biopsy of suspicious edges for peripheral extension should be performed.

4. *Imaging procedures,* especially contrast-enhanced CT and MRI as outlined in previously discussed diagnostic procedures, are currently recommended (15d,15e) (Table 21-1).

   a. Both CT and MRI can be applied effectively to clinical problems of primary and nodal SCC. Each modality is precise in graphic delineation of deep tissue anatomy and is based on questions raised.

   b. CT and MRI are effective in finding occult primary tumors when neck nodes are the presenting features and can direct biopsy as an alternative to blind biopsy of Waldeyer's ring.

   c. Iodinated contrast-enhanced CT and MR can define the size of the tumor more accurately than can clinical impressions. With T2 weighted images, MRI can be used to determine tumor extent and offers the advantage of three-dimensional multiplanar images.

   d. Iodinated contrast-enhanced CT and MRI are especially useful to visualize deep invasion and reconstruct three-dimensionally areas not accessible to clinical evaluation, particularly selected blind spots.

   e. Iodinated contrast-enhanced CT and MRI are particularly useful for assessing nodes. The radiologic criteria are size, nodes greater than 1.5 cm, or lymph nodes with central necroses (mixed density on CT or mixed intensity on MRI) regardless of size. Imaging has changed clinical staging 15% to 20% of the time.

   f. CT or ultrasound-guided biopsy establishes pathologic diagnosis firmly. False-positive results due to inflammation can be ruled out.

   g. Posttreatment baseline is essential for follow-up.

   h. Clinical evaluation can be difficult if there is fibrosis but CT and MRI can diagnose recurrent tumor when it is not possible by direct inspection and palpation at least 25% of the time, that is, submucosal recurrence and high nodal relapse at base of skull and parapharyngeal area.

5. *Chest x-ray* is recommended for metastasis detection.

6. *Blood cell count* and *liver function* studies are routine.

7. *Bone scanning* is of value only for symptomatic patients.

8. *Arteriography* is diagnostic of chemodectomas (carotid body or glomus jugulare tumors) and also allows the delineation of disease extent. It is valuable when combined otolaryngologic-neurologic resections are contemplated.

PRINCIPLES OF TREATMENT

General (10,30,35)

1. The goals of treatment in head and neck oncology have been well summarized (39) as: (1) eradication of cancer; (2) maintenance of adequate physiologic function; and (3) achievement of socially acceptable cosmesis.

   a. Eradication of cancer implies both eradication of clinically demonstrable disease (definitive treatment) and eradication of microscopic subclinical disease (elective treatment). The decision to use elective (prophylactic) treatment in any case is based on probability considerations that weigh the likelihood of microscopic disease against the likelihood of treatment complications and the ability to salvage the patient if the cancer relapses in the site of suspected spread against the morbidity of elective therapy in patients without disease.

   b. Maintenance of adequate physiologic function requires careful evaluation of dysfunction already present and of dysfunction likely to follow treatment in each of the four major functional categories: (1) *special senses* (vision, hearing, balance, taste, smell); (2) *mastication-deglutition* (mandible, teeth, tongue, saliva, palate, pharynx, larynx); (3) *respiration* (larynx, trachea); and (4) *speech* (larynx, tongue). Careful evaluation will enable an optimal treatment choice assuring high tumor control with least functional deficit.

   c. Acceptable cosmesis requires necessary but sufficient surgery, within tolerance irradiation and plastic surgical and prosthesis rehabilitation. The patient should be informed of treatment outcome and of treatment alternatives. Ultimately, the patient's desires must be respected.

2. The goals of treatment can only be achieved through a multidisciplinary approach involving the otolaryngologic surgeon, plastic surgeon, radiation oncologist, chemotherapist, pathologist, radiologist, dentist, nutritionist, nurse oncologist, and social worker. Each responsible oncologist must evaluate the tumor and the patient prior to any treatment. After joint consultation, a firm but flexible comprehensive program is formulated and cooperatively applied.

3. Treatment decisions are mainly based on an appraisal of the patient's tumor, but the patient often plays an important role (39). Emphasis is given to host factors such as: (1) age and general condition; (2) comorbidity; (3) habits and life-style; (4) occupation; and (5) patient's desires.

4. Surgery and radiation therapy are the major curative modalities. Chemotherapy may be potentially effective as an adjuvant to these modes and add to cure rates.

5. Small primary lesions (T1 and T2) with negative cervical nodes are generally best treated with one modality. Small lesions with involved nodes may need both surgery and irradiation for control of neck disease; the treatment sequence is dictated by the choice of therapy for the primary focus. If the primary is to be irradiated definitively, then both sides of the neck are also given 5,000 cGy prior to neck dissection. If the primary is to be surgically excised, then a neck dissection is also done and postoperative irradiation (6,000 cGy) may be indicated (27).

6. *Large primary lesions* (T3 and T4) and/or extensive cervical node disease usually need both surgery and irradiation. The sequencing of modes has not been optimized in this circumstance, but many centers favor postoperative irradiation (18,27,97,116).

7. Special sites such as nasopharynx are surgically inaccessible and are always irradiated.

8. *Follow-up* at regular intervals to detect early recurrence, extension, or complications is important. Patients can be salvaged and problems often corrected if they are detected early.

Surgery (10,21,23,35)

1. Biopsy: An unequivocal histopathologic diagnosis is mandatory in all cases. Although exfoliative cytology and needle aspiration are occasionally useful, definitive diagnosis requires incisional or excisional biopsy of the primary lesion. Any incisions through normal tissue must be well-planned and performed only by experienced oncologic surgeons. Injudicious biopsies of cervical nodes performed via poorly situated incisions complicate subsequent therapy and may compromise the patient's outlook (21).

2. "The success of surgical resection is directly correlated with encompassing en block resection" (10). Piecemeal tumor removal risks recurrence. Adequate wound exposure is required to facilitate total tumor removal. When cervical nodes are to be resected, an incontinuity procedure, removing the primary lesion and neck nodes in one tissue block is preferred. Many standardized operative procedures are described (14,23), but each case needs individualization. Technical decisions often need to be made during the surgical procedure and require considerable experience and skill.

3. Wide resection margins are necessary, though often unattainable in the head and neck. Small margins (0.5 to 2 cm) are sometimes acceptable but require intraoperative frozen section histologic study for confirmation of total tumor removal. Inadequate or positive margins require postoperative irradiation rather than waiting for recurrence.

4. The extremes to which surgical resection can be taken in any case are based on considerations relative to the likelihood for cure and the probability for physiologic-cosmetic rehabilitation of the patient.

5. Reconstructive procedures are essential. Pedicle flaps and grafts may be required to close surgical defects (37).

Radiation Therapy (13,28,31,38a)

1. Preservation of function and cosmesis depends on the selective effect of irradiation to leave muscle, nerves, bones, and major vessels intact. The major advantage of irradiation is its ability to eradicate cancers without undue complications.

2. The complexity of modern radical radiation therapy requires that it be administered only by specially trained and experienced radiation therapists who have full dosimetric and physics support facilities.

3. A variety of irradiation techniques are available and the appropriate choice for an individual patient must be made. Customization of treatment techniques is essential. External megavoltage irradiation is the cornerstone of modern treatment in most patients. Interstitial irradiation (radium, iridium, or gold) is important as a dose booster technique for accessible lesions, especially in the oral cavity. Although it is arguable, a number of authors have indicated interstitial irradiation increases head and neck radiocurability compared with external irradiation alone for T1,T2 cancers, i.e., 92% versus 65% (38b). Neck nodes can be boosted to high-dose levels with interstitial implants. The electron beam provides an excellent ancillary technique for boosting doses to superficial regions in the head and neck area. Occasionally, the peroral cone technique (using orthovoltage irradiation) is appropriate, but generally orthovoltage techniques have no place in radical irradiation. Wang has reported 5-year results using intraoral cones of 75% to 100% depending on site and stage (38).

4. Radiation dose selection is based on tumor size and clinical circumstances. Subclinical microscopic cancer requires 5,000 cGy in 5 weeks; small lesions (T1) require 6,000 to 6,500 cGy; intermediate lesions (T2) require 6,500 to 7,000 cGy; and large lesions (T3 and T4) generally need greater than 7,000 cGy, and even then prospects for permanent control are not great. Dose escalation beyond 7,500 cGy with external irradiation techniques is fraught with complications. Such high doses can only be achieved with interstitial irradiation as a component of the treatment plan. A schema for combined interstitial and external irradiation for a variety of sites is shown in Table 21-4 (10a).

5. The shrinking-field technique, with dose delivery to each region according to the amount of cancer present in that region, must be used to achieve high doses. The primary site receives the highest dose, peripheral areas (including neck nodes) receive a lower dose, but never less than 4,500 cGy in 4-½ weeks.

6. The use of *brachytherapy* or *interstitial implantation* of radioactive seeds in fine plastic threads evenly placed by the radiation oncologist to afford a uniform distribution of dose allows high concentrated doses to small volumes. One-thousand centigrays/d can be delivered using low dose rates and are equivalent to 1000 cGy a week of external irradiation given as 200 cGy daily fractions. The manner in which these two techniques are combined is shown in Table 21-4.

7. Fractionation: There is strong evidence to support the concept that continuous irradiation compared with split-course schedules (7,28,28a) yields superior results, as evidenced in a report by Amdur (1c) i.e.,5-year actuarial disease-free survival of 88% versus 44%, respectively. Hyperfractionation is currently gaining favor and has been investigated both by the European Organization for Research and Therapy for Cancer (EORTC) (17a) andthe Radiation Therapy Oncology Group (RTOG) (9d) with promising results in prospective randomized studies. Cox et al. (9e) reported increasing the total dose with multiple daily fractions (1.15 Gy bid) improved response rates, i.e., 67 Gy to 77 Gy for 24% to 44%. Horiort et al. (17b) reported the EORTC trial comparing 70 Gy with 2 Gy fractions to 80 Gy (1.15 Gy bid) improved 3-year survival from 43% to 59%.

8. Regression Patterns: Analysis of regression patterns has therapeutic implications with regard to the planning of salvage surgery. It is advisable to wait for a 2- to 3-month post-irradiation follow-up for nodes < 6 cm whereas longer intervals could be advised for bulky

Table 21-4. Treatment Decisions for Combining Interstitial and External Irradiation *

	Interstitial Alone (Gy)	External Beam + Interstitial (Gy)
TX— No visible or palpable tumor	60	NR
TX—Palpable induration or nodularity	70	NR
TX—Tumor at margins; gross residual	75	50 + 30
Early —<1cm	65	Not recommended
Early —1-3 cm	NR	30/2 wk + 35
Moderately advanced — 3-5 cm	NR	30/2 wk + 40
Advanced	NR	50 ± 35
Postoperative irradiaiton therapy, negative margins	NR	60 to 65/6 to 7 wk
Preoperative irradiation therapy, fixed nodes	NR	50/6 wk

* Irradiation policies for oral tongue cancer at the University of Florida.
NR = not recommended.
From Million in DeVita et al. (10a), with permission.

nodes based on differences in achieving complete regressions at the end of therapy versus waiting 4-8 weeks; that is, 62% versus 80% for primaries and 32% versus 76% for nodes (5a).

Chemotherapy (Table 21-5)

1. The role of chemotherapy in the treatment of SCCHN is still evolving. Chemotherapy has become standard treatment for metastatic disease or for locally recurrent disease for which radiation therapy and surgical treatments are no longer possible. The rationale for the use of chemotherapy relates to its possible enhancement of local disease control and eradication of micromestastases. Hematogenous metastases from SCCHN, once regarded as rare, are now recognized as a significant cause of treatment failure, especially in patients with advanced (T3 or T4, N2 or N3) disease. Such advanced tumors have a metastasis rate of 20% to 35% (78,95,165,230,245). Local failure above the clavicles is even more common with such advanced lesions (50% to 80%) (10,18,34,35).
2. The ability of chemotherapy to improve local control

and to eradicate metastatic foci from head and neck cancer has not been proven, but is under active clinical investigation. Its effectiveness has been limited by the advanced stage and poor nutrition of most patients referred for chemotherapy. Its use at an earlier stage as an adjuvant to surgery and/or radiation therapy may offer improved survival.

3. Many single agents are active in head and neck cancer. *Methotrexate* has been the most widely used drug and is considered a standard for judging new regimens. Response rates (>50% reduction in tumor volume) of 40% to 50% are seen in advanced lesions (235B). Use of high-doses methotrexate with leucovorin rescue has not been shown to be more effective and adds cost and risk of toxicity in noncompliant patients. *Cisplatin* produces response rates of 30% to 40% in advanced head and neck cancers (224a,235b). Other active agents are *bleomycin, cyclophosphamide, vinblastine,* and *doxorubicin,* which give response rates of 20% to 40% when used singly (224a). Complete disappearance of all known tumor is unusual with single drugs and the responses last only an average of 3 months.

Table 21-5. Recent Drug Combination: Response to Chemotherapy

Dosage and Schedule	Response Rate (%) Total	Response Rate (%) Complete	Duration of Response (mo)	Reference
Cisplatin, 5-FU	70	27	11.3 (if CR) 6.5 (if PR)	19a
Cisplatin, 5-FU	53	13	6.5 (survival)	27b
Doxorubicin, cyclophosphamide	46	0	6.5	8
Methotrexate, 5-FU	39	18	6.5	32a
Methotrexate, 5-FU	65	13	3.6	31c
Cisplatin, bleomycin Methotrexate/leucovorin, 5-FU	52	18	16 (survival CR) 9 (survival CR)	22b
Cisplatin, bleomycin methotrexate, 5-FU	50	4	3.5	37a
Bleomycin, vincristine methotrexate, cisplatin	74	21	6	9c

5-FU = 5 flourouracil; CR = complete response; PR = partial response.

4. Combinations of drugs achieve higher response rates than a single agent. Response rates of 50% to 90% have been reported, but complete responses (CR) are less than 30% (224a,235b). Despite these high response rates, there is no convincing evidence that duration of response or survival are improved (245). Combinations containing cisplatinum give the highest response rates. Cisplatinum has been successfully combined with infusion 5-FU as well as with other agents known to have activity such as bleomycin/methotrexate/vincristine in various combinations (224a,235b). The best results using these regimens are in patients with no prior therapy.

5. The low benefit from chemotherapy in patients with head and neck cancer who have had previous surgery and/or radiation therapy may occur for several reasons. The blood supply has been disrupted by the previous treatment. The patient may be in poorer overall health due to poor nutrition and coexistent lung disease and other medical illness. Previous irradiation, especially, makes the patients more susceptible to excessive oral mucosal toxicity from 5-FU, bleomycin, and methotrexate. These factors have led to investigations of chemotherapy as a first-line modality before planned irradiation or surgery in advanced head and neck cancers. This is called neoadjuvant or induction chemotherapy.

   The regimens used are similar to those used for recurrent and metastatic disease. These include platinum combinations with 5-FU and/or bleomycin, methotrexate, or vincristine (224a). To date, there has only been prolongation of survival for complete responders. While a majority of patients do have tumor shrinkage from induction chemotherapy, the prognostic significance of this response is still under investigation (228a).

6. The use of chemotherapy as an adjuvant after locoregional treatment has been disappointing (246,249).

   Laramore et al. (20b) report on the efficacy of sequential chemotherapy as an adjuvant to standard surgery and postoperative irradiation in locally advanced but operable cancer conducted by the Head and Neck Intergroup of six major cooperative groups. Resectable cancers of the oral cavity, oropharynx, hypopharynx, or larynx were randomized to either 3 cycles of CisPt + 5-FU followed by 50-60 Gy or radiation alone. There was no difference in the 4-year actuarial survival rate of 44% in the RT arm versus 48% in RT/CT arm with similar local regional failure rate of 29% versus 26%, respectively. The one gain that unfortunately did not translate into improved survival was overall decrease in the incidence of distant metastases to 15% in CT/RT arm compared to 23% in the RT arm (p = 0.03) confirming both SWOG and VA studies using induction chemotherapy (20b).

7. Neoadjuvant chemotherapy prior to definitive surgery, although producing high induction response rates of 50-90%, have not translated into improved survival rates (see Combined Modalities section that follows) (1a,34a,17c).

Combined Modalities

1. A multimodal assessment of each patient has been emphasized, but every patient does not require combining surgery, irradiation, and chemotherapy. *Small primary lesions* (T1 and T2) with a clinically negative neck are best managed with one modality; combining modes under these conditions results in overtreatment with an unnecessary risk for complications.

2. *Large primary lesions* (T3 and T4) or involvement of cervical lymphatics may require a planned combined approach, and currently the most frequent multimodal treatment is high-dose preoperative or postoperative irradiation and radical surgery. Although surgical techniques may need some modification when radiation therapy is given (5), the treatment team must guard against imposing "a plurality of minor efforts that may, in themselves, be defeatist" on the patient (10). When using a multimodal approach, it is crucial not to de-emphasize each modality to such an extent that the final result fails to achieve the outcome that could be possible with a single modality. Usually at least one modality (surgery or irradiation) has to be radical if a combined approach is to succeed (18,26,27,34).

3. The surgeon should not rely on postoperative radiation to eradicate *gross residual disease* (18,34). Potentially curative surgical treatment must remove all gross disease, and in the same way, although preoperative radiation therapy or chemotherapy may shrink a tumor, any modification of surgical technique must recognize that such shrinkage does not always imply that the scope of the surgical procedure can be reduced.

4. *Irradiation therapy* is highly effective in controlling microscopic, subclinical disease in surgically undisturbed tissues, but 5,000 cGy in 5 weeks is required (11,12,46). Postoperatively, surgically disturbed areas of subclinical disease require at least 6,000 cGy and possibly 7,000 cGy to highly contaminated sites (27,28,34).

5. The value of *chemotherapy* before or after radiation or surgery has not been determined. Results of studies on postsurgical or postirradiation adjuvant chemotherapy have been disappointing and arguments for initial chemotherapy have been made (224a,228a). Presurgical or preirradiation chemotherapy for advanced lesions is currently an area of intense investigation, but is not recommended as a routine procedure. Thorough recent reviews by Al Saraf (1a) and Taylor (34a) on this subject indicate that improved response rates do not translate into improved survival. A number of investigations have recently reported a variety of chemotherapy schedules with cisplatin (1b), and with other agents (31d) — with essentially the same theme — improved, impressive CR rates of 75%, 81%, and 78%, respectively, but in the latter British Clinical Trial with 10-year follow-up, only 25% of patients are alive. These authors caution achieving a final high CR *does not automatically* mean improved survival. Attempting subset analyses on the large national head and neck contract using induction chemotherapy of cisplatin

and bleomycin, Jacobs and Makuch (17c) noted the odd site that had a better survival compared with standard surgery and irradiation. These observations may indicate a direction for further study.

SPECIAL CONSIDERATIONS OF TREATMENT

Metastatic Neck Nodes (21,225-227,231,233,236)

The management of cervical lymphatics, whether overtly involved or not, is an integral part of managing the head and neck cancer patient. The incidence of lymph node metastasis in a variety of head and neck sites at presentation and subsequent conversion rate is shown in Table 21-6 (27a).

1. *Clinically involved nodes* are best managed by radical neck dissection (RND) or by modified neck dissection, but it is increasingly recognized that recurrences within the operative field and in the contralateral neck are common and exceed 40% if more than one node is histologically positive (226,228,230,240).
2. *Adjunctive irradiation* to both sides of the neck significantly reduces this failure pattern and should be considered in all patients with more than one positive node (18,27,240).
3. If the *primary lesion is managed radiotherapeutically*, then both sides of the neck receive 5,000 cGy in 5 weeks with either RND or modified neck dissection 4 to 6 weeks later (13,28).
4. If the *primary lesion is resected*, usually RND is also performed in continuity and irradiation to 6,000 cGy is given (28).
5. *Bilateral RND* may be required for bilateral disease and all such patients should receive adjunctive irradiation.

6. *Cervical nodes that are inoperable* due to fixation to base of skull, cervical spine, or prevertebral muscle or that are attached to the carotid vessels should receive preoperative irradiation followed by resection if they become mobile.
7. Under certain circumstances, *irradiation alone* may be adequate for the control of palpably involved nodes, although larger doses are necessary and neck fibrosis often results. A single node 1 to 2 cm in diameter receiving at least 6,500 cGy and completely regressing within 6 weeks of completion does not require resection. A 2 to 3 cm node receiving 7,000 cGy and completely regressing also is unlikely to recur (236,241). Electron beam boosts or interstitial implants are important technical "finesses" to achieve these high doses.
8. Unknown primary tumors: Despite the absence of a known primary, it has been recognized for decades that definitive treatment with surgery and/or irradiation can yield a 5-year survival from 25% to 50% depending on other factors in this heterogenous group of patients (11a,26b). For example, if the nodal stage is considered, the initial response and long-term neck control for N1, N2A, N2B, N3A, and N3B are 83%, 93%, 61%, 50%, and 33% (local control), respectively, and 83%, 71%, 67%, 44%, and 50% (long-term control), respectively (26b). An aggressive curative approach is worthwhile.
9. Hyperthermia is a promising new investigational mode that when added to irradiation has shown improved response in both nonrandomized and randomized studies according to Overgaard (30a).

Table 21-6. Incidence of Lymph Node Metastasis By Site of Primary In Head and Squamous Cell Carcinoma

Site	Percentage N+ at Presentation	Percentage N0 Clinically, N+ Pathologically	Percentage N0- > N+ with No Neck Treatment
Floor of mouth	30-59	40-50	20-35
Gingiva	18-52	19	17
Hard palate	13-24	-	22
Buccal mucosa	9-31	-	16
Oral tongue	34-65	25-54	38-52
Nasopharynx	86-90	-	19*-50
Anterior tonsillar pillar/	39-56	-	10-15
retromolar trigone	37-56	-	16-25
Soft palate/uvula	58-76	-	22†
Tonsillar fossa	50-83	22	-
Base of tongue	50-71	66	-
Pharyngeal walls	31-54	16-26	33
Supraglottic larynx	52-72	38	

- No data.
* T1N0 patients only.
† Patients received preoperative irradiation.
N = nodes.
From Mendenhall et al. (27a). Copyright ©; printed by permission of John Wiley & Sons, Inc.

Elective (Prophylactic) Treatment

Elective treatment of cervical lymphatics is controversial, due to the complexity of factors involved in the treatment decision (237,239). One must balance the likelihood of microscopic nodal involvement (depending on primary tumor site, T stage, and macroscopic and microscopic pathology) and the possibility of subsequent salvage (determined by, among other things, closeness of follow-up and patient reliability) against the morbidity-mortality of elective treatment. Irradiation therapy is highly effective in eradicating subclinical disease from surgically undisturbed neck lymphatics and 5,000 cGy in 5 weeks produces no detectable long-term sequelae (12,20,37). In a homogenous population with nasopharyngeal cancers stage I, Lee (22a) noted a failure rate of 0% versus 30% depending on the use of elective neck irradiation or its absence in treatment, respectively. In general, T1 primary lesions (except nasopharynx) with clinically negative nodes do not require prophylactic neck treatment. Well-differentiated T2 lesions of the oral cavity also do not usually receive elective neck treatment. T1 and T2 glottic lesions do not require neck treatment. For all other situations consideration should be given to elective cervical node treatment.

Surgical Complications (1,35,229)

Rehabilitation, plastic surgical reconstruction, and provision of prostheses are essential when wide resections are performed (9a). Immediate postoperative complications include wound infection, fistula formation, sloughing of skin flaps — especially at trifurcation points, exposure and rupture of carotid artery, aspiration when the airway remains connected to the food passage, peptic ulceration and gastritis with hematemesis, and pulmonary embolism. In experienced hands, the incidence of such complications is low. Local complications are more common if preoperative irradiation is used, and surgical techniques (especially skin incisions) need modification in such patients (5). Delayed surgical problems relate mainly to physiologic problems with deglutition, speech and tracheitis sicca following laryngectomy. Shoulder disability following RND and chronic neck pain also occur.

Radiation Complications (6,13,28,29,38a)

Dryness of the mouth (xerostomia) is universal in patients receiving greater than 5,000 cGy to major salivary glands; it lasts for months but tends to improve and become less bothersome after 1 to 2 years. Loss of taste is also universal but usually returns within 12 months. Dental caries can be severe but are totally preventable with comprehensive dental care involving oral hygiene, fluoride treatment, and conservative dental management (19). Osteoradionecrosis of the mandible is a major complication often precipitated by dental extraction following high-dose irradiation (> 6,000 cGy) to the mandible (8a). Dental extractions before and particularly after irradiation are to be avoided. Mandibular necrosis should be managed conservatively and patiently with antibiotics and maintenance of oral hygiene. The majority of patients will heal after some months and following sequestration of dead bone. Surgery for this complication is always major, involving resection of all bone receiving greater than 5,000 cGy. Soft tissue necroses invariably heal if the bone is not exposed. Complex radionecrotic problems may benefit

from hyperbaric oxygen therapy (16). Spinal cord tolerance has been widely recommended to be 50Gy and most protocols recommend not exceeding 45 Gy (22). In a recent evaluation, Marcus *et al.* (26c) challenged the tolerance dose after reviewing the records of 1112 patients treated to their cervical spinal cord to a variety of doses. The risk is zero or very small even with doses up to 55 Gy if fractional doses are kept to 1.2 to 2.0 Gy daily. Schultheiss (32b) analyzed the clinical data critically and indicated 50 Gy in 2 Gy fractions is a conservative estimate of spinal cord tolerance.

The "Interfraction Interval" as a major determinant of late effects with hyperfractionated radiotherapy in head and neck cancers is an important observation. This RTOG study by Cox *et al.* (9c*) demonstrates that interfraction intervals > 4.5 hours versus < 4.5 hours heightens both acute and late effects. Estimates of late toxicity at 1, 2, and 3 year intervals were 5.5%, 9.8%, and 15.4% with intervals > 4.5 hours versus 7.7% at all time periods < 4.5 hours.

Patterns of Failure

Second Malignant Tumors

The development of second malignant tumors (SMT) in head and neck cancer patients, for whom surgery and irradiation successfully have controlled the locoregional disease, has emerged as a major clinical concern (13,20,22b,91). Second malignant tumors have been reported in as many as 33% of patients with oral cavity, 37% with oropharyngeal, and 21% with laryngeal cancers (22c,22d,23a).

An RTOG database analysis of 928 head and neck cancer patients illustrated the risks of developing second malignant tumors (SMTs): 10% at 3 years, 15% at 5 years, and 28% at 8 years after treatment (9c).

Because 90% of patients with head and neck cancer smoke or drink alcohol, it is not surprising that the most prevalent sites for SMTs are the upper aerodigestive tract and lung, which reflects the diffuse effects of these carcinogens on wide areas of the mucosa, termed field cancerization or condemned mucosa syndrome (32e).

Patients with early-stage disease have the highest risk of developing SMTs and, because the prognosis for SMTs is poor, endeavors aimed at prevention should be a priority. Pharmacologic intervention (chemoprevention) as an adjunct to smoking cessation programs, is currently under investigation, using vitamin A and its analogs, which include the retinoids and carotenoids (22e,22f). In a small, randomized study of 100 treated head and neck cancer patients, 13 cis retinoic acid (50 to 100 mg/m^2/d) decreased SMT incidence to 4% versus 22% in the controls at median follow-up of 29 months. The total failure rate was also lower in the 13 cis retinoic acid group, i.e., 31% versus 52% and a trend emerged in favor of cis retinoic acid group in disease-free survival (17).

Types of Local-Nodal Recurrence

More than 75% of head and neck cancer patients who fail treatment do so first above the clavicles either in the primary region, neck nodes, or in both (18,64,68,78,97,165,176). Some primary sites remain notoriously difficult to control despite aggressive approaches: these include the base of the tongue, pharyngeal walls (lateral and posterior), and the postcricoid regions. In any site, T3 or T4 lesions have a high propensity to recur locally even following multimodal approaches. Recurrence at the primary site re-establishes the potential for cervical lymphatic failure (reseeding) irrespective of whether the neck was initially treated. Not surprisingly, the single most common failure pattern is the recurrent primary with a neck metastasis (34,68,78,97).

Metastatic Relapse

Increasingly aggressive locoregional therapy does improve disease control above the clavicles but has little effect on survival (95,230). As extensive T3, T4, N2, N3 diseases are controlled, the longer survival unmasks an unexpectedly high incidence of hematogenous metastases most commonly to lung but also to bone and elsewhere. Patients with large primary lesions and bilateral cervical nodes have an incidence of distant disease as high as 40% if they survive long enough from their locoregional disease (230).

Intercurrent Disease

Intercurrent disease is also an important factor in ultimate outcome. A high self-destructive element is found in these patients as a group. Many are socially maladjusted, often unable to modify their life-style, and continue heavy drinking and smoking. Alcohol-related deaths, chronic lung disease, accidents, suicide, and other illnesses account for 10% to 30% of deaths, depending on the reported series.

RESULTS AND PROGNOSIS

1. *Five-year survival rates*: A comprehensive listing of all head and neck sites offering 5-year determinate survival rates by each stage based on a review of the literature can be found in Table 21-7. These rates are independent of modality and are an overview using conventional methods of treatment. A 5-year follow-up is adequate for most sites, since recurrences occur within the first 2 years and rarely after 4 years (45,64,71,74,85,96, 114,161). Generally, for most sites 5-year survival for stage I is 75% to 90%; for stage II survival is 40% to 70%; for stage III survival is 20% to 50%; and for stage IV, 10% to 30%.
2. *The RTOG track record*: The RTOG has a large series of head and neck protocols and registry. Analysis of 1,000 cases has allowed the generation of response rate and survival data. For early T stages (T1, T2 and N0 and N1 nodal disease), the CR rate is 80% to 95%, while advanced T3, T4 stages and N2 and N3 nodes have only a 30% to 50% CR rate, (see Table 21-8) (26a).
3. *Surveillance, Epidemiology and End Result group data*: (1a)
   a. Based on 5,435 cases, the 5-year survival rate for oral cavity and pharynx is 43% and 51%, observed and relative, respectively, and at 10 years is 38% and 41%, respectively. Seventy-eight percent of 5-year survivors also survive to 10 years.
   b. Blacks do poorer than whites — 31% versus 54% survival at 5 years.
   c. There has been an overall decrease in mortality rates (13.9% from 1970 to 1985). The adjusted years of life lost decreased from 23.1% in 1970 to 19.9% in 1985.
4. *The Effects of Local-Regional Control on Distant Metastatic Dissemination in Carcinoma of the Head and Neck*: Leibel et al. (22a*,22a**) provide compelling evidence that improved local-regional control decreases dissemina-

tion and metastases and does translate into better overall survival. Using the large RTOG database in head and neck cancers (22a**), they report the incidence of distant metastases only 24% for NED patients versus 36% for patients with persistence of cancer at 5 years and the corresponding 5-year survival is 47% compared to 16%. When analyzed by subgroups, this observation applies to earlier Stage T1-T3N0 patients but not advanced T3-4 N2-3 sites, except for hypopharynx and nasopharynx. The explanation for this is that when cancers are very advanced locally with a high degree of nodal involvement, they probably are metastatic at the time of presentation. Most stimulating is the concept put forward to explain these events. Based on experimental and biological evidence, they explicate that failure to control the primary tumor leads to increased rates of metastatic dissemination because recurrent tumors develop more cell clonogens capable of metastasizing that are phenotypically and genotypically distinct (22a*). Based on these biological considerations, they hypothesize improved local-regional control at several anatomic sites is likely to decrease the ultimate rate of metastatic disease.

Prognostic Factors

Important prognostic factors are:
* anatomic site of primary
* T stage
* cervical node status
* associated diseases (comorbidity)

CLINICAL INVESTIGATIONS

1. The need for *predictive assays* for tumor radiocurability has been the subject of research since the 1960s, when it was very actively pursued in cervix cancer. Interest in this subject has been reawakened by new concepts and new techniques developed in the past decade by radiobiologists (31b). Based on the concepts that tumors cells are the target of therapy and that the *in vitro* sensitivity of stem cells reflects their *in vivo* sensitivity, Brock *et al.* (9) developed a special multicellular chamber using a cell-adhesive technique; cells were irradiated and incubated for 2 weeks, followed by staining; their optical density was read with an image analysis system. As explained, a survival curve parameter was calculated at 2 Gy (S2) based on the analyses of Fertil and Malaise (10e,10f) and Deacon *et al.* (9f), who found that S2 is a reliable descriptor of a low-dose region of the survival curve. Applying this technique to SCCHN patients who have been followed for more than 1 year, Peters *et al.* (31a) showed the recurrence rate to be a slightly higher failure pattern for those with an S2 value greater than 0.4, as compared with those with a value less than 0.3. Although the primary cultures are generally slightly more resistant for recurrent tumors, the difference is not statistically significant; the plotted recurrences virtually reconstitute the range of cell survival at 2 Gy (0.2 to 0.5, without much evidence of clustering). This has been a major clinical-radiobiologic effort, and it needs to be encouraged because predictive assays are essential in determining the potential biologic basis of the combined treatment modalities.

Table 21-7. Determinate* 5-Year Survival in Head and Neck Cancer

Anatomic Site of Primary	Overall 5-year Survival (%)	5-Year Survival According to Stage-Grouping (%)				References
		I	II	III	IV	
ORAL CAVITY						
Mobile tongue	45	80	60	30	15	40,43,44,45,47,50,51,54, 61,66
Floor of mouth	50	80	70	60	30	40,47,49,50,55,57,58,63
Buccal mucosa	45	75	65	30	15	41,48,57,60
Retromolar trigone	60	75	70	60	30	20,25,48,53
Lower gingiva	65	75	60	50	30	10,35,42,53,57
Lip	85	90	85	70	60	10,15,35,40a
OROPHARYNX						
Tonsil	45	90	60	40	15	71,73,75,80,81a,84,87a,89b, 90a,91,92
Base of tongue	30	60	40	20	10	69,71,73a,83,85,89a,91
Pharyngeal wall	20	50	30	20	10	35,77,77a,89-91
Soft palate	50	85	60	30	15	70,71,87,91
NASOPHARYNX	45	60	40	30	15	35,153,161,163,164-166,168- 171,174
LARYNX						
Glottic	85	95	85	60	35	117-121,126,128-130,136, 141,149
Supragolttic	55	65	65	55	40	109,114,115,122,132,135, 136,138,143,150
HYPOPHARYNX						
Pyriform sinus	25	30	20	15	5	89-90,93-97a,99,102, 103,106
Postcricoid	20	ID	ID	ID	ID	10,35
MAXILLARY SINUS	25	- 35 -		- 15 -		35,176,178,183,189-191

* Excludes patients dead of intercurrent disease.

ID = insufficient data.

2. *Adjuvant aggressive multiagent chemotherapy* is being studied. Intensive efforts are being directed toward the evaluation of pretreatment chemotherapy with 1 to 3 cycles (1b,34a,243). Cisplatin is the most intensively investigated agent with other agents and irradiation.

3. *Potential improvements in radiation therapy* include the use of high-density irradiation such as neutrons or pimesons (214). To date, the major advantage for neutrons has been in salivary gland tumors (15c).

4. *Hyperfractionation* or accelerated fractionation with multiple daily doses of radiation, is being studied and early results appear promising (9d,17a,37b,235). CHART—continuous, hyperfractionated, accelerated radiotherapy in head and neck—has been studied by Saunders *et al.* (32'). Further updating their experience

in advanced T3T4 squamous cell cancers in the upper aerodigestive passages, they note a 90% complete regression for primary and nodes compared to 62% using historical controls with conventional fractionation. This demanding regimen is given t.i.d. (8 a.m., 4 p.m., 8 p.m.) on 12 consecutive days at 1.4–1.5 Gy fractions to a total dose of 50.4 Gy–54 Gy.

5. *Hyperthermia* is a promising new investigational mode when added to irradiation. According to Overgaard *et al.* (30a) hyperthermia has shown improved response in both randomized and non-randomized studies.

6. Through study of hypoxic cell radiosensitizers, a major research effort has been devoted to overcoming the hypoxic cell fraction. Most studies (RTOG, EORTC, Medical Research Council) have been negative using misonidazole (7). The one positive note by Overgaard

Table 21-8. Results of RTOG Registry

Stage T, N (AJC)	Total evaluation	%CR	% dead	Estimated survival rates 1-Year	2-Year	3-Year
T$_2$ N$_0$ (II)	249	95	40	83	71	62
T$_1$ N$_1$ (III)	10	90				
		>88	46	87	63	55
T$_2$ N$_1$ (III)	38	87				
T$_3$ N$_0$ (III)	80	79	59	73	48	37
T$_3$ N$_1$ (III)	38	61	76	45	31	19
T$_1$ N$_2$ (IV)	9	78				
		>7	60	65	35	31
T$_2$ N$_2$ (IV)	34	68				
T$_1$ N$_3$ (IV)	7	57				
		>57	57	54	37	37
T$_2$ N$_3$ (IV)	23	57				
T$_3$ N$_2$ (IV)	30	70	83	53	20	11
T$_3$ N$_3$ (IV)	33	49	82	55	20	17
T$_4$ N$_0$ (IV)	36	75	64	71	48	26
T$_4$ N$_1$ (IV)	14	64	64	54	27	22
T$_4$ N$_2$ (IV)	22	41	77	41	13	2
T$_4$ N$_3$ (IV)	45	31	76	31	22	11

RTOG = Radiation Therapy Oncology Group; T = tumor; N = node; AJC = American Joint Committee; CR = complete response.
From Marcial et al. (26a), with permission.

(30b) in a Danish Head and Neck Cancer Study found that in patients with hemoglobin of less or more than 14g%, the survival improved from 26% to 40%, respectively. This has been refuted, however, by RTOG investigators (10c). (SR 2508 is currently being explored in clinical trials [22a]).

SPECIFIC HEAD AND NECK SITES

The major sites on subdivision of head and neck are illustrated in Fig. 21-3 and constitute the substance and sequence of the remainder of the chapter. Anatomic landmarks are provided by horizontal and vertical lines as shown in Fig. 21-3.

CANCER OF THE ORAL CAVITY

PERSPECTIVE

Oncoanatomically, the oral cavity extends from the skin-vermilion junction anteriorly to the posterior border of the hard palate above and the circumvallate papillae below. Subdivisions within the oral cavity are anterior two thirds of tongue, lip, buccal mucosa, lower alveolar ridge, upper alveolar ridge, retromolar trigone, floor of mouth, and hard palate (3).

The oral cavity is not only anatomically the logical starting point for application of the general principles previously outlined, but also in many respects tumors in this region present in capsular form all the problems encountered in head and neck oncology. Despite the apparently good prospects for early diagnosis, early lesions are too often not recognized as cancers by the general practitioner and dental surgeon.

EPIDEMIOLOGY AND ETIOLOGY

Epidemiology

Oral carcinoma is among the most common aerodigestive cancers. The lip is the most common site and the tongue is

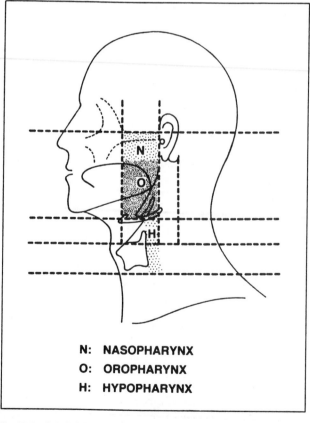

N: NASOPHARYNX

O: OROPHARYNX

H: HYPOPHARYNX

Fig. 21-3. Subdivisions of the pharynx. This figure illustrates the 3 subdivisions of the pharynx. All the lines indicated can be accurately located on the surface by reference to palpable structures: zygomatic arch, external auditory canal, mastoid process, hyoid bone, thyroid cartilage, cricoid cartilage.

only slightly less common (2). The floor of mouth is also a common site. Cancer of the oral cavity is predominantly a disease of men (80%) and occurs at a median age of 55 to 65 years (2).

Etiology

1. Cigarette smoking, pipe smoking, tobacco chewing, and heavy alcohol intake are etiologic factors.
2. Poor oral hygiene and chronic trauma from broken teeth or poorly fitting dentures are also important factors.
3. In females, the Plummer-Vinson syndrome (iron deficiency anemia, glossitis, achlorhydria, koilonychia) may be important.
4. Tertiary syphilis of the tongue (gumma) was significant in the preantibiotic era.
5. Sunlight is an important cause of lip cancer.
6. Unusual cultural habits such as betel nut chewing or reversed smoking in India are well-recognized etiologies of oral cancer.

DETECTION AND DIAGNOSIS

Clinical Detection

1. *Premalignant changes* rarely produce symptoms, and diagnosis rests with the physician's or dentist's awareness and examination. Leukoplakia (white patch) occurs mostly on the lower lip, floor of mouth, buccal mucosa, lateral tongue border, and retromolar region (59,62,65). Less often emphasized is erythroplasia (red patch) — a velvety red lesion of the floor of mouth, lateral tongue border, and soft palate (high-risk sites) (56,59,62). Ninety percent of such lesions are either invasive carcinoma, carcinoma *in situ*, or severe epithelial dysplasia (56) and must always be regarded seriously.
2. Carcinoma usually presents as a *chronic, nonhealing ulcer* and pain is paradoxically rare in early lesions.
3. *Localized pain* is a late symptom indicating deep invasion, perineural involvement, or bone involvement.

4. *Cervical node* presentations are uncommon and, when present, the submandibular or jugulodigastric nodes are enlarged.

Diagnostic Procedures

1. *Inspection* and *palpation* are important first steps. The malignant ulcer is typically raised, centrally ulcerated, and has indurated edges and an infiltrated base.
2. *Biopsy* is mandatory. A negative biopsy should be repeated if clinical index of suspicion is high.
3. *Imaging modality*: Both CT and MRI are useful for staging of advanced carcinomas (Table 21-9) (8).

CLASSIFICATION

Histopathology

1. SCC accounts for 90% to 95% of cancers of the oral cavity usually well- or moderately well-differentiated (15). Unusual variants of SCC may occur: verrucous carcinoma on buccal mucosa or alveolar ridges, and spindle cell SCC, usually as a recurrence following unsuccessful surgery or irradiation.
2. Adenocarcinomas of minor salivary gland origin may be encountered.

TNM Staging

See Table 21-10 (3,17b) and Fig. 21-4 for nodal involvement, distant metastasis, and stage grouping.

Patterns of Spread

Patterns of Local Spread

1. *Tongue* lesions usually arise along the lateral border and infiltrate into tongue muscle, sometimes deeply, demonstrable only by palpation. Extension into base of tongue may occur and carries a bad prognosis. Involvement may extend into floor of mouth, leading in advanced cases to total fixation of the tongue. Exophytic growths show less infiltration.

Table 21-9. Imaging Modalities for Evaluating Carcinoma of the Oral Cavity, Lips and Oropharynx

MODALITY	DIAGNOSIS AND STAGING CAPABILITY	RECOMMENDED ROUTINE STAGING PROCEDURE
Primary tumor and nodes		
CT	Extent of primary tumor and nodal involvement Primary site, nodes	Yes
MRI	Offers 3-D views of primary site and nodes	Yes
Plain films (mandible, soft tissue views)	Gross bone invasion	No
Orthopantomography	Mandibular, hard palate invasion	No
Metastatic		
Chest x-ray films	Look for metastases/second primary tumor	Yes
Radionnuclide Studies	Look for metastases if suspected	Yes

* Metastatic work-up for clinically suspected metastases.
CT = computed tomography; MRI = magnetic resonance imaging.
From Bragg et al. (8), with permission.

Table 21-10.   TNM Classification and Stage Grouping of the Lip, Oral Cavity and Oropharynx

TNM Classification		Stage Grouping			
T1 ≤ 2 cm		Stage 0	Tis	N0	M0
T2 > 2 to 4 cm		Stage I	T1	N0	M0
T3 > 4 cm		Stage II	T2	N0	M0
T4 Adjacent structures		Stage III	T3	N0	M0
			T1	N1	M0
N 1 Ipsilateral single ≤ 3 cm			T2	N1	M0
			T3	N1	M0
N 2 *a) Ipsilateral single > 3 to 6 cm					
*b) Ipsilateral multiple ≤ 6 cm		Stage IV	T4	N0,N1	M0
*c) Bilateral, contralateral ≤ 6 cm			Any T	N2,N3	M0
			Any T	Any N	M1
N 3 > 6 cm					

* New category.
T = tumor; N = node; M = metastasis.
From AJC/UICC (3,17b), with permission.

2. *Floor of mouth* cancers typically arise in the anterior segment to one or the other side of midline and have a deceptive spread pattern to the mandibular periosteum and then along the bone, often for significant distances. Actual bone invasion is a serious event, as is invasion into base of tongue via its inferior surface. Large lesions may fungate into submental skin.

3. *Buccal mucosa* lesions often arise at the occlusal level and typically spread superficially to involve large segments of mucosa. Deep invasion posteriorly leads to pterygoid muscle involvement and trismus — a serious sign. Extension may occur into anterior tonsillar pillar and soft palate. Deep invasion may occur through buccinator muscle into skin of the cheek. Verrucous carcinoma

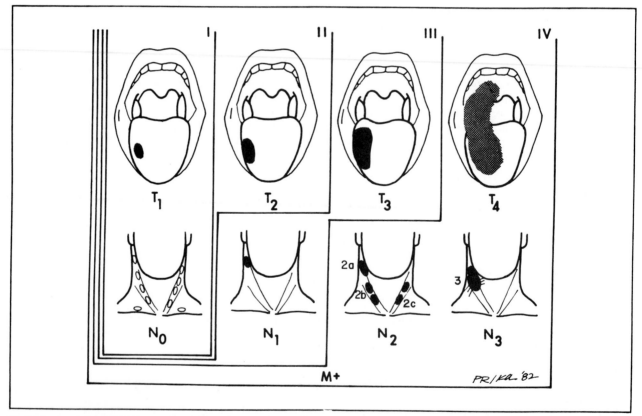

Fig. 21-4. Anatomic staging for cancer of the oral cavity. Tumor (T) categories: The primary tumor is largely characterized by size and then by extension to other sites. The diameters are ≤2 cm, >2 cm, ≤4 cm, and >4 cm for T1, T2, and T3 lesions. Massive tumors expanding into contiguous sites became T4. Node (N) categories: The size, number, and laterality relative to the primary tumor are factors in staging cervical nodes. The diameters are ≤3 cm, >3 ≤6 cm, and >6 cm for N1, N2, and N3. Bilateral or contralateral nodes <6 cm are N2C. Stage grouping: The T category is the major determinant of stage. N1 nodes are equivalent to T3 (stage III) and N2 and N3 nodes as well as M1, along with T4 lesions constitute stage IV.

— a well-differentiated squamous lesion presenting as a warty mucosal growth — may infiltrate deceptively deeply.

4. *Alveolar ridge* carcinomas commonly arise from gingival mucosa in the premolar or molar regions, more commonly from the lower than the upper jaw. Bone invasion is early and superior lesions may extend into maxillary sinus.

5. The *retromolar trigone* is a triangular area behind the last lower molar tooth, and carcinomas in this area may spread posterolaterally into the pterygoid muscles producing trismus. Invasion of ascending mandibular ramus may occur.

6. *Hard palate* carcinomas are rare and adenocarcinoma is more common than SCC (207). Spread is along periosteum and bone invasion may occur.

7. Carcinomas of the *lip* usually arise on the lower lip and infiltrate orbicularis oris muscle early, but they usually have an indolent course with slow progression. Spread along the lip may produce involvement of the entire vermilion margin.

Metastatic Behavior

With the exception of glottic carcinoma, oral cancers have the lowest incidence of cervical metastases of all head and neck sites (10,35). Lip carcinoma produces nodal disease in fewer than 15% of patients (10,57) and is virtually the only head and neck site to involve submental nodes. The remainder of oral cavity carcinomas have nodal disease at diagnosis in 35 to 45% of patients (48,232). Submandibular and jugulodigastric are the commonly affected nodes.

Hematogenous metastases from oral carcinoma occur with a frequency of 15 to 20%, mostly from poorly differentiated, locally advanced lesions having cervical node involvement at presentation (57,230).

Staging Work-up (Table 21-9)

T Work-up

Careful inspection, palpation, and measurement are the first steps. Assessment of the mandible for invasion by the use of plain films and orthopantograms is necessary. CT provides good visualization of the pterygoid region to assess invasion.

(N) Work-up

Bimanual palpation of submental and submandibular regions is necessary. Both sides of the neck should be checked down to clavicles. The number, size, and mobility of enlarged nodes should be noted.

(M) Work-up

Chest films, complete blood cell count (CBC), and Sequential Multiple Analysis (SMA-12) are routine. Specific symptoms need specific work-up (CT or plain chest tomograms, bone scan, liver scan).

PRINCIPLES OF TREATMENT (Table 21-11)

Primary Tumor

Premalignant lesions are best excised and attention directed to removal of inciting factors (smoking, alcohol, poor teeth, denture trauma).

A small primary lesion is best managed by either surgery or irradiation therapy alone. Large lesions (T3 and T4) usually require both modalities and surgery may have to be radical, especially if mandibular periosteum or bone are involved.

Neck Nodes

Overt nodal disease is treated surgically with either radical or modified radical neck dissection (21,227,228). Adjunctive irradiation to the neck is usually indicated if nodes are positive, especially if more than one node is involved, if

Table 21-11. Carcinoma of the Oral Cavity/Oropharynx			(10a,28,35,59a,81',86)
STAGE	SURGERY	RADIATION THERAPY	CHEMOTHERAPY
I $T_1 N_0 M_0$	Radical resection or	CRT 60-65 Gy	NR
II $T_2 N_0 M_0$	Radical resection or	CRT 65-70 Gy	NR
III $T_3 N_0 M_0$ $T_{any} N_1 M_0$	Radical resection and	ART preop v postop 50-60 Gy	IC III CCR
IV $T_4 N_{2,3} M_0$	Unresectable	DRT 50-70 Gy	IC II
Local relapse	RT for surgery relapse	Surgery for RT relapse	IC II CCR
Metastic	NR	NR	IC II
RT = radiation therapy; CRT = curative; ART = adjuvant; DRT = definitive; NR=not recommended; IC II= investigational chemotherapy, phase I/II clinical trials; IC III= investigational chemotherapy, phase II/III clinical trials; CCR = concurrent chemotherapy and radiation.			
PDQ: NR except for IC I,II,III and CCR			

disease is extranodal, or if a modified dissection was done. Under these conditions, both sides of the neck should be irradiated, with 6,000 cGy to the dissected side and 5,000 cGy to the undisturbed side (27).

Radiation therapy is preferred to surgery for elective treatment because of better cosmetic and functional results. Approximately 36% to 40% of initially node-negative patients with primary lesions of the tongue, floor of mouth, buccal mucosa, and retromolar trigone will eventually relapse in the neck, and consideration should be given to elective neck treatment for T2 or larger primary lesions (51,234). Lip lesions do not usually require elective neck treatment (10).

Surgery

Premalignant and small invasive lesions (< 1 cm) are generally easiest to treat by local excision. Larger T1 and T2 lesions are also effectively managed by surgery but resection must be adequate and may include hemiglossectomy for tongue carcinoma or resection of floor of mouth and marginal mandibular resection for a floor of mouth carcinoma. Inadequate margins require re-excision or irradiation and one should not merely wait for the recurrence. Large primary lesions (T3 and T4) treated surgically require radical procedures such as hemiglossectomy, hemimandibulectomy, and incontinuity radical neck dissection (commando procedure). Frozen section check of margins is an important procedure in head and neck surgery, where 3 to 4 cm margins are rarely possible (92). Involved neck nodes are best managed by radical or modified neck dissection. Fixed nodes should receive preoperative irradiation (5,000 cGy to both sides of the neck and 6,000 cGy to the node) in an attempt to mobilize the node and to eradicate extracapsular spread.

Irradiation Therapy

Radiotherapy is highly effective as a sole modality for T1 and T2 lesions within the oral cavity. For lesions in the anterior oral cavity (oral tongue, floor of mouth, buccal mucosa, lip), radioactive implantation is an integral part of irradiation and external irradiation alone produces significantly inferior results (44,45,48,64). A common approach is to combine external irradiation (5,000 cGy to primary and neck) with interstitial implantation (3,000 cGy to primary alone). Permanent eradication of the primary lesions occurs in 80 to 85% of T1 and T2 lesions that are radically irradiated (45,48,53,60,64). Many of the local failures can be salvaged surgically.

Combined Modalities

Both surgery and irradiation are commonly required under three circumstances.

1. a large primary (managed surgically) with clinically negative nodes (managed radiotherapeutically)
2. a small primary (managed radiotherapeutically) with neck nodes (managed surgically)
3. *massive disease* in which both modalities are directed to the same region (primary and/or neck)

In the first circumstance, the treatment sequence is surgery followed by irradiation; in the second, the sequence is irradiation followed by surgery; and in the third, the sequence is variable and usually dictated by the radicality of surgery. (Radical surgery should not be preceded by irradiation or

poor healing may occur.) When both modalities are directed to massive disease, at least one treatment must be radical.

RESULTS AND PROGNOSIS

Overall survival for oral cavity carcinoma, except lip, is between 40% and 65%, depending on site. Early primary lesions fare well, but advanced local disease has a poor outlook. Cervical node status is a significant survival determinant for all sites.

All treatment modalities can produce disability. Surgery may interfere with speech, mastication, and deglutition and irradiation can produce severe xerostomia, dental caries, and mandibular necrosis.

CANCER OF THE OROPHARYNX

PERSPECTIVE

This anatomic region includes the anterior tonsillar pillar, soft palate, uvula, tonsillar fossa and tonsil, base of tongue, and pharyngeal walls (lateral and posterior).

The oropharynx occupies a central position in the aerodigestive decussation. Tumors in this region, as well as their treatment, can have profound effects on all the basic aerodigestive functions: mastication, deglutition, respiration, and phonation. The oropharynx is relatively inaccessible surgically and operation in this site is both radical and formidable. The prognosis for oropharyngeal carcinoma remains relatively poor.

EPIDEMIOLOGY AND ETIOLOGY

Epidemiology

1. These tumors are among the more common head and neck cancers, superseded only by laryngeal carcinomas.
2. Tonsil is the most common primary site.
3. Males are affected more often than females in a ratio of 4:1 and median age is 55 to 65 years (68,73,84).

Etiology

Smoking and heavy alcohol consumption are especially prevalent in this patient population (68,72,85,86).

DETECTION AND DIAGNOSIS

Clinical Detection

1. *Sore throat* or *pain on swallowing* are the most common symptoms. Referred otalgia is also common.
2. Enlargement of *cervical nodes* is a presenting complaint in 20% to 30% (71,72,76).
3. Fetor oris, dyspnea, dysphagia, hoarseness, dysarthria, hypersalivation, fungation through suprahyoid skin are indicators of advanced massive disease.

Diagnostic Procedures

1. Inspection, including an indirect mirror examination, is essential.
2. Palpation should never be omitted. Carcinoma of the base of the tongue may not be apparent visually but obvious on palpation.

3. Biopsy is essential.

4. Imaging: CT and MRI are useful in detecting occult primaries and defining anatomic extensions three-dimensionally (Table 21-9).

CLASSIFICATION

Histopathology

1. More than 90% of carcinomas are *SCC* (15). Well-differentiated lesions are uncommon.

2. *Lymphoepithelioma* may occur in tonsil and base of tongue and is a variant of SCC (15).

3. The soft palate may be the site of *Queyrat's erythroplasia*, a velvety red patch of *in situ* or microinvasive SCC (82).

4. Minor salivary gland carcinomas (usually adenoid cystic or mucoepidermoid) may be encountered.

5. *Lymphoma of Waldeyer's ring* is discussed in Chapter 18, "Malignant Lymphomas."

TNM Classification

See Table 21-10 and Fig. 21-5 for nodal involvement, distant metastases, and stage grouping.

Patterns of Spread

Local Spread Patterns

1. Carcinoma of the *tonsil* commonly extends downwards across the glossotonsillar sulcus into the base of the tongue. Such extension should always be ruled out, for it carries a relatively poor prognosis, especially if the tongue base is significantly infiltrated (74,82). Extension superiorly into soft palate is also common but less ominous. Large lesions may move forward into buccal mucosa or backward into oropharyngeal wall. Trismus indicates deep infiltration into pterygoid muscles.

2. Carcinoma of the *base of the tongue* tends to infiltrate anteriorly into tongue muscle, creating deep necrotic clefts in the base of the tongue, sometimes visible as air-filled cavities on a lateral x ray (13). Advanced lesions spread into the anterior two thirds of the tongue and floor of mouth, producing total fixation of the tongue. Downward extension is via valleculae, epiglottis, and lateral glossoepiglottic ligaments into supraglottic larynx and pyriform sinus.

3. Soft palate carcinomas tend to infiltrate widely within the soft palate, often involving uvula and spreading contralaterally. Anterior extension is via anterior tonsillar pillar into buccal mucosa. Posterolateral extension into the pterygoid muscles produces trismus.

4. Pharyngeal wall carcinomas spread longitudinally into nasopharynx and hypopharynx. Anterior extension leads to involvement of tonsillar fossa, base of tongue, pyriform sinus, aryepiglottic folds, and paraglottic larynx. Posterior extension is limited by prevertebral fascia. These lesions may spread laterally and directly into the neck around the carotid sheath and create circumstances conducive to internal rupture of the carotid artery.

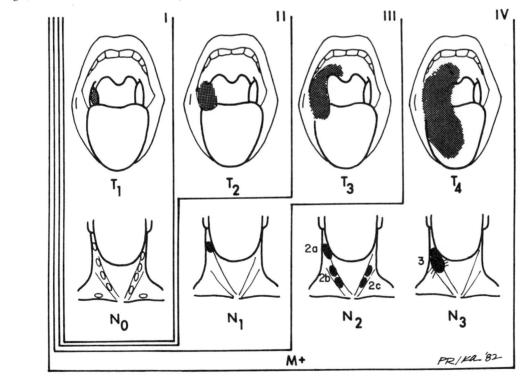

Fig. 21-5. Anatomic staging for cancer of the oropharynx. Tumor (T) categories: The primary tumor is largely characterized by size and then by extension to other sites. The diameters are ≤2 cm, >2cm, ≤4 cm, and >4 cm for T1, T2, and T3 lesions. Massive tumors expanding into contiguous sites become T4. Node (N) categories: The size, number, and laterality relative to the primary tumor are factors in staging cervical nodes. The diameters are ≤3 cm, >3 ≤6 cm, and >6 cm for N1, N2, and N3. Bilateral or contralateral nodes <6 cm are N2C. Stage grouping: The T category is the major determinant of stage. N1 nodes are equivalent to T3 (stage III) and N2 and N3 nodes as well as M1, along with T4 lesions constitute stage IV.

Metastatic Behavior

Oropharyngeal carcinoma has a high propensity to *cervical nodal involvement*. *Tonsillar* and *base of tongue* lesions have palpable metastatic nodes at diagnosis in 60% to 70% cases (80,83,232). *Pharyngeal wall* lesions have involved nodes in 50% to 60% (68,89), and *soft palate* carcinoma has metastasized in 40% to 50% (87). The most common involved nodes are jugulodigastric (tonsillar node). Bilateral nodal disease is not rare. Retropharyngeal node involvement, though clinically not detectable, is common.

Hematogenous metastases have been documented in tonsillar and base of tongue primaries in 10% to 20% of cases (71,77,80,83-85). Lung is the most common site. Pharyngeal wall carcinoma metastasizes less often and soft palate lesions rarely produce hematogenous dissemination. Most hematogenous metastases from oropharyngeal carcinoma occur in patients with massive primary disease and/or massive or bilateral cervical node deposits.

Staging Work-up

1. *T work-up*: Inspection and palpation are important early steps. Examination under anesthesia is recommended for full evaluation. Lateral soft tissue x-ray and CT scanning provide important information.
2. *N work-up*: Careful neck palpation for nodal disease is essential.
3. *M work-up*: Chest x-ray, CBC, and SMA-12 are routine.

PRINCIPLES OF TREATMENT (Table 21-11)

Anatomic and tumor factors dictate the use of irradiation therapy in early lesions and a combined surgical-radiotherapeutic approach in many of the more advanced cases. Anatomically, the oropharynx is relatively inaccessible and adequate surgical exposure usually requires mandibular osteotomy (Trotter's procedure). Conservative approaches through the oral cavity or via lateral submandibular pharyngostomy rarely allow complete removal of tumor (73,92). If disease approaches the mandible a hemimandibulectomy may be necessary. Involved cervical nodes may require a composite resection, often involving a hemimandibulectomy (commando procedure). There is little evidence that these heroic procedures applied for relatively early disease offer any survival advantage over radiation therapy (52,92,233). If cure is a goal in advanced disease, then radical surgery combined with irradiation offers the best prognosis (18,26,69,77,87).

Tumors in the oropharynx tend toward widespread regional infiltration and lymphatic dissemination, often toward surgically inaccessible nodes such as Rouviere's. Total tumor clearance, even by procedures such as pharyngolaryngectomy and radical neck dissection, is unusual and irradiation therapy has a better chance for eradication of widespread but often subclinical regional disease.

Surgery (68,69,73,92)

1. Surgery is recommended in the multimodal approach to advanced but resectable disease (T3 and some T4). Surgical techniques are *radical*, usually requiring mandibular osteotomy, sometimes hemimandibulectomy. Conservative approaches are likely to leave considerable subclinical disease (positive resection margins). Laryngectomy is often necessary to avoid potentially fatal aspiration or to remove disease extension (86,92). Pharyngeal wall lesions often require pharyngolaryngectomy. Intraoperative frozen section analysis of resection margins is necessary (92).
2. Radical or modified neck dissection is necessary if nodes are palpably involved. Bilateral nodal disease is surgically approached by radical dissection on the most advanced side and modified dissection on the contralateral side (10).
3. Reconstruction is essential and preferably should be one-stage to avoid undue delay in delivering postoperative radiation therapy.
4. Irradiation therapy is recommended in addition to surgery for all advanced oropharyngeal carcinoma (18).

Radiation Therapy (67,71,75,76,78,81,89)

1. Irradiation therapy alone is the treatment of choice for all early oropharyngeal carcinomas (T1 and T2). With the exception of T1, N0 lesions where only ipsilateral jugulodigastric nodes need to be treated (79), radiation portals must be large and include not only the primary but all neck lymphatics as well. Pharyngeal wall lesions require irradiation to Rouviere's nodes at the base of skull. Lower cervical nodes down to both clavicles need treatment whether or not clinically involved.
2. For T1 lesions, 6000 to 6500 cGy is adequate to control more than 90% of lesions; T2 disease requires 7,000 cGy for the same local control (81,88,91). More advanced disease is difficult to eradicate with irradiation therapy alone. Doses of 7,500 cGy (or higher) have been reported to control a significant proportion of pharyngeal wall and tonsil T3 and T4 lesions albeit at high complication rates (74,75,81,88). Massive base of tongue cancer is rarely controlled by any acceptable radiation dose (83,85).
3. Elective neck irradiation is recommended for all but the smallest primaries and 5,000 cGy is adequate. Involved nodes need boost doses with electron beams or radioactive implants. If the primary is controlled but nodes fail to regress, then radical or modified neck dissection is necessary.

RESULTS AND PROGNOSIS

Overall 5-year survival is approximately 33% (71,84,85,91). Survival according to anatomic site of primary, T stage, and N stage is given in Table 21-7. Tonsil and soft palate have the best prognosis and pharyngeal wall and base of tongue have a very serious outlook. The mortality in oropharyngeal cancer is due to regionally recurrent or uncontrollable disease (68,75,84,85,90). More radical locoregional treatment produces better freedom from disease above the clavicles, but with longer survival, cryptic metastatic disease becomes evident (13,78). Patients also have a high risk of developing other aerodigestive primary carcinomas or bronchogenic carcinoma due to epithelial field carcinogenesis secondary to smoking. Among survivors, the disabilities produced by treatment can be serious.

CANCER OF THE HYPOPHARYNX

PERSPECTIVE

Anatomically, this area includes the pyriform sinuses, the postcricoid region, and the lower posterior pharyngeal wall. Cancers in this region are among the most lethal of head and neck tumors. Diagnosis is usually late, local disease is advanced, nodal metastases are common, and treatment can be both mutilating and debilitating.

EPIDEMIOLOGY AND ETIOLOGY

Epidemiology

1. Pyriform sinus is the most common site for a primary lesion in this region.
2. The ratio of disease in males exceeds females by 2:1; the median age is 50 to 60 years.

Etiology

1. Heavy tobacco use and alcohol consumption are common antecedent factors.
2. In women, the Plummer-Vinson syndrome (iron deficiency anemia, gastric achlorhydria, and koilonychia) is a predisposing factor, especially for postcricoid carcinoma.

DETECTION AND DIAGNOSIS

Clinical Detection

1. *Odynophagia* (pain on swallowing) is a common presentation. Referred otalgia is also common.
2. *Dysphagia* is a later symptom.
3. *Hoarseness* indicates laryngeal involvement.
4. *Fetor oris*, difficulty in swallowing saliva, and dyspnea are advanced manifestations.
5. *Cervical mass* is often the only symptom.

Diagnostic Procedures

1. *Indirect laryngoscopy* to visualize the lesion.
2. *Direct laryngoscopy*, *esophagoscopy*, and *biopsy* are essential.
3. Imaging by CT and MRI are most valuable for diagnosing tumor extentions (Table 21-12) (8).

CLASSIFICATION

Histopathology

Virtually all lesions are SCC, usually moderately to poorly differentiated (15).

TNM Classification

See Table 21-13 (17b) and Fig. 21-6 for nodal involvement, distant metastasis, and stage grouping.

Patterns of Spread

Local Spread Patterns

1. *Pyriform sinus* lesions arising on the lateral wall invade thyroid cartilage early. Lesions arising on the medial pyriform sinus are intimately related to larynx and invade that organ directly through the aryepiglottic fold, entering the paraglottic larynx. Superior spread may lead to invasion of the oropharyngeal wall or base of tongue and inferior spread may occur into the cervical esophagus.
2. *Postcricoid carcinoma* spreads into the arytenoid region of the larynx, grows circumferentially around the cricopharyngeal region to encircle the upper esophagus, and may spread downward through the esophagus for considerable distances.

Metastatic Behavior

Early cervical node metastases are a hallmark of these lesions. Two-thirds to three-fourths of all patients have palpable nodes at diagnosis, usually jugulodigastric (96,100,102,232). Hematogenous metastases are not uncommon. They become manifest in up to 30% of patients and are usually delayed until the time of local recurrence (95,97,104).

Table 21-12.   Imaging Modalities for Evaluation Carcinoma of the Larynx and Hypopharynx

MODALITY	DIAGNOSIS AND STAGING CAPABILITY	RECOMMENDED ROUTINE STAGING PROCEDURE
Primary tumor and nodes		
CT	Extent of primary tumor and nodal involvement	Yes
MRI	Offers 3-D views, extent of invasion	Optional
Xeroradiographs and lateral soft tissue views	Survey primary site. Look for gross cartilage destruction	No
Barium swallow	Detect, stage hypopharyngeal carcinomas	No
Laryngography	Stage primary laryngeal hypopharyngeal tumor	No
Metastatic		
Chest x-ray films	Look for metastases, second primary	Yes
Radionnuclide studies	Look for metastases if suspected	Yes

Metastatic work-up for clinically suspected metastases.
CT = computed tomography; MRI = magnetic resonance imaging.
Adapted from Bragg et al. (8).

Table 21-13. TNM Classification and Stage Grouping of the Hypopharynx				
TMN Classification	**Stage Grouping**			
T1 One subsite	Stage 0	Tis	N0	M0
T2 > One subsite or adjacent site, without larynx fixation	Stage I	T1	N0	M0
T3 With larynx fixation	Stage II	T2	N0	M0
T4 Invades cartilage, neck, etc.	Stage III	T3	N0	M0
		T1	N1	M0
		T2	N1	M0
N1 Ipsilateral single ≤ 3 cm		T3	N1	M0
N2 *a) Ipsilateral single > 3 to 6 cm	Stage IV	T4	N0,N1	M0
*b) Ipsilateral multiple ≤ 6 cm		Any T	N2,N3	M0
*c) Bilateral, contralateral ≤ 6 cm		Any T	Any N	M1
N3 > 6 cm				

* New Category
T = tumor; N = node; M = metastasis.
From AJC/UICC (17b), with permission.

Staging Work-up

T Work-up
1. Tomograms and plain films may be helpful, but *contrast studies*—laryngogram and barium swallow—are recommended.
2. CT may define the lesion.
3. *Direct laryngoscopy* and *esophagoscopy* should always be done.

N Work-up
Careful *bilateral evaluation* of nodes including geographic mapping, size, number, and mobility is necessary.

M Work-up
Chest x-ray, CBC count, and SMA-12 are routine.

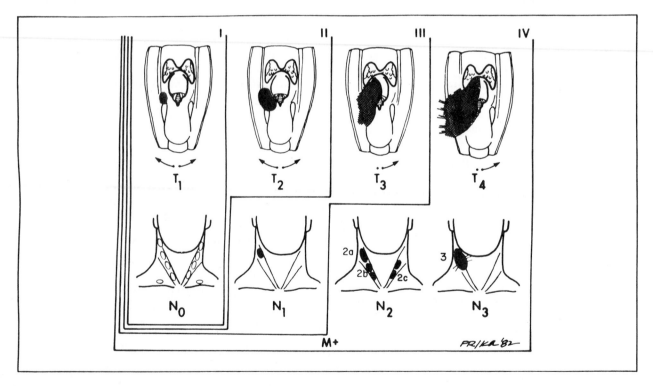

Fig. 21-6. Anatomic staging for cancer of the hypopharynx. Tumor (T) categories: The number of sites and the mobility of the vocal cords, rather than size are the crucial factors. The sites are listed as pharyngoesophageal junction (postcricoid area), pyriform sinus, and posterior pharyngeal wall. The difference between T1 and T2 is extension to more than one site. When the hemilarynx becomes fixed the lesion is T3. Extension into adjacent structures (e.g., cartilage or soft tissues of the neck) is T4. Node (N) categories: The size, number, and laterality relative to the primary tumor are factors in staging cervical nodes. The diameters are ≤3 cm, >3 ≤6 cm, and >6 cm for N1, N2, and N3. Bilateral or contralateral nodes <6 cm are N2C. Stage grouping: The T category is the major determinant of stage. N1 nodes are equivalent to T3 (stage III) and N2 and N3 nodes as well as M1, along with T4 lesions constitute stage IV.

PRINCIPLES OF TREATMENT (Table 21-14)

The uncommon small lesions (T1, early T2) may be adequately managed by irradiation therapy (96,103) or by surgery (93,94). Occasionally conservation surgery is possible (partial pharyngolaryngectomy) (103). The majority of patients, however, require *combined radical surgery* and *radical radiation therapy* if they are candidates for a curative approach (95,96,98,101) (Table 21-14). Palliation in this region is usually also radical if it is to be beneficial.

The preferred approach is radical pharyngolaryngectomy, radical neck dissection for involved nodes, and a one-stage reconstruction followed within 6 weeks by external megavoltage irradiation to 6000 to 6500 cGy (18,27,95). Preoperative irradiation is an alternative approach (96,98,105).

Postcricoid carcinomas pose serious problems by virtue of their direct downward spread and their metastasis to tracheoesophageal nodes, often down into superior mediastinum. Surgery to remove all disease often requires multistage reconstruction, delaying irradiation.

RESULTS AND PROGNOSIS

Early lesions with negative nodes have 5-year survivals higher than 70% (102,103). The majority of cases are, however, advanced and overall survival rarely exceeds 25% in any series (Table 21-7). Postcricoid carcinomas fare more poorly than pyriform sinus lesions. Superradical measures above the clavicles achieve better locoregional control, but longer median survival times unmask hematogenous metastases and 5-year outcomes are little improved compared to conservative measures (95). Systemic therapy will be needed to improve the grim prognosis.

CANCER OF THE LARYNX

PERSPECTIVE

Carcinomas of the larynx are the most common malignant tumors encountered in head and neck oncology. They arise from the epithelial lining of the laryngeal mucous membrane. A clear distinction must be made between lesions arising in the supraglottic larynx (epiglottis, aryepiglottic folds, arytenoids, false cords) and in the glottic larynx (true vocal cord). Subglottic carcinomas are rare. Carcinomas of the larynx, especially glottic lesions, usually are not to life-threatening, and major therapeutic decisions revolve on preservation of laryngeal function. The larynx is an organ of phonation and serves as an air passage and as a sphincter guarding the airway. Treatment decisions depend on the cancer and on the anticipated effect of treatment on each of the three laryngeal functions. Conservation laryngeal surgery has emphasized the importance of the larynx as an airway and a sphincter. Loss of voice due to disease or treatment is a serious handicap, but an ineffective airway or an inefficient sphincter may be fatal.

EPIDEMIOLOGY AND ETIOLOGY

Ninety percent of carcinomas of the larynx occur in males, with a peak incidence in the sixth and seventh decades (124). Glottic carcinoma accounts for 60% to 65% of all laryngeal cancer, the remainder arising in the supraglottis except for a small number (5%) of subglottic primary sites (124,136,148). Laryngeal carcinomas are uncommon among nonsmokers (151) and tobacco is incriminated as an etiologic factor.

DETECTION AND DIAGNOSIS

Clinical Detection

1. *Hoarseness* that persists is the cardinal manifestation of glottic carcinoma; it is much less common with supraglottic carcinoma.
2. *Sore throat* is the common presentation for supraglottic carcinoma.
3. *Referred otalgia* is not uncommon with supraglottic lesions.
4. *Dyspnea* occurs with advanced exophytic carcinomas.
5. *Dysphagia* implies very advanced disease.
6. *Cervical lymphadenopathy*, especially jugulodigastric, may be a presentation of supraglottic carcinoma but virtually never of glottic carcinoma.

STAGE	SURGERY		RADIATION THERAPY	CHEMOTHERAPY
Table 21-14. TREAMENT DECISIONS: Carcinoma of the Hypopharynx (10,28,35,103a)				
I $T_1 N_0 M_0$	Partial/total laryngo-pharyngectomy and RND	or	CRT 65-74 Gy	NR
II $T_2 N_0 M_0$	Partial/total laryngo-pharyngectomy and RND	and	DRT 65-74 Gy	NR
III $T_3 N_1 M_0$	Total laryngo-pharyngectomy	and	ART post-op 65-70 Gy	IC II CCR
IV $T_4 N_{2,3} M_0$	Total laryngo-pharyngectomy with reconstructive surgery	and	ART post-op 65-70 Gy	IC II CCR
Local relapse	RT for surgical relapse		Surgery for RT relapse	IC II
Metastatic	NR		Occasionally	IC II
RT = radiation therapy; CRT = curative; DRT = definitive; ART = adjuvant; NR = not recommended; RCT = recommended chemotherapy; CCR = concurrent chemotherapy and radiation; RND = radical node dissection; IC II= investigtional chemotherapy, phase I/II clinical trials.				
PDQ: RCT = IC II; CCR = Pt + RT.				

Diagnostic Procedures

1. *Indirect laryngoscopy* is essential in all cases of hoarseness.
2. *Direct laryngoscopy* visualizes the lesion accurately.
3. *Biopsy* is mandatory.
4. *Radiologic studies* include a lateral soft tissue x-ray of the neck, frontal laryngeal tomogram, laryngogram, and more recently high resolution CT scanning and MRI. A chest film is necessary for detecting metastases (Table 21-12).

CLASSIFICATION

Histopathology

More than 90% of laryngeal carcinomas are SCC (15). Leukoplakia of the laryngeal mucosa often accompanies carcinoma and a wide spectrum of borderline premalignant epithelial changes may be encountered, sometimes without clear evidence of invasion (15,125,131). Most SCCs of the true cord are well- or moderately well-differentiated. Supraglottic carcinomas tend to be less differentiated. Verrucous carcinoma is a clinicopathologic variant of squamous carcinoma and is characterized by a warty growth showing an extremely well-differentiated pattern (15). Occasionally adenocarcinomas of minor salivary gland origin are encountered.

TNM Classification

See Table 21-15 (3,17b) and Figs. 21-7 and 21-8 for nodal involvement, distant metastasis, and stage grouping.

Patterns of Spread

Local Spread Patterns

1. *Supraglottic carcinoma*: Whole larynx coronal section studies disclose a variety of typical intralaryngeal spread patterns determined to a significant degree by various anatomic subcompartments within the organ (epilarynx, paraglottic space, preepiglottic space, Reinke's space, anterior subglottic triangle, anterior commissure tendon) (112,123,125a,139,146,147). Common patterns include:

- epiglottis to preepiglottic space
- epiglottis to aryepiglottic fold
- aryepiglottic fold to pyriform sinus
- false cord to paraglottic space to preepiglottic space
- false cord to ventricle to true cord

Extension to the anterior commissure at the origin of the thyroepiglottic ligament may lead to thyroid cartilage invasion.

2. *Glottic carcinoma*: One-half of all true cord cancers involve only the anterior third of the cord, and 75% occur in the anterior two-thirds of the cords (124). The anterior commissure is involved in about 15% (134). Anterior subglottic extension may be difficult to detect. Several mechanisms may be responsible for cord fixation and all imply deep invasion. Most commonly, thyroarytenoid muscle invasion is responsible for a fixed cord, but other mechanisms include lateral crico-arytenoid muscle invasion, cricoarytenoid joint involvement, transverse arytenoid muscle invasion, and perineural infiltration (146).

Metastatic Behavior

Cervical node involvement is rare with glottic carcinoma (less than 10% incidence) and occurs only when the disease spreads from the cord into the supraglottic region (124,148).

Primary supraglottic carcinoma has a significant propensity to cervical metastases and 45% to 55% of patients have nodal disease at presentation (109,116,124,137,143,148). The first node involved is usually the jugulodigastric.

Staging Work-up

T Work-up

1. *Direct laryngoscopy* under general anesthesia is important in all cases.
2. *Lateral soft tissue x-rays* of the neck, frontal tomograms, contrast laryngograms, and fluoroscopy may be helpful but are limited in the information they yield on depth of invasion (133).

Table 21-15.   TNM Classification and Stage Grouping of the Larynx

TNM Classification		Stage Grouping			
Glottis		Stage 0	Tis	N0	M0
T1	Limited/mobile				
T1a	One cord	Stage I	T1	N0	M0
T1b	Both cords				
T2	Extends to supra- or subglottis/impaired mobility	Stage II	T2	N0	M0
T3	Cord fixation	Stage III	T3	N0	M0
T4	Extends beyond larynx, cartilage invasion		T1	N1	M0
Supra- and subglottis			T2	N1	M0
T1	Limited/mobile		T3	N1	M0
T2	Extends to subsite glottis/mobile				
T3	*Cord fixation, post cricoid, pyriform sinus, pre-epiglottic space	Stage IV	T4	N0, N1	M0
			Any T	N2, N3	M0
T4	Extends beyond larynx, cartilage invasion		Any T	Any N	M1
All regions					
N1	Ipsilateral single ≤ 3 cm				
N2	*a) Ipsilateral single > 3 cm				
	*b) Ipsilateral multiple ≤ 6 cm				
	*c) Bilateral, contralateral ≤ 6 cm				
N3	> 6 cm				

* New category.
T = tumor; N = node; M = metastasis.
From AJC/UICC (3,17b), with permission.

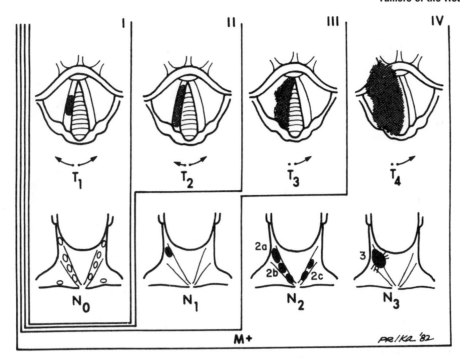

Fig. 21-7. Anatomic staging for cancer of the glottis. Tumor (T) categories: The categories are similar to those for hypopharynx. T1 lesions are confined to one or both vocal cords. Tumor extending to the supraglottis or subglottis and/or impairment of cord mobility constitutes T2. Fixation of the vocal cord is T3 and massive tumors extending beyond the larynx are T4. Nodal (N) categories: The size, number, and laterality relative to the primary tumor are factors in staging cervical nodes. The diameters are ≤3 cm, >3 ≤6cm, and >6 cm for N1, N2, and N3. Bilateral or contralateral nodes <6 cm are N2C. Stage grouping: The T category is the major determinant of stage. N1 nodes are equivalent to T3 (stage III) and N2 and N3 nodes as well as M1, along with T4 lesions constitute stage IV.

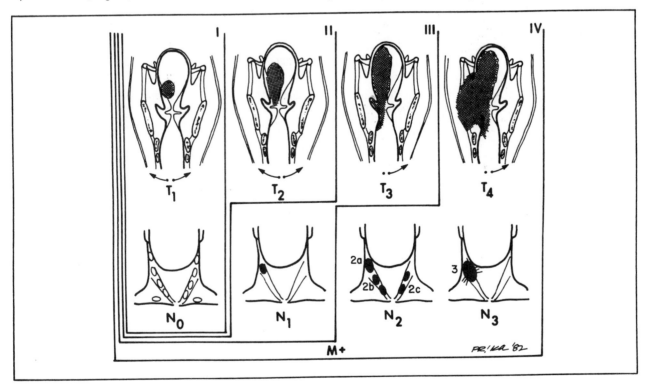

Fig. 21-8. Anatomic staging for cancer of the supraglottis. Tumor (T) categories: The key factors are local extension and cord mobility. The sites within the supraglottis are: false cords (ventricular bands), arytenoids, epiglottis, aryepiglottic folds. T2 tumors involve more than one site or extend to the vocal cords but do not fix the mobility of the cords. T3 lesions are associated with fixed cord. Massive tumors extending beyond the larynx or invading cartilage are T4 Node (N) categories: The size, number, and laterality relative to the primary tumor are factors in staging cervical nodes. The diameters are ≤3 cm, >3 ≤6cm, and >6 cm for N1, N2, and N3. Bilateral or contralateral nodes <6 cm are N2C. Stage grouping: The T category is the major determinant of stage. N1 nodes are equivalent to T3 (stage III) and N2 and N3 nodes as well as M1, along with T4 lesions constitute stage IV.

3. *High resolution CT scanning* promises better evaluation of invasion patterns (140).

N Work-up

Systematic palpation of cervical nodal areas.

M Work-up

This consists of a chest film. CBC count and SMA-12 are routine and specific symptoms need specific investigation.

PRINCIPLES OF TREATMENT

Treatment selection depends on the site and extent of the lesion. Early lesions (T1 or T2, N0, M0) are curable by total laryngectomy, but in the majority of such patients this would constitute overtreatment, producing unnecessary disability. In early laryngeal carcinoma, the treatment goals include preservation of a functioning larynx. In advanced disease, the organ is usually sacrificed.

Supraglottic Carcinoma (109,114,132,144,148) (Table 21-16)

Treatment must be directed at the primary lesion and at cervical lymphatics. Small primary lesions (T1 or T2) are treated equally well by irradiation or supraglottic laryngec-tomy (horizontal partial laryngectomy). Large primary lesions are best managed with total laryngectomy, often in combination with radiation therapy. RND is generally the best management for clinically positive lymph node metasta-ses. Elective neck treatment can be given either by neck dissection or radiation therapy. The large number of treat-ment options requires careful evaluation of each patient's suitability for any procedure and a cooperative interaction between members of the treatment team.

1. *Surgery* by supraglottic laryngectomy controls more than 80% of T1 and T2 supraglottic carcinomas (109,132), but the surgeon and patient must be prepared for total laryngectomy should the partial procedure prove technically impossible. Positive margins require postoperative irradiation. Large primary lesions usually need total laryngectomy (142). Palpable nodes are best managed by radical or modified neck dissection.

2. *Radiation therapy* permanently eradicates disease at the primary site of T1 and T2 lesions in more than 75% of patients (13,113,114,148). Local control is better for T1 lesions (85% to 95%) than for T2 lesions (73% to 80%). Doses ranging from 6600 to 7000 cGy are neces-sary (13,114). Patients who relapse following irradia-tion may be salvaged by total laryngectomy, though

Table 21-16. TREATMENT DECISIONS: Carcinoma of the Supraglottic Larynx and Larynx (10,28,35,123a,135b)

STAGE	SURGERY		RADIATION THERAPY	CT
Supraglottic Larynx				
I $T_1 N_0 M_0$	Supraglottic/partial laryngectomy spare vocal cord	or	CRT 60-65 Gy	NR
II $T_2 N_0 M_0$	Supraglottic laryngectomy and radical neck dissection	and/or	CRT 65-70 Gy	NR
III $T_{1-3} N_1$ $T_3 N_0$	Radical laryngectomy	and/or	CRT 65-70 Gy	and CCR Induction
IV $T_4 N_{2,3} M_0$	Radical laryngectomy plus radical pharyngectomy with reconstructive surgery if possible	and	ART postop 65-70 Gy	and CCR Induction
Local relapse	RT for surgical relapse		Surgery for RT relapse	and IC II
Metastatic	NR		Occasionally	IC II

PDQ: RCT - CCR Induction with CisPt + 5-FU prior to DRT. (31b*)

STAGE	SURGERY	RADIATION THERAPY	CT
Larynx			
I $T_1 N_0 M_0$	Laryngofissure/hemilaryng ectomy	Definitive RT preferred 60-65 Gy	NR
II $T_2 N_0 M_0$	Hemilaryngectomy or total laryngectomy	Definitive RT preferred 60-70 Gy	NR
III $T_3 N_1 M_0$	Radical laryngectomy and radical neck dissection	Definitive RT or postop 65-70 Gy	CCR Induction
IV $T_4 N_1 M_0$	Radical laryngectomy and radical neck dissection	Definitive RT or postop RT 65-70 Gy	CCR Induction
Relapse	Salvage RT	Salvage surgery	IC II
Metastatic	NR	Possibly	IC II

RT = radiation therapy; CRT = curative; DRT = definitive; NR = not recommended; RCT = recommended chemotherapy; CCR = concurrent chemotherapy and radiation; IC II = investigational chemotherapy, phase I/II clinical trials.

rarely by horizontal laryngectomy (107,145). More advanced supraglottic carcinomas are rarely controlled at the primary site by irradiation alone, though selected cases with more exophytic lesions have been reported to achieve 40% to 50% local control (113,114). More often, these patients have respiratory distress and cervical metastases, and are managed surgically. Radiation therapy is often added preoperatively or postoperatively (110,111). The treatment of choice for subclinical neck disease is radiation therapy.

Glottic Carcinoma (113,119,121,126,136,148,149) (Table 21-16b)

Glottic carcinoma only rarely requires treatment directed to the cervical lymphatics. Early glottic carcinomas (TIS, T1, or T2) are equally well treated by irradiation or by various conservation surgical procedures (cord stripping, cordectomy, or vertical hemilaryngectomy, as indicated). Fixed cord lesions do less well with irradiation, though local control has been achieved in selected patients. Cartilage invasion contraindicates radiation therapy as the primary modality.

1. *Surgery* is generally used for T3 and T4 primary lesions as well as for involved neck nodes. Radiation therapy is recommended as an adjunct. Postsurgical stomal recurrence occurs with subglottic extension and can be prevented by irradiation that includes the tracheal stoma (148).
2. *Radiation therapy* achieves local control of TIS, T1, or T2 glottic carcinomas in more than 75% of patients (119,120,121). Prospects for local control are better for TIS and T1 lesions (equal to or greater than 85%) than for T2 lesions (75% to 80%) (127). Doses of 6000 to 6600 cGy are adequate (13,119, 120). Care must be taken not to underdose the anterior commissure region when it is involved (134). Selected T3 cases may be irradiated (124), but cartilage destruction indicating extensive disease rarely contollable by irradiation, indicates surgery (108). Million (127a) covers in masterful style the management of laryngeal cancer from its earliest to its most advanced stage. The current approach to treatment is based on a thorough analysis of various dose/time fractionation regimens.

RESULTS AND PROGNOSIS

Prognosis in supraglottic carcinoma is mainly determined by cervical node status and in glottic carcinoma by cord mobility. *Supraglottic carcinoma* without cervical metastases has a 5-year survival of 70% to 80%; with cervical node disease the survival falls to 30% to 50% (124,143,148). *Glottic carcinoma* has a 5-year survival of 80% to 90% in the absence of cord fixation, but falls to 50% to 60% with cord fixation (139,147). In institutions following a policy of radiation therapy for early laryngeal cancer, significantly more T1 and T2 patients retain a functional larynx (70% to 80%) than if surgery is the first line of treatment (40% to 60%) (13,109,123a,135a).

CANCER OF THE NASOPHARYNX

PERSPECTIVE

The protean clinical manifestations of nasopharyngeal carcinoma (NPC) can lead to prolonged misdiagnosis; thus, a high index of suspicion is required. Although it is rare, NPC is actively under investigation because of its association with EBV.

EPIDEMIOLOGY AND ETIOLOGY

This disease is uncommon in white populations (2% of all head and neck cancer) (2). The age distribution is bimodal, with a small peak in adolescence and young adulthood and the major peak occurring between aged 50 and 70 years (153). This disease is not associated with tobacco consumption. A strikingly high incidence of NPC is found among the southern Chinese, where it accounts for 13% to 20% of all cancer and up to 57% of all head and neck cancer (159,171). This high incidence is fairly definitely linked to environment and customs rather than genetics (159). EBV is incriminated as a carcinogen or cocarcinogen in the majority of patients (white and Asian) with NPC (152,158,160,167). High titers of IgG and IgA antibodies to EBV antigens are present in the vast majority of NPC patient sera (158,167).

DETECTION AND DIAGNOSIS

Clinical Detection

1. *Common presentations* are lymphadenopathic (cervical node with unknown primary), otologic (due to Eustachian obstruction), and nasal.
2. *Atypical pain* due to trigeminal involvement or base of skull destruction can be a perplexing diagnostic problem.
3. Cranial nerve involvement occurs in 15% of cases and most commonly involves nerves V and/or VI (156,172). Involvement of cranial nerves II to VI results from superior extension of cancer through foramen lacerum into the middle cranial fossa. Less commonly involved are nerves IX to XII and/or the sympathetic nerves (Horner's syndrome). Involvement of these lower nerves is due to retropharyngeal (Rouviere) node metastasis. Nerves VII and VIII are rarely affected.

Diagnostic Procedures

1. Nasopharyngoscopy with a nasopharyngeal mirror or via fiber optic nasopharyngoscope is mandatory whenever the diagnosis of NPC is a possibility.
2. Biopsy is necessary.
3. Lateral skull films may be strikingly informative in showing a posterosuperior soft tissue bulge impinging on the airway.
4. Anti-EBV antibodies.
5. Imaging is best performed by contrast enhanced CT and MRI. CT is superior for bone destruction and MRI for soft tissue extentions (Table 21-17) (8).

CLASSIFICATION

Histopathology

Ninety percent of these lesions are SCCs or its variants (15,156). NPC has a tendency toward poor differentiation and unusual growth patterns. A profusion of terms has developed (keratinizing carcinoma, nonkeratinizing carcinoma, anaplastic carcinoma, undifferentiated carcinoma, lymphoepithelioma, transitional cell carcinoma) that are of doubtful significance. The World Health Organization recommends the following nomenclature (15,168):

- keratinizing SCC (<30%)
- nonkeratinizing carcinoma (50% to 70%)
- lymphoepithelioma (25%)
- Salivary gland carcinoma (5%)

Nonkeratinizing carcinoma and lymphoepithelioma are variants of SCC

TNM Classification

See Table 21-18 (3,17b) and Fig. 21-9 for nodal involvement, distant metastasis, and stage grouping.

Patterns of Spread

1. *Superior*: Via foramen lacerum into cavernous sinus (the petrosphenoidal crossway) with involvement of cranial nerves II to VI and erosion of skull base.
2. *Anteriosuperior*: Into infratemporal fossa and foramen ovale to involve mandibular division of nerve V.
3. *Lateral*: Into medial ostium of the Eustachian tube, producing obstruction and obstructive serous otitis media with conductive deafness (actual spread along the Eustachian tube is exceptionally rare).
4. *Posterior*: Into prevertebral muscle, producing pain upon flexion or extension of the head.
5. *Anterior*: Into nasal cavity and then paranasal sinuses.
6. *Inferior*: Into oropharyngeal wall and soft palate.

Metastatic Behavior

1. NPC is notorious for early and extensive *cervical node disease*, especially if the histology is lymphoepithelioma. Seventy percent to 85% of NPC patients have palpable nodes at diagnosis (153,158,232). Nodal disease is bilateral or contralateral in 40% to 50% of all cases (232). The most common nodal group is the jugulodigastric, followed by the upper posterior cervical group deep to the upper end of the sternomastoid. Retropharyngeal nodes of Rouviere are commonly affected, but usually not detected. Nodal disease can be extensive while the primary lesion is small.

2. Hematogenous metastases are a significant problem—an overall incidence of 25% in most series (161,165, 168,170). Patients with bilateral cervical nodes have up to a 40% likelihood of developing distant disease. Paradoxically, bone is a more common site than lung.

Staging Work-up

T Work-up

Careful neurologic examination of all cranial nerves is performed. Lateral skull films often reveal the characteristic tumor pattern. Radiologic views of the base of the skull allow evaluation of foramina. CT scanning allows excellent visualization of the nasopharynx and is becoming indispensable in the work-up.

N Work-up

Careful palpation and measurement of all cervical nodal sites is performed. Horner's syndrome, hoarseness, and hemiatrophy of the tongue all indicate Rouviere's node involvement.

M Work-up

Chest x-ray, CBC count, and SMA-12 are routine. Specific symptoms need specific investigation (e.g., bone scan and x-rays for bone pain).

The value of anti-EBV antibody titers in staging has not been delineated, but evidence suggests that higher titers correlate with more advanced disease (167).

PRINCIPLES OF TREATMENT

1. The inaccessibility of the nasopharynx, the proximity of the tumors to the skull base and to cranial nerves and the widespread lymphatic involvement dictate radiation therapy rather than surgery as the procedure of choice (Table 21-19). Irradiation techniques for NPC are especially complex and should only be undertaken by experienced radiation therapists.
2. There is *no place for small-volume irradiation* in the primary treatment of NPC. Radiation fields encompass structures from the base of the skull to clavicles, and use

Table 21-17. Imaging Modalities for Evaluating Carcinoma of the Nasopharynx

MODALITY	DIAGNOSIS AND STAGING CAPABILITY	RECOMMENDED ROUTINE STAGING PROCEDURE
Primary tumor and nodes CT	Extent of primary tumor and nodal involvement	Yes
MRI	Offers 3-D views of primary site and nodes	Yes
Plain films nasopharynx (lateral soft tissue view) based view skull	Gross screening: gross skull base destruction	Optional
Conventional tomography	Bone destruction skull base; suggest soft tissue extent of primary	No
Nasopharyngography	Superficial extent	No
Metastatic x-ray films	Look for metastases, second primary	Yes
Radionnuclide studies	Look for metastases if suspected	Yes

CT = chemotherapy; MRI = magnetic resonance imaging.
Adapted from Bragg et al. (8).

Table 21-18. TNM Classification and Stage Grouping of the Nasopharynx

TNM Classification		Stage Grouping			
T1	One subsite	Stage 0	Tis	N0	M0
T2	> One subsite	Stage I	T1	N0	M0
T3	Invades nose/oropharynx	Stage II	T2	N0	M0
T4	Invades skull/cranial nerve	Stage III	T3	N0	M0
			T1	N1	M0
N1	Ipsilateral single ≤ 3 cm		T2	N1	M0
			T3	N1	M0
N2	Ipsilateral single > 3 to 6 cm				
	Ipsilateral multiple ≤ 6 cm	Stage IV	T4	N0,N1	M0
	Bilateral, contralateral ≤ 6 cm		Any T	N2,N3	M0
			Any T	Any N	M1
N3	> 6 cm				

T = tumor; N = node; M = metastasis.
From AJC/UICC (3,17b).

is made of a shrinking-field pattern to deliver highest doses to gross disease (13,165,167,173).

3. *Keratinizing* and *nonkeratinizing* carcinomas require 6500 cGy for T1 and T2 lesions, and 7000 cGy for T3 and T4 disease. *Lymphoepithelioma* needs 6000 cGy for T1 or T2, and 6500 cGy for T3 and T4 (13,159,165).
4. Neck nodes require electron beam or interstitial boosts.

5. Occasionally, neck dissection may be indicated for persistent lymphadenopathy if the primary is controlled and distant metastases are absent.

RESULTS AND PROGNOSIS

The overall 5-year survival is 45% (161-166,168). Prognosis is related to T stage, N stage, and histology (161,162,163a,165,

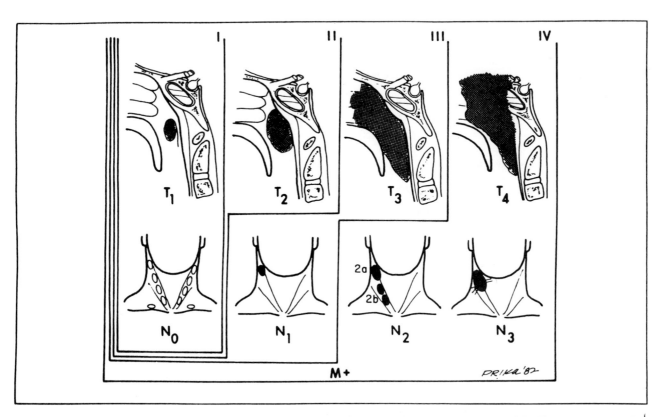

Fig. 21-9. Anatomic staging for cancer of the nasopharynx. Tumor (T) categories: The categories are based on sites of involvement, extension beyond the nasopharynx and skull or cranial nerve involvement. The sites are: posterosuperior wall, lateral wall, including the fossa of Rosenmuller, and the inferior wall consisting of the superior surface of the soft palate. T2 tumors involve more than one site within the nasopharynx, whereas extension into the nasal cavity or oropharynx constitutes T3. Skull base or cranial nerve involvement is T4. Nodal (N) categories: The size, number, and laterality relative to the primary tumor are factors in staging cervical nodes. The diameters are ≤3 cm, >3 ≤6cm, and >6 cm for N1, N2, and N3. Bilateral or contralateral nodes <6 cm are N2C. Stage grouping: The T category is the major determinant of stage. N1 nodes are equivalent to T3 (stage III) and N2 and N3 nodes as well as M1, along with T4 lesions constitute stage IV.

Table 21- 19. TREATMENT DECISIONS: Carcinoma of the Nasopharynx (10a,28,35,168a)

STAGE	SURGERY	RADIATION THERAPY	CHEMOTHERAPY
I $T_1 N_0 M_0$	NR	CRT, 65-70 Gy	NR
II $T_2 N_0 M_0$	NR	CRT, 65-70 Gy	NR
III $T_{1-3} N_1 M_0$	NR	CRT, 70-75 Gy	IC III
$T_3 N_0 M_0$			
IV $T_4 N_{2,3} M_0$	NR	DRT, 70-75 Gy	IC III
$T_{any} N_{any} M_0$			
N_0	NR	RT, 50 Gy	NR
N_{1-3}	NR	DRT, 60-70 Gy	IC III
Relapse and recurrence	NR	Occasionally PRT with introcavitary source	IC II
RT = radiation therapy; DRT = definitive; CRT = curative; NR = not recommended; IC II = investigational chemotherapy, phase I,II clinical trials; IC III = investigational chemotherapy, phase II,III clinical trials.			
PDQ: NR - IC III (31b*)			

168). Survival decreases from 50% to 60% for T1 lesions to 10% to 20% for T4 lesions. Patients without palpable nodes have a 50% to 75% survival; with palpable nodes, prognosis falls to 20% to 40% (155,161,166,174). Lymphoepithelioma has a better prognosis (60% to 65%) than SCC (40% to 45%) (162,165). As radiation techniques have improved, local control has also improved, but hematogenous metastases have been unmasked. Currently, 40% of all failures relapse at the primary site only, while 60% are metastatic failures (161,165). Integration of chemotherapy into the treatment program, especially for locally advanced disease, is increasingly a necessity.

Disabilities produced by radiation therapy includ xerostomia, dental caries, otitis media, trismus, soft tissue necrosis, pituitary dysfunction, and cranial nerve dysfunction. Cervical cord myelopathy should be avoided by careful technique.

CANCER OF NASAL FOSSA AND PARANASAL SINUSES

PERSPECTIVE

The ease with which cancers spread from one region to another within the nasal-paranasal cavities demands consideration of this region as an oncoanatomic unit. Cancer in this area progresses insidiously, masquerading as chronic sinusitis. Diagnosis is often delayed until the lesion is well advanced.

NASAL FOSSA: EPIDEMIOLOGY AND ETIOLOGY

This is a rare disease. Males are affected more commonly than females (3:1) and median age is 50 to 60 years (175,178,184). Chronic sinusitis and/or nasal polyps precede the disease in 10% to 20% of cases (179). A higher-than-expected incidence of adenocarcinoma is found in furniture workers (179).

DETECTION AND DIAGNOSIS

1. *Presenting symptoms* are unilateral nasal obstruction or epistaxis.

2. *Diagnostic procedures* include direct inspection with nasal speculum, fiberoptic nasal exam, and biopsy.

CLASSIFICATION

Histopathology

Eighty-five percent of carcinomas in the nasal fossa are SCC (175). Transitional cell carcinoma is a poorly differentiated variant of SCC.

Minor salivary gland adenocarcinomas may occur (adenoid cystic or mucoepidermoid) and malignant melanoma may also be encountered. The nasal cavity is also the site of origin for the extremely rare esthesioneuroblastoma.

TNM Classification

No accepted staging classification has been proposed.

Patterns of Spread

Local Spread Patterns

The most common site of origin is on the middle or inferior turbinate. The septum, vestibule, floor, and choanae may also be originating. Spread is along the walls of the nasal cavity and disease easily enters the maxillary sinus, and posteriorly, the nasopharynx. Bone destruction is demonstrable radiographically in about 30% of cases (178,184).

Metastatic Behavior

Cervical nodes are rarely involved (less than 15%) and usually only with locally advanced disease (177,178). Jugulodigastric and submandibular are the common nodal sites. Hematogenous spread is exceptionally rare.

Staging Work-up

T workup only is necessary. This involves careful assessment of both nasal cavities and *all paranasal sinuses*. Radiologic assessment is crucial: facial bone x-rays and views of maxillary, frontal, and ethmoid sinuses should be studied. Anteroposterior tomograms are necessary. CT is invaluable for optimal assessment.

PRINCIPLES OF TREATMENT (178,187,188)

Surgery and irradiation are equally effective for smaller lesions. Large lesions require a combined approach.

1. *Radiation therapy* is preferred for small lesions because of better cosmetic results. Lesions of the septum may be treated by radiation implants. Lesions invading bone are best treated surgically.
2. *Surgery* is used for lesions invading the bone.

RESULTS AND PROGNOSIS

Reported 5-year survivals are usually between 55% and 85% (175,178,188), depending on stage. Small lesions limited to one region (e.g., turbinate) have cure rates in excess of 90% (175).

MAXILLARY SINUS

Ethmoid, frontal, and sphenoid sinus cancers are rare and will not be considered. General information is contained in reference 35.

EPIDEMIOLOGY AND ETIOLOGY

Maxillary sinus lesions account for 80% to 90% of all paranasal sinus cancers (10,35). The disease is somewhat more common in males. There is sometimes a history of long-standing sinusitis.

DETECTION AND DIAGNOSIS

Clinical Detection

1. Early lesions masquerade as *sinusitis*. Any sinusitis showing bone sclerosis or destruction must be fully investigated, including biopsy.
2. *Typical presentations* include nasal obstruction, bloody nasal discharge, unilateral sinusitis, loosening of teeth, poor fitting of dental plates, and paresthesia of anterior cheek. Diplopia and epiphora indicate orbital invasion.
3. Inspection of oral cavity may show tumor extension into upper alveolus and hard palate. Palpation of the infraorbital ridge for irregularity is important.

Diagnostic Procedures

1. *Biopsy* of accessible lesions and/or antrostomy-biopsy are essential.
2. Imaging: Sinus films, tomograms, and *CT scans* are used to evaluate soft tissue swelling and bone destruction (24,36) (Table 21-20) (8).

CLASSIFICATION

Histopathology

More than 85% of these lesions are SCCs with various degrees of differentiation (15). Minor salivary gland adenocarcinomas are also encountered.

TNM Classification (Table 21-21) (3,17b)

Ohngren's line, joining the medial canthus of the eye with the angle of the mandible, is used to divide the maxillary sinus into an anteroinferior portion (the infrastructure) and a posterosuperior portion (the suprastructure) (3,180).

See Table 21-21 (3,17b) and Fig. 21-10 for nodal involvement, distant metastasis, and stage grouping.

Patterns of Spread

Local Growth Patterns

Lesions of the *suprastructure* tend to break through the floor of the orbit, involve infraorbital nerve, and displace the eye, causing diplopia. Extension superomedially leads to involvement of the ethmoid sinuses. Posterior extension leads to involvement of the pterygoid plates, muscles, infratemporal fossa, and skull base.

Infrastructure lesions erode through the floor of the sinus and appear as fungations on the superior maxillary alveolus, gingivobuccal sulcus, and hard palate. Anterior extension erodes through the zygomatic bone to the skin of the cheek.

Table 21-20. Imaging Modalities for Evaluating Carcinoma of the Paranasal Sinus

MODALITY	DIAGNOSIS AND STAGING CAPABILITY	RECOMMENDED ROUTINE STAGING PROCEDURE
Primary tumor and nodes		
CT	Extent of primary tumor and nodal involvement	Yes
MRI	Offers 3-D views of primary site and nodes	Yes
Conventional tomography	Good for detail of bone destruction; suggestive of extent of soft tissue invasion and likelihood of brain and orbital spread	No
Orthopantomography	Good for bone detail, hard palate, and maxillary alveolar ridge	No
Angiography	Occasionally for diagnosis (e.g. juvenile angiofibroma); usually for adjunctive therapy (eg arterial infusion of chemotherapeutic agent)	No
Metastatic		
x-ray films	Look for metastases, second primary	Yes
Radionnuclide studies	Look for metastases if suspected	No

CT = computed tomography; MRI = magnetic resonance imaging.
Adapted from Bragg et al. (8).

Table 21-21. TNM Classification and Stage Grouping of the Maxillary Sinus

TNM Classification		Stage Grouping			
T1	Antral mucosa	Stage 0	Tis	N0	M0
T2	Infrastructure, hard palate, nose	Stage I	T1	N0	M0
T3	Cheek, floor of orbit, ethmoid, posterior wall of sinus	Stage II	T2	N0	M0
		Stage III	T3	N0	M0
T4	Orbital contents and other adjacent structures		T1	N1	M0
			T2	N1	M0
			T3	N1	M0
N1	Ipsilateral single ≤ 3 cm	Stage IV	T4	N0,N1	M0
N2	*a) Ipsilateral single > 3 to 6 cm		Any T	N2,N3	M0
	*b) Ipsilateral multiple ≤ 6 cm		Any T	Any N	M1
	*c) Bilateral, contralateral ≤ 6 cm				
N3	> 6 cm				

* New category
T = tumor; N = node; M = metastasis.
From AJC/UICC (3,17b), with permission.

Metastatic Behavior

Cervical node involvement is uncommon (10% to 15%); when it occurs it is usually to the ipsilateral submandibular node (184). Distant metastases are uncommon and usually appear with massive, locally recurrent disease.

Staging Work-up

T Work-up

Full assessment of all potential directions of spread (superior, inferior, medial, and lateral) is essential. Sinus films, tomograms, (anteroposterior and lateral) are traditional, but CT scanning provides incomparably more data and is recommended in all cases (24).

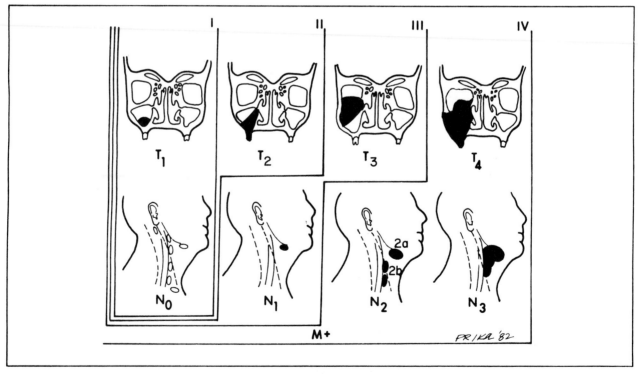

Fig. 21-10. Anatomic staging for cancer of the maxillary sinus. Tumor (T) categories: depth of penetration and extension to adjacent structures are the key criteria. T1 tumors are limited to the mucosa. T2 tumors erode bone inferiorly, while T3 tumors erode bone more extensively but do not extend into adjacent regions. T4 tumors invade surrounding structures including the orbit, cribiform plate, posterior ethmoids, nasopharynx, base of skull. Node (N) categories: The size, number, and laterality relative to the primary tumor are factors in staging cervical nodes. The diameters are ≤3 cm, >3 ≤6cm, and ≥6 cm for N1, N2, and N3. Bilateral or contralateral nodes <6 cm are N2C. Stage grouping: The T category is the major determinant of stage. N1 nodes are equivalent to T3 (stage III) and N2 and N3 nodes as well as M1, along with T4 lesions constitute stage IV.

N Work-up

Careful palpation of neck, especially of submandibular region, is necessary. Bimanual palpation often helps.

M Work-up

Chest films, CBC count, and SMA-12 are routine.

PRINCIPLES OF TREATMENT

1. While it is possible to cure a portion of early lesions with surgery alone, (181,186) or with irradiation alone (183,184), the most fruitful approach for most cases is a *combined surgical-radiotherapeutic* program (182,183,185,188) (Table 21-22). The argument of preoperative or postoperative irradiation is unsettled (182). Preoperative radiation therapy has some theoretic advantages and is the recommended approach. Preirradiation sinus drainage by fenestration of the palate or transnasal antrostomy is recommended for most patients in to deal with infected necrotic tumor (184). Patients with pyrexia or zygomatic bone involvement should always be treated with this procedure. This is followed by 6,000 cGy of external megavoltage irradiation to include all known disease extension. Orbital shielding is only applied when there is absolutely no breakthrough of the orbital floor. Maxillectomy follows 4 to 6 weeks after completion of irradiation. Orbital exenteration may be needed.

2. If residual disease remains following surgery, additional irradiation may be given via radium mold inserted into the surgical defect.

3. Neck dissection is added for involved nodes.

4. *Reconstruction* is important for appearance, speech, and eating. Prosthetic devices may be required.

RESULTS AND PROGNOSIS

Overall 5-year survival is 20% to 30%. The mortality of this disease is largely due to locally recurrent disease leading to base of skull and intracranial invasion (178,184,186).

TUMORS OF THE EAR

PERSPECTIVE

Tumors of the external and middle ear complex are rare but pose serious management problems The lesions often masquerade as chronic inflammatory or degenerative diseases, which resultis in delayed diagnosis. Important tumors in this region are carcinomas and chemodectomas.

CLASSIFICATION

No universally accepted classification has been proposed. A useful subdivision classified these lesions in terms of their site of origin.
- carcinoma of the auricle
- carcinoma of the external auditory canal
- carcinoma of the petromastoid (origin in the middle ear — mastoid complex)

Carcinoma of the auricle is a variant of skin cancer with a correspondingly excellent outlook. Carcinomas of the auditory canal and of the petromastoid have a poor prognosis, largely due to delay in diagnosis, their proximity to vital structures, and a tendency toward conservative therapeutic measures. More than 85% of the mortality of ear cancer is due to local recurrence leading to intracranial extension (189,191,193).

PRINCIPLES OF TREATMENT

Small lesions limited to the auditory canal can be managed by surgery or irradiation therapy. However, most patients require an aggressive combined surgical-radiotherapeutic approach. Radical resection, which may involve resection of the temporal bone, followed by irradiation therapy, is the treatment of choice for most patients (190,192).

Table 21-22. TREATMENT DECISIONS: Carcinoma of the Maxillary Sinuses (10,28,35,188a)			
STAGE	SURGERY	RADIATION THERAPY	CT
I $T_1 N_0$	Complete resection of maxillary sinus sparing eye if possible	ART Optional postop	NR
II $T_2 N_0$	Surgical decompression before RT; complete resection of maxillary sinus except for externation of orbit	ART 50-60 Gy Preop and/or postop	NR
III $T_3 N_0$	Surgical decompression before RT complete resection of maxillary sinus except for exteration	ART 50-60 Gy Preop and/or postop	IC II
IV $T_4 N_3$	Unresectable	DRT 70 Gy	IC II
Relapse after treatment	NR	NR	IC II
For N_0	NR	NR	NR
For $N_1 N_2$	Radical neck dissection if primary controlled	Postop RT	IC II
RT = radiation therapy; ART = adjuvant; DRT = definitive; NR = not recommended; CT = chemotherapy; IC II = investigational chemotherapy, phase I/II clinical trials.			
PDQ: NR - IC II (31b*)			

CHEMODECTOMA

PERSPECTIVE

Chemodectomas of the temporal bone (glomus jugulare tumors) are locally destructive, nonmetastasizing neoplasms arising from glomus bodies along the course of the Jacobson's nerve (tympanic branch of the glossopharyngeal) or the Arnold's nerve (auricular branch of the vagus). Histologically, these tumors are similar to carotid body tumors and are characterized by an exceedingly high vascularity. No universally accepted classification has been proposed.

DETECTION AND DIAGNOSIS

1. *Clinical presentations* include deafness, pulsatile tinnitus, otalgia, facial paralysis, and otorrhea. Symptoms are usually of several years standing. Females are more commonly affected than males, and the median age is 50% to 60 years (196,199,203).
2. *Diagnosis* demands a high index of suspicion. Otoscopy is abnormal in 90% (195,203), revealing a pulsating red ear drum or a polypoid mass in the external canal. *Petrous tomograms* are essential to evaluate bone destruction. *Carotid arteriography* is diagnostic in most cases (202,204) and reveals a characteristic vascular blush best visualized with subtraction techniques. *Biopsy* may be hazardous because of extreme bleeding and is not necessary in most cases.

PRINCIPLES OF TREATMENT

Treatment for lesions arising in the tympanic cavity (glomus tympanicum) without significant extension is surgical excision (195,198,203). Lesions arising in the jugular bulb (glomus jugulare) are best managed by radiation therapy. Doses of 4500 to 5000 cGy produce prolonged growth delay and probably permanent control in most patients (196,200,201, 205). Radiation therapy will usually improve tinnitus, otalgia, and otorrhea (197,200,205). Hearing is rarely restored and cranial nerve palsies are usually permanent. Surgical resection for glomus jugulare lesions is done in some centers and good results have been reported with this formidable procedure (195,203).

RESULTS AND PROGNOSIS

Prognosis for survival is excellent; fewer than 10% of patients die from this disease within 5 years of diagnosis (199,200,205). However, recurrences are not rare and often are delayed by 5, 10, or more years (194-196). At least 10% of patients will have a second chemodectomy in the head and neck region (202).

TUMORS OF THE SALIVARY GLANDS

PERSPECTIVE

Salivary gland tumors are a perplexing subgroup of head and neck neoplasms. Their diverse histologic structure, variation of origin site, relatively poor correlation between histopathology and clinical behavior, and long natural history all pose therapeutic problems.

EPIDEMIOLOGY AND ETIOLOGY

Both sexes are equally affected and the disease may occur at any age. Median age is 40 to 50 years (15). Radiation exposure is the only known etiologic factor.

Eighty percent of salivary tumors occur in the parotid gland and of these, two thirds are benign; 10% of tumors occur in the submandibular gland; about one half are benign. The sublingual glands are extremely rare sites of origin of salivary tumors and in this site most lesions are malignant. Minor salivary glands account for 10% of salivary tumors; two thirds of these are malignant (213,223,224).

DETECTION AND DIAGNOSIS

Clinical Detection

1. *Parotid lesions* present as a swelling in the parotid area. Clinical features suggestive of parotid malignancy include rapid growth of lesion, local pain, facial palsy, tenderness, attachment to surrounding structures, trismus, and palpable cervical nodes.
2. *Submandibular lesions* present as a painless, firm mass.
3. *Minor salivary lesions* may occur anywhere along the mucosa of the aerodigestive tract and usually present as nodular surface growths often without ulceration. Hard palate is the most common site.

Diagnostic Procedures

1. Tumor may masquerade as acute infection; the character of salivary discharge should be noted and a culture taken.
2. Bimanual examination should be performed for parotid, submandibular, and sublingual lesions to locate site of primary and exclude calculi.
3. Imaging: Plain x-ray and sialogram may be helpful in major gland lesions, but have been supplanted by CT and/or MRI (Table 21-23) (8).
4. Needle aspiration cytology is accurate in a high proportion of cases and may be done.
5. *Incisional biopsies* are generally *not* performed. Parotid lesions can be diagnosed by *superficial lobectomy —* frozen section examination. Submandibular gland lesions need excision and frozen section evaluation.
6. Minor salivary gland tumors are diagnosed by standard biopsy.

CLASSIFICATION

Histopathology

Outside the parotid gland the most common salivary cancer is adenoid cystic carcinoma, followed by mucoepidermoid carcinoma (15). Malignant mixed tumors and acinic cell carcinomas are rare outside the parotid. Mucoepidermoid carcinoma is subclassified into a low-grade variant that behaves similarly to a benign lesion, and a high-grade fully malignant variant (207,222,223).

TNM Classification (3,217)

Each T category is subdivided into (a) no local extension; and (b) local extension. Local extension is clinical or macroscopic

Table 21-23. Imaging Modalities for Evaluating Carcinoma of the Major Salivary Gland

MODALITY	DIAGNOSIS AND STAGING CAPABILITY	RECOMMENDED ROUTINE STAGING PROCEDURE
Primary tumor and nodes		
CT	Extent of primary tumor and nodal involvement	Yes
MRI	Offers 3-D views of primary site and nodes	Yes
Plain films of face, mandible	Show bone involvement or other etiology for mass	No
Sialography	Mass intrinsic, extrinsic; some suggestion of benign vs. malignant	No
Pleuridirectional tomography	Invasion of facial canal or temporal bone	No
Metastatic		
Chest x-ray films	Look for metastases, second primary	Yes
Radionuclide studies	Look for metastases if suspected	No

CT = computed tomography; MRI = magnetic resonance imaging.
Adapted from Bragg et al. (8).

evidence of invasion of skin, soft tissues, bone, or nerve. For classification purposes, microscopic evidence alone of local extension is not a criterion.

See Table 21-24 (3,17b) and Fig. 21-11 for nodal involvement and distant metastases.

Patterns of Spread

Local Growth Patterns

Parotid gland cancers arise in the superficial lobe (lateral to facial nerve) in 90% of cases (213,219,223). Local growth is by expansion and infiltration of parotid gland. Facial nerve paralysis is virtually diagnostic of malignancy. Large lesions involve skin and may erode the mandible. Deep lobe lesions may present as an oropharyngeal growth or with involvement of the lower four cranial nerves (218). Adenoid cystic carcinoma in all sites has a tendency to involve peripheral nerves and to spread centrally in a perineural pattern.

Submandibular and *sublingual growths* spread beyond the gland early and enter surrounding tissues.

Metastatic Behavior

The incidence of cervical node metastases according to histologic subtype is malignant mixed tumor, 25%; adenoid cystic carcinoma, 15%; and high-grade mucoepidermoid carcinoma, 50% to 60% (210,212,220-223). Hematogenous metastases are not uncommon and have been documented with incidences for malignant mixed tumor of 33%, adenoid cystic carcinoma 40% to 50%, and high-grade mucoepidermoid of 33% (15,221,223).

Table 21-24. TNM Classification and Stage Grouping of the Salivary Gland

TNM Classification		Stage Grouping			
T1	< 2 cm	Stage I	T1a	N0	M0
			T2a	N0	M0
T2	> 2 to 4 cm Categories divided: (a) no extension (b) extension	Stage II	T1b	N0	M0
			T2b	N0	M0
			T3a	N0	M0
T3	> 4 to 6 cm	Stage III	T3b	N0	M0
			T4a	N0	M0
T4	> 6 cm		Any T (except T4b)	N1	M0
N1	Ipsilateral single ≤ 3 cm	Stage IV	T4b	Any N	M0
			Any T	N2,N3	M0
N2	*a) Ipsilateral single > 3 to 6 cm *b) Ipsilateral multiple ≤ 6 cm *c) Bilateral, contralateral ≤ 6 cm		Any T	Any N	M1
N3	> 6 cm				

* New category.
T = tumor; N = node; M = metastasis.
From AJC/UICC (3,17b), with permission.

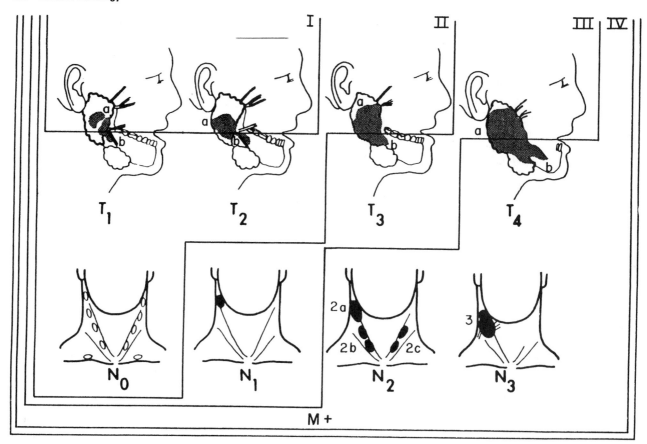

Fig. 21-11. Anatomic staging for cancer of the salivary glands. Tumor (T) categories: The size and extensions into adjacent tissue are the determinants of T category. The sizes are ≤2 cm, >2 ≤4, >4 ≤6 cm, <6 cm for T1, T2, T3, and T4. Depending on the absence (a) or presence (b) of local extension (e.g., facial nerve, skin, bone) each T category is subdivided into "a" or "b". Nodal (N) categories: The size, number and laterality relative to the primary tumor are factors in staging cervical nodes. The diameters are ≤3 cm, >3 ≤6 cm, and >6 cm for N1, N2, and N3. Bilateral or contralateral nodes <6 cm are N2C. Stage grouping: The T category is the major determinant of stage. N1 nodes are equivalent to T3 (stage III) and N2 and N3 nodes as well as M1, along with T4 lesions constitute stage IV.

Staging Work-up

T Work-up

Careful inspection, palpation, and cranial nerve evaluation are the first steps. Sialograms for parotid or submandibular lesions may be indicated. Tomograms and CT scans are useful.

N Work-up

Careful palpation of cervical nodal regions with measurement of size, documentation of number, and fixation of nodes are included in the workup.

M Work-up

Chest x-ray, CBC count, and SMA-12 are routine.

PRINCIPLES OF TREATMENT (Table 21-25)

Surgery (208,213,219,222,224)

1. Surgery is the primary treatment for all salivary gland tumors. For parotid lesions an attempt is made to spare the facial nerve.
2. For low-grade malignancies, neck dissection is reserved for those with palpable nodes. In high-grade lesions, elective neck dissection is indicated.

Radiation Therapy

Irradiation is used for residual, recurrent, and inoperable salivary gland cancers. All high-grade malignancies, including adenoid cystic carcinoma, should receive postoperative irradiation (215).

Neutron beam irradiation is highly effective in locoregional control of advanced salivary gland tumors and is under active investigation (15c,206,216).

RESULTS AND PROGNOSIS

Five-year survivals according to histology are malignant mixed tumor, 40% to 50%; high-grade mucoepidermoid carcinoma, 42%; and adenoid cystic carcinoma, 69%. Adenoid cystic carcinoma has a prolonged natural history and lengthy survival is possible even with overt metastatic disease (209-211,219). In one series (221), survival fell from 69% at 5 years to 40% at 10 years and 22% at 20 years. A number of large series of patients (>1000 patients) are being reported from mainland China, establishing a 5-year and 10-year survival rate of 47% to 33%, respectively, using radiation doses of 58 to 65 Gy (154). Continuous schedules are superior to split-course therapy (169). Of great interest are the excellent results obtained by Wang and Goodman (223a) for

Table 21-25. TREATMENT DECISION: Carcinoma of the Parotid Gland (10,28,35,218a)

STAGE	SURGERY	RADIATION THERAPY	CT
I $T_1 N_0$	Excisional biopsy including either, or both, superficial and deep lobes	NR	NR
II $T_2 N_0$	Excisional biopsy including either, or both, superficial and deep lobes	ART 60-65 Gy for intermediate and high grade; neck nodes 50-60 Gy	NR
III $T_3 N_{0,1}$	Radical resection of parotid; radical resection of neck nodes, unless fixed	CRT-Neutrons (28 Gy neutron dose); 65-70 Gy or mix of photons and electrons; unilateral neck nodes 50-60 Gy	IC I
IV $T_4 N_{2,3}$	Radical resection of parotid; radical resection of neck nodes, unless fixed	DRT-Neutrons (28 Gy neutron dose); For perineural invasion extend fields to cover nerve paths to base of skull Boost fields to residuum 70 Gy	IC I
Relapse	Radical resection, if possible; if nodes palpable, radical neck dissection	PRT 65-70 Gy as for stage IV disease	IC I

RT = radiation therapy; ART = adjuvant; CRT = curative; DRT = definitive; PRT = palliative; NR=not recommended; IC I= investigational chemotherapy, phase I clinical trials.
PDQ: NR (31b*)

unresectable salivary gland tumors with accelerated b.i.d. photon schedule and a variety of boosting techniques for a total of 65–70 Gy. Their 5-year actuarial local control rate for parotid tumor was 100% and survival rate was 65%; for minor salivary gland tumor the local control rate was 78% and the survival rate was 93%.

Recommended Reading

Ackerman and del Regato's book (10) is the best comprehensive introduction to this subject (pp 226-377). The two volumes edited by Thawley et al. (35) constitute an excellent, though formidable, textbook. Less intimidating though excellent texts are those of Million and Cassissi (28), and McQuarrie et al. (23b). The surgical perspective is well presented by Freund (14), and Lore (23). Radiation therapy perspectives are presented by Fletcher (13), Moss and Cox (30), Perez and Brady (31), and Wang (38a). The pathology of head and neck cancer is comprehensively presented by Gnepp (15). A recent *Seminars in Oncology* series devoted to head and neck cancers, edited by Brady (1988) summarizes and updates the RTOG clinical trials involving thousands of cases and different scientific questions to optimize radiation treatment (7). An assortment of critical questions and essays on "Head and Neck Oncology, Clinical Management" appear in an edited volume by Kagan and Miles (1989) (18c).

REFERENCES

General References

1. Aguilar, N.V.; Olson, M.L.; Shedd, D.P. Rehabilitation of deglutition problems in patients with head and neck cancer. Am. J. Surg. 124:489-492; 1972.
1a. Al-Sarraf, M. Head and Neck Cancer: Chemotherapy Concepts. Semin Oncol. Vol. 15, (1): 70-85; 1988.
1b. Al-Sarraf, M.; Tapazoglou, E.; Ensley, J.F.; Ahmad, K.; Jacobs, J.R. et al. Significant loco-regional control of advanced head and neck cancer (HN-CA) with concurrent cisplatin and radiotherapy (RT) after initial response to induction chemotherapy (CT). In: Proc Am Soc Clin Oncol. 9:173;1990. Abstract.
1c. Amdur, R.J.; Parson, J.T.; Mendenhall, M.W.; Million, R.R.; Cassisi, N.J. Split-course versus continuous-course irradiation in the postoperative setting for squamous cell carcinoma of the head and neck. Int. J. Rad. Oncol Biol Phys. 17:279-286;1989.
2. American Cancer Society. Cancer statistics, 1989. CA. 39:3-20; 1989.
3. American Joint Committee on Cancer. Manual for Staging for Cancer. 3rd ed. Philadelphia, PA: J.B. Lippincott Co; 1988.
4. Arthur, K.; Farr, H.N. Prognostic significance of histologic grade in epidermoid carcinoma of the mouth and pharynx. Am. J. Surg. 124:489-492; 1972.
5. Ballantyne, A.J. Surgical modifications necessary after radiation therapy in treatment for head and neck cancer. In: Neoplasia of head and neck. Chicago, IL: Year Book Medical Publishing; 85-96:1974.
5a. Bataini, J-P. The ESTRO Regaud lecture: Head and neck cancer and the radiation oncologist. Radiother and Oncol. 21:1-10; 1991.
6. Bedwinek, J.M.; Shukovsky, L.J.; Fletcher, G.H.; et al. Osteonecrosis in patients treated with definitive radiotherapy for squamous cell carcinomas of the oral cavity and naso- and oropharynx. Radiology. 119:665-667; 1976.
7. Brady, L.W. Davis, L.W. Head and neck cancer. Treatment of head and neck cancer by radiation therapy. Semin Oncol. 15:29-38;1988.
8. Bragg, D.G.; Rubin, P.; Youker, J.E. Oncologic Imaging. Elmsford, NY: Pergamon Press; 1985.
8a. Bragg, D.G.; Shidria, H.; Chu, F.C.H.; et al. The clinical and radiographic aspects of radiation osteitis. Radiology. 97:103-111; 1970.
8b. Brandsma, J.L.; Steinberg, B.M.; Abramson, A.L.; Winker, B. Presence of human papillomavirus type 16 related sequences in verrucous carcinoma of the larynx. Cancer Res. 46:2185-2188; 1986.
9. Brock, W.A.; Baker, F.L.; Wike, J.L.; Sivon, S.L.; Peters, L.J. Cellular radiosensitivity of primary head and neck squamous cell

carcinomas and local tumor control. Int. J. Rad. Oncol. Biol. Phys. 18:1283-1287; 1990.

9a. Bull, T.R.; Myers. E. Plastic Reconstruction in the Head and Neck. London, UK: Butterworths; 1986.

9b. Cognetti, F.; Pinnaro, P.; Carlini, P.; *et al.* CABO treatment (cisplatin, methotrexate, bleomycin, vincristine) in advanced or recurrent squamous cell carcinoma of the head and neck. J. Exp. Clin. Cancer Res. 3:411-417; 1984.

9c. Cooper, J.S.; Pajak, T.F.; Rubin, P.; *et al.* Second malignancies in patients who have head and neck cancer: incidence, effect on survival and implications based on the RTOG experience. Intl. J. Radiat. Oncol. Biol. Phys. 17(3):449-456; 1989.

9c*. Cox, J.D.; Pajak, Y.F.; Marcial, V.A.; *et al.* ASTRO plenary: Interfraction interval is a major determinant of late effects, with hyperfractionated radiation therapy of carcinomas of upper respiratory and digestive tracts: Results from Radiation Therapy Oncology Group protocol 8313. Int. J. Radiat. Oncol. Biol. Phys. 20:1191-1196; 1991.

9d. Cox, J.D.; Pajak, T.F.; Marcial, V.A.; Hanks, G.E.; Mohiuddin, M.; Fu, K.K.; Byhardt, R.W.; Rubin, P. Dose-response for local control with hyperfractionated radiation therapy in advanced carcinomas of the upper aerodigestive tracts: preliminary report of Radiation Therapy Oncology Group protocol 83-13. Int. J. Rad. Oncol. Biol. Phys. 18:515-522; 1990.

9e. Dabelsteen, E.; Clausen, H. Tumor-associated carbohydrate antigens. J. Oral Pathol. Med. 16:196-198; 1987.

9f. Deacon, J.; Peckham, M.J.; Steel, G.G. The radioresponsiveness of human tumors and the initial slope of the cell survival curve. Radiother. Oncol. 2:317-323;1984.

10. del Regato, J.A.; Spjut, H.J.; Cox, J.D. Ackerman and del Regato's Cancer: Diagnosis, Treatment and Prognosis. 6th edition. St. Louis, MO: C V Mosby; 226-377:1985.

10a. DeVita, V.T.; Hellman, S.; Rosenberg, S.A. Cancer Principles and Practice of Oncology, 3rd ed. Philadelphia, PA: J.B. Lippincott Co; 1989.

10b. Eisenberg, E.; Murphy, G.F.; Krutchkoff, D.J. Involucrin as a diagnostic marker in oral lichenoid lesions. Oral Surg. Oral Med. Oral Pathol. 64:313-319; 1987.

10c. Fazekas, J.T.; Scott, C.; Marcial, V.; Davis, L.W.; Wasserman, T.; Cooper, J.S. The role of hemoglobin concentration in the outcome of misonidazole-sensitized radiotherapy of head and neck cancers: based on RTOG trial #79-15. Int. J. Rad. Oncol. Biol. Phys. 17:1177-1182;1989.

10d. Fernandez, B.; Lund, J.; Meyers, F. Epithelial membrane antigen expression in benign and malignant squamous epithelium of the head and neck. Otolaryngol. Head Neck Surg. 97:288; 1987.

10e. Fertil, B.; Malaise, E.P. Inherent cellular radiosensitivity as a basic concept for human tumor radiotherapy. Int. J. Rad. Oncol. Biol. Phys. 7:621-629;1981.

10f. Fertil, B.; Malaise, E.P. Intrinsic radiosensitivity of human cell lines correlated with radioresponsiveness of human tumors: analysis of 101 published survival curves. Int. J. Rad. Oncol. Biol. Phys. 11:1699-1707;1985.

11. Fletcher, G.H. Basic principles of the combination of irradiation and surgery. Intl. J. Radiat. Oncol. Biol. Phys. 5:2091-2096; 1972.

11a. Fletcher, G.H. Controversial issues in the management of cervical metastases. Int. J. Rad. Oncol. Biol. Phys. 19: 1101-1102; 1990.

12. Fletcher, G.H. Elective irradiation of subclinical disease in cancers of the head and neck. Cancer 29:1450-1454; 1972.

13. Fletcher, G.H. Textbook of Radiotherapy. 3rd ed. Philadelphia, PA: Lea & Febiger; 1980:229-443.

14. Freund, H.R. Principles of Head and Neck Surgery. 2nd ed. New York,NY: Appleton-Century-Crofts; 1979.

15. Gnepp, D.R. Pathology of the Head and Neck. New York, NY: Churchill Livingstone; 1988.

15a. Goldsmith, M.M.; Cresson, D.H.; Arnold, L.A.; Postma, D.S.; Askin, F.B.; Pillsbury, H.C. Part I: DNA flow cytometry as a prognositic indicator in head and neck cancer. Otolaryngol. Head Neck Surg. 96:307; 1987.

15b. Grabel-Pietrusky, R.; Hornstein, O.P. Flow cytometric measurement of ploidy and proliferative activity of carcinomas of the oropharyngeal mucosa. Arch. Dermatol. Res. 273:121-128; 1982.

15c. Griffin, T.W.; Pajak, T.F.; Laramore, G.E.; *et al.* Neutron versus photon irradiation of inoperable salivary gland tumors: results of an RTOG-MRC cooperative randomized study. Intl. J. Radiat. Oncol. Biol. Phys. 15(5):1085-1090; 1988.

15d. Harnsberger, H.R.; Dillon, W.P. Imaging tumors of the central nervous system and extracranial head and neck. In: Holleb, A.I., ed. Imaging in Cancer. New York, NY: American Cancer Society, Inc.; 1987:89-102.

15e. Harnsberger, H.R.; Dillon, W.P. The Radiologic Role in Diagnosis, Staging, and Follow-up of Neoplasia of the Brain, Spine and Head and Neck. Seminars in Ultrasound CT and MR. Vol 10: (6):431-452;1989.

16. Hart, G.B.; Mainous, E.G. The treatment of radiation necrosis with hyperbaric oxygen (OHP). Cancer 37:2580-2585; 1976.

17. Hong, W.K.; Lippman, S.M.; Itri, L.; Karp, D.D.; Lee, J.S. Prevention of second malignant tumors (SMTs) in head and neck cancer with 13-cis-retinoic acid (13cRA): placebo-controlled, double-blind randomized trial. Proc Am Soc Clin Oncol. 9: 17;1990.Abstract.

17a. Horiot, J.C.; van den Bogaert, W.; Ang, K.K.; van der Schueren, E.; Bartelik, H.; Gonzalez, D.; de Pauw, M.; van Glabbeke, M. European Organization for Research on Treatment of Cancer trials using radiotherapy with multiple fractions per day: a 1978-1987 survey. Front. Radiat. Ther. Oncol. 22:149-161; 1988.

17b. International Union Against Cancer (UICC). TNM Classification of Malignant Tumors. 4th ed. New York, NY: Springer-Verlag; 1987: 83-88.

17c. Jacobs, C.; Makuch, R. Efficacy of adjuvant CT for patients with resectable head and neck cancer: a subset analysis of the head and neck contracts program. 8; (5): 838-847;1990.

18. Jaram, B.; Strong, E.W.; Shah, J.; *et al.* Elective postoperative radiation therapy in stages III and IV epidermoid carcinoma of the head and neck. Am. J. Surg. 149:580-584; 1980.

18a. Jenson, A.B.; Lancaster, W.D.; Hartman, D.P.; Shaffer, E.L. Frequency and distribution of papillomavirus structural antigens in verrucae, multiple papillomas, and condylomata of the oral cavity. Am. J. Pathol. 107:212-218; 1982.

18b. Johnson, T.S.; Williamson, K.D.; Cramer, M.M.; *et al.* Flow cytometric analysis of head and neck carcinoma DNA index and S-fraction from paraffin embedded sections: Comparison with malignancy grading. Cytometry. 6:461-470; 1985.

18c. Kagan, A.R.; Miles, J., ed. Head and Neck Oncology: Clinical Management. Elmsford, NY: Pergamon Press; 1989.

19. Keys, H.M.; McCashland, J.P. Techniques and results of a comprehensive dental care program in head and neck cancer patients. Intl. J. Radiat. Oncol. Biol. Phys. 1:859-866; 1976.

19a. Kish, J.A.; Weaver, A.; Jacobs, J.; *et al.* Cisplatin and 5-flurouracil infusion in patients with recurrent and disseminated epidermoid cacer of the head and neck. Cancer. 53:1819-1824; 1984.

20. Kogelnik, H.D.; Fletcher, G.H.; Jesse, R.H. Clinical course of patients with squamous cell carcinoma of the upper respiratory and digestive tracts with no evidence of disease 5 years after initial treatment. Radiology. 115:423-427; 1975.

20a. Kokal, W.A.; Gardine, R.L.; Sheibani, K.; Zak, I.W.; Beatty, J.D.; Riihimaki, D.U.; Wagman, L.D.; Terz, J.J. Tumor DNA content as a prognostic indicator in squamous cell carcinoma of the head and neck region. Am. J. Surg. 156:276; 1988.

20b. Laramore, G.E.; Scott, C.B.; Al-Saraff, M.; *et al.* Adjuvant chemotherapy for resectable squamous cell carcinomas of the head and neck; Report on Intergroup Study 0034. Int. J. Radiat. Oncol. Biol. Phys. 23(4):705-714; 1992.

21. Larson, D.L.; Ballantyne, A.J.; Guillamondegui, O.M., eds. Cancer in the Neck. Evaluation and Treatment. New York: Macmillan; 1986.

22. Lederman, M. The anatomy of cancer with special reference to tumors of the upper air and food passages. J. Laryngol. Otol. 78:181-208; 1964.

22a. Lee, A.W.M.; Sham, J.S.T.; Poon, Y.F.; Ho, J.H.C. Treatment of stage I nasopharyngeal carcinoma: analysis of the patterns of relapse and the results of withholding elective neck irradiation. Int. J. Rad. Oncol. Biol. Phys. 17:1183-1190; 1989.

22a*. Leibel, S.A.; Ling, C.C.; Kutcher, G.J.; *et al.* The biological basis for conformal three-dimensional radiation therapy. Int. J. Radiat. Oncol. Biol. Phys. 21:805-811; 1991.

22a**. Leibel, S.A.; Scott, C.B.; Mohiuddin, M.; *et al.* The effect of local-regional control on distant metastatic dissemination in carcinoma of the head and neck: Results of an analysis from the RTOG head and neck database. Int. J. Radiat. Oncol. Biol. Phys. 21:549-556; 1991.

22b. Lester, E.P.; Johnson, C.M.; Lester, A.K.; *et al.* Head and neck advanced squamous carcinoma: treatment with cis-platinum, bleomycin, and sequential methotrexate/5-fluorouracil (abstract C-707). Proc. Am. Soc.Clin. Oncol. 3:182; 1984. Abstract.

22c. Licciardello, J.T.W.; Spitz, M.R.; Hong, W.K. Multiple primary cancer in patients with cancer of the head and neck: second cancer of the head and neck, esophagus and lung. Intl. J. Radiat. Oncol. Biol. Phys. 17(3):467-476; 1989.

22d. Lippman, S.M.; Hong, W.K. Second malignant tumors in head and neck squamous cell carcinoma: the overshadowing threat for patients with cancer of the head and neck: second cancer of the head and neck, esophagus and lung. Intl. J. Radiat. Oncol. Biol. Phys. 17(3):691-694; 1989.

22e. Lippman, S.M.; Kessler, J.K.; Meyskens, F.L., Jr. Retinoids as preventive and therapeutic anticancer agents (part I). Cancer Treat. Rep. 71(4):391-405; 1987.

22f. Lippman, S.M.; Kessler, J.K.; Meyskens, F.L.; Jr. Retinoids as preventive and therapeutic anticancer agents (part II). Cancer Treat. Rep. 71(5):493-515; 1987.

23. Lore, J.M. An Atlas of Head and Neck Surgery. Philadelphia, PA: W B Saunders, Co; 1988.

23a. McDonald, S.; Haie, C.; Rubin, P.; *et al.* Second malignant tumros in patients with laryngeal carcinoma: diagnosis, treatment and prevention. Intl. J. Radiat. Oncol. Biol. Phys. 17(3):457-465; 1989.

23b. McQuarrie, D.G.; Adams, G.L.; Shous, A.R.; Browne, G.A. Head and neck cancer. Clinical decisions and management principles. Chicago, IL: Year Book Medical Publishers; 1986.

24. Mancuso, A.A.; Hanafee, W.N. Computed tomography of the head and neck. Baltimore, MD: Williams and Wilkins; 1982.

25. Maor, M.H.; Hussey, D.H.; Fletcher, G.H.; *et al.* Fast neutron therapy for locally advanced head and neck tumors. Intl. J. Radiat. Oncol. Biol. Phys. 7:155-163; 1981.

26. Marcial, V.A.; Hanley, J.A.; Ydrach, A.; *et al.* Tolerance of surgery after radical radiotherapy of carcinoma of the oropharynx. Cancer. 46:1910-1912; 1980.

26a. Marcial, V.A.; Pajak, T.F.; Kramer, S.; Davis, L.W.; Stetz, J.A.; Laramore, G.E.; Jacobs, J.R.; Al-Sarraf, M.; Brady, W. Radiation Therapy Oncology Group (RTOG) studies in head and neck cancer. Semin in Oncol. 15(1):39-60;1988.

26b. Marcial-Vega, V.A.; Cardenes, H.; Perez, C.A.; Devineni, V.R.; Simpson, J.R.; Fredrickson, J.M.; Sessions, D.G.; Spector, G.G.; Thawley, S.E. Cervical metastases from unknown primaries: radiotherapeutic management and appearance of subsequent primaries. Int. J. Rad. Oncol. Biol. Phys. 19: 919-928; 1990.

26c. Marcus, R.B.; Million, R.R. The incidence of myelitis after irradiation of the cervical spinal cord. Int. J. Rad. Oncol. Biol. Phys. 19(1): 3-8;1990.

27. Marcus, R.B.; Million, R.R.; Cassisi, N.J. Postoperative irradiation for squamous cell carcinomas of the head and neck: an analysis of time-dose factors related to control above the clavicles. Intl. J. Radiat. Oncol. Biol. Phys. 5:1943-1949; 1979.

27a. Mendenhall, W.M.; Million, R.R.; Cassisi, N.J. Elective neck irradiation in squamous cell carcinoma of the head and neck. Head Neck Surg. 3:15-20; 1980.

27b. Merlano, M.; Tatarek, R.; Grimaldi, A.; *et al.* Phase I-II trial with cisplatin and 5-FU in recurrent head and neck cancer: an effective outpatient schedule. Cancer Treat. Rep. 69:961-964; 1985.

28. Million, R.R.; Cassisi, N.J., eds. Management of Head and Neck Cancer. A Multidisciplinary Approach. Philadelphia, PA: J B Lippincott Co; 1984.

28a. Million, R.R.; Cassisi, N.J.; Clark, J.R. Cancer of the head and neck. In: DeVita, V.T., Jr.; Hellman, S.; Rosenberg, S.A. eds. Cancer: Principles and Practice of Oncology. 3rd ed. Philadelphia, PA: JB Lippincott Co.; 1989:488-590.

29. Mira, J.G.; Wescott, W.B.; Starcke, E.N.; *et al.* Some factors influencing salivary function when treating with radiotherapy. Intl. J. Radiat. Oncol. Biol. Phys. 7:535-541; 1981.

30. Moss, W.T. ; Cox, J.D., eds. Radiation Oncology: Rationale, Technique, Results. 6th ed. St. Louis, MO: C V Mosby Co; 1989.

30a. Overgaard, J. The current and potential role of hyperthermia in radiotherapy. Int. J. Rad. Oncol. Biol. Phys. 16:535-550; 1989.

30b. Overgaard, J.; Hansen, H.S.; Andersen, A.P.; Hansen, M.H.; Horgensen, K.; Sandberg, E.; Berthlesen, A.; Hammer, R.; Pedersen, M. Misonidazole combined with split-course radiotherapy in the treatment of invasive carcinoma of the larynx and pharynx (final report from the DAHANCA 2 study). Int. J. Rad. Oncol. Biol. Phys. 16:1065-1069;1989.

31. Perez, C.A.; Brady, L.W. Principles and practice of radiation oncology, 2nd ed. Philadelphia, PA: J B Lippincott Co; 1992:610-805.

31a. Peters, L.J.; Brock, W.A.; Chapman, J.D.; Wilson, G. Predictive assays of tumor radiocurability. Amer. J. Clin. Oncol. 1:275-287; 1988.

31b. Peters, L.J.; Chapman, D.J.; Withers, H.R. Conclusions: prediction of tumor treatment response. In: Prediction of Tumor Treatment Response. Elmsford, NY: Pergamon Press; 1988:317-320.

31b*. Physicians' Data Query. Head and Neck Cancer. Nat'l Cancer Inst; Bethesda, MD; January 1992.

31c. Pitman, S.W.; Kowal, C.D.; Bertino, J.R. Methotrexate and 5-fluorouracil in sequence in squamous head and neck cancer. Semin. Onocl. 10(suppl. 2):15-19; 1983.

31d. Price, L.A.; Hill, B.T. Lack of survival advantage in patients with advanced oral cavity tumors despite achieving a high response rate to initial combination chemotherapy without cisplatin and a high final complete remission rate after definitive local therapy. Proc Am Soc Clin Oncol. 9: 177; 1990. Abstract.

32. Saunders, J.B. de C.M.; Davis, C.; Miller, E.R. The mechanisms of deglutition (second stage) as revealed by cine-radiography. Ann. Otol. Rhinol. Laryngol. 60:897-916; 1951.

32'. Saunders, M.I.; Dische, S.; Grosch, E.J.; *et al.* Experience with CHART. Int. J. Radiat. Oncol. Biol. Phys. 21:871; 1991.

32a. Scherlacher, A.; Jaske, R.; Lehnert, M. Therapie rezidivierender plattenepitheljarzinome (rPECHN) im HNO-Bereich mit einem sequentiellen methrexat-(MTX)/5-fluorouracil (5-FU-protokoll. Laryngol. Rhinol. Otol. (Stuttg) 64:58-61; 1985.

32b. Schultheiss, T.E. Spinal cord radiation "tolerance": doctrine versus data. Int. J. Rad. Oncol. Biol. Phys. 19 (1):219;1990.

32c. Shabana, A.H.M.; Lubenko, A.; Ivanyi, L. Expression of blood group H antigen by normal, benign, and carcinoma cells of the oral epithelium: immunohistochemical study using monoclonal antibody RS13. Oral Surg. Oral Med. Oral Pathol. 62:532-537; 1986.

32d. Silverberg, E.; Lubera, J.A. Cancer statistics, 1989. CA. 39(1):3-20; 1989.

32e. Slaughter, D.P.; Southwick, H.; Smejkal, W. "Field cancerization" in oral stratified squamous epithelium: clinical implications of multicentric origin. Cancer. 6:963-968; 1953.

32f. Squire, C.A. Smokeless tobacco and oral cancer: a cause for concern? CA. 34:242-247; 1984.

33. Strauss, M.B. Familiar medical quotations. Boston, MA: Little Brown and Co; 1968.

34. Suen, J.Y.; Newman, R.K.; Hannahs, K.; *et al.* Evaluation of the effectiveness of postoperative radiation therapy for the control of local disease. Am. J. Surg. 140:577-579; 1980.

34a. Taylor, S.G. Chemotherapy in the combined modality treatment of head and neck cancer. In: Kagan, A.R., Miles, J. eds. Head and Neck Oncology: Clinical Management. Elmsford, NY: Pergamon Press; 1989: 166-170.

35. Thawley, S.E.; Panje, W.R.; Batsakis, J.G.; Lindberg, R.D., eds. Comprehensive Management of Head and Neck Tumors. vols. I & II. Philadelphia, PA: WB Sanders Co; 1987.

35a. Tytor, M.; Franzen, G.; Olofsson, J. DNA pattern in oral cavity carcinomas in relation to clinical stage and histological grading. Pathol. Res. Pract. 182:202-206; 1987.

36. Unger, J.M. Handbook of Head and Neck Imaging. New York, NY: Churchill Livingstone; 1987.

37. Vasconez, L.O.; McCraw, J.B., eds. Symposium on myocutaneous flaps. Clin. Plast. Surg. 7:1-134; 1980.

37a. Vogl, S.E.; Komisar, A.; Kaplan, B.H.; *et al.* Sequential methotrexate and 5-flourouracil with bleomycin and cisplatin in the chemotherapy of advanced squamous cancer of the head and neck. Cancer. 57:706-710; 1986.

37b. Wang, C.C. Clinical Radiation Oncology: Indications, Techniques and Results. Littleton, MA: PSG Publishing Company, Inc.; 1988.

38. Wang, C.C. How essential is interstitial radiation therapy to curability of head and neck cancer? Int. J. Rad. Oncol. Biol. Phys. 18: 1535; 1990.

38a. Wang C.C. Radiation Therapy for Head and Neck Neoplasms. Indications, Techniques and Results. Boston, MA: John Wright; 1983.

38b. Wendt, C.D.; Peters, L.J.; Delclos, L.; Ang, K.K.; Morrison, W.H.; Maor, M.H.; Robbins, K.T.; Byers, R.M.; Carlson, L.S.; Oswald, M.J. Primary radiotherapy in the treatment of stage I and II oral tongue cancers: importance of the proportion of therapy delivered with interstitial therapy. Int. J. Rad. Oncol. Biol. Phys. 18:1287-1292;1990.

39. Westbrook, K.C. Evaluation of patients with head and neck cancer. In: Neoplasia of Head and Neck. Chicago, IL: Year Book Medical Publishers.; 1974:39-46.

Specific References

Oral Cavity

40. Ange, D.W.; Lindberg, R.D.; Guillamondegui, O.M. Management of squamous cell carcinoma of the oral tongue and floor mouth after excision biopsy. Radiology. 116:143-146; 1975.

40a. Baker, S.R.; Krause, C.J. Carcinoma of the lip. Laryngoscope. 90:19; 1980.

41. Bloom, N.D.; Spiro, R.H. Carcinoma of the cheek mucosa. A retrospective analysis. Am. J. Surg. 149:556-559; 1980.

42. Byers, R.M.; Newman, R.; Russell, N.; et al. Results of treatment for squamous carcinoma of the lower gum. Cancer. 47:2236-2238; 1981.

43. Calley, C.D.; Spiro, R.H.; Strong, E.W. Changing trends in the management of squamous carcinoma of the tongue. Am. J. Surg. 148:449-452; 1984.

44. Chu, A.; Fletcher, G.H. Incidence and causes of failures to control by irradiation to the primary lesions in squamous cell carcinomas of the anterior two-thirds of the tongue and floor of mouth. Am. J. Roentgenol. 117:502-508; 1973.

45. Decroix, Y.; Ghossein, N.A. Experience of the Curie Institute in treatment of cancer of the mobile tongue: I. Treatment policies and results. Cancer. 47:496-502; 1981.

46. Decroix, Y.; Ghossein, N.A. Experience of the Curie Institute in treatment of cancer of the mobile tongue: II. Management of the neck nodes. Cancer. 47:503-508; 1981.

47. Delclos, L.; Lindberg, R.D.; Fletcher, G.H. Squamous cell carcinoma of the oral tongue and floor of mouth. Am. J. Roentgenol. 126:223-228; 1976.

48. Fayos, J.V.; Lampe, I. Treatment of squamous cell carcinoma of the oral cavity. Am. J. Surg. 124:493-500; 1980.

49. Guillamondegui, O.M.; Oliver, B.; Haden, R. Cancer of the floor of the mouth. Selective choice of treatment and analysis of failure. Am. J. Surg. 140:560; 1980.

50. Hamberger, A.D.; Fletcher, G.H.; Guillamondegui, O.M.; et al. Advanced squamous cell carcinoma of the oral cavity and oropharynx treated with irradiation and surgery. Radiology. 119:433-438; 1976.

51. Kondo, M.; Hashimoto, S.; Dokiya, T.; et al. Local control of squamous cell carcinoma of the mobile tongue: an experience of different modalities. Intl. J. Radiat. Oncol. Biol. Phys. 12:755-760; 1986.

52. Kremen, A.J. Cancer of the tongue — a surgical technique for a primary combined en bloc resection of tongue, floor of mouth, and cervical lymphatics. Surgery. 30:227-240; 1951.

53. Lo, K.; Fletcher, G.H.; Byers, R.M.; et al. Results of irradiation in the squamous cell carcinomas of the anterior fancial pillar — retromolar trigone. Intl. J. Radiat. Oncol. Biol. Phys. 13:969-974; 1987.

54. Marks, J.E.; Lee, F.; Freeman, R.B.; et al. Carcinoma of the oral tongue: a study of pertinent selection and treatment results. Laryngoscope. 91:1548-1558; 1981.

55. Marks, J.E.; Lee, F.; Smith, P.G.; Ogura, J.H. Floor of the mouth cancer: patient selection and treatment results. Laryngoscope. 93:473; 1983.

56. Mashberg A.; Garfinkel, L. Early diagnosis of oral cancer: the erythroplastic lesion in high risk sites. CA. 28:297-303; 1978.

57. Mendelson, B.C.; Hodgkinson, D.J.; Woods, J.E. Cancer of the oral cavity. Surg. Clin. North Am. 57:585-596; 1977.

58. Mendenhall, W.M.; VanCise, W.S.; Bova, F.J.; Million, R.R. Analysis of time-dose factors in squamous cell carcinoma of the oral tongue and floor of mouth treated with radiation therapy alone. Intl. J. Radiat. Oncol. Biol. Phys. 7:1005; 1981.

59. Moore, C.; Catlin, D. Anatomic origins and locations of oral cancer. Am. J. Surg. 114:510-513; 1967.

60. Pop, L.A.M.; Eijkenboom, W.W.; deBoer, M.F.; et al. Evaluation of treatment results of squamous cell carcinoma of the buccal mucosa. In: J. Radiat. Oncol. Biol. Phys. 16:483-487; 1989.

61. Schleuning, A.J.; Summers, G.W. Carcinoma of the tongue: review of 220 cases. Laryngoscope. 82:1446-1454; 1972.

62. Shafer, W.G. Oral carcinoma in situ. Oral Surg. 39:227-238; 1975.

63. Shaha, A.R.; Spiro, R.H.; Shah, J.P.; Strong, E.W. Squamous carcinoma of the floor of the mouth. Am. J. Surg. 148:455-458; 1984.

64. Vermund, H.; Gollin, F.F. Role of radiotherapy in the treatment of cancer of the tongue. A retrospective analysis on TNM-staged tumors treated between 1948 and 1968. Cancer. 32:333-345; 1973.

65. Waldron, C.A.; Shafer, W.G. Leukoplakia revisited. A clinico-pathologic study of 3,256 oral leukoplakias. Cancer. 36:1386-1392; 1975.

66. Wawro, N.N.; Babcock, A.; Ellison, L. Cancer of the tongue. Experience at the Hartford Hospital from 1931 to 1963. Am. J. Surg. 110:455-461; 1970.

Oropharynx

67. Cardinale, F.; Fisher, J.J. Radiation therapy of carcinoma of the tonsil. Cancer. 39:605-608; 1977.

68. Cunningham, M.P.; Catlin, D. Cancer of the pharyngeal wall. Cancer. 20:1859-1866; 1967.

69. Dupone, J.B.; Guillamondegui, O.M.; Jesse, R.H. Surgical treatment of advanced carcinomas of the base of the tongue. Am. J. Surg. 136:501-503; 1978.

70. Esche, B.A.; Haie, C.M.; Gerbaulet, A.P.; et al. Interstitial and external radiotherapy in carcinoma of the soft palate and uvula. Intl. J. Radiat. Oncol. Biol. Phys. 15:619-625, 1989.

71. Fayos, J.V. Carcinoma of the oropharynx. Radiology. 138:675-681; 1981.

72. Fleming, P.M.; Matz, G.H.; Powell, W.J.; et al. Carcinomas of the tonsil. Surg. Clin. North Am. 56:125-136; 1976.

73. Fletcher, G.H.; Lindberg, R.D. Squamous cell carcinomas of the tonsillar area and palatine arch. Am. J. Roentgenol. 96:574-587; 1966.

73a. Gardner, K.E.; Parsons, J.T.; Mendenhall, W.M., Million, R.R., Cassisi, N.J. et al. Time-dose relationships for local tumor control and complications follwing irraidiaton of squamous cell carcinoma fo the base of tongue. Intl. J. Radiat. Oncol. Biol. Phys. 13:507-510; 1987.

74. Gelinas, M.; Fletcher, G.H. Incidence and causes of local failure of irradiation in squamous cell carcinoma of the facial arch, tonsillar fossa and base of the tongue. Radiology. 108:383-387; 1973.

75. Kaplan, R.; Million, R.R.; Cassisi, N.J. Carcinoma of the tonsil: results of radical irradiation with surgery reserved for radiation failures. Laryngoscope. 87:600-607; 1977.

76. Lederman, M.; Mould, R.F. Radiation treatment of cancer of the pharynx: with special reference to telecobalt therapy. Br. J. Radiol. 41:251-274; 1968.

77. Marks, J.E.; Freeman, R.B.; Lee, F.; et al. Pharyngeal wall cancer: an analysis of treatment results, complications, and patterns of failure. Intl. J. Radiat. Oncol. Biol. Phys. 4:587-593; 1978.

77a. Marks, J.E.; Smith, P.G.; Sessions, D.G. Pharyngeal wall cancer: a reappraisal after comparison of treatment methods. Arch. Otolaryngol. 111:79; 1985.

78. Moez-Mendez, R.T.; Fletcher, G.H.; Guillamondegui, O.M.; et al. Analysis of the results of irradiation in the treatment of squamous cell carcinomas of the pharyngeal walls. Intl. J. Radiat. Oncol. Biol. Phys. 4:579-585; 1978.

79. Murthy, A.R.; Hendrickson, F.R. Is contralateral neck treatment necessary in early carcinoma of the tonsil? Intl. J. Radiat. Oncol. Biol. Phys. 6:91-94; 1980.

80. Perez, C.A.; Ackerman, L.V.; Mill, W.B.; et al. Malignant tumors of the tonsil. Am. J. Roentgenol. 114:43-58; 1972.

81. Perez, C.A.; Lee, F.A.; Ackerman, L.V.; et al. Carcinoma of the tonsillar fossa. Significance of dose of irradiation and volume treated in the control of the primary tumor and metastatic neck nodes. Intl. J. Radiat. Oncol. Biol. Phys. 1:817-827; 1976.

81a. Rammuler, D.; Medina, J.E.; Byers, R.M.; et al. Treatment of choice for squamous carcinoma of the tonsillar fossa. Head Neck Surg. 7:206; 1985.

82. Rider, W.B. Epithelial cancer of the tonsillar area. Radiology. 78:760-764; 1962.

83. Rollo, J.; Rozenbom, C.V.; Thawley, S.; *et al.* Squamous carcinoma of the base of the tongue: a clinicopathologic study of 81 cases. Cancer 47:333-342; 1981.

84. Scanlon, P.W.; Devine ,K.D.; Wollner, L.B.; *et al.* Cancer of the tonsil: 131 patients treated in the 11-year period 1940 through 1960. Am. J. Roentgenol. 100:894-903; 1967.

85. Scanlon, P.W.; Soule, E.H.; Devine, K.D.; *et al.* Cancer of the base of the tongue. 116 patients treated radiotherapeutically in the 11-year period 1952 through 1962. Am. J. Roentgenol. 105:26-36; 1969.

86. Sessions, D.G.; Stallings, J.O.; Brownson, R.J.; *et al.* Total glossectomy for advanced carcinoma of the base of the tongue. Laryngoscope. 83:39-50; 1973.

87. Seydel, A.G.; Scholl, H. Carcinoma of the soft palate and uvula. Am. J. Roentgenol. 120:603-607; 1974.

87a. Shrewsbury, D.; Adams, G.L.; Duvall, A.J. III; *et al.* Carcioma of the tonsillar region: a comparison of radiaiton thrpay with combined preoperative radiaiton and surgery. Otolaryngol. Head Neck Surg. 89:979; 1981.

88. Shukovsky, L.J.; Fletcher, G.H. Time-dose and tumor volume relationships in the irradiation of squamous cell carcinoma of the tonsillar fossa. Radiology. 107:621-626; 1973.

89. Talton, B.M.; Elkon, D.; Kim, J-A.; *et al.* Cancer of the posterior hypopharyngeal wall. Intl. J. Radiat. Oncol. Biol. Phys. 7:597-599; 1981.

89a. Thawley, S.E.; Simpson Marks, J.R. Preoperative irradiation and surgery for carcinoma of the base of tongue. Ann. Otol. Rhinol. Laryngol. 92:485; 1983.

89b. Tong, D.; Laramore, G.E.; Griffin, T.W.; *et al.* Carcinoma of the tonsillar region: results of external irradiation. Cancer. 49:2009; 1982.

90. Wang, C.C. Radiotherapeutic management of carcinoma of the posterior pharyngeal wall. Cancer. 27:894-896; 1971.

90a. Wang, C.C. Local control of oropharyngeal carcinoma after two accelerated hyperfractionation radiation therapy schemes. Intl. J. Radiat. Oncol. Biol. Phys. 14:1143-1146; 1988.

91. Weller, S.A.; Goffinet, D.R.; Goode, R.L.; *et al.* Carcinoma of the oropharynx. Results of megavoltage radiation therapy in 305 patients. Am. J. Roentgenol. 126:236-247; 1976.

92. Whicker, J.H.; DeSanto, L.W.; Devine, K.D. Surgical treatment of squamous cell carcinoma of the tonsil. Laryngoscope. 84:90-97; 1974.

Hypopharynx

93. Barton, R.T. Surgical treatment of carcinoma of the pyriform sinus. Arch. Otolaryngol. 97:337-339; 1973.

93a. Bataini, P.; Brugere, J.; Bernier, J.; *et al.* Results of radical radiotherapeutic treatment of carcinoma of the pyriform sinus — experience of the Institut Curie. Intl. J. Radiat. Oncol. Biol. Phys. 8:1277; 1982.

94. Bordette, W.J.; Jesse, R. Carcinoma of the cervical esophagus. J. Thorac. Cardiovasc. Surg. 63:41-52; 1972.

95. Byers, R.M.; Krueger, W.W.O.; Saxton, J. Use of surgery and postoperative radiation in the treatment of advanced squamous cell carcinoma of the pyriform sinus. Am. J. Surg. 138:597-599; 1979.

96. Byhardt, R.W.; Cox, J.D. Patterns of failure and results of preoperative irradiation vs. radiation alone in carcinoma of the pyriform sinus. Intl. J. Radiat. Oncol. Biol. Phys. 6:1135-1141; 1980.

97. Carpenter, R.J.; DeSanto, L.W.; Devine, K.D.; *et al.* Cancer of the hypopharynx: analysis of treatment and results in 162 patients. Arch. Otolaryngol. 102:716-721; 1976.

97a. El-Badawi, S.A.; Goepfert, H.; Fletcher, G.H.; *et al.* Squamous cell carcinoma of the pyriform sinus. Laryngoscope 92:357; 1982.

98. Goldman, J.L.; Silverstone, S.M.; Roffman, J.D.; *et al.* High dosage pre-operative radiation and surgery for carcinoma of the larynx and laryngo-pharynx — a 14-year program. Laryngoscope. 82:1869-1882; 1972.

99. Keane, T.J.; Hawkins, N.V.; Beale, F.A.; Cummings, B.J.; Harwood, A. R.; *et al.* Carcinoma of the hypopharynx: results of primary radical radiation therapy. Intl. J. Radiat. Oncol. Biol. Phys. 9:659; 1983.

100. Lederman, M. Cancer of the pharynx. A study based on 2,417 cases with special reference to radiation treatment. J. Laryngol. Otol. 81:151-172; 1967.

101. Marchetta, F.C.; Sako, K.; Holyoke, E.D. Squamous cell carcinoma of the pyriform sinus. Am. J. Surg. 114:507-509; 1967.

102. Martin, S.A.; Marks, J.E.; Lee, J.Y.; *et al.* Carcinoma of the pyriform sinus: predictors of TNM relapse and survival. Cancer. 46:1974-1981; 1980.

103. Million, R.R.; Cassisi, N.J. Radical irradiation for carcinoma of the pyriform sinus. Laryngoscope 91:439-450; 1981.

104. Razack, M.S.; Sako, K.; Marchetta, F.C.; *et al.* Carcinoma of the hypopharynx: success and failure. Am. J. Surg. 134:489-491; 1977.

105. Strong, M.S.; Vaughan, C.W.; Kayne, H.L.; *et al.* A randomized trial of preoperative radiotherapy in cancer of the oropharynx and hypopharynx. Am. J. Surg. 136:494-500; 1978.

106. Wang, C.C.; Schulz, M.D.; Miller, D. Combined radiation therapy and surgery for carcinoma of the supraglottis and pyriform sinus. Am. J. Surg. 124:551-554; 1972.

Larynx

107. Ballantyne, A.J.; Fletcher, G.H. Preservation of the larynx in the surgical treatment of cancer, recurrent after radiation therapy. Am. J. Roentgenol. 99:336-339; 1967.

108. Ballantyne, A.J.; Fletcher, G.H. Surgical management of irradiation failures of nonfixed cancers of the glottic region. Am. J. Roentgenol. 120:164-168; 1974.

109. Bocca, E. Supraglottic cancer. Laryngoscope. 85:1318-1326; 1975.

110. Constable, W.C.; Marks, R.D.; Robbins, J.P.; *et al.* High-dose preoperative radiotherapy and surgery for cancer of the larynx. Laryngoscope. 82:1861-1868; 1972.

111. Cummings, C.W. Complications of laryngectomy and neck dissection following planned preoperative radiotherapy. Ann. Otol. Rhinol. Laryngol. 86:745-750; 1977.

112. Dayal, V.S.; Hahir, H.; Stone, P. Pre-epiglottic space. An anatomic study. Arch. Otolaryngol. 95:130-133; 1972.

112a. Department of Veterans Affairs Laryngeal Cancer Study Group. Induction chemotherapy plus radiation compared with surgery plus radiation in patients with advanced laryngeal cancer. N. Engl. J. Med. 324:1685-1690; 1991.

113. Fletcher, G.H.; Linberg, R.D.; Hamberger, A.; *et al.* Reasons for irradiation failures in squamous cell carcinoma of the larynx. Laryngoscope 85:987-1003; 1975.

114. Ghossein NA, Bataini JP, Ennuyer A, *et al.* Local control and site of failure in radically irradiated supraglottic cancer. Radiology. 12:187-192; 1974.

115. Goepfert, H.; Jesse, R.H.; Fletcher, G.H.; *et al.* Optimal treatment for the technically resectable squamous cell carcinoma of the supraglottic larynx. Laryngoscope. 85:14-32; 1977.

116. Goepfert, H.; Zaren, H.A.; Jesse, R.H.; *et al.* Treatment of laryngeal carcinoma with conservative surgery and postoperative radiation therapy. Arch. Otolaryngol. 104:576-578; 1978.

117. Harwood, A.R. Cancer of the larynx: the Toronto experience. J. Otolaryngol. 11(suppl. 11): 3-21; 1982.

118. Harwood, A.R.; Beale, F.A.; Cummings, B.J.; *et al.* T3 glottic cancer: an analysis of dose-time-volume factors. Intl. J. Radiat. Oncol. Biol. Phys. 6:675-680; 1980.

119. Harwood, A.R.; Hawkins, N.V.; Rider, W.D.; *et al.* Radiotherapy of early glottic cancer. I. Intl. J. Radiat. Oncol. Biol. Phys. 5:473-476; 1979.

120. Harwood, A.R.; Tierie, A. Radiotherapy of early glottic cancer. II. Intl. J. Radiat. Oncol. Biol. Phys. 5:447-472; 1979.

121. Hawkins, N.V. VIII. The treatment of glottic carcinoma: an analysis of 800 cases. Laryngoscope 85:1485-1493; 1975.

122. Henry, J.; Balikdjian, D.; Storme, G.; *et al.* Radiotherapy in the treatment of T3-T4 supraglottic tumors. Laryngoscope 85:1682-1688; 1975.

123. Kirchner, J.A. Growth and spread of laryngeal cancer as related to partial laryngectomy. In: Alverti, P.W.; Bruce, D.P., eds. Centennial Conference on Laryngeal Cancer. New York, NY: Appleton Century Crofts; 1976:51-59.

124. Lederman, M. Cancer of the larynx, part I: natural history in relation to treatment. Br. J. Radiol. 44:569-578; 1971.

125. Lederman, M. Keratosis of the larynx. J. Laryngol. Otol. 77:651-659; 1963.

125a. Maguire, A.; Dayal, V.S. Supraglottic anatomy, the pre- or peri-epiglottic space? In: Alberti, P.W.; Bryce, D.P., eds. Centennial Conference on Laryngeal Cancer. New York, NY: Appleton Century Crofts; 1976:26-33.

126. Marks, R.D.; Fitz-Hugh, G.S.; Constable, W.C. Fourteen years

experience with cobalt-60 radiation therapy in the treatment of early cancer of the true vocal cords. Cancer. 28:571-576; 1971.

127. Mendenhall, W.M.; Parsons, J.T.; Million, R.R.; et al. Tl-T2 squamous cell carcinoma of the glottic larynx treated with radiation therapy: relationship of dose-fractionation factors to local control and complications. Intl. J. Radiat. Oncol. Biol. Phys. 15:1267-1273; 1988.

127a. Million, R.R. The larynx. . .so to speak: Everything I wanted to know about laryngeal cancer I learned in the last 32 years. Int. J. Radiat. Oncol. Bio. Phys. 23(4):691-704; 1992.

128. Mills, E.E.D. Early glottic carcinoma: factors affecting radiation failure, results of treatment, and sequelae. Intl. J. Radiat. Oncol. Biol. Phys. 5:811-817; 1979.

129. Mittal, B.; Rao, D.V.; Marks, J.E.; Perez, C.A. Role of radiation in the management of early vocal cord carcinoma. Intl. J. Radiat. Oncol. Biol. Phys. 9:997-1002; 1983.

130. Nass, J.M.; Brady, L.W.; Glassburn, J.R.; et al. Radiation therapy of glottic carcinoma. Intl. J. Radiat. Oncol. Biol. Phys. 1:867-872; 1976.

131. Norris, C.M.; Peale, A.R. Keratosis of the larynx. J. Laryngol. Otol. 77:635-647; 1963.

132. Ogura, J.H.; Sessions, D.G.; Spector, G.H. Conservation surgery for epidermoid carcinoma of the supraglottic larynx. Laryngoscope 85:1808-1815; 1975.

133. Olofsson, J.; Renouf, J.H.P.; VanNostrand, A.N.P. Laryngeal carcinoma: correlation of roentgenography and histopathology. A study based on whole organ, serially sectioned laryngeal carcinoma specimens. Am. J. Roentgenol. 11:526-539; 1973.

134. Olofsson, J.; Williams, G.T.; Rider, W.D.; et al. Anterior commissure carcinoma. Primary treatment with radiotherapy in 57 patients. Arch. Otolaryngol. 95:230-239; 1972.

135. Peters, L.T.; Thomas, H.D. Dose-response relationship for supraglottic laryngeal carcinoma. Intl. J. Radiat. Oncol. Biol. Phys. 9:421-442; 1983.

135a. Pfister, D.G.; Strong, E.; Harrison, L.; et al. Larynx preservation with combined chemotherapy and radiation therapy in advanced but resectable head and neck cancer. J. Clin. Oncol. 9:850-859; 1991.

136. Putney, F.J.; Chapman, C.E. Carcinoma of the larynx: analysis of 311 cases treated surgically. Ann. Otol. Rhinol. Laryngol. 81:455-464; 1972.

137. Razack, M.S.; Silapasvang, S.; Sako, K.; et al. Significance of site and nodal metastases in squamous carcinoma of the epiglottis. Am. J. Surg. 138:588-596; 1979.

138. Robbins, T.K.; Davidson, W.; Peters, L.J.; Goepfert, H. Conservation surgery for T2 and T3 carcinomas of the supraglottic larynx. Arch. Otolaryngol. Head Neck Surg. 114:421-426; 1988.

139. Russ, J.E.; Sullivan, C.; Gallager, H.S.; et al. Conservation surgery of the larynx: a reappraisal based on whole organ study. Am. J. Surg. 138:588-596; 1979.

140. Sagel, S.S.; Aufderheide, J.F.; Aronberg, D.J.; et al. High resolution computed tomography in the staging of carcinoma of the larynx. Laryngoscope. 91:292-300; 1981.

141. Schwaibold, F.; Scariato, A.; Nunno, M.; Wallner, P.E.; Lustig, R.A.; et al. The effect of fraction size on control of early glottic cancer. Intl. J. Radiat. Oncol. Biol. Phys. 14:451-454; 1988.

142. Shrala, U.; Paavolainen, M. The problem of advanced supraglottic carcinoma. Laryngoscope. 85:1633-1642; 1975.

143. Smith, R.R.; Caulk, R.; Frazell, E.; et al. Revision of the clinical staging system for cancer of the larynx. Cancer 31:72-80; 1973.

144. Som, M.L. Conservation surgery for carcinoma of the supraglottis. J. Laryngol. Otol. 84:655-678; 1970.

145. Sorensen, H.; Hansen, H.S.; Thomsen, K.A. Partial laryngectomy following irradiation. Laryngoscope. 90:1344-1349; 1980.

146. Tucker, G. The anatomy of laryngeal cancer. In: Alberti, P.W.; Bryce, D.P., eds. Centennial conference on laryngeal cancer. New York, NY: Appleton Century Crofts; 1976:11-25.

147. Tucker, G.F.; Alsonso, W.A.; Tucker, J.A.; et al. The anterior commissure revisited. Ann. Otol. Rhinol. Laryngol. 82:625-636; 1973.

148. Vermund, H. Role of radiotherapy in cancer of the larynx as related to the TNM system of staging. A review. Cancer. 25 485-504; 1970.

149. Wang, C.C. Treatment of glottic carcinoma by megavoltage radiation therapy and results. Am. J. Roentgenol. 120:157-163; 1974.

150. Weems, D.H.; Mendenhall, W.M.; Parsons, J.T.; et al. Squamous cell carcinoma of the supraglottic larynx treated with surgery and/or radiation therapy. Intl. J. Radiat. Oncol. Biol. Phys. 13:1483-1487; 1988.

151. Wynder, E.L.; Bross, I.J.; Day, E. A study of environmental factors in cancer of the larynx. Cancer 9:86; 1956.

Nasopharynx

152. Coates, H.L.; Pearson, G.R.; Neel, H.B.; et al. Epstein-Barr virus-associated antigens in nasopharyngeal carcinoma. Arch. Otolaryngol. 104:427-430; 1978.

153. Dickson, R.I. Nasopharyngeal carcinoma: an evaluation of 209 patients. Laryngoscope. 91:333-354; 1980.

154. En-Pee, Z.; Pei-Gun, L.; Kuang-Long, C.; Ying-Fu, C.; Min-Dian, C.; Xiang-Fa, Z.; Xun-Xing, G. Radiation therapy of nasopharyngeal carcinoma: prognostic factors based on a 10-year follow-up of 1302 patients. Int. J. Rad. Oncol. Biol. Phys. 16:301-306; 1989.

155. Fu, K.K. Prognostic factors of carcinoma of the nasopharynx. Intl. J. Radiat. Oncol. Biol. Phys. 6:523-526; 1980.

156. Godtfredsen, E. Ophthalmologic and neurologic symptoms of malignant nasopharyngeal tumors. Acta Psychiatrica Neurol. Scand. (suppl) 34:1-323; 1944.

157. Henderson, B.E.; Louis, E.; Jing, J.S.H.; et al. Risk factors associated with nasopharyngeal carcinomas. New Engl. J. Med. 295:1101-1106; 1976.

158. Henle, G.; Henle, W. Epstein-Barr virus-specific IgA and IgG serum antibodies an outstanding feature of nasopharyngeal carcinoma. Br. J. Cancer. 17:1-7; 1976.

159. Ho, J.H. An epidemiologic and clinical study of nasopharyngeal carcinoma. Intl. J. Radiat. Oncol. Biol. Phys. 4:183-198; 1978.

160. Ho, H.C.; Ng, M.N.; Kwan, H.C.; et al. Epstein-Barr virus-specific IgA and IgG serum antibodies in nasopharyngeal carcinoma. Br. J. Cancer. 34:655-660; 1976.

161. Hoppe, R.T.; Goffinet, D.R.; Bagshaw, M.A. Carcinoma of the nasopharynx. Eighteen years' experience with megavoltage radiation therapy. Cancer. 37:2605-2612; 1976.

162. Hoppe, R.T.; Williams, J.; Warnke, R.; et al. Carcinoma of the nasopharynx — the significance of histology. Intl. J. Radiat. Oncol. Biol. Phys. 4:199-205; 1978.

163. Hsu, M.M.; Huang, S.C.; Lynn, T.C.; et al. The survival of patients with nasopharyngeal carcinoma. Otolaryngol. Head Neck Surg. 90:289; 1982.

163a. Lee, A.W.M.; Poon, Y.F.; Foo, W.; et al. Retrospective analysis of 5037 patients with nasopharyngeal carcinoma treated during 1976-1985: Overall survival and patterns of failure. Int. J. Radiat. Oncol. Biol. Phys. 23(2):1992.

164. Marcial, V.A.; Hanley, J.A.; Chang, C.; et al. Split-course radiation therapy of carcinoma of the nasopharynx. Results of a national collaborative clinical trial of the Radiation Therapy Oncology Group. Intl. J. Radiat. Oncol. Biol. Phys. 6:409-414; 1980.

165. Mesic, J.B.; Fletcher, G.H.; Goepfert, H. Megavoltage irradiation of epithelial tumors of the nasopharynx. Intl. J. Radiat. Oncol. Biol. Phys. 7:447-453; 1981.

166. Meyer, J.E.; Wang, C.C. Carcinoma of the nasopharynx. Factors influencing results of therapy. Radiology. 100:385-388; 1971.

167. Moench, H.C.; Phillips, T.L. Carcinoma of the nasopharynx. Review of 146 patients with emphasis on radiation dose and time factors. Am. J. Surg. 124:515-518; 1972.

168. Perez, C.A.; Ackerman, L.V.; Mill, W.B.; et al. Cancer of the nasopharynx. Factors influencing prognosis. Cancer 24:1-17; 1969.

169. Rong-Xi, L.; Qi-Xin, T.; Yi-Wen, H.; Yu-Ping, L.; Xiao-De, M.; Zi-Hing, Hu. Comparison of continuous and split-course radiotherapy for nasopharyngeal carcinoma. Int. J. Rad. Oncol. Biol. Phys. 16:307-310; 1989.

170. Scanlon, P.W.; Rhodes, R.E.; Woolner, L.B.; et al. Cancer of the nasopharynx. Am. J. Roentgenol. 99:313-325; 1967.

171. Shu-Chen, H. Nasopharyngeal cancer: a review of 1,605 patients treated radically with cobalt-60. Intl. J. Radiat. Oncol. Biol. Phys. 6:401-407; 1980.

172. Thomas, J.E.; Waltz, A.G. Neurologic manifestations of nasopharyngeal malignant tumors. JAMA. 192:95-98; 1965.

173. Urdanetta, N.; Fischer, J.J.; Vera, R.; et al. Cancer of the nasopharynx. Review of 43 cases treated with supervoltage radiation therapy. Cancer. 37:1707-1712; 1976.

174. Wang, C.C.; Meyer, J.E. Radiotherapeutic management of carci-

noma of the nasopharynx. An analysis of 170 patients. Cancer. 28:566-570; 1971.

Nasal Fossa and Paranasal Sinuses

175. Bosch, A.; Vallecillo, L.; Frias, Z. Cancer of the nasal cavity. Cancer. 37: 1458-1463; 1976.
176. Cheng, V.S.T.; Wang, C.C. Carcinomas of the paranasal sinuses, a study of 66 cases. Cancer. 49:3038-3041; 1977.
177. Ellingwood, K.E.; Million, R.R. Cancer of the nasal cavity and ethmoid/sphenoid sinuses. Cancer. 43:1517-1526; 1979.
178. Frazell, E.L.; Lewis, J.S. Cancer of the nasal cavity and accessory sinuses. A report of the management of 416 patients. Cancer. 16:1293-1301; 1963.
179. Hadfield, E.H.; Macbeth, R.G. Adenocarcinoma of ethmoids in furniture workers. Ann. Otol. Rhinol. Laryngol. 80:699-702; 1971.
180. Harrison, D.F.N. Critical look at the classification of maxillary sinus carcinomata. Ann. Otol. Rhinol. Laryngol. 87:3-9; 1978.
181. Harrison, D.F.N. Problems in surgical management of neoplasms arising in the paranasal sinuses. J. Laryngol. Otol. 90:69-74; 1976.
182. Jesse, R.H. Preoperative vs postoperative radiation in the treatment of squamous carcinoma of the paranasal sinuses. Am. J. Surg. 110:552-557; 1965.
183. Kurohara, S.S.; Webster, J.H.; Ellis, F.; et al. Role of radiation therapy and of surgery in the management of localized epidermoid carcinoma of the maxillary sinus. Am. J. Roentgenol. 114:35-42; 1972.
184. Lederman, M. Cancer of the upper jaw and nasal chambers. Proc. R. Soc. Med. 62:65-72; 1969.
185. Lederman, M. The treatment of tumours of the upper jaw. Br. J. Radiol. 42:561-581; 1969.
186. Lee, F.; Ogura, J.H. Maxillary sinus carcinoma. Laryngoscope. 91:133-139; 1981.
187. Parsons, J.T.; Mendenhall, W.M.; Mancuso, A.A.; et al. Malignant tumors of the nasal cavity and ethmoid and sphenoid sinuses. Intl. J. Radiat. Oncol. Biol. Phys. 14:11-22; 1988.
188. Perlman, A.W.; Abadir, R. Carcinoma of the maxillary antrum: the role of preoperative irradiation. Laryngoscope 84:400-409; 1974.

Ear Carcinoma

189. Conley, J.; Schuller, D.E. Malignancies of the ear. Laryngoscope. 86:1147-1163; 1976.
190. Lederman, M. Malignant tumours of the ear. J. Laryngol. Otol. 79:85-119; 1965.
191. Lewis, J.S. Cancer of the ear. A report of 150 cases. Laryngoscope. 60:551-579; 1960.
192. Wang, C.C. Radiation therapy in the management of carcinoma of the external auditory canal, middle ear or mastoid. Radiology. 116:713-715; 1975.
193. Wilson, J.S.P.; Blake, G.B.; Richardson, A.E.; et al. Malignant tumors of the ear and their treatment. II. Tumors of the external auditory meatus, middle ear cleft, and temporal bone. Br. J. Plast. Surg. 27:77-91; 1974.

Chemodectoma

194. Cole, J.M. Glomus jugulare tumor. Laryngoscope. 87:1244-1258; 1977.
195. Glasscock, M.E.; Jackson, C.G.;, Dickins J.R.E.; et al. The surgical management of glomus tumors. Laryngoscope. 89:1640-1651; 1979.
196. Kim, J.; Elkon, D.; Liu, M.; et al. Optimum dose of radiotherapy for chemodectomas of the middle ear. Intl. J. Radiat. Oncol. Biol. Phys. 6:815-819; 1980.
197. Lees, C.D.; Levine, H.L.; Geven, E.G.; et al. Tumors of the carotid body. Experience with 41 operative cases. Am. J. Surg. 142:362-365; 1981.
198. McCabe, B.F.; Fletcher, M. Selection of therapy of glomus jugulare tumors. Arch. Otolaryngol. 89:182-185; 1969.
199. Moore, G.R.; Robbins, J.P.; Seale, D.L.; et al. Chemodectomas of the middle ear. A comparison of therapeutic modalities. Arch. Otolaryngol. 98:330-335; 1973.
200. Newman, H.; Rowe, J.F.; Phillips, T.L. Radiation therapy of the glomus julare tumor. Am. J. Roentgenol. 118:663-669; 1973.
201. Simko, T.G.; Griffin, T.N.; Gerdes, A.J.; et al. The role of radiation therapy in the treatment of glomus jugular tumors. Cancer. 42:104-106; 1978.

202. Spector, G.J.; Ciralsky, R.; Maisel, R.H.; et al. Multiple glomus tumors in the head and neck. Laryngoscope. 85:690-696; 1976.
203. Spector, G.J.; Fierstein, J.; Ogura, J.H. Comparison of therapeutic modalities of glomus tumors in the temporal bone. Laryngoscope. 86:690-696; 1976.
204. Spector, G.J.; Sobol, S.; Thawley, S.E.; et al. Glomus jugulare tumors of the temporal bone. Patterns of invasion in the temporal bone. Laryngoscope 89:1628-1639; 1979.
205. Tidwell, T.J.; Montague, E.D. Chemodectomas involving the temporal bone. Radiology. 116:147-149; 1975.

Salivary Glands

206. Catteral M. The treatment of malignant salivary gland tumors with fast neutrons. Intl. J. Radiat. Oncol. Biol. Phys. 7:1737-1738; 1981.
207. Coates, H.L.; Devine, K.B.; De Santo, L.W.; et al. Glandular tumors of the palate. Surg. Gynecol. Obstet. 140:589-593; 1975.
208. Chong, G.C.; Beahrs, O.H.; Wollner, L.B. Surgical management of acinic cell carcinoma of the parotid gland. Surg. Gynecol. Obstet. 138:65-68; 1974.
209. Conley, J.; Hamaker, R.P. Prognosis of malignant tumors of the parotid gland with facial paralysis. Arch. Otolaryngol. 101:39-41; 1975.
210. Cummings, C.W. Adenoid cystic carcinoma (cylindroma) of the parotid gland. Ann. Otol. Rhinol. Laryngol. 86:280-292; 1977.
211. Ellis, E.R.; Million, R.R.; Mendenhall, W.M.; et al. The use of radiation therapy in the management of minor salivary gland tumors. Intl. J. Radiat. Oncol. Biol. Phys. 15:613-617; 1988.
212. Eneroth, C.M.; Hjertman, L.; Moberger, G. Mucoepidermoid carcinoma of the palate. Acta Otolaryngol. (Stockh) 70:408-418; 1970.
213. Foote, F.W.; Frazell, E.L. Tumors of the major salivary glands. Cancer. 6:1065-1133; 1953.
214. Griffin, T.W.; Pajak, T.F.; Laramore, G.E.; et al. Neutron vs photon irradiation of inseparable salivary gland tumors: results of an RTOG-MRC cooperative randomized study. Intl. J. Radiat. Oncol. Biol. Phys. 15:1085-1090; 1988.
215. Guillamondegui, O.M.; Byers, R.M.; Luna, M.A.; et al. Aggressive surgery in treatment for parotid cancer: the role of adjunctive postoperative radiotherapy. Am. J. Roentgenol. 123:49-54; 1975.
216. Kaul, R.; Hendrickson, F.; Cohen, L.; et al. Fast neutrons in the treatment of salivary gland tumors. Intl. J. Radiat. Oncol. Biol. Phys. 7:1667-1671; 1981.
217. Levitt, S.H.; McHugh, R.B.; Gomez-Martin, O.; et al. Clinical staging system for cancer of the salivary gland: a retrospective study. Cancer. 47:2712-2724; 1981.
218. Nigro, M.F.; Spiro, R.H. Deep lobe parotid tumors. Am. J. Surg. 134:523-527; 1977.
219. Rafla, S. Malignant parotid tumors: natural history and treatment. Cancer. 40:136-144; 1977.
220. Spiro, R.H.; Huvos, A.G.; Strong, E.W. Acinic cell carcinoma of salivary origin. A clinicopathologic study of 67 cases. Cancer. 41:924-935; 1978.
221. Spiro, R.H.; Huvos, A.G.; Strong, E.W. Adenoid cystic carcinoma: factors influencing survival. Am. J. Surg. 138:579-583; 1979.
222. Spiro, R.H.; Huvos, A.G.; Strong, E.W. Cancer of the parotid gland. A clinicopathologic study of 288 primary cases. Am. J. Surg. 130:452-459; 1975.
223. Spiro, R.H.; Koss, L.G.; Hajdu, S.L.; et al. Tumors of minor salivary origin. A clinicopathologic study of 492 cases. Cancer. 31:117-129; 1973.
223a. Wang, C.C.; Goodman, M. Photon irradiation of unresectable carcinomas of salivary glands. Int. J. Radiat. Oncol. Biol. Phys. 21:569-576; 1991.
224. Woods, J.E.; Weiland, L.H.; Chong, G.C.; et al. Pathology and surgery of primary tumors of the parotid. Surg. Clin. North Am. 57:565-573; 1977.

Cervical Node Metastases

224a. Amrein, P. Current chemotherapy of head and neck cancer. J. Oral and Maxillofacial Surg. 49(8):864-70;1991.
225. Barkley, H.T.; Fletcher, G.H.; Jesse, R.H.; et al. Management of cervical lymph node metastases in squamous cell carcinoma of the tonsillar fossa, base of tongue, supraglottic larynx, and hypopharynx. Am. J. Surg. 124:462-467; 1972.

226. Beahrs, O.H.; Barber, K.W. The value of radical dissection of structure of the neck in the management of carcinoma of the lip, mouth, and larynx. Arch. Surg. 85:65-72; 1962.

227. Bocca E. Conservative neck dissection. Laryngoscope. 85:1511-1515; 1975.

228. Chu, W.; Strawitz, J.G. Results in suprahyoid, modified radical, and standard radical neck dissections for metastatic squamous cell carcinoma: recurrence and survival. Am. J. Surg. 136:512-515; 1978.

228a. Fornstiere, A. Randomized trials of induction chemotherapy. A critical review. Heme-Onc. Cl. Na. 5(4):725-36;1991.

229. Jesse, R.H.; Ballantyne, A.J.; Larson, D. Radical or modified neck dissection: a therapeutic dilemma. Am. J. Surg. 136:516-519; 1978.

230. Kalnins, I.K.; Leonard, A.G.; Sako, K.; et al. Correlation between prognosis and degree of lymph node involvement in carcinoma of the oral cavity. Am. J. Surg. 134:450-454; 1977.

231. Lee, J.G.; Krause, C.J. Radical neck dissection: elective, therapeutic, and secondary. Arch. Otolaryngol. 101:656-659; 1975.

232. Lindberg, R. Distribution of cervical lymph node metastases from squamous cell carcinoma of the upper respiratory and digestive tracts. Cancer. 29:1446-1449; 1972.

233. Martin, H.; Valle, B.; Ehrlich, H.; et al. Neck dissection. Cancer. 4:441-499; 1951.

234. Mendenhall, W.M.; Million, R.R. Elective neck irradiation for squamous cell carcinoma of the head and neck. An analysis of time-dose factors and causes of failure. Intl. J. Radiat. Oncol. Biol. Phys. 12:741-747; 1986.

235. Parsons, J.T.; Mendenhall, W.M.; Cassisi, N.J.; et al. Hyperfractionation for head and neck cancer. Intl. J. Radiat. Oncol. Biol. Phys. 14:649-659; 1988.

235a. Peppard, S.B.; Al-Sarraf, M.; Powers, W.E. et al. Combination of cisplatinum, oncovin, and bleomycin (COB) prior to surgery and/or radiotherapy in advanced untreated epidermoid cancer of the head and neck. Laryngoscope. 90:1273-1280;1980.

235b. Pints and Jacobs. Chemotherapy for Recurrent and Metastatic Head and Neck Cancer. Hematology-Oncology Clinics of N.A. 5(4):667-86;1991.

236. Schneider, J.J.; Fletcher, G.H.; Barkley, T.H. Control by irradiation alone of nonfixed clinically positive lymph nodes from squamous cell carcinoma of the oral cavity, oropharynx, supraglottic larynx, and hypopharynx. Am. J. Roentgenol. 123:42-48; 1975.

237. Shear, M.; Hawkins, D.M.; Farr, H.W. The prediction of lymph node metastases from oral squamous carcinoma. Cancer. 37:1901-1907; 1976.

238. Spiro, R.H.; Alfonso, A.E.; Farr, H.W.; et al. Cervical node metastasis from epidermoid carcinoma of the oral cavity and oropharynx. A critical assessment of current staging. Am. J. Surg. 128:562-567; 1974.

239. Statley, C.J.; Herzon, F.S. Elective neck dissection in carcinoma of larynx. Otolaryngol. Clin. North Am. 3:543-553; 1970.

240. Strong, E.W. Preoperative radiaton and radical neck dissection. Surg. Clin. North Am. 49:271-276; 1969.

240a Taylor, S.G. Integration of chemotherapy into the combined modality therapy of head and neck squamous cancer. Int. J. Rad. Oncol. Biol. Phys. 13:779-783;1987.

241. Wizenberg, M.J.; Bloedorn, F.G.; Weiner, S.; et al. Treatment of lymph node metastases in head and neck cancer. A radiotherapeutic approach. Cancer 29:1455-1462; 1972.

Chemotherapy

242. Brown, A.W.; Blorn, J.; Butler, W.M.; et al. Combination chemotherapy with vinblastine, bleomycin, and cis-diammine-dichloroplatinum II in squamous cell carcinoma of the head and neck. Cancer. 45:2830-2835; 1980.

243. Clark, J.R.; Fallon, B.G.; Frei, E. Induction chemotherapy as initial treatment for advanced head and neck cancer; a model for multidisciplinary treatment of solid tumors. In: DeVita, V.T.; Hellman, S.; Rosenberg, S.A., eds. Important Advances in Oncology; 1987. Philadelphia, PA: J BLippincott; 1987:175-195.

244. Glick, J.H.; Marcial, V.; Richter, M.; et al. The adjuvant treatment of inoperable stage II and IV epidermoid carcinoma of the head and neck with platinum and bleomycin infusions prior to definitive radiotherapy. An RTOG pilot study. Cancer 47:1919-1924; 1980.

245. Lustig, R.A.; DeMare, P.A.; Kramer, S. Adjuvant methotrexate in the radiotherapeutic management of advanced tumors of the head and neck. Cancer. 37:2703-2708; 1976.

246. Peppard, S.B.; Al-Sarraf, M.; Powers, W.E.; et al. Combination of cisplatinum, oncovin, and bleomycin (COB) prior to surgery and/or radiotherapy in advanced untreated epidermoid cancer of the head and neck. Laryngoscope. 90:1273-1280; 1980.

247. Randolph, V.L.; Vallejo, H.; Spiro, R.H.; et al. Combination therapy for advanced head and neck cancer. Induction of remissions with diamminedichloroplatinum II, bleomycin, and radiation therapy. Cancer. 41:460-467; 1978.

248. Rossi, A.; Molinari, R.; Boracchi, P.; et al. Adjuvant chemotherapy with vincristine, cyclophosphamide, and doxorubicin after radiotherapy in local-regional nasopharyngeal cancer: results of a 4-year multicenter randomized study. J. Clin. Oncol. 9:1401-1410; 1988.

249. Taylor, S.G. Integration of chemotherapy into the combined modality therapy of head and neck squamous cancer. Intl. J. Radiat. Oncol. Biol. Phys. 13:779-783; 1987.

250. Vokes, E.E.; Choi, K.C.; Schilsky, R.L.; et al. Cisplatin, fluorouracil, and high-dose leucovorin for recurrent or metastatic head and neck cancer. J. Clin. Oncol. 6:618-626; 1988.

Brent DuBeshter, M.D., Gynecologic Oncology
Jeffrey Lin, M.D., Gynecologic Oncology

Cynthia Angel, M.D., Gynecologic Oncology
Colin A. Poulter, M.D., Radiation Oncology

Chapter 22

GYNECOLOGIC TUMORS

In today's world, the physician must make his commitment not just to individual life, but to the institution of life.

Norman Cousins (5)

PERSPECTIVE

Most gynecologic cancers are curable. Many factors are responsible for this fortunate evolution in the history of medical care for women. The role of surgery, still central to the management of most gynecologic neoplasia, has been greatly enlarged since the first cancer operations for cervical cancer and ovarian neoplasia in the mid to late 1800s. The development of enhanced radiation technology and knowledge of radiation biology has also been a major factor. Since the mid-1950s, when chemotherapy for gynecologic malignancies made a dramatic entrance with the discovery that methotrexate could cure metastatic choriocarcinoma, a broad base of experience in the chemotherapy of gynecologic cancer has also been developed.

Cancer is the second most common cause of death in women, and gynecologic cancers play a significant part (69). Up until the menarche, gynecologic neoplasia is very rare, and even after the beginning of the reproductive years, is still uncommon. Lymphomas are the principal cancer affecting young females, and remain so up through the mid-twenties. Ovarian cancers, usually nonepithelial, are the fifth most frequently occurring tumor in this age group (69).

A dramatic shift in cancer incidence occurs as women reach their late twenties and early thirties. Uterine cancer, principally arising in the cervix, had been the fifth most common malignancy of women in their earlier twenties, but later in the decade, it moves dramatically into first place; breast cancer also makes a major appearance. Uterine cancer will affect 100 women per 1,000,000 whereas breast cancer affects 84 per 1,000,000 (69).

It is particularly ironic that cancer of the cervix affects so many women in their reproductive years. The discovery of the Papanicolaou smear in 1941 and its refinements over the years (21,29) provide the means whereby almost all cervical carcinoma can be detected far earlier in the neoplastic or preoplastic process, to the point where almost all would be preventable or curable if every woman had an annual Pap smear. Unfortunately, only 10% to 15% of women in the United States obtain a Pap smear each year.

After the reproductive years and the menopause, the incidence of endometrial cancer and epithelial ovarian cancer rises sharply. These two malignancies demonstrate quite different biologic behavior, despite close anatomic and func-

tional relationship. Cancers of the endometrium usually present early in the history of the disease, with irregular bleeding; this often results in early diagnosis and high cure rates. Just the opposite is true with ovarian cancer; while it presents in the same general age group, it has no early symptoms, is difficult to detect, and is diagnosed in late stages where cures are difficult to achieve.

Nowhere is the importance of early diagnosis more clearly evident than in the comparison of uterine and ovarian cancer death rates in the last 50 years (69). In 1930, uterine cancer (endometrial and cervical) was the most common cause of death in women. Death rates have dropped more than two thirds since then, and now are roughly equivalent to those for ovarian cancer. The principal reasons for the decline in uterine cancer deaths have been the availability of the Papanicolaou smear and the accessibility of the endometrial cavity to diagnostic currettage. However, cancer of the ovary, without a clear means of early diagnosis, remains the fourth leading cause of cancer deaths in women, causing more than 12,500 deaths per year in the United States (69).

There are eight types of gynecologic cancer. The following sections are arranged in descending anatomical order: ovary, fallopian tube, endometrium, uterine sarcomas, gestastional trophoblastic tumors, cervix, vagina, and vulva.

Some similarities in cancer detection, diagnosis, and treatment will become apparent. At the same time, each of these cancers behave quite differently from one another in a number of ways. Therefore, each patient requires optimal individualization of treatment.

CERVICAL CARCINOMA

EPIDEMIOLOGY AND ETIOLOGY

Epidemiology

1. In the United States, there are 12,900 new cases of invasive cervical cancer annually. This disease is responsible for approximately 7,000 deaths per year (69). Although the mean age at diagnosis is 52 years, cervical cancer may be found in women between the ages of 17 and 90 years (27).

2. There are a variety of histologic subtypes of cervical carcinoma. Squamous cell carcinoma is the most frequently seen and accounts for 80% to 90% of invasive cervical cancers. The following epidemiologic data are mainly applicable to this subtype.

3. The incidence of cervical cancer is inversely related to socioeconomic status. This may account for the interracial differences observed. In 1985, the probability of a newborn white female developing invasive cervical cancer during her lifetime was 0.7%. The probability for a black female was 1.6% (28).

4. Sexual behavior seems to have an impact on cervical cancer development. Risk increases with early age of first coitus, total number of sexual partners, and number of sexual partners before age 20 years. Females who engage in intercourse shortly after their menarche may be at highest risk (28).

5. Cervical cancer is often associated with a history of sexually transmitted diseases, including gonorrhea, syphilis, herpes simplex, trichomonas, and chlamydia. If a woman has ever had genital warts, her risk of developing cervical cancer increases threefold (28)

6. Sexual habits of the male partner may also increase a woman's risk of developing carcinoma of the cervix. A "high risk male" has been characterized as one who has a history of genital carcinoma, venereal disease, a prior wife with cervical cancer, low socioeconomic status, or multiple sex partners (58).

7. Immunologic status can change the risk of developing cervical carcinoma. Chronically immunocompromised renal transplant patients have a higher incidence of preinvasive and invasive cervical neoplasia (35).

8. Elderly postmenopausal women (age > 60 years) who become less active or sexually inactive and are not being annually screened by Papanicolaou (PAP) smears account, in our experience, for an increasing percentage of advanced-stage (IIB and III) cervix cancer.

Etiology

1. Normal endocervical epithelium is columnar and mucin-producing. Vaginal epithelium is squamous and glycogenated. The point at which these two types of epithelium meet is known as the squamocolumnar junction. At approximately 24 weeks' gestation, the original squamocolumnar junction of the female fetus is most commonly found on the cervical portio. Later in life, the new squamocolumnar junction migrates up into the canal as squamous metaplasia takes place. Metaplasia is most active in utero, during adolescence, and during the first pregnancy (62). Most cervical cancers originate in this transformation zone where metaplasia occurs.

2. Cervical carcinomas were often seen in women who had a history of venereal disease; therefore, attempts were made to identify a potential infectious agent or cocarcinogen. In the 1970s, much effort was expended to prove that infection with herpes virus type II could lead to cervical neoplasia. Although a clear correlation between the two entities was established, a cause-and-effect relationship could not be proven.

3. Human papilloma virus (HPV) is now thought to play an important role in the pathogenesis of cervical carcinoma. Approximately 45 different HPV viruses have

been categorized by DNA sequencing (21). All degrees of cervical intraepithelial neoplasia and invasive cancers have been associated with HPV infections.

4. HPV types 6 and 11 are usually found in benign condylomata acuminata, low-grade dysplasias, and laryngeal papillomas. HPV types 16, 18, 31, 33, 35, and 39 are associated with high-grade dyplasias and carcinomas. In addition to this association, actual HPV DNA has been found in the cervical neoplasia cell genome. Although HPV has not definitively been shown to cause cervical cancer, research in this area remains promising.

DETECTION AND DIAGNOSIS

Screening

1. In the 1940s, Papanicolaou introduced exfoliative cytology as a method of screening for cervical carcinoma. The PAP smear has become a standard screening procedure in the United States.

2. Optimal cytologic samples include a cervical scrape and endocervical sampling. In the past, endocervical mucous aspiration was cumbersome: the standard endocervical sample was obtained by using a moist, cotton-tipped applicator. More recently, an endocervical brush has been developed and has been shown to provide superior samples (46a).

3. Although PAP smears have proven beneficial in diagnosing preclinical cervical disease, certain pitfalls of this screening technique should be outlined. False-negative rates in the 20% to 50% range have been reported (29). This is often due to physician sampling error, inadequate fixation, and inaccurate reporting by the cytopathologist. In an invasive carcinoma, the malignant cells may be masked by cellular debris and inflammatory cells. If a gross lesion is seen, cervical biopsy (not cytology) should be performed (28). Table 22-1 contains the current recommendations of the American College of Obstetricians and Gynecologists regarding frequency of PAP smear screening (14).

4. Molecular techniques for identification of human papilloma virus (HPV) DNA are highly sensitive and specific but their usefulness in the diagnosis and management of squamous cell carcinoma of the cervix has not been established (19a).

Diagnosis

1. Cervical intraepithelial neoplasia and early invasive carcinomas of the cervix are usually asymptomatic and discovered only with routine screening. An abnormal PAP smear should be evaluated by colposcopy. Neoplastic epithelium has distinct patterns that may be recognized with the magnification of the colposcope (9). Cervical biopsy may be guided by the colposcopic findings. At times, the abnormal epithelium is not evident on the cervical portio, and colposcopy is inadequate. In these situations, diagnostic cone biopsy may be required.

2. The most common complaint is abnormal vaginal bleeding including postcoital bleeding, postmenopausal bleeding, or irregular menses. As the tumor increases in size, the patient may complain of vaginal discharge. In more advanced cases, the patient may have pelvic pain or urinary symptoms.

Table 22-1. ACOG Suggested Frequency of Cytologic Screening for Cervical

Patient population	Frequency
≥ 18 years / or any age sexually active	Initial smear
High risk: early sexual intercourse, multiple partners	Annually
Low risk: Late sexual intercourse, single partners	After 2 successive negative smears; 3-5 year risk of abnormality is small. Decision of patient and physician
Diethylstilbestrol exposed	Onset of menstruation or 14 years or symptomatic (whichever occurs first) every 6 months -- annually
S/P hysterectomy	Vaginal smears 3-5 yearly
S/P therapy for preinvasive / invasive malignancy	Every 3 months for 2 years then every 6 months
Postmenopausal Sexually active Sexually inactive	 Annually Every other year

ACOG = American College of Obstetrics and Gynecology; S/P = salpingo-oophorectomy.

3. Examination of the patient with cervical cancer may reveal an isolated, friable lesion on the cervix. In more advanced cases, the cervix may be replaced with an exophytic tumor. Sometimes, the cervix appears normal on speculum examination, but palpation reveals an expanded, firm, "barrel-shaped" cervix. Finally, the tumor may cause ulceration of the cervix; in these cases, the cervix may be impossible to identify and a crater may be found at the top of the vagina, extending out onto the vaginal fornices.

4. Local spread beyond the cervix to the parametrial tissues is best appreciated on rectovaginal examination. The tumor may involve the vagina walls. Sometimes, it invades the base of the bladder or rectum.

5. When the patient has systemic disease, an enlarged, supraclavicular lymph node may be appreciated. Rarely, patients present with lung metastases.

6. The diagnosis of cervical cancer is made by biopsy. Tissue pathology is required prior to staging and treatment planning.

7. Imaging procedures (Table 22-2) (20): Computed tomography (CT) and magnetic resonance imaging (MRI) are more commonly used for determining depth of invasion and extension to sidewalls. MRI identifies cancer as an intense signal and can more readily determine fat invasion of parametria (2). According to Hricak, MR can distinguish late effects in pelvic soft tissue as fibrosis, necrosis or edema from pelvic recurrent cancer (41a).

CLASSIFICATION

Histopathology

1. The major histologic subtypes of cervical carcinoma are listed in Table 22-3 (20). Squamous cell lesions are seen most frequently (50). Within this group are keratinizing and nonkeratinizing cancers. At this point, there is no evidence to support a difference in prognosis between the two types.

2. Adenocarcinoma occurs in 10% to 20% of cases; there is evidence that the incidence is increasing (68). These cancers originate in the endocervical canal and often are of greater volume at diagnosis. Optimum treatment of adenocarcinomas is controversial. Recent reports suggest a combination of surgery and irradiation is superior to either method alone (18,79).

3. Clear cell carcinomas of the vagina and cervix are associated with diethylstilbestrol (DES) exposure in utero, initially described in 1971 (38). The risk of developing cancer is small — estimated to be one in 1,000 to one in 10,000 (38). More commonly, benign abnormalities such as adenosis (glandular epithelium located in the vagina), and cervical changes (transverse ridges, "cock's comb") are seen.

4. Small cell carcinomas of the cervix are of neuroendocrine origin. These cancers are very aggressive and are often widely disseminated at the time of diagnosis (75). The prognosis for patients treated with conventional therapy, even at an early stage, is dismal (66). Borrowing from the literature concerning small cell bronchogenic carcinomas, some authors have advocated the addition of combination chemotherapy and radiation to traditional therapy (36,55a).

5. Other rare cervical malignancies include verrucous carcinoma, adenoid basal cell carcinoma, adenoid cystic carcinoma, and glassy cell carcinoma. Cervical sarcomas are rare also.

Staging

1. Recently, the staging system for cervical carcinoma has been changed. The most commonly used system is that proposed by the International Federation of Gynecology and Obstetrics (FIGO). In 1985, the system was changed to take into account tumor volume in early-stage disease. Table 22-4 and Fig. 22-1 outline the current system.

2. The FIGO staging system for cervix cancer is based on a clinical staging. Allowable staging procedures include physical examination (usually examination under anesthesia) with cystoscopy and proctoscopy. Radiologic studies, which may be used include an intravenous (IV) pyelogram, barium enema, chest x-ray, and skeletal x-rays.

Table 22-2. Imaging Procedures for Detection and Diagnosis of Carcinoma of the Cervix

METHOD	CAPABILITY	RECOMMENDED FOR USE
Primary tumor and regional nodes		
CT	Detects liver metastases > 1 cm in size; detects lymphadenopathy > 15 mm in size; detects extension of tumor locally to pelvic sidewall	Patients with high clinical stage
MRI	Detects soft tissue extent	Optional
Urography	Detects parametrial extension of tumor-producing hydronephrosis; screens for unsuspected urinary tract disease	Routine
Barium enema	Detects serosal invasion of primary tumor; screens for diverticulosis, adenomatous polyps	Patients with colonic symptoms or guaiac-positive stool
Biopsy	Confirms lesion detected by radionuclide scans, CT scans, or lymphangiograms	Patients with suspicious lesions
Metastatic		
Chest radiography	Detects soft tissue nodules > 15 mm; detects acute/chronic pulmonary disease	Routine
Skeletal radiography	Confirms suspicious findings on radionuclide scans	When radionuclide scan is equivocal
Liver sonography	Detects metastatic deposits > 15 mm.	Patients with elevated liver enzyme levels
Radionuclide bone	Sensitive assessment of bone metastases	Operative candidates, patients with elevated alkaline phosphatase or bone pain

CT = computed tomography; MRI = magnetic resonance imaging.
Adapted from Bragg et al. (20).

Table 22-3. Histologic Classification of Uterine Cervix Carcinoma

Type	INCIDENCE (%)
Squamous Carcinoma	
Large cell keratinizing	22 ⎫
Large cell nonkeratinizing	57 ⎬ 75-85
Small cell nonkeratinizing	6 ⎭
Adenocarcinoma	
Endocervical	
Endometrioid	10-15
Clear cell	
Others	
Mixed epithelial carcinoma	
Adenosquamous	2-5
Glassy cell	
Neuroendocrine	
Carcinoid	
Small cell	

From Bragg et al. (20), with permission.

Table 22-4. Comparison of FIGO and AJC Stagings of Carcinoma of the Cervix

FIGO		Site	AJC (1)
Stage	IA1	Microinvasive carcinoma with minimal stromal invasion	$T_{1a} N_0 M_0$
	A2	measurable invasion ≤ 5mm	
Stage	IB	Invasive cancer confined to the cervix > 5 mm	$T_{1b} N_0 M_0$
Stage	IIA	Extension to vagina (not lower one third)	$T_{2a} N_0 M_0$
Stage	IIB	Extension to parametrium	$T_{2b} N_0 M_0$
Stage	IIIA	Extension to lower one third of vagina	$T_{3a} N_0 M_0$
Stage	IIIB	Extension to pelvic side wall/hydronephrosis	$T_{1-3b} N_1 M_0$ $T_{3b} N_0 M_0$
Stage	IVA	Extension to bladder/rectum/beyond true pelvis	$T_4 N_{any} M_0$

T = tumor; N = node; M = metastasis.

FIGO (83) = International Federation of Gynecology and Obstetrics; AJC(1) = American Joint Committee on Cancer Staging.

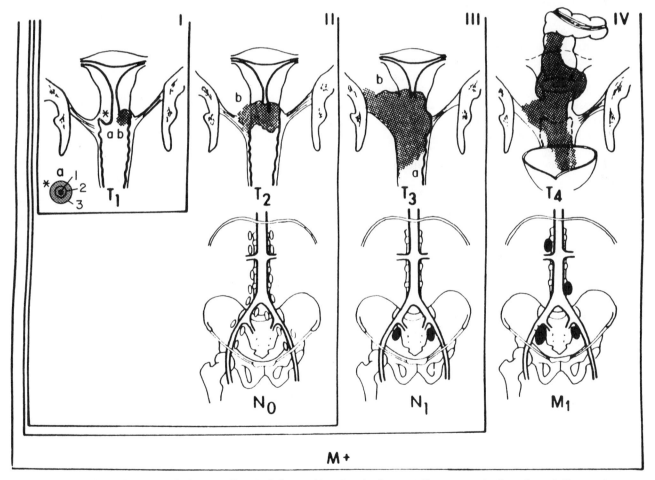

Fig. 22-1. Anatomic staging for cervical cancer. Key: 1 = Submental lymph nodes (cancer of larynx, anterior floor of mouth, lip, anterior two-thirds of tongue, gums, and mucosa of cheek. 2 = Submaxillary nodes (same sites as above). 3 = Superficial cervical nodes (cancer of nasopharynx). 4 = Superor deep cervical nodes (cancer of nasopharynx, oral cavity, pharynx, or larynx). 5 = Jugular chain nodes (cancer of the thyroid and nasopharynx). 6 = Spinal accessory nodes (cancer of the nasopharynx, oral cavity, pharynx, thyroid). 7 = Supraclavicular nodes (cancer of the thyroid, pyriform sinus, upper esophagus, primary below clavicle).

3. Lymphangiography and more sophisticated radiographic examinations, including CT scan and MRI have been used to further determine the extent of disease (1a). Suspicious, enlarged para-aortic nodes should be sampled by fine needle aspiration (FNA). It is important to note that information obtained by these ancillary studies does not alter the FIGO stage; however, it may affect treatment (Table 22-5) (40,52).

4. Although these studies may detect nodal metastases, nearly 28% of patients with stage III disease have occult para-aortic metastases not detected by radiographic means (19) (Table 22-5).

5. Surgical staging remains controversial in the evaluation and treatment of cervical carcinoma patients. The controversy is based on the risk of the surgical procedure and the number of patients with para-aortic disease who can be cured. Initially, a transabdominal approach was taken. Combined with extended field radiotherapy, this approach resulted in unacceptable morbidity due to bowel complications (80).

   Currently, an extraperitoneal approach is used and associated morbidity has been greatly reduced (47,62,78). Extended field radiotherapy prolongs survival and can cure some patients with para-aortic metastases (42). Therefore, since the morbidity with an extraperitoneal approach is acceptable, surgical staging may be justified in those patients at risk for para-aortic nodal spread.

6. In patients who have para-aortic metastases, a scalene node biopsy may be helpful in detecting occult systemic disease. Five percent to 30% of patients with positive para-aortic nodes will have supraclavicular metastases (22). Certainly, if a patient has an enlarged supraclavicular node, FNA should be performed to rule out systemic disease prior to initiating extensive radiation therapy.

7. Overexpression of the c-myc oncogene has been reported to be associated with poorer prognosis in invasive cervix cancer (80a).

PRINCIPLES OF TREATMENT

A multidisciplinary approach entailing cooperation between the gynecologic oncologist and radiation oncologist is essential to planning and for managing patients. Prior to any decision-making process, the pathologist and diagnostic imager actively participate in tumor classification and the staging process. Clinical trials are always encouraged. Table 22-6 summarizes the treatment decisions by stage.

Cervical Dysplasia and Carcinoma in situ

Cervical intraepithelial neoplasia I — III is usually treated with local methods. These include cryotherapy, electocautery, excision, conization, and laser therapy. Hysterectomy has also been used to treat cervical dysplasias and carcinoma in situ. The recurrence rate following cone biopsy is approximately 3% compared with a recurrence rate of about 1% following hysterectomy (46). Since almost 97% of women can be cured with cone biopsy, routine hysterectomy for pre-invasive disease is not warranted (9).

Invasive Cervical Carcinoma

Both surgery and radiation therapy are effective in the treatment of cervical carcinoma. The choice of treatment modality depends on the size and stage of the lesion, as well as the patient's general medical condition. Traditionally, chemotherapy is reserved for women with systemic disease. More recently, chemotherapy has been administered as a radiation sensitizer during primary treatment with radiotherapy. Finally, a new role for chemotherapy in a neoadjuvant setting is currently being investigated.

Surgery

Surgery is limited to early cancers in stages I and IIA. It may also be used in previously irradiated patients with recurrent disease. The different types of total abdominal hysterectomy are Intrafascial, Extrafascial Type I, Modified Radical Type II, and Radical Type III.

Stage Ia: Preclinical Cervical Carcinomas

1. Stage Ia cervical carcinoma is divided into two groups. Stage IA_1 represents those lesions in which there is minimal microscopically evident stromal invasion. Often, the depth of invasion is less than 1mm and is not measurable. Such patients may be treated with a standard, extrafascial hysterectomy. If childbearing is of concern, a cone biopsy may be adequate therapy (38), providing the specimen has clear margins.

2. Stage IA_2 lesions are treated in several ways, based on certain histologic variables. In the previous staging system, FIGO was not specific in its definition for microinvasion. Definitions and interpretations varied. In 1974, the Society of Gynecologic Oncologists (SGO)

Table 22-5. **Incidence of Lymph Node Involvement in Carcinoma of the Cervix**

Stage	Lymph nodes (%) Involved by Stage Para-aortic	Pelvic
I	5-8	11-30
IIA	7-18	23-33
IIB	17-33	23-33
IIIA	33	37-50
IIIB	19-46	37-50
IV	25-57	52

Adapted from Marcial (52) and Hoskins et al. (40).

(6,57,59')

Table 22-6. Multidisciplinary Treatment Decisions by Stage for Cervical Carcinoma

Stage	Surgery	Radiation Therapy	Chemotherapy
IA (T_{1a}, N_0) microinvasive	Total hysterectomy or Conization in select group	CRT Intracavitary RT mainly Pt. A: 70 Gy; Pt.B: 50 Gy	NR
IB* invasive (T_{1b}, N_0) IIA (T_{2a}, N_0)	Radical hysterectomy plus Pelvic node dissection extrafascial and/or	CRT Combined intracavitary and external RT Pt. A: 75 Gy; Pt. B: 55 Gy Para-aortic: 45 Gy	CCR
IIB (T_{2b}, N_0) IIIA,B (T_3, N_1, M_0) IV (T_4, N_0, M_0)	NR, surgical staging NR, surgical staging Exenteration for central locations	CRT Combined external, intracavitary and vaginal RT Pt. A: 80 Gy, Pt. B: 60 Gy Para-aortic: 45 Gy	CCR IC II
IV (T_{any}, N_{any}, M_+) Metastatic	NR	PRT	IC II

*Bulky or barrel-shaped cervix, Stages I-IIA preoperative irradiation and extrafascial hysterectomy.

RT = radiation therapy; CRT = curative; DRT = definitive; PRT = palliative; NR = not recommended; IC II = investigational chemotherapy, phase I/II clinical trials; CCR = concurrent chemotherapy and radiation. PDQ: NR - CCR = hydrozyurea, 5-FU/cisplatin or mitomycin C.

recommended a definition for microinvasive cervical cancer. This has been widely adopted and used in determining treatment. The definition of a microinvasive lesion is one in which neoplastic epithelium invades the stroma to a depth of less than or equal to 3 mm beneath the basement membrane and in which lymphatic or blood vascular involvement is not demonstrated.

3. The risk of lymph node metastases in lesions that have less than 3 mm of invasion is less than 1% (70). Therefore, those patients with stage Ia_2 disease who fulfill the SGO criteria for microinvasion can be treated with extrafascial hysterectomy. Cone biopsy (with clear margins) also can be used if childbearing potential is desired; however, this conservative treatment has not been extensively evaluated.

4. Because the incidence of lymph node metastases is significant in lesions with 3 to 5 mm invasion, more radical treatment is indicated. Although reports vary, about 8% of these patients are found to have lymph node metastases (56). Therefore, stage IA_2 patients who do not meet SGO criteria for microinvasion should be treated with a modified radical hysterectomy and pelvic lymphadenectomy.

5. Any stage IA patient who is a poor surgical candidate may be treated with radiotherapy.

Stage IB: Lesions of Greater Dimensions than Stage IA

1. In general, Stage IB patients may be treated with radical hysterectomy and pelvic lymphadenectomy. During a radical hysterectomy, the uterus, cervix, surrounding parametrial tissues, cardinal ligaments, and upper vagina are removed. The ovaries may be left in situ in young women.

2. Many gynecologic oncologists limit radical hysterectomy as primary treatment to patients with small cervical tumors. Patients with bulky cervical cancers, that is, lesions greater than 4 cm in size or barrel-shaped cervices are candidates for combined therapy. They are treated with preoperative external beam and intracavitary

irradiation followed by a standard, extrafascial hysterectomy. Retrospective studies suggest a lower recurrence rate in patients treated with combined therapy (32).

3. Radiation therapy can be an alternate effective treatment with minimal morbidity. The Gynecologic Oncology Group (GOG) is conducting a prospective, randomized trial comparing irradiation alone versus irradiation plus adjuvant extrafascial hysterectomy in these patients.

4. In a large surgico-pathologic staging study of clinical Stage IB patients, adverse factors are capillary-lymphatic space involvement, increasing tumor size and increasing depth of stromal invasion (26a).

Stage IIA: Cervical Carcinoma Involving the Upper Vagina

Appropriate surgical treatment for stage IIA cervical carcinomas is radical hysterectomy with pelvic/para-aortic lymphadenectomy. Lesion size may influence the choice of primary surgery versus primary irradiation.

Persistent or Recurrent Disease

1. If the carcinoma recurs after treatment with radiation therapy, the patient may be a candidate for surgery. The recurrence must be central and confined to the cervix, uterus, bladder, and rectum. Patients with disease that extends to the sidewall or patients with distant metastases cannot be salvaged by surgery.

2. Pelvic exenteration (removal of uterus, cervix, bladder, rectum, with subsequent urostomy and colostomy) may be performed. In selected cases, an anterior exenteration (removal of bladder, anterior vagina, cervix, and uterus) may be acceptable if the tumor is confined to the cervix and upper vagina. Cure rates for patients undergoing exenterative surgery range from 20% to 45% (11).

Radiation Therapy

Radiotherapy has been very effective in the treatment of cervical carcinoma. All stages may be treated with irradiation. This form of treatment is nearly always used in patients with stages higher than stage IIA. Approximate cure rates include

80% for stage I, 60% for stage II, 30% for stage III, and 10% for stage IV (4). Treatment plans are designed individually based on the clinical (and surgical) stage of the disease. Most commonly, patients are treated with combinations of external beam and intracavitary radiation therapy. We advocate the customization of radiation dose to extent or stage of disease similar to the MIR policies of treatment.

External Beam

External beam radiotherapy (supravoltage) is usually limited to the pelvis and includes tissues between the obturator foramina and the lower common iliac lymph nodes. Various portals for external beam irradiation can be designed. In addition, extended field radiation (including the para-aortic lymph nodes) may be used if initial evaluation reveals para-aortic metastases or when occult disease is suspected.

Intracavitary Irradiation

1. Intracavitary irradiation is also important in the treatment of cervical carcinoma. A hollow, metal tube (tandem) is placed into the endocervical canal and uterus. Two hollow vaginal colpostats are also placed in the vaginal fornices. Cesium sources are then placed in the hollow devices. The dose distribution is pear-shaped, with the largest dose in the area of the upper vagina, cervix, and parametria. The importance of intracavitary irradiation in bettering results in cervix cancer can be found in two reports. Marcial et al. (51a) compare 1 versus 2 or more intracavitary brachytherapy applications and Lanciano et al. (46b) note the impact on local control in more advanced Stage IIIB cases when intracavitary brachytherapy is not an integral part of the treatment plan. In Marcial's report, the 5-year actuarial survival for all stages is 66% for > 2 intracavitary applications versus 59% for one application. More striking is the impact on local control within field recurrences for all stages being 17% versus 30% and in Stage III the differences were 34% versus 53%, respectively. This is also confirmed in advanced Stage IIIB patients by Lanciano et al. (46b) who used intracavitary therapy with external irradiation and provided an improved 4-year survival rate of 65% versus 50%. As anticipated, parametrial dose is a strong correlate with end results.

2. The total dose given is usually described in relation to two reference points. Point A is 2 cm lateral and 2 cm superior to the external cervical os. Theoretically, point A represents the area where the uterine artery crosses the ureter. Point B is 3 cm lateral to point A and corresponds to the pelvic sidewall (iliac lymph nodes). In general, 7,500 to 8,500 cGy are delivered to point A and 4,500 to 6,500 cGy are delivered to point B. Dose calculations have standardized with adoption of Pt A (paracervical) and Pt B (pelvic sidewall) according to ICRU Handbook #38, 1985 (42a) and references point doses to anterior rectal wall and posterior bladder wall. The gradual introduction of computer reconstruction of isodose curves for both internal and external radiation sources will allow for more accurate determination of effective tumor doses and tolerable normal issue dose/volumes.

3. High-dose rate versus low-dose rate intracavitary brachytherapy for carcinoma of the cervix is reviewed by Fu and Phillips (31). Nonrandomized studies — which are in the majority — and the few randomized studies suggest similar survival, local control, and complication rates using fractionated high-dose-rate compared with protracted low-dose-rate. The 5-year survival results and local control rates reported in cervical cancers using HDBT equal those achieved with low dose rate brachytherapy (LDBT). This observation is confirmed in the experience of Chen et al. (23a) in treating approximately 400 patients with carcinoma of the cervix in a comparative study of HDRBT versus LDRBT following external irradiation. The techniques used in different institutions vary, and the danger with high-dose rate techniques is that one usually adopts a large fraction size (e.g., 4 to 5 Gy) with multiple fractions, usually 1 to 2 each week throughout the course of external irradiation. The FIGO annual summary report of 1987 (15) shows comparable results: there is no great difference in complications, with the exception of the Shigemutsu et al. series (67), one of the pioneers of this technique. Joslin demonstrated that higher control rates do mean higher complication rates, usually in rectum and bladder (44).

4. For medically inoperable patients, a single intracaviary insertion with tandem and ovoids for 8000 cGy vaginal surface (5000 mg hr) dose has been found effective in carcinoma-in-situ and Stage IA (32a).

Interstitial Radiotherapy

Interstitial implants also may be of benefit in the treatment of cervical carcinoma. Adequate treatment of the tumor is dependent on the geometry of the tumor and surrounding tissues. At times, adequate radiotherapy cannot be obtained with standard intracavitary applicators. With interstitial therapy, a template is placed on the vulva and hollow needles are inserted through the template into the tumor and surrounding tissues. After confirming adequate placement, iridium-192 is inserted into the needles. This device is particularly useful in patients with bulky parametrial disease, as well as for those who have vaginal recurrences following surgical therapy for cervical carcinoma.

Para-aortic versus Pelvic Irradiation

Rotman et al. (64) report on a large Radiation Therapy Oncology Group (RTOG) study that clearly demonstrates that para-aortic field irradiation added to pelvic irradiation results in a moderate incremental gain of approximately 10% in local control and a decrease of 5% in distant metastases; this translates to an overall 11% gain in 5-year survival from 55% to 66% in stage IB and IIB cervical cancer. Fletcher (31) presents the trials and tribulations of pursuing the concept of extended fields in cervical carcinoma. The complication rate increased with doses more than 45 Gy, but is also due to the larger volume included in para-aortic fields. The vexing issue of using extended field irradiation for known positive periaortic nodes in cervix cancer is addressed by Vigliotti et al. (76a). They argue persuasively that 28% of their series are alive, free of disease with a 32% actuarial survival rate. The favorable set of periaortic node-positive patients have small nodes < 2 cm in size, pelvic disease that can be reasonably controlled with standard radiation techniques, and the disease extending no higher than 3 cm. A European Organization on Research and Treatment of Cancer (EORTC) trial (34) showed no difference in relapse-free survival, but this was attributed to the inclusion of advanced stage III patients. Reasons for the RTOG success was in altering patterns of failure: cancer-related deaths occurred in only 20% of the para-aortic field patients versus 34% for those receiving pelvic irradiation only. The caveat remains, however, that if surgical exploration is done, there is a large difference in complications, i.e., 17% versus 2% without laparotomy (64).

Radiation Therapy Combined with Other Treatment Modalities

1. In an attempt to improve survival, several investigators have added chemotherapeutic agents as radiosensitizers to standard radiation treatment. The addition of hydroxyurea has improved response and survival rates (41,60). Other agents such as mitomycin C and 5-FU (74) and cisplatin (24) have been investigated and seem to provide a radiation-sensitizing effect. A high response rate was noted in a small series of cancer cervix cases using 5-FU, mitomycin C infusion with 30 Gy with the majority being complete responses (CRs) (13). The GOG has an ongoing, prospective, randomized trial comparing hydroxyurea versus cisplatin/5-FU as radiosensitizers in advanced-stage cervical carcinoma.
2. In patients with bulky or barrel-shaped stage IB cervix cancers, radiation therapy may be combined with surgery. This approach still remains somewhat controversial. Some retrospective studies conclude that radiation therapy and surgery are equally effective in the treatment of these cancers (52a,77); however, other investigators have found a lower recurrence rate in those patients treated with the combined approach (32,74a). The GOG currently is evaluating both approaches in a prospective, randomized trial.

Postoperative Radiotherapy Following Radical Hysterectomy

Poor prognostic indicators have been identified in patients undergoing radical hysterectomy for early cervix cancer. These include nodal metastases, positive margins, deep cervical invasion, and involvement of the parametrial tissues. Many authors recommend postoperative external beam irradiation (4,500 to 5,000 cGy) in these circumstances. Morbidity is acceptable (43); however, a clear survival benefit has not been demonstrated (55). The GOG is presently conducting a prospective, randomized trial investigating the benefit of postoperative radiation therapy in patients with large, deeply invasive tumors.

Chemotherapy

1. In the past, chemotherapy was reserved for patients with advanced or recurrent disease not amenable to surgical intervention or radiation therapy. In general, results with chemotherapy have been poor. This is often attributed to the fact that by the time chemotherapy is used, the patient has already been treated with surgery and/or radiotherapy. When recurrences develop in a previously irradiated field, it is difficult to obtain therapeutic tissue levels of chemotherapeutic agents (at the site of recurrence) due to the decreased blood supply.
2. Recently, chemotherapy has been introduced into primary therapy as an adjunct to surgery or radiotherapy.

Advanced or Recurrent Disease: (Table 22-7) (40)

Multiple agents have been evaluated for efficacy in patients with advanced or recurrent disease. With single agents, response rates vary from 6% to 40%. The single agent with the most activity is cisplatin (72,73). Different combinations of drugs have been evaluated. However, a randomized trial by the Southwest Oncology Group (SWOG) revealed no advantage of combination drugs over cisplatin alone (17). Standard administration is cisplatin 50 mg/m^2 every 3 weeks. There is some enthusiasm for combination chemotherapy, with a response rate of 69% for MVAC and 45% for mitomycin C/bleomycin/cisplatin (51,71).

SPECIAL CONSIDERATIONS OF TREATMENT

Cervical Cancer in Pregnancy

1. Cervical carcinoma complicates one in 2,200 pregnancies (33). Abnormal PAP smears should be evaluated with colposcopy and biopsies. Cone biopsy may be necessary if the PAP smear reveals malignant cells and invasive cancer cannot be diagnosed with colposcopically directed biopsies.
2. Treatment options depend on disease stage at diagnosis, the gestational age of the fetus, and the wishes of the patient. Patients with stage IA disease diagnosed on cone biopsy can be followed to term and undergo definitive therapy after delivery.
3. In patients with invasive cancer diagnosed before 20 weeks' gestation, the patient should be treated without regard to the fetus. Treatment modality is dependent on disease stage. Therapy can be delayed in those patients who are diagnosed after 20 weeks' gestation until fetal maturity is established. At that time, delivery is effected (usually by Cesarean section) and treatment is started.

Table 22-7. Combination Chemotherapy in Treatment of Cervical Carcinoma

Regimen	No. Evaluable Patients	Responses (%)	Complete Responses (%)
Doxorubicin/methotrexate	59	66	22
	24	28	0
AC	13	45	29
Doxorubicin and cisplatin	19	31	10
Mitomycin C and bleomycin	33	36	15
Mitomycin C, vincristine, and bleomycin	91	51	15
MOB-III	14	43	29
VBP	33	66	18
CABO	15	66	20

From Hoskins et al. (40), with permission.

4. The overall prognosis for pregnant patients with cervical carcinoma does not differ from that of nonpregnant women (33,48).

Cervical Stump Carcinoma

Following subtotal hysterectomy, patients may develop a carcinoma in the cervical stump. Currently an infrequent occurrence, this situation provides some treatment dilemmas. When the cancer is limited to the cervix (stage I), a surgical approach may be taken. More advanced disease should be treated with radiotherapy. External beam irradiation may be given effectively but placement of an intracavitary tandem is hindered by a short endocervical canal. Interstitial irradiation may be of some benefit in this situation.

Cervical Carcinoma Found at Simple Hysterectomy

1. Rarely, cervical cancer is detected in the hysterectomy specimen obtained in the treatment of benign disease. This often results from incomplete evaluation prior to surgery. Patients may be treated with postoperative radiotherapy or reoperation.
2. With postoperative pelvic irradiation, survival of patients with presumed stage IA disease is 100%; those with invasive cancer and clear surgical margins have nearly an 80% 5-year survival (37). In a series of patients who underwent reoperation (consisting of lymphadenectomy, radical parametrectomy, and upper vaginectomy), 73% of patients had surgical findings that obviated additional radiation therapy (56).

RESULTS AND PROGNOSIS

Long-Term Survival

Survival of patients treated between 1979 and 1981 are reported in the FIGO annual report (72). Table 22-8 (59) illustrates that overall survival for all stages approaches 55%. The comparison of results by irradiation and surgery for stage I cervix cancer are similar (Table 22-9). Usually, however, the more medically compromised and older patients are treated by radiation therapy; this lowers survival because of host factors.

Survival After Surgery

Radical surgery has been effective in the treatment of cervical carcinomas. Fig. 22-2 shows the 5-year survival statistics of all stages of squamous and adenocarcinomas treated with surgery alone. For stage I disease, cure rates approach 85% (12).

Table 22-8. Five-Year Survival by Stage for Cervical Carcinoma

Stage	No. Patients Treated	Five-yr Survival (%)
I	10,791	78.1
II	11,599	57.0
III	8623	31.0
IV	1377	7.8
No stage	9	——
Total	32,428	55.0

From Petterson (59), with permission.

Survival After Radiation Therapy

Radiation therapy is effective in the treatment of cervical carcinoma; it is superior to a surgical approach in higher-stage disease. Fig. 22-2 illustrates the 5-year survival for all stages treated with irradiation alone.

Complications

In a thorough analysis of more than 1200 cervical cancer patients followed for a minimum of 5 years, Perez *et al.* (57a) offer accumulated dose correlations and TDF guidelines for optimizing tumor control while minimizing complications. The pelvic failure rate decreases independent of stage as a function of dose to Pt A (<60 Gy, 60–90 Gy, > 90 Gy); the local recurrences in Stage IIB are 66.7%, 23.4%, 3.5%, respectively. Of greatest concern with normal tissues are

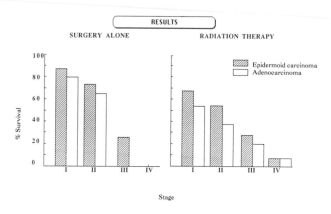

Fig. 22-2. Cervical cancer results: 5-year survival by stage. From Pettersson (12), with permission.

Table 22-9. Five-year Survival for Stage I Cervical Carcinoma with Surgery or Radiation Therapy

No. Patients	Surgery % Survival	Reference	No. Patients	Radiation Therapy % Survival	Reference
189	86.3	26	549	91.5	30
266	90.0	25	312	85.0	57
110	90.0	16	197	83.0	53
55	92.3	61	48	91.1	61

severe small bowel, rectosigmoid, and bladder injury, which, when added together, rarely exceed a 10% complication rate, and major sequelae are usually less than 5%. However, they are dose related and the rectosigmoid complications for similar doses are 2 to 4% for 60–80 Gy, 7 to 8% for 80–95 Gy, and 13% for > 95 Gy. The tolerance doses T5/5 from their data can be revised to small bowel < 60 Gy, rectosigmoid < 75 Gy, bladder 80 Gy provided small volumes are irradiated. These authors deserve praise for the painstaking detail they have given to determining and displaying their data and their literature review.

Impact of Local Regional Control on Distant Metastases

The identification of more effective therapeutic strategies designed to completely eradicate the primary tumor at the time of initial therapy is providing a strong rationale for clinical studies using 3-D conformal radiation therapy (26b).

CLINICAL INVESTIGATIONS

Chemotherapy Used as a Radiosensitizer

Hydroxyurea added to standard radiation therapy has been shown to increase response rates and survival (41,59a,60). Mitomycin C/5-FU and cisplatin/5-FU also have been shown to be effective in combination with irradiation (24,74). The GOG is presently undertaking a prospective, randomized trial comparing hydroxurea and radiotherapy versus cisplatin/5-FU and radiotherapy in patients with advanced cervical carcinomas.

Neoadjuvant Chemotherapy

Recently, combination chemotherapy used as primary treatment prior to radical surgery has been described (45,65,65a). In these cases, a modified VPB regimen was administered. The patients subsequently underwent radical hysterectomy with pelvic lymphadenectomy. This approach was not limited to early-stage disease. Early reports are promising, but further investigation is necessary.

INTRA-ARTERIAL INFUSION OF CHEMOTHERAPY

Several investigators have reported the use of intra-arterial infusion of various chemotherapeutic agents (49,54). Results have not shown an improvement over other methods of administration. The GOG is currently evaluating this method in selected institutions.

ENDOMETRIAL CARCINOMA

EPIDEMIOLOGY AND ETIOLOGY

1. Endometrial carcinoma is the most prevalent cancer of the female genital tract in the United States. Although 34,000 new cases are diagnosed annually, early diagnosis and effective treatment reduce the death rate to approximately 3,000 women annually for this disease (135).
2. The majority of patients are postmenopausal, with a median age at diagnosis of 61 years (108). However, 2.9% to 14.4% of patients with endometrial cancer are less than 40 years of age (95,101). Therefore, premeno-

pausal women at high risk for endometrial carcinoma who have abnormal uterine bleeding or long periods of amenorrhea should have histologic evaluation of the endometrium.
3. Risk factors for endometrial carcinoma are well defined. Obesity is associated with up to a tenfold increase in relative risk for endometrial cancer (106). A relative increase in free estrogen occurs in obese women due to a decrease in sex hormone-binding globulin and increased aromatization of circulating androgens, such as androstenedione, into estrone (137). In premenopausal women, this increase in estrone may produce anovulation, which allows incessant estrogen stimulation of the endometrium, a known factor in the development of both endometrial hyperplasia and carcinoma. An increased incidence of endometrial carcinoma also has been noted in women using either sequential oral contraceptives or menopausal estrogen replacement without progestins. The relative risk of developing endometrial cancer is increased by 1.7% to 8.0% in women on conjugated estrogens alone (103); however, the addition of adequate progestin treatment decreases the relative risk to 0.3% (102). Estrogen-secreting tumors may be associated with both endometrial hyperplasia and carcinoma (10). Nulliparous women and women with long periods of uninterrupted ovarian function are at slightly increased risk for endometrial carcinoma. Anovulation, from whatever etiology, also increases risk for endometrial carcinoma (102,103). Approximately 20% to 30% of untreated women with polycystic ovarian syndrome develop endometrial hyperplasia (137).
4. Heredity may be a factor in development of endometrial cancer, as women with a family history of breast, ovarian, or colon cancer are at higher risk for development of endometrial cancer. An autosomal dominant mechanism has been proposed (121).
5. Various forms of endometrial hyperplasia are recognized as precursors of endometrial carcinoma; these develop in the same hyperestrogenic hormonal milieu as well-differentiated adenocarcinomas of the endometrium (10,86). The presence of cytologic atypia within the hyperplasia increases the risk of developing endometrial carcinoma from 1.6% to 23% (110).

DETECTION AND DIAGNOSIS

Detection

1. The most common symptom is abnormal uterine bleeding, which occurs in more than 90% of patients. Postmenopausal bleeding is always abnormal and uterine sampling is mandatory. However, only 15% to 20% of patients with postmenopausal bleeding have endometrial cancer (11). In premenopausal women, menometrorrhagia may be noted.
2. Other symptoms rarely occur in the absence of uterine bleeding.
3. Rarely, an abnormal PAP smear suggests the presence of endometrial cancer in an asymptomatic patient. Normal endometrial cells can appear in vaginal pool PAP smears; although this may warrant further evaluation in postmenopausal women, the only finding on

PAP reliably associated with carcinoma is atypical endometrial cells (149). The presence of malignant endometrial cells on cervical cytology is associated with more advanced stage (97a).

4. Routine screening of asymptomatic postmenopausal women by endometrial sampling has been used to detect occult carcinoma. With aspiration curettage, occult endometrial carcinoma was detected in 0.6% of screened women in one study (109). The value of screening asymptomatic patients at risk still is being evaluated.

5. An elevated CA-125 antigen may also suggest the presence of an endometrial carcinoma. Although generally used in following patients with ovarian cancer, the CA-125 assay is elevated in patients with advanced endometrial carcinoma and may be useful in detection of recurrent disease (98,119).

Diagnosis

1. Fractional dilatation and curettage (D&C) of the uterus has been the standard diagnostic method for endometrial carcinoma. However, outpatient suction curettage provides diagnostic information comparable with fractional D&C, and has a false-negative rate of less than 3% (11). Other techniques, such as endometrial brush lavage, aspiration and vaginal smears are much less accurate and reliable in making a diagnosis (Table 22-10) (145).

2. Hysteroscopy with directed endometrial biopsy or curettage may further decrease the false-negative rate associated with D&C (127).

3. Occasionally, the distinction between a primary adenocarcinoma of the cervix or an endometrial carcinoma with cervical extension (stage II) is difficult. Cervical adenocarcinomas will more frequently contain intracytoplasmic mucin and will stain mucicarmine or Alcian-blue positive, whereas endometrial adenocarcinomas stain positive for mucin in 9% of patients (128). On immunohistochemical stain for carcinoembryonic antigen (CEA), endocervical primary tumors will be positive more often than will be endometrial carcinomas (89). Additionally, if the uterine corpus is enlarged and the cervix normal-size, then an endometrial primary is the more likely diagnosis.

4. Routine tests in the evaluation of a patient with endometrial carcinoma include chest x-ray, complete blood cell count, and evaluation of hepatic and renal function. If a pelvic mass is present, CT scan and barium enema are often performed. MRI is investigational, but it may, by signal intensity, predict depth of invasion into myometrium (2,20) (Table 22-11).

5. Endometrial carcinoma typically spreads by invasion of the myometrium with tumor infiltration of the lymphatics within the myometrium. Tumor may also extend into the lower uterine segment and through the endocervix. Tumor embolization in the myometrial and cervical lymphatics may result in pelvic and para-aortic lymph node involvement. Intraperitoneal spread (IP) of disease may result from transtubal spread of tumor or from transmural invasion of the myometrium. Less frequently, hematogenous dissemination can occur with pulmonary or hepatic metastases.

CLASSIFICATION AND STAGING

Histopathology (Table 22-12)

Endometrial hyperplasia is characterized by proliferation of endometrial glands, with or without atypia, with a relative decrease in endometrial stroma. Often, a well-differentiated, superficial adenocarcinoma of the endometrium will be difficult to distinguish from atypical endometrial hyperplasia. In the absence of myometrial invasion, an invasive adenocarcinoma is best differentiated from atypical hyperplasia by stromal invasion. Stromal invasion may be demonstrated by infiltration of atypical glands into the stroma, which produces a desmoplastic response (111).

Endometrial carcinoma may present with a variety of histologic subtypes (Table 22-12).

1. *Endometrioid adenocarcinoma* is the most common subtype; such tumors may contain isolated foci of other subtypes. Discernible atypical endometrial glands with varying degrees of stromal or myometrial invasion are seen histologically (10).

2. *Papillary serous carcinoma* is a more virulent subtype, with a high rate of recurrence even in stage I disease (100). This tumor may have an increased tendency to

Table 22-10. Accuracy of Diagnostic Methods for Endometrial Carcinoma

Method	No. Carcinomas	Accuracy (%)
Vaginal and ectocervical smear	1,433	42.2
Endocervical aspiration	454	72.9
Endometrial lavage	206	81.6
Endometrial brush	278	17.4
Gravlee jet-washer	328	83.0
Vabra aspirator	40	97.5
Endometrial biopsy	456	90.6

From Vuopala (145), with permission.

Table 22-11. Imaging Procedures for Detection and Diagnosis of Endometrial Carcinoma

METHOD	CAPABILITY	RECOMMENDED FOR USE
Primary tumor and regional nodes		
CT	Accurate staging information; assesses myometrial invasion. Not known to be accurate in detecting lymph node spread	All patients except those with clinical stage I grade 1 tumor, or clinical stage IV.
MRI	Not yet investigated. Potentially useful in local tumor staging	Unknown
Urography	Detects ureteral obstruction, bladder invasion; screens for unsuspected renal anomaly	All operative candidates
Barium enema	Detects serosal implantation of peritoneal spread; screens for diverticulosis, adenomatous polyps	Patients with colonic symptoms or guaiac positive stool
Biopsy	Confirms lesions detected by radionuclide scan, CT scans, or lymphangiogram	Patients with suspicious lesions
Metastatic		
Chest radiography	Detects soft tissue nodules > 15 mm; detects acute pulmonary disease	Routine
Skeletal radiography	May confirm suspicious findings on radionuclide scans (low probability in low-stage disease)	Only when radionuclide scan is positive
Liver sonography	Detects metastatic deposits > 15 mm (low probability unless liver enzymes elevated)	If enzymes elevated High grade/stage tumor
Radionuclide bone scan	Sensitive assessment of bone metastases	Only in patients with skeletal pain

CT = computed tomography; MRI = magnetic resonance imaging.
Adapted from Bragg et al. (20).

spread IP, resembling metastatic ovarian carcinoma. Histologically, this tumor has a high degree of cytologic anaplasia with a papillary growth pattern and may have psammoma bodies. Although papillary serous tumors may resemble papillary carcinoma of the endometrium, the latter has little cytologic atypia and does not behave as aggressively (107).

3. *Clear cell carcinoma* is characterized by large, anaplastic cells with clear cytoplasm. These tumors tend to be of

Table 22-12. Histological Classification of Uterine Tumors

	INCIDENCE (%)	
Adenocarcinoma		
Grade I	40	
Grade II	}	60
Grade III	40	
Adenocanthoma	}	20
Adenosquamous carcinoma	7	
Clear cell carcinoma	5	
Papillary carcinoma	5	
Secretory adenocarcinoma	1.5	
Mucinous adenocarcinoma		

high grade and even patients with stage I disease have a poor prognosis (88).

4. *Adenocarcinoma of the endometrium* may also be admixed with squamous elements (10). Adenocarcinoma with squamous metaplasia is termed adenoacanthoma and has a prognosis similar to typical adenocarcinoma. Adenosquamous carcinoma contains a malignant squamous component interspersed within the adenocarcinoma component. The poor prognosis associated with adenosquamous carcinoma relative to typical adenocarcinoma is best correlated to the grade of the adenocarcinomatous component in adenosquamous carcinoma (10,82).

5. *Mucinous adenocarcinomas of the endometrium* represent 9% of endometrial adenocarcinomas (10). Although small amounts of mucin may be found in as many as 92% of endometrioid adenocarcinomas (129); mucinous adenocarcinoma is diagnosed when more than 50% of the tumor is positive for intracytoplasmic mucin.

6. *Metastatic tumors to the endometrium* most commonly arise from primary tumors of the cervix or adnexa, and may pose a diagnostic problem. Breast cancer occasionally metastasizes to the endometrium (10).

7. *Progesterone receptors (PR)* have been shown to be important prognosticators in Stage I and II patients, that is, PR levels of 100 had a 3-year disease-free survival of

93% compared with 36% for <100 (107a). Good correlation of histopathologic grade using immunochemical staining for both estrogen and progesterone receptors has been shown with FIGO grade as well as survival (87a).

8. *Oncogene expression* and fraction of sphere have recently been found to be prognostic indicators (105a).

Histologic grading of *endometrial adenocarcinomas* in the FIGO system is based on architectural criteria (Table 22-12). The proportion of solid sheets of tumor relative to a glandular pattern determines the grade. However, for clear cell and papillary serous tumors, grade is assessed by nuclear criteria rather than architectural pattern (10). Tumor grade based on curettings may underestimate tumor grade in the hysterectomy specimen in 15% to 20% of patients (96).

Anatomic Staging

1. Until recently, the FIGO staging for endometrial carcinoma was based on clinical examination, followed by D&C. However, clinical staging underestimates disease extent in 15% to 51% of patients (11,92). Additionally, grade and histologic subtype in the hysterectomy specimen often differs from the results of the curettings. Several significant prognostic factors can only be identified after laparotomy and surgical-pathologic staging evaluation. These prognostic factors correlate well to recurrence risk and include deep myometrial invasion, the presence of gross IP disease, positive lymph nodes, lymphatic or vascular space invasion by tumor, or positive peritoneal cytology (94,97). The determination of grade or occult extension of tumor to the cervix are also important risk factors for recurrence and are better assessed by hysterectomy. Surgical staging allows more accurate determination of which patients with stage I disease will benefit from postoperative adjuvant radiotherapy.

2. The current FIGO staging for endometrial cancer, outlined in Table 22-13 (83) based on surgicopathologic findings (Fig. 22-3).

3. Results from the large GOG studies support the validity of a staging system based on operative findings. In evaluating apparent clinical stage I disease, which represents approximately 75% of endometrial carcinoma (108), 22% of patients had disease outside the uterus (94). In predicting recurrence risk, positive pelvic or para-aortic nodes have the highest positive predictive value; deep myometrial invasion and high grade are also significant (97). In predicting metastatic disease to the regional lymph nodes, deep myometrial invasion and adnexal metastases had the highest correlation with positive nodes. Of these positive nodes, only 10% were grossly positive (94). The correlation of anatomic stage, histopathologic grade, and depth of myometrial invasion associated with positive pelvic and para-ortic lymph nodes is shown in Table 22-14 (94). With deep muscle invasion and high grade tumors, nodal spread is 20–60% in pelvic and 10–30% in paraortic nodal regions (117b).

PRINCIPLES OF TREATMENT

Table 22-15 summarizes multidisciplinary treatment decisions; the vast majority of cases are treated by surgery and/or irradiation. Chemotherapy and hormones are used for advanced and metastatic disease stages.

Surgery

1. Surgical removal of the uterus and ovaries continues to be the mainstay of treatment for endometrial carcinoma. Frequently a curative procedure, hysterectomy may also be indicated for palliation in patients with advanced disease.

2. Appropriate steps at the time of surgical exploration include peritoneal cytology, extrafascial hysterectomy, bilateral salpingo-oophorectomy, selective bilateral pelvic and para-aortic lymph node sampling, and omental biopsy. Adequate surgical staging will determine whether the patient should receive no adjuvant therapy,

---

Table 22-13. Comparison of FIGO and AJC Stagings of Carcinoma of the Endometrium

FIGO	Site	AJC
Stage 0	In situ	**Tis**
Stage I	Confined to corpus A. limited to endometrial B. < 50 % myometrium C. > 50 % myometrium	$T_1N_0M_0$
Stage II	Extension to cervix A. endocervix glandular B. stromal	$T_2N_0M_0$
Stage III	Extension beyond uterus/within true pelvis A. serosa/adrexa/+cytology B. vaginal metastases C. pelvic/paraaortic nodes	$T_3N_1M_0$
Stage IVA	Extension to mucosa of bladder/rectum/beyond true pelvis	$T_4N_0M_0$
Stage IVB	Distant metastasis	$T_{any}\,N_{any}M_1$

T = tumor; N = node; M = metastasis.
FIGO (83) = International Federation of Gynecology and Obstetrics;
AJC (1) = American Joint Committee on Cancer Staging.

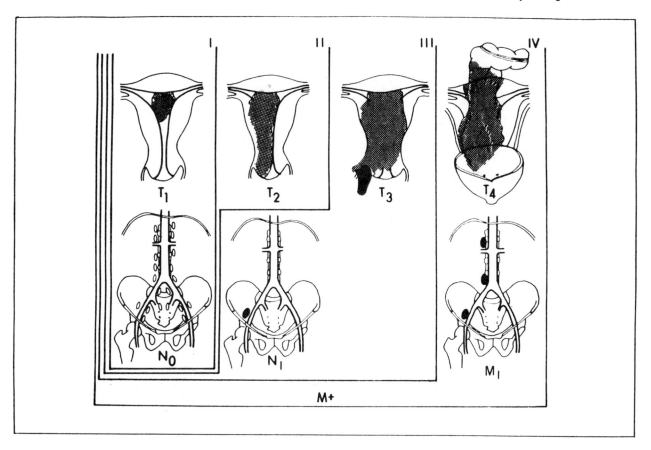

Fig. 22-3. Anatomic staging for endometrial carcinoma.

pelvic irradiation, pelvic and para-aortic irradiation, whole abdominal irradiation, systemic chemotherapy, or hormone therapy.

Radiation Therapy

1. Radiation therapy is an important component of the treatment plan in many endometrial carcinoma patients. In selected patients, radiotherapy alone may be curative. In addition, adjuvant pelvic radiotherapy is frequently used to decrease the risk of recurrence fol-

lowing surgery. Radiotherapy may also be indicated for palliation in patients with metastatic disease.

2. Primary treatment with irradiation is used in medically infirm patients who are not candidates for surgery (112,147). Most studies report a decrease in survival from 85% to 65% when irradiation alone is used compared with surgery or surgery and adjuvant radiotherapy for stage I carcinoma (11). Adjuvant pelvic radiotherapy for stage I carcinoma has been performed preoperatively for patients with poor prehysterectomy

Table 22-14. Factors Associated with Increased Frequency of Metastasis to Regional Lymph Nodes in Carcinoma of the Endometrium

Factor	Positive Pelvic Nodes (%)	Positive Para-Aortic Nodes (%)
Clinical stage		
I	7	3
II (cervix involved)	36	8
Grade	3	2
I	9	6
II	18	11
III		
Myometrial invasion		
Minimal or superficial	5	3
Moderate	6	1
Deep	25	17

From Creasmen et al. (94), with permission.

Table 22-15. Multidisciplinary Treatment Decisions by Stage for (6,57,120a)
Endometrial Carcinoma

Stage	Surgery		Radiation Therapy		Chemotherapy
I (T_1, N_0)	TAH BSO Selected pelvic and para-aortic nodal sampling	and/or	ART preop or postop 45-50 Gy Intracavitary or external RT		NR
II (T_2, N_0)	TAH BSO Pelvic and para-aortic nodal sampling	and/or	ART preop or postop 45-50 Gy external plus intracavitary 30-40 Gy to vagina		NR
III (T_3, N_0, N_{1a})	TAH BSO Pelvic and para-aortic nodal sampling	and/or	ART or DRT intracavitary and external to higher doses 60-65 Gy if only RT	and	HT
IV (T_4, N_0, N_{1a})					
V (T_{any}, N_{1b}, M_+)	NR		PRT	and	HT IC II

RT = radiation therapy; ART = adjuvant; PRT = palliative; DRT = definitive; NR = not recommended;
HT = hormonal therapy; IC II = investigational chemotherapy, phases I/II clinical trials; TAH BSO = total
abdominal hysterectomy, bilateral salpingo oophorectomy.
PDQ: NR - HT = hydroxyprogesterone, medroxyprogesterone, megesterol

prognostic features (e.g., poorly differentiated tumors, cervical involvement) as well as postoperatively, based on surgical-pathologic findings (131). As no randomized trials using preoperative versus postoperative radiotherapy have been performed, no single technique is definitively superior (11,93,138). However, postoperative radiotherapy has several advantages; the selection of patients for adjuvant radiotherapy is based on more accurate findings than clinical examination; extended field pelvic irradiation to the para-aortic lymph nodes or whole abdominal irradiation can be used if indicated; and patients suitable only for chemotherapy or hormonal therapy can be identified (93).

Technique

Many radiation techniques have been used, including preoperative packing of the uterus with Heymans' capsules, tandem placement, preoperative external pelvic irradiation, postoperative external pelvic irradiation, and postoperative vaginal cylinder brachytherapy.

Heymans' capsules: This type of brachytherapy involves placement of afterloading capsules into the uterine cavity and is used predominantly in patients being treated solely with radiotherapy, usually in conjunction with whole pelvic external beam irradiation (4,000 to 5,000 cGy) (147,148). Heymans' capsules are best suited to patients with a large uterine cavity, whereas a tandem with vaginal ovoids may be superior with small uteri or in cases with cervical extension (148), as uterine packing treats only the corpus.

Tandem and ovoids: The vaginal apex and parametria are best treated by this brachytherapy technique, so external pelvic irradiation is necessary if radiation therapy is the sole treatment modality. Currently, this method is used predominantly in patients with stage IIB tumors (142). Vaginal cylinders using HDR brachytherapy can be readily substituted for LDR brachytherapy that requires hospitalization (121a).

External beam pelvic irradiation: Postoperative external beam radiotherapy of 4,500 to 5,000 cGy to a pelvic field is advocated for grade 3 tumors, deep myometrial invasion, or vascular space involvement in patients with adequate surgical staging (11,81,93,117,141). Postoperative pelvic irradiation decreases vaginal recurrences significantly, although a survival benefit has not been demonstrated conclusively (11,117).

Extended field (para-aortic) radiotherapy: With more advanced stages, adjuvant radiotherapy may include the para-aortic area if tumor involvement of this area occurs. If pelvic or para-aortic nodes are the only site of extrauterine disease, then 67% of patients with positive pelvic nodes and 42% to 47% of patients with positive para-aortic nodes may survive 5 years (99,125). Patients with microscopic disease only in lymph nodes have a much better response to 5,000 cGy to the para-aortic area than do patients with gross disease (67% versus 17%) (124).

Whole abdominal irradiation: This technique has been used to treat patients with metastatic intra-abdominal disease when the maximal diameter of residual tumor is less than 2 cm. One pilot study using 2,600 to 2,800 cGy by moving-strip technique to the abdomen with a pelvic boost demonstrated a 5-year survival of 80% (104). Studies are under way to confirm the efficacy of this modality. Patients with large residual disease tend to have a much poorer response to whole abdominal radiotherapy; major complications such as intestinal perforation occur at a rate of 3% to 6% (104,114).

IP chromic phosphate (^{32}P) suspension has been used with some success in the treatment of patients with malignant peritoneal cytology (136); complication rates were markedly increased when IP^{32}P, a ß emitter, was used in conjunction with pelvic radiotherapy (74).

Chemotherapy

1. *Cytotoxic chemotherapy* treatment of endometrial carcinoma is limited to patients with an unresectable recurrence within a previously irradiated field. Also, patients with systemic disease in either a recurrent or primary setting are suitable chemotherapy candidates. The efficacy of hormonal therapy in advanced or recurrent endometrial cancer treatment has also delayed the development of significantly effective chemotherapy.

2. Doxorubicin has been used successfully in some advanced or recurrent endometrial cancer with a 37% total response rate. However, the mean duration of response was only 7.4 months (140). Doses used were 40 to 60 mg/m² doxorubicin IV every 3 weeks (93).

3. *Cisplatin* also is an effective agent for advanced or recurrent endometrial carcinoma. Total response rates from 20% to 42%, with approximately a 5-month duration of response, have been reported (133,139). Recently, carboplatin has been used as a substitute for cisplatin with less toxicity and with similar efficacy (115).

4. *Multidrug combination chemotherapy* has also been used for recurrent endometrial cancer. Unfortunately, results are difficult to interpret, as many of the preliminary studies combined cytotoxic agents with progestins, which have a response rate of about 30% when used alone (93). Table 22-16 lists commonly used combinations (59); currently, it is unclear whether multiagent combination chemotherapy is superior to single-agent therapy. Mean duration of response is uniformly less than 1 year.

Hormonal Therapy

1. Progestational agents are known to be effective in reversing endometrial hyperplasia; additionally, these agents have a long efficacious record in recurrent or advanced endometrial carcinoma treatment. Standard progestational agents include: hydroxyprogesterone (Delalutin), medroxyprogesterone (Provera) and megestrol (Megace) (120a).

2. Tumors that contain high levels of estrogen and progesterone receptors are more likely to respond to progestin therapy (11); receptor-positive tumors are more likely to be well differentiated (120).

3. Recent reports demonstrate an 11% response rate to progestational agents (hydroxyprogesterone caproate, megesterol acetate, or dimethyl-dehydroxy progesterone). Hormonal therapy with any of these agents is equally effective, yielding better and longer responses in well-differentiated tumors of small volume (123).

4. The use of progestins as an adjuvant to surgery with or without radiotherapy has not been demonstrated to be of value and were of no benefit in clinical trials in Stage I disease (113,116,120a).

5. Hormonal treatment may be the modality of choice in those cases of advanced or recurrent disease with positive estrogen or progesterone receptors, good differentiation, or with a late recurrence (11). In large, more anaplastic tumors, chemotherapy may be more appropriate. Progestin therapy is very well tolerated, even over prolonged administration periods.

6. Tamoxifen, an antiestrogen, may be of benefit for patients progressing on progestin therapy or in an alternating schedule with a progestin. Response rate in pretreated patients is 20% (126).

Summary of Treatment by Stage (Table 22-15) (85)

Endometrial hyperplasia with atypia:
1. Hysterectomy by vaginal or abdominal route.
2. Progestin therapy for 3 to 6 months in medically infirm patients and in those desiring preservation of fertility. Resampling of endometrium during and after therapy is required.
3. After exclusion of invasive cancer, the endometrium may also be ablated with neodymium-yttrium aluminum garnet laser via hysteroscopy in poor surgical candidates (84).

Stage I (A,B,C): Surgical staging with extrafascial hysterectomy, bilateral salpingo-oophorectomy, selective pelvic and para-aortic lymph node sampling, peritoneal washings, and a thorough exploration of the abdomen is performed. Adjuvant pelvic radiotherapy may be given postoperatively if there are high risk factors for recurrence. In patients who are extremely poor surgical candidates, primary radiotherapy may be used.

Stage II (A,B): Hysterectomy and oophorectomy with surgical staging as outlined above are appropriate; adjuvant pelvic radiotherapy postoperatively is often given. For patients with gross cervical involvement by tumor, radical hysterectomy with node sampling or preoperative radiotherapy followed by extrafascial hysterectomy in 4 to 6 weeks is frequently used, although hysterectomy with node sampling followed by irradiation also is an option (105,146).

Stage III (A,B,C): Hysterectomy and oophorectomy with surgical staging is performed. All gross tumors that can be resected with minimal morbidity are removed to enhance the efficacy of postoperative radiotherapy. If there is pelvic node involvement, adjuvant pelvic external irradiation is given; if para-aortic nodes contain metastatic disease, extended field

Table 22-16. Multiagent Chemotherapy in Treatment of Endometrial Carcinoma

REGIMEN	Total Response (%)	CR (%)	Reference
Melephelan/5-FU/medroxyprogesterone acetate	86	--	91
	48	20	122
Doxorubicin/cyclophosphamide/5-FU/megesteral acetate	37	16	90
Ace	63	38	118
	31	0	132
CAP	45	10	144
Cisplatin/doxorubicin	60	8	143

CR : complete response.

pelvic irradiation is given. If there is IP spread, whole abdomen radiotherapy with a pelvic boost may be the best adjuvant therapy in selected cases. For patients not suitable for adjuvant radiotherapy, systemic therapy with progestins or chemotherapy is appropriate.

Stage IV (A,B): Hysterectomy and oophorectomy with staging may be performed. With disease outside the abdomen, treatment is largely palliative. In stage IV disease patients — based on extensive abdominal tumor — cytoreductive surgery may be appropriate. Adjuvant therapy is individualized by disease distribution and may be a combination of chemotherapy or radiotherapy.

Recurrences: The type of prior treatment and site of recurrence determine which treatment options are appropriate. The distribution of recurrences for endometrial carcinoma is as follows: local, 50%; distant metastases, 28%; and both local and distant disease 22%. Patients who received pelvic radiotherapy in either a primary or adjuvant setting tend to have recurrence outside the irradiated field. In nonirradiated patients, treatment failure may often be noted at the vaginal apex, parametrium, or in the pelvic and para-aortic lymph nodes. Seventy-six percent of recurrences occur within the first 3 years after treatment (81).

With local recurrence in unirradiated patients, pelvic radiotherapy may be used; in patients previously irradiated, local central recurrence may be treated by pelvic exenteration in selected instances. Hormonal therapy or chemotherapy may be used alone or in combination in patients with distant disease (11). In patients with small-volume distant recurrence confined to the abdomen, whole abdominal radiotherapy also has been used (104,114).

RESULTS AND PROGNOSIS

Table 22-17 summarizes 5-year survival rates as a function of stage, tumor grade, and depth of invasion.

Stage I Carcinoma

Survival results using the 1988 revision of the FIGO staging system are currently unavailable. However, using clinical staging, 5-year survival in stage I endometrial carcinoma is 79% (131). Recurrence rate in surgical stage I patients is 15% (97). Negative prognostic factors are deep myometrial invasion and moderate to poor differentiation of tumors which can skew results, i.e., 84% for superficial, well-differentiated stage I to 69% for deeper invasion, poor differentiation (97).

Stage II Carcinoma

Cervical extension of tumor does worsen prognosis; there is a 5-year survival of 29% to 77% in most series (87,105).

Stage III - IV Carcinoma

5-year survival with positive pelvic nodes or para-aortic nodes may be as high as 67% and 42%, respectively, when treated by hysterectomy, node sampling, and postoperative external irradiation (125). Preliminary reports of treatment of IP disease are promising but lack long-term follow-up (104). Survival for stage IV disease is only about 10% (7).

Tumor Differentiation

Survival rates are excellent for well-differentiated tumors and decrease with further foci or differentiation into grade 2, but especially for grade 3. There has been only modest improvement before and after 1965; this indicates that chemotherapy has not impacted on survival for high-grade tumors.

Depth of Invasion

Superficial invasion has a high curability, similar to that when there is no invasion of the myometrium. The prognosis worsens for deep invasion and usually correlates with high-grade cancers and lymph node metastases.

System Treatment of Advanced and Recurrent Disease

Multiple systemic therapies have been used to treat patients with endometrial cancer. Although progestins have been standard initial treatment for metastatic disease for the past 30 years, they are effective in only 20% of patients, and several large randomized trials have failed to demonstrate any benefit in the adjuvant setting (117a).

GESTATIONAL TROPHOBLASTIC NEOPLASMS

PERSPECTIVE

Gestational trophoblastic neoplasms have a number of distinguishing features that have fascinated physicians for centuries. Tumors of this type were rarely curable prior to the advent of effective chemotherapy and were particularly tragic, as those afflicted were young women in their reproductive years. Fortunately, today the vast majority of patients with gestational trophoblastic neoplasms can be cured, as both effective treatment and a reliable tumor marker for monitoring treatment, human chorionic gonadotropin (CG), are available. Nevertheless, because of the rarity of this type of tumor, some confusion still exists regarding its appropriate classification and management.

Table 22-17. Five-Year Survival for Endometrial Carcinoma by Stage, Tumor Differentiation, and Depth of Invasion

Stage	%	TUMOR DIFFERENTIATION			DEPTH OF INVASION		
		Grade	<1965 (%)	>1965 (%)	Depth	<1965 (%)	>1965 (%)
I	75.1	I	62-88	79-100	No	67-100	79-93
II	57.8						
III	30.0						
IV	10.6	II	52-82	54-96	Superficial	70-86	72-95
No stage	63.5						
		III	14-80	30-75	Deep	34-56	27-81
Total	67.7						

From Petterson (59), with permission.

EPIDEMIOLOGY AND ETIOLOGY

The spectrum of gestational trophoblastic neoplasia (GTN) includes molar pregnancy (both complete and partial), invasive mole, choriocarcinoma, and placental site trophoblastic tumor. Approximately one half of patients with choriocarcinoma develop it following a molar gestation, with the remaining cases occurring after a nonmolar pregnancy.

1. There are wide geographic and ethnic variations in the incidence of molar pregnancy. Some of the highest rates are reported from Asia (China, 1:150 pregnancies, Indonesia, 1:85) and the lowest in industrialized nations such as the United States (1:1700) (157). In the United States, molar pregnancy is one half as frequent among black women as other women (163).

2. Maternal age is an important risk factor for molar pregnancy; the highest risk is for women over age 40 years and there is somewhat increased risk for women under age 20. Nevertheless, the single most important risk factor is a prior history of a molar gestation. Although patients with a past history of molar pregnancy have a 20 to 40 fold increase in risk, the odds are still good (70%) that a subsequent pregnancy will be normal (161).

3. The chromosomal aberrations identified with molar gestations give important insight into the etiology of this disease. Complete moles are most frequently 46XX, with the entire genome composed of paternal chromosomes. In contrast, partial moles are triploid (69 XXY) (171). The relationship of these chromosomal aberrations to both maternal and paternal age have not been well defined.

DETECTION AND DIAGNOSIS

Complete mole: Abnormal vaginal bleeding occurs in virtually all patients with molar pregnancy (155).

1. Although excessive uterine size is a classic feature, this occurs in only 50% of patients with complete moles.

2. Currently, the majority of patients are diagnosed when bleeding or uterine enlargement with absent fetal heart tones prompts investigation by ultrasound, the extremely reliable diagnostic method of choice.

3. Other presenting signs associated with complete molar pregnancies include large ovarian cysts (theca-lutein), preeclampsia, and hyperemesis.

4. Occurrence of preeclampsia in the first trimester of pregnancy is virtually pathognomonic of a molar gestation.

5. Although not diagnostic of molar gestations, the hCG level is usually higher in molar than in nonmolar gestations.

Partial mole: Vaginal bleeding is a common symptom in patients with partial molar pregnancies also, but excessive uterine size and large ovarian cysts are distinctly uncommon with partial moles so that the diagnosis is seldom suspected.

1. Most cases are diagnosed after pathologic review following evacuation of what was presumed to be an incomplete abortion (154).

2. Other contrasting features of complete and partial molar gestations are shown in Table 22-18.

Invasive mole: Invasive mole is most frequently diagnosed during gonadotropin follow-up of a molar gestation. The diagnosis is made when either a plateau or increase in serum

Table 22-18. Features of Molar Gestations

	Complete Mole	Partial Mole
Pathology		
Hydropic Villi	Diffuse	Focal
Trophoblastic		
Hyperplasia	Diffuse	Focal
Embryonic Tissue	Absent	Present
Karyotype	46XX(95%);46XY	69XXY;69XYY
Malignant Potential	20%	10%
Clinical Features	33%	10%
Excessive Uterine Size	Usually	Unusual
HCG Titer	>50,000	<50,000

Adapted from Morrow, CP and Townsend, DE (eds). Synopsis of Gynecologic Oncology. Churchhill Livingstone, New York, NY (11) and Berek and Hacker (3), with permission.

hCG occurs during the follow-up period, although a new pregnancy must be excluded.

1. Approximately 20% of patients with a molar gestation will develop invasive mole, but the risk is only 5% to 10% for patients with partial moles.

2. Importantly, patients with molar gestations can be stratified into low- and high-risk categories on the basis of clinical and laboratory parameters. Those who have large-for-dates uteri or a preevacuation serum hCG level higher than 100,000 mIU/mL (high-risk molar pregnancy) have about a 50% risk of developing invasive mole.

3. Patients without these and other high risk features have less than a 5% risk. Invasive mole can occur also following spontaneous abortion, tubal pregnancy, or any gestational event. In these cases the diagnosis is usually made when a serum hCG is obtained in conjunction with ultrasound to evaluate abnormal vaginal bleeding, the most frequent presenting symptomatology.

Metastatic GTN: Although invasive mole occasionally can be found in metastatic sites such as the lung, generally when metastases occur the histology, if obtained, is choriocarcinoma.

1. The most frequent symptoms in patients with metastatic gestational trophoblastic disease are abnormal vaginal bleeding and abdominal pain. As this tumor can spread hematogenously the lung, liver, and brain can all be involved by tumor.

2. Persistent cough, hemoptysis, stroke, hemianopsia, and other symptoms reflecting the metastatic sites can occur as the initial symptomatology. A serum hCG should be obtained in any woman in the reproductive age range

Table 22-19. Histologic Classification of Gestational Trophoblastic Disease

- **Placental site tumor**

- **Hydatidiform mole (complete and partial)**

- **Invasive hydatidiform mole (chorioadenoma destruens)**

- **Choriocarcinoma**

From World Health Organization (8), with permission.

who has a metastatic tumor without a known primary if histology is unavailable.

CLASSIFICATION AND STAGING

Histopathologic Classification (Table 22-19) (8)

1. Complete mole is characterized histologically by hydropic villi, trophoblastic hyperplasia, and the absence of fetal vessels. In contrast, partial moles often have evidence of fetal development and there is an admixture of villi, some with hydropic change and some without.
2. Invasive mole appears similar to complete mole histologically, but in addition invades the myometrium.
3. Choriocarcinoma consists predominantly of cytotrophoblast and syncytiotrophoblast and does not have chorionic villi.
4. Placental site tumors are composed of intermediate trophoblast; there are no villi. These tumors are notable for low hCG production not reflective of tumor burden.

Anatomic Staging (Table 22-20)

One commonly used clinical classification of GTN is shown in Table 22-20 (165). Other common methods of classification are based on a number of clinical features related primarily to tumor bulk at diagnosis.

The number of classifications developed is reflective of differing views regarding the best method to classify these tumors. The FIGO system shown in Table 22-20 is elegant in its simplicity but fails to take into account a number of known risk factors (151,158,168).

PRINCIPLES OF TREATMENT

Surgery

1. A complete or partial mole in a patient desirous of further childbearing is best treated by suction evacuation of the uterus. In patients with large uteri this procedure can be formidable and accompanied by excessive blood loss.
   a. Other disease complications include trophoblastic embolization to the lung, causing respiratory failure, preeclampsia, thyroid storm, disseminated intravascular coagulation, and, rarely, torsion or rupture of a theca-lutein cyst.
   b. In patients who have completed childbearing, a hysterectomy may be performed with the mole left in situ.
   c. Theca-lutein cysts should be left intact at the time of hysterectomy unless removal is otherwise indicated, as they invariably involute over several months following removal of the molar pregnancy.

Table 22-20. FIGO Staging for Gestational Trophoblastic Tumors

Stage I	Confined to Uterine Corpus
Stage II	Metastases to Pelvis
Stage III	Metastases to Lungs
Stage IV	Distant Metastases

d. Gonadotropin follow-up is mandatory even after hysterectomy as patients are still at risk for development of metastases.
2. Patients with nonmetastatic GTN who are finished with childbearing should also be offered hysterectomy, since removal of the tumor reduces the number of courses of chemotherapy required to achieve remission compared with patients who retain their uterus (169,172).
3. Although placental site tumors have been successfully treated with D&C, some authorities recommend hysterectomy when this diagnosis is confirmed because of the uncertain risk for extrauterine spread and the tumors' insensitivity to current chemotherapy (168).
4. Isolated metastases in the lung, brain, or other sites that have become resistant to chemotherapy can be managed successfully with surgical removal.

Radiotherapy

1. The role of radiotherapy in the management of patients with GTN is limited. Some investigators (169) advocate hepatic irradiation (3,000 cGy) for patients with metastases to this site, but patients with liver involvement can be managed successfully with chemotherapy alone (174).
2. In patients with cerebral metastases, whole brain irradiation (3,000 cGy) is generally recommended, although intrathecal chemotherapy has been used successfully and craniotomy may still be required for bleeding (150).

Chemotherapy (Tables 22-21 and 22-22) (6)

Gestational trophoblastic neoplasms are, with the exception of placental site tumors (160), exquisitely sensitive to a variety of chemotherapeutic agents. Methotrexate and actinomycin D have been used extensively and are about equal in activity. More recently, etoposide has been found to be highly effective against this tumor and consequently has been incorporated into a number of treatment regimens (151,173).

1. Nonmetastatic and low-risk metastatic GTN can be managed successfully with single-agent chemotherapy (158a) using either methotrexate (152), actinomycin D (167), or etoposide (Table 22-22) (164).
2. High-risk metastatic GTN should be treated aggressively with combination chemotherapy. Until recently, the standard regimen consisted of MAC (153). However, several authorities (151,156,162,170) currently recommend a new regimen that appears to be superior, EMA-CO, for treatment of these patients. Randomized trials will be required to define the optimal regimen for treatment of this group of patients, who should be managed in centers experienced with some of the life-threatening complications that can occur during treatment (159).

FOLLOW-UP OF PATIENTS WITH GESTATIONAL TROPHOBLASTIC NEOPLASMS (Table 22-23) (6)

1. Surveillance of patients treated for gestational trophoblastic disease is mandatory. Fortunately, these tumors produce hCG (with the exception of placental site tumor), which can be measured accurately in the serum and is close to an ideal tumor marker.
2. Patients with either a complete or partial mole should undergo weekly serum hCG measurement until a nor-

Table 22-21. Management of Single-Agent Chemotherapy for Gestational Trophoblastic Disease

- Chemotherapy as noted in Table 22-22.
  - Repeated at 7-10 day intervals depending on toxicity
  - Contraception begun (oral if not contraindicated)

- Drug continued as above until human chorionic gonadotropin titer is normal

- Chemotherapy changed if:
  - Titer rises (tenfold or more)
  - Titer plateaus
  - Evidence of new metastsis

- Laboratory values — chemotherapy not repeated unless:
  - White Blood Cell Count > 3,000/mm^3
  - Polymorphonuclear leukocyted (polys) > 1,500/mm^3
  - Platelets > 100,000/mm^3
  - Blood urea nitrogen (BUN), serum glutamic-oxaloacetic transaminase (SGOT), serum glutamic-pyruvic transaminase (SGPT) essentially normal

- Toxicity mandating postponement of chemotherapy
  - Severe oral or gastrointestinal ulceration
  - Febrile course (usually present only with leukopenia)

- Remission defined as 3 consecutive normal weekly human chorionic gonadotropin titers

From Disaia and Creasman (6), with permission.

mal level is reached. Following three normal levels, monthly serum hCG measurements are obtained for 12 months.

3. The follow-up for those with invasive mole or choriocarcinoma is similar to that for patients with a molar pregnancy. However, in cases where remission was difficult to achieve (required more than three or four courses of chemotherapy) the period of serum hCG follow-up should be extended to 2 years, as late recurrences have been reported (21).

RESULTS AND PROGNOSIS

Currently, patients undergoing evacuation of a molar pregnancy have an excellent prognosis, both in terms of their outlook for future fertility and with respect to the available treatment should an invasive mole or choriocarcinoma develop.

1. The majority of patients (80%) with a molar pregnancy have no further sequelae following evacuation of the mole. The remaining 20% will develop either nonmetastatic or metastatic GTN which will require chemotherapy.

2. Virtually all patients with nonmetastatic disease will be cured (172), although some (< 5%) may require hysterectomy or uterine resection to remove a focus of resistant tumor. Patients with low-risk metastatic GTN also have an excellent prognosis.

3. Currently, about 20% of patients with high-risk metastatic GTN will die of the disease (159,168). This group of patients usually is comprised of those with extensive lung metastases, or spread to the brain or liver (158). Until recently liver metastases connoted a poor outlook, but it is hoped the development of new chemotherapeutic regimens (173) and the recognition of those patients who require intensive therapy from the outset will lead to further success in the treatment of this disease.

Table 22-22. Single-Agent Chemotherapy for Gestational Trophoblastic Disease by Risk Factors

- **Methotrexate 20-25 mg**
  IM every day for 5 days
  (repeat every 7 days if possible)

- **Actinomycin D 10-12 μ g/kg**
  IV every day for 5 days
  (repeat every 7 days if possible)

- **Methotrexate 1 mg/kg**
  IM on days 1,3,5, and 7; and
  folinic acid (citrovorum factor) 0.1 mg/kg
  IM on days 2,4,6, and 8
  (repeat every 7 days if possible)

IM = intramuscularly; IV = intravenously.

From Disaia and Creasman (6), with permission.

Table 22-23. Remission and Follow-up in Treatment of Gestational Trophoblastic Neoplasia

- **Three consecutive normal weekly hCG assays**

- **hCG titers every 2 weeks for 3 months**
  - **Then monthly for 3 months**
  - **Then every 2 months for 6 months**
  - **Then every 6 months**

- **Frequent chest film and pelvic exam**

- **Contraception for 1 year**

hCG = human chorionic gonadotrophin.
From Disaia and Creasman (6), with permission.

SARCOMA OF THE UTERUS

EPIDEMIOLOGY AND ETIOLOGY

1. Sarcomas, which represent 3% of all malignant tumors of the uterus (191), are derived from pure mesenchymal tissue or mixtures of epithelial and mesenchymal tissue.
2. Of mesenchymal tumors, benign uterine leiomyomata are far more common than uterine sarcomas.
3. Approximately 2.4% to 17% of women with uterine sarcomas have a history of prior pelvic irradiation (179,181,184,191). Mixed mesodermal tumors are most often associated with prior irradiation (184,188).
4. Mean age at diagnosis is 58 to 60 years. Women with endometrial stromal sarcomas and leiomyosarcomas (LMS) tend to be younger than those with mixed mesodermal tumors (179,188,191).
5. Unlike endometrial carcinomas uterine sarcomas are not associated with nulliparity or obesity.

DETECTION AND DIAGNOSIS

1. Common presenting symptoms and signs are abnormal uterine bleeding, abdominal pain, tumor prolapse through the cervical os, and an enlarging uterus.
2. Uterine sarcoma can only be differentiated from the more common endometrial adenocarcinoma by obtaining an adequate histologic sample, usually by D&C.
3. Diagnosis of the sarcoma by D&C or biopsy prior to hysterectomy is difficult for leiomyosarcomas and stromal sarcomas; only 4% of stromal sarcomas and leiomyosarcomas are identified preoperatively compared with 91% of mixed mesodermal tumors (199).
4. A PAP smear is rarely diagnostic of uterine sarcoma.

CLASSIFICATION AND STAGING

Histopathology

1. Histology is an important prognostic factor in uterine sarcoma; mitotic activity and grade strongly influence the natural history of the tumor (Table 22-24).

2. Histologic classification is most often by the system proposed by Ober (185). Homologous tumors contain malignant cells native to the uterus; heterologous tumors are derived from mesenchymal elements normally found outside the uterus. Mixed tumors have more than one malignant element.

LMS: 26% to 38% of uterine sarcomas are of the LMS type (179,199). Occurring often in premenopausal women, LMS are not associated with prior pelvic irradiation (180b). Often LMS is diagnosed after hysterectomy for a presumed leiomyomatous uterus. Histologically, the smooth muscle cells have increased atypia, pleomorphism, and cellularity. The degree of atypia and mitotic activity are used to differentiate LMS from lesser smooth muscle tumors; tumors exceeding ten mitoses per 10 high-power fields are classified as malignant (3,198).

Mixed mesodermal tumors represent 33% to 67% of all uterine sarcomas (179,185). These tumors are composed of an admixture of a sarcomatous stromal component and malignant epithelium. The epithelial component frequently is adenocarcinoma; however, squamous carcinoma also may be seen (3). The mesenchymal component may be a fibrosarcoma, rhabdomyosarcoma, or an endometrial stromal sarcoma component. Carcinosarcomas are often categorized with mixed mesodermal tumors and exhibit similar biologic behavior (178).

Endometrial stromal sarcoma: Only 13% of uterine sarcomas are of the endometrial stromal type (179,199). Histologically, increased numbers of endometrial stromal cells are seen with varying degrees of atypia and pleomorphism. High-grade stromal sarcomas have ten or more mitoses per 10 high-power fields, while low-grade stromal sarcomas have fewer than ten (3). Low-grade tumors were formerly termed endolymphatic stromal myosis, which is descriptive of their predilection to extend into lymphatic or vascular channels within the uterus. These low-grade sarcomas have a protracted natural history and may recur very late (187).

Table 22-24.   Histologic Classification of Uterine Sarcomas

- **Endometrial stroma**
  - **Endolymphatic stromal myosis**
  - **Endometrial stromal sarcoma**

- **Endometrial glands and stroma**
  - **Mixed Mullerian sarcomas**
    - **Homologous**
    - **Heterologous**

- **Myometrium**
  - **Leiomyosarcoma**
  - **Other smooth muscle neoplasms (rare but generally benign behaving)**
    - **Leiomyoblastoma**
    - **Metastasizing leiomyoma**
    - **Leiomatosis peritonealis disseminata**
    - **Intravenous leiomyomatosis**

- **Arising in other Sites as well as the uterus (rare)**
  - **Rhabdomyosarcoma**
  - **Osteosarcoma**
  - **Chondrosarcoma**
  - **Liposarcoma**

Rhabdomyosarcoma: Of the very rare, pure, heterologous sarcomas, these are the most common. Rhabdomyoblasts are seen on histology. This tumor more commonly arises from the vagina and vulva and has a grave prognosis (182).

Staging

1. Uterine sarcomas are generally staged by the FIGO system for carcinoma of the endometrium.
2. Thorough abdominal exploration including inspection of peritoneal surfaces and pelvic and para-aortic lymph node sampling are important determinants of the exact disease extent. In stages I and II disease, lymph node metastases occur in 15% to 45% (176). Tumor extent at initial diagnosis is the most important predictor of prognosis, and patients with lymph node metastases have a poor outlook. Approximately 50% to 60% of patients present with clinical stage I or II disease (179,191); LMSs more commonly present with early disease than do other sarcomas, accounting for their slightly higher overall survival (191).

PRINCIPLES OF TREATMENT

Surgery

1. Surgical evaluation of the pelvis and abdomen with removal of the uterus, fallopian tubes, and ovaries with pelvic and para-aortic lymph node sampling, omental biopsy, and peritoneal washings is currently the standard treatment for all stages of disease. In early disease (stages I and II), adjuvant radiation or chemotherapy does not improve survival over surgery alone (177,179,180,186,190,199).
2. More extensive surgery such as exenteration has been proposed for locally advanced disease but little data exist regarding this approach; exenteration for select patients with local pelvic recurrence may be an option (189). Local treatment for recurrence is unlikely to be successful, as distant metastases occur in more than 80% of cases with a pelvic recurrence (190).
3. Hysterectomy for advanced disease is largely palliative but can control hemorrhage from the uterine tumor.

Radiation Therapy

1. Radiation therapy as primary treatment for the uterine sarcoma has been used with poor results (190). External pelvic radiotherapy with brachytherapy can be used for palliation in medically infirm patients with advanced disease.
2. Adjuvant postoperative pelvic irradiation has been used; this decreases failure rates within the pelvis but does not improve absolute survival (190,199). In patients receiving adjuvant radiotherapy, the distant sites of failure are most often the upper abdomen and lung.

Chemotherapy

1. Chemotherapy has been used often following surgery because most patients are at substantial risk for recurrence. Adjuvant doxorubicin has been used postoperatively to try to improve the 50% 5-year survival of patients with disease confined to the uterus; however, a randomized trial demonstrated no benefit for doxorubicin in this context (186). Doxorubicin has a total response rate of 19% when used for advanced or recurrent disease; adding vincristine, cyclophosphamide, or dactinomycin does not improve the response rate (183). Responses usually are less than 1 year duration and do not influence 2-year survival. A large nonrandomized study demonstrated improved survival and a lower local failure rate in patients with mixed mullerian tumors following postoperative external and intracavitary radiation therapy (186a).
2. In mixed mesodermal tumors newer agents such as ifosfamide have been used in phase II trials for advanced or recurrent tumor and produce a total response rate of 32% (194). One nonrandomized study appears to show benefit for adjuvant therapy with cisplatin and doxorubicin (180a). Cisplatin has also been used to treat advanced or recurrent mixed mesodermal tumors with a total response rate of 18%; the duration of response may be longer than that seen with doxorubicin (196). Doxorubicin and cisplatin in combination may also produce a better response rate than doxorubicin alone (192).

Hormonal Therapy

1. Estrogen and progesterone receptors are present in 55% of patients with uterine sarcoma (195). The rate of positivity for receptors does not vary with histologic type. Conflicting data exist regarding whether receptor positivity is predictive of improved short-term survival (193,195).
2. Although progestins have been reported to suppress tumor growth in sarcoma cells in vitro and in athymic mice (197), they have not been of benefit in clinical practice (193,195). Only in low-grade endometrial stromal sarcoma is there an indication of significant response with progestin therapy (187).

RESULTS AND PROGNOSIS

1. Survival is largely dependent on disease extent (Table 22-25) (191). When controlled for stage, there is little difference in survival rates between histologies, excluding low-grade endometrial stromal sarcomas (179,191). Overall 5-year survival for all stages is 17% to 27% (77,191,199); for clinical stage I disease and for stage II - IV disease, 5-year survival is 54% and 11%, respectively (191). Currently, adjuvant therapy does not improve 5-year survival; however, it may increase disease-free survival and provide palliation.

CARCINOMA OF THE FALLOPIAN TUBE

EPIDEMIOLOGY AND ETIOLOGY

1. Carcinoma of the fallopian tube is an uncommon malignancy that accounts for 0.3% to 1.1% of all female genital tract cancers (201,202,204,208,211,212).
2. Slightly more than 1,200 cases have been reported; it is this paucity of information that makes its natural history and management unfamiliar.
3. The median age at diagnosis in most series is between 55 and 60 years.

Table 22-25. Five-Year Survival for Uterine Sarcomas by Stage, Treatment, and Pathologic Type

Stage	Cell Type	Surgery	5-year Survival (%) Surgery and Radiation Therapy	Radiation Therapy
I	Mixed mesodermal sarcoma	52	48	29
	Leiomyosarcoma	49	77	33
	Endometrial stromal sarcoma	47	88	50
II-IV	Mixed mesodermal sarcoma	5	16	0
	Leiomyosarcoma	0	13	0
	Endometrial stromal sarcoma	0	33	0

Adapted from Salazar et al. (191).

4. The clinical course of fallopian tube carcinoma is often similar to epithelial ovarian carcinoma, but there are several significant differences.

DETECTION AND DIAGNOSIS

1. Unlike epithelial ovarian carcinoma, fallopian tube carcinoma is often symptomatic.
2. The three most common symptoms and signs are abnormal vaginal bleeding (30% to 53%), a pelvic mass (12% to 70%), and abdominal or pelvic pain (26% to 49%) (201,202,204,208,212).
3. Pelvic pain is more common in tubal carcinoma than in ovarian carcinoma. As the tumor in the fallopian tube enlarges, pain results from the peristaltic contractions of a hollow viscus.
4. The classic triad of pelvic pain, a palpable mass, and profuse watery discharge (hydrops tubae profluens) is a relatively infrequent occurrence (0% to 14% of patients) (202,204,208). The lack of specificity of these findings and the rarity of tubal carcinoma make accurate preoperative diagnosis very difficult.
5. Fallopian tube carcinoma often may be mistaken for an ovarian neoplasm, uterine leiomyomata, hydrosalpinx, or a tubo-ovarian abscess — all of which are more common than tubal carcinoma. In several series, the diagnosis of fallopian tube carcinoma was considered prior to exploratory laparotomy in only 0% to 13% of patients (202,204,212). In 18% of patients, the diagnosis of tubal carcinoma was made incidentally only after histologic examination of the fallopian tubes (202).
6. Occasionally, fallopian tube carcinoma is detected on PAP smear. In previous series, it was estimated that as many as 60% of patients had cervical cytology suggestive of tubal carcinoma (211); more recent reports have a rate of positive cytology of 0% to 20% (201,212).
7. Pelvic ultrasound may demonstrate tubal carcinoma, but it is often mistaken for an ovarian tumor. Tubal carcinomas most often appear as a complex fusiform mass on ultrasound (213).
8. While laparotomy is necessary for definitive diagnosis of primary tubal carcinoma, there still can be uncertainty on gross examination. Metastatic disease from the ovary or endometriosis is more common than primary tubal carcinoma and can sometimes be difficult to distinguish from tubal carcinoma.

CLASSIFICATION

Histopathology

1. Benign neoplasms can arise from the fallopian tube and are usually of mesodermal origin. These tumors include leiomyomata, adenomatoid tumors, and teratomas. Malignant neoplasms resemble serous adenocarcinoma of the ovary and may assume papillary, alveolar, or medullary growth patterns. These tumors rarely contain mucin but may have associated benign or malignant squamous components (205).
2. Hu's criteria for diagnosing tubal carcinoma specify that most of the tumor must be in the fallopian tube with involvement of the tubal mucosa in a papillary pattern. There must also be a clearly defined transition between normal and malignant epithelium in the tube (203). Metastases to the fallopian tube from ovarian carcinoma are generally extramucosal.
3. No uniform grading sytem exists, but most incorporate assessment of architectural abnormalities and nuclear atypia. Two thirds of tumors are poorly differentiated (200,203,212); early-stage, poorly differentiated tumors clearly have a much poorer prognosis than well-differentiated tumors (200).

Anatomic Staging

1. Tubal carcinomas spread transmurally. Tumor gradually extends from tubal mucosa to serosa. Spread may also occur via the ostia into the endometrial or intraperitoneal cavity.
2. Lymphatic spread is common to both para-aortic and pelvic lymph nodes; however, the exact frequency of nodal spread at initial diagnosis is unclear because surgical staging has not been performed uniformly in previous series.
3. Staging systems commonly used:
   - modification of FIGO ovarian cancer staging (Table 22-26) (201)
   - Schiller and Silverberg system (209)

Table 22-26. Comparison of FIGO and AJC Stagings of Carcinoma of the Ovary

FIGO	SITE	AJC
Stage 1	Limited to ovaries	T1
Stage IA	One ovary, capsule intact	T1a
Stage IB	Both ovaries, capsule intact	T1b
Stage IC	Capsule ruptured, tumor on surface, malignant cells in ascites or peritoneal washings	T1c
Stage II	Pelvic extension	T2
Stage IIA	Uterus, tube(s)	T2a
Stage IIB	Other pelvic tissues	T2b
Stage IIC	Malignant cells in ascites or peritoneal washings	T2c
Stage III	Peritoneal metastasis beyond pelvis and/or regional lymph node metastases	T3 and/or N1
Stage IIIA	Microscopic peritoneal metastases	T3a
Stage IIIB	Macroscopic peritoneal metastases <2 cm	T3b
Stage IIIC	Peritoneal metastasis > 2 cm and/or regional lymph node metastases	T3c and or/ N1
Stage IV	Distant metastasis (excludes peritoneal metastasis)	M1

FIGO = International Federation of Gynecology and Obstetrics; AJC = American Joint Committee on Cancer Staging; T = tumor; N = node; M = metastasis.

4. Survival correlates well to both staging systems. It is interesting that fallopian tube carcinoma manifests earlier than ovarian carcinoma, in part because of the more severe symptoms associated with tubal carcinoma. In most series, about 70% of patients with tubal carcinoma present with disease confined to the pelvis (stage I or II) with only 30% stage III or IV; with ovarian cancer the ratio is reversed (202,204,208).

PRINCIPLES OF TREATMENT

Surgery

1. Exploratory laparotomy with total abdominal hysterectomy, bilateral salpingo-oophorectomy, omentectomy, peritoneal washings with a thorough evaluation of all peritoneal surfaces, and pelvic and para-aortic lymph node sampling should be performed to fully evaluate the patient for IP or lymphatic metastases.
2. Surgical cytoreduction to minimize residual tumor may be of benefit in prolonging mean survival (202).
3. Adjuvant chemotherapy or radiotherapy is used generally for tumors demonstrating any invasion of the fallopian tube.

Radiation Therapy

1. Early series, which used pelvic radiotherapy only, produced no benefit in either early or advanced tubal carcinoma.
2. Whole abdomen irradiation or intraperitoneal ^{32}P has been reported to reduce recurrence rates in patients with stage III disease (210). This approach in earlier-stage cases needs further investigation.

Chemotherapy

1. Although previously only anecdotal data existed regarding the efficacy of alkylating agent chemotherapy in the treatment of fallopian tube carcinoma, recent reports of treatments using CAP combination chemotherapy have demonstrated response rates and 5-year survival superior to single-agent therapy and non-cisplatin-based combination chemotherapy regimens (206,210). Response rates in patients with advanced disease may be as high as 81% (206).
2. Although the value of second-look laparotomy has not been defined, it is generally used to assess response to chemotherapy treatment.

RESULTS AND PROGNOSIS

Overall, the 5-year survival for fallopian tube carcinoma is 22% to 40% (201,202,207). In patients with stage I cancer, survival estimates range from 55% to 74% (200,208) However, as most series reported include patients treated over a 20-year span, current results using modern adjuvant therapy with cisplatin-based combination chemotherapy probably will improve survival.

OVARIAN CANCER

EPIDEMIOLOGY AND ETIOLOGY
(214,215,217,233,263,271,342)

1. In the United States female population, ovarian cancer ranks fifth in absolute mortality among cancer-related deaths (12,000/yr). There are 20,000 new cases of ovarian cancer diagnosed annually, the majority of which occur in advanced stages (III or IV). Of all females currently born in the United States, about 1.4% will develop ovarian cancer within their lifetime (217,263).
2. Epithelial ovarian cancers are diagnosed most frequently in the sixth and seventh decades of life, at a median age of 59 years.
3. While most epithelial ovarian cancers occur in the perimenopausal or postmenopausal woman, malignant germ cell tumors and low malignant potential epithelial carcinomas tend to occur in younger women. Management is more difficult in these patients who are usually concerned with preserving fertility (271).

4. Epidemiologic risk factors are relatively weak, making identification of a high-risk group difficult. Increased risk is associated with nulliparity, talc use, a family history of ovarian cancer, or non-white race. A decrease in risk is noted with multiparity, prior hysterectomy (342), oral contraceptive use (233), European descent, and an early first pregnancy. The low frequency of ovarian cancer and the nonspecific nature of ovarian cancer symptoms make screening and early diagnosis difficult. The incidence of ovarian cancer is about 12 of 100,000 women annually.

5. Genetic factors play a part in the risk of developing epithelial ovarian cancer, and several tumor registries for familial ovarian cancer have been established. The pedigrees of these families demonstrate mother-daughter, sister-sister (first-degree relatives) relationships (286a). These data suggest that the gene for familial ovarian cancer is autosomal dominant with variable penetrance. A reasonable argument has been made for prophylactic bilateral oophorectomy in female members of afflicted kindreds after they have completed childbearing. However, metastatic cancer histologically identical to ovarian cancer has subsequently developed in patients who have undergone prophylactic oophorectomy, so that its protective value is unclear (215,308). In some families, a relationship also exists between breast and ovarian carcinoma.

6. The etiology of ovarian cancer is unclear. Support for the "incessant ovulation" theory is based on data regarding the protective effects of pregnancy and oral contraceptives.

7. Perineal talc use and asbestos exposure have both been weakly linked to development of epithelial ovarian cancer.

8. Conflicting data linking ovarian cancer with childhood mumps exist. A slightly increased risk for ovarian cancer is present in women with type A blood.

Biology

Potential serum tumor markers for ovarian cancer:
- alpha - fetoprotein (AFP)
- human chorionic gonadotropin (ßCG)
- lactate dehydrogenase (LDH)
- CEA
- CA-125
- lipid-associated sialic acid protein
- NB-70K

DETECTION AND DIAGNOSIS (Table 22-27)

1. Early diagnosis is difficult due to lack of early symptoms.

2. Clinical presentation ranges from completely asymptomatic to a myriad of vague abdominal complaints that all too often are attributed to diseases of the gastrointestinal (GI) or biliary tract. The symptoms of ovarian cancer according to site are:
   - abdomen: Abdominal pain, dyspepsia, bowel obstruction, and increasing abdominal girth
   - pelvis: pelvic pain, abnormal vaginal bleeding, dyspareunia, and constipation
   - thorax: dyspnea and pleuritic pain
   - general: cachexia and fatigue

   Although detection of an ovarian mass in an asymptomatic patient is common, with careful questioning the patient will often disclose other vague abdominal complaints that become manifest with ovarian cancer.

   Physical examination may also demonstrate presence of ascites (fluid wave), cul-de-sac nodularity, an omental cake, pleural effusion, groin or supraclavicular lymphadenopathy, or virilization.

3. A palpable ovary in a postmenopausal patient may suggest an ovarian neoplasm (219). A normal postmenopausal ovary measures no more than 2.0 cm in

Table 22-27. Imaging Procedures for Detection and Diagnosis of Ovarian Carcinoma

METHOD	CAPABILITY	RECOMMENDED FOR USE
Primary tumor and regional nodes		
CT	Accurate staging information; assesses myometrial invasion. Not known to be accurate in detecting lymph node spread	Following patients on chemotherapy
MRI	Not yet investigated. Potentially useful in local tumor staging	Unknown
Urography	Detects ureteral obstruction, bladder invasion; screens for unsuspected renal disease	Routine
Sonography	May detect unsuspected tumor. Displays overall bulk of primary tumor in pelvis/abdomen. Sensitive to ascites but not small peritoneal implants	Postoperative follow-up; evaluation of suspected ovarian mass
Biopsy	Confirms lesions detected by ultrasound, CT	Patients with suspicious lesions

CT = computed tomography; MRI = magnetic resonance imaging.
Adapted from Bragg et al. (20).

diameter. Transvaginal ultrasonography may elucidate an ambiguous pelvic examination (313). In fact, for postmenopausal patients with a simple cyst less than 5 cm in diameter, the risk of malignancy is low (259,320).

4. Various laboratory and radiologic tests may suggest the presence of an otherwise occult ovarian malignancy. A PAP smear occasionally has malignant cells with psammoma bodies suggestive but not diagnostic of an ovarian malignancy. An IV pyelogram or barium enema may demonstrate extrinsic compression by a pelvic mass. Chest x-ray may disclose a pleural effusion.

5. Route cul-de-sac aspiration to detect malignant cells shed by ovarian cancer has been evaluated as a screening tool. However, discomfort and the potential for causing leakage from an encapsulated tumor have precluded widespread use.

6. Noninvasive diagnostic imaging techniques (ultrasound, CT, MRI) may detect an ovarian malignancy during evaluation of other medical or surgical problems. These tests may provide information regarding the likelihood that a pelvic mass is malignant (259,274,320), but usually exploration is required for definitive diagnosis (2) (Table 22-27). Complex adnexal mass, ascites, cul-de-sac nodules, omental disease, pelvic or para-aortic lymphadenopathy, pleural effusion, and/or large adnexal mass are evidence for malignancy.

7. A number of tumor antigens may be elevated with ovarian cancer. Unfortunately, all these assays have limited value for screening because of the low frequency of ovarian cancer and the lack of specificity (353).

8. CA-125 assay is most useful to follow response to therapy and detect persistent disease prior to surgical reassessment of epithelial ovarian cancer (283,296,309, 310,323,338). Some have used CA-125 assays in the preoperative evaluation of persistent adnexal masses; patients with elevated CA-125 may be triaged to facilities experienced in ovarian cancer management and, in particular, primary cytoreductive surgery (287). When combined with other antigens (13) CA-125 can be used to screen high-risk patients, i.e., familial history (330).

9. AFP and ßCG are extremely useful in following response to therapy and in detecting persistent disease in the germ cell tumors that are antigen-positive, such as endodermal sinus tumor, embryonal carcinoma, and choriocarcinoma (324,346,347).

10. In metastatic adenocarcinoma of unknown primary, an underlying ovarian malignancy may be discovered at laparotomy in 20% of patients (277).

11. Ultimately, the diagnosis of ovarian cancer depends on obtaining an adequate histologic specimen, which usually entails exploratory laparotomy with ovarian resection. If an ovarian malignancy is confirmed, disease extent must be determined accurately and surgical removal of all possible tumor must be undertaken.

CLASSIFICATION AND STAGING

Histopathology

The classification of ovarian neoplasms is based on the histologic origin of the neoplasm within the ovary (Table 22-28) (247).

Germinal epithelium: These tumors originate from the ovarian surface and comprise 80% of all ovarian malignan-

cies. They occur predominantly in the postmenopausal period, and comprise a large variety of histologic subtypes (Table 22-28). These tumors may have benign, low malignant potential, or frankly malignant histology.

1. *Serous carcinoma*: Serous tumors are usually cystic; they account for 50% of epithelial malignancies. Bilateral involvement occurs in up to one third of cases (287). Psammoma bodies (calcific concretions) are often found. Primary papillary peritoneal carcinoma also originates from the peritoneal surface epithelium and closely resembles papillary serous carcinoma. Borderline tumors are also common. Serous cystadenocarcinomas may have a CA-125 level higher than 35 U/mL in 82% of cases (222).

2. *Mucinous carcinoma*: Comprising 15% of epithelial carcinomas, bilateral tumors occur in only 5% to 10% of cases. Large cysts are often filled with thick, mucinous debris. Cells in mucinous cystadenocarcinomas of the ovary closely resemble mucin-producing cells from the colon. Mucin leakage from benign mucinous cystadenomas, borderline tumors, or frank mucinous cystadenocarcinoma can lead to the syndrome of pseudomyxoma peritonei, in which chronic IP mucin accumulation occurs.

3. *Endometrioid adenocarcinoma*: Most are cystic and resemble endometrial carcinoma. Synchronous carcinoma of the endometrium is found in 15% of cases. This type of tumor may arise from areas of endometriosis (326).

4. *Clear cell adenocarcinoma*: Previously known as mesonephroid carcinoma, clear cell adenocarcinoma is composed of clear cells containing glycogen. "Hobnail" cells are characteristic. Although a greater proportion of cases are stage I, the prognosis is worse stage for stage than other epithelial cancers, with an overall 5-year survival of only 34% (277). This tumor also is found frequently in association with endometriosis.

5. *Brenner tumor*: Usually benign, this tumor is typically solid on gross examination, and is bilateral in about 5% of cases. Composed microscopically of epithelial nests (resembling urothelium) surrounded by a fibrous stroma, this tumor can cause stimulation of the endometrium, which can lead to abnormal uterine bleeding.

Germ cell tumors: These neoplasms constitute approximately 15% of all primary ovarian tumors.

1. *Dysgerminoma*: 40% of all malignant germ cell tumors are dysgerminomas, the most common histologic type. Dysgerminomas commonly occur in the second to third decade of life and have a predilection for lymph node metastases (249). As with gonadoblastomas, dysgerminomas are associated with dysgenetic gonads. At presentation, the majority of dysgerminomas are confined to the ovary. In stage I tumors, the bilaterality rate is approximately 10% to 15%. Microscopic examination reveals germ cells within fibrous trabeculae, often accompanied by a lymphocytic infiltrate. Serum LDH may often be elevated in these tumors; AFP and ßCG are usually negative. It is important to differentiate pure dysgerminomas from mixed germ cell tumors with a dysgerminomatous component, which are not radiosensitive and do not have quite as favorable a prognosis.

2. *Endodermal sinus tumor*: This is a more aggressive histologic subtype than dysgerminoma. Histologically, the

Table 22-28.   Histologic Classification of Ovarian Neoplasms

Common epithelial tumors (85%-90%)
- Types
  - Serous (tubal type; approximate frequency: 50% of epithelial carcinomas)
  - Mucinous (cervical type; 10%)
  - Endometrioid (endometrial type; 20%)
  - Clear cell (4%)
  - Unclassified / undifferentiated (15%)

- Differentiation
  - Benign: cystadenoma
  - Borderline malignancy/low malignant potential (applies mainly to serous and mucinous type)
  - Malignant
    Cystadenocarcinoma, grades 1,2, 3

Stromal tumors
- Specialized stroma: sex cord stromal tumors (3% - 8%)
  - Granulosa-theca (estrogen producing, about 3% - 6% of malignant ovarian tumors)
  - Sertoli-Leydig (virilizing, rare)
- Nonspecialized stroma: Mixed mesodermal tumor, lymphoma, leiomyosarcoma

Germ cell tumors (2% - 4%)
- Dysgerminoma (1% - 2%)
- Embryonic differentiation
  - Benign cystic teratoma
  - Malignant teratoma (AFP-, βhCG-negative)
- Extraembryonic differentiation
  - Endodermal sinus tumor/embryonal carcinoma (AFP-positive)
  - Choriocarcinoma (rare, βhCG-positive)

Secondary (metastatic) carcinomas

AFP = α-fetoprotein; βhCG = beta-human chorionic gonadotropin.
From Dembo (247), with permission.

tumor resembles fetal yolk sac structures with a reticular pattern, often accompanied by Schiller-Duval bodies. These tumors generally secrete AFP. These tumors were highly lethal prior to the advent of modern combination chemotherapy. Bilateral tumors in early disease are rare (11).

3. *Embryonal cell carcinoma:* These rare tumors are most commonly diagnosed in adolescent female patients. These tumors often secrete both ßCG and AFP. Bilaterality is rare. Histologically, large, primitive germ cells with considerable mitotic activity and nuclear atypia are seen with syncytiotrophoblastic giant cells (10). This is a very aggressive tumor with a clinical course similar to endodermal sinus tumor.

4. *Immature teratoma:* Most ovarian teratomas are cystic and benign. The malignant variety accounts for 1% of all teratomas. Although immature teratoma is generally unilateral, the contralateral ovary may contain a benign cystic teratoma. Immature teratomas are graded 0 to 4 on the basis of an estimate of the quantity of immature embryonal tissue present as well as the mitotic index. Histologically, any combination of both mature and fetal tissues may be seen. High-grade, immature teratomas may approach endodermal sinus tumors in aggressiveness.

5. *Nongestational choriocarcinoma:* This is a relatively rare germ cell tumor; a component of choriocarcinoma is often noted in mixed germ cell tumors and often in immature teratomas. ßCG is often produced by these tumors. Histologically, both syncytiotrophoblasts and cytotrophoblasts are seen.

6. *Polyembryoma:* This rarest germ cell tumor is composed of embryoid bodies.

7. *Mixed germ cell tumors:* These tumors are composed of at least two different germ cell histologies. Dysgerminoma is the most common component, followed by immature teratoma, endodermal sinus tumor, and embryonal cell carcinoma. Like most germ cell tumors, the majority present as stage I; the rate of bilaterality approaches 0% unless there is a dysgerminomatous component (280).

8. *Struma ovarii:* This tumor is a variant of ovarian teratoma composed mostly of thyroid acini. Clinical symptoms of thyroiditis can occur.

9. *Carcinoid tumors:* These may arise from benign cystic teratomas. Most ovarian carcinoids are metastases from an intestinal primary.

Sex cord tumors:

1. Granulosa cell tumors
   a. Occur predominantly in perimenopausal women; however, occasional tumors occur in adolescent females.

b. Are often associated with estrogen production. In postmenopausal women this may produce postmenopausal bleeding; in prepubertal females this may cause pseudoprecocious puberty. Virilization rarely occurs.

c. Large granulosa cell tumors and tumor spill convey a worse prognosis.

d. Histologically, microfollicular arrangement of cells with Call-Exner bodies are characteristic.

e. Late recurrences after 5 years' follow-up are not uncommon (345).

f. Juvenile granulosa cell tumors generally occur in pubertal females. Most patients have stage I tumors. Bilaterality occurs in less than 5%.

2. *Thecoma:* Occurs mainly in perimenopausal females and is composed of both thecal and spindle-shaped fibroblasts. Most present as stage I tumors. Thecomas may produce both estrogens and androgens and can cause endometrial hyperplasia or, rarely, virilization.

3. *Sertoli-Leydig's cell tumors:* rare tumors originating from the sex cord of the ovary. They occur most frequently in the third decade of life and are bilateral in 3% of patients. They often secrete androgens, frequently producing virilization. Histologically, tubular cells are seen with Leydig's cells in the intervening stroma.

4. *Gonadoblastoma:* benign tumors with cells derived from sex cords and germ cells. They are often associated with gonadal dysgenesis. However, gonadoblastomas may be accompanied by malignant germ cell tumors, especially dysgerminomas. Histologically, cellular nests of germ cells and sex cord derivatives separated by connective tissue stroma are seen.

5. *Leydig's cell/hilus cell's tumor:* develop from the hilum of the ovary. They can often produce testosterone and cause mild virilization. Eosinophilic Reinke crystalloids are seen between Leydig's cells.

Staging (Table 22-26 and Fig. 22-4)

1. Ovarian cancer spreads by IP, lymphatic, and locally invasive pathways. Lymphatic pathways may extend from the abdominal retroperitoneum to the groin via the inguinal/femoral canals or across the diaphragm to the pleural space. IP spread of tumor begins with extension of tumor through the ovarian capsule, allowing implantation of tumor throughout the abdomen. IP metastases show a predilection for the omentum and diaphragm, but no organ is spared, and concomitant ascites are frequent. Parenchymal disease of the liver is rare. The incidence of positive lymph nodes at surgical exploration has been reported to be 25% Stage I, 50% in Stage II, and 74% in Stage II and IV (232a).

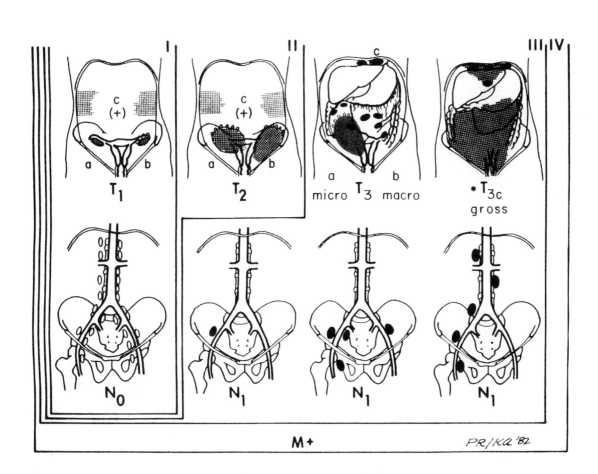

Fig. 22-4. Anatomic staging for ovarian cancer.

2. Clinical examination is frequently inaccurate in assessing the extent of ovarian cancer. The work-up of a patient with suspected ovarian carcinoma is designed to exclude diseases of other organs that may mimic ovarian tumors. Procedures useful for the work-up and staging of ovarian cancer are: Colonoscopy or barium enema; abdominal CT scan or sonogram if presence of mass is uncertain; chest x-ray with possible thoracentesis if there is effusion; and staging laparotomy. Often, a thorough evaluation of the colon is helpful in excluding a primary colon cancer when abdominal carcinomatosis is discovered. Proper surgical staging reflects known patterns of spread and entails a thorough abdominal exploration (usually through a vertical midline abdominal incision) with cytologic washings of the upper abdomen, including the diaphragm, infracolic omentectomy, pelvic and para-aortic lymph node sampling, and often random peritoneal biopsies. As older series suggest, failure to evaluate these areas, in particular the retroperitoneal spaces and the upper abdomen, may lead to significant understaging (290). The principal staging systems used are the FIGO staging for ovarian cancer (Table 22-26 and Fig. 22-4). The American Joint Commission on Cancer Staging uses the tumor (T), node (N), metastasis (M) staging system.

PRINCIPLES OF TREATMENT

The modern management of ovarian cancer is based primarily on maximal surgical resection of tumor, followed by adjuvant chemotherapy or radiotherapy. Initial laparotomy provides an accurate histologic diagnosis, precisely defines disease extent, and allows the opportunity for primary cytoreductive surgery. Table 22-29 presents a concise tabulation of multidisciplinary decisions in treatment choices and combinations according to stage.

Surgery

1. For early ovarian cancer, surgery is the mainstay of therapy. With encapsulated, well-differentiated epithelial carcinomas and many germ cell tumors, *unilateral adnexectomy* is adequate with appropriate staging biopsies. Following conservative surgery, adjuvant chemotherapy may be indicated and still allows preservation of fertility. For borderline epithelial carcinoma, surgical resection with adequate staging is the principal treatment, as cytotoxic chemotherapy is of unproven benefit.

2. *Surgical intervention* in the treatment of ovarian cancer may be for a specific purpose, such as the relief of GI, urinary, or biliary tract obstruction. It may also be for a purely cytoreductive purpose with aggressive surgical resection of tumor and structures that tumor has invaded in an attempt to reduce the tumor volume. Residual tumor following primary cytoreductive surgery has been demonstrated to be an important predictor of response to chemotherapy and disease-free survival in numerous retrospective studies (244,264,265,268,272).

3. In the past decade, the extent of surgical resection to achieve maximal cytoreduction has been expanded. Although various definitions exist regarding what constitutes *optimal cytoreduction*, most studies use a residual tumor diameter of less than 0.5 to 2.5 cm. While data supporting primary surgical cytoreduction are substantial, the question remains whether an inability to perform optimal cytoreduction merely reflects a more aggressive tumor (282,291). Gynecologic surgeons have developed techniques to remove extensive pelvic tumor previously deemed unresectable by taking advantage of the retroperitoneal free spaces. Tumor may be removed from a viscus by serosal stripping or surgical resection of the structure with the tumor attached. While bowel resection for optimal cytoreduction is well accepted,

				(6,246a,306a)
Table 22-29. Multidisciplinary Treatment Decisions by Stage for Ovarian Carcinoma				
Stage	Surgery	Radiation Therapy		Chemotherapy
IA,B (T_1,N_0 M_0)	Oophorectomy with tumor resection, radical HBSO,			
IC	omentectomy	Intraperitoneal radioisotopes	or	MAC
II (T_2, N_0, M_0)	Oophorectomy with tumor resection, radical HBSO, and omentectomy Excise adhesions Biopsy diaphragm and pelvis	DRT whole abdomen/pelvic 25 Gy/50 Gy	or	MAC
III (T_3,N_1,M_0)	Cytoreductive surgery	DRT whole abdomen/pelvic	or	MAC
IV (T_{any},N_{any}, M_+)	Debulking optional	PRT	and	MAC
Relapse and recurrence	Second look	PRT	and	IC II

RT = radiation therapy; DRT = definitive; PRT = palliative; RCT = recommended chemotherapy;
HBSO = hysterectomy and bilateral salpingo-oophorectomy; MAC = multiagent chemotherapy phase III clinical trials; IC II = investigational chemotherapy, phase I,II clinical trials.
PDQ: RCT - MAC = CP,CC,HCAP,CAP.

recent reports suggest that resection of portions of the genitourinary tract, diaphragm, involved lymph nodes, and splenectomy are well tolerated (226). Successful cytoreduction to an optimal state can be achieved in approximately 80% of stage III and stage IV epithelial ovarian cancers at centers experienced in this modality (307). However, there is as yet no randomized study proving that radical surgery including peritoneal stripping and bowel resection for the purpose of complete cytoreduction improves survival (310b). Complications of extensive cytoreduction include prolonged operating time, increased blood loss, anastomotic complications, increased frequency of pulmonary embolus, and potential vascular injury (238).

4. *Second-look laparotomy*: Second-look laparotomy is another surgical intervention commonly used in the management of ovarian cancer. In the strictest sense, second-look laparotomy is only for surgical reassessment of tumor status after obtaining a clinical CR following adjuvant therapy. Originally, second-look laparotomy was used to determine the treament duration with alkylating agents; however, prolonged treatment with alkylating agents has been abandoned because of the risk of inducing acute nonlymphocytic acute leukemia (262). In ovarian cancer, response rates for patients with stage III or IV carcinoma who have been optimally cytoreduced by surgery can be as high as 40% to 92% (307). Second-look laparotomy may demonstrate a pathologic CR in which no microscopic tumor can be detected on multiple random biopsies and peritoneal washings. Previously, patients with a pathologic CR did not undergo any further treatment.

   a. Recurrence: Unfortunately, in all but early-stage ovarian cancer, recurrence after even a CR to adjuvant therapy is all too common. Recurrence rates after a negative second-look laparotomy range from approximately 20% to 57% (227,234,319). Some authors suggest that patients with negative second-look laparotomies, after treatment with cisplatin-based adjuvant chemotherapy, are more likely to have recurrences than those treated with agents other than cisplatin (319). In view of the high rate of recurrence after a negative second-look laparotomy, many have advocated using additional therapy such as IP radiocolloids postoperatively (339). Others have suggested replacing second-look laparotomy with statistical predictive models based on historical or pathologic findings for assessment of tumor persistence or recurrence (234).

   b. Most authorities have found stage IV status, high tumor grade, old age, poor performance status, suboptimal tumor residual after primary cytoreductive surgery, or extensive initial volume of metastatic disease within the abdomen to be predictive of a poor outcome regardless of the results of second-look laparotomy (227,234,236,256,273,319).

   c. In view of all these deficiencies, many have argued against routine second-look laparotomy because no studies demonstrate any survival benefit (234,236,256,273,310a). Persistently elevated CA-125 values may indicate tumor persistence, even when tumor is inapparent on physical or radiologic examination (296). In addition, although there are currently salvage regimens with reasonable response rates, further study is needed to determine whether there is any survival benefit to initiating salvage therapy at the time of second-look versus waiting to begin salvage treatment after clinical recurrence or perhaps when CA-125 levels increase or are still elevated 6 months after treatment (239,321,324,330). Patients with stage I or stage II disease who have been adequately staged and appropriately treated with adjuvant therapy may not benefit from routine second-look laparotomy, as the recurrence rate in this subcategory of patients is relatively low. In early-stage patients treated appropriately, the rate of persistent disease in patients without symptoms is only 5%, as documented with second-look laparotomy data (341).

5. *Secondary cytoreductive surgery*: The value of a secondary cytoreductive procedure, either as an adjunct for macroscopically positive second-look procedure or as a planned therapeutic modality prior to salvage chemotherapy or radiotherapy is highly controversial. Initial reports suggest a prolongation of disease-free survival after secondary cytoreduction in those with residual tumor less than 1.5 cm (228). Whether this is related to overall tumor burden or improved responsiveness to salvage therapy is unknown. Other studies that examined the role of secondary cytoreductive surgery after primary chemotherapy for refractory ovarian carcinoma suggested no benefit (293,340). Again, the success of salvage therapy seems highly dependent on the amount of residual tumor at the conclusion of the second-look operation.

Radiotherapy for Ovarian Carcinoma

Radiotherapy is an accepted treatment option in select cases following primary cytoreductive surgery or as salvage therapy for patients with tumor persistence. Radiation may be delivered externally, as in the form of whole abdomen radiation therapy with or without a boost to the pelvis. Additionally, radiation can be delivered via radiocolloids instilled into the peritoneal cavity.

Radiocolloids ^{32}P: In early-stage ovarian cancer, a variety of randomized studies have demonstrated a role for intraperitoneal ^{32}P. A pure ß-emitter with a half-life of 14.3 days, ^{32}P has replaced ^{198}Au as the radiocolloid of choice based on equal efficacy and a low complication rate. While its role as an adjuvant for high-risk, early-stage disease is well established, its use in the treatment of microscopic or small (< 5 mm) residual disease at the time of reassessment is under study (311,331). IP ^{32}P is administered once in a dose of 10 to 15 mCi. Complications include bowel obstruction, radiation enteritis, and bowel perforation; however, these are infrequent (7%) (311). The use of ^{212}Pb, a high-energy, superficially penetrating alpha-emitter has also been examined (317).

External irradiation (whole abdomen radiation therapy, Fig. 22-5): Although chemotherapy is the adjuvant modality of choice for advanced epithelial ovarian cancer in most U.S. centers, external beam radiotherapy to the whole abdomen has also been used very effectively following initial cytoreductive surgery (246). Generally, patients receive whole

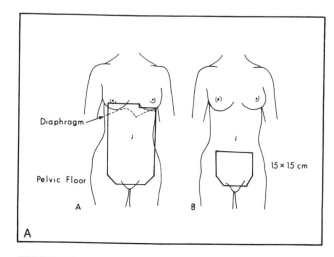

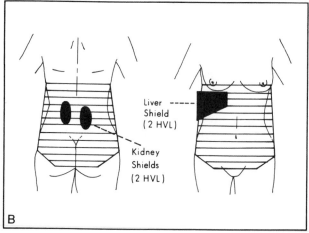

Fig. 22-5. (A,B) Principles of treatment: whole abdominal irradiation techniques for ovarian cancer.

abdomen irradiation with a pelvic boost. Initially abdominal irradiation was delivered by a moving strip technique; however, open field techniques appear equally efficacious, simpler, and safer (248). Most centers deliver 2,200 to 3,200 cGy to the whole abdomen with this technique. Whole abdomen radiotherapy has also been used as a salvage regimen for persistent ovarian cancer. Short-term survival rates range from 0% to 45% with a major complication rate as high as 30% (278). Microscopic or small macroscopic residual carcinoma, low grade, and low age all seem to improve the chances of salvage (267,278,292,329).

Chemotherapy for Ovarian Cancer

Chemotherapy is currently the predominant approach to treating ovarian carcinoma. Virtually all patients with epithelial ovarian cancer, except those with completely resected borderline carcinomas or well-differentiated, encapsulated stage I ovarian carcinomas, receive some form of adjuvant chemotherapy. Chemotherapy is the most commonly used adjuvant modality for ovarian cancer and ovarian cancer is one of the more responsive solid tumors (Table 22-30) (352a).

1. *Alkylating agents* such as hemisulfur mustard were first used in the 1950s for palliative treatment of advanced epithelial ovarian carcinoma by both IP and IV routes (261,327). Subsequent clinical trials demonstrated response rates between 35 and 65%, for alkylating agents such as melphalan, chlorambucil, and cyclophosphamide, but median survival was only 8 to 19 months despite patients surviving prolonged treatment (352). Concern developed regarding the incidence of acute nonlymphocytic leukemia in patients treated with prolonged administration of alkylating agents. Most studies showed the relative risk of developing acute nonlymphocytic leukemia in patients on long-term alkylating agent therapy to be increased 21 to 175 times. The onset of leukemia generally is 4 to 5 years after diagnosis of the carcinoma. This increase in relative risk seems to be related to the total dose of alkylating agents

Table 22-30. Results of Controlled Trials With Combination Chemotherapy for Ovarian Cancer

Year (Reference)	Drugs	No. Patients	Complete Response (%)	Median PFI (mos)	Median Survival (mos)
1978 (352)	Melphalan	39	16	--	17
	HexaCAF	41	33	--	29
1982 (243)	Cyclophosphamide	19	5.2	7.4	16.5
	Cisplatin/cyclophosphamide	21	23.8	27.6	40+
1986 (297)	ACe	120	26	7.7	15.7
	CAP	107	51	13.1	19.7
1987 (266)	Cisplatin	173	20.2	8.7	19.4
	Cisplatin/cyclophosphamide	174	20.7	12.9	21.4
	CAP	169	26.0	14.6	23.8
1989 (298)	Cisplatin/cyclophosphamide	176	30.2	22.7	31.2
	CAP	173	32.8	24.6	38.9

received and most patients who developed acute nonlymphocytic leukemia received alkylating agents for more than 2 years (242,284,300). In advanced disease, subsequent randomized clinical trials demonstrated increased response rates and increased median survivals with multidrug combination chemotherapy when compared with single-agent alkylating agents, particularly those incorporating cisplatin into the regimen (243,285,352). Currently, alkylating agents are most often used as adjuvant therapy for early epithelial ovarian carcinoma.

2. *Doxorubicin* when used alone has a response rate comparable with single-agent alkylators. Initial clinical trials found improved response rates when doxorubicin was combined with other agents (299). However, more recent trials comparing cisplatin-based regimens with and without doxorubicin find no significant difference in efficacy (231,298). In addition, the dose-related cardiotoxicity of doxorubicin, alopecia, and the potential for extravasation injury make it a less attractive agent. Administering doxorubicin encapsulated in liposomes via an IP route may decrease systemic toxicity and allow delivery of high-dose doxorubicin tumor cells by endocytosis (245).

3. *Cisplatin* or its analogs are the single most effective agents in the treatment of ovarian carcinoma. The first reported use of cisplatin in ovarian carcinoma was in 1976 for patients who failed primary chemotherapy (349). Cisplatin does not seem to share cross-resistant characteristics with alkylating agents and has a different spectrum of toxicity. Toxicity includes renal damage, ototoxicity, peripheral neuropathy, severe emesis, and hypomagnesemia. Cisplatin has been combined with other agents following cytoreductive surgery for the treatment of advanced epithelial carcinoma and in salvage regimens for recurrent or persistent disease (Table 22-30). However, several studies suggest that single-agent cisplatin for advanced disease may be comparable with cyclophosphamide-cisplatin or CAP (266). An analysis of 34 publications and five unpublished reports of 5,016 patients suggests that cisplatin combination chemotherapy has yielded results superior to either single-agent cisplatin or an effective alkylator (347,348). Cisplatin dose intensity may also play a significant role in response rates because high-dose cisplatin (200 mg/m^2) has produced responses in patients otherwise refractory to treatment with cisplatin; unfortunately, neurotoxicity of this dose is severe (316). Cisplatin analogs such as carboplatin and tetraplatin may prove equally efficacious, and with their lower toxicity may allow greater dose intensification. High-dose carboplatin (800 mg/m^2/cycle) has been used in phase II trials as a salvage regimen for refractory ovarian carcinoma with some success (258,301,303,316,347,348). In SWOG study 8412, carboplatin 300 mg/m^2/cycle and cyclophosphamide 600 mg/m^2/cycle was compared with cisplatin 100 mg/m^2/cycle and cyclophosphamide 600 mg/m^2/cycle for a total of six courses in a randomized prospective fashion; no differences were noted in pathologic CR rates or median survival and there was significantly less nephrotoxicity, neurotoxicity, and emesis in the carboplatin arm. The role of carboplatin and other

analogs in the treatment of ovarian cancer is still under investigation. IP cisplatin also has been used for both primary therapy and in salvage therapy. In patients with small residual abdominal disease, IP cisplatin allows high levels of cisplatin to be delivered to the tumor. A recent report by Kirmani *et al.* (279) indicates IP consolidation of IV induction chemotherapy (etoposide) has lead to a 87% CR with 31 months follow-up.

Cisplatin and its analogs also have considerable activity in the treatment of germ cell tumors (232,348).

4. Hexamethylmelamine, although structurally similar to nitrogen mustard, does not exert its antineoplastic effect by alkylation of DNA; the exact mode of action is currently unknown. Hexamethylmelamine has been used as a single agent for salvage therapy in ovarian epithelial carcinoma, and in various combinations with cyclophosphamide, doxorubicin, and cisplatin. Objective responses can be obtained in previously cisplatin-or alkylating agent-refractory epithelial tumors (288,304,314). Hexamethylmelamine is an oral agent generally given over 2 week periods; its chief toxicity is GI and it has a potential for peripheral neuropathy.

5. *Etoposide* is a congener of podophyllotoxin, an agent that causes metaphase arrest during mitosis. Several studies report using etoposide in combination or as a single agent in patients failing alkylating therapy (250). In doses of 100 to 200 mg/m^2/cycle in combination with cisplatin there can be responses in previous cisplatin failures, this suggests some synergy between etoposide and cisplatin (221). Severe bone marrow suppression is the dose-limiting toxicity, especially in pretreated patients (235).

6. A wide variety of other agents have been used, including 5FU, methotrexate, and actinomycin D, in many combinations. Agents such as ifosfamide, a cyclophosphamide analog are being used in current clinical trials as salvage therapy with a response rate of 21% (334). Ifosfamide toxicities include nephrotoxicity, neurotoxicity with possible metabolic encephalopathy, and granulocytopenia; hemorrhagic cystitis has been largely eliminated with the addition of the uroprotector mesna (260,322). Taxol, a derivative from the bark of the western yew, is an antitumor drug with efficacy against epithelial ovarian cancer; it induces microtubule aggregation during mitosis. Given by continuous infusion over 24 hours, taxol produced a 32% response rate in heavily pretreated patients (318). Its principle toxicity is severe granulocytopenia and alopecia. Rarely, patients also describe anaphylactic reactions and cardiac rhythm disturbances (251,318).

Hormonal Therapy for Ovarian Cancer

Levels of estrogen and progesterone receptors in epithelial ovarian tumors may be obtained at the time of initial surgery or second-look laparotomy; however, the status of these receptors has no particular value in assessing the likelihood of response to hormonal therapy for refractory ovarian carcinoma. Most studies involve the use of tamoxifen or megesterol acetate as salvage therapy for patients who have previously failed first or second-line chemotherapy. Patients' tolerance of either tamoxifen 10 mg. orally bid, or megesterol acetate 160 to 800 mg orally qd, is generally good and prolonged stabilization of the disease may be obtained. In the GOG study, a 10% response rate was obtained with a mean duration of response of 8 months (224,294,325).

Immunotherapy for Ovarian Cancer

Biologic response modifiers such as bacillus Calmette-Tuerin, tumor necrosis factor, *Corynebacterium Parbum*, or alpha-interferon have been used in several clinical trials singly and with salvage chemotherapy. Some studies suggest improved response rates to chemotherapy (216,229,230,240,343). Currently, the use of biologic response modifiers is confined to clinical research trials.

Multidisciplinary Treatment of Epithelial Ovarian Carcinoma (Table 22-29)

Early stage (stage I and stage II):

1. Staging laparotomy, generally through a vertical, midline, abdominal incision, including peritoneal washings of the entire abdomen, infracolic omentectomy, abdominal hysterectomy, bilateral salpingonophorectomy, and careful exploration of all peritoneal surfaces should be performed. The retroperitoneum should be evaluated by pelvic and para-aortic lymph node sampling to avoid the possibility of understaging the patient. As many as 8% of apparently stage I tumors may have lymph node metastases (11). In apparent stage II disease, 5% to 42% of patients had positive retroperitoneal nodes (350). It is particularly important if IP ^{32}P is to be the adjuvant treatment used because ^{32}P has been shown to be inadequate for treatment of retroperitoneal disease (311).

2. In encapsulated stage IA or stage IB disease that is not poorly differentiated, adjuvant chemotherapy and radiotherapy may not be of benefit. All other patients with stage I and stage II disease are at higher risk for recurrence and require adjuvant treatment. In these situations both melphalan for 1 year and IP ^{32}P appear equally efficacious (351). Whole abdomen radiation therapy has also been used; however, concern regarding its toxicity limits its use for this indication. Currently, there are trials to evaluate short-term, intensive cisplatin combination chemotherapy as adjuvant treatment for early-stage disease.

Advanced epithelial ovarian carcinoma (stages III, IV):

1. Stage III disease with optimal cytoreduction (0.5 to 2.0 cm maximal residual diameter): These patients also require appropriate staging laparotomy with maximal effort toward primary surgical cytoreduction. The feasibility of cytoreduction at major centers is approximately 30% to 80%. Additional treatment is necessary and includes combination chemotherapy. Randomized trials comparing cisplatin-based combination chemotherapy with single-agent therapy have demonstrated the superiority of the former in producing more CRs and lengthening disease-free survival (220,243,352) (Table 22-30). However, it is unclear whether this translates into differences in long-term survival. Currently, the most widely accepted regimen is cyclophosphamide 500 to 1,000 mg/m²/cycle and cisplatin 50 mg/m²/course for 6 to 8 courses. Data from salvage regimens on patients with small disease at second-look laparotomy (275,302) suggest that increasing dose intensity and IP delivery of cisplatin may improve response rates (312). However, there are no randomized studies demonstrating conclusively that this is true for primary adjuvant chemotherapy. Additionally, carboplatin shows good activity in salvage regimens and will probably replace cisplatin in primary chemotherapy regimens due to its superior therapeutic index (301).

2. Whole abdomen radiation therapy with pelvic boost may also be curative, particularly in patients with minimal tumor residual and low tumor grade (85,269). Randomized studies comparing adjuvant radiotherapy to adjuvant melphalan initially discouraged physicians from recommending whole abdomen irradiation (332). On careful review, some of these may not be justified because toxicity of whole abdomen radiotherapy can be minimized by the open field technique (246,329). Toxicities of whole abdomen irradiation include bowel obstruction, hepatitis, enterocutaneous fistula, and hemorrhagic cystitis.

3. Second-look laparotomy is still the most sensitive method of assessing response to treatment in patients who have achieved a clinical CR. Although no survival benefit has been demonstrated for this procedure, it does provide information that is useful for assessing response to investigational treatments and prognosis.

4. Stage III and stage IV ovarian carcinoma with suboptimal tumor residual: A combination chemotherapy regimen similar to those used in patients with optimal cytoreduction is appropriate. Response rates are decreased, with little chance of CR. The therapeutic advantage obtained with cisplatin combination therapy relative to alkylating agents may be reduced (346).

5. Radiation therapy generally is not indicated, as virtually all patients (88%) demonstrate either tumor persistence or rapid recurrence (268).

   Second-look surgery for optimal secondary cytoreduction is performed in approximately 38% of patients (228).

6. Stage IV epithelial ovarian carcinoma: While tumor burden for patients with stage IV disease may not be significantly higher than with stage IIIC, 5-year survival is 4.8% and is poorer than with stage III (305). However, in the common scenario of abdominal carcinomatosis with a malignant pleural effusion, the same therapies may be used as those for stage III, suboptimally cytoreduced patients. Chemotherapy may reduce symptomatic pleural effusion; occasionally chemical pleurodesis is necessary for relief of dyspnea. Second-look laparotomy is performed less frequently because the chance for a pathologic CR after adjuvant chemotherapy is very limited and many patients will eventually relapse, regardless of the results of second-look surgery (234).

7. Persistent, progressive, or recurrent epithelial ovarian carcinoma: This is usually discovered by clinical examination, chest x-ray, abdominal CT scan or surgical reassessment. Alternatively, persistent elevations in CA-125 levels may strongly suggest persistent disease (296,309,323).

   Salvage, or second-line chemotherapy may be beneficial, particularly in patients with small residual tumor, after a second-look laparotomy. Patients with persistent disease previously treated with cisplatin may respond to high doses of cisplatin or IP cisplatin with either etoposide or cytarabine (275,302,312,333). Carboplatin, tamoxifen, and ifosfamide may be used successfully as single agents for salvage chemotherapy (301). Hexamethylmelamine has also been used most often in combination with other agents(306).

Hormonal therapy with tamoxifen or megestrol acetate may provide prolonged stabilization of disease in patients unable to tolerate salvage chemotherapy or radiotherapy.

SPECIAL CONSIDERATIONS OF TREATMENT

Germ Cell Tumors

These tumors frequently affect women of reproductive age. Since many present at early stage, preservation of fertility is often possible, even when adjuvant chemotherapy is necessary. Therapeutic approaches vary according to disease stage, tumor histology, and the reproductive desires of the patient.

Treatment by Histologic Type

1. *Dysgerminoma:* Since dysgerminomas often disseminate by lymphatics, lymph node sampling definitely should be included as part of appropriate staging. In stage Ia, 10-year survival with unilateral adnexal removal is above 90%, which is comparable with survival with hysterectomy and bilateral salpingo-onophorectomy (337). Since the rate of bilaterality in stage I disease is approximately 10% to 15%, careful evaluation, including possible biopsy of the contralateral ovary, is necessary for conservative treatment. Recurrences after conservative treatment can be treated successfully with either radiation therapy or chemotherapy. Like testicular seminomas, ovarian dysgerminomas are exquisitely radiosensitive. Response rates to combination chemotherapy such as VAC and VBP are also excellent, and normal ovulation usually resumes after therapy. Currently, adjuvant therapy for advanced disease is chemotherapy or whole abdomen irradiation. The optimal combination is still under study: vinblastine, vincristine, actinomycin D, cisplatin, and etoposide all show good activity against dysgerminomas.

2. *Endodermal sinus tumor (EST):* Adjuvant chemotherapy is indicated in all cases of EST, as survival rates with surgery alone in stage I cases are dismal. Conservative surgery with adjuvant chemotherapy is possible in most stages. VAC was the first successful regimen used, with about 75% survival (257). Other series do not report such a favorable survival rate with VAC. Better results with acceptable toxicity were demonstrated with regimens using VBP. Survival rates with VBP in excess of 90% in early-stage disease and 70% to 80% with advanced disease have been reported (345). Chronic toxicity of VBP include vasculitis with Raynaud's phenomenon paresthesias and a questionable increase in coronary artery disease and paresthesias (315). Response to adjuvant chemotherapy can often be assessed by serial evaluation of serum AFP values. It is unclear whether second-look laparotomy is appropriate for germ cell tumors, particularly those tumors in which ß-CG or AFP is elevated and can be used as a tumor marker (255).

Embryonal carcinoma: This aggressive tumor is treated in the same fashion as EST.

Immature teratomas: High-grade, immature teratomas require adjuvant chemotherapy even for early-stage disease. Chemotherapy regimens are similar to those for EST.

Nongestational choriocarcinoma: Surgical management is the same as for other nondysgerminomatous germ cell tumors. Adjuvant chemotherapy regimens are similar to those used in the treatment of high-risk, metastatic GTN.

Polyembryoma: Current therapy is the same as for the other nondysgerminomatous germ cell tumors.

Mixed germ cell tumor: The majority of these tumors present as stage I. Surgery and adjuvant chemotherapy are identical to those for endodermal sinus tumor.

Struma ovarii: Only 5% of struma ovarii are malignant; treatment with ^{131}I is effective.

EARLY EPITHELIAL OVARIAN CANCER

If future childbearing is of great concern, conservative surgery can be performed for encapsulated, well-differentiated stage Ia ovarian epithelial carcinomas. Adjuvant chemotherapy does not improve the prognosis of patients treated by surgery alone and unilateral salpingo-ophorectomy produces equivalent results to hysterectomy and bilateral salpingo-ophorectomy in well-staged patients. Pregnancy should be attempted expeditiously, and consideration should be given to eventual removal of the remaining ovary after childbearing is completed.

EPITHELIAL TUMORS OF LOW MALIGNANT POTENTIAL

1. Also known as borderline carcinoma, these tumors were first described in 1929 by Taylor (335) as appearing histologically malignant but having an indolent natural history.
2. Borderline carcinoma comprises approximately 20% of invasive ovarian epithelial carcinomas (218).
3. In 1973, Hart and Norris (270) defined specific criteria for the diagnosis of both mucinous and serous borderline carcinoma based on excessive stratification, nuclear atypia, and absence of ovarian stromal invasion. Approximately 50% of patients present with stage I disease (223,237).
4. Intraoperative diagnosis of low malignant potential tumors by frozen section can be difficult, particularly when trying to distinguish between a mucinous cystadenoma and a borderline mucinous tumor. Appropriate staging for invasive cancer should be done.
5. Treatment of reproductive-age women desirous of childbearing with stage IA tumors may be a unilateral salpingo-oophorectomy, with no change in survival (336).
6. The cornerstone of therapy is surgical resection of all gross tumor; chemotherapy and radiotherapy are of unproven benefit even in advanced disease. Adjuvant therapy is clearly unwarranted for stage I tumors (241). It is not surprising that cytotoxic therapy is not very effective, because the cell cycle for many borderline carcinomas does not differ much the normal cell cycle. For advanced-stage disease, cytotoxic chemotherapy may be of value in incompletely resected disease. Recurrent disease may be best treated with further cytoreductive surgery. Some authorities suggest that

patients who have persistent disease after chemotherapy do poorly (252).

7. The value of second-look laparotomy is not well established for advanced disease; it is probably not indicated for early disease.

8. The GOG is currently investigating the role of adjuvant chemotherapy for advanced disease. Because of the indolent nature of these tumors, this study will require many years to complete.

Sex Cord Tumors of the Ovary

Granulosa cell tumors

1. Eighty-five percent of cases present in stage I with survival with surgery alone in excess of 90%.

2. Unilateral adnexectomy is adequate for stage IA tumors because bilaterality is rare.

3. Staging and appropriate surgical resection should be performed as initial therapy. Radiotherapy may be of benefit for cases with tumor spill or in advanced disease. VAC chemotherapy has also been used. Results are ambiguous, since trials with advanced disease are limited due to its rarity.

Thecoma. These tumors are almost never malignant and are unilateral in 97% of patients (223). Most of these tumors present as stage I and unilateral oophorectomy is adequate treatment.

Sertoli-Leydig's cell tumors: Conservative surgery may be appropriate for females with stage Ia tumors desirous of childbearing. For other stages, hysterectomy and bilateral oophorectomy and cytoreductive surgery are recommended. Patients with residual tumor generally receive whole abdominal radiation or can be treated with VAC chemotherapy.

Gonadoblastoma: Although these are benign tumors, they may be accompanied by a malignant germ cell tumor, most frequently dysgerminoma. Management is based on the presence or absence of these germ cell tumors and whether the patient has dysgenetic gonads with a Y chromosome, in which case removal of both gonads is indicated.

Leydig's cell tumor or hilus cell tumor: Always unilateral and benign, they require only surgical resection.

SMALL CELL CARCINOMA OF THE OVARY

This is a rare variant of epithelial ovarian carcinoma and usually is accompanied by paraendocrine hypercalcemia. It affects younger women, with a mean age of occurence of 23 years. Small cell carcinoma is highly lethal; chemotherapy regimens utilized include cisplatin, vinblastine, bleomycin, doxorubicin, and etoposide. These regimens are marginally effective for advanced disease (328).

OVARIAN CANCER DURING PREGNANCY

Ovarian cancer is rare during pregnancy, occurring once in 19,000 to 25,000 pregnancies. Cancers account for 2% to 5% of persistent adnexal masses during pregnancy. The detection of an ovarian tumor is more difficult during pregnancy as examination of the adnexae is difficult with the enlarging uterus. Additionally, the vague, nonspecific abdominal discomfort that is often a symptom of ovarian cancer is masked by similar symptoms derived from obstetric problems. Sonography is helpful for the evaluation of potential ovarian tumors. Generally, exploratory laparotomy should be deferred until the midsecond trimester, when there is a reduced rate of pregnancy loss. For unilateral, low-grade epithelial carcinoma or stage I germ cell tumors, patients may undergo unilateral adnexectomy. A variety of chemotherapeutic agents can be given postoperatively with successful pregnancy outcomes. However, the long-term effects of chemotherapy on the offspring are unknown.

RESULTS AND PROGNOSIS

Appropriate assessment of disease extent is crucial to appropriate selection of adjuvant therapy. Table 22-31 presents recent survival statistics of invasive ovarian cancers from FIGO. Five-year survival rates are illustrated for major prognostic factors and include anatomic stage, pathology, age, grade, and residuum of tumor postlaparotomy (Fig. 22-6). Most patients

Table 22-31. Distribution by Stage and 3- and 5-year Survival of Carcinoma of the Ovary. Patients Treated in 1979-1981.

STAGE	Patients treated No.	Patients treated (%)	3-year survival No.	3-year survival (%)	5-year survival No.	5-year survival (%)
I	2,230	(26.1)	1,780	(79.8)	1,624	(72.8)
II	1,313	(15.4)	794	(60.5)	608	(46.3)
III	1,946	(22.8)	515	(26.0)	335	(17.2)
IIIA	199	(2.3)	83	(41.7)	61	(30.7)
IIIB	303	(3.6)	119	(39.3)	96	(31.7)
IIIC	891	(10.4)	199	(22.3)	128	(14.4)
IV	1,391	(16.3)	141	(10.1)	67	(4.8)
No stage	268	(3.1)	85	(31.7)	58	(21.6)
Total	8,541	(100.0)	3,706	(43.4)	2,977	(34.9)

From Petterson (306), with permission.

STAGE   AGE   PATHOLOGY

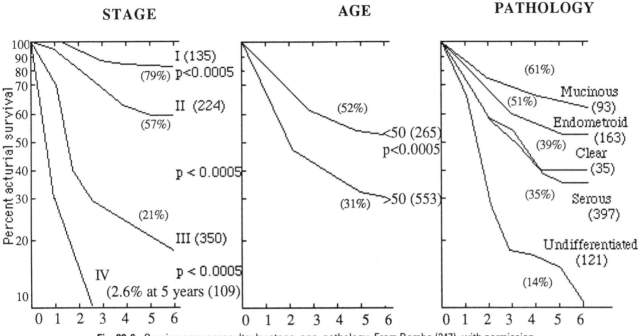

Fig. 22-6. Ovarian cancer results: by stage, age, pathology. From Dembo (247), with permission.

have widespread disease at the time of diagnosis and partly as a result of this, yearly mortality in ovarian cancer is approximately 65% of the incidence rate. Long-term follow-up of suboptimally debulked Stage II and Stage IV patients reveals a 5-year survival rate of less than 10% even with platinum-based combination therapy (297a). An excellent and final review by the late Alon Dembo of his life's work in ovarian cancer presents a summary of decades of clinical investigation using a combination of whole abdominal radiation therapy and chemotherapy (246a).

Survival in early-stage epithelial ovarian carcinoma: For stage I epithelial carcinoma, GOG studies demonstrate the ability of adjuvant melphalan to decrease the recurrence rate to 6% and also demonstrate no benefit in adjuvant pelvic irradiation (276). Subsequent randomized studies demonstrated that survival for stage IA, IB grade I or II ovarian epithelial carcinoma was in excess of 90% without additional treatment. Patients with stage I poorly differentiated tumor, stage IC, and stage II cancers can be treated with either melphalan or ^{32}P with the expectation that 80% will be disease-free at 2 years (215). Current studies are randomizing patients to platinum-based combination chemotherapy or IP ^{32}P for this high-risk subgroup of patients with early ovarian cancer. Using whole abdomen irradiation for consolidation after induction chemotherapy and cytoreductive surgery, Haie *et al.* (269) report 3- and 6-year survival of 60% and 33%, respectively.

Survival in advanced epithelial ovarian cancer (stages III and IV): After appropriate staging and attempts at optimal primary cytoreductive surgery, patients may receive either adjuvant chemotherapy or radiation therapy. Patients with advanced disease may have a 50% total response rate with a CR rate of approximately 20% to first-line chemotherapy. Long-term survival ranges from 4% to 16% (215). Long-term survival, 5 years or more, in stage III cancer is best correlated with no minimal residual tumor postsurgical resection (Table 22-32).

Adjuvant whole abdomen radiotherapy, like combination chemotherapy, may produce reasonable survival rates in patients with small-volume residual disease; Dembo (246) reported up to 28% 10-year survival with disease residual less than 2 cm, however it dropped to 67% for larger lesions and 38% for small excresions (269). Combination chemotherapy regimens containing cisplatin have been shown to produce higher response rates and, in some studies, have produced a statistically significant prolongation of survival compared to drug regimens without cisplatin. A recent meta-analysis addressing this comparison in 1400 patients revealed a strong trend in favor of platinum-containing combinations with respect to response, but not survival. This analysis suggests that the combination confers to a 15% survival advantage out to the eighth year over the use of single-agent platinum (215b). Another recent meta-analysis of cyclophosphamide and cisplatin with or without doxorubicin in patients with stage III disease showed a 6% survival advantage at 2 years for the addition of doxorubicin (299a). The dose intensity of cisplatin appears to be particularly important.

Combinations in common use include:

CP: cyclophosphamide + cisplatin
CC: cyclophosphamide + carboplatin
H-CAP: hexamethylmelamine + cyclophosphamide + doxorubicin + cisplatin (260,295a)

Survival in germ cell tumors, stromal tumors: Survival in patients with germ cell tumors is excellent. For dysgerminomas, surgery with appropriate adjuvant chemotherapy or radiotherapy produces cure rates of about 90% for all stages (215). Survival with stage I disease should approach 100% (337). Fertility can often be preserved with conservative surgery and chemotherapy. Even for nondysgerminomatous germ cell tumors there is reasonable survival with surgery and adjuvant chemotherapy regimens using vinblastine, etoposide, cisplatin and bleomycin; overall long-term cure rates can be as high as 86%, and in stage I patients, 95% (345). Most stromal tumors present as early-stage cancer, and when

Table 22-32.   **Long-Term Survival in Stage III Ovarian Carcinoma by Size of Gross Residual Tumor**

Author	Reference	Treatment	Residual Tumor (% Survival)		
			None	Minimal	Macro
Beilinson et al	(225)	Chemotherapy	100	53	30
Wharton et al	(344)	Chemotherapy		40	14
Dembo	(246)	Radiation	48	43	18
Martinez et al	(289)	Radiation	68	54	20
Lambert & Berry	(281)	Chemotherapy		35	16
Louis et al	(286)	Chemotherapy	66	16	7
Neijt et al	(295)	Chemotherapy	71	57	30
Fuks et al	(254)	Chemotherapy & Radiation	38	20	20

From Fuks (253), with permission.

treated with adequate surgical resection, they have an excellent prognosis as well.

CLINICAL INVESTIGATIONS (85)

1. IP versus IV chemotherapy as first-line treatment for patients with optimally debulked stage III ovarian carcinoma have been studied (GOG, SWOG).
2. Biologic response modifiers have been used to augment chemotherapy with the addition of alternate cytotoxic modalities such as lethal monoclonal antibody conjugates, immunologic adjuvants, lymphokines, and tumor necrosis factor.
3. Whole abdomen irradiation with and without multiagent chemotherapy needs to be assessed in a variety of settings and doses. Prophylaxis after negative second-look operations needs thorough testing.
4. New predictive assays for selecting either chemotherapy and/or irradiation are being explored in different body sites.
5. High dose chemotherapy with autologous bone marrow transplant and use of protective agents to reduce toxicity of Cisplatin are currently under study (290a).
6. Taxol, a unique antimitotic cytotoxic agent has demonstrated objective response rate between 21%–36% in three Phase II trials in recurrent and refratory ovarian cancer (251a).

VAGINAL CARCINOMA

EPIDEMIOLOGY

1. Vaginal cancer is one of the rarest gynecologic malignancies, constituting only 1% to 2% of malignant neoplasms of the female genital tract.
2. Metastatic involvement of the vagina, particularly by cervical or vulvar carcinoma, occurs much more frequently than primary vaginal cancer. Also, the FIGO staging system requires that tumors involving both the vagina and cervix or the vagina and vulva be classified as primary cervical or vulvar carcinoma, respectively.
3. Vaginal cancer is predominantly a disease of postmenopausal women; in a recent series, more than 60% of patients were over aged 60 years (363).
4. A prior history of invasive cervical carcinoma or cervical carcinoma in situ has been noted in about one third of patients with vaginal carcinoma (364).
5. Although vaginal intraepithelial neoplasia (VAIN) is a precursor of invasive carcinoma, the risk of progression in patients treated appropriately for VAIN is less than 5% (354,361).
6. The role of HPV in the genesis of vaginal cancer, as well as cancer of the cervix and vulva, is the focus of current research (362,365,367). In contrast to squamous cell carcinoma of the vagina, which affects predominantly postmenopausal women, clear cell vaginal carcinoma, which has been linked to maternal diethylstilbestral exposure, occurs in young women, with a peak incidence at age 19 years.

DETECTION AND DIAGNOSIS

1. Although many patients present with irregular vaginal bleeding or discharge, almost onehalf of patients in a recent series were asymptomatic or had the tumor discovered on routine examination (365).
2. Symptoms referable to the GI or genitourinary tract may be the presenting complaint in some patients and may reflect involvement by the vaginal cancer.
3. The majority of vaginal cancers are located in the upper onethird of the vagina on the posterior wall. This site can be hidden by the speculum blade, so careful inspection of all vaginal surfaces is mandatory during examination.
4. Routine cytologic testing of the vagina should be continued even for patients who have previously undergone hysterectomy, particularly if the hysterectomy was performed for intraepithelial or invasive carcinoma of the cervix.
5. Biopsy is the cornerstone of diagnosis and usually can be performed in the office without anesthesia.

CLASSIFICATION

Histopathology

1. Squamous cell carcinoma constitutes 85% of primary vaginal cancers, with adenocarcinoma, melanoma, and other histologic subtypes making up the remainder (Table 22-33).
2. The majority of nonsquamous vaginal cancers are adenocarcinomas. Endometrioid, mucinous, papillary, and clear cell variants have been reported. Vaginal adenocarcinomas occur in younger patients (mean age, 41 years) than do squamous cell carcinomas (366).
3. Sarcoma botryoides occurs primarily in children less than 5 years old, and is characterized grossly by a polypoid mass resembling a bunch of grapes and microscopically by crowded rhabdomyoblasts in a distinct subepithelial cambium layer (10).
4. Melanoma accounts for only 3% of vaginal malignancies; it is usually located in the distal third of the vagina. Microscopy demonstrates pleomorphic cells laden with melanin, although pigmentation may be absent in the amelanotic variety. Progression of pre-existing melanosis to malignant melanoma of the vagina has been reported (360).
5. Endodermal sinus tumor of the vagina is similar histologically to its ovarian counterpart, with typical Schiller-Duval bodies.

Staging

1. Staging studies for evaluation of a patient with vaginal carcinoma are:
   - examination under anesthesia, cystoscopy, proctoscopy
   - chest x-ray
   - CT scan of abdomen and pelvis
   - barium enema
   - endocervical and endometrial biopsy

A thorough search should be performed to exclude metastatic involvement of the vagina from another site.

2. The FIGO staging system is shown in Table 22-34. Because of the rarity of vaginal cancers, surgical staging has not been reported so that the risk of pelvic and periaortic node involvement according to stage is unknown.
3. TNM staging is shown in Table 22-34 and Fig. 22-7.

Table 22-33. Histologic Classification of Malignant Tumors of the Vagina

- Metastatic (e.g., cervical, endometrial, ovarian)
- Squamous cell carcinoma
- Adenocarcinoma - clear cell
- Endodermal sinus tumor
- Malignant melanoma
- Sarcoma botryoides
- Lymphoma
- Carcinoid
- Rhabdomyosarcoma

PRINCIPLES OF TREATMENT

Multidisciplinary treatment decisions are summarized in Table 22-35. They include surgery and radiation therapy.

1. Vaginal carcinoma spreads predominantly by direct extension and by lymphatic embolization.
2. The lymphatic drainage of the distal vagina differs from the proximal, so that inguinal lymph nodes are at risk with distal cancers, while pelvic lymph node metastases occur with proximal lesions.
3. The close proximity of the bladder and rectum complicate treatment, whether by radiotherapy or surgery.

Surgery

1. *Vaginal intraepithelial neoplasia*: Wide local excision or partial or complete vaginectomy is effective treatment for localized VAIN (17). Alternative modes of therapy, particularly well-suited to multifocal VAIN are 5-FU and carbon dioxide laser vaporization (359). Brachytherapy is also extremely effective and is applicable to patients not suited for surgical treatment.
2. *Stage I* cancers located in the upper vagina may be treated by radical hysterectomy and vaginectomy in suitable patients, such as those with clear cell carcinoma. However, the majority of patients with

Table 22-34. Comparison of FIGO and AJC Stagings of Carcinoma of the Vagina

FIGO	Site	AJC
Stage I	Confined to vaginal mucosa	T1
Stage II	Submucosal infiltration into parametrium, not extending to pelvic wall	T2
Stage III	Tumor extending to pelvic wall	T3
Stage IV	Tumor extension to bladder or rectum or metastasis outside true pelvis	T4

FIGO (83) = International Federation of Gynecology and Obstetrics;
AJC(1) = American Joint Committee on Cancer Staging.

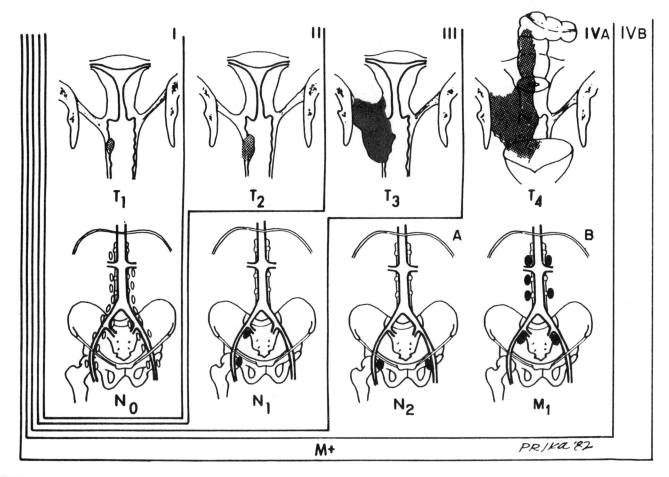

Fig. 22-7. Anatomic staging for vaginal carcinoma.

squamous cell carcinomas are elderly so that radiotherapy is the predominant treatment for vaginal carcinoma.

3. *Stage II-IV:* Virtually all advanced vaginal cancers are best treated with radiotherapy. Pelvic exenteration is reserved for central failures following radiation treatment.

Radiation Therapy

1. The majority of vaginal cancers are treated by radiation therapy. Distal vaginal cancers require that the inguinal nodes be incorporated in the treatment field. Early lesions can be managed with brachytherapy alone, while more advanced tumors are treated with external beam followed by a brachytherapy implant (363).

Table 22-35. Multidisciplinary Treatment by Stage for Vaginal Carcinoma (357,364a)

Stage	Surgery	External Radiation	Brachytherapy	Chemotherapy
0	Excision for localized disease	-	CRT 70 Gy surface dose	NR
1 (T_1, N_0) Superficial (> 0.5 cm thick)	Wide local resection/ total vaginectomy (upper 1/3)	-	CRT Interstitial irradiation, 60-70 Gy	NR
Larger lesions		CRT 40-50 Gy whole pelvis	Interstitial implant 30-40 Gy	NR
II (T_2, N_0)	NR	CRT 40-50 Gy whole pelvis	Same as above	NR
III (T_{1-3}, N_0)	NR	CRT 50 Gy whole pelvis optional (10-20 Gy through reduced fields)	Interstitial implant, 20-30 Gy (if tumor regression is optimal)	NR
IV (pelvis only)	NR	Same as above	Same as above	NR

RT = radiation therapy; CRT = curative; NR = not recommended.
PDQ: NR

Chemotherapy

1. Due to the rarity of vaginal cancer, no large series using chemotherapy have been reported. Regimens similar to those for cervical cancer generally are used.
2. The role of neoadjuvant chemotherapy is currently being investigated (358). Endodermal sinus tumors are extremely sensitive to chemotherapy and may be managed successfully in some instances without surgery (356).

RESULTS AND PROGNOSIS

1. The 5-year survival for vaginal carcinoma is worse on a stage-for-stage basis than for cervical carcinoma (Table 22-36 [306], Fig. 22-8).
2. Vaginal melanoma has an extremely poor prognosis; less than 25% of patients survive in most series. Preoperative radiotherapy may improve these results (355).

VULVAR CARCINOMA

PERSPECTIVE

The vulva is prone to a number of malignancies, which, by virtue of their location, should be amenable to early diagnosis and treatment. Unfortunately, the extensive lymphatics in this region contribute to nodal metastases even with early lesions (380), and in the past, both patient and physician procrastination have led to delays in diagnosis. Nevertheless, over the past 2 decades significant advances have been made in the management of vulvar malignancy. The predominant approach to therapy of vulvar carcinomas has been surgical, but more individualized surgical treatment and the incorporation of radiotherapy and chemotherapy in certain situations have reduced the morbidity associated with treatment of both early and advanced vulvar malignancies (385,400a).

EPIDEMIOLOGY AND ETIOLOGY

1. Carcinoma of the vulva is an infrequent malignancy, accounting for 5% of female genital malignancies and 0.3% of all cancers in the United States in women. Only one or two women per 100,000 per year in the United States will be afflicted, with approximately 2,500 new cases annually (404).
2. This is a disease of postmenopausal women, with a peak incidence in the sixth and seventh decades of life (aver-

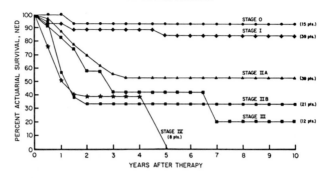

Fig. 22-8. Vaginal carcinoma results (by stage): actuarial disease free survival for irradiation. From Perez *et al.* (363), with permission.

age age, 63 years) (384,393). In contrast, the median age for vulvar carcinoma in situ is 47 years (375).
3. Although vulvar dystrophies are commonly found in association with vulvar carcinoma, they infrequently progress to invasive carcinoma if left untreated. In a recent series, 10% of patients with vulvar carcinoma in situ progressed to vulvar carcinoma. The risk of progression was higher for older patients (375).
4. A prior history of leukoplakia or inflammation of the vulva, as well as other urogenital malignancies has been associated with vulvar carcinoma. From 2% to 38% of patients previously had or will develop another primary malignancy in the lower genital tract, frequently the cervix (373,389).
5. Previously suspected associations with obesity and heart disease, which commonly afflict patients in this age group, have not been confirmed in recent case control studies. Prior reports have noted an association with a number of venereal infections, such as lymphogranuloma venereum, syphilis, herpes, and more recently, HPV. Currently, the only clinically important association is with HPV.
6. Condyloma acuminata is found in 5% to 10% of patients with vulvar carcinoma. The role of specific subtypes of HPV in the etiology of vulvar malignancies is as yet undetermined (399).

DETECTION AND DIAGNOSIS

1. The majority of patients seek medical attention due to itching or the discovery of a lump. Less frequent symptoms include bleeding, discharge, or dysuria (11).
2. Unfortunately nearly 60% of patients have had symptoms for 10 months before seeking attention (381).
3. Inspection and biopsy of any lesion on the vulva is the cornerstone of early diagnosis (Table 22-2).
4. Biopsy is easily performed under local anesthesia in the office with a Keyes dermatologic punch. Excisional biopsy of small lesions also is readily performed.
5. Although cytology of the vulva can be performed, it is infrequently used because of the ease of performing a definitive biopsy.
6. The application of toluidine blue stain was used frequently in the past to assess early vulvar lesions. Unfortunately, both false-positive and false-negative results have limited the use of this method for selection of a biopsy site.

Table 22-36. Five-Year Survival by Stage for Vaginal Carcinoma

Stage	No. Patients	(%) 5-yr Survival
I	163	53
II	168	43
III	141	28
IV	64	12

From Petterson (306), with permission.

7. Careful inspection of the vulva with a colposcope or even a magnifying glass following the application of 3% acetic acid has replaced the use of toluidine blue in assessing preclinically apparent lesions of the vulva.

8. A biopsy is warranted with virtually all ulcerated, discolored (red, white, pigmented), or exophytic lesions of the vulva. Although isolated condyloma acuminata may be treated without biopsy, persistence or confluence warrant biopsy to confirm the diagnosis. Similarly, multiple herpetiform ulcers do not need biopsy unless they persist.

CLASSIFICATION

Histopathology

1. The majority (86%) of vulvar carcinomas are squamous. The tumor is usually solitary and located on the labia majora or minora, although the clitoris is involved in approximately 10% of cases. Multifocal lesions occur in 10% of patients (Table 22-37) (392).

2. Most invasive squamous cell carcinomas of the vulva are well differentiated. An increased risk of nodal spread with poorly-differentiated carcinomas (recognizable by absence of keratin formation) has been noted by some investigators (380,396). Additional factors thought to be of prognostic significance are size of the lesion and lymph vascular space involvement (369).

3. Other less frequent vulvar malignancies include melanoma, leiomyosarcoma and other sarcomas, basal cell carcinoma, and both adenocarcinoma and squamous carcinoma of Bartholin's gland. Treatment is dependent on the histology identified.

Anatomic Staging

Table 22-38 and Fig. 22-9 show anatomic staging for vulvar cancer.

Tumor (T) categories: The size and extent of invasion determine the category. Whether the diameter of the tumor is greater than or less than 2 cm determines the T category for early stages: a tumor less than 2 cm is T1; larger than 2 cm is

T2. Extension into the urethra and vulva (T3) versus the upper urethra and bladder (T4) are determinants in advanced disease.

Node (N) categories: The presence of unilateral or bilateral metastases determines the N category.

Stage grouping: Each T category from T1 to T4 determines stage I and IV. N1 and N2 categories are equivalent to T3 and T4. M0 and M1 determine stage IVA versus IVB.

Lymph node involvement: The risk of lymph node spread has been correlated best to the lesions depth of invasion (Table 22-39). However, in superficial carcinomas the points selected for measurement of depth of invasion in previous reports have varied and are somewhat arbitrary (395). Tumor thickness, which can be measured more consistently, also has been reported (370,396) to correlate extremely well to the risk of nodal metastasis and is probably the preferred method of evaluating superficially invasive vulvar carcinomas. As expected, lymph node spread is associated with a poorer prognosis.

PRINCIPLES OF TREATMENT

Vulvar carcinoma spreads predominantly via the lymphatics. The pattern of drainage, from the vulva to the inguinal and femoral nodes, and thence to the pelvic lymph nodes, has been well studied (376,402). The prior belief that direct spread to the pelvic lymph nodes from carcinomas involving the clitoral region or Bartholin's gland has not been substantiated. Pelvic node involvement is rare in the absence of groin node spread (376). In addition, in well-lateralized lesions, the risk of spread to the contralateral groin is less than 1% in the absence of ipsilateral nodal involvement (3). Although most agree that surgery has played and will continue to play a major role in therapy of vulvar carcinoma, views differ on the type and extent of surgical treatment necessary to achieve a cure while minimizing the morbidity of therapy. In the past, the standard surgical approach involved a radical vulvectomy and bilateral inguinal-femoral lymphadenectomy in conjunction with an extraperitoneal pelvic lymphadenectomy. In those cancers involving the rectum or bladder, a pelvic exenteration was added to this extensive procedure. Better understanding of the spread pattern of vulvar carcinoma and the incorporation of radiotherapy has allowed a more individualized approach to management. It is hoped that the use of various chemotherapeutic agents as radiosensitizers will further improve current therapy of patients with advanced cancers. Table 22-40 summarizes standard approaches by stage of advancement.

Surgery

Stage 0 Vulvar Carcinoma in situ

1. In a recent study, the median age for women with vulvar intraepithelial neoplasia (VIN) was 40 years (375). As the potential for lymphatic spread with in situ disease is nil, a variety of locally ablative therapeutic methods can be used. Wide local excision is appropriate for the majority of lesions. Because VIN is multifocal in over one half of patients, even wide local excision can involve most of the vulva. Therefore, skinning vulvectomy with skin grafting has been used for widespread multifocal lesions (378). Of importance is the finding of occult early foci of invasion, usually less than 1 mm, in up to

Table 22-37. Histologic Classification of Vuvlar Neoplasms

Tumor Type	Percent	
Epidermoid	86.2	
Melanoma	4.8	
Sarcoma	2.2	
Basal cell	1.4	
Bartholin's gland		
Squamous	0.4	
Adenocarcinoma	0.6 }	
	} 1.2	
Adenocarcinoma	0.6 }	
Undifferentiated	3.9	

From Plentl and Griedman (392), with permission.

Table 22-38. TNM* and Staging Classifications of Carcinoma of the Vulva

TNM		Staging (FIGO)† 1988		
T Primary Tumor		Stage 0 Tis	Carcinoma in situ; intraepithelial carcinoma	
Tis	Preinvasive carcinoma (carcinoma in situ)	Stage I	T1 N0 M0	Tumor confined to the vulva and/or
T 1	Tumor confined to the vulva and/or *perineum*—2 cm or less in diameter			*perineum*—2 cm or less in greatest dimension. *No nodal metastases.*
T 2	Tumor confined to the vulva and/or *perineum*—more than 2 cm in diameter	Stage II	T2 N0 M0	Tumor confirmed to the vulva and/or *perineum*—more than 2 cm in greatest dimension. *No nodal metastases.*
T 3	Tumor of any size with adjacent spread to the urethra, vagina, anus or all of these	Stage III	T3 N0 M0	Tumor of any size with the following:
T 4	Tumor of any size infiltrating the bladder mucosa or the rectal mucosa or both, including the upper part of the urethral mucosa or fixed to the anus		T3 N1 M0	(1) Adjacent spread to the lower urethra, the vagina, the anus, and/or the following:
			T1 N1 M0	(2) *Unilateral regional lymph node metastases*
N Regional Lymph Nodes				
N 0	No nodes palpable	Stage IVA	T1 N2 M0	Tumor invades any of the following:
N 1	*Unilateral regional lymph node metastases*		T2 N2 M0	Upper urethra, bladder mucosa, rectal
N 2	*Bilateral regional lymph node metastases*		T3 N2 M0	mucosa, pelvic bone, and/or *bilateral regional node metastases*
			T4 any N M0	
M Distant Metastases		Stage IVB any T, any N, M1		*Any distant metastases, including pelvic lymph nodes*
M 0	No clinical metastases			
M 1	Distant metastases (*including pelvic lymph node metastases*)			

Creasman WT: Obstet Gynecol 75:287, 1990.
Italicized words indicate changes from the pre-1988 definitions.
*TNM = Tumor–Nodes–Metastases.
†FIGO = International Federation of Gynecology and Obstetrics.
From Herbst (384a), with permission.

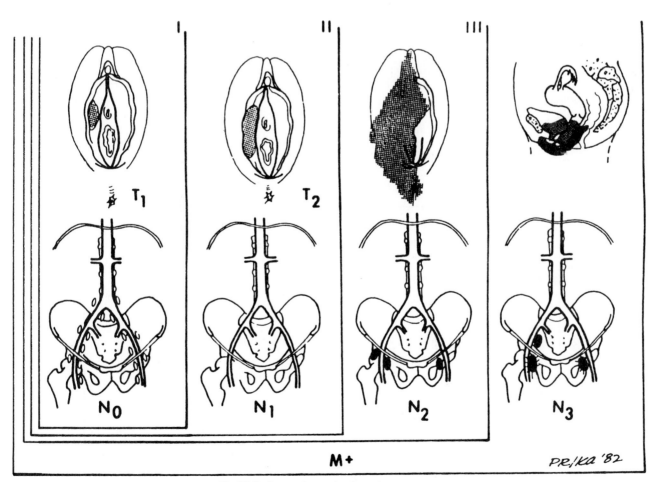

Fig. 22-9. Anatomic staging for vulvar cancer.

Table 22-39. Incidence of Lymph Node Metastases in Vulvar Cancer

Stage	% Lymph Nodes	Thickness (mm)	Number (%)
1	11	<1	1/36 (3)
2	26	2	5/64 (8)
3	64	3	11/67 (16)
4	89	4	24/77 (31)
		5	21/64 (33)

Depth	Number	Positive Nodes (%)
<1	148	0 (0)
1.1-2	147	10 (7)
2.1-3	117	10 (9)
3.1-4	65	17 (26)
4.1-5	48	12 (25)
>5	32	12 (38)

Adapted from Sedlis et al. (396), Hacker et al. (384), Dvoretsky et al. (379), Ross and Ehrmann (395), Berek and Hacker (3).

20% of patients being treated for VIN. Chafe *et al.* (372) reported on 69 patients with biopsy-proven vulvar carcinoma in situ treated by surgical excision. Unsuspected invasion was found in 13 patients (19%), and four patients (6%) had invasion greater than 1 mm in depth. Irregular raised lesions were more likely to harbor occult foci of invasion. As the carbon dioxide laser has also been used with success (401) in the local ablation of VIN by vaporization, great care and multiple representative biopsies, particularly of irregular raised lesions, are mandatory prior to laser treatment, to detect occult foci of early invasion. The optimal therapy, given these data, may be combined laser vaporization and excision. Topical therapy with 5-FU has been reported but should not be used due to the low cure rate (60%) and significant morbidity associated with this type of treatment (397).

2. Paget's disease of the vulva is also an intraepithelial carcinoma that can be treated with wide local excision. In contrast to Paget's disease of the breast, only 20% of patients have an associated underlying adenocarcinoma. It is important to be aware of the increased risk of other synchronous malignancies that occur in association with Paget's disease of the vulva, so that appropriate screening is performed (400). Recurrences are common after local excision and are usually managed by re-excision.

Stage I Vulvar Carcinoma

1. This group encompasses all patients with lesions less than 2 cm in diameter confined to the vulva without lymph node metastasis. The depth of invasion or tumor thickness is not part of the staging system but is critical in determining the risk of lymph node metastasis (Table 22-39). Although some investigators have advocated omitting lymph node dissection in patients with invasion less than 1 mm (3), metastases, although rare, have been reported in this situation, so we currently omit groin dissection only in patients with tumors less than 0.75 mm thick without multifocal invasion. The recent

Table 22-40. Multidisciplinary Treatment Decisions by Stage for Vulvar Carcinoma (6,57,390a)

Stage	Surgery	Radiation Therapy	Chemotherapy
0 (T_{is})	Wide local excision	NR	NR
I (T_1, N_0) <2 cm size, <5 mm invasion	Modified hemivulvectomy, BIL	NR	NR
II ($T_2, N_{0/1}$)	RV, BIL	ART pelvic/inguinal if node (+)	NR
III ($T_3, N_{0/1}$) ($T_{1/2}, N_1$)	RV, BIL	ART pelvic/inguinal if node (+)	CCR
IV ($T_4 N_{any}$) (T_{1-3}, N_3)	CCR, RVBIL	CCR	IC II

RT = radiation therapy; ART = adjuvant; NR = not recommended; CCR = concurrent chemotherapy and radiation; RV = radical vulvectomy; BIL = bilateral inguinal lymphadenectomy; IC II = investigational chemotherapy, phases I/II clinical trials.
PDQ: NR - CCR - RT + 5-FU + Mito-C.

modification of the FIGO staging system, which uses surgical rather than clinical assessment of lymph node status, mandates surgical assessment of regional lymph nodes in all suitable patients at risk for lymph node metastases.

2. A modified radical vulvectomy, which leaves normal structures intact but removes the tumor with a wide margin, has been reported by several recent investigators (370,377) to be a safe and less disfiguring method of treating the primary lesion.

3. Lymph node metastasis can be expected in 11% of tumors this size, so that 11% of patients considered stage I by the prior FIGO staging will now be upstaged to stage III or IV.

4. In lesions on the lateral aspect of the vulva, it is rare for nodal metastases to occur to the contralateral groin unless the ipsilateral nodes are involved. The safety of omitting a contralateral groin dissection when the ipsilateral nodes are free of tumor is currently being studied by the GOG. This approach has been suggested because of the low risk of contralateral nodal spread in the absence of ipsilateral nodal involvement. The outcome is frequently disastrous for the rare patient who develops a contralateral groin node metastasis (3), so that this approach should not be used unless part of a protocol treatment.

5. The use of separate groin incisions has dramatically reduced the morbidity associated with en bloc radical vulvectomy and groin dissection. Initial concern regarding the risk of recurrence in the skin bridge left between the vulva and groin has not been born out by investigators (384) who have used this approach.

6. A superficial groin lymphadenectomy (lymph nodes above the cribriform fascia overlying the femoral vessels) has been used by Disaia *et al.* (377), who recognized the rarity of deep femoral lymph node metastasis in the absence of superficial femoral lymph node involvement. Unfortunately, frozen section assessment of all of the superficial groin nodes can be difficult and cases of deep femoral node metastasis in the absence of superficial node involvement have been reported. This approach is perhaps most applicable to patients with tumors less than 3 mm in thickness, whose risk of positive nodes is less than 16% (379). Fortunately, the use of separate groin incisions has reduced the morbidity of lymph node dissection so that the recommended approach to stage I vulvar carcinoma is currently a modified radical vulvectomy with bilateral groin dissection through separate incisions. Wide local excision with ipsilateral groin dissection is acceptable treatment for those patients with well lateralized superficial tumors less than 3 mm thick.

Stage II

1. This stage incorporates those cases with a lesion greater than 2 cm in diameter confined to the vulva, without lymph node metastasis.

2. A modified radical vulvectomy (radical local excision) with bilateral groin dissection through separate incisions is the preferred approach to management of these patients. A standard radical vulvectomy may be necessary in some patients because of the size or location of the tumor.

3. Lymph node metastasis can be expected in 25% of patients with tumors this size, so that 25% of patients considered stage II by the prior FIGO staging system will now be upstaged to stage III or IV.

4. The safety of omitting groin dissection and substituting elective groin radiation is currently under study by the GOG in patients without clinically suspicious groin nodes. Given the low morbidity associated with groin dissection through separate incisions, this approach, if shown to be efficacious, may be best applied to those patients with multiple medical problems. However, radical vulvar surgery is generally very well tolerated, even in the medically infirm.

Stage III

1. Patients with lesions extending to the lower vagina, urethra, or anus or those with unilateral groin lymph node metastasis are included in this stage.

2. A modified or full radical vulvectomy with bilateral groin dissection (en bloc in those with suspicious nodes) is the preferred surgical approach. The distal urethra can be sacrificed if necessary without loss of continence.

3. In the past, some patients with stage III vulvar cancer required pelvic exenteration combined with radical vulvectomy and groin dissection to adequately excise the lesion. Although up to 50% of patients were cured with this approach (371), more recently several investigators have used preoperative radiation therapy combined with less extensive excision with equally good results (368,383).

Stage IV

1. Stage IVA includes patients with tumor involvement of the upper urethra, bladder or rectal mucosa, or pelvic bone, or with bilateral lymph node metastasis. Stage IVB includes those with distant or pelvic lymph node metastasis.

2. A radical vulvectomy and groin dissection is appropriate therapy for those patients whose tumor can be adequately encompassed by this type of resection. Otherwise, preoperative radiotherapy combined with radical local excision is preferred over pelvic exenteration in conjunction with radical vulvectomy because the cure rate seems comparable and patients are spared the morbidity of a permanent stoma. Suspicious groin nodes should be excised prior to radiotherapy because of the poor results obtained in this situation with radiotherapy alone (391).

3. Even when patients present with distant metastases, which is infrequent, treatment of the primary lesion by either surgical excision or radiotherapy should be considered for palliation.

Radiation Therapy

1. Radiotherapy has begun to play an increasing role in the management of vulvar malignancy. During the orthovoltage era, the limited tolerance of the vulva to curative doses of radiation precluded its widespread use, especially since the results with surgery were reasonably good. The advent of megavoltage equipment, which spares the skin from the full radiation dose, has allowed a greater role for managing vulvar malignancies with irradiation. Currently, radiotherapy is used postopera-

tively for patients with close margins or positive nodes, pre-operatively for patients with advanced cancers that would otherwise require pelvic exenteration, and for treatment of recurrences not amenable to curative resection. In addition, patients not suitable for any type of surgical resection can be treated definitively with irradiation (382).

2. In the past, patients with positive groin nodes were candidates for pelvic lymphadenectomy. Several recent series have confirmed the finding that pelvic lymph node metastases are rare unless three or more groin nodes are involved by tumor (376,386). In the GOG study comparing pelvic lymphadenectomy with pelvic irradiation for patients with one or more positive groin nodes, a survival advantage for radiation treatment was noted for patients with two or more positive groin nodes. Therefore pelvic radiotherapy is preferred to pelvic lymphadenectomy for patients with positive groin nodes (386). If there are no metastases in the contralateral groin, then radiotherapy administered to the involved hemipelvis can be considered.

3. Boronow (368) and others have investigated the role of preoperative radiotherapy in patients with advanced vulvar cancers that would ordinarily only be resectable by pelvic exenteration. Boronow used primarily brachytherapy and 65% (17 of 26) of patients were rendered disease-free without an exenterative procedure, but six patients (23%) developed fistula to either the GI or genitourinary tract. By delivering 4,400 to 5,400 cGy to the tumor via external beam before local resection Hacker *et al.* (383) were able to achieve tumor control without any fistulas in 62% of patients for periods ranging from 15 months to 10 years. More recently, radiation therapy in conjunction with chemotherapy has been used based on the encouraging results achieved with this type of multimodal therapy in anal carcinomas (398). It is hoped that this type of therapy will allow a reduction in radiation dose (3,000 cGy) with equal tumor regression, thereby minimizing the morbidity of radiation treatment.

4. Recurrences limited to the perineum or groin can be managed with radiotherapy. Prempree and Amornmarn (394) reported on 21 patients with recurrent vulvar carcinoma managed by irradiation alone. The cure rate was best (100%) for six patients with disease limited to the vagina and introitus, although even 50% (two of four) of those with limited groin recurrences were salvaged. The results of treating extensive recurrences with irradiation alone were not good, so that combined treatment with chemotherapy, irradiation, and surgery needs to be explored for these patients.

Chemotherapy

1. Although agents active against other squamous cell carcinomas (i.e., cisplatin, bleomycin, and methotrexate) have been used for patients with metastatic vulvar carcinoma, unfortunately responses are few and of short duration (7).

2. At present, chemotherapy plays a greater role as a radiation sensitizer in managing advanced vulvar carcinoma. Whether or not this approach will improve cure rates is currently unknown.

RESULTS AND PROGNOSIS

For vulvar carcinoma in situ and early cancers, the results with limited resection as outlined herein have been good. VIN is 100% curable.

For invasive cancers, the prognosis is best determined by the lesion size and whether there has been metastatic involvement of lymph nodes. Survival according to stage and lymph node status prior to the recent change in FIGO staging is given in Table 22-41. As yet, no survival results have been published with the revised FIGO staging system, although improved survival in stage I and II patients is expected based on the exclusion of those cases with positive nodes.

Inguinal nodes: The value of elective irradiation of the pelvic lymph nodes was demonstrated by Homesley and associates (386,386a), who reported on a randomized study involving 114 patients with invasive squamous cell carcinoma of the vulva and positive inguinal lymph nodes treated with radical vulvectomy and a bilateral groin lymphadenectomy. The patients were randomized to receive pelvic irradiation (4500 cGy to 5000 cGy in 5 to 6 weeks) in addition to the inguinal regions or observation only. No irradiation was given to the central vulvar area. Of 59 patients randomized to irradiation, the 53 who were treated had a 68% 2-year survival rate. In contrast, the nonirradiated group had a 54% survival rate. The benefit of radiation therapy was noted only in patients with two or more positive nodes.

Table 22-41. Survival Versus FIGO Stage in Vulvar Carcinoma

STAGE	SURGERY and RADIATION THERAPY
1	90
2	77
3	51
4	18
OVERALL	70

FIGO = International Federation of Gynecology and Obstetrics.

Less Frequent Vulvar Malignancies

1. Vulvar melanoma is the second most common neoplasm of the vulva, but accounts for only 3% to 7% of all melanomas in women (10). The prognosis correlates well to either the Clark or Breslow classifications, which both in effect quantify tumor thickness. In contrast to squamous carcinoma, the most common sites affected are the labia minora and clitoris. In the past, radical vulvectomy and groin dissection with pelvic lymphadenectomy were recommended. Recognizing the probable prognostic nature of lymphadenectomy, many authors currently recommend wide local excision for lesions less than 0.75 mm from the skin surface, and wide local excision with groin dissection for deeper lesions. The outlook for patients with lymphatic metastasis is poor, with no survivors in one recent series (387).

2. Verrucous carcinoma of the vulva is a variant of squamous cell carcinoma that can be treated with wide local excision because of its indolent nature and infrequent lymphatic metastases (3). Radiation therapy is contraindicated because this type of tumor displays more aggressive behavior following irradiation.

3. Carcinoma of Bartholin's gland is frequently misdiagnosed as a Bartholin's cyst or abscess. The physician should be cautious when an older woman has a Bartholin's cyst, and biopsy or excision should be performed. Management is similar to that for squamous cell carcinoma of the vulva (388,403).

4. Adenoid cystic carcinoma of Bartholin's gland comprises only 10% of all Bartholin's gland carcinomas and is managed in a similar fashion (374).

5. Basal cell carcinomas can occur on the vulva, usually involving the labia majora, and are treated by wide local excision.

6. Leiomyosarcoma is the most frequently encountered sarcoma involving the vulva, and wide local excision is the initial treatment of choice (10).

Recommended Reading

In addition to classic textbooks by Disaia and Creasman (6) and Morrow and Townsend (11), several recent multiauthored textbooks provide a comprehensive view of gynecologic oncology for the student. The recent texts by both Hoskins (7a), Knapp (8a), and Berek (3) provide a timely and thorough review of the field. Other recommended multiauthored texts include those edited by Gusberg (7) and by van Nagell (12a). Several textbooks are available dealing with the pathologic (10) and radiotherapeutic (11a) aspects of this field, and are highly recommended.

REFERENCES

General References

1. American Joint Committee on Cancer Staging and End-results Reporting. Manual for Staging of Cancer (3rd ed). Philadelphia, PA: J.B. Lippincott Co.; 1988.
2. Balfe DM, Heiken JP, McClennan BL. Oncologic imaging for carcinoma of the cervix, ovary and endometrium. In: Bragg DG, Rubin P, Youker JE (eds). Oncologic Imaging. Elmsford, NY: Pergamon Press, Inc.; 1985, pp 439-476.
3. Berek JS, Hacker NF (eds). Practical Gynecologic Oncology. Baltimore, MD: Williams & Wilkins; 1989.
4. Campodonico I., Escudero P, Suarez E. Carcinoma of the cervix uteri. In: Pettersson F, Kolstad P, Ludwig H., Ulfelder H. (eds). Annual report of the results of treatment in gynecologic cancer. Stockholm: Tryckeri Balder, AB; 1985.
5. Cousins N. Medical ethics: Is there a broader view? J Am Med Assoc 241:2711-2712; 1979.
6. DiSaia PJ, Creasman WT. Clinical gynecologic oncology. London, UK: C.V. Mosby, Co.; 1981.
7. Gusberg SB, Shingleton HM, Deppe G: Female genital cancer. New York NY: Churchill-Livingstone; 1988.
7a. Hoskins WJ, Perez CA, Young RC (eds). Principles and Practice of Gynecologic Oncology. Philadelphia, PA: J.B. Lippincott Co.; 1992.
8. International Histologic Classification of Tumors, nos. 1-20. Geneva, Switzerland: World Health Organization; 1978.
8a. Knapp RC, Berkowitz RS (eds). Gynecologic Oncology. 2nd ed. New York, NY: McGraw-Hill, Inc. Health Professions Div.; 1992.
9. Kolstad P, Stafl A. Atlas of Colposcopy. Baltimore, MD: University Park Press; 1972.
10. Kurman RJ (ed). Blaustein's Pathology of the Female Genital Tract, Third Edition. New York, NY: Springer-Verlag; 1987.
11. Morrow CP, Townsend DE (ed). Synopsis of Gynecologic Oncology. New York, NY: Churchill Livingstone; 1987; p 62.
11a. Perez CA, Brady LW (eds). Principles and Practice of Radiation Oncology. 2nd ed. Philadelphia, PA: J.B. Lippincott Co.; 1992.
12. Pettersson F (ed). Annual report on the results of treatment in gynecologic cancer, Radiumhemmet, Stockholm, Sweden; 1988.
12a. VanNagell, Jr., J.R. (ed). Modern Concepts of Gynecologic Oncology. Boston, MA: Wright PSG; 1982.

Specific References

Carcinoma of the Cervix

13. Ali, M.; Kalra, J.; Seltzer, V.; Molho, L.; Cortes, E. Simultaneous chemo-radiotherapy for advanced squamous cell carcinoma of the female genital tract - 4-year follow-up. Proceedings of the American Society of Clinical Oncology 9:167; 1990.
14. American College of Obstetricians and Gynecologists. ACOG Techincal Bulletin, No. 81; 1984.
15. Annual report on the results of treatment in gynecological cancer. In: Pettersson, F.; ed. Twentieth volume statements of results obtained in patients treated in 1979-1981, inclusive 5-year survival up to 1986.Stockholm, Sweden: International Federation of Gynecology and Obstetrics; 1987, 20:52.
16. Artman LE, et al. Radical hysterectomy and pelvic lymphadenectomy for Stage IB carcinoma of the cervix: 21 years experience. Gynecologic Oncology 28:8-13; 1987.
17. Baker, L., Boutselis, J., Alberts, D., Surwit, E.A. and Hilgers, R. Combination chemotherapy for patients with disseminated carcinoma of the uterine cervix. Proc. ASCO 4:120; 1985.
18. Berek, J.S., Castaldo, T.W., Hacker, N.F., Petrilli, E.S., Lagasse, L.D., and Moore, J.G. Adenocarcinoma of the uterine cervix. Cancer 48:2734-2741; 1981.
19. Berman, M., Keys, N., Creasman, W. and DiSaia, P. Survival and patterns of recurrence in cervical cancer metastatic to paraaortic lymph nodes. Gynecologic Oncology 19:8; 1984.
19a. Bourhis J, Le MG, Barrois M, et al. Prognostic value of c-myc proto-oncogene overexpression in early invasive carcinoma of the cervix. J Clin Oncol 8(11):1789-1796; 1990.
20. Bragg DG, Rubin P, Youker JE. Oncologic Imaging. New York, NY. Pergamon Press; 1985.
21. Broker, T.R. Structure and genetic expression of papillomaviruses. Obstetrics and Gynecology Clinics of North America 14(2):329-348; 1987.
22. Buchsbaum, J.H. and Lifshitz, S. The role of scalene lymph node biopsy in advanced carcinoma of the cervix uteri. Surgery. Gynecology and Obstetrics 143:246; 1976.
23. Cavanagh D, Praphat H, Ruffolo EH. Carcinoma of the uterine cervix: some current views. Obstet Gynecol Ann 10:193-236; 1981.
23a. Chen M-S, Lin F-J, Hong C-H, et al. High-dose-rate afterloading technique in the radiation treatment of uterine cervical cancer: 399 cases and 9 years experience in Taiwan. Int J Radiat Oncol Biol Phys 20:915-920; 1991.
24. Choo, Y.C., Choy, T.K., Wong, L.C. and Ma, M.K. Potentiation

of radiotherapy by cis-dichlorodiammine platinum (II) in advanced cervical carcinoma. Gynecoloqic Oncology. 24:143; 1986.

25. Creasman WT, Soper JT, Clarke-Pearson D: Radical hysterectomy as therapy for early carcinoma of the cervix. Am J Obstet Gynecol, 155:964-969; 1986.

26. Currie WC: Operative treatment of carcinoma of the cervix. J Obstet Gynecol Brit Commonwealth, 78:385-405; 1971.

26a. Delgado G, Bundy B, Zaino R, et al. Prospective surgical-pathological study of disease-free interval in patients with stage IB squamous cell carcinoma of the cervix: A Gynecologic Oncology Group study. Gyn Oncol 38(3):352-357; 1990.

26b. Fagundes H, Perez CA, Grigsby PW, Lockett MA. Distant metastasis after irradiation alone in carcinoma of the uterine cervix. Int J Radiat Oncol Biol Phys 24(2):197-204; 1992.

27. Ferenczy A, Winkler B. Carcinoma and metastatic tumors of the cervix. In: Kurman RJ (ed): Blaustein's Pathology of the Female Genital Tract, Third edition. New York, NY: Springer-Verlag; 1987.

28. Ferenczy A, Winkler B. Cervical intraepithelial neoplasia. In: Kurman RJ (ed): Blaustein's Pathology of the Female Genital Tract, Third edition. New York, NY:Springer-Verlag; 1987.

29. Fetherston, W.C. False-negative cytology in invasive cancer of the cervix. Clinical Obstetrics and Gynecol. 26 (4): 929-937; 1983.

30. Fletcher GH: Cancer of the uterine cervix. Janeway Lactive. Am J Roentgerol Radium Ther Nucl Med 111:225; 1971.

31. Fu, K.K.; Phillips, T.L. High-dose-rate versus low-dose-rate intracavitary brachytherapy for carcinoma of the cervix. Int. J. Radiat. Oncol. Biol. Phys. 19:791-796; 1990.

32. Gallion, H.H., van Nagell, J.R., Jr., Donaldson, E.S., Hanson, M.B., Powell, D.E., Maruyama, Y., and Yoneda, J. Combined radiation therapy and extrafascial hysterectomy in the treatment of Stage IB barrel-shaped cervical cancer. Cancer 56:262-265; 1985.

32a. Grigsby PW, Perez CA. Radiotherapy alone for medically inoperable carcinoma of the cervix: Stage IA and carcinoma in situ. Int J Radiat Oncol Biol Phys 21(2):375-378; 1991.

33. Hacker, N.F., Berek, J.S., Lagasse, L.D., Charles, E.H., Savage, E.W., and Moore, J.G. Carcinoma of the cervix associated with pregnancy. Obstetrics and Gynecology. 59:735; 1982.

34. Haie, C.; Pejovic, M.H.; Gerbaulet, A.; Horiot, J.D.; Pourquier, H.; Delouche, J.; Heinz, J.F.; Brune, D.; Fenton, J.; Pizzi, G.; Bey, P.; Brossel, R.; Pillement, P.; Volterrani, F.; Chassagne, D. Is prophylactic para-aortic irradiation worthwhile in the treatment of advanced cervical carcinoma? Results of a controlled clinical trial of the EORTC radiotherapy group. Radiat. Oncol. 11:101-112; 1988.

35. Halpert, R., Fruchter, R.G., Sedlis, A., Butt, K., Boyce, J.G. and Sillman, F.H. Human papillomavirus and lower genital neoplasia in renal transplant patients. Obstetrics and Gynecology 68:251; 1986.

36. Hatch, K.D. Cervical cancer. In: Berek, J.S. and Hacker, N.F. Practical Gynecologic Oncology. Baltimore: Williams and Wilkins; 1989.

37. Heller, P.B., Barnhill, D.R., Mayer, A.R., Fontaine, T.P., Hoskins, W.J. and Park, R.C. Cervical carcinoma found incidentally in the uterus removed for benign indications. Obstetrics and Gynecology 67:187- 190; 1986.

38. Herbst, A.L., Cole, P., Colton, T., Robboy, S.J., and Scully, R.E. Age-incidence and risk of diethylstilbestrol-related clear cell adenocarcinomas of the vagina and cervix. Am. J. Obstetrics Gynecology 12(1):43-50; 1977.

39. Herbst, A.L., Ulfelder, H., and Poskanzer, D.C. Adenocarcinoma of the vagina; association of maternal stilbestrol therapy with tumor appearance in young women. New Enqland Journal of Medicine 284:878; 1971.

40. Hoskins, W.J.; Perez, C.; Young, R.D. Gynecologic tumors. In: DeVita, Jr., V.T.; Hellman, S.; Rosenberg, S.A. (eds). Cancer: Principles and Practice of Oncology, 3rd ed. Philadelphia, PA: J.B. Lippincott Co.; 1989, p 1115.

41. Hreshchyshyn, M.M., Aron, B.S., Boronow, R.C. et al. Hydroxyurea or placebo combined with radiation to treat stage IIIb and IV cervical cancer confined to the pelvis. International Journal of Radiation Oncology Biol Phys 5:317; 1979.

41a. Hricak H. Cancer of the uterus: The value of MRI pre-and post-irradiation. Int J Radiat Oncol Biol Phys 21:1089-1094; 1991.

42. Hughes, R.R., Brewington, K.C., Hanjani, P., et al. Extended field

irradiation for cervical cancer based on surgical staging. Gynecoloqic Oncology 9: 153-161; 1980.

42a. ICRU Report #38. Dose and Volume Specification for Reporting Intracavitary Therapy in Gynecology. Bethesda, MD: International Congress of Radiological Units and Measurements; 1985.

43. Jacobs, A.J., Perez, C.A., Camel, H.M., and Kao, M-S. Complications in patients receiving both irradiation and radical hysterectomy for carcinoma of the uterine cervix. Gynecoloqic Oncology 22: 273; 1985.

44. Joslin, C.A.F. Brachytherapy: a clinical dilemma. Int. J. Radiat. Oncol. Biol. Phys. 19: 801-802; 1990.

45. Kim, D.S., Moon, H., Hwang, Y.Y., Cho, S.H. Preoperative adjuvant chemotherapy in the treatment of cervical cancer stage Ib, IIa, and IIB with bulky tumor. Gynecoloqic Oncol. 29: 321-332; 1988.

46. Kolstad, P. and Klem, V. Long term followup of 1121 cases of carcinoma-in-situ. Obstetrics and Gynecology 48:125; 1976.

46a. Kristen GB, Holund B, Grinsted P. Efficacy of the cytobrush versus cotton swab in true collection of endocervical cells. Acta Cytol 33:849-851; 1989.

46b. Lanciano RM, Martz K, Coia LR, Hanks GE. Tumor and treatment factors improving outcome in stage IIIB cervix cancer. Int J Radiat Oncol Biol Phys 20:95-100; 1991.

47. LaPolla, J.P., Schlaerth, J.B., Gaddis, O, Jr., and Morrow, C.P. The influence of surgical staging on the evaluation and treatment of patients with cervical carcinoma. Gynecologic Oncology 24: 194; 1986.

48. Lee, R.B., Neglia, W., Park, R.C. Cervical carcinoma in pregnancy. Obstetrics and Gynecol. 58(5): 584-589; 1981.

49. Lifshitz, S., Railsback, L.D. and Buchsbaum, H.J. Intraarterial pelvic infusion chemotherapy in advanced gynecologic cancer. Obstetrics and Gynecology. 52: 476; 1978.

50. Lohe, K.J., Burghardt, E., Hillemanns, H.G., Kaufmann, C., Ober, K.G., and Zander, J. Early squamous cell carcinoma of the uterine cervix. Gynecoloqic Oncology 6:31-50; 1978.

51. Long, H.J.; Cross, W.G.; Wieand, H.S. MVAC: a highly active combination chemotherapy regimen in advanced/recurrent cancer of the uterine cervix and vagina. Proceedings of the American Society of Clinical Oncology 9:158; 1990.Abstracts.

51a. Marcial LV, Marcial VA, Krall JM, Lanciano RM, et al. Comparison of 1 vs 2 or more intracavitary brachytherapy applications in the management of carcinoma of the cervix with irradiation alone. Int J Radiat Oncol Biol Phys 20:81-86; 1991.

52. Marcial, V.A. The cervix. In: Moss, W.T.; Cox, J.D., eds. Radiation oncology rationale, technique, results. St. Louis, MO: C.V. Mosby Co.: 1989:516.

52a. Mendenhall WM, McCarty PJ, Morgan LS, et al. Stage IB or IIA-B carcinoma of the intact uterine cervix > 6 cm in diameter: Is adjuvant extrafascial hysterectomy beneficial? Int J Radiat Oncol Biol Phys 21:899-904; 1991.

53. Montan GS, Fowler WC, Jr, Baria MA, Alton LA, Mack Y. Analysis of results of radiation therapy for stage IB carcinoma of the cervix. Cancer, 60:0059-0064; 1987.

54. Morrow, C.P.; DiSaia, P.J.; Mangan, C.F. and Lagasse, L.D. Continuous pelvic arterial infusion with bleomycin for squamous carcinoma of the cervix recurring after irradiation therapy. Cancer Treatment Reports 61: 1403; 1977.

55. Morrow, P., Shingleton, H.M., Averette, H.E., Webb, M.J., Masterson, J.G., Morely, G.W., and Webb, M.J. Panel report. Is pelvic irradiation beneficial in the postoperative management of stage Ib squamous cell carcinoma of the cervix with pelvic node metastases treated by radical hysterectomy and pelvic lymphadenectomy? GYnecoloqic Oncology 10: 105; 1980.

55a. O'Hanlon KA, Goldberg GL, Jones JG, et al. Adjuvant therapy for neuroendocrine small cell carcinoma of the cervix: Review of the literature. Gynecol Oncol 2:167-172; 1991.

56. Orr JW, Jr, Ball G C, Soong S J, et al. Surgical treatment of women found to have invasive cervix cancer at the time of total hysterectomy. Obstetrics and Gynecology 68:353-356; 1986.

57. Perez CA, Camel HM, Kuske, R.R., Kao, M-S.: Radiation therapy alone in the treatment of carcinoma of the uterine cervix: A 20-year experience. Gynecol Oncol, 23:127-140; 1986.

57a. Perez CA, Fox S, Lockett MA, et al. Impact of dose in outcome of irradiation alone in carcinoma of the uterine cervix: Analysis of two different methods. Int J Radiat Oncol Biol Phys 21:885-898; 1991.

58. Peters, R.K., Thomas, D., Hagan, D.G., Mack, T.M. and

Henderson, B.E. Risk factors for invasive cervical cancer among Latinas and nonLatinas in Los Angeles County. Journal of the National Cancer Institute Nov 77(5): 1063-77; 1986.

59. Petterson F. ed. Annual Report on the Results of Treatment in Gynecologic Cancer Vol 19, Stockholm, Sweden: International Federation of Gynecology and Obstetrics; 1985.

59. Physician's Data Query. Cervical cancer. National Cancer Institute: Bethesda, MD; January 1992.

59a. Piver MS. Invasive cervical cancer in the 1990s. Sem Surg Oncol 6(6):359-363; 1990.

60. Piver, M.S., Barlow, J.J., Vongtama, V., Blumenson, L. Hydroxyurea: A radiation potentiator in carcinoma of the uterine cervix. American Journal of Obstetrics and Gynecology 147: 803-808; 1983.

61. Piver MS, et al. Radical hysterectomy and pelvic lymphadenectomy versus radiation therapy for small(< 3 cm) stage IB cervical carcinoma. Am J Clin Oncol 11(1):21-24; 1988.

62. Potish, R.A., Twiggs, L.B., Okagaki, T., Prem, K.A. and Adcock, L.L. Therapeutic implications of the natural history of advanced cervical cancer as defined by pretreatment surgical staging. Cancer 56:956; 1985.

63. Reid, R. Preinvasive disease. In Practical Gynecologic Oncology. Berek, J.S. and Hacker, N.F. (eds). Williams and Wilkins: Baltimore; 1989.

64. Rotman, M.; Choi, K.; Guze, C.; Marcial, V.; Hornback, N.;John, M. Prophylactic irradiation of the para-aortic lymph node chain in Stage IIB and bulky Stage IB carcinoma of the cervix. Initial treatment results of RTOG 7920.Int. J. Radiat. Oncol. Biol. Phys. 19:513-522; 1990.

65. Sardi, J.E., diPaola, G.R., Giaroli, A., Sananes, C., Rueda, N.G., Cachau, A., Vighi, S. and Burlando, S. Results of phase II trial with neoadjuvant chemotherapy in carcinoma of the cervix uteri. Gynecologic Oncology 31:256-261; 1988.

65a. Sardi J, Sananes C, Giaroli A, et al. Neoadjuvant chemotherapy in locally advanced carcinoma of the cervix uteri. Gyn Oncol 38(3):486-493; 1990.

66. Sheets, E.E., Berman, M.L., Hrountas, C.K., Liao, S.Y., DiSaia, P.J. Surgically treated, early-stage neuroendocrine small-cell cervical carcinoma. Obstetrics and Gynecology 71:10-14; 1988.

67. Shigematsu, Yl; Nishiyama, K.; Masaki, N.; Inoue, T.; Miyata, Y.; Ikeda, H.; Ozeki, S.; Kawamura, Y.; Kurachi, K. Treatment of carcinoma of the uterine cervix by remotely controlled afterloading intracavitary radiotherapy with high dose rate: a comparative study with a low-dose rate system. Int. J. Radiat. Oncol. Biol. Phys. 9:351-356; 1983.

68. Shingleton, H.M., Gore, H., Bradley, D.H., and Soong, S-J. Adenocarcinoma of the cervix. I. Clinical evaluation and pathologic features. American Journal of Obstetrics and Gynecology 139:799; 1981.

69. Silverberg E, Boring CC, Squires TS. Cancer statistics; 1990. CA-A Cancer Journal for Clinicians 40:9-26; 1990.

70. Simon, N.L., Gore, H., Shingleton, H.M., Soong, S.J., Orr, J.W., Jr., Hatch, K.D. Study of superficially invasive carcinoma of the cervix. Obstetrics and Gynecology 68:19-24; 1986.

71. Smith, H.O.; Stringer, C.A.; Kavanagh, J.J.; Gershenson, D.M.; Edwards, C.L., Wharton, J.T. Treatment of advanced or recurrent squamous cell carcinoma of the uterine cervix with mitomycin c, bleomycin and cisplatinum chemotherapy. Proceedings of the American Society of Clinical Oncology 9:163; 1990. Abstract.

72. Thigpen, J.T., Shingleton, H., Holmsley, H.D., Lagasse, D.L., and Blessing, J.A. Cisplatinum in treatment of advanced or recurrent squamous cell carcinoma of the cervix: A phase II study of the Gynecologic Oncology Group. Cancer 48:899; 1981.

73. Thigpen, J.T., Vance, R., Balducci, L., and Blessing, J.A. Chemotherapy in the management of advanced or recurrent cervical and endometrial carcinoma. Cancer 48:658; 1981.

74. Thomas, G., Dembo, A., Beale, F., Bean, H., Bush, R., Herman, J., Pringle, J., Rawlings, G., Sturgeon, J., Fine, S., Black, B. Concurrent radiation, mitomycin C and 5-flourouracil in poor prognosis carcinoma of the cervix: preliminary results of a Phase I- II study. International Journal of Radiation Oncology Biol Phys 10:1785-1790; 1984.

74a. Thoms Jr WW, Eifel PJ, Smith TL, et al. Bulky endocervical carcinoma: A 23-year experience. Int J Radiat Oncol Biol Phys 23(3):491-500; 1992.

75. Van Nagell, J.R., Jr., Donaldson, E.S., Wood, E.C. et al. Small cell carcinoma of the cervix. Cancer 40:2243; 1979.

76. van Nagell, J.R., Jr., Greenwell, N., Powell, D.F., Donaldson, E.S., Hanson, M.B., and Gay, E.C. Microinvasive carcinoma of the cervix. American Journal of Obstetrics and Gynecology 145:981; 1983.

76a. Vigliotti AP, Wen B-C, Hussey DH, et al. Extended field irradiation for carcinoma of the uterine cervix with positive periaortic nodes. Int J Radiat Oncol Biol Phys 23(3):501-510; 1992.

77. Weems DW, Mendenhall WM, Bova FJ, et al. Carcinoma of the intact uterine cervix, Stage Ib-IIa- b, > 6 cm in diameter: Irradiation alone vs. preoperative irradiation and surgery. International Journal of Radiation Oncol and Biol. Phys. 11:1911-1914; 1985.

78. Weiser, E.B., Bundy, B.N., Hoskins, W.J., Heller, P.B., Whittington, R.R., DiSaia, P.J., Curry, S.L., Schlaerth, J. and Thigpen, J.T. Extraperitoneal versus transperitoneal selective paraaortic lymphadenectomy in the pretreatment surgical staging of advanced cervical carcinoma (A Gyecologic Oncology Group study). Gynecologic Oncology 33:283-289; 1989.

79. Weiss, R.J. and Lucas, W.E. Adenocarcinoma of the uterine cervix. Cancer 57:1996-2001; 1986.

80. Wharton, J.T., Jones, H.W., III, Day, T.G. Jr., Rutledge, F.N. and Fletcher, G.H. Preirradiation celiotomy and extended field irradiation for invasive carcinoma of the cervix. Obstetrics and Gynecology 49:33; 1977.

80a. Wright TC, Richart RM. Role of human papillomavirus in the pathogenesis of genital tract warts and cancer. Gyn Oncol 37(2):151-164; 1990.

Carcinoma of the Endometrium

81. Aalders, J.; Abeler, V.; Kolstad, P. et al. Postoperative external irradiation and prognostic parameters in stage I endometrial cancer. Obstet Gynecol. 56:419-426; 1980.

82. Alberhasky, R.C.; Connelly, P.J.; Christopherson, W.M. Carcinoma of the endometrium. IV. Mixed adenosquamous carcinoma. Am J Clin Path. 77:655-664; 1982.

83. Announcements: FIGO stages - 1988 revisions. Gynecol Oncol. 35:125-127; 1989.

84. Baggish, M.S.; Ba Hoyannis, P. New techniques for laser ablation of the endometrium in high-risk patients. Am J Obstet Gynecol. 159:287-92; 1988.

85. Berek, J.S.; Dembo, A.; Markham, M.; Ozols, R. Ovarian Cancer. In: American Society of Clinical Oncology Educational Booklet. Published by ASCO and the Bostrom Corporation; Chicago, IL; 1990, pp 3-25.

86. Bockhman, J.V. Two pathogenic type of endometrial carcinoma. Gunecol Oncol 15:10-17; 1983.

87. Boothby, R.A.; Carlson, J.A.; Neiman, W. et al. Treatment of stage II endometrial carcinoma. Gynecol Oncol. 33:204-208; 1989.

87a. Carcangiu ML, Chambers JT, Voynick IM, et al. Immunohistochemical evaluation of estrogen and progesterone receptor content in 183 patients with endometrial carcinoma. Part I: clinical and histologic correlations. Am J Clin Path 94(3):247-254; 1990.

88. Christopherson, W.M.; Alberhasky, R.C.; Connelly, P.J. Carcinoma of the endometrium. I. A clinicopathologic study of clear-cell carcinoma and secretory carcinoma. Cancer 49:1511-1523; 1982.

89. Cohen, C.; Schulman, G.; Budgeon, L.R. Endocervical and endometrial adenocarcinoma: an immunoperoxidase and histochemical study. Am J Surg Pathol. 6:151-157; 1982.

90. Cohen, C.J.; Bruckner, H.W.; Deppe, G. et al. Multidrug treatment of advanced and recurrent endometrial carcinoma: a gynecologic oncology group study. Obstet Gynecol. 63:719-726; 1984.

91. Cohen, C.J.; Deppe, G.; Bruckner, H.W. Treatment of advanced adenocarcinoma of the endometrium with melphalan, 5-fluorouracil, and medroxyprogesterone acetate. Obstet Gynecol. 50:415-420; 1982.

92. Cowles, T.A.; Magrina, J.F.; Masterson, B.J. et al. Comparison of clinical and surgical staging in patients with endometrial carcinoma. Obstet Gynecol. 66:413-416; 1985.

93. Creasman, W.T. ed. Endometrial cancer. Clin Obset Gynecol. 13:751-767; 1986.

94. Creasman, W.T.; Morrow, C.P.; Bundy, B.N. et al. Surgical pathologic spread patterns of endometrial cancer: a gynecologic oncology group study. Cancer 60:2035-2041; 1987.

95. Crissman, J.A.; Azoury, R.S.; Barnes, A.E. *et al.* Endometrial carinoma in women 40 years of age or younger. Obstet Gynecol. 57:699-704; 1981.

96. Daniel, A.G.; Peters, W.A. Accuracey of office and operating room curettage in the grading of endometrial carcinoma. Obstet Gynecol. 71:612-614; 1988.

97. Disaia, P.J.; Creasman, W.T.; Boronow, R.C. *et al.* Risk factors and recurrent patterns in stage I endometrial carcinoma. Am J Obstet Gynecol. 151:1009-1015; 1985.

97a. DuBeshter B, Warshall DP, Angel CA, *et al.* Endometrial carcinoma: The relevance of cervical cytology. Obstet Gynecol 77:458-462; 1991.

98. Duk, J.M.; Aalders, J.F.; Fleuren, G.J. *et al.* CA 125: a useful marker in endometrial carcinoma. Am J Obstet Gynecol. 155:1097-1102; 1986.

99. Feuer, G.A.; Calanog, A. Endometrial carcinoma: treatment of positive para-aortic nodes. Gynecol Oncol. 27:104-109; 1987.

100. Gallion, H.H.; Van Nagell, J.R.; Powell, D.F. *et al.* Stage I serous papillary carcinoma of the endometrium. Cancer. 63:2224-2228; 1989.

101. Gallup, D.G.; Stock, R.J. Adenocarcinoma of the endometrium in women 40 years of age of younger. Obstet Gynecol. 64:417-420; 1984.

102. Gambrell, Jr., R.D. Role of hormones in the etiology and prevention of endometrial and breast cancer. Acta Obstet Gynecol Scand. 106:37-46; 1982.

103. Gambrell, R.D.; Bagnell, C.A.; Greenblatt, R.B. Role of estrogens and progesterone in the etiology and prevention of endometrial cancer: review. Am J Obstet Gynecol. 146:696-707; 1983.

104. Greer, B.E.; Hamberger, A.D. Treatment of intraperitoneal metastatic adenocarcinoma of the endometrium by the whole-abdomen moving strip technique and pelvic boost irradiation. Gynecol Oncol. 16:365-373; 1983.

105. Grigsby, P.W.; Perez, C.A.; Camel, H.M. *et al.* Stage II carcinoma of the endometrium: results of therapy and prognostic factors. Int J Rad Oncol Biol Phys. 11:1915-1923.

105a. Gurpide E. Endometrial cancer: Biochemical and clinical correlates. JNCI 83(6):405-416; 1991.

106. Hartz, A.; Fishcer, M.; Cassell, E. *et al.* Obesity and endometrial cancer. Intern Med. 6:61-65; 1985.

107. Hendrickson, M.; Martinez, A.; Ross, J. *et al.* Uterine papillary serous carcinoma: a highly malignant fomr of endometrial adeno-carcinoma. Am J Surg Path. 6:93-108; 1982.

107a. Ingram SS, Rosenman J, Heath R, *et al.* The predictive value of progesterone receptor levels in endometrial cancer. Int J Radiat Oncol Biol Phys 17(1):21-27; 1989.

108. Kauppila, A.; Gronroos, M.; Nieminen, V. Clinical Outcome in Endoemtrial Cancer. Obstet Gynecol. 60:473-480; 1980.

109. Koss, L.G.; Schreiber, K.; Oberlander, S.G. *et al.* Detection of endometrial carcinoma and hyperplasia in asymptomatic women. Obstet Gyncol. 64:1-11; 1984.

110. Kurman, R.J.; Kaminski, P.F.; Norris, J.F. The behavior of endometrial hyperplasia: a long-term study of "untreated" mycoplasia in 170 patients. Cancer 56:403-412; 1985.

111. Kurman, R.J.; Norris, H.J. Evaluation of criteria for distinguishing atypical endometrial hyperplasia from well-differentiated carcinoma. Cancer. 49:2547-2559; 1982.

112. Landgren, R.C.; Fletcher, G.H.; Delclos, L. *et al.* Irradiation of endometrial cancer in patients with medical contraindication to surgery or with unresectable lesions. Am J Roentgenol. 126:148-154;1976.

113. Lewis, G.C.; Glaek, N.H.; Mortel, R. *et al.* Adjuvant progestogen therapy in the primary definitive treatment of endometrial cancer. Gynecol Oncol. 12:368-376;1974.

114. Loeffler, J.S.; Rosen, E.M.; Niloff, J.M. *et al.* Whole abdominal irradiation for tumors of the uterine corpus. Cancer. 61:1332-1335; 1988.

115. Long, H.J.; Pfeifle, D.M.; Weiland, S. *et al.* Phase II evaluation of carboplatin in advanced endometrial carcinoma. J Natl Cancer Inst. 80:276-279; 1987.

116. MacDonald, R.R.; Thorogood, J.; Mason, M.C. A randomized trial of progestogens in primary treatment of endometrial carcinoma. Br J Obstet Gynecol. 95:166-174; 1988.

117. Mandell, L.; Nori, D.; Anderson, L. *et al.* Postoperative vaginal radiation of endometrial cancer using a remote after-looking technique. Int J Rad Oncol Biol Phys. 11:473-478; 1985.

117a. Moore TD, Phillips PH, Nerenston SR, Cheson BD. Systemic treatment of advanced and recurrent endometrial carcinoma: Current status and future directions. J Clin Oncol 9:1071-1088; 1991.

117b. Morrow CP, Bundy BN, Kurman RJ, *et al.* Relationship between surgical-pathological risk factors and outcome in clinical stage I and II carcinoma of the endometrium: A Gynecologic Oncology Group study. Gyn Oncol 40:55-65; 1991.

118. Muggia, F.M.; Chia, G.; Reed, L.F. *et al.* Doxorubicin-cyclophos-phamide: effective chemotherapy for advanced endometrial adenocarinoma. Am J Obstet Gynecol. 128:314-319;1977.

119. Niloff, J.M.; Klug, T.L.; Schaetzl, E., *et al.* Elevation of serum CA 125 in carcinomas of the fallopian tube, endometrium and endocervix. Am J Obstet Gynecol. 148:1057-1058; 1984.

120. Palmer, D.C.; Muir, I.M.; Alexander, A.I. The prognostic importance of steroid receptors in endometrial carcinoma. Obstet Gynecol. 72:388-392; 1988.

120a. Physician's Data Query. Cancer of the Endometrium. National Cancer Institute: Bethesda, MD; January 1992.

121. Piver, M.D. (ed) Ovarian Malignancies, Diagnostic and Therapeutic Advances, New York, NY: Churchill, Livingstone; 1987.

121a. Piver MS, Hempling RE. A prospective trial of postoperative vaginal radium/cesium for grade 1-2 less than 50% mypometrial invasion in surgical stage I endometrial adenocarcinoma. Cancer 66(6):1133-1138; 1990.

122. Piver, M.S.; Lele, S.B.; Patsner, B. *et al.* Melphalan, 5-fluorouracial, and medroxyprogesterone acetate in metastatic endometrial carcinoma. Obstet Gynecol. 67:261-264; 1986.

123. Podratz, K.C.; O'Brien, P.C.; Malkasian, G.D. *et al.* Effects of progestational agents in the treatment of endometrial carcinoma. Obstet Gynecol. 66:106-110; 1985.

124. Potish, R.A. Radiation therapy of periaortic node metastases in cancer of the uterine cervix and endometrium. Radiology. 165:567-570; 1987.

125. Potish, R.A.; Twiggs, L.B.; Adcock, L.L. *et al.* Paraaortic lymph node radiotherapy in cancer of the uterine corpus. Obstet Gynecol. 65:251-256; 1985.

126. Quinn, M.A.; Campbell, J.J. Tamoxifen therapy in advanced/recurrent endometrial carcinoma. Gynecol Oncol. 32:103; 1989.

127. Raeinet, C. ed. Endometrial Cancers, 56th Cancer Workshop, Grenoble; 1985. New York, NY: Karger; 1986:67-74.

128. Ross, J.C.; Eifel, P.F.; Cox, R.S. *et al.* Primary mucinous adenocarcinoma of the endometrium: a clinicopathologic and histochemical study. Am J Surg Pathol. 7:715-728; 1983.

129. Ross, J.C.; Kempson, R.L.; Eifel, P.F. *et al.* Primary mucinous adenocarcinoma of the endometrium: a clinicopathologic and histochemical study. Am J Surg Path. 7:715-729; 1983.

130. Rutledge, F. The role of radical hysterectomy in adenocarcinoma of the endometrium. Gynecol Oncol. 2:331-336;1977.

131. Sause, W.T.; Fuller, D.B.; Smith, W.G.; Johnson, G.H.; Plenk, H.P.; Menlove, R.B. Analysis of preoperative intracavitary cesium application versus postoperative external beam radiation in Stage I endometrial carcinoma. Int J Rad Oncol Biol Phys. 18:1011-1019; 1990.

132. Seski, J.C.; Edwards, C.L.; Gershenson, D.M. *et al.* Doxorubicin and cyclophosphamide chemotherapy for dessminated endometrial cancer. Obstet Gynecol. 58:88-91; 1981.

133. Seski, J.C.; Edwards, C.L.; Herson, J. *et al.* Cisplatin chemotherapy for disseminated endometrial cancer. Obstet Gynecol. 59:225-228; 1982.

134. Shepherd, J.H. Revised FIGO staging for gynecological cancer. Br J Obstet Gynecol. 1989:889-892.

135. Silverberg, E.; Lubera, J.A. Cancer Statistics; 1989. CA-A Cancer. 34:12-13; 1989.

136. Soper, J.T.; Creasman, W.T.; Clarke-Pearson, D.L. *et al.* Intraperitoneal chromic phosphate P32 suspension therapy of malignant peritoneal cytology in endometrial carcinoma. Am J Obstet Gynecol. 153:191-196; 1985.

137. Speroff, L.; Glass, R.H.; Kase, N.G. Clinical gynecologic endocrinology and infertility, 4th ed. Baltimore, MD: Williams and Wilkins, Co.; 1989.

138. Surwit, E.A.; Joelsson, I.; Einhorn, N. Adjunctive radiation therapy in the management of stage I cancer of the endometrium. Obstet Gynecol. 58:590-595; 1981.

139. Thigpen, J.T.; Blessin, J.A.; Homersley, H. *et al.* Phase II trial of cisplain on first line chemotherapy in patients with advanced or

recurrent endometrial carcinoma: a gynecologic oncology group study. Gynecol Oncol. 33:666-670; 1984.

140. Thigpen, W.T.; Buchsbaum, W.J.; Mangan, C. *et al.* Phase II trial of adriamycin in the treatment of advanced or recurrent endometrial cancer: a gynecologic oncology group study. Cancer Treat. 63:21-27;1979.

141. Torrisi, J.R.; Barnes, W.A.; Popescu, G. *et al.* Postoperative adjuvant external-beam radiotherapy in surgical stage I endometrial carcinoma. Cancer 64:1414-1417; 1989.

142. Trimble, E.L.; Jones, H.W. Management of stage II endometrial adenocarcinoma. Obstet Gynecol. 71:323-326; 1988.

143. Trope, C.; Johnson, J.E.; Simonsen, E. *et al.* Treatment of recurrent endometrial adenocarcinoma with a combination of doxorubicin and cisplatin. Am J Obstet Gynecol. 149:379-381; 1984.

144. Turbow, M.M.; Thorbon, J.; Ballon, S. *et al.* Chemotherapy of advanced carcinoma with platinum, adriamycin, and cyclophosphamide, Proc Am Assoc Cancer Res. 1:108-112; 1982.

145. Vuopala S: Diagnostic Accuracy and Clinical Applicability of Cytological and Histological Methods for Investigating Endometrial Carcinoma. Acta Obstet Bynecol Scand (Suppl)70:1-72; 1977.

146. Wallin, T.E.; Matkasian, G.D.; Gaffey, T.A. *et al.* Stage II cancer of the endometrium: a pathologic and clinical study. Gynecol Oncol. 18:1-17; 1984.

147. Wang, M.L.; Hussey, D.H.; Vigliotti, A.P. *et al.* Inoperable adenocarcinoma of the endometrium: Radiation therapy. Radiology. 165:561-565; 1987.

148. Wollin, M.; Kagan, A.R.; Kwan, D.K. Radiation dose calculations in endometrial cancer treatment with Heyman capsules or Tandem. Gynecol Oncol. 13:37-43; 1982.

149. Zucker, P.K.; Kasdon, E.J.; Feldstein, M.L. The validity of pap smear parameters as predictors of endometrial pathology in menopausal women. CAncer 56:2256-2263; 1985.

Gestational Trophoblastic Neoplasia

150. Athanassiou, A.; Begent, RHJ; Newlands, E.S.; Parker, D.: Central nervous system of choriocarcinoma. Cancer. 52:1728-1735; 1983.

151. Bagshawe KD: Treatment of high-risk choriocarcinoma. J Reprod Med 29:813-820; 1984.

152. Berkowitz RS, Goldstein DP: Methotrexate with citrovorum factor rescue for nonmetastatic gestational trophoblastic neoplasia. Obstet Gynecol 54:725-728; 1979.

153. Berkowitz RS, Goldstein DP and Bernstein MR: Modified triple chemotherapy in the management of high-risk metastatic gestational trophoblastic tumors. Gynecol Oncol 19:173-181; 1984.

154. Berkowitz RS, Goldstein DP, and Bernstein MR: Natural history of partial molar pregnancy. Obstet Gynecol 66:677-681; 1983.

155. Berkowitz RS, Goldstein DP, DuBeshter B, and Bernstein MR: Management of complete molar pregnancy. J Reprod Med 32:634-639; 1987.

156. Bolis G, Bonazzi C, Landoni F, *et al.* EMA/CO regimen in high-risk gestational trophoblastic tumor (GTT). Gynecol Oncol 31:439-444; 1988.

157. Buckley JD: The epidemiology of molar pregnancy and choriocarcinoma. Clin Obstet Gynecol 27:153; 1984.

158. DuBeshter B, Berkowitz RS, Goldstein DP, and Bernstein MR: Analysis of treatment failure in high-risk metastatic gestational trophoblastic disease. Gynecol Oncol 29; 199-207; 1988.

158a. DuBeshter B, Berkowitz RS, Goldstein DP, Bernstein MR. Management of low risk metastatic gestational trophoblastic tumors. J Reprod Med 36:36-39; 1991.

159. DuBeshter B, Berkowitz RS, Goldstein DP, Bernstein MR: Metastatic gestational trophoblastic disease: experience at the New England Trophoblastic Disease Center. Obstet Gynecol 69:390; 1987.

160. Finkler NJ, Berkowitz RS, Driscoll SG, *et al.* Clinical experience with placental site trophoblastic tumors at the New England Trophoblastic Disease Center. Obstet Gynecol 71:854; 1988.

161. Goldstein DP, Berkowitz RS, and Bernstein MR: Reproductive performance after molar pregnancy and gestational trophoblastic tumors. Clin Obstet Gynecol 27:221-227; 1984.

162. Gordon AN, Gershenson DM, Copeland LJ, *et al.* High-risk metastatic gestational trophoblastic disease: further stratification into two clinical entities. Gynecol Oncol 34:54-56; 1989.

163. Hayashi K, Bracken MB, Freeman, Jr, DH, Hellenbrand K.

Hydatidiform mole in the United States; 1970-1977): A statistical and theoretical analysis. Am J of Epidemiology 115:67-77; 1982.

164. Jones WB: Current management of low-risk metastatic gestational trophoblastic disease. J Reprod Med 32:653-657; 1987.

165. Jones, W.B. Treatment of chorionic tumors. Clin. Obstet. Gynecol. 18:247-265; 1975.

166. Jones WB, Lewis JL: Late recurrences of gestational trophoblastic disease. Gynecol Oncol 20:83-91; 1985.

167. Petrilli ES, Twiggs LB, Blessing JA, Teng NN, and Curry S: Single dose actinomycin-D treatment for nonmetastatic gestational trophoblastic disease. Cancer 60:2173-2176; 1987.

168. Soper JT, Clarke-Pearson D, and Hammond CB: Metastatic gestational trophoblastic disease: prognostic factors in previously untreated patients. Obstet Gynecol 71:338; 1988.

169. Soper JT, Hammond CB: Role of surgical therapy and radiotherapy in gestational trophoblastic disease. J Reprod Med 32:663-668; 1987.

170. Surwit EA: Management of high-risk gestational trophoblastic disease. J Reprod Med 32:657-662; 1987.

171. Szulman AE, Surti U: The syndromes of hydatidiform mole I. Cytogenetic and morphologic correlations. Am J Obstet Gynecol 131:664. 1978.

172. Twiggs LB, Savage JE: Nonmetastatic gestational trophoblastic disease: a curable disease. Contemp Ob Gyn 61-69 May; 1987.

173. Wong LC, Choo YC, Ma HK: Etoposide, methotrexate, and bleomycin in drug resistant gestational trophoblastic tumor (GTT). Gynecol Oncol 31:439-444; 1988.

174. Wong LL, Choo YC, and Ma HK: Hepatic metastases in gestational trophoblastic disease. Obstet Gynecol 67:107; 1986.

175. Wong LC, Choo YC, and Ma HK: Primary oral etoposide therapy in gestational trophoblastic disease an update. Cancer 58:14-17; 1986.

Sarcomas of the Uterus

176. Chen SS: Propensity of retroperitoneal lymph node metastasis in patients with stage I sarcoma of the uterus. Gynecol Oncol 32:215-217; 1989.

177. Covens AL, Nisker JA, Chapman WB, *et al.* Uterine sarcoma: An analysis of 74 cases. Am J. Obstet Gynecol 156:370-374; 1987.

178. Doss LL, Lorens AS, Henriquez EM: Carcinosarcoma of the uterus: A 40-year experience from the state of Missouri. Gynecol Oncol 18:43-53; 1984.

179. George M, Pejovic MH, Kramar A, *et al.* Uterine sarcomas: Prognostic factors and treatment modalties — study on 209 patients. Gynecol Oncol 24:58-67; 1986.

180. Hannigen EV, Freedman RS, Rutledge RN: Adjuvant chemotherapy in early uterine sarcoma. Gynecol Oncol 15:56-64; 1983.

180a. Larson B, Silfversward C, Nilsson B, *et al.* Mixed mullerian tumours of the uterus — prognostic factors: A clinical and histopathologic study of 147 cases. Radiother and Oncol 17(2):123-132; 1990.

180b. Leibsohn S, d'Ablaing G, Mishell DR, Schlaerth JB. Leiomyosarcoma in a series of hysterectomies performed for presumed uterine leiomyomas AMJ Obstet Gynecol 162:968-976; 1990.

181. Meredith RF, Eisert DR, Kaka Z, *et al.* An excess of uterine sarcomas after pelvic irradiation. Cancer 58:2003-2007; 1986.

182. Montag TW, D'Ablaing G, Schlaerth JB, *et al.* Embryonal rhabdomyosarcoma of the uterine corpus and cervix. Gynecol Oncol 25:171-194; 1986.

183. Muss HB, Bundy B, DiSaia PF, *et al.* Treatment of recurrent or advanced uterine sarcoma: A randomized trial of doxorubicin versus doxorubicin and cyclophosphamide. Cancer 55:1648-1653; 1985.

184. Norris JH, Taylor HB: Postirradiation sarcomas of the uterus. Obstet Gynecol 26:689-693; 1965.

185. Ober WB: Uterine sarcomas. Histogenesis and taxonomy. Ann NY Acad Science 75:568-585, 1959.

186. Omura GA, Blessing JA, Major F, *et al.* A randomized clinical trial of adjuvant adriamycin in uterine sarcoma: A Gynecologic Oncology Group Study. J Clin Oncol 3:1240-1245; 1985.

186a. Peters WA, Rivkin SE, Smith MR, *et al.* Cisplatin and adriamycin combination chemotherapy for uterine stromal sarcomas and mixed mesodermal tumors. Gyn Oncol 34(3):323-327; 1989.

187. Piver MS, Rutledge FN, Copeland L, *et al.* Uterine endolym-

phatic stromal myosis: A collaborative study. Obstet Gynecol 64:173-178; 1984.

188. Podczaski ES, Woomert CA, Stevens CW, *et al.* Management of malignant mixed mesodermal tumors of the uterus. Gynecol Oncol 32:240-244; 1989.

189. Reid GC, Morley GW, Schmidt RW, *et al.* The role of pelvic exenteration for sarcomatous malignancies. Obstet Gynecol 74:80-84; 1989.

190. Salazar OM, Bonfiglio TA Patten SF, *et al.* Uterine sarcomas: analysis of failures with special emphasis on the use of adjuvant radiation therapy. Cancer 42:11611170; 1978.

191. Salazar, O.M.; Bonfiglio, T.A. Patten, S.F.; *et al.* Uterine sarcomas: natural history, treatment, prognosis. Cancer 42:1152-1160;1978.

192. Seltzer V, Kaplan B, Vogl S, *et al.* Doxorubicin and cisplatin in the treatment of advanced mixed mesodermal uterine sarcoma. Cancer Treat Rep 68:1389-1390; 1984.

193. Soper JT, McCarty Jr KS, Hinshaw E, *et al.* Cytoplasmic estrogen and progesterone receptor content of uterine sarcomas. Am J Obstet Gynecol 150:342-348; 1984.

194. Sutton GP, Bessing JA, Rosenstein N, *et al.* Phase II trial of ifosfamide and mesna in mixed mesodermal tumors of the uterus (A Gynecologic Oncology Group study). Am J Obstet Gynecol 161:309-312; 1989.

195. Sutton BP, Stehman FB, Michael H, *et al.* Estrogen and progesterone receptors in uterine sarcomas. Obstet Gynecol 68:709-714; 1986.

196. Thigpen JT, Blessing JA, Orr JW, *et al.* Phase II trial of clsplatin in the treatment of patients with advanced or recurrence mixed mesodermal sarcomas of the uterus: A Gynecologic Oncology Group study. Cancer Treat Rep 70:271-274; 1986.

197. Tseng L, Tseng JK, Mann, WJ, *et al.* Endocrine aspects of human uterine sarcoma: A preliminary study. Am J Obstet Gynecol 155:95-101; 1986.

198. van Dinh T, Woodruff JD: Leiomyosarcoma of the uterus. Am J. Obstet Gynecol 144:817-823; 1982.

199. Wheelock JB, Krebs HB, Schneider V, *et al.* Uterine sarcoma: Analysis of prognostic variables in 71 cases. Am J. Obstet Gynecol 151:1016-1022; 1985.

Carcinoma of the Fallopian Tube

200. Asmussen M, Kaern J, Kjoerstad K, *et al.* Primary Adenocarcinoma Localized to Fallopian Tubes: Report on 33 Cases. Gynecol Oncolog 30:183-186; 1988.

201. Dodson MG, Ford, JH, Averette HE: Clinical Aspects of Fallopian Tube Carcinoma. Obstet Gynecol 36:935-939; 1970.

202. Eddy GL, Copeland LJ, Gershenson DM, *et al.* Fallopian Tube Carcinoma. Obstet Gynecol 64:546-552; 1984.

203. Hu CY, Taylor ML, Hertz AT. Primary Carcinoma of the Fallopian Tube. Am J Obstet Gynecol. 59:58-67; 1950.

204. Maxson WZ, Stenman FB, Ulbright TM, *et al.* Primary Carcinoma of the Fallopian Tube: evidence for Activity of Cisplatin Combination Therapy. Gynecol Oncol. 26:305-313; 1987.

205. Moore DH, Woosley JT, Reddick RL, *et al.* Adenosquamous carcinoma of the fallopian tube: A Clinicopathologic Case Report with Verification of the Diagnosis by Immunohistochemical and Ultrastructural Studies. Am J Obstet Gynecol. 157:903-905;1987.

206. Peters WA, Andersen WA, Hopkins MP. Results of Chemotherapy in Advanced Carcinoma of the Fallopian Tube. Cancer. 68:836-838; 1989.

207. Raju KS, Barker GH, Wiltshaw E. Primary Adenocarcinoma of the Fallopian Tube: Report on 22 Cases. Br J Obstet Gynecol. 88:1124-1130; 1981.

208. Roberts JA, Lifshitz S. Primary adenocarcinoma of the Fallopian Tube. Gynecol Oncol. 13:301-308; 1982.

209. Schiller HM, Silverberg SG. Staging and Prognosis in Primary Carcinoma of the Fallopian Tube. Cancer. 28:389-395; 1971.

210. Schray MF, Podratz, KC, Malkasian DG. Fallopian Tube Cancer: The Role of Radiation Therapy. Radiother Oncol. 10:267-275; 1987.

211. Sedlis A. Carcinoma of the Fallopian Tube. Surg Clin North Am. 58:121-129; 1978.

212. Tamimi HK, Figge DC. Adenocarcinoma of the Uterine Tube: Potential for Lymph Node Metastases. Am J Obstet Gynecol. 41:132-137; 1981.

213. Yamamoto K, Katoh S, Nakayama S, *et al.* Ultrasonic evaluation of the Fallopian Tube Carcinoma. Gynecol Obstet Invest. 25:202-208; 1988.

Ovarian Carcinoma

214. American Cancer Society. Cancer Statistics; 1989. CA. 1:3-39; January 1989.

215. Piver MS, ed. Ovarian Malignancies. Diagnostic and Therapeutic Advances. New York, NY: Churchill Livingstone; 1987.

215a. Young RC, Fuks Z, Hoskins WJ. Cancer of the ovary. In: DeVita Jr, VT, Hellman S, Rosenberg SA (eds): Cancer: Principles and Practice of Oncology (3rd ed). Philadelphia, PA: JB Lippincott Co.; 1989: 1162-1196.

215b. Advanced Ovarian Cancer Trialist Group. Chemotherapy in advanced ovarian cancer: An overview of randomised clinical trials. Brit Med J 303(73):884-893; 1991.

216. Alberts DS, Moon TE, Stephens RA, *et al.* Randomized study of chemoimmunotherapy for advanced ovarian carcinoma: a preliminary report of a Southwest Oncology Group study. Cancer Treat Rep. 63:325-331;1979.

217. Annegers JR, Strom H, Decker DG, *et al.* Ovarian cancer: incidence and case-control study. Cancer. 43:723-729; 1979.

218. Aure JC, Hoeg K, Kolstad P. Clinical and histologic studies of ovarian carcinoma: long-term followup of 990 cases. Obstet Gynecol. 37:1-9; 1981.

219. Barber HR, Graber EA. The PMPO Syndrome. Obstet Gynecol. 38:921-922; 1971.

220. Barlow JJ, Diver MS. Single agent vs combination chemotherapy in the treatment of ovarian cancer. Obstet Gynecol. 49:609-611; 1977.

221. Barlow JJ, Lele S. Etoposide Plus Cisplatin: A new active, chemotherapeutic combination in patients with stage III-IV ovarian adenocarcinoma. J Surg Oncol. 32:43-45; 1986.

222. Bast RC, King TL, St. John E, *et al.* A radioimmunoassay using a monoclonal antibody to monitor the course of epithelial ovarian cancer. N Engl J Med. 309:883-887; 1983.

223. Barnhill D, Heller PB, Brzozowski P, *et al.* Epithelial ovarian carcinoma of low malignant potential. Obstet Gynecol. 65:53-59; 1985.

224. Beecham J, Blessing J, Creasemen W, *et al.* Tamoxifen is effective on second-line therapy for certain patients with advanced chemotherapy-resistant epithelial ovarian cancer: a Gynecologic Oncology Group study. Am Soc Clin Oncol. 1988. Abstract no. 522.

225. Belinson JL, McClure M, Ashikaga T, Krakoff IJ. Treatment of advanced and recurrent ovarian carcinoma with cyclophosphamide, doxorubicin, and cisplatin. Cancer. 54; 1983-1990; 1984.

227. Berek JS, Hacker NF, Lagasse LD. Second-look laparotomy in stage III epithelial ovarian cancer: Clinical variables associated with disease status. Obstet Gynecol. 64:207-212; 1984.

226. Berek JS, Hacker NF, Lagasse LD, *et al.* Lower urinary tract resection as part of cytoreductive surgery for ovarian cancer. Gynecol Oncol. 13:87-92; 1982.

228. Berek JS, Hacker NF, Lagasse LD, *et al.* Survival of patients following secondary cytoreductive surgery in ovarian cancer. Obstet Gynecol. 61:189-193; 1983.

229. Berek JS, Knapp RC, Hacker NF, *et al.* Intraperitoneal immunotherapy of epithelial ovarian carcinoma with cornebacterium parvum. Am J Obstet Gynecol. 159:1003-1010; 1985.

230. Berek JS, Welander CE, Montz FJ, *et al.* Treatment of ovarian cancer with intraperitoneal cisplatin and alpha-2b interferon. Am Soc Clin Oncol. 1988. Abstract no. 531.

231. Bertelsen K, Jakobsen A, Andersen JE, *et al.* A randomized study of cyclophosphamide and cis-platinum with or without doxorubicin in advanced ovarian carcinoma. Gynecol Oncol. 28:161-169; 1987.

232. Bolis G, Colleoni R, Colombo N, Franchi M, Mangili G, Pecorelli S, Torri V, Zanaboni F. Advanced epithelial ovarian cancer: randomized trial dose-intensive regimens with weekly cisplatin plus cyclophosphamide or adriamycin. Clin Oncol. 9:169; 1990. Abstract.

232a. Burghardt E, Girardi F, Lahousen M, *et al.* Patterns of pelvic and paraaortic lymph node involvement in ovarian cancer. Gyn Oncol 40(2):103-106; 1991.

233. Cancer and Steroid Hormone Study for CDC and NIHCD. The reduction in risk of ovarian cancer associated with oral contraceptive use. N Engl J Med. 316:650-655; 1987.

234. Carmichael JA, Shelley WE, Brown LB, *et al.* A predictive index

of cure versus no cure in advanced ovarian carcinoma patients — replacement of second-look laparatomy as a diagnostic test. Gynecol Oncol. 27:269-278; 1987.

235. Chambers SK, Chambers JT, Kohorn EI, et al. Etoposide plus cisdiamminedichloroplatinum as salvage therapy in advanced epithelial ovarian cancer. Gynecol Oncol. 27:233-240; 1987.

236. Chamber SK, Chambers JT, Kohorn EI, et al. Evaluation of the role of second-look surgery in ovarian cancer. Obstet Gynecol. 72:404-408; 1988.

237. Chambers JT, Merino NJ, Kohorn EI, et al. Borderline ovarian tumors. Am J Obstet Gynecol. 159:1088-1094; 1988.

238. Chen SS, Bochner R. Assessment of morbidity and mortality in primary cytoreductive surgery for advanced ovarian carcinoma. Gynecol Oncol 20:190-195; 1985.

239. Cole, L.A, Nam, J.H, Schwartz, P.E, Chambers, J.T. Urinary gonadotropin fragment (UGF), a complementary marker to CA125 in the management of ovarian cancer. Clin Oncol. 9:164; 1990. Abstract.

240. Creasman WT, Gall SA, Blessing JA, et al. Chemoimmuno therapy in the management of primary stage III ovarian cancer: a Gynecologic Oncology Group study. Cancer Treat Rep. 63:319-323; 1979.

241. Creasman WT, Park RC, Norris JG, et al. Stage I borderline ovarian tumors. Obstet Gynecol. 59:93-96; 1982.

242. Decker DG, Fleming TR, Malkasian GD, et al. Cyclophosphamide plus cisplatinum in combination: treatment program for stage III or IV ovarian carcinoma. Obstet Gynecol. 60:481-487; 1982.

243. De Gramont A, Remes P, Krulik M, et al. Acute leukemia after treatment for ovarian cancer. Oncology. 43:165-172; 1986.

244. Delgado G, Oram DH, Petrilli EG. Stage III epithelial ovarian cancer: The role of maximal surgical reduction. Gynecol Oncol. 18:293-297; 1984.

245. Delgado G, Potkul RK, Treat JA, et al. A phase I/II study of intraperitoneally administered doxorubicin entrapped in cardiolipin liposomes in patients with ovarian cancer. Am J Obstet Gynecol. 160:812-819; 1989.

246. Dembo AJ. Abdominopelvic radiotherapy in ovarian cancer. Cancer. 55:2285-2290; 1985.

246a. Dembo AJ. Epithelial ovarian cancer: The role of radiotherapy. Int J Radiat Oncol Biol Phys 22:835-846; 1992.

247. Dembo AJ. In: Cox, JD (ed). The ovary. In: Radiation Oncology: Rationale, Technique, Results. St. Louis, MO: CV Mosby Co. 583. 1989.

248. Dembo AJ, Bush RS, Beak FA, et al. Randomized clinical trial of moving strip versus open field whole abdominal irradiation in patients with invasive epithelial cancer of the ovary. Int J Radiat Oncol Biol Phys. 5:1933-1942; 1979.

249. DePalo G, Pilotti S, Kenda R, et al. Natural history of dysgerminoma. Am J Obstet Gynecol. 143:799-807; 1987.

250. Edmonson JH, Decker DG, Malkasian GD, et al. Phase II evaluation of VP16-213 (NSC-14540) in patients with advanced ovarian carcinoma resistant to alkylating agents. Gynecol Oncol. 6:7-9; 1978.

251. Einzig AI, Trump DL, Sasloff J, et al. Phase II pilot study of taxol in patients with malignant melanoma. Proc Am Soc Clin Oncol. 7:249; 1988. Abstract.

251a. Einzig AI, Wiernik PH, Sasloff J, et al. Phase II study of taxol (T) in patients with advanced ovarian cancer. Proc of Am Assoc Canc Res 31:A-1114, 187; 1990.

252. Fort MG, Pierce VK, Saigo PE, et al. Evidence for the efficacy of adjuvant therapy in epithelial ovarian tumors of low malignant potential. Gynecol Oncol. 32:269-272; 1989.

253. Fuks Z. Questioning current policies for the curative management of ovarian carcinoma. ASTRO Refresher Course no. 310; 1988.

254. Fuks Z, Rizel S, Biran S. Chemotherapeutic and surgical induction of pathological complete remission and whole abdominal irradiation for consolidation does not enhance the cure of stage III avarian carcinoma. J Clin Oncol. 6; 1988.

255. Gershenson DM, Copeland LF, Del Junco G, et al. Second-look laparatomy in the management of malignant germ cell tumors of the ovary. Obstet Gynecol. 67:789-793; 1986.

256. Gershenson DM, Copeland LJ, Wharton JT, et al. Prognosis of surgically determined complete responders in advanced ovarian cancer. Cancer. 55:1129-1135; 1985.

257. Gershenson DM, Del Junco G, Henson J, et al. Endodermal sinus tumor of the ovary: the M.D. Anderson Experience. Obstet Gynecol. 61:194-202; 1983.

258. Gobel, U, Bamberg, M, Pelzer, V, Wolf, A, Mecke und, H, Harms, D. for the GPO Study Group. Prognosis in pure dysgerminoma and dysgermino containing mixed germ cell tumors of the ovary after combined modality treatment. Clin Oncol. 9:162; 1990. Abstract.

259. Goldstein SR, Subramanyam B, Snyder JR, et al. The postmenopausal cystic adnexal mass: the potential role of ultrasound in conservative management. Obstet Gynecol. 73:8-10; 1989.

260. Goren MP, Wright RK, Pratt CB, et al. Potentiation of ifosfamide neurotoxicity, hematologic toxicity and tubular nephrotoxicity by prior cisplatin therapy. Cancer Res. 47:1457-1460; 1987.

260a. Greco FA, Johnson DH, Hainsworth JD. A comparison of hexamethylmelamine (altretamine), cyclophosphamide, doxorubicin, and cisplatin (H-CAP) vs. cyclophosphamide, doxorubicin, and cisplatin (CAP) in advanced ovarian cancer. Cancer Treatment Rev 18(Suppl A):47-55; 1991.

261. Green TH. Hemisulfur mustard in the palliation of patients with metastatic ovarian carcinoma. Obstet Gynecol. 13:383-393; 1959.

262. Greene MH, Boice JD, Greer BE, at al. Acute nonlymphocytic leukemia after therapy with alkylating agents for ovarian cancer. N Engl J Med. 307:1416-1421; 1982.

263. Greene MH, Clark JW, Blayney DW. Epidemiology of ovarian cancer. Semin Oncol. 11:209-226; 1984.

265. Griffiths CT, Parker LM, Fuller AJ. Role of cytoreductive surgical treatment in the management of advanced ovarian cancer. Cancer Treat Rep. 63:235-240;1979.

264. Griffiths CT. Surgical resection of tumor bulk in the primary treatment of ovarian carcinoma. NCI Monog. 42: 101-104; 1975.

266. Gruppo Interegionale Cooperative Oncologic Ginecologia: Randomized comparison of cis-platin with cyclophosphamide/cisplatin and cyclophosphamide/doxorubicin/cisplatin in advanced ovarian cancer. Lancet. II(No. 8555): 353-358; 1987.

267. Hacker NF, Berek JS, Burnison CM, et al. Whole abdominal radiation as salvage therapy for epithelial ovarian cancer. Obstet Gynecol. 65:60-66; 1985.

268. Hacker NF, Berek JS, Lagasse LD, et al. Primary cytoreductive surgery for epithelial ovarian cancer. Obstet Gynecol. 61:413-420; 1983.

269. Haie C, Pejovic-Lenfant M.H, George M, Michel G, Gerbaulet A, Prade M, Chassagne D. Whole abdominal irradiation following chemotherapy in patients with minimal residual disease after second look surgery in ovarian carcinoma. Int J Radiat Oncol Biol Phys.17:15-21; 1989.

270. Hart WR, Norris HJ. Borderline and malignant mucinous tumors of the ovary. Cancer. 31:1031; 1973.

271. Hartge P, Schiffman MH, Hoover R, et al. A Case-control study of epithelial ovarian Cancer. Am J Obstet Gynecol. 161:10-16; 1989.

272. Heintz APM, Oosterom AT, Trimbos JB, et al. The treatment of advanced ovarian carcinomas (I): Clinical variables associated with prognosis. Gynecol Oncol. 30:347-358; 1988.

273. Heintz APM, Oosterom AT, Trimbos JB, et al. The treatment of advanced ovarian carcinoma (II): uterral reassessment operations during chemotherapy. Gynecol Oncol. 30:359-371; 1988.

274. Herrman UJ, Locher G, Goldhirsch A. Sonographic patterns of ovarian tumors: prediction of malignancy. Obstet Gynecol. 69:777-781; 1987.

275. Howell SB, Zimm S, Markman M, et al. Long-term survival of advanced refractory ovarian carcinoma patients with small-volume disease treated with intraperitoneal chemotherapy. J Clin Oncol. 5:1607-1612; 1987.

276. Hreshchyshyn MM, Park R, Blessing, JA, et al. The Role of adjuvant therapy in stage I ovarian cancer. Am J Obstet Gynecol. 138:139-144; 1979.

277. Jenison EL, Montay AG, Griffiths CT, et al. Clear cell adenocarconima of the ovary: A clinical analysis and comparison with serous carcinoma. Gynecol Oncol. 32:65-71; 1989.

278. Kersh CR, Randall ME, Constable WC, et al. Whole abdominal radiotherapy following cytoreductive surgery and chemotherapy in ovarian carcinoma. Gynecol Oncol. 31:113-120; 1988.

279. Kirmani, S.; McVey, L.; Goel, R.; Kim, S.; Howell, S.B. Intraperitoneal cisplatin/etoposide for consolidation of pathologic complete response in ovarian carcinoma. Clin Oncol. 9:167; 1990. Abstract.

280. Kurman RJ, Norris JG. Malignant mixed germ cell tumors of the ovary: A clinical and pathologic analysis of 30 cases. Obstet Gynecol. 48:579-589; 1976.

281. Lambert HE, Berry RJ. High dose cisplatin compared with high dose cyclophosphamide in the management of advanced epithelial ovarian cancer (FIGO stages III and IV): report from the North Thames Cooperative Group. Brit Med J. 290:889-893; 1985.

282. Landesman R, Silver RT. Cytoreductive surgery. Obstet Gynecol. 64:148-149; 1984.

283. Lavin PT, Knapp RC, Malkasiam G, et al. CA 125 for the monitoring of ovarian carcinoma during primary therapy. Obstet Gynecol. 69:223-227; 1987.

284. Levin L, Hryniuk WM. Dose intensity analysis of chemotherapy regimens in ovarian carcinoma. J Clin Oncol. 5:756-767; 1987.

285. Littleton RE, Homesly HD, Richards F. Leukemogenesis related to chemotherapy of ovarian carcinoma: a review with three new case reports. Gynecol Oncol. 19:268-277; 1984.

286. Louis KG, Ozols RF, Myers CE, Ostechega Y, Jenkins J, Howser D, Young RD. Long-term results of a cisplatin-containing chemotherapy regimen for the treatment of advanced ovarian carcinoma. J Clin Oncol. 4:1579-1585; 1986.

286a. Lynch HT, Fitzsimmon ML, Conway TA, et al. Hereditary carcinoma of the ovary and associated cancers: A study of two families. Gynecol Oncol 36:48-55; 1990.

287. Malkasian GD Jr, Knapp RC, Lavin PT, et al. Preoperative evaluation of serum CA-125 levels in premenopausal and postmenopausal patients with pelvic masses: Discrimination of benign from malignant disease. A J Obstet Gynecol. 159:341-346; 1988.

288. Manetta A, MacNeill C, Lyler J, et al. Hexamethylmelamine for advanced ovarian cancer. Society of Gynecologic Oncologists; 1989. Abstract no. 88.

289. Martinez A, Schray MF, Howes AE, Bagshaw MA. Postoperative radiation therapy for epithelial ovarian cancer: the curative role based on a 24 year experience. J Clin Oncol. 3:901-911; 1985.

290. McGowan L, Lesher LP, Norris HJ, et al. Misstaging of ovarian cancer. Obstet Gynecol. 65:568-571; 1985.

290a. McGuire WP, Rowinsky EK. Old drugs revisited, new drugs, and experimental approaches in ovarian cancer therapy. Sem Oncol 18(3):255-269; 1991.

291. Moore, GE. Debunking debulking. Surg Gynecol Obstet. 150:395-396; 1980.

292. Morgan L, Chafe W, Mendenhall W, et al. Hyperfractionation of whole abdomen radiation therapy: salvage treatment of persistent ovarian carcinoma following chemotherapy. Gynecol Oncol. 31:122-134; 1988.

293. Morris M, Gershenson DM, Wharton JT. Secondary cytoreductive surgery in epithelial ovarian cancer: Non-responders to first-line therapy. Gynecol Oncol. 33:1-5; 1989.

294. Myers AM, Moore GE, Major FJ. Advanced ovarian carcinoma: response to antiestrogen therapy. Cancer. 48:2368-2370; 1981.

295. Neijt JP, ten Bokkel Huinink WW, van der Berg ME, van Oosterom AT, Willemse PH, Heintz AP, van Lent M, Trimbos J, Bouma J, Vermorken JB, Ban Houwelinger JC. Randomized trial comparing two combination chemotherapy regimens (CHAP 5 v CP) in advanced ovarian carcinoma. J Clin Oncol. 5:1157-1168; 1987.

295a. Neijt JP, ten Bokkel, Huinink WW, van der Burg ME, et al. Long-term survival in ovarian cancer: Mature data from the Netherlands Joint Study Group for ovarian cancer. Eur J Cancer 27(11):1367-1372; 1991.

296. Niloff JM, Bast RC, Schaetzl EM, et al. Predictive value of CA 125 antigen levels in second-look procedures for ovarian cancer. Am J Obstet Gynecol. 151:981-986; 1985.

297. Omura GA, Blessing JA, Ehrlich CE, et al. A randomized trial of cyclophosphamide and doxorubicin with or without cisplatin in advanced ovarian cancer: a Gynecologic Oncology Group study. Cancer. 57:1725-1730; 1986.

297a. Omura GA, Brady MF, Homesley HD, et al. Long-term follow-up and prognostic factor analysis in advanced ovarian carcinoma: The Gynecologic Oncology Group experience. J Clin Oncol 9(7):1138-1150; 1991.

298. Omura GA, Bundy BN, Berek JS, et al. Randomized trial of cyclophosphamide plus cisplatin with or without doxorubicin in ovarian carcinoma: a Gynecologic Oncology Group Study. J Clin Oncol. 7:457-465; 1989.

299. Omura GK, Morrow CP, Blessing JA, et al. A randomized comparison of melphalan versus melphalan plus hexamethylmelamine versus Adriamycin plus cyclophosphamide in ovarian carcinoma. Cancer. 51:783-789; 1983.

299a. Ovarian Cancer Meta-Analysis Project. Cyclophosphamide plus cisplatin versus cyclophosphamide, doxorubicin, and cisplatin chemotherapy of ovarian carcinoma: A meta-analysis. J Clin Oncol 9(9):1668-1674; 1991.

300. Ozols RF. The case for combination chemotherapy in the treatment of advanced ovarian cancer. J Clin Oncol. 3:1445-1446; 1985.

301. Ozols, RF, Ostchega Y, Curt G. High-dose carboplatin in refractory ovarian cancer patients. J Clin. Oncol. 5:197-201; 1987.

302. Ozols RF, Ostchega Y, Myers CE, et al. High-dose cis-platin in hypertonic saline in refractory ovarian cancer. J Clin Oncol. 3:1246-1250; 1985.

303. Pater J. Cyclophosphamide/cisplatin versus cyclophosphamide/carboplatin in macroscopic residual ovarian cancer. Initial results of a National Cancer Institute of Canada Clinical Trials Group. 9:155; 1990. Abstract.

304. Pater JL, Carmichael JA, Krepart GV, et al. Second-line chemotherapy of stage II-VI ovarian carcinoma: a randomized comparison of melphalan to melphalan and hexamethylmelamine in patients with persistent disease after doxorubicin and cisplatin. Cancer Treat Rep. 71:277-281; 1987.

305. Patsner B, Mann WJ. High-dose (120 mg/m2) intravenous cisplatinum chemotherapy in refractory ovarian adenocarcinoma. Am Soc Clin Oncol. 534; 1988. Abstract.

306. Petterson F. ed. Annual report of the result of treatment in gynecologic cancer. vol. 20. Stockholm, Sweden: International Federation of Gynecology and Oncology. 1988.

306a. Physician's Data Query. Ovarian Carcinoma. National Cancer Institute: Bethesda, MD; January 1992.

307. Piver MS, Baker T. The potential for optimal (<2 cm) cytoreductive surgery in advanced ovarian cancer at a tertiary medical center: a prospective study. Gynecol Oncol. 24:1-8; 1986.

308. Piver MS, Mattlin CJ, Tsukaday, et al. Familial ovarian cancer registry. Obstet Gynecol. 64:195-199; 1984.

309. Podczaski E, Whitney C, Manetta A, et al. Use of CA 125 to monitor patients with ovarian epithelial carcinomas. Gynecol Oncol. 33:193-197; 1987.

310. Potter ME, Moradi M, To AC, et al. Value of serum CA 125 levels: does the result preclude second look? Gynecol Oncol. 33:201-203; 1989.

310a. Potter ME, Hatch KD, Soong S, et al. Second look laparotomy and salvage therapy: A research modality only. Gynecol Oncol 44:3-9; 1992.

310b. Potter ME, Partridge EE, Hatch KD, et al. Primary surgical therapy of ovarian cancer: How much and when. Gyn Oncol 40(3):195-200; 1991.

311. Potter ME, Partridge EE, Shingleton HM, et al. Intraperitoneal chromic phosphate in ovarian cancer: risks and benefits. Gynecol Oncol. 32:314-318; 1989.

312. Reichman B, Markman M, Hakes T, et al. Intraperitoneal cisplatin and etoposide in the treatment of refractory recurrent ovarian carcinoma. J Clin Oncol. 7:1327-1332; 1989.

313. Rodriguez MH, Platt LD, Medearis AL, et al. The use of transvaginal sonography for evaluation of postmenopausal ovarian size and morphology. Am J Obstet Gynecol. 159:810-814; 1989.

314. Rosen GF, Lurain JR, Newton M. Hexamethylmelamine in ovarian cancer after failure of cisplatin-based multiple-agent chemotherapy. Gynecol Oncol. 27:173-179; 1987.

315. Roth BJ, Greist A, Kubilis PS, et al. Cisplatin-based combination chemotherapy for disseminated germ cell tumors: Long term followup. J Clin Oncol. 6:1239-1247; 1988.

316. Rothenberg, M.L.; Ozols, R.F.; Glatstein, E.; Myers, C.E.; Young, R.C. Dose-intensive induction therapy for advanced epithelial ovarian cancer: cyclophosphamide, high dose cisplatin, and abdominal radiation. Am Soc of Clin Oncol. 9:169; 1990. Abstract.

317. Rotmensch J, Atcher RW, Schlenker R, et al. The effect of the ~-emitting radionuclide Lead-212 on human ovarian carcinoma: a potential new form of therapy. Gynecol Oncol. 32:236-239; 1989.

318. Rowinsky ED, Donhaver RC, Roshenshein NB, et al. Phase II study of taxol in advanced ovarian epithelial malignancies. Proc Am Soc Clin Oncol. 7:136; 1988. Abstract.

319. Rubin SC, Hoskins WJ, Hakes TB. Recurrence after negative second-look laparotomy for ovarian cancer: analysis of risk factors. Am J Obstet Gynecol. 159:1094-1098; 1988.

320. Rulin MC, Preston AL. Adnexal mass in postmenopausal women. Obstet Gynecol. 70:578-581; 1987.

321. Rustin G.J.S. Nelstrop A. Stilwell J. Lambert J. Sexton S. Savings obtained by CA 125 measurements during therapy for ovarian carcinoma. Am Soc Clin Oncol. 9:165; 1990. Abstract.

322. Sarosy G. Ifosfamide-pharmacologic overview. Semin Oncol. 16:2-8; 1989.

323. Schilthuis MS, Aalders JG, Bouona J, et al. Serum CA 125 levels in epithelial ovarian cancer: Relation with findings at second-look operations and their role in the detection of tumor recurrence. Br J Obstet Gynecol. 94:202-207; 1987.

324. Schwartz, P.E.; Hayden, C.; Chambers, J.; Kohorn, E.I.; Chambers, S. New criteria for tumor markers in detecting occult ovarian cancer following clinically successful initial therapy. Am Soc Clin Oncol. 9:164; 1990. Abstract.

325. Schwartz PE, Keating G, MacLusky N, et al. Tamoxifen therapy for advanced ovarian cancer. Obstet Gynecol. 59:583-588; 1982.

326. Scully RE, Richardson G, Barlow JF. The development of malignancy in endometriosis. Clin Obstet Gynecol. 9:389;1966.

327. Seligmen AM, Rutenberg AM, Persky L, and Friedman OM. Effect of 2-choloro-2' hydroxydiethyl sulfide on carcinomatosis with ascites. Cancer. 5:359-360;1952.

328. Senekjian EK, Weiser PA, Talerman A, et al. Vinblastine, cisplatin, cyclophosphamide, bleomycin, doxorubicin, and etoposide in the treatment of small cell carcinoma of the ovary. Cancer. 64:1183-1187; 1989.

329. Shray M, Martinez A, Cox R, et al. Radiotherapy in epithelial ovarian cancer: Analysis of prognostic factors based on long-term experience. Obstet Gynecol. 62:373-382; 1983.

330. Skates, S.; Singer, D. The potential benefit due to early detection of ovarian cancer using CA 125. Proc Am Soc Clin Oncol. 9:162; 1990. Abstract.

331. Smirz LR, Stehman TB, Ulbright TM, et al. Second-look laparotomy after chemotherapy in the management of ovarian malignancy. Am J Obstet Gynecol. 152:661-668; 1985.

332. Smith JP, Rutledge RN, Delclos L. Postoperative treatment of early cancer of the ovary: A random trial between postoperative irradiation and chemotherapy. NCI Monog. 42:149-153;1975.

333. Soper JT, Wilkinson, RH, Bandy LC, et al. Intraperitoneal chronic phosphate p32 as salvage therapy for persistent carcinoma of the ovary after surgical restaging. Am J Obstet Gynecol.156:1153-1158; 1987.

334. Sutton G, Blessing J, Berman M, et al. Phase II trial of ifosfamide and mesna in refractory epithelial ovarian carcinoma. Society of Gynecologic Oncologists; 1989. Abstract.

335. Taylor HC. Malignant and semimalignant tumors of the ovary. Surg Gynecol Obstet. 48:702; 1929.

336. Tazelaar HD, Bostwick DG, Ballon SC, et al. Conservative treatment of borderline ovarian tumors. Obstet Gynecol. 66:417-422; 1985.

337. Thomas GM, Dembo AJ, Hacker NJ, et al. Current therapy for dysgerminoma of the ovary. Obstet Gynecol. 70:268-275; 1987.

338. Vardi JR, Tadros GH, Foemmel R, et al. Plasma lipid-associated sialic acid and serum CA 125 as indicators of disease status with advanced ovarian cancer. Obstet Gynecol. 74:379-383; 1989.

339. Varia M, Rosenman J, Venkattraman S, et al. Intraperitoneal chromic phosphate therapy after second-look laparotomy for ovarian cancer. Cancer. 61:919-927; 1988.

340. Vogl SE, Seltzer V, Calanog A. "Second-effort" surgical resection for bulky ovarian cancer. Cancer. 54:2220-2225; 1984.

341. Walton L, Ellenberg SS, Major F, et al. Results of second-look laparotomy in patients with early stage ovarian carcinoma. Obstet Gynecol. 7:770-773; 1987.

342. Weiss NS, Harlow BL. Why does hysterectomy without bilateral oophorectomy influence the subsequent incidence of ovarian cancer? Am J Epidemiol. 124:856-858; 1986.

343. Welander CE. Use of interferon in the treatment of ovarian cancer as a single agent and in combination with cytotoxic drugs. Cancer. 59:617-619; 1987.

344. Wharton JT, Edwards CL, Rutledge FN. Long-term survival after chemotherapy for advanced epithelial ovarian carcinoma. Am J Obstet Gynecol. 148:997-1005; 1984.

345. Willemse PH, Aalders JG, Bouma J, et al. Long-term survival after vinblastine, bleomycin, cisplatin treatment in patients with germ cell tumors of the ovary: an update. Gynecol Oncol. 28:268-277; 1987.

346. Williams, CJ, Mead GM, Macbeth FR, et al. Cisplatin combination chemotherapy versus chlorambucil in advanced ovarian carcinoma: mature results of a randomized trial. J Clin Oncol. 3:1455-1462; 1985.

347. Williams CJ, Stewart LA, Parmar MKB, Guthrie D. An overview of chemotherapy in advanced ovarian carcinoma (FIGO III and IV). Proc Am Soc Clin Oncol. 9:160; 1990.

348. Williams S.D, Blessing J, Hatch K, Homesley H. Chemotherapy of advanced ovarian dysgerminoma: trials of the Gynecologic Oncology Group (GOG). Proc Am Soc Clin Oncol. 9:155; 1990. Abstract.

349. Wiltshaw E, Kroner T. Phase II study of cis-dichloro-diammineplatinum (II) (NSC-119875) in advanced adenocarcinoma of the ovary. Cancer Treat Rep. 60:55-60;1976.

350. Wu PC, Qu JY, Lang JH, et al. Lymph node metastasis of ovarian cancer: A preliminary survey of 74 cases of lymphadenectomy. Am J Obstet Gynecol. 155:1103-1108; 1986.

351. Young, RC. Initial therapy for early ovarian carcinoma. Cancer. 60:2042-2049; 1987.

352. Young RC, Chabner BA, Hubbard SP, et al. Advanced ovarian adenocarcinoma: a prospective clinical trial of Melphalan versus combination chemotherapy. N Engl J Med. 299:1261-1266;1978.

352a. Young RC, Walton LA, Ellenberg SS. Adjuvant therapy in stage I and stage II epithelial ovarian cancer: Results of two prospective randomized trials. N Engl J Med. 322(15):1021-1027; 1990.

353. Zurawski VR, Broderick SF, Pickens P, et al. Serum CA 125 levels in a group of nonhospitalized women: relevance for the early detection of ovarian cancer. Obstet Gynecol 69:606-611; 1987.

Carcinoma of the Vagina

354. Benedet JL, Saunders BH. Carcinoma in situ of the vagina. Am J Obstet Gynecol. 148:695; 1984.

355. Bonner JA, Peres-Tamayo C, Reid GC, Roberts JA, and Morley GW. The management of vaginal melanoma. Cancer. 62:2066-2072; 1988.

356. Collins HS, Burke TW, Heller PB, Olson TA, Woodward JE, and Park RC. Endodermal sinus tumor of the infant vagina treated exclusively by chemotherapy. Obstet Gynecol. 73:507-509; 1989.

357. Disaia PJ, Creasman WT. Invasive cancer of the vagina and urethra in clinical gynecologic oncology. St. Louis, Mo: CV Mosby Co; 1986; 241.

358. Evans LS, Kersh R, Constable WC, and Talylor PT, Concomitant 5-fluorouracil, mitomycin-C, and radiotherapy for advanced gynecologic malignancies, Int J Radiat Oncol Biol Phys. 15:901-906; 1988.

359. Krebs HB. Treatment of vaginal intraepithelial neoplasia with laser and topical 5-fluorouracil. Obstet Gynecol. 73:657-660; 1989.

360. Lee RB, Buttoni L, Dhru K, and Tamimi H. Malignant melanoma of the vagina: a case report of progression from preexisting melanosis. Gynecol Oncol. 19:238-245; 1984.

361. Lenehan PM, Meffe F, Lickrish GM. Vaginal intraepithelial neoplasia: biologic aspects and management. Obstet Gynecol. 68:333-337; 1986.

362. Ostrow RS, Manias DA, Clark BA, Fukushima M, Okagaki T, Twiggs LB, and Faras AJ. The analysis of carcinomas of the vagina for human papillomavirus DNA. Int J of Gynecol Pathol. 7:308-314; 1988.

363. Perez CA, Camel M, Galakatos AE, Grigsby PW, Kuske RR, Buchsbaum G, and Hederman MA. Definitive irradiation in carcinoma of the vagina: long-term evaluation of results. Int J Radiation Oncology Biol Phys. 15:1283-1290; 1988.

364. Peters WA, Kumar NB, Morley GW. Carcinoma of the vagina. Cancer. 55:892; 1985.

364a. Physician's Data Query. Vaginal Cancer. National Cancer Institute: Bethesda, MD; January 1992.

365. Rubin SC, Young J, Mikuta JJ. Squamous carcinoma of the vagina: treatment, complications, and long-term follow-up. Gynecol Oncol. 20:346-353; 1985.

366. Sulak P, Barnhill D, Heller P, Weiser E, Hoskins W, Park R, and Woodwoard J, Nonsquamous cancer of the vagina. Gynecol Oncol. 29:309-320; 1988.

367. Weed JC, Lozier C, Daniel SJ. Human papilloma virus in multifocal, invasive female genital tract malignancy. Obstet Gynecol. 62:832; 1983.

Carcinoma of the Vulva

368. Boronow RC. Therapeutic alternative to primary exenteration for advanced vulvo-vaginal cancer. Gynecol Oncol. 1:223; 1973.

369. Boyce J, Fruchter RG, Kasambilides E, *et al.* Prognostic factors in carcinoma of the vulva. Gynecol Oncol. 20:364-377; 1985.

370. Burrell MO, Franklin EW, Campion MJ, *et al.* The modified radical vulvectomy with groin dissection: an eight year experience. Am J Obstet Gynecol. 159:715-22; 1988.

371. Cavanagh D, Shepherd JH. The place of pelvic exenteration in the primary management of advanced carcinoma of the vulva Gynecol Oncol. 13:318; 1982.

372. Chafe W, Richards A, Morgan L and Wilkinson E. Unrecognized invasive carcinoma in vulvar intraepithelial neoplasia (VIN). Gynecol Oncol. 31:154-162; 1988.

373. Choo YC, Morley GW. Double primary epidermoid carcinoma of the vulva and cervix Gynecol Oncol 9:324-333; 1980.

374. Copeland LJ, Sneige N, Gershenson DM *et al.* Adenoid cystic carcinoma of bartholin gland. Obstet Gynecol. 67:115-119; 1986.

375. Crum CP, Liskow A, Petras P, Keng WC and Frick HC. Vulvar intraepithelial neoplasia (severe atypia and carcinoma in situ). Cancer. 54:1429-1434; 1984.

376. Curry SL, Wharton JT, Rutledge F. Positive lymph nodes in vulvar squamous carcinoma. Gynecol Oncol. 9:63; 1980.

377. Disaia PJ, Creasman WT, Rich WM. An alternate approach to early cancer of the vulva. Am J Obstet Gynecol. 133:825-830; 1979.

378. Disaia P, Rich WM. Surgical approach to multifocal carcinoma in situ of the vulva. Am J Obstet Gynecol. 140:136-145; 1981.

379. Dvoretsky PM, Bonfiglio TA, Helmkamp FH, *et al.* The pathology of superficially invasive, thin vulvar squamous cell carcinoma. Int J Gynecol Pathol. 3:331-342; 1984.

380. Figge DC, Tamimi HK, Greer BE. Lymphatic spread in carcinoma of the vulva. Am J Obstet Gynecol. 152:387-394; 1985.

381. Franklin EW, Rutledge FD. Epidemiology of epidermoid carcinoma of the vulva. Obstet Gynecol. 39:165; 1972.

382. Frishbier HJ, Thomsen K. Treatment of cancer of the vulva with high energy electrons. Am J Obstet Gynecol. 111:431-435; 1971.

383. Hacker NF, Berek JS, Juillard GJF, Lagasse LD. Preoperative radiation therapy for locally advanced vulvar cancer. Cancer. 54:2056; 1984.

384. Hacker NF, Leuchter RS, Berek JS, *et al.* Radical vulvectomy and bilateral inguinal lymphadenectomy through separate groin incisions. Obstet Gynecol. 58:574-579; 1981.

384a. Herbst AI. Premalignant and malignant disease of the vulva. In: Herbst AI, Mishell Jr, DR, Stenchener, MA, Droegemueller W, (eds): Comprehensive Gynecology, 2nd ed. St Louis, MO: Mosby Yearbook; 1990:989-1018.

385. Hoffman MS, Roberts WS, Lapolla JP, and Cavanagh D. Recent modification in the treatment of invasive squamous cell carcinoma of the vulva. Obstet Gynecol Surv. 44:4; 227-233; 1989.

386. Homesley HD, Bundy BN, Sedlis A, Adcock L. Radiation therapy versus pelvic node resection for carcinoma of the vulva with positive groin nodes. Obstet Gynecol. 68:733-740; 1986.

386a. Homesley HD, Bundy BN, Sedlis A, *et al.* Assessment of current International Federation of Gynecology and Obstetrics staging of vulvar carcinoma relative to prognostic factors for survival (a Gynecologic Oncology Group study). Am J Ob Gyn 164(4):997-1004; 1991.

387. Jaramillo Ba, Ganjei P, Averette HE, Sevin B, Lovecchio JL. Malignant melanoma of the vulva. Obstet Gynecol. 66:398-401; 1985.

388. Leuchter RS, Hacker NF, Voet RL, *et al.* Primary carcinoma of the Bartholin Gland: A report of 14 cases and review of the literature. Obstet Gynecol 60:361; 1982.

389. Mabuchi K, Bross DS, Kessler II. Epidemiology of cancer of the vulva: A case control study. Cancer 55:1843-1848; 1985.

390. Microinvasive cancer of the vulva. Report of the ISSVD Task Force. J Reprod Med 29:454-456; 1984.

390a. Physician's Data Query. Vulvar Cancer. National Cancer Institute: Bethesda, MD; January 1992.

391. Pirtoli L, Rottoli ML. Results of radiation therapy for vulvar carcinoma. Acta Radiol Oncol 21:45-48; 1982.

392. Plentl AA, Griedman EA. Lymphatic system of the female genitalia. Philadelphia, PA: WB Saunders Co; 1971.

393. Podratz KC, Symmonds RE, Taylor WF, *et al.* Carcinoma of the vulva: Analysis of treatment and survival. Obstet Gynecol 61:63-74; 1983.

394. Prempree T, Amornmarn R. Radiation treatment of recurrent carcinoma of the vulva. Cancer 54:1943-1949; 1984.

395. Ross MG, Ehrmann RL. Histologic prognosticators in stage I squamous cell carcinoma of the vulva. Obstet Gynecol 70:774; 1987.

396. Sedlis A, Homesley H, Bundy BN, *et al.* Positive groin lymph nodes in superficial squamous cell vulvar cancer. Am J Obstet Gynecol 156:1159; 1987.

397. Sillman FH, Sedlis A, Boyce JG. A review of lower genital intraepithelial neoplasia and the use of topical 5-fluorouracil. Obstet Gynecol Surv 40:190-220; 1985.

398. Sishy B. The use of radiation therapy combined with chemotherapy in the management of squamous cell carcinoma of the anus and marginally resectable adenocarcinoma of the rectum. Int J Radiat Oncol Biol Phys 11:1587-1593; 1985.

399. Sutton GP, Stehman FB, Ehrlich CE, Roman A. Human papillomavirus deoxyribonucleic acid in lesions of the female genital tract: Evidence for type 6/11 in squamous carcinoma of the vulva. Obstet Gynecol 70:564; 1987.

400. Taylor PR, Stenwig JT, Klausen H. Paget's disease of the vulva. Gynecol Oncol 3:46; 1975.

400a. Thomas GM, Dembo AJ, Bryson CP, *et al.* Changing concepts in the management of vulvar cancer. Gynecol Oncol 42:9-21; 1991.

401. Townsend DE, Levine RU, Richart, RM, *et al.* Management of vulvar intraepithelial neoplasia by carbon dioxide laser. Obstet Gynecol 60:49; 1982.

402. Way S. The anatomy of the lymphatic drainage of the vulva and its influence on the radical operation for carcinoma. Annals of the Royal College of Surgeons of England. 3:187; 1948.

403. Wheelock JB, Goplerud DR, Dunn LF, Oates JF. Primary carcinoma of the bartholin gland: A report of ten cases. Obstet Gynecol 63:820-824; 1984.

404. Young JL, Percy CL, Asire AS. Surveillance, Epidemiology and End Results: Incidence and Mortality Data, 1973-1977. NCI Monogr. 57:982; 1981.

James W. Keller, M.D., Radiation Oncology
Deepak M. Sahasrabudhe, M.D.,
Medical Oncology

Craig. S. McCune, M.D., Medical Oncology

Chapter 23

UROLOGIC AND MALE GENITAL CANCERS

He who masters the two sciences of the pulse and the urine will possess almost all that is necessary for diagnosis and prognosis. Conversely, he who knows only one of these two sciences will be prone to a thousand errors, for in the study of disease, the science of urines is as valuable as that of the pulse.

Johannes Acutarius (3)

PERSPECTIVE

Since the last edition of this textbook, there have been a number of advances in the field of genitourinary cancers. The cure of testicular cancer with chemotherapy was being realized at that time. Subsequently, many studies have documented its effectiveness; there has been more precise identification of poor prognostic factors; and refinement of chemotherapy has occurred, producing more tolerable side effects.

Similarly the role of chemotherapy in advanced bladder cancer, previously considered a refractory site, has been established. The effect of combination chemotherapy has prompted studies of invasive bladder cancer in an attempt to improve results of cystectomy alone and as an adjuvant to radiation therapy with emphasis on bladder preservation. The effect of bacillus Calmette Guerin on superficial bladder cancer is also producing exciting results.

The search for a cure for prostate cancer and tests to detect early-stage disease continues. There is a current trend to surgery, especially since Walsh described the nerve-sparing procedure that preserves potency in the majority of cases (131). However, what we now consider early stages (A and B) is frequently proven to have extracapsular extension (stage C) by the pathologist after radical prostatectomy. A recent consensus conference on prostate cancer concluded that radiation therapy and radical prostatectomy were competitive, definitive modalities for early-stage disease. The problem in selecting patients for surgery who will not have unfavorable features, and the role of post-operative irradiation in this subset needs to be defined. However, much work remains to demonstrate convincingly cures in this disease, which has a broad natural history.

Renal cell cancer always has been considered one of the cancers most resistant to chemotherapy and a worthy opponent for any new agent. The excitement in treatment of this cancer comes from studies using biologic response modifiers. It is hoped the early results and clues with interferon (IFN), interleukin-2 (IL-2), and vaccines can lead to further innovative strategies and a breakthrough in successful treatment.

Equally important to advances in multimodal therapy are the diagnostic advances used in urologic oncology. Detection, diagnosis, and the staging of genitourinary malignancies have undergone dramatic changes. Refinement of mag-

netic resonance imaging (MRI) and computerized tomography (CT) technologies has allowed accurate diagnosis and determination of tumor and extent of renal, bladder, and prostate cancer. The most exciting advances have occurred in screening for prostatic cancer, in which transrectal ultrasound has detected twice as many cancers as did digital examination and the use of fine needle, automatic-firing biopsy gun under ultrasound guidance permits acquisition of multiple biopsy specimens on an outpatient basis with low morbidity and high accuracy. Tumor markers have great potential, both for diagnosis and monitoring response. Treatment of urologic cancers is in the forefront, with the wide use of a radioimmunoassay for prostate-specific antigen (PSA). An elevated PSA may be an indication for prostate biopsy. Human chorionic gonadotrophin (hCG) B subunit and a-fetoprotein (AFP) currently are used for monitoring tumor response in selected testicular cancers. PSA is used for early detection of recurrence in prostate cancers after radical prostatectomy or radiation therapy. These three markers are essential for best tumor management.

Neoplasms in the urinary tract and in the male genital tract are among the most commonly encountered malignancies. It is estimated that they will account for approximately 33% of new cancer cases in the male in 1992 (1a). All modes of cancer therapy are used in the care of patients with these neoplasms, including hormones and chemotherapy. A collaborative approach to diagnosis and therapy is essential if optimal care and maximum survival are to be realized. These goals are best achieved by accurate pretreatment tumor staging.

KIDNEY CANCER

EPIDEMIOLOGY AND ETIOLOGY

Epidemiology (1a)

1. It is estimated that 26,500 cases of kidney cancer will be diagnosed in the United States in 1992. The male:female ratio is 1.6.
2. During this same period, 10,700 patients will die of renal cancer for an incidence:death ratio of 2.5, reflecting the grave prognosis in most cases.

419

3. The disease is uncommon before age 40 years (the average age at time of diagnosis is 55 to 60 years).

Etiology (31)

1. Renal cancer has been said to be associated with a number of environmental factors, but the most convincing is cigarette smoking.
2. Patients with von Hippel-Lindau syndrome are at increased risk for renal carcinoma, frequently bilateral.
3. The data for trace elements, e.g., cadmium and lead, and radiation exposure other than Thorotrast (an alpha emitter) are not strong. Low dietary intake of vitamin A has been implicated.

Biology

The data generated by chromosomal analysis of renal cancer patients suggest that lesions on the short arm of chromosome 3 (3p) are important (4a).

DETECTION AND DIAGNOSIS

Detection

1. *Presenting symptoms and signs*: The most frequent traditional presentations are hematuria (56%), pain (38%), palpable mass (36%), weight loss and fatigue (27%), fever (11%), varicocele (2%), and incidental (6%). It is not uncommon for renal carcinoma to be diagnosed incidently due to the more frequent use of ultrasound and CT and MRI scans for other regions.
2. *Metastases*: Other presentations may be signs and symptoms related to metastases to lung, mediastinum, bone, skin, liver, and brain (29,40).

   Unusual metastatic sites include iris, epididymis, gallbladder, nailbed, and corpus cavernosum (40).

3. *Paraneoplastic signs*: Renal cell carcinoma has been referred to as the "internist's cancer" since it can be quite indolent, with no traditional localizing symptoms or signs. Indeed, 30% of patients may have associated paraneoplastic syndromes, including: (a) anemia, (b) erythrocytosis, (c) thrombocytosis, (d) hypertension, (e) hypercalcemia, (f) gynecomastia, (g) Cushing's syndrome, (h) nephrotic syndrome, (i) amyloidosis, (j) polymyositis, and (k) dermatomyositis and hepatic dysfunction without metastases (Stauffer's syndrome) (14,40).

Diagnostic Procedure

1. *Urinalysis* will demonstrate red blood cells in over half the cases, but this is hardly specific.
2. Currently, *urine cytology* is also performed, but the yield for renal cell carcinoma is much less than for bladder carcinoma.
3. *Intravenous pyelogram* (IVP) has long been the traditional method for detecting mass lesions in the kidney and continues to be used frequently. The test does not differentiate cystic lesions from solid tumors well and depends on good bowel preparation to maximize its usefulness. The presence of mottled central calcifications or peripheral calcifications are more suggestive of a solid mass lesion than a cyst.
4. *Ultrasound* is most helpful in differentiating a cystic lesion from a solid tumor.
5. *CT* scan is currently the most sensitive and specific test available (90% accuracy) (10). With contrast enhancement, it readily distinguishes cysts from solid tumor accurately, and also helps with staging by defining capsular extension, nodal metastases, renal vein invasion, and bony and hepatic metastases (4) (Table 23-1).

Table 23-1. Imaging Methods for Evaluation of Carcinoma of the Kidney

METHOD	CAPABILITY	RECOMMENDED FOR USE
Primary tumor and regional nodes		
CT	Most useful test for TNM staging information	Always
MRI	Promising role for tumor detection and staging	Unknown
Ultrasound	Useful to exclude simple cysts and confirm solid tumor; limited staging information available, less sensitive and less specific than CT for tumor extent	Not usually
Urography	Best screening test available; limited ability for precise staging Lacks specificity	Yes
Arteriography	Limited diagnostic and staging information compared with CT. Arteriography is required for embolization therapy	No
Venography	Useful if CT indeterminate for renal vein/cava involvement	No
Biopsy -- (CT, US, fluoroscopy)	Percutaneous biopsy requires US, CT, or fluoroscopy. Open biopsy rarely needed. Not necessary for T stage confirmation May be useful to confirm metastases and determine operability	No
Metastatic		
Chest radiography	Limited usefulness unless tomography used for detection of metastases	Yes
Skeletal radiography	Limited usefulness except to confirm positive bone scan for metastases	No

CT = computed tomography; TNM = tumor, node, metastasis; MRI = magnetic resonance imaging; US = ultrasound.
Modified from Bragg (11).

6. *Renal angiography*: Prior to CT, this was the most frequently used test to evaluate a renal mass seen on IVP. It is still used occasionally to obtain information about vascular anatomy prior to surgery, or for renal artery embolization prior to nephrectomy in an attempt to reduce blood loss and operating time because renal carcinomas are extremely vascular (Table 23-1).

7. *MRI* is competitive with CT and gives similar if not more information, with a similar accuracy, 96%. It has the advantage of demonstrating vascular invasion better, of visualizing renal hilar nodes, and constructing images in the coronal and sagittal planes as well as in the transverse planes. Patients allergic to iodinated contrast media are ideal for MRI, as are those in whom CT was indeterminate. The disadvantages include higher cost, some degree of motion artifact, and poor definition of calcification (4).

8. *Biopsy*: fluoroscopic, ultrasound, or CT-guided.

CLASSIFICATION AND STAGING

Histopathology

The terms renal cell carcinoma, renal adenocarcinoma, clear cell carcinoma, hypernephroma, and Grawitz tumor are synonymous. Beside the clear cell variety, such tumors are granular and spindle cell (Table 23-2). They frequently arise in the cortex of the gland and are believed to originate from the proximal convoluted tubule cell. Approximately 45% are well differentiated, 36% moderately, and 18% poorly differentiated. Renal adenomas are believed to be small renal carcinomas. Other grading systems also have been used (15). Renal oncocytomas are benign adenomas also originating from the epithelium of the proximal tubule (15). Renal angiomyolipoma is a benign hamartoma consisting of fat, smooth muscle, and abnormal blood vessels (4). Cancers of the renal pelvis are transitional cell types, similar to cancers of the ureter, bladder, and urethra (Table 23-2).

Anatomic Staging

Table 23-3 and Fig. 23-1 show anatomic staging according to tumor, node, metastasis (TNM) classification. The T categories have been simplified and redefined based on tumor size, i.e., 2.5 cm. T1 and T2 are based on less than or more than 2.5 cm in size; T3 and T4 are now based on local extension of primary tumor. N category is defined as other sites, based on size: 2-5 cm, more than 5 cm metastases (M1). Any sign of

nodal disease reflects the potential for advancement, therefore T4 disease is similar to N1 and N2; N3 disease is equivalent to metastases.

Staging Work-up (15,40)

Staging tests are performed to assess local disease extent for surgical resection and to search for evidence of distant metastases. Laboratory tests aid in this differential, as well as provide data on renal function and possible paraneoplastic syndromes.

1. *Blood tests* include complete blood cell counts (CBC), differential and platelet count, blood urea nitrogen (BUN), creatinine, electrolytes, serum calcium, and liver enzyme measurements.

2. *CT* is the test of choice because it defines extrarenal extension, lymph node spread, and vascular invasion, as well as extension to surrounding abdominal structures.

3. *MRI* may eventually replace CT as the preferred procedure. MRI has a staging accuracy of 96% with no errors in assessment of venous and lymph node involvement. In a small study comparing CT and MRI, the latter proved to be superior (4). Tumor tissue is brighter and has a higher intensity signal than renal tissue on T2 images. Through coronal plane imaging, the renal vein and inferior vena caval invasion is better seen than on CT. The negative predictive value for venous invasion and surrounding organs is 98% and 99%, respectively. Iodinated contrast enhancement, however, is more cost effective and MRI is advised when CT is equivocal for venous organ involvement such as adrenal and lymph nodes.

4. *Ultrasound* (color flow Doppler ultrasound) may be useful for detecting presence of tumor thrombosis in renal vein and inferior vena cava. Ultrasonography also may be used to distinguish between a cystic or solid lesion.

5. *Chest x-ray* is certainly important in evaluating a common site of metastasis. CT of the chest is increasingly used because it is more sensitive to small metastatic lesions.

6. *Bone scan* is performed only if the patient has bone symptoms or an elevated serum alkaline phosphatase.

7. *Optional tests* are renal arteriography and venacavagram. IVP is frequently the initial diagnostic test that leads to the detection of a renal mass.

PRINCIPLES OF TREATMENT

Multidisciplinary Treatment Decisions (Table 23-4)

The prognosis of renal cell carcinoma is related to tumor grade, the presence of perinephric fat invasion, renal vein-vena caval extension, regional node involvement, and distant metastases (32). These are more or less reflected in the staging tests. It has been repeatedly demonstrated that venous extension is less serious than node metastases (24). The kidneys are retroperitoneal organs with their own separate capsule. They are surrounded by fat and loose areolar tissue, which is enclosed in a specialized fascia termed renal fascia or Gerota's fascia. Although a cancer may penetrate the renal capsule into the fat, Gerota's fascia acts as another barrier to contain it. Typical stages at presentation are approximately stage I, 20% to 40%; stage II, 10% to 20%; stage III, 10% to

Table 23-2. Histologic Classification for Kidney Tumors	
	INCIDENCE (%)
Renal Parenchyma	
Adenocarcinoma (hypernephroma)	80-90
- Clear cell	
- Granular cell	
- Spindle cell	
Other	rare
Renal Pelvis	
Transitional cell	90
Squamous cell	7
Adenocarcinoma	<3

Table 23-3. TNM Classification and Stage Grouping for Kidney Tumors

TNM Classification		Stage Grouping			
	Stage				
T1 ≤ 2.5 cm/limited to kidney	**I**	Stage I	T1	N0	M0
T2 > 2.5 cm/limited to kidney	**II**	Stage II	T2	N0	M0
T3 a) Perinephric invasion	**IIIA**	Stage III	T1	N1	M0
b) Major veins			T2	N1	M0
T4 Invades beyond Gerota's	**IV**		T3a	N0, N1	M0
fascia			T3b	N0, N1	M0
		Stage IV	T4	Any N	M0
N1 Single ≤ 2 cm	**IIIB**		Any T	N2, N3	M0
N2 Single > 2 cm ≤ 5 cm,			Any T	Any N	M1
N3 Multiple ≤ 5 cm					
> 5 cm					

T = tumor; N = node; M = metastasis.
From AJC (1)/UICC (2).

20%; and stage IV, 30% to 50% (41). Both the primary and metastatic lesions are generally quite vascular, a fact of extreme importance to the surgeon. The natural history of this cancer is less broad and more predictable than prostate cancer, but three points are important: (1) spontaneous regression has been noted in this disease, but overall it is probably less than 1%; (2) recurrences may be quite late, as much as 30 years after initial "curative" nephrectomy (27); and (3) an occasional patient may live for some time even after metastatic disease has been found (40). These

observations have suggested host immune interaction, which is now being supported by response to biologic response modifiers.

Surgical resection is the only proven curative therapy for kidney cancer. Overall survival rates at 5 years are approximately 35% to 45% (39). A selection process in most series is based in part on the staging tests performed and medical operability. There has not been a recent surgical series based on systematic staging that included MRI or CT of the chest and abdomen.

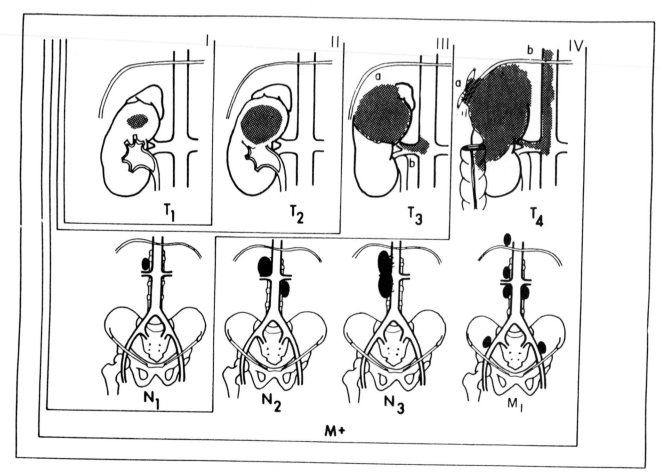

Fig. 23-1. Anatomic staging for renal carcinoma (see Table 23-3).

(6,32a)

Table 23-4.   Multidisciplinary Treatment Decisions by Stage for Kidney Tumors

Stage	Surgery	Radiation Therapy	Chemotherapy
$T_1 T_2 N_0$	Radical nephrectomy	NR	NR
$T_{3a} N_0$	Radical nephrectomy	ART, optional 50-55 Gy	NR
$T_{3b} N_0$	Radical nephrectomy	ART, optional 50-55 Gy	NR
$T_{any} N_1 N_2$	Radical nephrectomy includes involved veins	ART, optional 50-55 Gy	NR
T_{3b}, N_{1-3}	Radical nephrectomy includes involved veins	ART, optional 50-55 Gy	NR
$T_4 M_0$	Palliative resection for bleeding	PRT	IC II or IM
M_+	Resect if solitary	PRT	IC II or IM
Relapse	NR	NR, PRT	. NR

RT = radiation therapy; ART = adjuvant; PRT = palliative; NR=not recommended; IM = immunotherapy;   IC II = investigational chemotherapy, phase I/II clinical trials.

PDQ: NR - IC II and IM (or Interferon + Interleukin 2)

Surgery

1. The cornerstone of renal cancer treatment is radical nephrectomy—removal of the kidney and Gerota's fascia, using either a thoracoabdominal, transperitoneal, or extraperitoneal approach, depending on the experience of the surgeon, the location in the kidney, and the size of the tumor. Early ligation of the renal vein pedicle to preclude tumor embolization is a principle of the operation (7,35).

2. Lymphadenectomy unquestionably defines the extent of nodal metastases; however, convincing data to support improved survival in stages III and IV disease from a randomized trial are not available. Nevertheless, a limited lymphadenectomy is generally performed (19).

3. Some authors have advocated simple nephrectomy and even partial nephrectomy for smaller tumors (13). The operative mortality varies from 2% to 6% (19). As mentioned above, nodal metastases are more serious than renal-vein and vena cava extension. Cure rates with disease confined to the kidney and only venous extension benefit from removal of the tumor thrombus; survival in this subset approaches that of early-stage disease (24).

4. Nephrectomy also may be a palliative procedure for relief of pain or persistent bleeding requiring transfusions, mass effect on adjacent abdominal organs producing disabling symptoms, and heart failure from arterioventricular shunting within the tumor; however, most cases can be managed by conservative means.

5. Nephrectomy in the face of metastatic disease to promote spontaneous regression of distant metastases is mentioned only to be condemned. The chance of this happening is less than 1% and the surgical mortality in this setting is approximately 6%.

6. Bilateral carcinomas occur in 2% to 3% of cases (15,19). Conservative surgery on the less involved kidney is indicated in the form of a partial in vivo or ex vivo nephrectomy if possible; bilateral radical nephrectomy and dialysis are the alternatives.

7. Renal transplantation generally is not a good option because the immunosuppressive therapy may be associated with cancer recurrence (15).

8. In patients with bilateral Stage I neoplasms (concurrent or subsequent), bilateral partial nephrectomy or unilateral partial nephrectomy with contralateral radical nephrectomy when technically feasible may be a preferred alternative to bilateral nephrectomy with dialysis or transplantation (30a).

Radiotherapy

The role of radiotherapy has been investigated both in the preoperative setting and postoperatively in patients with unfavorable features, or as the sole modality.

Radiation dose: The radiation oncologist is handicapped in this area by the tolerance of the small bowel, stomach, liver, spinal cord, and opposite kidney and ultimately is able to administer a dose between 45 to 50 Gy. This is hardly enough for microscopic disease in most sites, and especially not for macroscopic or extensive disease. In general, it is ineffective as a sole curative modality. A number of authors have praised the effectiveness of radiation in this disease (8,34). However, randomized studies do not support its benefit.

Preoperative radiation:

1. Van der Werf-Messing administered 30 Gy in 3 weeks followed by nephrectomy and compared this with nephrectomy alone; there was no difference in survival, but local control was improved (43)

2. Juusela *et al*. (20) administered 33 Gy in 3 weeks in a similar study; the 5-year survival in the irradiated group was 47% versus 63% in the nephrectomy-only group, which was not significant.

Postoperative irradiation: Two randomized studies used postoperative radiation therapy versus nephrectomy alone. Finney (16) administered 55 Gy in 5-½ weeks and could not demonstrate improved survival or local control. Similarly, Kjaer *et al*. (22) treated patients with stages II and III disease to a total dose of 50 Gy in 2.5 Gy fractions at 4 fractions per week. A recent encouraging report from Israel claimed an improved 5-year and 10-year survival in those patients receiving postoperative irradiation, i.e., 50% and 40% with radiotherapy and 40% and 32% without radiotherapy, respectively (23). Again, adjuvant irradiation did not improve survival or local control; indeed, the complication rate in the combined arm prompted early closure of the study. One could argue that there still might be a role in some subsets of stages II and III patients who have been thoroughly staged with CT scans of the abdomen and chest, and bone scans, however, the above data are not encouraging (8,42). Certainly, radiation therapy may be effective for the relief of pain, and bone and central nervous system (CNS) metastases.

Chemotherapy

Hormones, especially progestational agents and androgens, have been tried as therapy in this disease for many years. Occasionally, one may see a dramatic improvement but, in general, the response rates are low and short-lived. Chemotherapy has had little impact. Active single agents include vinblastine and the nitrosoureas but there have been only 10% to 20% response rates. Numerous combinations have been tried, but none are better than single agents (12,44).

Immunotherapy

Immunologic approaches to the treatment of renal carcinomas have recently been successful, particularly in three categories (25) (Table 23-5).

IFN: This new class of drugs has been evaluated extensively and produces response in 15% to 20% of metastatic renal cancer cases. Patients most likely to respond are those with small pulmonary metastases and a good performance status (30).

IL-2 and lymphokine-activated killer (LAK) cells: When lymphocytes are cultured with the T-cell growth factor, IL-2, cell populations expand (LAK cells) that are cytotoxic for tumor cells but not for normal cells. When this unique lymphoid cell population is reinfused to patients along with IL-2, regression occurs in 16% to 33% of metastatic renal carcinoma patients (17).

Active specific immunotherapy with vaccines: For the purpose of inducing cell-mediated immunity directed at cell surface antigens of tumor cells, vaccines have been made from patients' tumor cells. Regression have been observed in 20% to 25% of patients (37).

Table 23-5. Response Rates of Renal Cell Carcinoma to Various Interferons, LAK Cells, IL-2

Interferon Type	Response Rate (%)
Hu IFN (Lc)	7—26
Hu IFN (Ly)	5—23
α A	18
rIFN-α	0—29
rIFN-ß	13
rIFNγ	35
LAK cells + IL-2	21

IFN = interferon; LAK = lymphokine-activated killer; IL-2 = interleukin-2.
From Linehan et al. (25), with permisson.

RESULTS AND PROGNOSIS

Results (Table 23-6) (25)

Table 23-6 and Fig. 23-2 summarize results and progress in improving 5- and 10-year survival rates by stage (6,21,25,36,39).

Stages I and I

Treatment for these stages is radical nephrectomy. Five- and 10-year survival rates vary from 50–90% to 20–65%. There does not appear to be any advantage for postoperative radiation therapy if the disease is truly pathologic stage I or stage II.

Stage III

Surgical resection is still the treatment of choice for this stage disease and it is important to appreciate that renal vein/

Table 23-6. Summary of Published Survival Rates in Renal Cell Carcinoma

Year	Length of Survival (years)	Survival (%) by Stage				
		I	II	III	IV	Ref
1969	5	66	64	42	11	36
	10	60	67	38	0	
1971	5	65	47	51	8	39
	10	56	20	37	7	
1979	5	56	100	50	8	7
	10	20	66	25	0	
1981	5	67	51	34	14	27
	10	56	28	20	3	
1982	5	—	—	0-53	0	13
	10	—	—	—	—	
1983	5	93	63	80	13	38
	10	—	—	—	—	
1985	5	91-100	—	—	18	5
	10	—	—	—	—	
1986	5	88	67	40	2	18
	10	66	35	15	—	

Adapted from Linehan et al. (25).

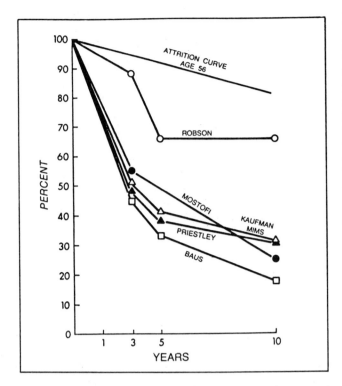

Fig. 23-2. Crude survival curves of several large series of renal carcinomas, treated surgically and followed-up for 10 years: Robson (36); Kaufman and Mims (21); Priestley (33a); Mostofi (29); the British Association of Urologic Surgeons (BAUS) (33a). From Kaufman and Mims (21), with permission.

inferior vena cava involvement has a better prognosis than does nodal spread (60% and 20%, respectively, at 5 years) (13,24). Should postoperative radiation therapy be given in these cases (25) (Table 23-7)? The controversy arises and continues if unfavorable features are found such as residual disease in the fossa, extension into the perinephric fat microscopically, adjacent nodal metastases, renal vein extension, transection of tumor during the surgery, or tumor spillage. There is no evidence that postoperative irradiation improves survival (16,22), but some argue that it is indicated based on improved local control (8,42). Adjuvant medroxyprogesterone in a randomized study of 136 M0 patients who underwent nephrectomy did not improve survival (33).

Stage IV

When the disease is advanced prognosis is dismal. Untreated patients have less than 5% survival at 3 years. A recent series of patients with metastatic disease (not necessarily from initial diagnosis) had a 48% survival at 1 year and 9% at 5 years. Disease-free interval, performance status, prior nephrectomy, and lung as the only site of metastasis were important prognostic factors (18,26). There is no standard therapy for this stage and hormonal therapy and chemotherapy are generally ineffective. Radiation therapy is used frequently for palliation when metastases occur in bone or brain and occasionally elsewhere (8). Biologic response modifiers are currently the most exciting strategy, but their final role is yet to be defined (12).

CLINICAL INVESTIGATIONS (24)

1. Biologic response modifiers are under investigation, more often in combination with each other than with chemotherapeutic agents, which are generally ineffective alone.
2. A widely tested combination, IL-2 and interferon alpha, is active but toxic (28). Lower doses can detoxify the regimen but also produce lesser response rates.
3. One confounding factor is spontaneous regressions can occasionally occur; one prospective surveillance series of 73 patients with advanced renal cell cancer illustrates this (30b).

BLADDER CANCER

EPIDEMIOLOGY AND ETIOLOGY

Epidemiology

It is estimated that there will be 51,600 new cases of bladder cancer diagnosed in the United States in 1992, 75% of which will be in males. The male predominance probably reflects exposure to industrial carcinogens and higher incidence of smoking. The expected cancer deaths from this disease during this same year will be 9,500 for an incidence:death ratio of 5.4 (1a). Most cases occur in the 50- to 70-year-old age group.

Etiology

Bladder cancer has been associated with a number of environmental factors including smoking, chemicals (especially ß-

Table 23-7. Treatment Results With and Without Adjuvant Radiation Therapy for Renal Cell Carcinoma

	5-YEAR SURVIVAL		
	Nephrectomy	Nephrectomy + RT	Reference
Preoperative RT	50	45	43
	63	47	20
Postoperative RT	44	36	16
	62	38	22

RT = radiation therapy.
From Linehan et al. (25), with permission.

naphthylamines, by-products of the aniline dye industry), metabolic defect in tryptophan metabolism, and infections (schistosomiasis) (85).

DETECTION AND DIAGNOSIS

Detection

The most frequent presentations of bladder cancer are:
- painless, microscopic or gross hematuria with or without clots, or dark urine resembling tea;
- urinary tract infections
- irritative symptoms such as urinary frequency, dysuria, and urgency (which usually signifies detrusor muscle involvement)

Obstructive symptoms are uncommon. Since only 5% of patients present with distant metastases, weight loss, fever, bone pain, or signs related to pulmonary or hepatic metastases are unusual.

Diagnostic Procedures (Table 23-8)

1. Diagnosis of bladder cancer is based on cytoscopy and transurethral biopsy of the bladder tumor (TURBT).
2. Urine cytology is often a helpful clue to diagnosis but only bladder biopsy localizes the disease. There is now renewed interest in urinary cytology and flow cytometric examination (to determine degree of aneuploidy) of bladder washings for detection of this disease.
3. There are rarely any physical findings to suggest this disease.
4. An abnormality seen on an IVP or CT scan of the abdomen will reveal a bladder-filling defect, leading to the diagnosis.
5. It is also not uncommon to find bladder cancer incidentally in patients being evaluated for prostate cancer.

CLASSIFICATION AND STAGING

Histopathology

For the most part, all bladder cancers are transitional cell carcinomas. Other less frequent types include squamous cell, adenocarcinomas, and sarcomas (Table 23-9).

Based on their degree of differentiation, bladder cancers traditionally have been graded as grade 1 (well differentiated); grade 2 (moderately well differentiated); and grade 3 (poorly differentiated). Broder initially described four grades, based on the degree of anaplasia and mitotic activity, but since grades 3 and 4 behave similarly, these three grades are most often used (85).

Table 23-8. Imaging Methods for Evaluation of Bladder Cancer

METHOD	CAPABILITY	RECOMMENDED FOR USE
Primary tumor and regional nodes		
CT	Sensitive to local invasion if macroscopic	No; only preoperatively
MRI	Provides three-dimensional view; limited for macroscopic	No
Ultrasound	Urothelial screening examination	Yes
Cystography	May demonstrate fixation of bladder wall, but insensitive to minimal invasion	No
(Transurethral) sonography	Capable of imaging local invasion	As alternative to CT
Retrograde ureteropyelography	Screens urothelium, evaluates suspicious urographic lesions	Yes
Percutaneous needle aspiration	Documents presence and character of tumor detected by other methods	Selected patients
Metastatic		
Chest imaging		
Plain films	Capable of detecting large lesions; preoperative screening technique	Yes
Radionuclide studies		
Bone scan	Sensitive to skeletal metastatses	No; only in patients clinically at risk for widespread metastases
Liver-spleen scan	Sensitivity for large intrahepatic metastases	No
Bone films	May document skeletal metastases (complements bone scan)	Only to document lesions detected by radionuclide scanning

CT = computed tomography; MRI = magnetic resonance imaging.
Modified from Bragg (11).

Table 23-9. Histologic Classification of Bladder Tumors

	INCIDENCE (%)
Papilloma	
Transitional cell carcinoma	
Grade 1 invasive papillary	85
Grade 2 in situ, papillary	
in situ, papillary/flat	
Grade 3 invasive	
Squamous cell carcinoma	
In situ	
Grade 1 invasive	10
Grade 2 invasive	
Grade 3 invasive	
Adenocarcinoma	
Carcinomas of mixed histologic types	
In situ	5
Invasive	
Undifferentiated carcinoma	
Sarcoma	<1

Anatomic Staging

The two most frequent staging systems are TNM and American Urologic System (2) (Table 23-10). Fig. 23-3 provides an anatomic diagram according to TNM classification. This is essentially a surgical-pathologic staging system. The differences in depth of invasion need either deep biopsies or cystectomy and radical nodal dissection to sample tissues adequately. The T categories are redefined but require endoscopic biopsy of tissue and reassessment by groups. N staging is similar to other systems. Lymph node metastases incidence by stage is presented in Table 23-11 (74).

Staging Work-up (Table 23-8)

1. *Cystoscopic examination*: The most important test is undoubtedly the cystoscopic examination with biopsy of any abnormalities, deep biopsies when appropriate to evaluate muscle invasion, random biopsies to evaluate for carcinoma in situ (CIS), bimanual palpation before and after removal of tissue to determine if stage T2 or T3, and bladder washings for flow cytometry and cytology. Careful mapping of the area diagrammatically is important for treatment planning and response/progression follow-up.

2. *IVP* is used to determine obstruction of the ureters, local extension, lymph node involvement, or other tumors of the pelvocalyceal system or ureters.

3. *Pelvic/abdominal CT scans* are helpful to search for nodal metastases, obstructed ureters, and bony and hepatic metastases. CT is limited in its ability to accurately assess depth of invasion or extent of perivesical invasion—it has an accuracy of 40% to 83% for distinguishing transmural intravesical lesions (T2 and B) from perivesical fat invasion (T3 or C). This test is neither very helpful in determining the extent of bladder wall penetration nor very sensitive to nodal metastases.

4. *MRI* is more accurate in bladder-wall invasion assessment, with an accuracy reaching 85% to 94%. Although it does not distinguish T1 versus T2 or A versus B, that is, mucosal versus muscle invasion, it improves assessment of deeper invasive lesions (T3 or C), tumor into perivesical fat is a diminished signal on T1-weighted image or adjacent viscera such as seminal vesicles, rectum, and adjacent muscles of pelvic wall (T4 or D). The sensitivity is 66% for fat invasion and 44% for organ involvement, but specificity is 100% and overall accuracy is 60%.

5. *Ultrasound* can detect tumors larger than 1.5 cm in 58% to 94% of cases; it is unreliable for staging. Transurethral ultrasound improves accuracy of diagnosis and staging, but further evaluation is needed.

6. *Lymph node assessment* with any of the three modalities, CT, MRI, or ultrasound, is disappointing until tissue characterization of cancerous versus normal nodes is realized. CT-guided needle biopsy of lymph nodes is advised for a high degree of certainty, but surgical assessment is the gold standard.

Table 23-10. TNM Classification, Stage Grouping, and American Urologic System for Bladder Tumors

	TNM Classification	American Urologic System	Stage Grouping			
Tis	In situ: "flat tumor"	0				
Ta	Papillary non-invasive	0	Stage 0	Tis	N0	M0
T1	Subepithelial connective tissue	A		Ta	N0	M0
T2	Superficial muscle (inner half)	B1	Stage I	T1	N0	M0
T3	Deep muscle or perivesical fat		Stage II	T2	N0	M0
T3a	Deep muscle (outer half)	B2	Stage III	T3a	N0	M0
T3b	Perivesical fat	C		T3b	N0	M0
T4	Prostate, uterus, vagina, pelvic wall, abdominal wall	D1	Stage IV	T4	N0	M0
				Any T	N1, N2, N3	M0
N1	Single ≤ 2 cm			Any T	Any N	M1
N2	Single > 2 cm ≤ 5 cm, multiple ≤ 5 cm	D2				
N3	> 5 cm					

T = tumor; N = node; M = metastasis.
Adapted from UICC (2a) / AJC (1).

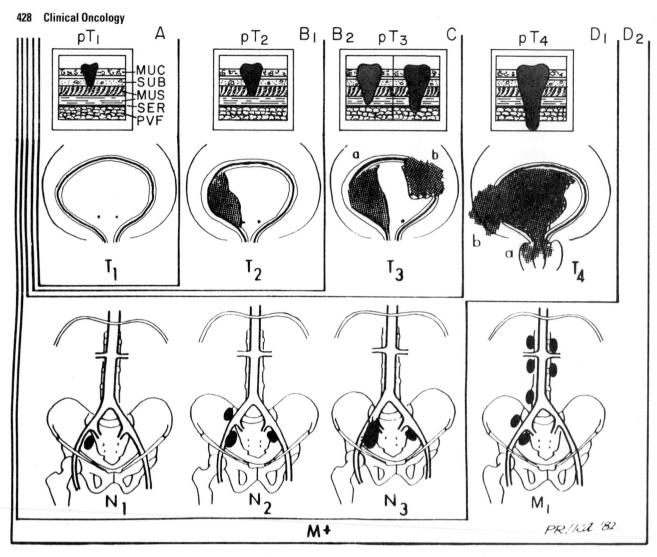

Fig. 23-3. Anatomic staging for bladder carcinoma (see Table 23-10).

7. *Bone scans, chest x-rays, chest CT scans, and blood test* that includes complete blood cell count (CBC), differential, blood urea nitrogen (BUN), creatinine, calcium, alkaline phosphatase to assess the amount of blood loss, renal function, and the common sites of metastases, which include the lung, bone, and liver are done. There are no good biochemical markers of bladder cancer.

PRINCIPLES OF TREATMENT

Multidisciplinary Treatment Decisions (Table 23-12)

Although bladder cancer was defined according to the above staging system, a more useful clinical stratification for treatment purposes is (1) superficial, (2) invasive, and (3) metastatic disease. At presentation approximately 75% of cases are superficial (tumor in situ [TIS], Ta, T1), 20% are invasive (T2, T3a, T3b, T4), and 5% are metastatic (86).

Superficial bladder cancer, that is, disease confined to the mucosa, is a heterogeneous entity, as suggested by the staging system. At the time of presentation, approximately 70% are Ta, 30% T1, and less than 10% TIS. These cancers are usually low grade (1 and 2), rarely become invasive (10%), but locally recur in approximately 50% of cases within 6 to 12 months; but most importantly, recurrences for the most part are the same low stage and grade. Besides grade and stage, the

Table 23-11. Incidence of Lymph Node Metastases by Stage

Stage	Patients with Lymph Node Metastases (%)
T0	0
Tis	11
T1	9
T2	25
T3a	61
T3b	41
T3	50
T4	60

From Skinner (74), with permission.

Table 23-12. Multidisciplinary Treatment Decisions by Stage for Bladder Tumors (68a,90)

Stage	Surgery	Radiation Therapy	Chemotherapy
T1 N0 0, A	Transurethral resection	NR Rarely when multiple DRT 60 Gy	Recurrent, multiple intravesical chemotherapy or immunotherapy (BCG)
T2 N0 B1 Low grade	Segmental cystectomy	Interstitial implantation	NR
T2 N0 B1 High grade	Radical cystectomy and/or Ileal loop	ART preop 20-45 Gy DRT, 60-70 Gy	MAC, CCR
T3a N0 B2 T3b N0 C	Radical cystectomy or Ileal loop	ART preop 45-50 Gy or DRT, 60-70 Gy	MAC, CCR
T4 N1,2,3 D1	Ileal diversion	PRT	MAC, CCR
Relapse	Surgical salvage for RT failure	RT for surgical failure	IC III

RT = radiation therapy; DRT = definitive; ART = adjuvant; PRT = palliative; RCT = recommended chemotherapy; CCR = concurrent chemotherapy and radiation; MAC = multiagent chemotherapy; IC III = investigational chemotherapy, phase II/III clinical trials.
PDQ: RCT - MAC/CCR - MVAC or MCV with RT 60 Gy or IC III - M-VAC, MEV, CisPt

degree of multicentricity and amount of CIS present are important predictors of the natural history. For example, Ta disease is usually grade 1 (95%), unifocal (66%), and has a local recurrence rate of 30% for a single focus, as compared with 65% if multifocal. Stage T1 disease is also unifocal (66%) but usually of higher grade (60% to 75% grade 2 and 24% to 40% grade 3). Recurrence for T1 disease is 50% if single focus and 70% when multiple . Extensive TIS, on the other hand, is a more serious finding because of the 85% local recurrence rate, but more importantly because of a 30% chance of becoming invasive, compared with Ta and T1 of a 5- to 10-year rate of progression to invasive disease (56,81,85). Hence, most patients with superficial bladder cancer will not die of their disease but have it controlled for long periods or cured with local therapies. One often speaks of "field changes" in the entire urothelium (urethra, bladder, ureters, and renal pelvis) and there is always the possibility, though low, of similar cancers developing in these other sites.

Invasive bladder cancer implies extension of cancer into the detrusor muscle and frequently subclinical metastatic disease because 50% of these patients die of distant metastases. The bladder does not have a serosa as such and disease invading the muscle does not encounter a significant barrier to retard spread into the fat, nodes, and surrounding structures.

The vagaries of clinical diagnostic staging in bladder cancer are obvious. How accurately determined is T2, T3a, T3b disease? Certainly, there are sites in the bladder that do not lend themselves to palpation even under anesthesia, and "deep" biopsies have to be deep enough to obtain muscle tissue, but not so deep as to produce perforation. In addition, our current noninvasive staging tests (CT and MRI) are not sensitive to these staging nuances. Hence the reason for placing all stages under the rubric of "invasive bladder cancer" for purposes of discussion and treatment; however, the problems with interpretation of the data must be considered. When surgical staging (not TURBT but radical cystectomy) and clinical staging are compared, approximately 40% of patients were understaged (pathologic stage > clinical stage), 20% were overstaged (pathologic stage < clinical stage), and

35% retained the same stage (pathologic stage - clinical stage) (69).

Table 23-12 presents a concise review of multidisciplinary treatment decisions by stage.

Surgery

1. The standard operations for bladder cancer are TURBT or radical cystectomy, which in males means a cystoprostatectomy and in females an anterior vaginectomy and anterior pelvic exenteration with the cystectomy.
   - TURBTs are obviously most helpful for localized, superficial bladder cancer.
   - partial cystectomy has been replaced by radical cystoprostatectomy by most urologists because it is a better cancer operation, removing en bloc any cancer and surrounding tissue.
2. Obviously, urinary diversion follows pari passu and is most often accomplished by implanting the ureters in an ileal loop; however, continent diversions that obviate an external appliance are gaining more acceptance, such as Kock pouch, or the Gilchrist or Camey procedures. Partial cystectomy for bladder cancer is now rarely performed and is only satisfactory in very limited situations.
3. Complications of radical cystectomy include impotence and the psychologic trauma and inconvenience of a ileal loop (85).

Radiation Therapy

Like surgery, radiation therapy is a modality for localized disease. As in so many other sites where radiation therapy and surgery are compared for effectiveness, exact comparisons have been fraught with difficulty because our noninvasive tests to define the disease extent are imprecise; hence we are frequently comparing clinical staging results for radiation therapy with pathologic staging results for surgery (86).

1. Definitive, high-dose radiation, local control results for invasive bladder cancer stage for stage are usually inferior to surgery by approximately 20%. Some of this

difference is accounted for by the difference between clinical and pathologic staging, but perhaps more important is the "field effect" of the cancer that irradiation cannot effectively control long term. Obviously, removal of the bladder removes the field, and prevents recurrence. Local failure rates after partial cystectomy also address this concept.

2. Radiation therapy is most often administered externally with high-energy accelerators. Interstitial irradiation, popularized by van der Werf Messing in Holland (83), has not been used often in the United States.

3. Intraoperative irradiation also has been used in an attempt to reduce injury to normal structures (62). Doses of external irradiation are in the 6000 to 6500 cGy range given in 180 cGy fractions.

4. Complications primarily include radiation proctocystitis. If the entire bladder is in the high-dose volume, bleeding fibrosis and contractures may negate the reservoir function of the bladder and necessitate cystectomy on this ground in about 5% to 10% of cases.

Drug Therapy (Table 23-13) (49a,55a,89,90)

1. *Superficial bladder cancer* is currently treated by intravesical drugs or biologics. Historically, thiotepa was one of the first agents used. More recently, mitomycin C and doxorubicin have been used. Lately however, bacillus Calmette-Guerin has been quite popular because of higher complete response (CR) rates (70%) in therapeutic situations and also, when given prophylactically, it reduces recurrences and progression to invasive disease (57a). Intravesical therapy is accomplished by instilling a certain amount of drug into the bladder through an urethral catheter and draining it out 1 to 2 hours later. This procedure is repeated every week, generally for a total of 4 to 8 weeks. Therapy is then continued monthly for 12 to 24 months in responding patients. Side effects include allergic reactions, bladder infection, irritability, and if the drug is absorbed and myelosuppressive (e.g., thiotepa), reduction in blood cell counts (56,81).

2. *Metastatic bladder cancer* was considered unresponsive to chemotherapy until recently. Cisplatin was one of the first agents to produce responses in patients with metastatic disease. Combination chemotherapy such as CMV, CISCA, and M-VAC have proven even more effective (78). Hormonal therapy currently plays no role in the management of bladder cancer.

Table 23-13. Combination Chemotherapy for Bladder Cancer

DRUGS	Response Rate (%)
Cisplatin combinations*	30
Methotrexate combinations*	29
Doxorubicin combinations*	17
Cisplatin + methotrexate	46
+ vinblastine (CMV)	56
M-VAC	67

* Combinations with cyclophosphamide, 5-FU, teniposide, bleomycin, vinca.

Adapted from Yagoda (89,90).

Treatment Decisions by Stage (Table 23-12)

Superficial Disease

Disease confined to the bladder mucosa has been managed with local therapy, either by repeated TURBT with or without fulguration, or by intravesical therapy. Usually Tl, Ta or focal TIS disease can be managed with TURBT and careful follow-up with cystoscopy. Superficial multifocal Ta, Tl, or TIS disease, especially if higher grade, requires more comprehensive local therapy which is best accomplished with TURBT and intravesical chemotherapy or biologics. Typical responses to chemotherapy include 35% to 70% CR with local control in 50% of cases. Recurrences are the norm and repeated cycles of treatment may be necessary. Intravesical therapy also has been used prophylactically to reduce the recurrence rate and prevent progression to invasive disease. Transition to invasive bladder cancer and the risk of tumors developing in the ureters or urethra is not frequent, but is another reason for close monitoring. Rarely, cystectomy may be indicated for superficial disease, especially TIS, if disease persists despite repeated attempts at eradication (56,81).

Invasive Bladder Cancer

Treatment strategies for invasive bladder cancer include: (a) radical cystectomy; (b) definitive irradiation; (c) preoperative irradiation; (d) postoperative irradiation; (e) chemotherapy followed by cystectomy; and (f) chemotherapy followed by irradiation. There are a variety of identifiable prognostic factors: stage, grade, tumor size, tumor configuration (papillary versus solid), ureteral obstruction, vascular invasion, anemia, and age.

1. The standard treatment remains *radical cystoprostatectomy*. As mentioned above, approximately 50% of patients with this disease (T2, T3a, T3b) will die of metastatic disease within 2 years, indicating occult distant spread at diagnosis. The 5-year survival with surgery alone is approximately 50%, with pathologic stage T2 doing better (60%), and pathologic stage T3a doing worse (30%). Local recurrences after surgery are less than 10% (85,87).

2. *Adjuvant preoperative radiation therapy*: Radiation therapy for invasive bladder cancer has been used adjuvantly by administering it preoperatively to improve surgical results (71,72). Underlying the concept of adjuvant preoperative radiation therapy is the hope that this strategy could downstage (pathologic stage < clinical stage) the disease, (for example, convert T3a to T2), as determined by the disappearance of palpable disease on examination under anesthesia, or no disease found in the pathologic specimen. Only one of three randomized studies demonstrated a benefit for this strategy over surgery alone (77). There is a belief that this strategy may be helpful for T3a stage patients *who respond to irradiation*, but it is currently impossible to define this favorable group preoperatively. Two different fractionation schemes have been used in the preoperative setting: (1) 2,000 cGy in five fractions with surgery to follow within 5 to 7 days, and (2) a conventional dose of radiation for microscopic disease (4500 cGy) administered at 180 to 200 cGy per fraction, with surgery to follow in approximately 4 weeks. When all invasive cancer is combined in series comparing surgery versus

preoperative radiation therapy, no improvement in local control or overall disease-free survival has been shown as one might expect with the stage heterogeneity and high rate of subclinical metastatic disease at presentation (67,77,85).

3. *Postoperative radiation therapy* has its advocates, and as in other sites the strongest argument has been tailoring treatment strategies to the precise pathologic stage. Most oncologists would agree that pT2 patients, grade 2 or less, have an excellent chance for cure, and hence do not require any more treatment. On the other hand, patients with pT4 or any positive nodes will have little chance of improved survival with adjuvant irradiation, and therefore, should go on to chemotherapy. But patients with pT2, grade 3, or pT3a or pT3b disease could benefit from postoperative radiation therapy. There have been no controlled studies, however, to substantiate these claims (65).

4. *Definitive radiation therapy* for invasive bladder cancer produces 5-year overall survivals of 30%, with higher values for T2 disease (40%) and lower for T3a (10%) (72,84). Because of the high rates of local failures, in spite of doses in the range of 6000 to 6500 cGy, and concern about the tolerance of surrounding structures and bladder preservation, interstitial and intraoperative radiation therapy have been used. Van der Werf-Messing (83) used interstitial therapy, generally favoring cases with cancers no more than 5 cm in diameter, with low-grade histologies (1 and 2), without vascular invasion or ureteral obstruction, and medically operable. Patients were given three fractions of 360 cGy external irradiation, followed by surgery and an implant, then 3000 cGy of external irradiation. Results for T2 and T3 disease were comparable with surgery. Van der Werf Messing has recently suggested giving 4000 cGy external irradiation followed in a week by an implant to deliver the biologic equivalent of 6500 cGy in 7 days for T2, T3 cases with poor prognostic factors. A recent update of her results indicates a 5-year survival of approximately 80% (84). Intraoperative radiation therapy also reduces normal tissue side effects. By its very nature there is again a selection bias in that patients must be operable and the disease must be confined to the bladder at the time of surgery and easily encompassed within an electron cone that fits into the bladder. Intraoperative irradiation is not commonly available and it is difficult to know at this juncture the role it will play in future invasive bladder cancer management (55,62)

5. *Chemotherapy*: With the recent good results of chemotherapy in disseminated disease, chemotherapy is being used for invasive bladder cancer (74a). Currently, there is a national study treating all eligible patients with M-VAC chemotherapy for three cycles followed by radical cystoprostatectomy. The chemotherapy could impact on the subclinical metastatic disease as well as the invasive bladder cancer. Bladder response is determined by cystoscopy and cystectomy. The results of this study will be most interesting and will be the basis for future studies. Similarly, with emphasis on bladder preservation, there has been an attempt to integrate chemotherapy and radiation therapy. There is concern

within the radiation oncology community that doxorubicin would produce added side effects; thus the chemotherapy selected for study by the Radiation Therapy Oncology Group has been MVC in the same doses and schedule as M-VAC. After two cycles the patients receive 4000 cGy of external irradiation and cisplatin, followed by a markedly reduced field, to boost the bladder tumor with a margin only, to 6500 cGy. Patients are evaluated by cystoscopy with biopsy and washings at the end of MCV chemotherapy, and after cisplatin and 4000 cGy of irradiation. If active disease persists at this point, cystectomy is done. Marks *et al.* (61) have reported on a small number of patients treated in this manner but with short follow-up. Intra-arterial cisplatin also has been used with radiation therapy and surgery (51). Gentler alternatives are intravenous infusion 5-FU and mitomycin C combined with irradiation which produces impressive response rates (70).

Metastatic Disease (Table 23-13)

Perhaps one of the biggest recent advances in bladder cancer therapy has been the recognition that chemotherapy has a role. Without chemotherapy, patients with unresectable or metastatic disease had a 2-year survival of less than 10%. Studies (80,89,90) in patients with advanced disease (N+, M+) demonstrated that cisplatin and methotrexate were the most active single agents, producing average responses of 30%, but CRs of less than 5%. This led to further studies using combinations such as M-VAC, CMV and CISCA (or CAP). Overall responses of 50% to 70% have been observed with CRs in 20% to 40%. Nonresponders usually have a short median survival (< 6 months), and partial responders do better (12 months). On the other hand, some of those who achieve a CR with chemotherapy alone or with chemotherapy and surgery are surviving disease-free for more than 4 years. This is a remarkable achievement. Positive prognostic factors include good performance status, nodal versus metastatic disease, and transitional cell histology versus mixed transitional with squamous or adenocarcinoma (60,79).

RESULTS AND PROGNOSIS

Results in bladder cancer are a direct reflection of stage and histopathologic grade. Radical cystectomy is commonly used and has been combined with either preoperative or postoperative irradiation.

1. Survival after radical cystectomy is shown as a function of depth of invasion and grade (Table 23-14) (63,68,75,76): Low-grade carcinomas have a 70% to 80% 5-year survival versus 35% to 40% for high-grade cancers. Superficial cancers are often low grade and have similar survivals, whereas, deeper, invading cancers commonly have less than a 50% survival rate. Depth of invasion is more accurately determined by surgery (pathologic stage rather than T stage), with 5-year survival rates higher for surgical versus comparable clinical stage (i.e., p2, 83% to 88%, versus T2, 30% to 60%).

2. Survival after radiation: the 5-year survival results are lower than with cystectomy, related to the comparism of clinical versus pathologic staged patients. Radiation may allow for organ preservation (Table 23-15).

Table 23-14. Therapeutic Results for Radical Cystectomy for Invasive Bladder Cancer*

5-Year Survival as a Function of Pathologic Stage		5-Year Survival as a Function Grade and Depth of Invasion		
Pathologic Stage	Survival (%)			Survival (%)
P0 P1 CIS	71-83	Grade		
		1 and 2	(Low-grade)	70-85
P2	83-88			
		3 and 4	(High-grade)	35-40
P3A	57-69			
		Depth of Invasion		
P3B	29-40	Ta, T1	(Noninvasive)	60-85
		T2, T3	(Invasive)	30-60
P4	27-36			

* Patients grouped by pathologic stage.
Adapted from Mathur et al. (63), Skinner and Lieskovsky (75,76), and Pearse (68).

3. Combining surgery and radiation is associated with 5-year survival of approximately 50% (Table 23-16). There is a need for a biologic marker to predict outcome, especially for chemoradiation regimens. The use of 5-FU plus cisplatin infusion during irradiation appears to improve local control, but has not clearly impacted on survival (58). Rotman *et al.* report 74% CR for the combination of 5-FU with and without mitomycin C and overall 5-year survival of 39% and 53.6% by actuarial life-table method (70).

4. More aggressive chemotherapy combinations are yielding better results. In a randomized study by Daniel *et al.* (50) patients were randomized to four cycles of VAC postcystectomy with lymphadenectomy or observation yielding promising results of 70% versus 30% frequency following response at 3 years and median survival of 4.2 years versus 2.5 years, respectively. When M-VAC is compared with cisplatin alone in a large, intergroup, randomized study, the combination produced a better response rate (33% vs 9%) and a median survival of 12.7 months versus 8.7 months for advanced and recurrent disease (59). M-VAC prior to cystectomy and lymphadenectomy led to downstaging in 72% of patients, i.e., 50% CR and 22% p1s or p1. Survival correlates with response - 80% of patients with CR are alive at a median follow-up of 19.5 months. In a series of 40 patients with localized muscle-invasive bladder carcinomas treated by MCV (methotrexate, cisplatin, and vinblastine) and 4,000 cGy radiotherapy by Fung *et al.* (51a), the 3-year actuarial survival rates were for T2 patients (89%) and for T3-4 patients (50%). The cur-

rent chemoradiotherapy regimen may have beneficial effects in the treatment of muscle-invasive bladder carcinoma. The efficacy of neoadjuvant chemotherapy remains to be proven by ongoing randomized trials.

CLINICAL INVESTIGATIONS

1. Predictive assays: A search for a marker to determine response to chemoradiation combinations is essential for bladder preservation. Possible candidates are DNA ploidy, s-phase fraction (57,59).
2. Bladder preservative protocols: MVC + RT → Cis PT + RT is yielding high tumor clearance rates between 66%–79%, allowing for bladder preservation. Cystectomy was performed in only 11/42 (26%) of eligible patients in RTOG protocols.

PROSTATE CANCER

EPIDEMIOLOGY AND ETIOLOGY

Epidemiology (1a)

It is estimated that 132,000 cases of prostate cancer will be diagnosed in the United States in 1992 surpassing lung cancer in men. During this same time 34,000 men are expected to die of this disease, for an incidence:death ratio of 3.9. It accounts for 12% (and is the second leading cause) of all cancer deaths in males. Black Americans continue to be diagnosed at a more advanced stage, and therefore, their survival is lower than whites.

Table 23-15. 5-Year Survival as a Function of Stage for Bladder Cancer*

	5-Year Survival (%) by Stage	
Series (reference)	T2,T3	T4
Bloom et al (47)	25	-
Miller & Johnson (64)	20	13
Goffinet et al (52)	28	8
Morrison (66)	33	-
Greiner et al (54)	28	10
Blandy et al (46)	34	9
Goodman et al (53)	38	7
Shipley et al (71)	39	6
Quilty & Duncan (88)	26	

* Full-dose radiation (5000-7000 cGy).

Table 23-16. Results for Radiation Therapy and Radical Cystectomy for Invasive Bladder Cancer

Series (Reference)	Stage	Preoperative Radiation Therapy	5-Year Survival
Boileau (48)	T2, T3	5,000 cGy	50
Batata (45)	T3, T4	2,000 cGy	35
van der Werf Messing (82)	T3	4,000 cGy	52
National Bladder Cancer Group (71)	T2-T4	4,000 cGy	52

Etiology

The cause of carcinoma of the prostate is unknown; however, indirect evidence suggests a relationship to sex hormones. Prostatitis and benign prostatic hypertrophy are not considered harbingers of cancer.

DETECTION AND DIAGNOSIS

Detection (103,106)

The detection of prostate cancer has changed over the years. It is usually detected as follows:

1. It may be discovered as a nodule or area of induration on a routine rectal examination.
2. There may be obstructive symptoms whereupon rectal examination reveals an abnormality.
3. Transurethral resection of the prostate for purposes of relieving the obstruction reveals adenocarcinoma in the tissue chips.
4. The patient displays a systemic presentation such as unexplained weight loss, fever, fatigue, anemia, and/or bone pain; with x rays of the bone demonstrate osteoblastic or lytic lesions.
5. There is elevated PSA or acid phosphatase.

Other signs or symptoms of prostate cancer include hematuria, urinary infection, azotemia, and edema of the legs and genitalia.

Diagnostic Procedures (Table 23-17)

1. *Routine physical examination*: Digital examination remains the most reliable clue for a diagnosis of prostate cancer. The most frequent abnormalities are enlargement, induration, and nodularity; the latter two are most suggestive of cancer. The gland may palpate normally, however, and biopsy results may still be positive.
2. *Transrectal ultrasound (TRUS)*: Perhaps the most important test in recent years to aid in the diagnosis of prostate

Table 23-17. Imaging Methods for Evaluation of Carcinoma of the Prostate

METHOD	DIAGNOSIS AND STAGING CAPABILITY	RECOMMENDED FOR USE
Primary tumor and regional nodes		
CT	Capable of imaging local tumor volume and extension. Capable of imaging pelvic lymph node metastases	No; selected patients at risk for extracapsular and/or lymph node metastases
MRI	Unknown; early reports indicate capability of seeing normal prostatic capsule, and may detect intraglandular tumor	Unknown
Urography	Screens urinary tract for obstruction or coexistent abnormalities.	Yes
Transrectal sonography	Capable of assessing tumor stage	Yes; high specificity
Lymphangiography	Capable of assessing nodes in external iliac, commmon iliac, and para-aortic groups	No; selected patients at risk for nodal metastases may benefit
Percutaneous aspiration biopsy	Documents presence and character of tumors seen by other methods	No; selected patients only
Metastatic		
Chest films	Detect hematogenous or lymphatic spread	Yes
Bone films	Detect lytic, blastic, or mixed metastases in advanced disease	No; confirms and follows bone scan findings
Radionuclide studies:		
Bone scan	Detects early skeletal metastases	Yes
Liver-spleen	Detects liver metastases	No; low-yield study
PSA	Useful to monitor response and recurrence	Yes

CT = computed tomography; MRI = magnetic resonance imaging; PSA = prostatic-specific antigen.
Modified from Bragg (11).

cancer has been TRUS. Abnormalities generally appear as hypoechoic (75%) or isoechoic lesions. TRUS can image small cancers in peripheral zones of the gland (two thirds of cancers) and when complemented by TRUS-directed needle biopsy at hypoechoic defects has improved accuracy over digital examination. There is, however, a 40% to 60% range of false-positives and negatives due to prostatic hyperplasia. It must be appreciated that the test is highly user and equipment dependent, and has a higher degree of specificity than palpation. Although not considered reliable for screening, it has enhanced our ability to detect small lesions and guide needle biopsies (116).

3. *Needle biopsy*: The ultimate diagnosis of cancer of the prostate rests on a biopsy that reveals adenocarcinoma. This can be accomplished with a transrectal or percutaneous transperineal needle biopsy, transurethral resection of the prostate, or open surgical biopsy. The most popular approach is transrectal ultrasound-guided automatic-firing biopsy gun.

Once the diagnosis is established, the patient is then staged.

Locoregional spread: Tests for detecting disease spread outside the gland to the periprostatic tissues, seminal vesicles, pelvic and retroperitoneal lymph nodes, bladder, and rectum are not especially sensitive or specific.

4. *Cystoscopy* can evaluate extension into the bladder or urethra.

5. *CT and MRI scans of the pelvis/abdomen*: MRI is better able than CT to detect prostate cancer extensions and offer three-dimensional views. In addition, the scans detect enlarged nodes, a biopsy can then be done guided by these scans using fine needle aspirates.

6. *Surgical staging with laparoscopic lymph node biopsies, formal pelvic lymphadenectomy* or lymph node sampling is the most unequivocal method for detecting nodal spread and usually is performed as a prelude to a radical prostatectomy. Only lymph node sampling is capable of detecting microscopic disease. A lymph node 1 cm in diameter could contain as many as 1 billion cells, the limit of our current resolution with scans.

Distant spread is evaluated by other tests (103).

7. *A bone scan* is quite sensitive for detecting metastatic disease, antedating changes shown on plain x rays by 6 months or more. The false-negative percentage is approximately 5%. Since a positive bone scan represents increased blood flow to the bone or new bone formation, degenerative joint disease, rheumatoid arthritis, Paget's disease, osteomyelitis, traumatic fractures, and primary and benign tumors of bone must be excluded.

8. *Plain x rays* of the "hot spots" on the bone scan may detect blastic changes to improve specificity of bone scan, and exclude the other conditions.

9. *Chest films*: Although prostate cancer spreads most frequently to bones and abdominal lymph nodes, occasionally metastases to the lungs or mediastinum occur. Therefore, a chest x ray is part of the metastatic work-up.

10. *Lymphangiography and IVPs* have been essentially replaced by contrast CT scans.

Over the years a variety of biochemical markers have been used with the hope of diagnosing and staging prostate cancer and for follow-up.

11. *Serum acid phosphatase (SAP)* was discovered in the 1930s to be elevated in this disease and has been subsequently extensively used. It is not specific for carcinoma but has some correlation with the tumor stage and grade.

12. *Prostatic acid phosphatase (PAP)* determined by radioimmunoassay was popular in the late 1970s. The assay detects that portion of total acid phosphatase produced by the prostate. It was once recommended as a screening test for carcinoma of the prostate but studies did not confirm its usefulness nor did it add much to acid phosphatase. Like acid phosphatase, elevation correlates to the disease stage: stage A, 7% to 14%; B, 21% to 30%; C, 23% to 64%; D1, 48% to 66%; and D2, 70% to 94% (129).

13. *PSA*: The search for the ideal prostate cancer tumor marker has now led to PSA. The test is based on a monoclonal antibody against prostate tissue. It was initially hoped that the antigen was specific for cancer; it is not, but is unique for prostate tissue. It is correlated with clinical stage related to tumor volume, and useful for monitoring response and recurrence. Stamey and Kabalin (129) found PSA elevated (>2.5 ng/mL) in clinical stages as follows: A-1, 38%; A-2, 57%; B, 95%; and C and D, 100%; the mean values and ranges increased with advancing stage. It can be elevated in benign prostatic hypertrophy (mean 24 ng/mL, range 9.5 to 44) and is more sensitive than PAP (128). The same authors noted that pelvic lymph nodes were negative if the PSA was less than 10 ng/mL; however, if the value was higher than 40 ng/mL, 63% of pelvic nodes were positive after surgical staging (128,129). It has proven valuable in follow-up after radical prostatectomy, radiation therapy, and hormonal manipulation.

All markers may be temporarily elevated after prostatic surgery, cystoscopy (1.5 to 4 times), catheterization, or needle biopsy (up to 134 times).

14. The issue of screening asymptomatic men for prostate cancer with tests other than digital rectal examination is controversial. Serum PSA and transrectal ultrasound are more sensitive and will increase the diagnostic yield of prostate cancer when used in combination with rectal exam. However, they are also associated with high false positive rates and may identify a greater number of medically insignificant tumors (97a).

STAGING AND CLASSIFICATION

Histopathology

Prostate cancers generally are adenocarcinomas. The rarer histologies are reviewed by Tannenbaum (130). Based on the degree of differentiation, they have traditionally been graded as grade 1 (well differentiated), grade 2 (moderately well differentiated), grade 3 (poorly differentiated).

After reviewing hundreds of cases from the Veterans Administration Cooperative Urologic Research Group, Gleason devised a system of grading based on "the degree of glandular differentiation and the growth pattern of the tumor in relation to the prostatic stroma" (Table 23-18) (Fig. 23-4) (104). He described five patterns and also noted that many cases had more than one pattern. The pattern that was most extensive was termed primary and the less prominent pattern

Table 23-18. Histologic Classification for Adenocarcinomas of the Prostate

		INCIDENCE (%)

GLEASON GRADING

Grade 1	Single, separate, uniform glands in close-packed masses with definite rounded limiting edges	
Grade 2	Single, separate, slightly less uniform glands, loosely packed. Definable but less sharp edge	
Grade 3A	Single, separate, very variable glands, may be closely packed but usually widely separated with ragged, poorly defined tumor edge	
3B	Like 3A but tiny glands or small cell clusters	
3C	Sharply and smoothly circumscribed, often rounded masses of papillary or loose cribriform tumor	
Grade 4A	Raggedly infiltrating "fused-glandular" tumor	
4B	Like 4A but large pale cells ("hypernephroid")	
Grade 5A	Sharply, smoothly circumscribed rounded masses of almost solid cribriform tumor, usually with some central necrosis ("comedocarcinoma")	
5B	Ragged masses of anaplastic carcinoma with only enough gland formation or vacuoles to insure that it is an adenocarcinoma	

Acinar adenocarcinoma	**95**
Transitional cell and ductal cell	**2**

Adapted from Gleason (104).

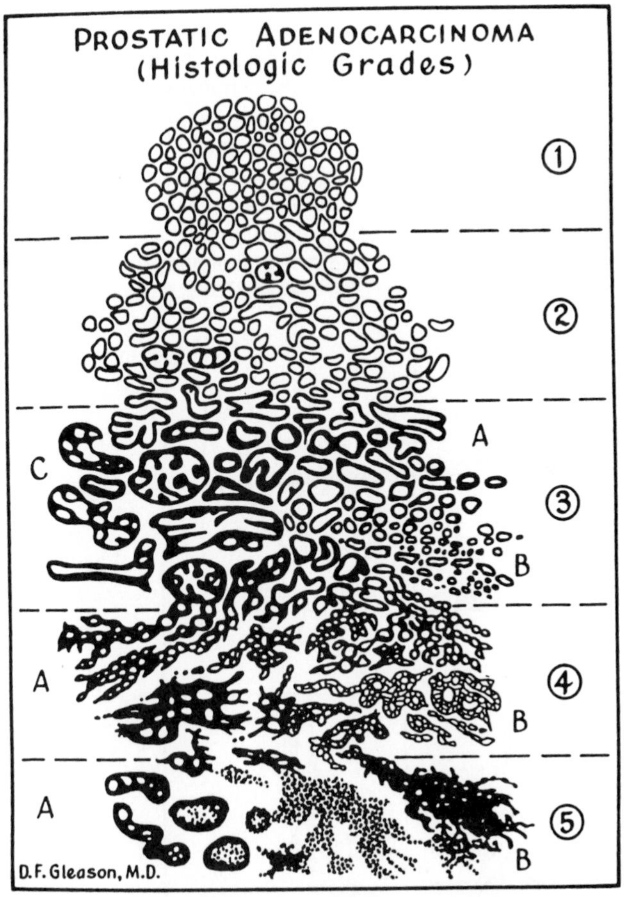

Fig. 23-4. Simplified outline drawing of histologic patterns, emphasizing degree of glandular differentiation and relation to stroma. All black in the drawing represents tumor epithelium and glands with no cytologic detail, except in 4B where tiny open structures represent clear "hypernephroid" cells. Modified from Gleason D.F. The Veterans Administration Cooperative Urological Research Group, In Urologic Pathology: The Prostate. Edited by M. Tannenbaum. Philadelphia, Lea & Febiger, 1977. Used with permission.

was termed secondary. He found there was better correlation with outcome if the patterns were added to give a "Gleason score" with a range from 2 to 10. Some investigators have assumed correlation to the other grading system: well-differentiated—usually Gleason grade 2 to 4; moderately well differentiated—Gleason grade 5 to 7; and poorly differentiated—7 to 10 Gleason score; although this is tidy, it may not be accurate. There still is controversy among pathologists as to the best grading system.

Anatomic Staging

The two most frequent staging systems used are the Jewett and TNM International Union Against Cancer (UICC). TNM classification is shown in Table 23-19 (2), and anatomic staging is illustrated in Fig. 23-5. The major difference between T1 and T2 (stages A and B) is presence of a nonpalpable versus a palpable nodule. Note the similar staging for bilateral spread as seen in T1a and T2a categories. Nodal staging is based on size for advancement for N1 and N2 to N3 and juxtaregional, common iliac, para-aortic and/or inguinal nodes (N4) are now M1 in metastatic. The American Joint Committee for Cancer Staging(1)/UICC(2) stage grouping is too complex and will probably not be used because it subdivides stages and compounds the issue by adding histopathologic grading, which are not Gleason categories. Instead, The American Urologic Association Cancer Staging is made equivalent to TNM categories.

Staging Work-up (103) (Table 23-17)

The stage correlates with prognosis and a staging work-up aids in the selection of treatment strategies. Determinations of CBC and differential, BUN, creatinine, alkaline phosphatase (usually included in sequential multiple analysis-12), as well as PSA should be done. The current recommended staging tests include:

1. *Rectal examination* to define local extent.
2. *Transrectal ultrasound* for local extension has a sensitivity approaching 90% and a specificity of 95%. For extracapsular penetration, overall accuracy is 90% but

Table 23-19. TNM Classification, Stage Grouping, and American Urologic System for Prostate Tumors

	TNM Classification	American Urologic System		Stage Grouping			
T1	Incidental	A					
T1a	≤ 3 foci	1	* Stage 0	T1a	N0	M0	G1
T1b	> 3 foci	2		T2a	N0	M0	G1
T2	Clinically or grossly, limited to gland	B	* Stage I	T1a	N0	M0	G2,3-4
				T2a	N0	M0	G2,3-4
T2a	≤ 1.5 cm	1	* Stage II	T1b	N0	M0	Any G
T2b	> 1.5 cm/ > one lobe	2		T2b	N0	M0	Any G
T3	Invades prostatic apex/beyond	C	* Stage III	T3	N0	M0	Any G
	capsule/bladder neck/seminal	1	* Stage IV	T4	N0	M0	Any G
	vesical/not fixed	2		Any T	N1, N2, N3	M0	Any G
T4	Fixed or invades other adjacent structures			Any T	Any N	M1	Any G
N1	Single ≤ 2 cm	D1					
N2	Single > 2 cm ≤ 5 cm, multiple ≤ 5 cm						
N3	> 5 cm						
M1		D2					

* new category
T = tumor; N = node; M = metastasis.
Adapted from UICC (2).

this is not universally agreed because detection of critical seminal vesicle invasion is only 77%.

3. *CT* is capable of distinguishing intracapsular disease (T2 and B) from the more extensive extracapsular penetration (T3 and T4 or C and D) with detection of seminal vesicle asymmetry and alteration of peripelvic fat planes. However, a significant false-negative and false-positive rate exists for the latter findings. CT scans of the pelvis and abdomen to evaluate pelvic and para-aortic adenopathy, evidence of hydronephrosis and, indirectly, renal function, bladder and/or rectal invasion, and extension into the seminal vesicles, are used more frequently. (CT is also useful for treatment planning if radiation therapy is selected.)

4. *MRI* has an 80% to 90% accuracy rate in prostatic cancer staging when multiplanar imaging is done with T2-weighted images that can identify signal alteration in periprostate fat or disruption of periprostatic venous

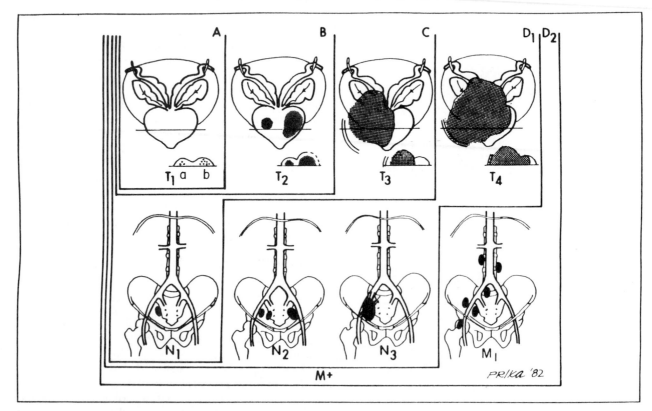

Fig. 23-5. Anatomic staging for carcinoma of the prostate (see Table 23-19).

plexus, which normally appears anterolaterally as a high-intensity signal or alteration of figure of eight seminal vesicle contours with an abnormally low signal. MRI has also been shown to be a potentially useful and accurate staging modality for extracapsular extension and nodal disease (108a).

5. *Lymph node staging* is comparable for CT/MRI with accuracies of 80% to 90% due to the inability to detect microdeposits (false-negatives) or inflammatory node enlargements (false-positives). The use of CT-guided fine needle aspiration biopsy increases accuracy to 95%, but surgical sampling is considered the gold standard.

6. *Pathologic staging* information for the pelvic lymph nodes, periprostatic tissue, and seminal vesicles is currently available from pelvic lymphadenectomies and radical prostatovesiculectomies.

7. *Nuclear DNA Ploidy* is an independent prognostic factor for progression and for cause-specific survival in patients with pathologic Stages C and D1 (103b).

Clinical stage at presentation has shifted in recent years to earlier disease and current approximations are: A, 23% to 25%; B, 30% to 34%; C, 16% to 20%; and D, 24% to 28% (120). The staging system currently used is somewhat misleading. Stage A1 disease progresses in a low percentage of cases: 16% at 4 to 8 years and 26% at 10 years. Note that in addition to being found in a small number of chips, stage I histologies are low grade. On the other hand, A2 tumors, ostensibly early stage, may be multifocal and/or may diffusely infiltrate the gland with more volume involvement than a B1 tumor. Stage A2 tumors progress in up to one third of cases at 4 years and one third have pelvic nodal metastases at presentation (103). Staging tests for periprostatic, seminal vesicle, and pelvic nodal involvement are lacking and understaging of stages A and B disease varies from 7% to 55% (93,115).

Pelvic lymph node involvement portends a poor prognosis and poor outcome in general for local therapeutic strategies, such as surgery and radiation therapy. Nodal disease is often correlated with tumor stage and grade (95,101,121) (Table 23-20).

Pelvic lymphadenectomy or modified pelvic lymph node dissection is often an important procedure prior to a radical prostatectomy. It is doubtful that either procedure has any therapeutic benefit, but each is pivotal in selecting patients for surgery and obtaining a homogeneous cohort of patients if comparing two localized therapies like surgery and irradiation.

PRINCIPLES OF TREATMENT

Multidisciplinary Treatment Decisions (Table 23-21)

It is important to appreciate the broad biologic potential and behavior pattern of prostate cancer; the high incidence:death ratio speaks to this issue. It has a slow growth rate and long doubling time. It is a disease of men over age 50 years with about one half the cases occurring in those older than 70 years. It has frequently been said that all men will develop prostate cancer if they live long enough. Hirst and Bergman (108) found an 80% incidence in the United State in men over the age of 90 years in a small autopsy series. During these same years other causes of death interdict the development of concise and clear prognostic formulae. A large Veteran's Administration (VA) study of patients with stage C prostate cancer who received hormonal therapy (75%) or placebo (25%) had a 49% 5-year survival and of those who died 80% were from other causes. Similarly stage D patients had a 24% 5-year survival, with 46% of those who died dying of other causes (97). Staging tests in these VA studies included (a) rectal examination (b) IVP, (c) chest, thoracic, lumbar and pelvic x rays, and (d) acid phosphatase measurement (119). The study points out that: (a) the natural history of the disease is broad; (b) intercurrent illness is a frequent cause of death in the population who has the disease; and (c) patients may do well for long periods with palliative or no therapy. These points make one cautious in interpreting the results of any treatment strategy. The similarities between prostate and breast cancer are obvious and 5-, 10-, and even 15-year follow-up is mandatory. We are learning more about prostate cancer and, rather than decry the broad natural history, some investigators are beginning to speak of a predictable and constant course. Numerous recent reports have appeared indicating PSA is a reliable measure of tumor response and also can be used to determine persistent, recurrent cancer as well as new metastases when previously normal levels become elevated (92,118,125).

Surgery

1. *Radical prostatectomy*: There has been renewed interest in radical prostatectomy since Walsh (131) described a modification of the operation that spares the

Table 23-20. Regional Node Involvement by Stage, Grade, and Tumor Size for Prostate Cancer

Preoperative Category	Positive Regional Nodes (%)	Positive Regional Node Differentiation (%)		
		Well	Moderate	Poor
		0-2	–	–
Stage A1		0-5	23-26	43-50
Stage A2	25	4-5	14-20	27-33
Stage B1		18-28	27	38-43
Stage B2	63	18-50	41-42	68-93
Stage C				
Size < 0.25	5			
2.5 - 7.9	34			
8 - 18 cc	72			

Adapted from Barzell et al. (95), Donahue et al. (101), and Middleton (121).

			(94,123b,132)
Table 23-21. Multidisciplinary Treatment Decisions for Prostate Cancer			
Stage	Surgery	Radiation Therapy	Chemotherapy
A or T1	Total prostatectomy	CRT - 60-65 Gy	NR
B or T2	Radical prostatectomy or	CRT - 66-70 Gy	NR
C or T3 , T4	Transurethral resection if or obstructed	DRT 66-70 Gy	HT if RT not used because of age or other reasons
D1 or N1,2,3	NR	DRT 66-70 Gy and	HT before RT
D2 or N3	NR	PRT and	HT
Relapse	NR	RT if surgical failure	HT preferred
Metastatic	NR	PRT	HT preferred
RT = radiation therapy; DRT = definitive; CRT = curative; PRT = palliative; HT = hormonal therapy; NR = not recommended; RCT = recommended chemotherapy.			
PDQ: RCT - HT-Leuporide, other LHRH agonist (zolodex) or estrogen (1 mgm/day)			

neurovascular bundles laterally and retains potency in the majority of individuals. (Prior to this modification impotency was associated with the surgery in 100% of cases.) This operation is usually performed by a retropubic approach in which the prostate gland, seminal vesicles, and portion of bladder neck are removed; it is usually preceded by pelvic lymph node sampling.

2. The major complications include incontinence (2% to 10%), impotence (7% to 44%, varying with age and stage), and operative deaths (0.5% to 3.6%). The procedure is used in medically operable patients with normal bones scans and acid phosphatase.

3. Patients with stage B1 disease are most often for this surgery (64%), followed by B2 (22%), A2 (10%), and A1 (4%) (93). Radical prostatectomy and preservation of the neurovascular bundles may be more difficult after repeated or extensive TURPs. Patients with high-grade tumors (Gleason score 8 to 10) are not usually good candidates, especially if the tumor is B2 stage or higher.

4. The presence of pelvic metastases precludes curative radical surgery as does clinical stage C disease. The incidence of local recurrence will increase when the disease is extracapsular and/or margins are positive (123a).

Radiation Therapy

Radiotherapy has played an increasingly important role in the treatment of prostate cancer. Initially it was used for patients considered medically inoperable or when the disease was considered to be outside the capsule (stage C) or locally restricted to the pelvis (stage D1) (114). More recently, it has played a role in the treatment of patients with stage A and B disease, with 5- and 10-year survivals comparable with radical prostatectomy.

1. The dose of radiation delivered is related to the volume of disease present: stage A, 60 Gy; stage B, 60 to 65 Gy; and stage C, 66 to 70 Gy (107).

2. Chronic complications of external irradiation have included radiation proctitis and cystitis in less than 10% and impotence in about 30% of patients, but this varies with age and the presence of vascular risk factors such as diabetes and hypertension.

3. The presence of pelvic metastases is a poor prognostic factor (pathologic stage D1) and irradiation of pelvic nodes in several studies, as opposed to only prostate irradiation, has not improved survival (94,103,106).

4. Radioactive implant of the prostate performed at the time of pelvic lymph node sampling has not produced improved survival or local control over external irradiation, but bladder, rectal, and small bowel complications were reduced as was impotency (111).

5. Radiation therapy also has been used for palliation of the pain of osseous metastases by radiating with involved fields or by hemibody irradiation (103,106,126).

6. The time factor has not received the same attention as dose, which also reflects the exponents attached to each in mathematical modeling of fractionation schedules. Lai *et al.* (114a) note no distinct effect on outcome by prolongation of the overall time in a prostate cancer stage A2, B1 C on RTOG protocols. They examined three subsets, that is, 7, 8-9 weeks, and found no major difference in local failure rates as long as a minimum dose of 65 Gy was delivered. The overall 5-year survival, the disease-free survival and local regional control within each stage, and each histologic grade range by Gleason score were not statistically different. Based upon the slow clinical regression of prostate cancers and lack of obvious effect of prolonging treatment time, it is postulated that prostate cancer behaves more like a late reacting tissue than most rapidly dividing cancers that are akin to early reacting tissues.

7. The low incidence of intestinal and urinary complications is a function of dose and volume factors. In analyses of approximately 1000 patients in two major RTOG prostate protocols presented by Lawton *et al.* (115a), severe intestinal complications (grade 3) occurred in 3.3% of patients and life-threatening morbidity (grade 4) such as bowel obstruction or perforation occurred in less than 0.6%. Urinary toxicity was moderate in 7.7% and major in less than 0.5% requiring surgery. The only significant

factor was the total radiation dose > 70 Gy with regard to complications. No difference in incidence was found when comparing pelvic and para-aortic and pelvic fields, but high doses (> 60 Gy) are usually delivered to cone down prostate fields. These authors note the very low incidence of major complications supports the use of external beam irradiation as an excellent alternative radical prostatectomy.

Drug Therapy (Tables 23-22 and 23-23) (96)

1. *Drug therapy* based on current results is purely palliative. The role of chemotherapy has yet to be established (Table 23-22).
2. *Hormonal therapy* is the mainstay of noncurative treatment based on the classical observations of Huggins and Hodges (109) that orchiectomy and/or administration of female hormones produced regression of prostate cancer. The three current strategies for reducing testosterone are orchiectomy, administration of female hormones (primarily, diethylstilbesterol), and luteinizing hormone-releasing hormone (LHRH) agonist with or without antiandrogens (121). The efficacy of one strategy over the other is not clear and selection is often based on side effects and cost (Table 23-23).
3. *Orchiectomy* is associated primarily with the psychologic side effects of emasculation, impotence, and hot flashes; however, the surgical procedure is fairly straightforward and there is little morbidity.

4. *Estrogens* have been associated with thromboembolic phenomena that can be life-threatening, but usually are fairly safe if there is no cardiovascular disease and if doses are kept below 3 mg/d diethylstilbestrol. Gynecomastia is frequently associated with estrogen administration, but can be avoided if the breasts are given low-dose irradiation *before* initiation (96); impotence, gastrointestinal distress, and hot flashes also are seen.
5. *LHRH agonist* reduces luteinizing hormone at the pituitary level, causing testosterone reduction. Antiandrogens block the androgen receptors. LaBrie *et al.* (113) in Quebec popularized the use of both drugs in the so-called "androgen blockage" regimen and reported higher responses and longer duration of response. Recently, a large cooperative, randomized, double-blind study in the United States found the combination of a LHRH agonist (leuprolide) and antiandrogen (flutamide) was associated with a longer progression-free survival and overall survival than the LHRH alone (99). In a randomized study, Crawford *et al.* (100) found the addition of an antiandrogen to leuprolide increased response from 38% to 51% but median time to progression and median survival were not different—25 to 27 months for both. Currently, this therapy is quite expensive, an obvious drawback. A depot LHRH agonist formulation (leuprolide acetate and goserelin acetate) has recently become available in the United States that requires an injection monthly rather than daily. These drugs have not been associated with thromboembolic complications, but impotence, hot flashes, gynecomastia, peripheral edema, and gastrointestinal distress are not uncommon. One can expect a 70% to 80% response to hormonal manipulation with a response duration of a few years. Second-line hormonal therapies such as megestrol, aminoglutethamide, and ketoconazole are associated with responses in about 40% of cases but duration of response is less than 6 months.

RESULTS AND PROGNOSIS

Results

Overall Survival

Overall survivals described in the literature for definitive irradiation or surgery are comparable. Despite some small, randomized studies that favor one mode, stage for stage

Table 23-22. Randomized Trials of Combination Chemotherapy Versus Single-Agent Chemotherapy in Prostatic Cancer

TREATMENT	SURVIVAL (%) CR + PR	MEDIAN SURVIVAL
5-FU	2	34 wk
FAC	2	25 wk
Cyclophosphamide	0	8 mo
CMF	1	5 mo
Lomustine	0	24 wk
CMF	3	26 wk

CR = complete response; PR = partial response.
Adapted from Eisenberger et al. (102).

Table 23-23. Effect of Endocrine Therapy on Hormonal Levels in Prostatic Cancer Patients

Therapy	Testosterone Levels First Week	Long-term	Duration	Luteinizing Hormone Levels	Estradiol Levels
Orchiectomy	Castrate	Castrate	Indefinite	Increased	Decreased
Estrogens	Decreased	Castrate	Reversible	Decreased	Increased
LHRH agonists	Increased	Castrate	Reversible	Increased, then decreased	Decreased
Progestational agents	Decreased	May rebound	Reversible	Decreased	Unknown
Pure antiandrogens	Increased	Increased	Reversible	Increased	Increased
Inhibitors of steroid synthesis	Castrate	Unknown	Reversible	Increased	Decreased

LHRH = luteinizing hormone-releasing hormone.
From Eisenberger et al. (102), with permission.

survival rate ranges are similar (i.e., stage A > 80%; Stage B > 70%; and Stage C > 40% to 50% (Table 23-24) (124). When patterns of failure or causes of death are identified, a large portion of failures are due to non-cancer-related aging disease (Fig. 23-6).

Early-Stage Disease (Stages A and B)

1. In 1987, a Consensus Conference meeting (122) in Washington DC concluded that radiation therapy and radical prostatectomy were equally effective (Table 23-24). Many Stage A cancers (A₁) are well differentiated and focally involved in gland (one of a number of cores or chips) and require no further treatment except in the younger age group (50-60 years of age). The generally quoted survivals at 5, 10, and 15 years for radiation therapy are approximately 80%, 60%, and 40%; disease-free survival is 10% to 20% lower. Surgery produces similar results, but some have suggested that the 15-year survival is better with surgery (110). There has been only one (highly criticized) study comparing radiation therapy with radical prostatectomy, and it favored surgery (123). Questions frequently raised about this paper include the end point (first treatment failure), the homogeneity of the patients (accuracy of staging), the manner in which some patients were made ineligible or carried after randomization, and the unexplained poor results in the radiation therapy arm in comparison with other studies. An important issue is that radiation therapy results are based primarily on clinically staged patients, whereas patients treated with radical prostatectomy are surgically staged and therefore knowledge of nodal, capsular penetration, and seminal vesicle spread is known; however, they are frequently reported according to pathologic stage and not clinical stage. Selection of patients for radical prostatectomy is not ideal, and in a recent series up to 55% of cases had unfavorable pathologic features predictive of progressive disease (disease at surgical margins, seminal vesicle invasion, or pelvic nodal metastases) (104a,115). When lymph node status is known to be negative on surgical staging, radiation treatment yields excellent and comparable results to radical prostastectomy. In a subset of RTOG patients with lymph node dissections, Hanks, Asbell, Krall *et al.* (106a) demonstrate comparable or better survival and local control rates with external irradiation in T1B, T2N0M0 prostate cancers when compared to radical prostatectomy. Irradiation patients with early prostate cancers who are surgically staged have a clinical local recurrence rate of 14% and a 10-year survival rate of 86%.

Table 23-24. Survival by Treatment and Stage for Prostate Cancer

Stage	Radiotherapy	5-yr Survival (%)
A	80-95	84
B	71-90	70-78
C	39-58	63

From Pilepich and Perez (124), with permission.

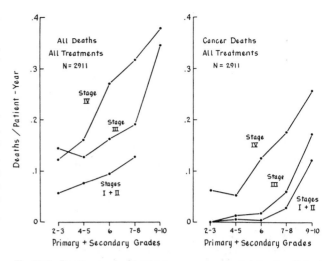

Fig. 23-6. Death rates for histologic scores, separately for the clinical stages. Note overlapping death rates. Modified from Gleason D.F. The Veterans Administration Cooperative Urological Research Group, In Urologic Pathology: The Prostate. Edited by M. Tannenbaum. Philadelphia, Lea & Febiger, 1977. Used with permission.

2. There has been concern in the urologic and radiation oncology community that a significant number (up to 93%) of biopsies taken from patients after 18 months demonstrate cancer cells and that this finding is correlated with the development of distant metastases (110,124a). Interesting and challenging questions must be answered in the next few years to select the most appropriate therapy for the stage and grade of disease and as yet undescribed subsets, and to determine which modality controls the disease for the longest time and which can cure.

Stage C

The standard treatment for stage C disease has been external radiation therapy. Survival results have been 60%, 40%, and 20% approximately at 5, 10, and 15 years (94,106) (Table 23-25). With appreciation that many of these cases have nodal involvement and that wide field irradiation to include pelvic nodes has not been successful and, therefore, treatment is palliative, other strategies are being investigated. In general, surgery has not played a role in this disease stage, although one study from the Mayo Clinic demonstrated that patients with stage C disease who underwent an immediate orchiectomy did better that those who did not (133). This observation has prompted combined-modality treatment. Combined surgery and irradiation has been used either when positive lymph nodes are encountered at exploratory laporotomy or when margins are positive. A number of series have shown postoperative irradiation can negate risk factors and prevent recurrence; results have been similar to more favorably contained cancers within the prostate capsule (112). The current approach is to combine radiation therapy with hormonal therapy, specifically LHRH agonist plus or minus antiandrogen. Current studies by the Radiation Therapy Oncology Group (RTOG) and other groups should clarify this issue.

Stage D

Treatment is primarily palliative and hormonal manipulation produces the best results, but possibly no prolongation of overall survival. As in most clinical situations, responders do better than non-responders and those with minimal disease better than those with severe disease (99). The timing

Table 23-25. Results of External Beam Therapy of Prostate Cancer: Weighted Averages of Collected Series

Stage	Survival (%)	5-Year NED Survival (%)	Free of Local Recurrence (%)	Survival (%)	10-Year NED Survival (%)	Free of Local Recurrence (%)	15-Year Survival (%)
A	86	80	94	62	51	97	
B	78	62	85	68	24	74	37
C	61	46	78	37	28	69	22

NED = no evidence of disease.

Adapted from Bagshaw (94) and Eisenberger et al. (102).

and type of treatments is individualized. Survival in stage D is not improved when therapy is initiated at the time of diagnosis in the asymptomatic patient versus withholding therapy until they become symptomatic. Predicting response to hormonal therapy is an important clinical question, but there is no reliable way of estimating the androgen-dependent cell population. Hence, all patients should be given a therapeutic trial even if they have high-grade lesions, low levels of PSA, or lack androgen receptors if measured. Radiation therapy has been used for palliation of osseous metastases, usually 3000 cGy in ten fractions. Hemibody (upper, lower, or mid) is also an effective method of managing diffuse disease (126).

Preservation of Potency: Surgery versus Radiation Therapy (Table 23-26)

Preservation of potency has been an important aspect of radiation therapy management in contradistinction to radical prostatectomy or hormonal therapy in which potency is sacrificed. The conservation of potency has varied in different series from 75% to 90%. Recently, Walsh (131) reported a 75% potency preservation (Table 23-27), with his nerve-preserving capsular resection of the prostate; his results indicate outcome similar to irradiation.

Effect of Local Control on Distant Metastatic Dissemination

Fuks, Leibel et al. (103a) provide compelling evidence that improved local regional control decreases dissemination and metastases and does translate into better overall survival. In

Table 23-26. Influence of Clinical Stage on Postoperative Potency in 320 Men with Prostate Cancer Followed for at Least 1 Year

Clinical Stage	Total (%)
A1	93
A2	72
B1N	92
B1	72
B2	56
Total	74

Adapted from Walsh (132).

prostate cancer, these authors demonstrate in a large mature series (679 patients) at 15 years, the actuarial distant metastases-free survival (DMFS) for local control is 77% compared to 24% for those who developed local relapses. The relative risk of metastatic spread subsequent to local failure is increased 4-fold compared to the risk without failure.

CLINICAL INVESTIGATIONS

Combined Modality and Salvage Therapy

Surgery and radiation therapy are being combined because each alone cannot cure specific subsets of patients with localized cancer. Surgery may cut across capsular invasion and seminal vesical involvement in stage C disease, leaving positive margins. Radiation therapy controls local progression but positive foci of disease have been found both on needle biopsy and with PSA levels months and years later. Protocols are being designed to determine whether using the other modality as an adjuvant on salvage improves survival.

Southwest Oncology Group (Intergroup): In clinically operable lesions (stages B and C) following radical prostectomy, patients were randomized to observation versus immediate irradiation. Depending on local examination, rising PSA levels, and bone scan, local irradiation or systemic treatment should be considered.

Hormonal Therapy and Radiation Therapy

RTOG is evaluating combinations of LHRH agonists (leuprolide) with and without flutamide concurrently in a tight sequence with irradiation to evaluate impact on local control.

Radiosensitizers such as SR 2508 (etanizadole) in conjunction with 66 Gy to prostate are advocated by Coleman et al. (98) who found a 71% CR in a small phase I/II study.

Radiation Prophylaxis of Osseous Metastases

An intriguing report of radiation therapy to ablate micro foci of metastatic prostate can be found in a report by Kaplan et al. (112) who note a decrease in lumbar spine metastases in patients who received irradiation to para-aortic fields versus pelvic fields only, i.e., 3% versus 15%, respectively. A recent RTOG hemibody irradiation (8Gy) study showed hemibody irradiation significantly delayed the appearance of new metastases and kept known lesions from progression and retreatment in prostate cancer patients. Use of hemibody irradiation deserves investigation as an adjuvant after definitive treatment of primary and lymph nodes (117).

Table 23-27. Walsh Potency Preservation: Influence of Age and Clinical Stage On Postoperative Potency in 320 Men Followed for at Least 1 Year

Clinical Stage	Age (years)					
	30-39	40-49	50-59	60-69	70-75	Total (%)
A1	—	100% (2/2)	90% (9/10)	100% (3/3)	—	93% (14/15)
A2	—	—	90% (9/10)	57% (4/7)	0% (0/1)	72% (13/18)
B1N	100% (2/2)	80% (4/5)	97% (30/31)	92% (11/12)	0% (0/1)	92% (47/51)
B1	—	79% (11/14)	82% (42/51)	65% (39/60)	20% (1/5)	72% (93/130)
B2	—	67% (2/3)	68% (15/22)	40% (8/20)	—	56% (25/45)
Total	100% (2/2)	79% (19/24)	85% (105/124)	64% (65/102)	14% (1/7)	74% (192/259)

From Walsh (131), with permission.

TESTICULAR CANCER

EPIDEMIOLOGY AND ETIOLOGY

Epidemiology

Testicular cancer accounts for 1% of all male cancers. However, it is the most common cancer between the ages of 15 to 35 years. It occurs more commonly in whites than in blacks. The estimated incidence of testicular cancer for 1992 is 6300 cases (1a).

Etiology

Cryptorchidism is the only known risk factor. Twelve percent of all testicular cancers occur in patients with cryptorchid testes. The risk of developing cancer in the cryptorchid testis is 40 times higher than in normally descended testis (136). Klinefelter's syndrome has been associated with mediastinal germ cell tumors. Mumps orchitis may also be a risk factor.

DETECTION AND DIAGNOSIS

Clinical Detection

Testicular cancer generally presents as a painless mass. Minor trauma to the testis often draws attention to the mass. Patients may also have symptoms related to metastases such as abdominal fullness, palpable mass, pain, lower extremity edema, left supraclavicular mass, and systemic symptoms such as fatigue. Gynecomastia can occur due to high levels of chorionic gonadotrophin. Extragonadal germ cell tumors can occur in the midline anywhere from the sacrum to the pineal body.

Diagnostic Procedures (Table 23-28)

The differential diagnosis of a testicular mass includes varicocele, hydrocele, hematocele, orchitis, and hernia. It is important to determine if the mass is intratesticular or extratesticular. Intratesticular masses are malignant unless proven otherwise, whereas, extratesticular masses are generally benign.

Optimal Work-up Should Include:

1. Complete history and physical examination with careful palpation of the testes, the supraclavicular lymph nodes, the abdomen for the presence of a mass, and the breasts for the presence of gynecomastia.
2. Scrotal ultrasound is the test of choice to distinguish between intratesticular and extratesticular location of the mass (150).
3. Routine blood tests (CBC, SMA-12, including lactate dehydrogenase).
4. Radioimmunoassay for AFP and ß-hCG. Eighty-five percent of patients will have elevation of at least one of the two markers. The half lives of AFP and ß-hCG are 5 days and 18 to 24 hours, respectively. After orchiectomy the rate of fall of the markers should follow an exponential pattern. A slower rate of fall indicates residual viable tumor. Ten percent of patients with early-stage seminomas can have elevated ß-hCG, whereas AFP is never elevated in pure seminomas. Therefore, patients with elevated AFP, regardless of the histology, should be treated as though they had a nonseminomatous germ cell tumor. Lactate dehydrogenase is not a specific marker for germ cell cancer.
5. Pelvic, abdominal, and chest CT scans, and, in selected cases, bipedal lymphangiography (Table 23-28) are used to uncover nodal or pulmonary metastases.

CLASSIFICATION AND STAGING

Histopathology (Table 23-29, Fig. 23-7) (157,158,159)

Ninety-six percent of testicular tumors are germ cell tumors. The remaining 4% are benign stromal tumors. Sixty percent of testicular germ cell cancers have only one histologic pattern and 40% contain a mixture of patterns. Seminomas are the most common tumors, accounting for 40% of all germ cell tumors. Embryonal carcinoma (20% to 25%), teratocarcinoma (5% to 10%), choriocarcinoma (1% to 3%), and yolk sac tumors (1%) comprise the rest (144). Seminomas and nonseminomas are thought to be derived from a single germ cell (157). It is important to determine if there are

Table 23-28. Imaging Methods for Evaluation of Testis Cancer

METHOD	DIAGNOSIS AND STAGING CAPABILITY	RECOMMENDED FOR USE
Primary tumor and regional nodes		
CT	Method of choice for staging and follow-up (chest and abdomen)	Always
MRI	Promising role for staging and follow-up	Unknown
Urography	Limited usefulness because of insensitivity in detecting small to moderate-sized retroperitoneal metastases	No
Ultrasound	A. Very useful for detection of occult testis cancer	A. Yes
	B. For staging and follow-up may be useful in thin patients with sparse retroperitoneal fat but is generally less sensitive and specific than CT	B. No
Lymphography	Limited usefulness in patients with positive CT scans or in patients with normal CT scans (clinical stage I) who are going to undergo elective treatment of the retroperitoneum	Recommended only for patients with clinical stage I disease for whom elective treatment of the retroperitoneum is not planned
Metastatic		
Chest radiography	Limited usefulness unless tomography is used for detection of metastases; however, whole lung tomography is less sensitive than chest CT	Yes
Radionuclide studies: routine imaging tests	Limited usefulness	No
Radioimmunoassay for β -HCG and AFP	Very useful for staging and follow-up; used in conjunction with available imaging tests; has decreased staging errors	Always
Labeled antibodies to β -HCG and AFP	Promising role for detecting occult metastases and residual tumor following therapy	Unknown
Biopsy (CT,US, fluoroscopy)	Percutaneous biopsy requires US, CT, or fluoroscopy. May be useful in some cases to confirm metastases, but usually is not necessary	No

CT = computed tomography; MRI = magnetic resonance imaging; β -HCG = beta-human chorionic gonadotropin; AFP = alpha-fetoprotein; US = ultrasound.
Courtesy of Bragg et al. (11).

Table 23-29. Comparison of Classifications of Testicular Germ-cell Tumor: AFIP versus WHO

AFIP	WHO
Tumors of one histologic type	**Tumors of one histologic type**
Seminoma (typical)	Seminoma
Spermatocytic seminoma	Spermatocytic seminoma
Anaplastic seminoma	
Embryonal carcinoma	Embryonal carcinoma
Polyembryoma	Polyembryoma
Adult teratoma	Teratoma
Mature	Mature
Immature	Immature
With malignant change	With malignant transformation
Embryonal carcinoma juvenile	Yolk sac tumor (embryonal carcinoma, juvenile type; endodermal sinus tumor)
Choriocarcinoma	Choriocarcinoma
Tumors of more than one histologic type	**Tumors of more than one histologic type**
Embryonal carcinoma with teratoma ("teratocarcinoma")	Embryonal carcinoma with teratoma ("teratocarcinoma")
Specify types	Choriocarcinoma and any other types (specify)
Specify types	Other combinations (specify)

AFIP = Armed Forces Institute of Pathology; WHO = World Health Organization.
Modified by permission from Mostofi and Price (158); and, adapted by permission from F.K. Mostofi et al. Histological typing of testis tumours. Geneva, World Health Organization, 1977 (International Histological Classification of Tumours No. 16).

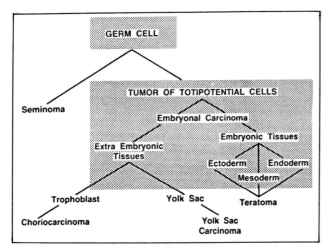

Fig. 23-7. A representation of the unified theory for the derivation of testicular tumors. Adapted, by permission, from F.K. Mostofi *et al.* Histological typing of testis tumours. Geneva, World Health Organization, 1977 (International Histological Classification of Tumours No. 16).

nonseminomatous elements in a germ cell tumor because treatment of pure seminomas and nonseminomas differs.

Anatomic Staging (Table 23-30, Fig. 23-8)

The Walter Reed system with modification is most commonly used. The modifications involve subdivisions of stages II and III on the basis of disease extent to identify poor-prognosis patients. As with other cancers, staging is done either noninvasively (clinical staging) or surgically (pathologic staging). Compare Walter Reed with AJC/UICC staging in Table 23-30; the TNM staging is shown in Fig. 23-8. The T categories after T1 have been redefined so that deeper invasion is presently defined in terms of testicular/scrotal layers. Down-staging has occurred: previous T3 is now T2; previous T4a is now T3, and previous T4b is now T4. The N categories are mainly characterized by size and number, rather than laterality. The stage grouping reflects T stage.

Subdivisions of Stage III Disease (as defined by Indiana University group [170])

Minimal Extent

1. Elevated markers only .
2. Cervical nodes (± nonpalpable retroperitoneal nodes).
3. Unresectable nonpalpable retroperitoneal disease.
4. Less than five pulmonary metastases per lung field AND largest less than 2 cm (± nonpalpable retroperitoneal nodes)

Moderate Extent

1. Palpable (>10 cm in diameter) abdominal mass only (no supradiaphragmatic disease).
2. Moderate pulmonary metastases; five to ten metastases per lung field and largest less than 3 cm OR solitary pulmonary metastasis of any size greater than 2 cm (± nonpalpable retroperitoneal disease).

Advanced Extent

1. Advanced pulmonary metastases: primary mediastinal germ cell tumor OR greater than 10 pulmonary metastases per lung field OR multiple pulmonary metastases with largest more than 3 cm (± nonpalpable retroperitoneal disease).
2. Palpable (> 10 cm in diameter) abdominal mass plus supradiaphragmatic disease.
3. Liver, bone, or CNS metastases.

Staging Work-up (Table 23-28)

After completion of the tests described under Diagnostic Procedures, the next step is a radical orchiectomy, which involves removal of the testis and the spermatic cord via an inguinal approach. Transscrotal biopsy is contraindicated because it is associated with a risk of contaminating scrotum and inguinal lymph nodes. It is important to obtain preoperative AFP and ß-hCG measurements and to measure the rate of decline postoperatively. In clinical stage I and stage

Stage	Walter Reed Hospital		AJC / TNM Classification	Stage Grouping
I	Tumor confined to one testis	T_1	Limited to body of the testis, incl rete	I
	No clinical or radiographic evidence of	T_2	> Tunica albuginea/epididymus	I
	spread beyond	T_3	Invasion of spermatic cord	II
		T_4	Invasion of scrotal wall	II
		N_1	Single homolateral ≥ 2 cm	III
IIA	As in stage I but minimal metastases to iliac or para-aortic lymph nodes	N_2	2-5 cm or multiple regional lymph nodes, if inguinal, mobile	IV
IIB	Clinical or radiographic evidence of metastases to femoral, inguinal, iliac, or para-aortic lymph nodes. No metastases above diaphragm or visceral organs	N_3	> 5 cm or fixed	IV
		M_1	Distant metastasis present	IV
III	Clinical or radiographic evidence of metastases above the diaphragm or other distant metastases to body organs			

Table 23-30. Comparison of Some Staging Systems for Testis Cancer

T = tumor; N = node; M = metastasis.

AJC (1)/UICC(2)

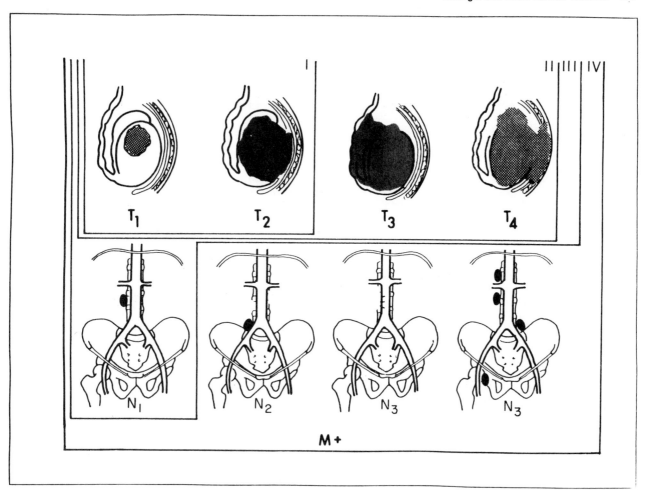

Fig. 23-8. Anatomic staging for carcinoma of the testis (see Table 23-30).

IIA nonseminomatous germ cell cancers some surgeons recommend retroperitoneal lymph node dissection (RPLND).

Most patients with testicular cancer are young and fertility is often an important consideration. At the time of diagnosis only about 6% to 40% of patients have sufficient sperm counts for cryopreservation of semen (139). Since chemotherapy and RPLND affect future fertility, patients should be counselled regarding sperm banking.

At the time of presentation most seminomas are an early stage: stage I, 64% to 77%; stage II, 19% to 29%; stage III, 3% to 8%. The distribution of non-seminomatous germ cell cancers is similar. RPLND previously was the standard staging/therapeutic operation once the diagnosis was established. It was found that approximately 10% to 15% of seminoma and 25% to 30% (140) of nonseminomatous cases with negative IVPs and/or lymphograms (and more recently CT scans) had microscopic disease in the retroperitoneal nodes. A formal and complete RPLND is a major operation and is associated with a high incidence (>75%) of infertility related to injury of the sympathetic chains bilaterally and resultant retrograde ejaculation. The role of adjuvant therapy in clinical stage I disease instead of surveillance has been controversial. It has been made somewhat easier by the high cure rates with chemotherapy in early-stage disease, and the recently described modified RPLND that preserves fertility.

Modified nerve-sparing techniques preserve antegrade ejaculation in 50% to 100% of patients (152).

PRINCIPLES OF TREATMENT

Testicular germ cell tumors are the most curable cancers. Radical orchiectomy establishes accurate histopathologic diagnosis and provides other information that may influence other diagnostic or therapeutic strategies, e.g., penetration of the tunica albuginea, lymphatic-vascular space invasion, spermatic cord involvement. The disease tends to spread in a predictable fashion to para-aortic, precaval, and renal hilar nodes, with subsequent spread to mediastinal and supraclavicular lymph nodes; hematogenous dissemination is rare, except in choriocarcinoma. Late sites of spread include the lungs, liver, and brain. Historically, seminoma has been separated from the other testicular cancers because of its radiosensitivity, and stage for stage there does not appear to be any difference among classical spermatocytic, or anaplastic seminoma. In the past 15 years we have learned that the nonseminomatous cancers are readily cured with platinum-based combination chemotherapy. Indeed seminoma, too, has been found to be curable with the same types of drugs. Radiotherapy has remained the standard treatment, however, for early-stage seminoma, but this primacy is being challenged in some surveillance clinical trials. The current multidisciplinary treatment decisions by stage are summarized for seminoma and nonseminoma in Table 23-31.

			(134,161,162b)

Table 23-31. Multidisciplinary Treatment Decisions by Stage for Testis Cancer

Stage	Surgery	Radiation Therapy	Chemotherapy
Seminoma			
I T1, 2 N0	Radical orchiectomy*	CRT - Para-aortic and ipsilateral iliac nodes (20-30 Gy)	NR
I T3-4b N0	Radical orchiectomy*	CRT - Para-aortic, ipsilateral iliac and inguinal nodes (20-30 Gy)	NR
IIA anyT, N1, 2	Radical orchiectomy*	CRT - Para-aortic and ipsilateral iliac (20-30 Gy) ± inguinal if T3-4b	NR
IIB anyT, N3	Radical orchiectomy*	CRT - Para-aortic and iliac (30-35 Gy) and elective mediastinal RT (20-25 Gy)	and/or MAC
III M1	Radical orchiectomy*	NR	MAC
Recurrence		PRT	MAC
Nonseminoma			
I	Rad Orchiectomy± RPLND	NR	at relapse MAC
II/III	Rad Orchiectomy (RPLND post MAC for residual disease)	NR	and MAC
Metastases	Excision of selected metastases (post-MAC)	NR	and MAC
Recurrence	Limited excision of recurrent disease (post-MAC)		and MAC

* Inguinal approach

RT = radiation therapy; CRT = curative; PRT = palliative; NR = not recommended; MAC = multiagent chemotherapy, phase III clinical trials; RPLND = retroperitonial lymphnode dissection.

PDQ: RCT - MAC = BEP,EP,PVB16,PVB16B

Surgery

1. Radical orchiectomy is performed by the inguinal approach for diagnosis.
2. The role of RPLND as a staging procedure in patients with stage I nonseminomatous germ cell testicular cancer is being redefined. Patients with clinical stage I nonseminomatous germ cell cancers can be monitored closely and treated at relapse, resulting in more than 98% cures. Many oncologists prefer the observe-and-treat-if-needed approach. In a large study, 27% of clinical stage I tumors had metastatic involvement of removed lymph nodes and were upstaged to pathological stage II (149a). A nerve-sparing RPL that preserves ejaculation in virtually every patient has been described in clinical stage I patients and appears to be as effective as the standard RPL dissection (137c).
3. Surgery is indicated for extirpation of residual disease after treatment of advanced-stage nonseminomatous germ cell cancers. The role of tumor-reductive surgery in seminomas is not well defined because surgery is technically difficult due to extensive fibrosis; radiation therapy is effective for the treatment of residual disease; and the incidence of occult viable cancer is low in lesions <less than 3 cm in diameter.

Radiation Therapy

1. Seminoma is very sensitive to fractionated irradiation. Typical doses for stage I disease are 20 to 30 Gy in 1.5 to 1.8 Gy fractions to the para-aortic and ipsilateral pelvic nodes ("hockey stick" field). Retroperitoneal nodes are prophylactically irradiated even with a negative lymphangiogram and/or CT scan because approximately 15% will have occult nodal spread that can be cured with irradiation (139'). The morbidity associated with this low-dose irradiation is minimal and usually mild anorexia, nausea, and diarrhea. Transient oligospermia occurs in almost all patients but usually recovers by 18 to 24 months. The dose of radiation to the remaining testicle varies from 25 to 100 cGy. Genetic effects have been difficult to document. Second malignancies have not been increased, but it should be noted that disease in the other testicle develops in 5% to 10% of cases (146,155,169).
2. Stage IIA disease is treated the same as stage I. However, the dose administered is 30 to 35 Gy. Mediastinal irradiation formerly was routine for stages I and II disease. This is no longer recommended because of the low incidence of mediastinal failures, the effectiveness of salvage chemotherapy, and the reduction in bone marrow reserve that occurs with abdominal and mediastinal irradiation (167).
3. The treatment of stage IIB disease has been controversial. Part of the problem is whether bulky disease should be defined as greater than 5 cm, greater than 10 cm or palpable. Many radiation therapists use the 10 cm cutoff and those greater than this are treated with chemotherapy.
4. Although radiation therapy was used in the past adjuvantly in stages I and II nonseminomatous cancers with good results, it has essentially been replaced by chemotherapy. Salvage radiation therapy is sometimes used in patients with refractory nonseminomatous neoplasms.

Chemotherapy

1. Cisplatin is the single most active agent in the treatment of germ cell cancers. All front-line and most salvage chemotherapy combinations include cisplatin. The most widely used frontline combination administered PVP-16B is shown (170).

 Cisplatin 20 mg/m2/d IV x 5 days q 3 wk x 4 cycles
 Etoposide 100 mg/m2/d IV x 5 days q 3 wk x 4 cycles
 Bleomycin 30 U/wk IV x 12 weeks.

 Adequate hydration, diuresis, and antiemetics are mandatory. Ondansetron, a selective 5HT3 receptor site antagonist, is very effective in controlling the acute and delayed nausea associated with cisplatin. The recommended dose of ondansetron is 0.15 mg/kg given intravenously 30 minutes before and 2 and 4 hr after cisplatin (137a).

2. Combination chemotherapy is the treatment of choice for stage IIB (large volume) and stage III seminoma, for selected cases of clinical stage I, all cases of stage IIB and stage III nonseminomatous germ cell cancers, and for all cases of extragonadal germ cell cancers (149).

3. Etoposide is myelosuppressive, therefore, patients should be watched closely for signs of infection and bleeding and treated promptly with antibiotics and given platelet transfusions if the platelet count is less than 20,000/cm. Testicular cancers are curable, therefore, patients should be treated on schedule except in the event of fever in association with leukopenia.

4. PDQ regimens include (162a):

 BEP: bleomycin + etoposide + cisplatin
 EP: etoposide + cisplatin
 PVB: cisplatin + vinblastine + bleomycin
 VPV: vinblastine + cisplatin + etoposide
 VAB VI: vinblastine + dactinomycin + bleomycin

Results

Seminoma (Table 23-32) : Orchiectomy is performed to establish the diagnosis. RPLND is not done for staging purposes in seminoma. The terms stage I and stage II accordingly refer to clinical stages, not pathologic.

1. *Stage I disease*: Radiation therapy results in a 95% cure rate as recent series corroborated (134,142,146a, 167,173). Three different groups have embarked on a surveillance-only policy in stage I patients after a radical orchiectomy and careful clinical staging usually with markers, IVP, chest x ray, lymphogram, and different combinations of ultrasonography and abdomino/pelvic and chest CT scans. These studies reported in abbreviated form, reveal between 4% and 15% relapses (160,162,168). This corresponds with the retroperitoneal node dissection data (153). The detection and treatment of relapses depends on the closeness of surveillance: most relapses occur in the first 2 years, but late relapses have been reported, which makes these studies premature. Certainly this approach is not suitable for routine practice; it is costly, labor intensive, and requires compliance. Many of the recurrences have been treated with radiation therapy, however, some have required chemotherapy.

2. *Stage II disease*: Tumor bulk is the most important prognostic factor. Patients with infradiaphragmatic disease less than 10 cm in diameter have 74% to 92% long-term disease-free survival compared with 54% to 73% for patients with bulky, i.e., larger than 10 cm, disease (156,172). Radiation therapy is the treatment of choice for stage IIA seminoma (138), whereas, current recommendations for stage IIB seminomas are combination chemotherapy.

3. Stage IIB and stage III disease: Cisplatin-based combination therapy is curative in 61% to 88% of patients (154). Occasionally, consolidation with radiation therapy is used for any residual retroperitoneal mass greater than 3 cm.

Nonseminomatous Germ Cell Tumors (Table 23-33) (170)

1. *Stage I disease*: The treatment of stage I disease is controversial (143). Treatment options are: (a) RPLND followed by close monitoring and chemotherapy to those who relapse; (b) close monitoring, without RPLND, and chemotherapy at relapse. (Close monitoring consists of monthly physical examination, AFP, ß-hCG, and chest x ray for the first year and every other month during the second year. CT scans of abdomen and pelvis are done every 2 months during the first year and less frequently during the second year); (c) two cycles of adjuvant chemotherapy, without RPLND, to all patients; and (d) two cycles of adjuvant chemotherapy, without RPLND, to selected patients who are at a higher risk of relapse.

Table 23-32. Results of Postorchiectomy Radiation Therapy in Stage I and Stage II Seminoma

Treatment Center	(Reference)	STAGE I 5-Year Survival	STAGE II 5-Year Survival (%)
Walter Reed Army Hospital	(155)	97	76
Royal Marsden Hospital	(145/161)	98	79
M.D. Anderson Hospital	(173/174)	95	88
Stanford Univ. Hospital	(139a)	100	
Ontario Cancer Institute	(167)		74
Massachusetts General Hospital	(138)	98	92
US Patterns of Care Study	(146)	98	
Cross Cancer Institute	(170)	98	70
Total		98	79

Table 23-33. Comparison of Results of Sequential PVB Studies in Nonseminomatous Germ Cell Tumors at Indiana University

Years	Patients with CR (%)	NED With Surgery (%)	Now NED (%)
1974-1976	70	11	57
1976-1978	65	17	73
1978-	63	21	80

CR = complete response; NED = no evidence of disease; PVB = cisplatin, vinblastine, bleomycin.
From Williams et al. (170). Reprinted by permission of the New England Journal of Medicine.

The rate of relapse for patients staged by RPLND is 10%; for clinically staged patients it is 25% to 30%. However, almost all patients who relapse can be cured by combination chemotherapy (163,165). Patients with primary tumors of embryonal histology, vascular or lymphatic invasion, extension to spermatic cord or scrotum, and a slow decline in markers, are at a higher risk of relapse (148). Such patients can be treated with adjuvant chemotherapy. Other patients at lower risk of relapse can be monitored closely. Treatment decisions have to be individualized. Regardless of the option used, the overall cure rate is higher than 95% (137).

2. *Stage II disease:* For clinical stage IIA disease, most surgeons perform RPLND. If tumor markers normalize after surgery, the patient is considered to have pathologic stage IIA disease. These patients can be treated with two cycles of adjuvant PVP-16B chemotherapy or monitored closely. After adjuvant chemotherapy the probability of relapse is less than 5% (171). Without adjuvant chemotherapy the probability of relapse is nearly 50%. However, nearly all patients can be salvaged with three to four cycles of chemotherapy (171). The overall cure rate is approximately 95% for stage IIA disease, regardless of the treatment option used.

3. *Stage IIB and stage III disease:* The standard treatment is four cycles of PVP-16B chemotherapy. For stage III minimal- or moderate-extent advanced disease (refer to Classification section above) three cycles of PVP-16B are as effective as four cycles (141). Approximately 70% of patients will achieve a CR. An additional 10% to 20% will have normalization of markers but have persistent radiographic abnormalities. These patients can be rendered free of disease by surgery. Twenty percent of patients will have viable microscopic cancer and the remaining 80% will have either fibrosis or mature teratoma. If viable cancer is found, two more cycles of chemotherapy are administered. If marker levels do not normalize after four cycles of chemotherapy, cytoreductive surgery is not curative. Such patients should be treated with salvage chemotherapy. The overall cure rate for stages IIB and III is approximately 80%.

Recommended Follow-up

The purpose of follow-up is to detect relapse and to monitor patients for short- and long-term, treatment-related toxicities. Greater than 95% of relapses occur within the first 2 years. Therefore, close monitoring is recommended for the first 2 years consisting of monthly history and physical examinations, routine laboratory tests, markers, and chest x rays during the first year and every other month during the second year. CT scans are done periodically. Semiannual follow-up is recommended after 2 years because late relapses can occur (166). Complications of chemotherapy include peripheral neuropathy, high-frequency hearing loss, Raynaud's phenomenon, thrombotic events, and bleomycin pulmonary toxicity (135). If alkylating agents are used there is increased risk of secondary leukemia and myelodysplastic syndromes (164).

Elevation of ß-hCG alone should not be considered reason for immediate salvage chemotherapy. Since most of these patients receive chemotherapy, they can have suppression of testosterone secretion by the remaining testis and appropriate elevations of luetinizing hormone (LH). Occasionally there can be cross-reactivity between LH and ß-hCG in the radioimmunoassay. It is prudent to administer testosterone 300 mg intramuscularly and repeat the ß-hCG assay 2 weeks later to rule out this cause of spurious elevation in ß-hCG. Persistently elevated ß-hCG connotes recurrence. Elevated AFP, in the absence of liver disease, is also indicative of recurrence. If CT scans of the abdomen and chest do not reveal the site of recurrence, the CNS and the remaining testis should be evaluated as they can be sanctuary sites.

CLINICAL INVESTIGATIONS

There are two types of clinical investigations. One involves minimizing the treatment-related toxicity without sacrificing the high cure rates and the other involves testing of newer drugs in the treatment of refractory germ cell cancer. The value of bleomycin in stage IIB disease is being determined by comparing PVP-16B and PVP-16. Ifosfamide (administered along with the uroepithelial protector mesna) and carboplatin are being evaluated in the treatment of germ cell tumors refractory to conventional chemotherapy. High-dose platinum-based chemotherapy followed by autologous bone marrow rescue is also being evaluated in phase II clinical trials (137a).

AFP and ß-hCG are useful markers. However, 15% of patients will have normal levels. Neuron-specific enolase (151) and placental alkaline phosphatase (147) are being evaluated as markers in the follow-up of these patients.

Recommended Reading

Best (6) gives a 10-year review of renal carcinoma. DeKernion and Mukamel (15) provide guidelines for selection of initial therapy. Stenzl and deKernion (40) give a review of surgical and histopathology of renal tumors. Chapters by Lai (23a) and Linehan (25) give good overviews of treatment of renal tumors. Pearse (68) deals with radiation oncology techniques for cancer of the urinary bladder and Richie *et al.* (69) give a comprehensive review of cancer of the bladder. Yagoda's book (90) *Bladder Cancer: Future Directions for Treatment* is a valuable resource. Whitmore (85), Parsons and Million (66a), and Richie (69) give an overview of bladder cancer and its treatment. Freiha *et al.* (103) provide a review of pathology, staging and treatment of carcinoma of the prostate. Lai *et al.* (114) give an up-to-date view of radiotherapy treatment. Walsh (131,132) covers radical prostatectomy and Grayhack *et al.* (105) report on hormonal therapy in carcinoma of the prostate.

For testicular seminoma, Babaian and Zagars (134) report the M.D. Anderson Experience and give treatment recommendations. Einhorn *et al.* (140,141) discuss the use of chemotherapy in disseminated germ cell tumors. Fung *et al.* (143) and Thomas and Williams (168a) give good reviews of treatment of testicular carcinoma. Also, Peckham's book (161) is a comprehensive view of the management of testicular tumors.

REFERENCES

General References

1. American Joint Committee on Cancer Staging and End Reporting. Manual for Staging Cancer, 3rd ed. Philadelphia, PA: JB Lippincott Co; 1988.
1a. Boring, C.C., Squires, T.S., Tong, T. Cancer Statistics, 1992. CA. 42:19-38; 1992.
2. International Union Against Cancer (UICC). TNM Classification of malignant tumors. 4th ed. New York, NY: Springer-Verlage; 1987:83-88.
3. Murphy, L.J. The History of Urology. Springfield: C.C. Thomas; 1972;127.

Specific References

Kidney Cancer

4. Amendola MA: Comparison of MR Imaging and CT in the Evaluation of Renal Masses. Crit Rev Diagn Imaging 1989; 29:117-150.
4a. Anderson, G.A., Lawson, R.K. Chromosomal defects in renal cell carcinoma. Urol. 39:473-477, 1992.
5. Bassil, B.; Dosoretz, D.E.; Prout, G.R. Jr. Validation of the tumor, nodes and metastatis classification of renal cell carcinoma. J. Urol. 134:450-454;1985.
6. Best BG: Renal Carcinoma: At Ten-Year Review 1971-1980. Br J Urol 1987; 60:100-102.
7. Boxer, R.J.; Waisman, J.; Leiber, M.M. *et al.* Renal Carcinoma: Computer Analysis of 96 Patients Treated by Nephrectomy. J. Urol. 122:598-601;1979.
8. Brady LW: Carcinoma of the Kidney — The Role for Radiation Therapy. Semin Oncol 1983; 10:417-421.
9. Bragg, D.G. State of the art of oncological imaging. Semin. Ultrasound CT and MR. 10: 453-466;1989.
10. Bragg, D.G.; Dodd, G.D. Imaging in Cancer: State of the Art. In. Imaging in Cancer. New York, NY: American Cancer Society; 1987.
11. Bragg, D.G.; Rubin, P. Youker, J.E. Oncologic Imaging. Elmsford, NY: Pergamon Pres; 1985.
12. Buzaid AC, Todd MB: Therapeutic Options in Renal Cell Carcinoma. Semin Oncol 1989; 16 (Suppl 1): 12-19.
13. Cherri, R.J.; Goldman, G.G.; Lindner, A. *et al.* Prognostic implications of vena caval extension of renal cell carcinoma. J. Urol. 128:910-912;1982.
14. Cronin RE, Kaehny WD, Miller PD, Stables DP, Gabow PA, Ostroy PR, Schrier RW: Renal Cell Carcinoma: Unusual Systemic Manifestations. Medicine 1976; 55:291-311.
15. deKernion JB, Mukamel E: Selection of Initial Therapy for Renal Cell Carcinoma. Cancer 1987; 60:539-546.

16. Finney R: An Evaluation of Postoperative Radiotherapy in Hypernephroma Treatment - A Clinical Trial. Cancer 1973; 32:1332-1340.
17. Fisher RI, Coltman CA, Doroshow JH, Rayner AA, Hawkins MJ, Mier JW, Wiernik P, McMannis JD, Weiss GR, Margolin KA, Gemlo BT, Hot DF, Parkinson DR, Paietta E: Metastatic Renal Cancer Treated with Interleukin-2 and Lymphokine-activated Killer Cells. Ann Int Med 1988; 108: 518-523.
18. Golimbu, M.; oshi, P.; Sperber, A. *et al.* Renal cell carcinoma: Survival and prognostic factors. J. Urology. 27:291-301;1986.
19. Gonick P: Surgical Therapy of Renal Adenocarcinoma. Semin Oncol 1983; 10:413-416.
20. Juusela H, Malmio K, Alfthan O, Oravisto KJ: Preoperative Irradiation in the Treatment of Renal Adenocarcinoma. Scan J Urol Nephrol 1977; 11:277-281.
21. Kaufman, J.J.; Mims, M. Tumors of the kidney. In: Current Problems in Surgery. M.M. Ravitch, E.H. Ellison, O.C. Julian, *et al.* (eds). Chicago, Ill.: Year Book Medical Publ., 1966:1-44.
22. Kjaer M, Frederiksen PL, Engelholm SA: Postoperative Radiotherapy in Stage II and III Renal Adenocarcinoma. A Randomized Trial by the Copenhagen Renal Cancer Study Group. Int J Radiation OncologY Biol Phys 1987; 13:665-672.
23. Kuten, A.; Stein, M.; Halpern, J.; Rubinov, R.; Cohen, Y.; Robinson, E. The Value of Postoperative Irradiation in Renal Cell Cancer: A Retrospective Study on 147 Patients. In: Proceedings of Am Soc Clin Oncol. Washington, D.C.: ASCO; 9:136:1990.Abstract.
23a. Lai, P.P. Kidney, renal pelvis, and ureter. In: Perez, C.A.; Brady, L.W., eds. Principles and Practice of Radiation Oncology. Philadelphia, PA: JB Lippincott Co; 1992:1025-1035.
24. Libertino JA, Zinman L, Watkins E: Long-Term Results of Resection of Renal Cell Cancer with Extension into Inferior Vena Cava. J Urol 1987; 137:21-24.
25. Linehan, W.M.; Shipley, W.U.; Longo, D.L. Cancer of the Kidney and ureter, In: Cancer Principles and Practice of Oncology. 3rd ed. V.T. DeVita, S. Hellman, S.A. Rosenberg, eds. Philadelphia, PA: J.B. Lippincott, Co.; 1989: 979-1007.
26. Maldazys JD, deKernion JB: Prognostic Factors in Metastatic Renal Carcinoma. J Urol 1986; 136:376-379.
27. McNichols, D.W.; Segrura, J.W.; DeWeerd, J.H. Renal cell carcinoma: Long-term survival and late recurrence. J. Urol. 126:17-23;1981.
28. Moran, R.; Richner, J.; Evers, P.; Senn, H.J. Interleukin-2 (rIL-2) and Interferon-alpha Combination Immunotherapy in Patients with Metastatic Renal Cell Carcinoma. In: Proceedings of Am Soc Clin Oncol. Washington, D.C.; ASCO; 9:141;1990. Abstract.
29. Mostofi, F.K. Pathology and Spread of Renal Cell Carcinoma. In: Renal Neoplasia. J.S. King, Jr (ed.). Boston, Mass. : Little Brown & Co.;1967:45-85.
30. Muss HB: The Role of Biological Response Modifiers in Metastatic Renal Cell Carcinoma. Sem Oncol 1988; 15:30-34.
30a. Novick, A.C.; Streem, S.; Montie, J.E.; *et al.* Conservative surgery for renal cell carcinoma: A single-center experience with 100 patients. J Urol 141(4):835-839;1989.
30b. Oliver, R.T.; Nethersell, A.B.; Bottomley, J.M. Unexplained spontaneous regression and alpha-interferon as treatment for metastatic renal carcinoma. Brit J Urol 1989; 63(2): 128-131.
31. Outzen HC, Maguire HC: The Etiology of Renal Cell Carcinoma. Semin Oncol 1983; 10:378-384.
32. Paulson DF: Prognostic Factors in Renal Adenocarcinoma. Prog Clin Biol Res 1988; 269:359-380.
33. Pizzocaro G, Piva L, di Fronzo G, Giongo A, Cozzoli A, Dormia E, Minervini S, Zanollo A, Fontanella U, Longo G, Maggioni A: Adjuvant Medroxyprogesterone Acetate to Radical Nephrectomy in Renal Cancer: 5 Year Result of a Prospective Randomized Study. J Urol 1987; 138: 1379-1381.
33a. Priestley, J.T. Survival Following Removal of Renal Neoplasms. JAMA. 113:902-906;1939.
34. Rafla S: Renal Cell Carcinoma. Natural History and Results of Treatment. Cancer 1970; 25:26-29.
35. Robson, C.J. Radical Nephrectomy for Renal Cell Carcinoma. J. Urol. 89:37-42;1963.
36. Robson CJ, Churchill BM, Anderson W: The Results of Radical Nephrectomy for Renal Cell Carcinoma. J Urol 1969; 101:297-301.
37. Sahasrabudhe, D.M.; deKernion, J.B.; Pontes, J.E.; Ryan, D.M.; O'Donnell, R.W.; Marquis, D.M.; Mudholkar, G.S.; McCune,

C.S. Specific Immunotherapy with Suppressor Function Inhibition for Metastatic Renal Cell Carcinoma. J Biol Resp Mod. 5:581-594;1986.

38. Seli, C.; Hinshaw, W.M.; Woodward, B.H. *et al.* Stratification of risk factors in renal cell carcinoma. Cancer. 52:899-903;1983.

39. Skinner DG, Colvin RB, Vermillion DC, Pfister RC, Leadbetter WF: Diagnosis and Management of Renal Cell Carcinoma. A Clinical and Pathologic Study of 309 Cases. Cancer 1971; 28:1165-1177.

40. Stenzl A, deKernion JB: Pathology, Biology, and Clinical Staging of Renal Cell Carcinoma. Semin Oncol 1989; 16 (Suppl 1): 3-11.

41. Thompson IM, Peek M: Improvement in Survival of Patients with Renal Cell Carcinoma — The Role of the Serendipitously Detected Tumors. J Urol 1988; 140:487-490.

42. Vaeth JM: cancer of the Kidney — Radiation Therapy and Its Indications in Non-Wilm's Tumors. Cancer 1973; 32:1053-1055.

43. van der Werf-Messing B: Carcinoma of the Kidney. Cancer 1973; 32:1056-1061.

44. Wright JC: Update in Cancer Chemotherapy: Genitourinary Tract Cancer, Part 1. J Natl Med Assoc 1987; 79:1249-1258.

Bladder Cancer

45. Batata, M.A.; Chu, F.C.H.; Hilaris, B.S., *et al.* Preoperative whole pelvis versus through pelvis irradiation and cystectomy for bladder cancer. Int. J. Rad Oncol. Biol. Phys. 7:1349-1355;1981.

46. Blandy, J.T.; England, H.R.; Evans, S.J.W. *et al.* T3 bladder cancer — the case for salvage cystectomy. Brit J Urol. 52:506-510; 1980.

47. Bloom, H.C.G.; Hendry, W.R.; Wallace, D.M. *et al.* Treatment of T3 bladder cancer: controlled trial of preoperative radiotherapy and radical cystectomy versus radical radiotherapy, second report and review, Brit. J. Urol. 54(2):136-151;1982.

48. Boileau, M.A.; Johnson, E.D.; Chan, R.C., *et al.* Bladder carcinoma: Results with preoperative radiation therapy and radical cystectomy. Urology. 16:569-576;1980.

49. Broders, A.C. Epithelioma of the genitourinary organs. Ann Surg. 574-580;1922.

49a. Coplen, D.E.; Marcus, M.D.; Myers, J.A. *et al.* Long-term follow-up of patients treated with 1 or 2, 6-week courses of intravesical bacillus Calmette-Guerin: Analysis of possible predictors of response free of tumor. J Uro 144(3): 652-657; 1990.

50. Daniels, J.R.; Skinner, D.G.; Russell, C.A.; Lieskovsky, G.; Boyd, S.D.; Nichols, P.; Kern, W.; Sakamoto, J.; Krailo, M.; Groshen, S. The Role of Adjuvant Chemotherapy Following Cystectomy for Invasive Bladder Cancer: A Prospective Comparative Trials. In: Proceedings of Am Soc Clin Oncol. Washington, D.C.: ASCO; 9:131;1990. Abstract.

51. Eapen L, Stewart D, Danjoux C, Genest P, Futter N, Moors D, Irvine A, Crook J, Aitken S, Gerig L, Peterson R, Rasuli P; Intraarterial cisplatin and concurrent radiation for locally advanced bladder cancer. J Clin Oncol 1989; 7:230-235.

51a. Fung, C.Y.; Shipley, W.U.; Young, R.H.; Griffin, P.P.; Convery, K.M.; Kaufman, D.S.; Althausen, A.F.; Heney, N.M.; Prout, Jr., G.R. Prognostic factors in invasive bladder carcinoma in a prospective trial of preoperative adjuvant chemotherapy and radiotherapy. J Clin Oncol. 9:1533-1542; 1991.

52. Goffinet, D.R.; Schneider, N.J.; Glastin, E.J. *et al.* Bladder cancer: results of radiation therapy in 384 patients. Rad. 117:149-153; 1975.

53. Goodman, G.B.; Hislop, D.G.; Bellwood, J.M., *et al.* Conservation of bladder function in patients with invasive bladder cancer treated by definitive irradiation and selective cystectomy. Int J. Rad Oncol Biol Phys. 7:559-573; 1981.

54. Greiner, R.; Skaleric, K.C.; Veraguth, P. The prognostic significance of ureteral obstruction in carcinoma of the bladder. Int J Rad Oncol Biol Phys. 2:1095-1100;1977.

55. Greven, K.M.; Solin, L.W.; Hanks, G.E. Prognostic factors in patients with bladder carcinoma treated with definitive irradiation. Cancer. 65:908-912;1990.

55a. Herr, H.W. Progression of stage T1 bladder tumors after intravesical bacillus Calmette-Guerin. J Urol. 145(1): 40-44; 1991.

56. Herr HW, Laudone VP: Intravesical therapy for superficial bladder cancer. In: Updates of Cancer: Principles and Practice of Oncology. Devita VT, Hellman S, Rosenbery SA. eds. Philadelphia, Pa: J.B. Lippincott, Co.: 2:1-10, 1988.

57. Jacobsen, A.-B.; Lunde, S.; Ous, S. *et al.* T2/T3 bladder carcinomas treated with definitive radiotherapy with emphasis on flow cytometric DNS ploidy values. Int J Rad Oncol Biol Phys. 17:923-930;1990.

57a. Lamm, D.L.; Blumenstein, B.A.; Crawford, E.D. *et al.* A randomized trial of intravesical doxorubicin and immunotherapy with Bacille Calmeta-Guerin for transitional-cell carcinoma of the bladder. New Engl J Med. 1991; 325: 1205-1209.

58. Lange, C.S.; Rotman, M. Chemo-radiation therapy of bladder cancer. Int J Rad Oncol Biol Phys. 19:817-820;1990.

59. Loehrer, P.J.; Elson, P.; Kuebler, J.P.; Crawford, E.D.; Tannock, I.; Raghavan, D.; Stuart-Harris, R.; Trump, D.; Einhorn, L.H. Advanced Bladder Cancer: A Prospective Intergroup Trial Comparing Single Agent Cisplatin (CDDP) Versus M-Vac Combination Therapy (INT 0078). In: Proceedings of Am Soc Clin Oncol. Washington, D.C.: ASCO; 9:132;1990. Abstract.

60. Logothetis CJ, Johnson ED, Chong C, Dexeus FH, Sella A, Ogden S, Smith T, Swanson DA, Babaiian RJ, Wishnow KI, Von Eschenbach A: Adjuvant Cyclophosphamide, Doxorubicin and Cisplatin chemotherapy for bladder cancer: An update. J Clin Oncol 6:1590-1596; 1988.

61. Marks LB, Kaufman SD, Prout GR, Heney NM, Griffin PP, Shipley WU: Invasive bladder carcinoma: Preliminary report of selective bladder conservation by transurethral surgery, upfront MCV (Methotrexate, Cisplatin, and Vinblastine) chemotherapy and pelvic irradiation plus Cisplatin. Int J Radiation Oncol Biol Phy 1988; 15:877-883.

62. Martinez A, Gunderson LL: Intraoperative radiation therapy for bladder cancer. Urol Clin of North Am. 1984; 11:693-698.

63. Mathur, V.K.; Krahn, H.P.; Ramsey, E.W. Total cystectomy for bladder cancer. J. Urol. 125:784;1981.

64. Miller, L.S.; Johnson, D.E. Megavoltage radiation for bladder carcinoma: alone, postoperative, or preoperative. In: Proceedings of Seventh National Cancer Conference. 3:771-782; 1987.

65. Mohiuddin M, Kramer S, Newall J, Parsons J, Wiley A: Combined pre and postoperative adjuvant radiotherapy for bladder cancer: Results of RTOG/Jefferson study. Cancer 1981; 61:255-262.

66. Morrison, R. The results of treatment of cancer of the bladder: a clinical, contribution of radiobiology. Clin Radiol. 76:67-78;1975.

66a. Parsons, J.T., Million, R.R. Bladder. In: Principles and Practice of Radiation Oncology, 2nd ed. Perez, C.A., Brady, L.W. eds. Philadelphia, PA: JB Lippincott Co; 1992: 1036-1058.

67. Parsons JT, Million RR: Planned preoperative irradiation in the management of clinical stage B2-C (T3) bladder cancer. Int J Radiation Oncol Biol Phys. 1988; 14:797-810.

68. Pearse HD: The urinary bladder. 6th ed. In: Moss, W.T.; Cox, J.D., (eds). Radiation Oncology, Rationale, Technique, Results. St Louis, MO, 1989; 433-467.

69. Richie JP, Shipley WU, Yagoda A: Cancer of the bladder. In: DeVita VT, Hellman S, Rosenberg SA (eds). Cancer Principles and Practice of Oncology. 3rd ed. Philadelphia, PA: JB Lippincott Co., 1989; 1008-1022.

70. Rotman, M.; Aziz, H.; Porrazzo, M.; Choi, K.N.; Silverstein, M.; Rosenthal, J.; Laungani, G.; Macchia, R. Treatment of Advanced Transitional Cell Carcinoma of the Bladder with Irradiation and Concomitant 5-Fluorouracil Infusion. Int J Radiat Oncol Biol Phys. 18:1131-1138;1990.

71. Shipley, W.U.; Coombs, L.J.; Prout, G.R. Jr. Preoperative irradiation and radical cystectomy for invasive cancer - patterns of failure and prognostic factors associated with patient survival and disease progression. J. Urol. 135:222A;1986.

72. Shipley WU, Kaufman SD, Prout GR: The role of radiation therapy and chemotherapy in the treatment of invasive carcinoma of the urinary bladder. Seminars Oncol 1988; 15:390-395.

73. Shipley, W.U.; Rose, M.A.; Perrone, T. *et al.* Full-dose irradiation for patients with invasive bladder carcinoma: clinical and pathological correlates of improved survival. J. Urol. 134:679-683;1985.

74. Skinner, D.G. Management of Invasive Bladder Cancer. In: Yagoda, A. ed. Bladder cancer: future directions for treatment. New York, NY: John Wiley and Sons; 1986:87.

74a. Skinner, D.G.; Daniels, J.R.; Russell, C.A. *et al.* The role of adjuvant chemotherapy following cystectomy for invasive bladder cancer: A prospective comparative trial. J Urol 145(3):459-467; 1991.

75. Skinner, D.G.; Liekovsky, G. Contemporary cystectomy with pelvic node dissection compared to preoperative radiation therapy

plus cystectomy in management of invasive bladder cancer. J Urol. 131:1069-1072;1989.

76. Skinner, D.G.; Liekovsky, G. Management of invasive and high grade bladder cancer. In: Skinner DG, Liekovsky G (eds). Diagnosis and Management of Genitourinary Cancer. Philadelphia, PA: W.B. Saunders, Co.; 1988; 295-312.

77. Spera JA, Whittington R, Littman P, Solin LJ, Wein AJ: A comparison of pre-operative radiotherapy regimen for bladder carcinoma. The University of Pennsylvania experience. Cancer 1988; 61:255-262.

78. Sternberg, C.N.; Yagoda, A.; Scher, H.I.; Watson, R.C.: MVAC (Methotrexate, Vinblastine, Doxorubicin, and Cisplatin) for advanced transitional cell carcinoma of the urothelium. J Urol 1988; 139:461-469.

79. Sternberg CN, Yagoda A, Scher HI et al: Methotrexate, Vinblastine, Doxorubicin, and Cisplatin for advanced transitional cell carcinoma of the urothelium: efficacy, and patterns of response and relapse. Cancer 64:2448-2458;1989.

80. Stoter, G.; Splinter, T.A.W.; Child, J.A. et al. Combination chemotherapy with cisplatin and methotrexate in advanced transitional cell carcinoma of the bladder, J. Urol. 137:663;1987.

81. Torti FM, Lum BL: The biology and treatment of superficial bladder cancer. J Clin Oncol 1984; 2:505-531.

82. van der Werf-Messing, B. Carcinoma of the urinary bladder T3NxMO treated by preoperative radiation followed by simple cystectomy. Int J. Radiat Oncol Biol Phys. 8:1849-1855;1982.

83. van der Werf-Messing B, Menon RS, Hop WCJ. Cancer of the urinary bladder category T2, T3 (NxMO) treated by interstitial radium implant: Second report. Int J Radiation Oncol Biol Phys 1983; 9:481-485.

84. van der Werf-Messing, B.H.P.; van Putten, W.L.J. Carcinoma of the Urinary Bladder Category T2,3NxM0 Treated by 40 Gy External Irradiation Followed by Cesium 137 Implant at Reduced Dose (50%). Int J Rad Oncol Biol Phys. 16:369-372;1989.

85. Whitmore WF: Bladder Cancer: An overview. CA 1988; 38:213-223.

86. Whitmore WF: Irradiation and/or surgery. Some areas of confrontation in urologic oncology. Am J Clin Oncol 1989; 7:595-606.

87. Wishnow KI, Dmochowski R: Pelvic recurrence after radical cystectomy without pre-operative radiation. J Urol 1988; 140:42-43.

88. Wuilty, P.M.; Duncan, W. Primary radical radiotherapy for T3 transitional cell cancer of the bladder: An Analysis of survival and control. Int. J. Rad Oncol Biol. Phys. 12:853-860;1986.

89. Yagoda, A. Chemotherapy of *urothelial* tract tumors. Cancer. 60:574-585;1987.

90. Yagoda, A. Chemotherapy for advanced bladder tumor. In: Yagoda, A. (ed). Bladder Cancer: Future Directions for Treatment. New York, NY: John Wiley and Sons; 1986; 87.

91. Zincke H, Sen SE, Hahn RG, Keating JP: Neoadjuvant chemotherapy for locally advanced transitional cell carcinoma of the bladder: Do local findings suggest a potential for salvage of the bladder? Mayo Clinic Proc 1986; 63:16-22.

Prostate Cancer

92. Ahmann, F.R.; Marx, P.; Ahmann, M. Predicting Response to Therapy in Metastatic Prostate Cancer with Serum Prostate Specific (PSA) Levels. In: Proceedings of Am Soc Clin Oncol. Washington, D.C.: ASCO; 9:134;1990. Abstract.

93. Alexander RB, McGuire MG, Epstein JI, Walsh PC: Pathologic stage is higher in older men with clinical Stage Bl adenocarcinoma of the prostate. J Urol 1989; 141:880-882.

94. Bagshaw MA: Potential for radiotherapy alone in prostate cancer. Cancer 1985; 55:2079-2085.

95. Barzell, W.; Bean, M.A.; Hilaris, B.S.; Whitmore, W.F. Prostatic Adenocarcinoma: Relationship of Grade and Local Extent of the Pattern of Metastases. J. Urol. 118:278-282;1977.

96. Brown DF, Rubenfeld S: Irradiation in preventing gynecomastia induced by estrogens. Urology 1974; 3:51-53.

97. Byar, D.P.; Corle, D.K. Hormone therapy for prostate cancer: Results of the Veterans Administration Cooperative Urological Research Group Studies. JNCI Monograph 7:165-170; 1988.

97a. Catalona, W.J.; Smith, D.S.; Ratliff, T.L. et al. Measurement of prostate-specific antigen in serum as a screening test for prostate cancer. N Engl J Med. 324(17):1156-1161; 1991.

98. Coleman, C.N.; Rose, M.A.; Noll, L.; Buswell, L.; Riese, N.; Johnson, D.; DeWolfe, W.; Richie, J. A Phase II Trial of the Radiation Sensitizer Etanidazole (ETA) [SR 2508] for Locally Advanced Prostatic Carcinoma. In: Proceedings of Am Soc Clin Oncol. Washington, D.C.: ASCO; 9:151;1990. Abstract.

99. Crawford ED, Eisenberger MA, McLeod DG, Spaulding JT, Benson R, Dorr FA, Blumenstein BA, Davis MA, Goodman PJ: A controlled trial of leuprolide with and without Flutamide in prostate carcinoma. New Engl J Med. 1989; 321:419-424.

100. Crawford, E.D.; Kasimis, B.S.; Gandara, D.; Smith, J.A.; Soloway, M.S.; Lange, P.H.; Lynch, D.F.; Al-Juburi, A.; Bracken, R.B.; Wise, H.A.; Heyden, N.; Bertagna, C. A Randomized Controlled Clinical Trial of Leuprolide and Anandron (LA) Versus Leuprolide and Placebo (LP) for Advanced Prostate Cancer. In: Proceedings of Am Soc Clin Oncol. Washington, D.C.: ASCO; 9:135;1990. Abstract.

101. Donahue, R.E.: Mani, J.H.; Whitesel, J.A.; Mohr, S. Pelvic Lymph Node Dissection. Urology. 20:559-565;1982.

102. Eisenberger, M.A.; Simon, R.; O'Dwyer, P.J. et al. A reevaluation of nonhormonal cytotoxic chemotherapy in the treatment of prostatic carcinoma. J. Clin. Oncol. 3:827-841;1985.

103. Freiha FS, Bagshaw MA, Torti FM: Carcinoma of the prostate: pathology, staging, and treatment. Curr Probl Cancer 1988; 12:335-397.

103a. Fuks, Z.; Leibel, S.A.; Wallner, K.E.; Begg, C.B.; Fair, W.R.; Anderson, L.L.; Hilaris, B.S.; Whitmore, W.F. The effect of local control on metastatic dissemination in carcinoma of the prostate: Long-term results in patients treated with ^{125}I implantation. Int J Radiat Oncol Biol Phys. 21:537-548; 1991.

103b. Gittes, R.F. Carcinoma of the prostate. N Engl J Med. 324(4):236-245; 1991.

104. Gleason DF: Veterans Administration Cooperative Urological Research Group: Histologic Grading and Clinical Staging of Prostatic Carcinoma. In: Tannenbaum M. (ed). Urologic Pathology: The Prostate. Philadelphia, PA: Lea and Febiger, 1977; 171-198.

104a. Graverson, P.H.; Nielsen, K.T.; Gasser, T.C.; et al. Radical prostatectomy versus expectant primary treatment in stages I and II prostatic cancer: A fifteen-year follow-up. Urology 36(6):493-498; 1990.

105. Grayhack, J.T.; Keeler, T.C.; Kozlowski, J.M. Carcinoma of the prostate: Hormonal Therapy. Cancer. 60:589-601;1987.

106. Hanks GE. The prostate In: Moss WT, Cox JD (eds). Radiation Oncology, Rationale, Technique Results. St. Louis, MO: CV Mosby Co.; 1988; 487-511.

106a. Hanks, G.E.; Asbell, A.; Krall, J.M.; Perez, C.A.; Doggett, S.; Rubin, P.; Sause, W.; Pilepich, M.V. Outcome for lymph node negative T-1b, T-2(A-2,B) prostate cancer treated with external beam radiation therapy in RTOG 77-06. Int J Radiat Oncol Biol Phys. 21:1099-1104; 1991.

107. Hanks GE, Martz KL, Diamond JJ: The effect of dose on local control of prostate cancer. Int J Radiation Oncology Biol Phy 1988; 15:1299-1305.

108. Hirst AE, Bergman T: Carcinoma of the prostate in men 80 or more years old. Cancer 1954; 7:136-41.

108a. Hricak, H.; Dooms, G.C.; Jeffrey, R.B. et al. Prostatic carcinoma: Staging by clinical assessment, CT, and MR imaging. Radiol. 162(2):331-336; 1987.

109. Huggins C, Hodges C, V.: Studies on prostatic carcinoma. I. The effect of castration, of estrogens and androgen invection on serum phosphatases in metastatic carcinoma of the prostate. Cancer Res 1941; 1:293-297.

110. Kabalin Jn, Hodge KK, McNeal JE, Freiha FA, Stamey TA: Identification of residual cancer in the prostate following radiation therapy: role of transrectal ultrasound guided biopsy and prostatic specific antigen. J Urol 1989; 142:326-331.

111. Kuban DH, El-Mahdi AM, Schellhammer PF: I-125 interstitial implantation for prostate cancer. What have we learned 10 years later? Cancer 1989; 63: 2415-20.

112. Kaplan, I.D.; Valdagni, R.; Cox, R.S.; Bagshaw, M.A. Reduction of Spinal Metastases After Preemptive Irradiation in Prostatic Cancer. Int J Radiat Oncol Biol Phys. 18:1019-1026;1990.

113. Labrie F, Dupont A, Belanger A: Complete androgen blockade for the treatment of prostate cancer In: DeVita VT, Hellman S, Rosenberg SA, (eds). Important Advances in Oncology. Philadelphia, Pa: JB Lippincott Co. 1985; 193-217.

114. Lai, P.P.; Perez, C.A.; Shapiro, S.J.; Lockett, M.A. Carcinoma of the Prostate Stage B and C: Lack of Influence of Duration of Radiotherapy on Tumor Control and Treatment Morbidity. Int J Radiat Oncol Biol Phys. 19:561-568;1990.

114a. Lai, P.P.; Pilepich, M.V.; Krall, J.M.; Asbell, S.O.; Hanks, G.E.; Perez, C.A.; Rubin, P.; Sause, W.T.; Cox, J.D. The effect of overall treatment time on the outcome of definitive radiotherapy for localized prostate carcinoma: The Radiation Therapy Oncology Group 75-06 and 77-06 experience. Int J Radiat Oncol Biol Phys. 21:925-934; 1991.

115. Lange PH, Ercole CJ, Lightner DJ, Fraley EE, Vessella R: The value of serum prostate specific antigen determinations before and after radical prostatectomy. J Urol 1989; 141:873-879.

115a. Lawton, G.E.; Won, M.; Pilepich, M.V.; Asbell, S.O.; Shipley, W.U.; Hanks, G.E.; Cox J.D.; Perez, C.A.; Sause, W.T.; Doggett, S.R.L.; Rubin, P. Long-term treatment sequelae following external beam irradiation for adenocarcinoma of the prostate: Analysis of RTOG studies 7506 and 7706. Int J Radiat Oncol Biol Phys. 21:935-940; 1991.

116. Lee F, Littrup PJ, Torp-Pederson ST, Mettlin, C, McHugh TA, Gray JM, Kumasaka GH, McLeary RD: Prostate Cancer: Comparison of transrectal US and digital rectal examination for screening. Radiology 1988; 168:389-394.

117. MacLennan, I.; Selim, H.; Rubin, P. Sequential Hemi-body Radiotherapy in Poor Prognosis Localized Adenocarcinoma of the Prostate Gland: A Preliminary Study of RTOG. Int J Radiat Oncol Biol Phys. 16:215-218;1989.

118. Meek, A.G.; Park, T.L.; Oberman, E.; Wielopolski, L. A Prospective Study of Prostate Specific Antigen Levels in Patients Receiving Radiotherapy for Localized Carcinoma of the Prostate. Int J Rad Oncol Biol Phys. 19:733-742;1990.

119. Mellinger, G.T.; Arduino, L.J.; Becker, L.E.; Berman, H.I.: Carcinoma of the prostate: A continuing cooperative study. J Urol 1964; 91:590-594.

120. Mettlin C, Natarajan N: End results for urologic cancers. Trends and interhospital differences. Cancer 1987; 60:474-479 (Supplement).

121. Middleton, R.G. Value of and indication for staging pelvic lymph node dissection. Presented at the NIH Consensus Development Conference, Management of Clinically Localized Prostate Cancer, Bethesda, Md. June 15-17; 1987.

122. National Institutes of Health Consensus Development Conference Statement, June 15-17, 1987: The management of clinically localized prostate cancer. J Urol 1987; 138:1369-1375.

123. Paulson DF, Lin GH, Hinshaw W, Stephani S: Radical surgery vs. radiotherapy for adenocarcinoma of the prostate. J Urol 1982; 128:502-504.

123a. Paulson, D.F.; Moul, J.W.; Walther, P.J. Radical prostatectomy for clinical stage T1-2N0M0 prostatic adenocarcinoma: Long-term results. J Urol. 144:1180-1184; 1990.

123b. Perez, C.A.; Fair, W.R.; Ihde, D.C. Carcinoma of the prostate. In: DeVita, V.T., Hellman, S., Rosenberg, S.A. (eds): Cancer: Principles and Practice of Oncology, 3rd ed. Philadelphia, PA: JB Lippincott Co.; 1989:1023-1058.

123c. Physician's Data Query. Prostatic Cancer. Nat'l. Cancer Inst., Bethesda, MD: January 1992.

124. Pilepich, M.V.; Perez, C.A. Does radiotherapy alter the course of genitourinary cancer? In: Genitourinary Cancer. I. ED Paulson, ed. Boston, Mass.: Martinus Nijhoff; 1982:215-238.

124a. Prestidge, B.R.; Kaplan, I.; Cox, R.S.; Bagshaw, M.A. The clinical significance of a positive post-irradiation prostatic biopsy without distant metastases. Int J Radiat Oncol Biol Phys. 24(3):403-408; 1992.

125. Russel, K.J.; Dunatov, C.; Haferman, M.D.; Griffeth, J.T.; Pollisar, L.; Pelton, J.G.; Cole, S.B.; Taylor, E.W.; Wiens, L.W.; Koh, W.J.; Austin-Seymour, M.M.; Griffin, B.R.; Russell, A.H.; Laramore, G.E.; Griffin, T.W. Rapid Decline of Post-Treatment Serum Prostate Specific Antigen(PSA) as a Predictor for Clinical Outcomes in Patients with Adenocarcinoma of the Prostate Treated With Primary External Beam Irradiation. In: Proceedings of Am Soc Clin Oncol. Washington, D.C.: ASCO; 9:136;1990. Abstract.

126. Salazar OM, Rubin P, Keller B, Scarantino C: Systemic (half-body) radiation therapy: response and toxicity. Int J Rad Oncol Biol Phys.1978; 4:937-950.

127. Shevlin, B.E.; Mittal, B.B.; Brand, W.N.; Shetty, R.M. The Role of Adjuvant Irradiation Following Primary Prostatectomy, Based on Histopathologic Extent of Tumor. Int J Rad Oncol Biol Phys. 16:1425-1430;1989

128. Stamey TA, Yang N, Hay AR, McNeal JE, Freiha FS, Redwin E: Prostate specific antigen as a serum marker for adenocarcinoma of the prostate. New Engl J Med. 1987; 317:909-916.

129. Stamey TA, Kabalin JN: Prostate specific antigen in the diagnosis and treatment of adenocarcinoma of the prostate. I. Untreated patients. J Urol 1989; 141:1070-1075.

130. Tannenbaum M: Histopathology of the prostate gland. In: Tannenbaum M ed. Philadelphia, Pa.: Lea and Febiger; Urologic Pathology: The Prostate 1977; 303-397.

131. Walsh PC: Nerve sparing radical prostatectomy for early stage prostate cancer. Semin Oncol 1988; 15:351-358.

132. Walsh, PC. Preservation of sexual function in the surgical treatment of prostatic cancer — an anatomic surgical approach. In: VT DeVita, Jr., S. Hellman, SA Rosenberg, eds. Important advances in oncology. Philadelphia, Pa.: JB Lippincott, Co.; 1988:165.

133. Zincke H, Utz DC, Benson RC, Patterson DE: Bilateral pelvic lymphadenectomy and radical retropubic prostatectomy for Stage C adenocarcinoma of prostate. Urology 1984; 24:532-539.

Testicular Cancer

134. Babaian J, Zagars GK: Testicular Seminoma: The M.D. Anderson Experience. An Analysis of Pathological and Patient Characteristics, and Treatment Recommendations. J Urol 1988; 139:311-314.

135. Barneveld PU, Sleijfer DT, van der Mark TU, et al.: Natural History of Bleomycin Induced Pneumonitis. Am Rev Resp Dis 1987; 135:48-51.

136. Batata MA, Chu FCH, Hilaris BS, Whitmore WF, Golbey RB: Testicular Cancer in Cryptorchids. CA 1982; 49:1023-1030.

137. Birch R, Williams SD, Cone A, Einhorn LH, Roark P, et al.: Prognostic Factors for Favorable Outcome in Disseminated Germ Cell Tumors. J Clin Oncol 1983; 3:400-407.

137a. Brown, E.R.; Nichols, C.R.; Kneebone, P., et al. Long-term outcome of patients with relapsed and refractory germ cell tumors treated with high-dose chemotherapy and autologous bone marrow rescue. Ann Int Med 117:124-128; 1992.

137b. De Mulder, P.H.M.; Seynaeve, C.; Vermorken, J.B.; van Liessum, P.A.; Mols-Jevdevu, Snezana; Allman, E.L.; Beranek, Paul; Verweij, Jaap. Ondansetron compared with high-dose metoclopramide in prophylaxis of acute and delayed cisplatin-induced nausea and vomiting. An Int Med 113: 834-840; 1990.

137c. Donohue, J.P.; Foster, R.S.; Rowland, R.G., et al. Nerve-sparing retroperitoneal lymphadenectomy with preservation of ejaculation. J Urol 144(2):287-292; 1990.

138. Dosoretz, D.E.; Shipley, W.U.; Blitzer, P.H. et al. Megavoltage irradiation for pure testicular seminoma: Results and patterns of failure. Cancer 48:2184-2190;1981.

139. Drasga RE, Einhorn LH, Williams DS, Patel DN, Stevens EE: Fertility After Chemotherapy for Testicular Cancer. J Clin Oncol 1983; 3:179-183.

139 . Duchesne, G.M.; Horwich, A.; Dearnaley, D.P. et al. Orchiectomy alone for stage I seminoma of the testis. Cancer 65(5):1115-1118; 1990.

139a. Earle, J.D.; Bagshaw, M.A.; Kaplan, H.S. Supervoltage radiation therapy of testicular tumors. Am J Roentgenol. 117:653-661;1973.

140. Einhorn, L.H.; Crawford, E.D.; Shipley, W.U.; Loehrer, P.J.; Williams, S.D.: Cancer of the Testes, In: Cancer Principles and Practice of Oncology, 3rd ed, DeVita VT, Hellman S, Rosenberg SA, eds. J.B. Lippincott, Co.: Philadelphia, Pa.: 1989: 1071-1098.

141. Einhorn LH, Williams SD, Loehrer PJ, Birch R, Drasga R, et al.: Evaluation of Optimal Duration of Chemotherapy in Favorable-Prognosis Dissmeniated Germ Cell Tumors: A Southeastern Cancer Study Group Protocol. J Clin Oncol 1989; 7:387-391.

142. Fossa SD, Aass N, Kaalhus 0: Radiotherapy for Testicular Seminoma Stage I: Treatment Results and Long Term Post-Irradiation Morbidity in 365 Patients. Int J Radiation Oncology Biol Phy 1989; 16:383-388.

143. Fung CY, Garnick MD: Clinical Stage I Carcinoma of the Testis: A Review. J Clin Oncol 1988; 6:734-750.

144. Hadu SI: Pathology of Germ Cell Tumors of the Testis. Seminars in Oncol 1979; 6:14-25.

145. Hamilton, C.; Horwich, A.; Peckham, M.J. et al. Radiotherapy for

Stage I seminoma testis: Results of treatment and complication. Radiother. 6:115-210;1986.

146. Hanks, G.E.; Herring, D.F.; Kramer, S. Patterns of care outcome studies: Results of the National Practice in Seminoma of the Testis. Int J Radiat Onco Biol. 7:141-147;1981.

146a. Hanks, G.E; Peters, T.; Owen, J. Seminoma of the testis: Longterm beneficial and deleterious results of radiation. Int J Radiat Oncol Biol Phys.; 24(5):913-919; 1992.

147. Horwich A, Tucker DF, Peckham MJ: Placenta Alkaline Phosphatase as Tumor Marker in Seminoma Using the H17E2 Monoclonal Antibody Assay. Br J Cancer 1985; 51:625-629.

148. Hoskin P, Dilly S, Easton D, Horwich A, Hendry UF, et al.: Prognostic Factors in Stage I Non-Seminomatous Germ-Cell Testicular Tumors Managed by Orchiectomy and Surveillance: Implications for Adjuvant Chemotherapy. J Clin Oncol 1986, 4:1031-1036.

149. Israel A, Bosl GJ, Golbey RB, et al.: The Results of Chemotherapy for Extragonadal Germ Cell Tumors in the Cisplatin Era: The MSKCC Experience. J Clin Oncol 1985; 1073-1078.

149a. Klepp, O.; Olsson, A.M.; Henrikson, H. et al. Prognostic factors in clinical stage I nonseminomatous germ cell tumors of the testis: Multivariate analysis of a prospective multicenter study. J Clin Oncol. 8(3):509-518; 1990.

150. Krone KD, Carroll BA: Scrotal Ultrasound. Radiol Clin North Am. 1985; 23:121-139.

151. Kuzmits R, Schernthaner G, Kirsch K: Serum Neuron-Specific Enolase: A Marker for Response to Therapy in Seminoma. Cancer 1987; 60:1017-1020.

152. Lange PH, Narayan P, Vogelzang NJ, et al.: Return of Fertility After Treatment for Nonseminomatous Testicular Cancer: Changing Concepts. J Urol 1983; 129:1131-1135.

153. Lindsey CM, Glenn JF: Germinal Malignancies of the Testis: Experience, Management and Prognosis. J Urol 1976; 116:59-62.

154. Loehrer PJ, Birch R, Williams SD, Greco FA, Einhorn LH: Chemotherapy of Metastatic Seminoma: The Southeastern Cancer Study Group Experience. J Clin Oncol 1987; 5:1212-20.

155. Maier, J.G.; Sulak, M.H. Radiation therapy in malignant testis tumors seminoma. Cancer. 32:11-116;1973.

156. Mason BR, Kearsley JH: Radiotherapy for Stage II Testicular Seminoma: The Prognostic Influence of Tumor Bulk. J Clin Oncol 1988; 6:1856-1862.

157. Mostofi FK: Pathology of Germ Cell Tumors of Testis: A Progress Report. Cancer (Suppl) 1980; 45:1735-1754.

158. Mostofi, F.K.; Price, E.B. eds. Tumors of the Male Genital System, Atlas of Tumor Pathology, Second series, fascicle 8, p. 7, Washington, D.C. Armed Forces Institute of Pathology.

159. Mostofi, F.K.; Sesterhenn, I.A.; Sobin, L.H. Histological typing of testis tumors. Geneva, Switzerland: World Health Organization; 1977 (International Histological Classification of Tumors, No. 16).

160. Oliver RTD: Long Term Follow-up of Single Agent Cisplatin in Metastatic Seminoma and Surveillance for Stage I Seminoma. Proc Am Soc Clin Oncol. 1988; 7:120. Abstract.

161. Peckham, M.J. Testicular tumors: Investigation and staging. In: The Management of Testicular Tumors. London: Edwin Arnold; 1981:89-101.

162. Peckham MJ, Hamilton CR, Horwich A, Hendry WF: Surveillance After Orchiectomy for Stage I Seminoma of the Testis. Brit J Urol 1987; 59:343-347.

162a. Physician's Data Query. Testicular Cancer. Nat'l. Cancer Inst., Bethesda, MD: January 1992.

163. Pizzocaro G, Zanoni F, Milani A, Savioni R, Piva L, et al.: Orchiectomy Alone in Clinical Stage I Nonseminomatous Testis Cancer: A Critical Appraisal. J Clin Oncol 1986; 4:35-40.

164. Redman JR, Vugrin D, Arlin ZA, et al.: Leukemia Following Treatment of Germ Cell Tumors in Men. J Clin Oncol 1984; 2:1080-1087.

165. Richie, J.P. Is Adjuvant Chemotherapy Necessary for Patients With Stage B1 Testicular Cancer? In: Proceedings of Am Soc Clin Oncol. 9:144;1990. Abstract.

166. Terebelo HR, Taylor HG, Brown A, et al.: Late Relapse of Testicular Cancer. J Clin Oncol 1983; 1:566-571.

167. Thomas GM, Rider UD, Dembo AJ, Cummings BJ, Gospodarowicz M, Hawkins NV, Herman JG, Keen, CW. Seminoma of the Testis: Results of Treatment and Patterns of Failure After Radiation Therapy. Int J Radiation Oncology Biol Phy 1982; 8: 165-174.

168. Thomas GM, Sturgeon JF, Alison R, Jewett M, Goldberg S, Sugar L, Rideout D, Gospodarowicz MK, Duncan U: A Study of Post-Orchiectomy Surveillance in Stage I Testicular Seminoma. J Urol 1989; 142:313-316.

168a. Thomas, G.M.; Williams, S.D. Testis. In: Perez, G.A., Brady, L.W. (eds). Principles and Practice of Radiation Oncology, 2nd ed. Philadelphia, PA: JB Lippincott Co.; 1992;1117-1130.

169. Willan, B.D.; McGowan, D.G. Seminoma of the testis: A 2-year experience with radiation therapy. Int J Radiat Oncol Biol Phys. 11:1769-1775;1985.

170. Williams SD, Birch R, Einhorn LH, Irwin L, Greco FA, Loehrer PJ: Treatment of Disseminated Germ Cell Tumors with Cisplatin, Bleomycin and Either Vinblasin or Etoposide. New Engl J Med. 316:1435-1440;1987.

171. Williams SD, Stablein DM, Einhorn LH, Muggia FM, Weiss RB, et al.: Immediate Adjuvant Chemotherapy vs. Observation with Treatment at Relapse in Pathological Stage II Testicular Cancer. N Engl J Med 1987; 317: 1433-1438

172. Zagars GK, Babaian RJ: The Role of Radiation in Stage II Testicular Seminoma. Int J Radiation Oncology Biol Phys.13:163-170;1987.

173. Zagars, G.K.; Babaian, R.J. Stage I testicular seminoma: Rationale for post-orchiectomy radiation therapy. Int J Radiat Oncol Biol Phys. 13:155-170;1987.

Jacob M. Rowe, M.D., Medical Hematology
George B. Segel, M.D., Pediatric Hematology and Oncology

Chapter **24**

THE LEUKEMIAS

Out, damned spot! Out, I say!

William Shakeapeare (1)

PERSPECTIVE

Over the past decade major advances have occurred in therapy for the leukemias. Although suppressive chemotherapy has markedly decreased the morbidity of chronic leukemias, this has not greatly altered patient survival. Allogeneic bone marrow transplantation (BMT) now offers a potential of cure for chronic myelogenous leukemia (CML). In contrast, improvement in therapy for acute leukemias, using either intensive chemotherapy or bone marrow transplantation, has resulted in an increase in the number of patients who have a remission of their disease, improvement in the survival of patients in remission, and the cure of some patients, both in the pediatric and adult age groups.

Advances in cytogenetic analysis and immunophenotyping have led to more precise characterization of leukemias (106, 113). Ongoing research in these areas, and the development of newer cytotoxic agents and biologic response modifiers, coupled with studies of in vitro drug sensitivities, are directed at identifying patients most suitable for the different therapeutic modes and are also an attempt at greater predictability of outcome.

The term "weisses blut," that is, white blood (now leukemia) was introduced by Virchow in 1845 (55) to describe patients with chronic leukemia and massive accumulations of white blood cells (WBCs) in the blood. Many patients with chronic leukemia have less dramatic increases in (WBC) count, and the total (WBC) count in patients with acute leukemia is more often normal or decreased.

Leukemias are neoplasias in which the two major defects are unregulated proliferation and incomplete maturation of hemopoietic or lymphopoietic progenitors. Leukemia originates in the marrow, although leukemic cells may infiltrate lymph nodes, liver, spleen, and other tissues. The principal clinical manifestation is a decrease of red blood cells (RBCs), granulocytes, and platelets in the blood as a result of suppression of normal hemopoiesis by the malignant process. In the chronic or well-differentiated leukemias, unregulated proliferation, accumulation of leukemic cells, and elevated WBC count dominate, although differentiation and maturation of the leukemic cells may be largely preserved. In acute leukemias, unregulated proliferation also occurs, but maturation of the leukemic progenitors is profoundly impaired.

Therapy of chronic leukemias is directed toward suppressing the excessive proliferation to reduce the accumulation of leukemic cells and to permit improvement in effective hemopoiesis, whereas in acute leukemias intensive treatment is used to obliterate the leukemic clone.

EPIDEMIOLOGY AND ETIOLOGY

Epidemiology (14,24,43)

The incidence rates of leukemia vary with the morphologic type. The frequency of a given type of leukemia is also dependent on age, sex, race, and locale. Highlights of the differences are noted under "Epidemiology" in the discussion of each leukemia. In broad terms, acute lymphocytic leukemia (ALL) is a disease of childhood; chronic lymphocytic leukemia (CLL) is a disease of the aged; acute myelogenous leukemia (AML) occurs with similar frequency at all ages; and CML occurs most frequently in middle life. Sex differences are slight except in CLL, where male predominance is more striking.

Etiology

Evidence from epidemiologic studies supports the causal role of both environmental and genetic factors in leukemia. However, a definite antecedent causal factor can be identified in only a small fraction of all cases.

Environmental factors:
1. Ionizing radiation: Studies in subjects exposed to large quantities of irradiation have provided firm evidence for its causal role in human leukemia (13,37). Leukemia after irradiation exposure has been documented most carefully by the Atomic Bomb Casualty Commission in Hiroshima and Nagasaki (8). Leukemogenesis has also been observed after therapeutic irradiation for such diseases as ankylosing spondylitis and Hodgkin's disease (12). Acute leukemia and CML may develop following irradiation. A latent period of several years is usual (8). Irradiation also has been shown to be a leukemogen in several animal species (51). The role of low-level irradiation, diagnostic x-rays, in the etiology of leukemia remains uncertain (39).

2. Chemicals and drugs: Benzene exposure has been associated most closely with subsequent development of leukemia (4,52). Phenylbutazone (38), arsenic (34), and chloramphenicol exposure (10) have also been related to the future development of leukemia. In most cases, bone marrow aplasia caused by drug exposure is the initial hemopathy; leukemia evolves later. Chemical leukemogens have been described in several animal species (47). Oral alkylating agents, especially melphalan, given to patients with solid tumors or multiple myeloma, have resulted in an increase in the incidence of AML in those patients (44,57). Combinations of chemotherapeutic regimens and radiation therapy such as MOPP and total nodal irradiation for advanced Hodgkin's disease increase the incidence of leukemia and second malignancies in survivors (45).

3. Marrow hypoplasia: Marrow hypoplasia may be related to the development of leukemia and may account for some cases of postirradiation leukemia. In both animals and humans, a marked reduction in hemopoietic cells in the marrow predisposes to later leukemic transformation. This has been particularly noteworthy in congenital (Fanconi's) aplasia and in paroxysmal nocturnal hemoglobinuria during its aplastic phase (15).

4. Environmental interactions: Environmental factors predisposing to leukemia can be multiple, interactive, and difficult to identify. An example is the apparent increase in leukemia in children only when they are exposed to multiple rather than single risk factors (20) or to prenatal influences (27). Such risk factors include maternal irradiation, in utero irradiation, early childhood viral diseases, and a maternal history of fetal wasting. Wide geographic and seasonal differences in incidence have been reported for different types of leukemia. These observations could point to as yet unidentified environmental factors in disease causation (29).

Genetic factors: The marked increase in leukemia frequency in the identical twin of a leukemia patient, in Down's syndrome, Bloom's syndrome, Fanconi's syndrome, Klinefelter's syndrome, and congenital aneuploidy has suggested a genetic predisposition to leukemia (41). In the latter five syndromes, the presence of a congenital chromosomal aberration may play a role in the development of leukemia (19). The propensity for in vitro viral transformation of fibroblasts grown from subjects with chromosomal abnormalities is compatible with such a concept (50). An increase in the frequency of leukemia in siblings could be related either to genetic or environmental factors. The failure to find an increase in leukemia incidence in spouses of leukemia patients or in time-space studies of large communities in the United States (21) suggests that horizontal transmission of leukemia does not occur in a manner akin to that of typical viral infections. On careful analysis, clusters of leukemia cases are often within the probability of chance occurrence. Studies in New Zealand (25) and in Japan (31) suggest a time-space clustering in childhood leukemia but not in adult leukemia; this warrants further evaluation. The 40 times increase in frequency of leukemia in infant identical twins as compared with siblings also points to a genetic influence on leukemia causation (40). The risk of leukemia in the second of identical twins falls after infancy, suggesting an interaction of developmental or envi-

ronmental factors with the hereditary predisposition to leukemia. The increased frequency of certain human lymphocyte antigen (HLA) or B-lymphocyte genotypes in individuals with ALL also supports genetic influences (9,16). Although all major types of leukemia have been found to occur in families, CLL is the most striking in this regard (25).

Viral factors: Overwhelming evidence has been garnered to implicate RNA viruses in the etiology of animal leukemia (11,30,33). It is possible that a similar etiologic agent has a role in human leukemia. Candidate viruses have been identified in human leukemic cells by electron microscopy (53). The discovery of RNA-dependent DNA polymerase reverse transcriptase, an enzyme capable of synthesizing DNA from an RNA template, provided a modus operandi for the oncogenicity of RNA viruses (48). Evidence is accumulating to link RNA viruses to leukemogenicity in human cells (54). These viruses are now referred to as retroviruses and have been shown to carry the gene for the enzyme, reverse transcriptase. In animal viruses, an oncogene is inserted in the viral genome and demonstrates its leukemogenic potential when the virus infects a host cell (7).

Immunologic factors: Several lines of evidence have suggested that immune deficiency may favor development of neoplasia and that development or progression of tumors may be related to host immune capabilities (5,17). Preliminary but intriguing relationships between immune alterations in relatives of leukemic patients have been reported (49). The role of immune mechanisms in the prevention or control of leukemia in humans is also an area of intense study (42).

Interacting factors: Like most diseases, the etiology of human leukemia may involve multiple host and environmental factors. Animal studies have indicated that irradiation (23) and chemically-induced (32) leukemia may be mediated through activation of a latent RNA virus, or may require other accompanying host insults. Japanese populations exposed to irradiation from atomic bomb detonations generally developed leukemia of a type characteristic of the subpopulation, albeit at an increased frequency. For example, ALL occurred predominantly in children, and the myelogenous leukemias had their own characteristic age distribution. CLL, known to be extremely rare in the Japanese, did not occur.

CLASSIFICATION

Morphologic, Histochemical, and Immunologic Assessment

Morphologic and histochemical characteristics of cells, observed on stained smears of blood and marrow, are the basis for classification of leukemia (18,22,28). Complete agreement has not been reached on the nosology of leukemia. One of the most widely used morphologic classifications is described by the French-American-British (FAB) group, which relates the morphology of leukemic cells to presumed normal hematopoietic counterparts (22,64,65,66). Certain types of AML (Ml-M7) have been described: Ml and M2 represent undifferentiated and differentiated myeloblastic leukemia; M3 designates promyelocytic leukemia; M4 and M5 refers to myelomonocytic and monocytic variants; M6, erythroleukemia; and M7, megakaryocytic leukemia. While this classification is particularly useful for clinical trials in which arbitrary distinctions may be used, the prevailing attitude is to consider

AML—wherein most of the interest in classification has focused—as a single disease with several forms of morphologic expression. This variation is not surprising; the disease affects the hemopoietic stem cell, which is normally capable of multivariate differentiation. Hence, partial differentiation of leukemic cells may allow one or another cell type to predominate.

Among the lymphocytic leukemias, immunologic characteristics, such as surface immunoglobulin and sheep cell receptors, are used for classification. A small proportion of cases are unclassifiable after histochemical and immunologic assessment. High resolution histochemistry and electron microscopic anatomic features have permitted identification of most of the cell types in this group (56). A classification of the major types of leukemia is shown in Table 24-1.

ACUTE MYELOGENOUS LEUKEMIA (AML)

EPIDEMIOLOGY AND PATHOGENESIS

Epidemiology

AML is seen with nearly equal frequency in all decades of life, although the frequency is increased somewhat in those over 40 years of age (Fig. 24-1) (46). There is a slight predominance in males (14,43)

Pathogenesis

Normal hemopoiesis: The pathogenesis of leukemia is best understood when it is considered in respect to normal hemopoiesis. Hemopoiesis is the process by which mature RBCs, neutrophils, eosinophils, basophils, monocytes, and platelets are made. Although it is a continuum, one can consider hemopoiesis as having five major levels (Fig. 24-2) (109a).

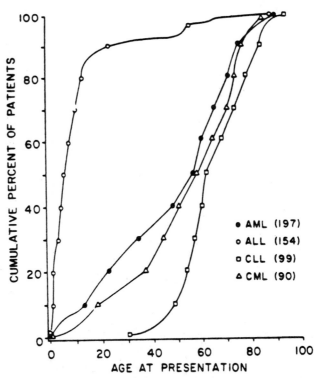

Fig. 24-1. Epidemiology: age at presentation. Cumulative percentage of subjects of a given age at the time of diagnosis for patients with acute myeloid (AML), acute lymphocytic (ALL), chronic myeloid (CML), and chronic lymphocytic (CLL) leukemias. The number of patients with each type of leukemia is shown in parentheses. From Rowe (46), with permission.

Table 24-1. Morphologic Categories of Myelogenous and Lymphocytic Leukemias

Acute or Poorly Differentiated Leukemia (incompletely differentiated cells predominate)	Chronic or Well-Differentiated Leukemia (cells morphologically similar to normal predominate)
Myelogenous	*Myelogenous*
1. Myeloblastic	1. Ph₁ positive (classical) — CML*
2. Myelomonocytic	a. Basophilic Ph₁ positive leukemia
3. Monocytic	2. Ph₁ negative — CML
4. Erythroid	3. Chronic myelomonocytic leukemia
5. Eosinophilic	4. Chronic monocytic leukemia
6. Megakaryocytic	
7. Progranulocytic	*Lymphocytic*
	1. B cell (classical — CLL**
Lymphocytic	2. T cell CLL
1. Common type (cALLa positive)†	a. Sezary cell
2. Null cell	3. Prolymphocytic
3. T cell	4. Lymphoma cell
4. B cell	5. Hairy cell
	6. Plasma cell

Undifferentiated

*Chronic myelogenous leukemia.
**Chronic lymphocytic leukemia.
†cALLa = Common acute lymphocytic leukemia antigen.
From Lichtman M.A. and Segel, G.B. (110a), with permission.

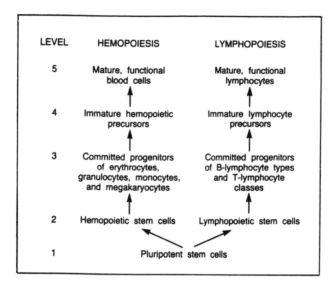

Fig. 24-2. Acute myelogenous leukemia etiology. Hemopoiesis versus lymphopoiesis. The functioning stem cell pool in mice is thought to be at level 1, the pluripotent cells. In healthy human beings, two stem cell pools may be operative; these are the cell pools at level 2. Cells at level 3 have become sensitive to specific cytopoietic hormone, such as erythropoietin, thrombopoietin, or neutropoietin. The committed progenitor cells at this level of differentiation are referred to as colony-forming units or cells, since they form colonies of cells in semisolid culture medium in the presence of the appropriate stimulating hormone. These hormones are capable of inducing proliferation and maturation of these committed progenitor cells so that they achieve level 4, at which the first morphologically identifiable precursors are present, such as myeloblasts and proerythroblasts, and, ultimately, level 5, the fully-matured blood cells. From Lichtman and Brennan (109a), with permission.

1. Level 1: The first and most primitive level is the pluripotent stem cell pool. This compartment of cells is capable of providing progenitors for lymphopoiesis and hemopoiesis. In healthy humans, it is uncertain if this pool of cells is functioning on a day-to-day basis, that is, whether it is the stem cell pool for hemopoiesis, or whether the common hemopoietic and lymphopoietic cell pools are separate stem cell pools.

2. Level 2: The second level of hemopoiesis is composed of two distinct stem cell pools: the common hemopoietic pool, capable of providing progenitors for the six types of blood cells and the common lymphopoietic stem cell pool, capable of providing progenitors for various lymphocyte classes and types.

3. Level 3: The common stem cell pools, by a process of differentiation, lead to the development of several committed progenitor cells. In hemopoiesis, these are committed unipotential progenitor cells for each of the six blood cell types. These committed progenitor cells each can be grown in semisolid medium and have been referred to as colony-forming cells (CFC), or colony-forming units (CFU), with a suffix for the cell line (e.g., CFU-N, for the cell that generates neutrophil colonies). Although less fully characterized, there are presumably committed progenitors for different types of B lymphocytes and subsets of T lymphocytes.

4. Level 4: The committed progenitors develop into the precursors of blood cells such as proerythroblasts, myeloblasts (granuloblasts), and megakaryoblasts.

5. Level 5: The precursor cells undergo a sequence of maturation until they become fully mature, functional blood cells. Fig. 24-3 (109) depicts the commitment and differentiation of the hemopoietic stem cell pool.

Leukemic hemopoiesis: AML results from the proliferation of cells derived either from a leukemic pluripotent or hemopoi-

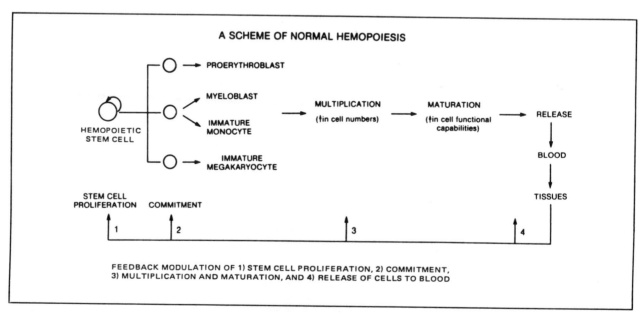

Fig. 24-3. Schematic depicting normal hemopoiesis in the etiology of acute myelogous leukemia. It presumes that the hemopoietic progenitor cell at level 2 in Fig. 28-2 acts as the stem cell pool for hemopoiesis. The regulatory mechanisms for the rate of stem cell proliferation and differentiation are unknown. Members of the hemopoietic progenitor cell pool become committed to one or another cell type. This corresponds to level 3 in Fig. 28-2. This, irrevocable to commitment, provides them with receptors and responsivity to hormones that further drive their multiplication, differentiation, and maturation into fully-differentiated cells. From Lichtman (109), with permission.

etic stem cell (105). An inability to mature or defective maturation is the primary abnormality in the cells. The growth fraction (percent of cells dividing), and the generation time of cells (the time to complete the cell mitotic cycle), is usually the same or less than that of normal primitive hemopoietic cells. Cell proliferation, when considered in absolute terms (total number proliferating) can be increased because of the marked increase in total number of primitive cells (83). Since the hemopoietic stem cell pool may be the site of injury in leukemia, erythropoiesis and thrombopoiesis, as well as granulopoiesis, are considered to be leukemic. Hence, defective erythropoiesis and thrombopoiesis of leukemic progenitor cells are present, as is inhibition of normal progenitor cells (105). The involvement of all blood cell lines (by nature of the lesion being in the hemopoietic stem cell pool) has been supported by studies of chromosome composition of cells in leukemia (132). In these studies, erythroblasts, megakaryocytes, and granulocyte precursors may each contain a similar chromosomal abnormality. Studies of the X-chromosome-linked isoenzymes, glucoae 6-phosphate dehydrogenase types A and B in black women with myelogenous leukemia, also support a clonal origin of the disease (151). A schematic representation of the defective hemopoiesis in myelogenous leukemia is shown in Fig. 24-4 (109).

Also see the section in this chapter on the pathogenesis of CML for further consideration of this topic.

DETECTION AND DIAGNOSIS

Clinical Detection

Principal findings in AML result from the absence of sufficient normal hemopoietic activity to maintain blood cell counts (72). In addition, less common disease manifestations may relate to the accumulation of leukemic blast cells in blood vessels and tissues. Onset may be very abrupt, but most cases have a prodromal period of 1 to 6 months, during which symptoms or signs are present.

Symptoms and signs may be attributed to:

1. *Anemia.* These include fatigue, dyspnea on exertion, palpations, or pallor.
2. *Neutropenia* (71): Local infections, for example, skin abscesses or systemic infections—usually acute—manifested by fever, chills, and symptoms relating to site, e.g., laryngitis, pneumonitis, meningitis, or septicemia may be present. Functional abnormalities of granulocytes also occur and contribute to infection onset (141).
3. *Thrombocytopenia:* These include petechiae and purpura, epistaxis, gingival bleeding, and gastrointestinal

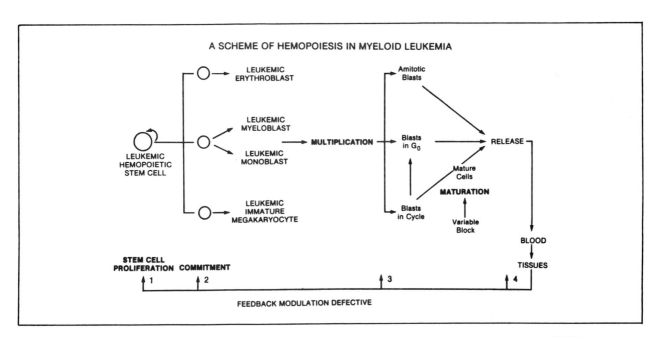

Fig. 24-4. Diagram depicting the current understanding of hemopoiesis in the etiology of acute myeloid leukemia (AML). The malignant process is believed to reside in the pluripotent or hemopoietic stem cell pool. These cell pools are represented at levels 1 and 2 in Fig. 28-2. This pool of cells is capable of multivariate commitment to leukemic erythroid, granulocytic, and megakaryocytic precursors. In most cases, granulocytic commitment predominates, and myeloblasts and promonocytes or their immediate derivatives are the dominant cell types. Multiplication of these precursors leads to the accumulation of leukemic blast cells in the marrow. The multiplying blast cells can take one of three paths. The leukemic cells may become amitotic (sterile), effete, and die. Alternatively, the blasts may stop dividing for prolonged periods (blasts in G_0) but have the potential to reenter the mitotic cycle. Third, the blasts may divide and undergo varying degrees of maturation. The maturation may lead to terminally differentiated cells such as red cells, segmented neutrophils, monocytes, or platelets. A severe block in maturation is characteristic of AML, whereas a high proportion of leukemic blast cells mature in chronic myelogenous leukemia. The disturbance in commitment and maturation in myelogenous leukemia is quantitative, and thus, many patterns are possible.

At least four major steps in hemopoiesis are regulated: stem cell proliferation, commitment to one of the three major hemopoietic cell lines (red blood cells, granulocytes, platelets), multiplication and maturation of early committed cells, and release of mature marrow cells to the blood. These control points are partially or totally defective in AML. From Lichtman (109), with permission.

(GI) or urinary tract bleeding. Functional abnormalities in leukemic platelets also may contribute to the hemorrhagic state (146).

4. *Other complaints*: Fatigue and malaise out of proportion to anemia are frequent. Occasionally, the sensation or awareness of an enlarged spleen is the initial symptom. Arthralgias and bone pain may also appear early in the disease, although this is more common in ALL. Fever is often related to the tumor itself at the time of diagnosis. An infection should always be considered in the presence of fever, and is usually the cause of fever later in the course of the disease and during treatment.

5. *Physical findings* may include pallor, petechiae, and purpura. The spleen is palpable in about 40% of cases. Hepatomegaly and lymphadenopathy are uncommon in AML. Leukemic infiltration of any organ may lead to signs or symptoms referable to AML. Localized tumors of myeloblasts, referred to as granulocytic sarcomas (myeloblastomas, chloromas), may develop in skin, paranasal sinuses, brain, or other sites (122). Rarely, this may precede evidence of leukemia in blood and marrow (107,150). Involvement of the cranial or spinal meninges is rare at the time of presentation. Unlike ALL, it is an infrequent complication even after disease progression.

Preleukemia or Myelodysplasia

The preleukemia syndrome includes several types of dyshemopoietic states, which combine blood cytopenias with hyperplastic and dysplastic hemopoiesis in marrow. The syndrome can terminate in AML after months or years. Preleukemia has been referred to by various terms, including, herald state of leukemia, refractory anemia, hyporegenerative anemia, and pancytopenia with hyperplastic marrow (84,112). The FAB group in 1982 subclassified preleukemia into five myelodysplastic syndromes (6). Essentially this classification subdivides different groups based on the number of blasts in the peripheral blood and marrow, and whether the bone marrow contains sideroblasts and the peripheral blood contains increased monocytes. It must be emphasized that these syndromes comprise a spectrum of clinical and laboratory abnormalities and expressions of the myeloid or hemopoietic stem cell disorder. Such patients often have different clinical findings at different times in their disease course and sometimes patients may present at a time when they have evolved into frank clinical AML.

Chromosomal abnormalities are common in myelodysplasia (68). Reported incidence for such abnormalities varies between 20% to 90%, but most studies report that the bone marrow of 40% to 60% of myelodysplastic patients contains a nonrandom karyotypic abnormality in the neoplastic clonal cells (35,36,138). The most common abnormalities in myelodysplasia are deletion of all portions of chromosome 5 (-5/5q-), chromosome 7 (-7/7q-), chromosome 20 (-20/20q), or additional chromosome 8 (8+). Additionally, unstable alterations such as ring chromosomes, dicentric chromosomes, and chromosome breaks also have been reported frequently in myelodysplasia. About 50% of patients ultimately die from leukemia. The pre-leukemic state itself has significant morbidity and mortality from infection and hemorrhage, and these events are correlated with the severity of the depression in granulocytes and platelets, as well as the functional disturbance in those cell

types. It is important to emphasize that some patients with early myelodysplasia (particularly patients with anemia, with or without ring sideroblasts), but without excessive number of blasts in their blood and bone marrow, do not progress into frank AML.

Several chronic myeloproliferative disorders may terminate in acute leukemia and, in that sense, are also preleukemic states. These include myeloid metaplasia, polycythemia vera, CML, and primary thrombocythemia. The term preleukemia, as it is currently used, refers principally to the dyshemopoietic states described at the beginning of this section that do not fall into the category of frank AML or a classic chronic myeloproliferative disease.

Pseudoleukemia

Several clinical situations can resemble leukemia. In patients with severe drug-induced hypoplastic neutropenia, removal of the drug can result in a wave of proliferation of normal immature granulocytes that can mimic progranulocytic leukemia in the marrow. Thus, neutropenia may be associated with a striking cohort of progranulocytes, if the marrow examination is performed during the early stage of hemopoietic recovery. The absence of anemia, thrombocytopenia, and blasts in the blood and the history of drug use are clues to the true diagnosis. Neutrophils return to the blood and the marrow appears normal a few days after the offending drug is discontinued.

Although acute leukemia occurs more frequently in children with Down's syndrome, these children also may undergo a profound transient myeloproliferative state during the neonatal period, which closely simulates AML. Increased blasts and a high WBC count may occur. The transient disorder disappears in weeks to months (85).

Diagnostic Procedures

1. *Blood cell counts* will uncover anemia and thrombocytopenia in nearly all cases of AML. Total leukocyte counts can be low, normal, or elevated to marked degrees. One third of cases have leukocyte counts less than 10,000/μL. Myeloblasts are present in the blood and usually compose more than 25% of leukocytes.

2. *Marrow aspiration* or biopsy usually shows an increase in leukemic blast cells; normal precursors are greatly reduced (72), although megakaryocytes are often more numerous in marrow biopsies than in aspirates from leukemic patients. Varying degrees of dyshemopoiesis are common in AML. Disorderly erythropoiesis, megaloblastoid erythroblasts, monocytic cells, and atypical megakaryocytes can be seen in many cases. Differentiation of myeloblasts from lymphoblasts may be difficult. Myeloblasts tend to be larger, have more numerous nucleoli, and may contain rodlike azure cytoplasmic inclusions (Auer rods). Histochemistry is very useful in differentiation. The myeloblast has peroxidase-positive granules and either no or light diffuse reactivity with periodic acid-Schiff stain (18,28). Cell inclusions, phi bodies—which are spindle-shaped rods—have been found by special histochemical methods and are thought to be pathognomonic of AML cells (99).

3. Chromosome studies using banding techniques reveal gross abnormalities in untreated patients with de novo AML in 50% to 60% of cases studied prospectively in

large groups (70). Smaller series from single institutions have reported clonal chromosomal abnormalities in 80% - 95% of newly diagnosed patients (153).

There are two major types of abnormality: first aneuploidy, in which there is either a gain (hyperdiploidy) or loss (hypodiploidy) in chromosome number from the normal 46; and second, an abnormality of chromosome structure in which the chromosome number is normal but chromosome abnormalities, detectable by standard methods, are present, such as unduly long chromosomes, ring forms, etc. In those patients having aneuploidy, the abnormalities are nonrandom, with a propensity for loss of chromosome number 7 or a gain of chromosome number 8 (131).

The most common structural abnormalities found in de novo AML are t (15;17) (q22;qll), and t (8;21) (q22;q22); rearrangement of 16q22, del (5q), del (7q), t (9;11) (p21;q23), del (llq), del (12p), del (9q), and del (20) (qll). In AML that follows a previous hematologic disorder or cytotoxic chemotherapy or radiotherapy, the abnormalities are del (7q), del (5q), t (1;3) (p36;q21), t (1;7(pll;pll), and t (2;11) (p21;q23) (70,89,131).

Several chromosomal abnormalities are associated with specific morphologic types of AML: t (9;22) with undifferentiated AML (M1); t (8;21) with classic myeloblastic morphology (M2); t (15;17) with promyelocytic AML (M3); t (9;11); and llq23 with monoblastic morphology (M5). Additionally, there appears to be an association between chromosomal abnormality and age. In younger patients more of the t (8;21) and t (15;17) abnormalities are seen, whereas the del (5q) and del (7q) are often seen in the older age group. The latter is also seen in secondary leukemias; this may represent chromosomal damage over a long period.

Chromosomal abnormalities that persist or appear when patients are in clinical remission usually predict a poor prognosis and short duration of remission

4. Metabolic alterations such as hyperuricemia (133), hypokalemia (121), and lactic acidosis (147) may occur. Other alterations in sodium, calcium, and phosphate concentrations, as well as blood pH, have been observed (124). Spurious alterations like hypoglycemia, hyperkalemia, and hypoxemia also may be reported by the laboratory as a result of leukemic cell metabolism and demise in vitro (102,191) .

CLASSIFICATION

Anatomic Staging

Anatomic classification is not applicable because of the nature of this disease.

Histopathology

Vertical (commitment) variants: The histopathology of AML is variable because the defect resides in the hemopoietic progenitor cell pool (105,109). The cell pool is capable of multivariate differentiation into erythroid cells (137), neutrophils, eosinophils (67), basophils (128), monocytes (90), and megakaryocytes (109). In the myelogenous leukemias, accentuated commitment to one of these cell lines can occur, leading to a large proportion of cells having a single phenotype. Neutrophilic and monocytic phenotypes are most common. These different types of leukemia can be thought of as vertical variants (Fig. 24-5a) (2).

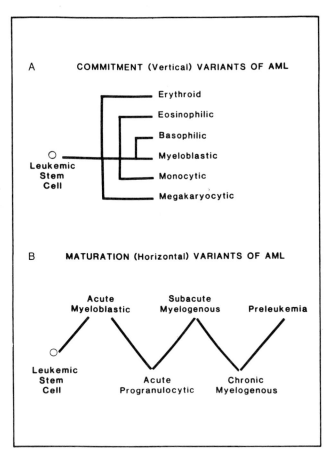

Fig. 24-5. Classification of acute myelogenous leukemia (AML). AML has a wide spectrum of morphologic expression and a wide spectrum in the maturation of leukemic cells into recognizable precursors. This phenotypic variation is a consequence of the leukemic lesion residing in a cell pool normally programmed to be capable of many different commitment decisions (a). The morphologic variants of AML can be considered point of commitment accumulate prominently (e.g., leukemic erythroblasts, leukemic monocytes). This represents the analogy of morphologic variants of AML to the normal, vertical commitment options of the hemopoietic stem cell pool (b). AML, progranulocytic leukemia, subacute leukemia, and chronic leukemia can be considered horizontal variants in which different blocks of maturation are present. This represents the analogy of morphologic variants of AML to the normal (horizontal) maturation stages of the hemopoietic cell pool. From Williams *et al.* (2), with permission.

Horizontal (maturation) variants: Different degrees of maturation also occur that can lead to a predominance of myeloblasts, progranulocytes or later stages of granulocytes or monocytes. These different types of leukemia can be thought of as horizontal variants (Fig. 24-5b).

Prognostic features: The pathogenesis and cytotoxic drug therapy of AML are the same regardless of the phenotypic variant present. Outcome is not greatly different for different morphologic types, although some studies have shown slightly different median survivals. Some studies suggest that the more differentiated the cells, the better the outcome (69, 74,139,154). Factors such as patient age, tumor burden at diagnosis, and the drug sensitivity of leukemic cells are more important than cell morphology in predicting survival.

Clinical manifestations of variants: Several morphologic variants of AML can have distinctive clinical features. Morphologic, histochemical, immunologic, and cytogenetic criteria for these distinctions have recently been standardized (78').

1. Monocytic leukemia is associated with leukemic cells that have morphologic or histochemical features (fluoride sensitive, ∞-naphthyl acetate esterase) similar to normal blood monocytes (119,140,143) . This AML variant is associated with a predisposition to tissue infiltrates (111), especially in gingival, cutaneous, and perirectal sites. Lymphadenopathy and meningeal involvement may also be seen. Lysozymuria (muramidasuria) is often striking and can be used to identify this variant.

2. Hypergranular progranulocytic leukemia is associated with leukemic progranulocytes that are heavily granulated, and in which a proportion of cells have single or multiple Auer rods. The peroxidase stain is intensely positive. A translocation between chromosomes 15 and 17 has been reported in a high proportion of cases (94). The frequency of disseminated intravascular coagulation is much greater than in other variants of AML (81,97).

3. Eosinophilic leukemia is associated with pulmonary and cardiac signs such as fibrosing endocarditis and heart failure (67,152).

4. Megakaryoblastic leukemia is an unusual variant that is associated with pancytopenia and undifferentiated blast cells in blood; and often there is evidence of atypical megakaryocytes in the marrow biopsy. The blast cells may contain platelet peroxidase or ultrastructural features of megakaryocytes. This disease is associated with marked marrow fibrosis (73). The disease referred to as acute myelofibrosis may, in many cases, be an example of megakaryocytic leukemia (125). Although the prognosis is often poor for patients with acute megakaryoblastic leukemia, standard treatment for AML is given, and in successful cases, the excessive marrow fibrosis may be normalized.

5. Erythroleukemia has distinctive marrow and blood cell morphology with bizarre, large, and extremely dyserythropoietic erythroblasts (137). The clinical course of this variant of AML may be protracted until the disease becomes more frankly like that of classic myeloblastic leukemia. There is a propensity for bone pain in this variant.

6. Some investigators have attempted to correlate remission duration with the morphologic cell type, such as briefer remissions in monocytic leukemias (80,101,120), fewer remissions in erythroleukemia, (63) or longer remissions in promyelocytic leukemia (63,88,120). However, these observations have not been uniformly observed (22,88,120,149).

PRINCIPLES OF TREATMENT

Decision to Treat

In most AML cases, treatment with cytotoxic drugs is necessary. In some cases of hypoaccumulative (smouldering, oligoblastic) leukemia, patients may have adequate granulocytes for sustained periods (130). RBC and platelets transfusions may be required periodically. In such patients, the risks of early, intensive drug therapy do not appear justified when compared with the natural course of the disease. Very aged patients tolerate aplasia poorly and have a reduced probability of remission. In such patients, treatment modalities and doses may require modification (62). Some patients in this category may not wish to be treated. Infants with neonatal myelogenous leukemia do not respond well to treatment and have an extremely poor prognosis (148).

Principles of Treatment

The cytotoxic drug treatment of AML and its variants rests on two premises (105):

1. Two competing clones of primitive hemopoietic cells are present in bone marrow—a leukemic and a normal or less leukemic clone; and,

2. Profound suppression of the leukemic cell population in marrow is required in AML to allow a clone change and thereby the opportunity for a return of normal or less leukemic hemopoiesis.

Chromosomal studies in leukemia support the first premise (105). In at least 50% of cases, a demonstrable chromosomal abnormality (qualitative or quantitative) is evident (131). During remission, the karyotype of mitotic cells is normal, which suggests replacement by a normal or a more-normal clone. With relapse, the original karyotypic abnormality reappears. These data suggest the presence of two competing clones. The second premise requires that intensive cytotoxic therapy be given (84a). This therapy induces severe marrow hypoplasia and severe cytopenias.

Although the risks to the patient are heightened during the first 4 weeks of treatment, the probability of a remission is greatly increased.

Chemotherapy

Induction therapy: Several types of drugs have proven useful in AML treatment (117). These include antimetabolites, especially cytarabine, and anthracycline antibiotics, especially daunorubicin. Addition of 6-thioguanine or other agents has not proved beneficial (87). Usually at least two drugs are used since this improves remission rates. A current recommended protocol calls for 3 days of an anthracycline antibiotic and 7 days of cytarabine. If the marrow is free of blast cells 1 week after such treatment, therapy is stopped. If it is not, another treatment cycle is given using a similar dose regimen. Up to one third of patients who achieve a complete remission (CR) may require two sequential courses of cytoreduction therapy. The patient is supported during the period of marrow aplasia in anticipation of a restitution of normal hemopoiesis. This restitution occurs in 50%-70% of patients after a period of 4 to 6 weeks (92,104).

"An exciting new development in induction or subsequent therapy for patients with AML relates to the development of maturational therapy of acute promyelocytic leukemia with all trans retinoic acid (TRA). Recent reports from China and France, and more recently the United States, have demonstrated a high rate of reponse in the patients with prompt resolution of the DIC (147a, 67a, 142a, 74b). Major cooperative group trials are now underway to fully establish the exact role in the treatment and maintenance of patients with this type of leukemia. Ultimately attempts will be made to extend the efficacy of this maturational agent or other types of hemopoietic stem cell disorders."

Hyperuricemia may result from increased nucleic acid degradation prior to, and particularly after, the start of therapy and can be controlled with allopurinol, reducing the risk of urate crystalluria and ureteral obstruction.

Consolidation therapy: If a remission is achieved, some type of continuing chemotherapy is usually used. While the duration and frequency of consolidation therapy remains controversial, it is clear that patients who have successfully completed one or more consolidation courses have a longer remission duration and increased survival (75,114,115,129,134). Drug regimens used for consolidation therapy may be similar to those used for induction therapy, or, in most instances, may use high doses of cytarabine either alone or in combination with an anthracycline antibiotic (143a).

Component Transfusion

Intensive chemotherapy of AML further reduces mature blood cells to levels incompatible with life. Transfusions of RBCs, platelets, or granulocytes invariably are required. The availability of blood components has been a key advance in the treatment of leukemia (123). RBC and platelet transfusions are readily available at all major medical centers. Many blood banks also can harvest leukocytes for transfusion (103).

1. *Platelet transfusion* is used to treat overt bleeding in the presence of thrombocytopenia and is also strongly recommended when the platelet count is less than 20,000/μL, especially if cutaneous bleeding or fever is present. The platelets are usually prepared from multiple, random donors. Administration of seven to ten units of random donor platelets per square meter body surface area results in a rise in platelet concentration of about 50,000/μL. In patients who become isoimmunized to random donor platelets, single-donor, HLA-matched platelets may be obtained from the general population or a sibling (135).

2. *Granulocyte transfusion* is reserved for patients who are severely neutropenic (< 500/μL), febrile, and who either have septicemia or have not responded to antibiotic therapy within 72 hours. Prophylactic use of granulocyte transfusion in severely granulocytopenic patients without evidence of infection has not proven beneficial, probably because of the limited number of granulocytes that one can transfuse successfully (135).

Antimicrobial Therapy

During the period of marrow aplasia induced by chemotherapy, infection is frequent. A high proportion of the infectious episodes are caused by gram-negative bacteria. Serologic studies suggest these have been resident in the patient's GI tract. Often an etiologic agent is not uncovered. For this reason, broad-spectrum, microbicidal antibiotic combinations such as aminoglycosides and semisynthetic penicillins are used. There is no unequivocal evidence that prophylactic antimicrobials are helpful in preventing life-threatening infections during the neutropenic period.

Those patients who require continuous, intensive chemotherapy may develop defects in cellular immunity that predispose them to infection by opportunistic microorganisms such as *Pneumocystis carinii* (pneumonia), fungi, and cytomegalovirus. The use of protected environments and prophylactic gut-cleansing antibiotics have not improved results of treatment (108,136).

With the advent of broad spectrum and effective antibacterial therapy, there has been marked decrease in the incidence and mortality from fungal infections. In fact, the majority of patients with AML receive amphotericin B at some point during their neutropenia.

Hemopoietic Growth Factors

A major potential advance in the supportive therapy of patients with acute leukemia is the recent development of colony stimulating factors (CSFs). These hemopoietic growth factors are peptide hormones that may dramatically alter the management of patients with cytopenias. These cytokines have added a new dimension to dose-intensive marrow-suppressive treatment regimens, with a potential that is yet to be fully realized. Due to the potential for cytokine-stimulation of the acute leukemia there was initially great hesitation in conducting clinical trials with granulocytemacrophage-(GM) or granulocyte-(G) colony stimulating factor (CSF) in acute leukemia. However, recent trials have suggested that this may not be a significant risk and several major trials have been completed or are ongoing to determine the exact role of colony stimulating factors in acute leukemia. One large randomized study, conducted in Japan, and most recently reported (122a), noted a marked reduction in documented infections, although it was not clear whether the actual incidence of febrile episodes was reduced. While a definitive role for cytokines in the management of patients with acute leukemia has not been fully established, these peptide hormones have enormous potential that should be more clearly defined in the coming years.

Radiotherapy

Rarely, granulocytic sarcomas may require local radiotherapy. Small total doses of irradiation (500 to 1,000 cGy) can relieve pain, reduce skin and mucosal infiltrates, and reverse spinal cord compression by myeloblastomas (82). Central nervous system (CNS) leukemia also occurs infrequently and can be treated with intrathecal chemotherapy and/or radiotherapy. This is far more common in lymphocytic leukemia (see section on ALL).

Bone Marrow Transplantation

Marrow cells obtained from an HLA-identical sibling have been administered intravenously (IV) to patients with AML who have been treated first with large doses of cyclophosaphamide and total body irradiation (TBI) (144,145) or with high doses of chemotherapy alone (e.g., busulfan and cyclophosphamide) (133a). Such a preparative regimen helps to reduce the leukemic cell load and impair the host's ability to reject the donor marrow cells. The dose of TBI should be large enough (~ 1,000 cGy) to suppress the immunologic capability of the recipient so that the BMT will not be rejected (145). A low dose rate of fractionated radiation treatments should be used to reduce pulmonary toxicity and avoid interstitial pneumonitis. Long-term survival of patients who received allogeneic transplants during advanced stage of their disease has been about 10%. This treatment mode is ideally available only to those patients with a histocompatible donor, usually a sibling or an identical twin. More recently, however, successful transplants have been performed in patients with nonrelated histocompatible donors (obtained through bone marrow registries of many thousands of donors) or from partially HLA-matched donors (60,61,100).

Three factors may result in failure of BMT: (1) recurrent leukemia; (2) graft versus host disease; and (3) uncontrollable infection such as viral interstitial pneumonitis (145). Usually the recurrent leukemia arises from the recipient's own marrow cells; however, rare cases have occurred in which the leukemic cells contained chromosome markers of the donor cell type (86,93).

Because of the limitation of donors available for allogeneic BMT and the age limit and the toxicity from this procedure, many studies are under way that evaluate the efficacy and indications for autologous BMT in AML. This method involves reinfusion of the patient's own bone marrow or rarely, peripheral blood stem cells, collected and cryopreserved while the patient is in CR. Prior to the reinfusion, the patient requires a preparative regimen consisting of high-dose chemotherapy with or without TBI. Early results suggest that autologous BMT of AML may be as good or better than conventional consolidation chemotherapy (95), although, to date, there have been few prospective clinical trials that have demonstrated this. At present, there is no unequivocal evidence that cleansing or purging the marrow ex vivo improves outcome. Allogeneic bone marrow transplantation in first remission can be considered in patients less than 40 years of age, if a histocompatible sibling is available as potential donor. In some studies, results from chemotherapy alone or high-dose chemotherapy with autologous bone marrow transplantation appear to be comparable to those allogeneic transplantation (74c,119a).

A major disadvantage of autologous BMT is the absence of graft versus leukemia effect, which is thought to play a major role in the long-term, disease-free survival seen in allogeneic transplant patients (95). The absence of graft versus leukemia effect is also likely to be the explanation for the high rate of relapse following syngeneic transplantation or transplantation using T-cell depletion.

Immunotherapy

In an attempt to reduce residual leukemic cells toward zero (98,116,142), or to retard the accumulation of small cones of cells, procedures to stimulate immune cytotoxicity have been explored. Protocols that include administration of bacillus Calmette-Guerin vaccine (active, nonspecific immunotherapy) have been studied. To date, there has been no convincing evidence of the efficacy of adjunctive immunotherapy. As mentioned above, the best evidence for the efficacy of any form of immunotherapy for AML comes from the data on the graft versus leukemia effect in allogeneic bone marrow transplantation.

Emotional Support

Emotional factors in the patient and the family and care of dying patients require skilled, compassionate health care providers. These include nurse practitioners, social workers, and physicians (96).

RESULTS AND PROGNOSIS

The median survival of untreated patients with AML is about 2 months. Intensive chemotherapy has increased the median survival to about 15 months. This increment results primarily from the prolongation of life in the 50% to 70% of subjects who have a remission after induction therapy. Occasionally, patients have a remission of several years (77). The longest remissions have been reported in studies that used intensive consolidation/intensification chemotherapy (74a,75,115,129). Most of these studies report 5-year disease-free survival rates of 10%-25% for adults in AML who have achieved CR.

Death is most commonly caused by infection (59). Hemorrhage has become a less frequent cause of death because of the efficacy of platelet transfusions. Leukocclusion in subjects with high leukemic blast cell counts in the blood can result in cerebral infarction, and patients with high blast counts are also prone to intracranial hemorrhage (91,110,118,191).

Intensive Chemotherapy with BMT

If the patient receives a bone marrow graft after induction of a first CR, the long-term survival may be as high as 45% to 65% (58,76,126). For patients in early first relapse or in second remission, bone marrow transplantation offers only a 20% to 30% long term survival, but is the only potentially curative therapy in such patients. In most studies, the outcome of BMT is related to patient age, with the best results in patients aged under 30 years (127,144). This is due, at least in part, to the ability of younger patients to recover from the transplant-related toxicity (graft-versus-host disease and infections). Recent clinical trials show little difference between patients over and under age 8 years if treated in first CR (Fig. 24-6) (78).

CLINICAL INVESTIGATIONS

Our understanding of and ability to manage AML has increased greatly in the last 20 years. Despite these advances, life has been lengthened only by 1 or 2 years for most patients. Better methods for the transfusion of adequate numbers of normal neutrophils and monocytes during marrow aplasia

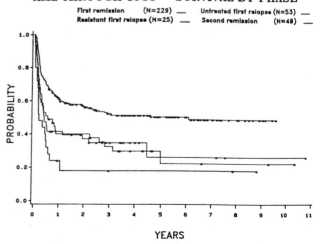

Fig. 24-6. Results of allogeneic bone marrow transplantation with acute myelogenous leukemia transplanted in different remission stages through 1985. From Clift *et al.* (78a), with permission.

prior to remission may increase the proportion of patients who enter remission. This advance will require improved techniques for the collection and storage of neutrophils. Marrow aplasia, the main goal of chemotherapy, can be achieved in most patients with AML. New cytotoxic drugs are not likely to improve further the treatment results but are being studied (58a,67a,114a). More intensive therapy during the remission period is being evaluated. Further advances in the treatment of AML are likely to depend on either new conceptual breakthroughs or innovative approaches.

The best results (40% to 50% long-term survival) in the treatment of AML have been obtained using allogeneic BMT in first remission. Unfortunately, this is only available for the minority of patients with AML.

CHRONIC MYELOGENOUS LEUKEMIA (CML)

EPIDEMIOLOGY AND PATHOGENESIS

Epidemiology

CML is uncommon before age 20 years and increases in frequency with each succeeding decade. There is a slight predominance of cases among males (14,43) (Fig. 24-1).

Pathogenesis

This disorder, like AML and other myelodysplastic syndromes, is a result of an abnormality in the hemopoietic stem cell pool, which in this case results in the accumulation of mostly mature or nearly mature granulocytic cells and often of megakaryocytes. Erythropoiesis usually is impaired. CML may result from a disorder in cell maturation with asynchronous development of the cytoplasm and nucleus (160,161,201). This results in decreased proliferation of the earliest granulocyte progenitors and increased proliferation of more mature marrow cells having an increased longevity. Hence, the predominant cells in the blood are mature or partially matured cells, such as segmented neutrophils and myelocytes. There may be mild functional impairment of mature neutrophils and platelets, but this impairment is not uniform or severe enough to lead to bleeding or infection. The Philadelphia chromosome (Ph[1]), a translocation of the long arms of chromosome 22 to another chromosome (most often chromosome 9), is present in marrow cells (Fig. 24-7) (1a,195,199). Evidence from studies in twins indicates that the translocation is an acquired abnormality (176). It is a highly specific abnormality of chromosomes in the leukemias because it is present in over 90% of cases with a clinical picture typical of CML (156,194) and since the molecular rearrangement involving the breakpoint cluster region (*bcr* on chromosome

Normal Configuration of Chromosomes 9 & 22

Rearranged Chromosomes 9(9q+) & 22(Ph)

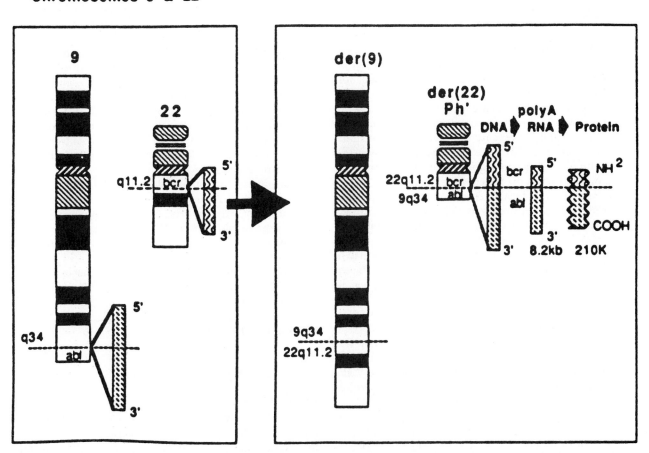

Fig. 24-7. Schematic representation of the translocation between chromosomes 9 and 22. Also shown are the molecular consequences of the Ph translocation — a hybrid DNA joining most of the C-*abl* gene to the 5' region of the *bcr* gene on chromosome 22, a hybrid mRNA of 8.2 kb and a hybrid protein of 210 kd. From Fialkow and Singer (1a), with permission.

22q11) and the proto-oncogene *c-abl* on chromosome 9 is present in a number of additional Ph[1] negative cases (163). The presence of the Ph[1] chromosomes in dividing erythroid, granulocytic and megakaryocytic cells has been taken as evidence for a common hemopoietic progenitor cell lesion (105). Other data support a clonal origin of the cells in CML (171,194). The Ph[1] chromosome usually is present in all metaphases, even after treatment. Thus, a normal hemopoietic clone is not overly evident in this disease, although recent evidence suggests that it may be overshadowed by the accumulation of the neoplastic clone. The disappearance of Ph[1]-negative cells now has been described after intensive treatment, treatment with interferon, or after standard treatment (159,172,202). In vitro studies also suggest that a dual population can exist (165).

Early studies in CML patients emphasized the absence of the Ph[1] chromosome in phytohemagglutinin-stimulated lymphocytes. Recent studies have reported that cells with features of lymphocytes, but containing monoclonal enzyme markers or chromosome markers, are present in some patients with CML (84,162,171,188,190). These reports suggest that the leukemic lesions in myelogenous leukemia are closer to the pluripotent stem cell (level 1, Fig. 24-2) than to the hemopoietic stem cell (level 2, Fig. 24-2). The evidence in this matter is contradictory and not as yet definitive; moreover, the lesion may exist at level 1, between levels 1 and 2, or at level 2 in different subjects. These considerations also apply to the pathogenesis of AML.

DETECTION AND DIAGNOSIS

Clinical Detection

The onset of CML usually is insidious. Occasionally, the disease will be discovered during routine medical evaluation, although most patients have symptoms.

1. Symptoms of malaise, fatigue, heat intolerance, sweating, easy bruising, discomfort in the abdomen, and early satiety or fullness because of splenic enlargement are most common (182). Rarely, the symptoms associated with a splenic infarction, gouty arthritis, or a urate renal stone may bring the patient to the physician.
2. *Physical findings* include enlargement of the spleen in 90% of cases. Hepatomegaly and lymphadenopathy are very uncommon. Easy bruising, purpura, gingival bleeding or CNS signs may occur occasionally, especially if the leukocyte count is markedly elevated. This may be related to poor platelet function and leukostasis. Rarely, a tumor of myeloblasts (granulocytic sarcoma) may be found as the initial sign of the disease.

Diagnostic Procedures

1. *Blood analysis* identifies leukocytosis as a constant feature (> 20,000/μL) that can reach extraordinary levels (> 500,000/μL). About one third of patients have WBC counts between 30,000 and 100,000/μL, and two thirds over 100,000/μL, at the time of diagnosis. Myeloblasts, promyelocytes, and nucleated RBCs are present in the blood. Myelocytes and segmented neutrophils predominate, in contrast to AML in which myeloblasts predominate. An increase in eosinophils may occur and an increase in the absolute basophil count is a constant finding. Mild or moderate anemia is often present,

depending on the level of leukocytosis (46). The platelet count usually is normal or elevated. Thrombocytopenia is a rare early finding.

The leukocyte alkaline phosphatase activity is low in most cases prior to treatment (198). The myeloid immaturity, basophilia, and low leukocyte alkaline phosphatase in CML help to distinguish it from a leukemoid reaction.

2. *The marrow* shows marked granulocytic and often megakaryocytic hyperplasia. The proportion of cells at each level of maturation is approximately normal. Cells engorged with glucocerebroside, morphologically identical to Gaucher cells, may be found in marrow (186). The reticulin fibers in marrow may be slightly increased. Only in rare cases is fibrosis prominent.
3. *A specific chromosome abnormality*: the Ph[1] chromosome, is present in the marrow cells of patients with CML (199). As mentioned earlier, this chromosome results from a translocation of the long of arm chromosome 22 to chromosome 9 (t [9;22] [q34;q11]), or more rarely to another chromosome (Fig. 24-7). It is present in virtually all of the metaphase cells in marrow, including erythroid, megakaryocytic, and granulocytic cells. Some define CML by the presence of this abnormality of chromosomes. However, the chromosomal abnormality has been identified in rare patients with other myeloproliferative diseases and in some patients with acute lymphoblastic or myeloblastic leukemia (185). These latter observations could represent cases of CML presenting as blastic transformations (162).

   Of the approximately 10% Ph1 chromosome-negative patients, some have a genomic rearrangement of the *bcr* region on chromosome number 22 and the proto-oncogene *c-abl* region on chromosome 9 at the molecular level without the morphologic appearance of the Ph[1] chromosome (163,168). This t(9;12) translocation is the molecular representation of the Ph[1] chromosome even in its absence. This in turn results in a fused abl-bcr gene and in the production of an abnormal tyrosine kinase protein which may be related to the disordered myelopoiesis found in CML (167a,178a).

   Other Ph1-negative patients with the clinical features of CML may have had disappearance of the Ph[1] chromosome, or have CML of a juvenile type characterized by a high fetal hemoglobin concentration and a particularly poor response to therapy.
4. *Metabolic alterations* are similar to those that can occur in AML. Hyperuricemia is common because of the high nucleic acid turnover (133).

CLASSIFICATION

Anatomic Staging

Anatomic staging is not applicable to this disease.

Histopathology

Morphologic variation of typical CML: Occasionally, eosinophils or basophils so predominate that the disease is referred to as eosinophilic (187) or basophilic (175,206) leukemia. This usually occurs later in the disease after an initial phase with cytologic characteristics of CML. This type of leukemia should be distinguished from eosinophilic or basophilic leukemia occurring de novo in which the Ph^1 chromosome is absent and the disease is more atypical (67,189).

Other variants of CML: Apparent CML in the elderly and very young may be atypical in its features. In some cases of CML, the Ph^1 chromosome is absent and the clinical and histopathologic features are atypical (169). Disorders referred to as chronic myelomonocytic leukemia (174) and subacute myelogenous leukemia (79,139) may resemble CML also. In these disorders, however, blast cells usually are more prominent, leukocyte counts may be only modestly elevated, the Ph^1 chromosome is absent, and thrombocytopenia is more common than in CML. These forms of the disease are more resistant to therapy (169).

Relationship to other myeloproliferative syndromes: Polycythemia vera and essential thrombocythemia are related to CML in that they have excessive proliferation and accumulation of hemopoietic cells, predominantly erythrocytes and platelets, respectively. Although granulocytic cell lines also are involved in the hyperproliferative state, their accumulation in blood is not as prominent as in CML. Thus, erythrocytosis is the hallmark of polycythemia vera, thrombocytosis of primary thrombocythemia, and granulocytosis of CML.

Myelofibrosis also has been described in the marrows of CML patients (181). The marrow fibroblasts of CML patients do not contain the Ph^1 chromosome and thus the fibroplasia is a secondary phenomenon. Agnogenic myeloid metaplasia (AMM) (idiopathic myelofibrosis) bears some similarities to CML, although usually the diagnostic distinctions are clear, based on the height of the leukocyte count (CML>>AMM), the marrow fibrosis on biopsy (AMM>>CML), and the RBC shape changes (AMM>>CML) (158). The myelofibrosis in myeloproliferative diseases, especially idiopathic myelofibrosis, has been related to the intramedullary release of platelet growth factor from megakaryocytes, which has been shown to stimulate fibroblast growth in culture (183).

Accelerated Phase of CML

Inevitably, patients with CML have an alteration in the nature of their disease. This change appears to be the result of a Ph^1-bearing clone evolving into a more malignant cell type (167,199). Four major superimposed chromosome abnormalities have been observed during the accelerated phase of CML. There may be no additional abnormality other than the Ph^1 chromosome, or there may be: (1) a second Ph^1 chromosome; (2) hyperdiploidy; or (3) isochromosome 17q; or (4) several other structural changes (199).

Any of several clinical patterns of metamorphosis may occur (155,197). The single hallmark of each pattern is the failure of busulfan or hydroxyurea to maintain good control of the disease, as it does during the chronic phase.

Dyshemopoietic phase: The most common type of accelerated phase is the transition into a more dyshemopoietic phase. Anemia and thrombocytopenia become more troublesome. Immature cells increase in blood and marrow. Increases in basophils may occur. Spleen size increases and recurrent splenic infarctions may occur. Fever and bone pain may be present; and extramedullary myeloblastic tumors may develop in skin, paranasal sinuses, epidural space, or elsewhere. This phase may last for months or transform into a more acute leukemia-like pattern.

Blastic crisis: In the most severe form of metamorphosis, the disease may rapidly develop into an acute leukemia (blastic transformation). A marked increase in blast cells is present in marrow, cytopenias are severe, and the patient may die within several weeks (162a). Most such blast transformations are morphologically and histochemically characteristic of AML. In about 25% of cases, the blast cells are morphologically, histochemically, and biochemically similar to lymphoblasts, usually of the T-cell type, rarely of the pre-B-cell type (157,170,173,190).

Acute basophilia: Rarely, a dramatic increase in basophils may occur and develop into a terminal acute basophilic leukemia (175).

Progressive fibrosis: Some patients develop progressive marrow fibrosis and pancytopenia (181). This marked fibrotic reaction in marrow is an uncommon form of metamorphosis in CML.

PRINCIPLES OF TREATMENT

Chronic-Phase CML

The treatment of CML is directed toward suppression of the excessive rate of hemopoiesis in the marrow and the spleen (165a). If this is accomplished, symptoms fade, spleen size is reduced, and the blood counts can be kept near normal. Functional capacity of cells is close enough to normal so that infection or bleeding are rare. No effort is made to make the marrow aplastic in the hope that a normal clone of hemopoietic cells will emerge, since, unlike AML, the risks outweigh the results that occur.

CML usually requires therapy at the time of diagnosis or soon after. Fever, sweating, fatigue, malaise, symptomatic splenomegaly, progressive anemia, and excessive leukocytosis (> 150,000/µL) are indications to use cytotoxic therapy.

Chemotherapy: Many drugs are effective in the treatment of CML; however, busulfan, an alkylating agent given orally, is commonly used (192c). The gradual reduction of the leukocyte count toward normal is accompanied by a reciprocal increase in RBC count, a decrease in spleen size, and a loss of symptoms. Hyperuricemia is almost always present and can be reversed with allopurinol. Maintenance therapy with busulfan is of no special benefit and increases the risk of side effects of the drug. Moreover, occasional patients have sustained beneficial effects from an initial course of therapy, although the disease usually progresses when treatment is discontinued. Treatment should be reinstituted when spleen size, WBC count, or symptoms warrant. A very low dose of busulfan may be required for patients with rapid regrowth of the tumor.

Hydroxyurea is an alternative drug for treatment of CML. It blocks DNA synthesis by inhibiting a ribonucleotide reductase and acts rapidly when compared with busulfan (157a). However, the dosage has to be adjusted frequently to the patient's leukocyte count and close monitoring is required. Hydroxyurea appears to be comparable to busulfan in treating CML and the median survival of treated patients is equivalent (202). This agent may be preferred to avoid the permanent reduction of residual normal marrow and pulmonary fibrosis associated with busulfan, particularly for those patients who are candidates for autologous or allogeneic bone marrow transplantation.

Interferon: Both alpha interferon (IFN-alpha) and gamma interferon (IFN-gamma) have been used successfully to treat chronic-phase CML. Response rates as high as 70% have been reported with IFN-alpha, and a small but significant proportion may show elimination of the Ph[1] chromosome-containing clone in the marrow (202). Survival of patients treated with IFN-alpha is as good or better than other treatments (202,202a). The results of IFN-gamma are less impressive, and more data are required for assessment of the role of both these agents in the CML treatment. Preliminary results using ß-IFN have been discouraging to date (196).

Marrow transplantation (177,204): In spite of an increase in the median survival from 1 ½ years for untreated patients to approximately 3 years for busulfan- or hydroxyurea-treated patients (202), CML remains a fatal disease. Marrow transplantation from a histocompatible donor is the only curative treatment for patients with CML (Table 24-2). The success rate for transplantation is lower in the accelerated phase and even more difficult to achieve if the patient has developed a blast transformation. The potential for long-term survival makes allogeneic marrow transplantation the treatment of choice in those patients who have a histocompatible marrow donor (164,192a,200a).

Leukapheresis and splenectomy: Chronic leukapheresis is not a practical means of primary treatment for most patients with CML (205). In some patients with high leukocyte counts (200,000 to 600,000/μL), leukapheresis may be helpful in rapidly reducing the leukocyte count and reversing the signs of hyperleukocytosis such as papilledema, retinal engorgement, priapism, stupor, and loss of well being. Hydroxyurea should be used with leukapheresis until the WBC count is under 100,000/μL. Splenectomy during the chronic phase of CML does not produce a change in the disease course (184). Moreover, the risk of severe thrombocytosis is present after splenectomy.

Radiotherapy: Radiotherapy to the spleen was an efficacious form of treatment; however, it is rarely used because of the increased efficacy of chemotherapy. Small daily doses of 25 to 50 cGy to the entire spleen produce a gradual descent in WBC counts. Marked reduction in blood counts occur after 500 to 1,000 cGy of spleen irradiation. Granulocytic sarcomas in soft tissues, brain, and paranasal sinuses, or osseous involvement may require localized radiation therapy.

Accelerated Phase of CML

Treatment at this disease stage is usually akin to that for acute leukemia. For the proportion of patients who have the lymphoid type of blast transformation, vincristine and prednisone should be used (192). Ideally, one should do histochemical, immunologic, or biochemical measurements to determine if the blast transformation is myeloid or lymphoid. If the myeloid type is present, drugs like cytarabine and daunorubicin can be used. The results of therapy in the myeloid blast transformation are poor. Remission occurs in a high proportion of the lymphoid type of blast transformation, although the remissions are short-lived (192,203). If remission is achieved, allogeneic BMT offers the only hope for long-term survival (192b).

RESULTS AND PROGNOSIS

Median survival in CML is about 3 ½ years (200). The range of survival is 1 to 12 years. Busulfan or hydroxyurea therapy has prolonged survival only slightly, but has made the chronic phase of the disease a less morbid experience. In most patients, good health is completely restored for several years by busulfan or hydroxyurea treatment. Busulfan has several serious adverse effects, such as marrow aplasia, pulmonary fibrosis, and an Addison's-disease-like syndrome, and it must be supervised carefully. It may also result in skin hyperpigmentation and infertility. Although the prognosis is difficult to predict at the time of diagnosis in an individual patient, it is likely to be worse the higher the blast cell percentage and in the presence of marked basophilia or eosinophilia, and thrombocytopenia (180).

After the onset of the accelerated phase, median survival is about 3 months for those with myeloid blast crises and about 5 months with lymphoid blast crisis.

Patients with CML can be divided into several prognostic groups based on their spleen size, platelet count, hematocrit, sex, and percentage of blood myeloblasts (200). Patients in prognostic group I have a median survival of approximately 5 ½ years, prognostic group II of 4 years and prognostic group III of 2 years. As noted, the use of chemotherapeutic agents such as busulfan and hydroxyurea has prolonged the median survival by 1 to 2 years, but no increase in long-term survival has been observed. BMT from a histocompatible donor is the only curative treatment for patients with CML, and hence is the treatment of choice if the patient has a histocompatible donor (usually a sibling). Long-term survival of 50% to 70% has been observed for patients transplanted in the chronic phase of CML (Table 24-2, Fig. 24-8) (166,166',178). However, the timing of transplantation is critical because of the high rate of transplant mortality (30% to 40%, and is influenced by the patient's age, prognostic group, and the success rate of transplantation, which is dependent on whether the bone marrow is syngeneic or allogeneic (Table 24-2) (191a).

Table 24-2. Results of Marrow Transplantation Treatment in CML

Disease Stage	Type of Transplant	Relapse Rate (%)	Survival >3 Years (% of Patients)
Chronic	Syngeneic	25	>90
	Allogeneic	10–30	55–70
Accelerated	Syngeneic	43	25
	Allogeneic	30–70	30
Blast crisis	Syngeneic	50	16
	Autologous	100	0
	Allogeneic	50–70	0–20
Second chronic phase	Allogeneic	15	35

From Fialkow, P.J. and Singer, J.W. (1a), with permission.

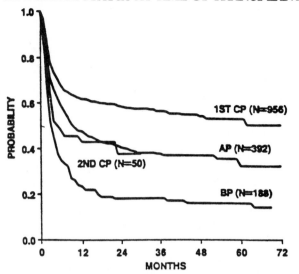

PROBABILITY OF SURVIVAL FOR CML BY DISEASE STATUS AT TIME OF TRANSPLANT

Fig. 24-8. Results of life table analyses demonstrating that chronic myelogenous leukemia recipients of human lymphocyte-identical sibling bone marrow transplant in first chronic phase (CP) have a significantly higher probability of survival (53%, 95% confidence interval [CI] = 4%) than patients transplanted in accelerated phase (AP) (32%, 95% CI = 6%) in second chronic phase (2ND CP) (25%, 95% C.I. = 23%) or in blast crisis (16%, 95% C.I. = 6%). Estimates of significance are based on the Lee-Desu (univariate) statistic.

As transplantation from unrelated donors and imperfect matches become more feasible, these may be useful for treatment of CML patients during the chronic phase and for later transplantation when the disease progresses to the accelerated phase (179). Although the chronic phase has been reestablished briefly, patients have deteriorated rapidly with this treatment, and its usefulness is limited in the accelerated and blastic phases when long-term survival beyond 3 years is 0% to 20% after BMT (Table 24-2).

CLINICAL INVESTIGATIONS

Marrow Transplantation

Allogeneic BMT has become the treatment of choice for patients with CML (164). Unfortunately, only 20% to 30% of patients have an available histocompatible donor to permit this treatment. Investigations using unrelated matched donors identified through histocompatibility registries, may increase the applicability of this treatment. Further transplantation from mismatched donors may be possible if the donor marrow can be purged of those cells mediating graft-versus-host disease or more effective treatment for graft-versus-host disease becomes available. Autologous marrow transplantation may return the patient to a chronic phase, which on occasion may be durable (196a).

Alpha and Gamma Interferon

Treatment with the interferons has highlighted the presence of a normal clone of residual stem cells in the marrow of

patients with CML. It remains to be seen whether elimination of the Ph[1] positive clone with such treatment can sustain the hegemony of the normal clone.

ACUTE LYMPHOCYTIC LEUKEMIA (ALL)

EPIDEMIOLOGY AND PATHOGENESIS

Epidemiology

Cancers are the second most frequent cause of death in children, and leukemia is the most common neoplasm in children. There are six new cases per 100,000 subjects per year (14). The mode of the incidence curve is at 4 years of age, after which it declines rapidly, and the disease is an uncommon type of leukemia after age 15 (Fig. 24-1). There is a slight predominance of cases in males (14,43).

Pathogenesis

ALL is regarded as a proliferation and accumulation of lymphoblasts originating in marrow and perhaps in extramyeloid lymphatic tissue. The normal homologue of the leukemic lymphoblast is not known. It is probable that the lesion is present in a primitive lymphoid progenitor cell pool, that may be placed at a pre-B-cell level 3 of lymphopoiesis in most cases (Fig. 24-2).

In humans, lymphopoiesis and hemopoiesis are independent; thus, the development of anemia, thrombocytopenia, and granulocytopenia in ALL results from the noxious effects of masses of leukemic lymphoblasts on normal hemopoietic stem cells. This view is supported by: (1) the absence in nonlymphoid hemopoietic cells of the chromosome abnormality present in 90% of patients with ALL; and (2) the rapid restitution in ALL of normal hemopoiesis after the reduction of marrow leukemic lymphoblasts by drugs.

DETECTION AND DIAGNOSIS

Clinical Detection (72)

As in AML, the most frequent manifestations of ALL result from the reduction of normal hemopoietic cells. Accumulation of leukemic blast cells in peripheral tissues may occasionally lead to symptoms referable to specific sites or organs.

1. *Symptoms* of malaise, lethargy, or fatigue are nearly always present. Anorexia, abdominal discomfort, or headache may be prominent. Fever and gingival, cutaneous, or nasal bleeding are present in as many as half the patients. Lymphadenopathy occurs, but is not unusually prominent. Liver, spleen, or testicular enlargement are more frequent in ALL than in other forms of leukemia and are a chief complaint. Unlike AML, symptoms of ALL are rarely present more than 6 weeks prior to diagnosis.

2. *Physical findings* including pallor, petechiae, purpura, and hepatosplenomegaly are frequent. Lymphadenopathy may be present. Leukemic cell accumulation in specific organs can lead to a variety of findings in individual cases (236). An example of this is leukemic meningitis (217).

Diagnostic Procedures

1. *Blood cell counts* will identify anemia and thrombocytopenia in nearly all patients. Granulocytopenia is often present. The total WBC count can be low or high, but blast cells are almost always found in the blood.

2. The *marrow* is replaced by leukemic lymphoblasts. Erythroid, granulocytic, and megakaryocytic cells are decreased markedly in number. Histochemical and immunologic studies may be required to aid in the classification of the leukemia. Periodic acid-Schiff staining material (glycogen) is present in lymphoblasts, whereas peroxidase staining of primary lysosomal granules does not occur (28). The presence of cytoplasmic or surface immunoglobulin or certain surface antigens may establish the lymphoid nature of the leukemia, the lymphocyte subtype, and the stage of ALL maturation (see below).

3. *Metabolic abnormalities*, especially hyperuricemia, may occur, as in AML. These abnormalities are directly related to the proliferation of leukemic cells (124,133,243).

Pseudoleukemia (Lymphoid)

Infectious mononucleosis has been mistaken for ALL, especially if a marrow aspirate is performed and the reactive lymphocytes are mistaken for lymphoblasts. In most cases, the classical clinical picture and the absence of anemia and thrombocytopenia should lead to caution and pursuit of a morphologic and serologic diagnosis of mononucleosis. Pertussis is associated with a lymphocytosis that is sometimes marked (50,000 to 100,000/μL). These cells are usually small and well differentiated. The clinical picture of whooping cough and the absence of other hematologic abnormalities also should prevent confusion. Rarely, the transient dyshemopoietic state in the neonate with Down's syndrome may be associated with lymphoblasts (214).

CLASSIFICATION

Anatomic Staging

Anatomic staging is not usually applicable to patients with leukemia. Leukemia is a disseminated disease and involves the marrow, blood, and other organs at the time of diagnosis. However, in ALL, two extramedullary areas—the CNS and testicles—are of importance in treatment and prognosis. It is important to determine if leukemic involvement of the meninges is present at the time of diagnosis. Such involvement, identified by cerebrospinal fluid examination, occurs frequently at diagnosis only in patients with high lymphoblast counts. Meningeal leukemia requires treatment of the CNS and is often associated with an unfavorable prognosis.

Testicular involvement usually occurs later in the natural history of ALL, and has been an important site of relapse in male patients with prolonged survival. Some investigators have suggested that bilateral testicular biopsy be done in patients in long-term remission before chemotherapy is discontinued.

Histopathologic Types of ALL

A number of morphologic classifications of ALL have been suggested to predict responsiveness to treatment and the prognosis (228,241). The most recent morphologic classification has divided the lymphoblasts in ALL into three types:

1. Type L1, has small cells with scant cytoplasm and indistinct nucleoli. About 85% of cases fall in this category.
2. Type L2, has large cells with more cytoplasm and prominent nucleoli. About 15% of cases fall in this category.
3. Type L3, has large cells with deep blue cytoplasm and vacuoles (Burkitt type). Less than 1% of cases are this type.

The L3 type has a poorer prognosis than the other two types of ALL.

Immunologic Classification

An alternative classification of ALL is based on the immunologic characteristic of lymphoblasts. About 20% of ALL cases have T-cell markers and 1% to 2% have B-cell characteristics with surface immunoglobulin. Of those with neither B-nor T-cell surface markers, 80% display the common ALL antigen (CALLA). These cases have been subclassified as "common type" because they react to antibody made from a surface antigen commonly found on ALL cells. More recent data indicate that these lymphoblasts are of B-cell origin because some contain cytoplasmic immunoglobulin or exhibit rearrangement of the heavy or light chain immunoglobulin genes (223). The presence of heavy chain or light chain immunoglobulin gene rearrangement, cytoplasmic immunoglobulin or surface immunoglobulin reflects the maturational stage of the leukemic B cell (Fig. 24-9) and may influence prognosis (see below). T lymphoblasts also may exhibit surface antigens reflecting early, Leu 9, T1, and T11, or later, T3, T4, T8, or T6 development (226). T-cell ALL is defined by the expression of the T-cell associated antigens CD2, CD7, CD5, or CD3 by the leukemic cells and is frequently associated with a constellation of clinical features including male sex, older age, leukocytosis, and mediastinal mass (232a,235a).

Cytogenetic Classification

Abnormalities in chromosome number or structure can now be identified in over 90% of patients with ALL (Table 24-3) (229). The abnormalities may primarily include diploidy and hyperdiploidy, or may include aneuploidy. Those patients with increased numbers of chromosomes in the lymphoblasts appear to have a better prognosis than those with decreased numbers or those with structural abnormalities such as translocations. More recently, bone marrow responses at day 7 has been shown to have prognostic significance (218a). The t translocation (9:22) is seen in those patients with ALL and a Ph¹ chromosome present at the time of diagnosis and is a poor prognostic feature. The t translocation (8:14) is observed in B-cell leukemias that also have immunoglobulin on the cell surface and fit the L3 or Burkitt morphologic classification. Such translocations may involve proto-oncogenes such as ber-abl (9:22) c-myc (8:14) which may play some role in the neoplastic transformation (225). The presence of hyperdiploidy (modal chromosome number >50) is associated with a more favorable prognosis. Ploidy analysis can be performed by flow cytometry, and a DNA index > 1.6 is associated with a more favorable prognosis (232b). Specific nonrandom chromosomol translocations appear to have prognostic significance (222a).

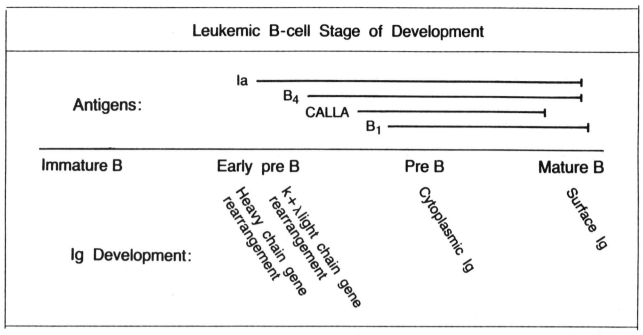

Fig. 24-9. Immunological differentiation of B cells. The surface antigen markers provide a very useful adjunct to the morphological diagnosis of acute lymphocytic leukemia and correlate well with maturational development of the B cell. CALLA = common acute lymphoblastic leukemia antigen; Ig = immunoglobulin.

Prognostic Factors at Diagnosis of ALL

The most favorable prognostic group consists of patients between 2 and 10 years of age with CALLA-reacting lymphoblasts and an initial WBC count less than 10,000/µL (216). The features that have been associated with a poor prognosis vary with the effectiveness of the available treatment and do not remain constant. However, in most series a WBC count greater than 20,000/µL, T-cell ALL with a mediastinal mass, surface immunoglobulin positive B-cell ALL, and chromosomal hypodiploidy are associated with an unfavorable prognosis (218a). In addition, failure to eradicate a leukemic clone as assessed by a marrow on the 14th day after therapy initiation is an unfavorable sign, and males tend to fare less well than females with ALL. It should be noted, however, that the T-cell immunophenotype is no longer considered an adverse prognostic sign in adult patients with ALL (222).

PRINCIPLES OF TREATMENT

Treatment of ALL is based on the premise that eradication of leukemic blast cells will allow regrowth and ascendancy of suppressed normal hemopoietic cells. This usually can be accomplished without the prolonged posttreatment marrow aplasia that occurs in AML because ALL cells are more sensitive to drugs than are AML cells. Moreover, cytocidal drugs (periwinkle alkaloids and glucocorticoids) used to reduce the body burden of leukemic lymphoblasts initially are less toxic to hemopoietic cells than are drugs used in AML. Thus, remission-inducing therapy carries less risk from cytopenias for ALL patients than it does in AML.

Chemotherapy

Induction therapy (208): Initial therapy with vincristine, prednisone, and either l-asparaginase or doxorubicin leads to

Table 24-3. Chromosomal Translocations and Deletions in Leukemic Lymphoblasts: Frequency and Associated Clinical Findings

Translocation	Breakpoint	Oncogene(s)	Immunophenotype	Frequency (%)	Features	Prognosis
t1;19 (50,61)	q23;13	—	Pre-B cytoplasmic m+	4–7	Mean age: 11 yr	1–4 yr
t4;11 (54,55,58)	q21;q23	*ets-1*	B-cell precurson + monocytic (biclonal)	5	Mean age <16 mo mkd. leukocytosis	< 1 yr
t8; 14 (65) t2;8 t8;22	q24;q32	*c-myc*	B-cell	5	FAB L3 (Burkitt) extramedullary, lymphomatous presentation	< 1 yr
t9;22 (7,50)	q34;q11	*abl, bcr-abl*	B-cell precursor T cell	4–6	Mean age: 9 yr	< 1 yr
t11;14 (50)	p13;q11.2	(TCR-B)	T4 + , T6 + , T8 + , T3 – , common thymocyte	5		1 yr
t(V;12) (V;p12) (50)	Variable	*k-ras2*	B-cell presursor, pre-B	2	Mean age: 5 yr	Poor
del 6q (65)	q23	*c-myb*	B-cell precursor	2	Mean age: 6 yr	< 1 yr
del 9p (64)	q15,q23	—	T-cell CALL		lymphomatous ALL	Poor

From Miller et al. (228), with permission.

CR in 95% of children with ALL. The addition of a fourth drug has not increased remission rates or duration of remission.

Intensification therapy: CR can occur with a modest proportional reduction in the total body leukemic cell population, for example, from 10^{12} to 10^9 leukemic blasts. To further reduce the body burden of leukemic cells, some therapists use additional cytoreductive therapy using drugs like cytarabine prior to starting maintenance therapy.

Maintenance therapy (208): Continued therapy prolongs the period of remission and is an essential part of ALL therapy. Antimetabolites, especially methotrexate used weekly, and 6-mercaptopurine used daily—with or without anthracyclines, alkylators and glucocorticoids—are the most effective agents to maintain remissions. The impact of the addition of delayed intensification is under clinical evaluation (233a).

Central Nervous System Prophylaxis

Systemic chemical treatment appears to be inadequate for certain anatomic locations, where the disease can recur when marrow and blood are apparently unaffected. These "sanctuary" sites include the CNS (231) pia-arachnoid and gonads (230). The need for prophylactic treatment of the CNS appears related to the prognostic features present at the time of diagnosis (227,232). In the worst prognostic group, leukemia recurs more frequently in the CNS with increasing length of remission (218), and CNS relapse exceeds 50% when chemotherapy is used without CNS prophylaxis. For these patients, cranial irradiation, combined with intrathecal methotrexate, is the preferred form of CNS prophylaxis. Cranial-spinal irradiation is not more effective, produces more hemopoietic injury, and can suppress longitudinal growth. The recommended dose for cranial irradiation is 1,800 cGy. The success of prophylactic CNS treatment has been confirmed by several studies (216, 227).

Intrathecal methotrexate alone is effective prophylaxis for patients other than the highest risk group, and CNS leukemia occurs in fewer than 5% of these children (227). Currently under investigation is whether CNS disease can be prevented in children with the best prognostic features without specific CNS treatment, using only intensive systemic chemotherapy (227,227a,232).

Most treatment centers attempt to tailor the CNS treatment to the severity of the disease to avoid the adverse neuropsychologic effects of CNS treatment. These late effects include primarily a variety of learning disabilities and a decrease in performance IQ (242). Further, an increase in the incidence of malignant brain tumors has been documented after treatment with cranial irradiation (207). A recent prospective study by Mulhern *et al.* (229a) comparing neuropsychologic performance in children surviving leukemia who received 18 Gy cranial irradiation plus intrathecal methotrexate (IT MTX), those who received 24 Gy cranial irradiation + IT MTX, and those who received IT MTX with no cranial irradiation revealed no statistically significant declines in Verbal, Performance, or Full Scale IQs for any of the three groups. Therefore, suggesting other etiologic factors need to be explored as the basis for late CNS changes such as ecologic factors and chemotherapy during the continuation phase of treatment.

Prophylactic irradiation of other sanctuary sites, for example, the liver, spleen, kidneys, and gonads, has not enhanced survival. Moreover, it increases the morbidity of treatment and compromises residual normal hemopoietic cells. Testicular biopsies at the end of treatment have been used to detect residual testicular decrease, which is found in approximately 10% of patients undergoing a biopsy. These patients are treated with testicular irradiation and additional chemotherapy.

Component Transfusion, Antimicrobial Therapy, Emotional Support

As in AML, transfusions of RBCs, platelets, or granulocytes may be required during remission induction, although the need for such support usually is less during the initial therapy. In patients treated for relapses of ALL, such support is needed more often (see AML). The use of prophylactic, poorly absorbable antibiotics to reduce intestinal flora and isolated environments usually is not warranted. Infection may be present prior to therapy or may develop in the early weeks of treatment, especially if neutropenia is severe. These infections are usually bacterial and do not influence the therapy outcome if they are treated with specific antimicrobial drugs. Supporting the emotional needs of the patient and family is a vital aspect of care and requires sensitive and concerned attention (209).

MARROW TRANSPLANTATION

Both allogeneic and autologous BMT have been used to treat patients with relapsed ALL. Allogeneic BMT requires a histocompatible sibling as a bone marrow donor and is available only to 20% to 30% of patients. For those patients with recurrent leukemia and no histocompatible sibling, HLA-matched unrelated donor, mismatched, and autologous BMT are alternative choices. Unfortunately, the latter treatments are not as effective as allogeneic BMT. Long-term survival may exceed 50% with allogeneic transplantation compared with less than 30% for conventional therapy and perhaps 15% to 20% for autologous BMT.

RESULTS AND PROGNOSIS

Childhood ALL (Fig. 24-10) (212a)

With therapy that includes induction, intensification, prophylactic CNS treatment, and maintenance, long remissions have become commonplace. The 3-year disease-free survival for all children with ALL exceeds 50% of patients, and this figure reaches 80% in those who have favorable prognostic signs (237) or are treated intensively (232). In these patients, chemotherapy has been stopped arbitrarily after 2 to 3 years. Seventy-five percent of such patients remain in remission indefinitely with no further treatment, and these patients likely are cured (219). Relapses were noted more frequently in males. One reason for this was the propensity for recurrence in the testicles (234). Some investigators have favored prolonging treatment beyond 3 years in males; whereas others have suggested performing bilateral testicular biopsies and continuing therapy if evidence of leukemia is found. Testicular irradiation is also used (237).

ALL patients who relapse can be treated successfully with vincristine, prednisone, and l-asparaginase. Eighty percent

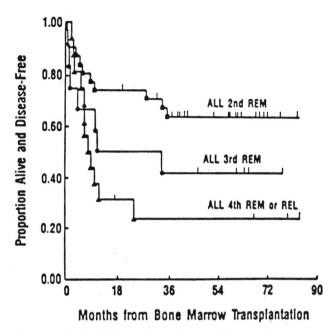

Fig. 24-10. Kaplan-Meier product estimates of disease-free survival at 5 years for patients with acute lymphoblastic leukemia in second complete remission (REM), third complete REM and fourth complete REM. REL = relapse. From Brochstein *et al.* (212a), with permission.

of patients will enter a second remission, which is nearly always shorter than the first remission (224). Although successive remissions can be induced, long-term survivals are rare. Allogeneic BMT is the preferred treatment for patients with recurrent ALL who have a histocompatible sibling. The results are best if the transplant is administered during a period of remission. Approximately 50% of transplanted patients are long-term survivors (240).

Adult ALL

In those over 15 years of age, ALL is less responsive to therapy and survival is shorter (123,220). Vincristine and prednisone, usually with the addition of daunorubicin or cyclophosphamide are used for remission induction. Intensive consolidation therapy with cytarabine and other drugs is used by some therapists. Maintenance treatment includes methotrexate, cyclophosphamide and an anthracycline. Seventy-five percent of patients enter a remission and CNS prophylaxis usually is used. The median survival in some series exceeds 3 years and there may be up to 20% of patients who are alive at 5 years (215,219a,221,222,224a,235). Because of the poor results and the low percentage of long-term survivors, neither the optimal continuation therapy nor the duration of such therapy in adult ALL is clear. Although bone marrow transplantation has been studied in this setting, it has not yet demonstrated any advantage over chemotherapy alone (221a).

The ALL cells of adults have been found to carry the Ph¹ chromosome in about 25% of cases. Ph¹ positive cells have also been found in about 2% of childhood cases. Several adults with Ph¹-positive ALL have developed the features of CML with Ph¹-positive cells, following remission of ALL after therapy with vincristine and prednisone. The prognosis for these patients is worse than Ph¹-negative ALL (162).

COMPLICATIONS OF TREATMENT

Neurotoxicity

Neurotoxicity can occur acutely from intrathecal methotrexate alone. Headache, visual complaints, lethargy, stupor, and other neurologic abnormalities can occur. This acute neurotoxicity is more often seen in older children and adults and results from excessive retention of methotrexate in the spinal fluid (211). Late neurologic side effects have been seen in patients receiving cranial irradiation and IV methotrexate (211). Moreover, prophylactic radiation therapy of the brain has been associated with lower IQ test scores than comparison groups (229).

Immunosuppression

Immunosuppression results from chemotherapy and may depress cellular immunity, thus opportunistic infections during remission are a serious threat. In one series, about 15% of leukemia deaths occurred during remission and were caused by fungal, viral, or protozoal infection (238). Prophylactic trimethaprim sulfamethoxazole to minimize the frequency of carinii pneumonia is often used.

Sequelae of Long-term Chemotherapy

Thus far, frequent serious sequelae from long-term chemotherapy for ALL have not been observed; however, the possibility that oncogenesis, immune deficiencies, and germ cell mutations will be enhanced must be carefully evaluated in survivors. In this regard, there are increasing numbers of reports of myeloproliferative diseases, especially AML, in patients treated for ALL (212,233).

Ovarian (239) and testicular development and function (210) seem to be preserved in children treated with chemotherapy.

CHRONIC LYMPHOCYTIC LEUKEMIA (CLL)

EPIDEMIOLOGY AND PATHOGENESIS

Epidemiology

Epidemiology is rare under the age of 35 and increases in frequency with succeeding decades (14,43) (Fig. 24-1). There is an excess of cases among males. Familial clustering, especially in siblings, is most notable of all leukemias (25,268). In rare cases, a similar chromosomal abnormality has been present in several family members (267).

Pathogenesis

CLL is a disorder in which increased proliferation of short- and long-lived lymphocytes and prolonged survival of long-lived lymphocytes can lead to an enormous accumulation of lymphocytes in marrow, blood, lymph nodes, liver, and spleen. The disorder may originate in marrow lymphoid tissue; however, abnormal proliferation occurs in lymph nodes and spleen also. About 95% of the cases of CLL have leukemic lymphocytes whose phenotype is that of B lymphocytes (254,315). CLL is a monoclonal proliferation in which the lymphocytes usually carry determinants for immunoglobulin M or immunoglobulin D on their surface (297). The surface membrane light chain type is either k or y. Glucose-6-phosphate dehydrogenase isoenzyme analysis has also supported the monoclonal nature of the disease. A small percentage of patients with CLL have cells that are capable of secreting monoclonal immunoglobulin.

The precise level of differentiation at which the leukemic lesion originates is unknown. It probably is at a level that corresponds to the common lymphopoietic progenitor cell, since a T-cell surface antigen CD5 may be present on a high proportion of CLL cells, despite their dominant phenotypic expression of B-cell markers. These B-cell markers include surface immunoglobulin, Fc receptors, mouse RBC rosette receptors, and complement receptors (248,259,284). A rare case of concomitant CML and CLL has shown the coexistence of two clones, the CML clone with the Ph[1] chromosome and the CLL clone without the chromosome marker (314). This finding also suggests that the CLL lesion is at the level of the common lymphopoietic progenitor cell.

Acquired abnormalities of T-cell function that appear later in the disease course may be important in pathogenesis. It has been suggested that excessive suppressor activity by T cells limits the immunoglobulin response of residual normal B cells in CLL, eventually leading to hypogammaglobulinemia (251,302,308). In later disease stages, T-cell function may be depressed by large accumulations of B cells or by an intrinsic defect (258).

In contradistinction, a proportion of patients with CLL have exaggerated delayed hypersensitivity reactions or may produce autoantibodies to RBCs or platelets.

Normal hemopoietic cell proliferation is felt to be impaired indirectly because of the noxious effects of massive accumulation of lymphocytes in marrow. Hence, varying degrees of blood cell cytopenias (anemia, neutropenia, and thrombocytopenia) can develop secondarily. The abnormality in humoral antibody production and the granulocytopenia that develop late in the disease from marrow replacement by CLL cells and chemotherapy often lead to serious difficulties with defenses against challenging microbes, resulting in serious infections.

DETECTION AND DIAGNOSIS

Clinical Detection (249,250)

A large proportion of patients are asymptomatic at the time of diagnosis. Thus, the disorder is often discovered while the patient is being evaluated for an unrelated medical problem.

1. *Symptoms* include malaise, fatigue, weight loss, excessive sweating, and abdominal discomfort or distention from organomegaly. Infections of skin and pneumonia can be initial events. Often, enlarged lymph nodes are discovered and lead to medical evaluation.
2. *Physical findings* frequently include enlargement of lymph nodes in any or all node-bearing areas. Splenomegaly and hepatomegaly are common. Nodular skin infiltrates or other cutaneous lesions can occur. If prominent, they should suggest a T-cell type of lymphocytic leukemia, since this type of tumor has a predilection for the skin.

Diagnostic Procedures

1. *RBC and platelet* counts may be normal or a slight anemia may be present. More severe anemia and thrombocytopenia may occur at the time of diagnosis, and their early presence is a poor prognostic finding (299). An absolute lymphocytosis is always present. The lymphocyte count is at least 8,000/μL. The CLL lymphocyte is small with scant cytoplasm, and is difficult to distinguish from the normal small lymphocyte by light microscopy (306). In 95% of cases, the CLL lymphocyte has monoclonal surface immunoglobulin as well as other B-cell markers that can be detected by appropriate laboratory tests.
2. *Marrow* is rarely necessary for the diagnosis of the disease. The marrow aspirate or biopsy shows a diffuse infiltration with small, well-differentiated lymphocytes. These cells account for 25% to 90% of marrow nucleated cells.
3. *Metabolic disturbances*, as a result of leukemic cell turnover, are unusual unless induced by an abrupt reduction in cell number by aggressive therapy (290). Hyperuricemia is uncommon, unlike other types of leukemia (133).

Immune Alterations

RBC autoantibodies can appear (positive Coombs' test), and hemolytic anemia, occasionally severe, can occur (296). Rarely, immune thrombocytopenia may also occur (256,265). Immunoglobulin levels can be very low, especially as the disease progresses (266,304,313). About 3% of patients may have cells that secrete monoclonal immunoglobulin and may have a paraprotein in the plasma (304).

CLASSIFICATION

Anatomic Staging

A staging of CLL patients has been suggested that correlates with the median survival of patients (Table 24-4) (299). These formal categorizations reveal that those with less evidence of disease at the time of diagnosis have a better prognosis. The presence of mild lymphocytosis represents minimal disease and is associated with a median survival of over 10 years. Lymphadenopathy, enlargement of spleen or liver, anemia, or thrombocytopenia at the time of diagnosis are indicators of a poor prognosis and foreshadow reduced longevity.

Table 24-4. Staging of Chronic Lymphocytic Leukemia*

Stage 0:	Blood lymphocytosis, 15,000 mm³; marrow, 40% lymphocytes
Stage I:	Lymphocytosis with lymphadenopathy
Stage II:	Lymphocytosis with enlarged spleen or liver. Lymphadenopathy is not necessarily present.
Stage III:	Lymphocytosis with anemia. Lymph nodes, liver, and spleen may or may not be enlarged. Anemia may be hemolytic or due to decreased red cell production.
Stage IV:	Lymphocytosis with thrombocytopenia (<100,000/mm³); anemia and lymphadenopathy. Hepatic and splenic enlargement may be present.

*After Rai *et al.* (299).
From Fialkow and Singer (1a), with permission.

Histopathology

B-cell CLL: This cell bears a close relationship to well-differentiated (lymphocytic) lymphoma. The lymph node histopathology is identical and can lead to a diagnosis of lymphoma by the pathologist if blood cell counts are not known. Studies of large numbers of patients have suggested that CLL with cells morphologically close to poorly differentiated lymphoma cells may have a more aggressive course (213). Cytochemistry may be helpful in distinguishing different cell types because CLL cells usually do not stain well with B-glucuronidase but lymphoma cells do (245). The reduction in B-glucuronidase and acid phosphatase appears to result from a marked diminution in lysosomes in CLL cells (264). Also, lymphoma cells in the blood usually are heavily coated with immunoglobulin (245,284).

Cases of CLL have been reported in which intracellular inclusions have been notable (291), and in some cases these have been shown to be intracellular crystalline immunoglobulin (262).

T-cell CLL: In less than 5% of cases of well-differentiated lymphocytic leukemia, the lymphocytes express a phenotype more closely related to T cells. The cells form rosettes with sheep RBCs and have T-cell surface markers but not B-cell markers. In these cases, there is a higher incidence of skin involvement, and splenomegaly and hepatomegaly are more frequent. The WBC count varies but the proportion of patients with counts over 100,000/μL may be greater than in B-cell CLL. Mediastinal lymphadenopathy has not been a prominent feature of the disease (252,292,312).

Prolymphocytic leukemia: This tumor appears to be a variant of CLL, although the prognosis is poor compared with CLL. The lymphocytes in most cases bear phenotypic markers of B cells. There is usually marked lymphocytosis, prominent splenomegaly (270), and scant lymphadenopathy. A proportion of the cells are usually larger than those in CLL and have a prominent nucleolus (247,270). There appears to be an intermediate group of patients with increased prolymphocytes who do not have the typical clinical course of prolymphocytic leukemia. These patients have a prognosis only slightly worse than classic CLL (279,280).

PRINCIPLES OF TREATMENT

Decision to Treat

Many patients, despite marked increases in lymphocyte counts in the blood and in marrow, and moderate lymph node and splenic enlargement, maintain adequate RBCs, neutrophils, and platelets and can indulge in their usual pursuits for years without difficulty. There is little evidence to suggest that treatment benefits such patients. In patients with active disease, in whom either anemia, thrombocytopenia, hypermetabolism, or enormous lymph node and splenic enlargement is present, an attempt to reduce the lymphocyte mass in marrow and tissue, reduce symptoms, and improve hemopoiesis is justified (249,250).

Chemotherapy

In patients who require treatment, alkylating agents are the most useful drugs. Chlorambucil or cyclophosphamide are used most commonly (274,287,307). Glucocorticoids are useful to treat Coombs'-positive hemolytic anemia. Recent observations suggest that in those patients with hepatosplenomegaly and cytopenias, the results of treatment are improved if alkylating agents and glucocorticoids are combined. Although a combination of an alkylating agent and corticosteroid has been the mainstay of CLL treatment for decades, several studies have now demonstrated significant activity of Fludarabine phosphate in previously treated CLL (261a). Keating, using a daily dose of 25–30 mg/m² for 5 days every 3–4 weeks in 75 previously treated patients, documented 56% objective response, 13% achieved a complete remission, 20% nodular partial remission (complete remission except for residual lymphoid nodules in bone marrow), and 23% had more than 50% reduction in measurable evidence of disease (281a); in previously untreated patients results have even been better (281a). High-dose chlorambucil-prednisone given monthly have been shown to be an effective alternative to daily therapy in most patients (303). Patients with advanced disease treated with monthly therapy for extended periods have a high frequency of salutary results. New experimental agents such as deoxycoformycin appear to have promising results for patients with advanced disease (271,282,289,294).

Radiotherapy

Irradiation of extracorporeal lymphocytes (257), spleen (255), thymus (301), and the whole body (277,278) has been used to ameliorate progressive CLL (247a). In subjects with a good hemopoietic response, evidence for a restitution of immunoglobulin synthesis was found after TBI (278,302a). However, data from cooperative group trials failed to confirm that TBI produced any CRs. An alternative to failed chemotherapy is use of TBI (10 cGy twice daily to total doses of 100 to 150 cGy) which produces high response rates (>50%) but prolonged thrombocytopenia can occur. Therefore, radiation therapy as a primary treatment for CLL is not as useful as chemotherapy. However, localized masses of lymphoid tissue, especially if they are compromising tubular structures or viscera, can be treated successfully by local irradiation.

Splenectomy and Leukapheresis

Splenectomy may be helpful in the treatment of CLL if autoimmune thrombocytopenia or anemia is not controlled by glucocorticoids, or requires persistent use of glucocorticoids. In situations where a markedly enlarged spleen produces cytopenias because of accelerated removal or excessive pooling of platelets or RBCs, surgical removal of the spleen can be useful (244,261).

Reduction of lymphocyte mass by leukapheresis has been shown to be possible and may result in improvement of anemia and thrombocytopenia in some patients (263). This treatment may be neither practical nor successful in many patients. Nevertheless, occasionally it has proven useful as an adjunct to chemotherapy. A recent randomized study of intravenous immunoglobulin (I.V. Ig: 400 mg/kg q 3 weeks for 1 year) in patients with CLL and hypogammglobulinemia produced significantly fewer bacterial infections and a significant delay in onset of first infection during the study period. However, routine chronic administration of I.V. Ig is expensive and the long-term benefit (more than 1 year) is unproven (314a).

RESULTS AND PROGNOSIS

Most patients die from the effects of the tumor, immunosuppression, and recurrent infections (Fig. 24-8). Because CLL is a disease of the elderly, carcinoma and other diseases may be superimposed. Occasionally, the cytologic character of the disease will change markedly and result in a terminal phase analogous to that seen in CML. This may take the form either of a blast crisis with poorly differentiated lymphoblasts emerging as the dominant cell type in marrow and blood (253,269) or a terminal syndrome (Richter's) manifested by malignant large cells coexisting with well-differentiated CLL cells in marrow, lymph nodes, and spleen (246,285). In addition, a variety of late transformations have been reported that may evolve into a more malignant lymphoproliferative disease or a superimposed event like the development of undifferentiated leukemia. The latter change may be related to therapy and the immunodeficiency state (317).

The survival rates by stage are presented in Fig. 24-11 (299) in three major groupings. Good median survival is shown in stage I chronic form (75%), in active phase (40%) for stage I, II, and blast crisis (stages III and IV), with which no long-term survival occurs and survival is limited to 2 to 4 years. Recent French cooperative group randomized studies support conservative measures and single drug therapy in early stages of the disease compared to combinations of agents (268a,268b).

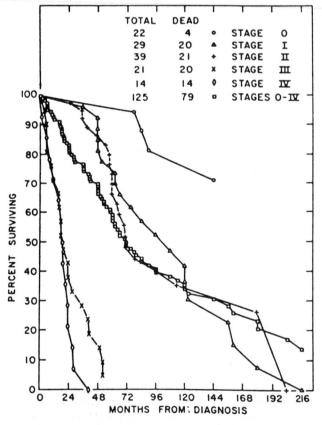

Fig. 24-11. Survival by Rai stage in 125 patients with chronic lymphocytic leukemia. From Rai *et al.* (299), with permission.

OTHER LYMPHOCYTIC LEUKEMIAS

Lymphosarcoma Cell Leukemia

Diffuse involvement of marrow and the presence of large numbers of circulating pathologic lymphocytes may accompany any histopathologic type of lymphoma (305). This pattern is seen most frequently with nodular, poorly-differentiated lymphoma. When lymphoma cell leukemia develops in the course of previously diagnosed lymphoma, it indicates disease progression. If lymphoma cell leukemia represents the initial presentation of a lymphoproliferative disorder, it often may be distinguished from classical ALL or CLL by the clinical features of the case and the morphology of the cells (305,316). Most lymphoma cells express phenotypes of B lymphocytes, as do cells in CLL. The cells are different in that the blood lymphocytes in CLL have receptors in mouse RBCs and have a light concentration of surface immunoglobulin, whereas the blood lymphocytes in cases of B-cell-derived lymphomas do not have receptors for mouse RBCs and have a large concentration of immunoglobulin on their surface (245,284). Some lymphomas express T-lymphocyte markers, (especially the lymphoblastic lymphoma), Sezary syndrome, and some of the immunoblastic lymphomas.

Hairy Cell Leukemia

This form of leukemia is manifested most commonly by bicytopenia or pancytopenia in 80% of cases and splenomegaly in 90% of cases (273a,311). The diagnosis is made by the identification in either blood, marrow, or spleen of a mononuclear cell with lymphocytic or histiocytic morphology and villous cytoplasmic projections as well as B-cell lymphoid immunologic markers. These "hairy" cells have a tartrate-resistant acid phosphate isoenzyme, a finding that is important for their identification (281). The blood may contain from 500 to 50,000 malignant cells/μL, although the total leukocyte count is elevated in only a small proportion of cases (~10%). The percentage of hairy or histochemically positive cells varies from rare to 90% in a given case. The disease may have a prolonged course. Cytopenias, if severe, are normally improved by splenectomy, which has been the traditional treatment of choice (273c). Recent advances in using either alpha-IFN (256a,298,300,314b) or deoxycoformycin (271,272,276,282a,310,310a) have shown a dramatic improvement in the results of chemotherapy in this disease with complete normalization of blood counts in the majority of patients (Table 24-5) (1a,276). Recent evidence suggests that fludarabine may be active in patients who are refractory to alpha interferon or pentostatin (280a). Cooperative trials are underway to evaluate the long-term results of these new agents and to explore the possibility of using these agents as an alternative to splenectomy. Because of the history of this disease, the results of these trials may not be known for another 10 to 15 years. Repeat marrow biopsy and careful evaluation of splenic histology after surgical removal may be required to verify the diagnosis.

Plasma Cell Leukemia

A leukemic disorder, in which the blood contains pathologic plasma cells, may develop in the course of classical multiple myeloma or as the initial feature of a myelomatous disorder (283,318). The diagnosis is made by the

Table 24-5. Treatment of Hairy Cell Leukemia

Regimen	Reference	Patients (No. Treated/ No. Evaluable)	Response Rate* (% of Patients)
Splenectomy	264,265	166/166	CR 42 PR 58
Human recombinant interferon 2 alpha (IFa) (3 – 12 × 10⁶ U/day for 4 – 6 mo, then 3 × weekly for 12 mo)	266	30/30	CR 30 PR 57
IFa (2 × 10⁶ U/m² 3 × weekly	267	22/21	CR 0 PR 43†
IFa (2 × 10⁶ U 3 × weekly for 18 mo or less)	268	135/128	CR 4 PR 77
Deoxycoformycin (5 mg/m² for 2 days every other week)	269	37/27	CR 59 PR 37
Deoxycoformycin (4 mg/m² every other week)	270	31/18	CR 83 PR 6

*CR = complete response; PR = partial response.
†PR rate low owing to early reporting of data.
From Fialkow and Singer (1a), with permission.

morphologic similarity of the circulating cells to plasma cells, the infiltration of marrow with neoplastic plasma cells, and the presence of any or all of the features of multiple myeloma (light chainuria, paraproteinemia, osteolysis, and pancytopenia). Circulating, malignant plasma cells may be present in a concentration of 2,000 to 15,000/μL. The percent of plasma cells in the blood may range from 20% to 95%. A higher frequency of hepatomegaly or splenomegaly also distinguishes this syndrome from typical multiple myeloma. The disease usually is fatal rapidly, although some responses to alkylating agents and glucocorticoids have been observed. The use of antimetabolites in a program like that used to treat AML may be warranted, but results are poor.

Sezary Cell Leukemia

This disorder is manifested by blood lymphocytosis, generalized erythroderma with exfoliation, lymphadenopathy, and hepatosplenomegaly (286,319). The tumor cell is a helper T lymphocyte (CD4+) and the cell has a folded nucleus by light microscopy and a characteristic cerebriform shape by electron microscopy. The skin also may have plaques and infiltrated lesions. Skin biopsies are very similar to those seen in mycosis fungoids in which epidermal accumulations of lymphocytes form Pautrier's microabscesses. Skin involvement has been treated with cutaneous chemotherapy and electron beam therapy, and various programs of systemic chemotherapy have been used with alkylating agents, glucocorticoids, and other drugs. There is no single best approach and the disease tends to resist therapy or to recur (275,288).

Recommend Reading

Both *Hematology* (2) and *Clinical Hematology* (3) provide a comprehensive look at the leukemias for the student.

REFERENCES

General References

1. Bartlett, J. Familiar Quotations. Boston, MA: Little, Brown and Co; 1955.
1a. Fialkow, PJ; Singer, JW Chronic leukemias. In: Cancer: Principles and Practice of Radiation Oncology. 3rd ed. DeVita, VT, Jr., Hellman,S, Rosenberg, SA, eds. Philadelphia, PA: JB Lippincott Co; 1836-1852; 1989.
2. Williams WJ; Beutler E; Erslev AJ; *et al.* Hematology. 4th ed. New York, NY: McGraw-Hill; 1990.
3. Wintrobe, MM; Boggs, DR; Bithell, R; *et al.* Clinical Hematology. Philadelphia,PA: Lea & Febiger; 1981.

Specific References

Epidemiology and Etiology of Leukemia

4. Aksoy, M; Erdem, S; Dincol, K. Leukemia in shoe workers exposed chronically to benzene. Blood. 44:837-841; 1974.
5. Balner, H. Immunosuppression and neoplasia. Rev Europ Etudes Clin et Biol. 15:599-604;1970.
6. Bennett, JM; Catovsky, D; Daniel, T; *et al.* (FAB) Co-operative group proposals for the classification of the myelodysplastic syndromes. Br J Haematol. 51:189-199; 1982.
7. Bishop, JM. The molecular biology of RNA tumor viruses: a physician's guide. Engl J Med. 303:675-682; 1980.
8. Bizzozero, O.J. Jr.; Johnson, K.G.; Ciocco, A. Radiation-related leukemia in Hiroshima and Nagasaki, 1946-1964. l. Distribution, incidence, and appearance times. New Engl J Med. 274:1095-1101; 1966.
9. Blattner, WA; Naiman, JL; Mann, DL; *et al.* Immunologic determinants of familial acute lymphocytic leukemia. Ann Intern Med. 89:173-176; 1978.
10. Brauer, MJ; Dameshek, W. Hypoplastic anemia and myeloblastic leukemia following chloramphenicol therapy. New Engl J Med. 277:1003-1005; 1967.
11. Bryan, WR; Moloney, JB; O'Connor, TE; *et al.* Viral etiology of leukemia. Ann Intern Med. 62:376-399; 1965.
12. Coleman, C.N.; Williams, C.J.; Flint, A.; *et al.* Hematologic neoplasia in patients treated for Hodgkin's disease. N Engl J Med. 297:1239-1252; 1977.
13. Cronkite, E.P.; Moloney, W.; Bond, V.P. Radiation leukemogenesis. Am J Med. 28:673-682; 1960.

14. Cutter, S.J.; Axtell, L.; Heise, H. Ten thousand cases of leukemia: 1940-1962. JNCI. 39:993-1026; 1967.

15. Dameshek, W. Riddle: what do aplastic anemia, paroxysmal nocturnal hemoglobinuria (PNH), and "hypoplastic" leukemia have in common? Blood. 30:251-254; 1967.

16. DeBruyere, M; Cornu, G; Hermans-Bracke, T; *et al.* HLA haplotypes and long survival in childhood acute lymphoblastic leukemia treated with transfer factor. Br J Haematol. 44:243-251; 1980.

17. Fairley, G.H. Immunity to malignant disease in man. In: Gilliland, I.; Frances, J., eds. Scientific Basis of Medicine. London, UK: Antholone Press; 1971.

18. Flandrin, G.; Bernard, J. Cytological classification of acute leukemias: a survey of 1,400 cases. Blood Cells. 1:7-15; 1975.

19. German, J. Oncogenic implications of chromosomal instability. Hosp Pract. 8:93-104; 1973.

20. Gibson, R.W.; Bross, I.D.; Graham, S. Leukemia in children exposed to multiple risk factors. N Engl J Med. 279:906-909; 1968.

21. Glass, A. Lack of time-space clustering of childhood leukemia in Los Angeles County, 1960-1964. Cancer Res. 29:1995-2001; 1969.

22. Gralnick, H.R.; Galton, D.A.G.; Catovsky, D.; *et al.* Classification of acute leukemia. Ann Intern Med. 87:740-753; 1977.

23. Gross, L. Attempt to recover filterable agent from x-ray induced leukemia. Acta Haematol (Basel). 19:353-361; 1958.

24. Gunz, FW. The leukemia-lymphoma problem. In: Zarafonetis, C.J.D., ed. International Conference Leukemia and Lymphoma Proceedings. Philadelphia, PA: Lea & Febiger; 1968.

25. Gunz, F.W.; Gunz, J.P.; Veale, A.M.O.; *et al.* Familial leukemia: a study of 909 families. Scand J Haematol. 15:117; 1975.

26. Gunz, FW; Spears, GFS. Distribution of acute leukemia in time and space: studies in New Zealand. Br Med J. 4:604-608; 1968.

27. Hakulinen, T; Hovi, L; Karkinen-Jaaskelainen, M; *et al.* Association between influenza during pregnancy and childhood leukemia. Br Med J. 4:265-267; 1973.

28. Hayhoe, FGJ. Acute leukemia: cellular morphology, cytochemistry, and fine structure. Clin Haematol. 1:49-94; 1972.

29. Hee, JAH. Epidemiological aspects of the preventon of leukemia. In: Raven, RW; Roe, JC, eds. The Prevention of Cancer, vol. 54. London, UK: Butterworth; 343-360: 1967.

31. Hirayama, T. An epidemiological study of leukemia in Japan, with special reference to the problem of time-space clustering. Gan Monogr. 7:5-30; 1969.

30. Heubner, RJ; Todaro, GJ. Oncogenes of RNA tumor viruses as determinants of cancer. Proc Natl Acad Sci USA. 64:1087-1094; 1969.

32. Igel, HJ; Huebner, RJ; Turner, HC; *et al.* Mouse leukemia virus activation by chemical carcinogens. Science. 166:1624-1626; 1969.

33. Kinkaid, R. Cancer viruses in primates. Science. 169:828-831; 1970.

34. Kjelsdsberg, C.R.; Ward, H.P. Leukemia in arsenic poisoning. Ann Intern Med. 77:935-937; 1972.

35. Knapp, R.H.; Dewald, G.W.; Pierre, R.V. Cytogenetic studies in 174 consecutive patients with preleukemic myelodysplastic syndromes. Mayo Clin Proc. 60:507-516; 1985.

36. Knowell, P.C. Cytogenetics of preleukemia. Cancer Genet Cytogenet. 5:265-278; 1982.

37. Lawrence, JS. Irradiation leukemogenesis. JAMA. 190:1049-1054; 1964.

38. Leavesley, GM; Stenhouse, NS; Dougan, L; *et al.* Phenylbutazone and leukemia. N Engl J Med. 302:1101-1105; 1980.

39. Linos, A; Gray, JE; Orvis, AL.; *et al.* Low-dose radiation and leukemia. New Engl J Med. 302:1101-1105; 1980.

40. Miller, RW. Deaths of childhood leukemia and solid tumors and other sibs in the United States, 1960-67. JNCI. 46:203-209; 1971.

41. Miller, RW. Genetics of leukemia: epidemiologic aspects. Jpn J Hum Genet. 13:100-103; 1968.

42. Morton, DL. Immunotherapy of cancer. Cancer. 30:1647-1655; 1972.

43. Patterns in cancer mortality in the United States: 1950-1967. NCI Monogr. No. 33; May 1971.

44. Pedersen-Bjergaard, J.; Nissen, N.I.; Sorensen, H.M.; *et al.* Acute nonlymphocytic leukemia in patients with ovarian carcinoma following long-term treatment with treosulfan. Cancer. 45:19-29; 1980.

45. Rosner, R; Grunwald, HW; Zarribi. MH. Acute leukemia as a complication of cytotoxic chemotherapy. Intl J Radiat Oncol Biol Phys. 5:1705-1708; 1979.

46. Rowe, JM. Clinical and laboratory features of the myeloid and lymphocytic leukemias. Am J Med Tech. 49:(2)103-109; 1983.

47. Ryser, H.J.F. Chemical carcinogenesis. N Engl J Med. 285:721-734; 1971.

48. Temin, HM; Baltimore, D. RNA-directed DNA synthesis and RNA tumor viruses. Adv Virus Res. 17:129-186; 1972.

49. Till, MM; Jones, LH; Pentycross, CR; *et al.* Leukemia in children and their grandparents: studies of immune function in 6 families. Br J Haematol. 29:575-586; 1975.

50. Todaro, GJ; Swift, MR. Susceptibility of human diploid fibroblast strains to transformation by SV40 virus. Science. 153:1252-1254; 1966.

51. Van Pelt, A.; Congdon, C.C. Radiation leukemia in guinea pigs. Radiat Res. 52:68-81; 1972.

52. Vigliani, E.C.; Saita, G. Benzene and leukemia. N Engl J Med. 271:872-876; 1964.

53. Viola, MV; Dalton, AJ; Mitchell, E; *et al.* Virus-like particles in a patient with chronic lymphocytic leukemia. N Engl J Med. 277:503-506; 1967.

54. Viola, MV; Frazier, M; Wiernick, PH; *et al.* Reverse transcriptase in leukocytes of leukemic patients in remission. N Engl J Med. 294:75-80; 1976.

55. Virchow, R. Weisses blut. Foriep's Notizen. 36:151-153; 1845.

56. Youness, E; Trujillo, JM; Ahearn, MJ; *et al.* Acute unclassified leukemia: a cliniopathologic study on the diagnostic implications of electron microscopy. Am J Hematol. 9:79-88; 1980.

57. Zarrabi, MH; Rosner, F. Acute myeloblastic leukemia following treatment for nonhemopoietic cancers. Am J Hematol. 7:357-367; 1979.

Acute Myelogenous Leukemia

58. Appelbaum, FR; Dahlerg, ES; Thomas, ED. *et al.* Bone marrow transplantation or chemotherapy after remission induction for adults in acute lung lymphoblastic leukemia. Ann Intern Med. 101:581-588; 1980.

58a. Arlin, Z.; Case, D.C.; Moore, J.; *et al.* Randomized multicenter trial of cytosine arabinoside with mitoxntrone or danorubicin in previously untreated adult patients with acute nonlymphocytic leukemia (ANLL): Lederle Cooperative Group. Leukemia 4(3):177-183; 1990.

59. Armstrong, D; Young, LS; Meyer, RD; *et al.* Infectious complications of neoplastic disease. Med Clin N Am. 55:729-745; 1971.

60. Ash, RC; Horowitz, MM; Bortin, M. Outcome of allogeneic marrow transplants from related donors other than HLA identical siblings: preliminary international bone marrow registry analysis. Exp Hematol. 16:470-473; 1988.

61. Beatty, PT; Clift, RA; Nickelson, EM. Marrow transplantation from related donors other than HLA-identical siblings. New Engl. J. Med. 313:765-771; 1985.

62. Bell, R; Rohatineraz, S; Slevin, ML.; *et al.* Short term treatment for acute myelogenous leukemia. Br Med J. 284:1221-1223; 1982.

63. Bennett, JM; Begg, C; Eastern Cooperative Oncology Group. Study of the cytochemistry of adult acute myeloid leukemia by correlation of subtypes with response and survival. Cancer Res. 41:4833-4837; 1981.

64. Bennett, JM; Catovsky, D; Daniel, T; *et al.* Criteria for diagnosis of acute leukemia megakaryocytic lineage (M7): report of the French-American-British Cooperative Group. Ann Intern Med. 103:460-462; 1985.

65. Bennett, JM; Catovsky, D; Daniel, T; *et al.* Proposals for classification of the acute leukemia. Br J Haematol. 33:451-456; 1976.

66. Bennett, JM; Catovsky, D; Daniel, T; *et al.* Proposed revised criteria for classification of acute myeloid leukemia: report of the French-American-British Cooperative Group. Ann Intern Med. 103:620-625; 1985.

67. Benvinisti, DS; Ultmann, JE. Eosinophilic leukemia. Ann Intern Med. 71:731-745; 1969.

67a. Berman, E.; Heller, G.; Santorsa, J.; *et al.* Results of a randomized trial comparing idarubicin and cytosine arabinoside with newly dignosed acute myelogous leukemia. Blood 77(8):1666-1674; 1991.

67b. Biondi A, Rumbaldi A, Alcalay M, *et al.* RAR-a gene rearrangements as a genetic marker for diagnosis and monitoring in acute promyelocytic leukemia. Blood 77: 1418-1422; 1991.

68. Bloomfield, CD. Chromosome abnormalities in secondary myeloid dysplastic syndromes. Scand J Haematol. 36:82-90; 1986.

69. Bloomfield, CD; Brunning, RD. Prognostic implications of cytology in acute leukemia in the adult: the case for subacute leukemia. Hum Pathol. 5:641-659; 1979.

70. Bloomfield, CD; del Chapelle, A. Chromosome abnormalities in acute nonlymphocytic leukemia: clinical and biological significance. Semin Oncol. 14:372-383; 1987.

71. Bodey, GP; Buckley, M; Sathe, YS; et al. Quantitative relationships between circulating leukocytes and infections in patients with acute leukemia. Ann Intern Med. 64:328-340; 1966.

72. Boggs, DR; Wintrobe, MW; Cartwright, GE. The acute leukemias. Medicine. 41:163-225; 1962.

73. Breton-Gorius, J; Reyes, F; Duhamel, G; et al. Megakaryoblastic acute leukemia: identification by the ultrastructural demonstration of platelet peroxidase. Blood. 51:45-60; 1978.

74. Brincker, H. Clinical classification and evaluation of treatment response in acute myeloid leukemia on the basis of difference of leukemic cell differentiation. Scand J Haematol. 11:383-390; 1973.

74a. Cassileth, PA; Begg, CB; Silber, R. et al. Prolonged unmaintained remission after intensive consolidation therapy in adult acute nonlymphocytic leukemia. Cancer Treat Rep. 71:137;1987.

74b. Castaigne S, Chomienne C, Daniel MT, et al. All-Trans-Retinoic acid as a differentiation therapy for acute promyelocytic leukemia. I. Clinical Results. Blood 76: 1704-1709; 1990.

74c. Champlin, R.; Gajewski, J.; Nimer, S.; et al. Postremission chemotherapy for adults with acute myelogenous leukemia: Improved survival with high-dose cytarabine and daunorubicin consolidation treatment. J Clin Oncol 8(7):1199-1206; 1990.

75. Champlin, R; Gale, RP. Acute myelogenous leukemia: recent advances in therapy. Blood. 69:(6)1551-1562; 1987.

76. Champlin, R; Ho, W; Gale, RP; et al. Treatment for acute myelogenous leukemia: a prospective controlled trial of bone marrow transplantation versus consolidation of chemotherapy. Ann. Intern. Med. 102:285-291; 1985.

77. Champlin, R; Jacobs, A; Gale, RP; et al. Prolonged survival in acute myelogenous leukemia without maintenance therapy. Lancet. 1:894-897; 1984.

78. Champlin, R.; Gale, R.P. Acute myelogenous leukemia: recent advances in therapy. Blood 69:1551-1562; 1987.

78'. Cheson, B.D.; Cassileth, P.A.; Head, D.R.; et al. Report of the National Cancer Institute-sponsored workshop on definitions of diagnosis and response in acute myeloid leukemia. J Clin Oncol 8(5):813-819; 1990.

78a. Clift, RA; Buckner, CD; Thomas ED, et al. The treatment of acute non-lymphoblastic leukemia by allogeneic marrow transplantation. Bone Marrow Transplant. 2:243-258; 1987.

79. Cohen, J.R.; Creger, W.P.; Greenberg, P.L.; et al. Subacute myeloid leukemia. Am J Med. 66:959-966; 1979.

80. Collins, SJ; Ruscetti, FW; Gallagher, RE; et al. Terminal differentiation of human promyelocytic leukemia cells induced by dimethyl sulfoxide and other polar compounds. Proc Natl Acad Sci USA. 75:2458-2460; 1978.

81. Daly, PA; Schiffer, CA; Wiernik, PH. Acute promyelocytic leukemia—clinical management of 15 patients. Am J Hematol. 8:347-359; 1980.

82. D'Angio, GJ; Evans, AE; Mitus, A. Roentgen therapy of certain complications of acute leukemia in childhood. AJR. 82:541-553; 1959.

83. Dormer, P; Lau, B; Williams, W. Kinetics of bone marrow cell production in human acute and chronic myeloid leukemias. Leuk Res. 4:231-237; 1980.

84. Dreyfus, B. Preleukemic states. Blood Cells. 2:33-45; 1976.

84a. Dutcher, JP; Wiernik, PH; Markus, S. et al. Intensive maintenance therapy improves survival in adult acute non-lymphocytic leukemia: an eight-year follow-up. Leukemia. 2:413;1988.

85. Engel, RR; Hammond, D; Eitzman, DV; et al. Transient congenital leukemia in 7 infants with mongolism. J Pediatr. 65:303-305; 1964.

86. Fialkow, PJ; Bryant, JU; Thomas, ED; et al. Leukemic transformation of engrafted human marrow cells in vivo. Lancet. 1:251-255; 1971.

87. Finnish Leukemia Group. The effect of thioguanine and the combination of daunorubicin, cytarabine and prednisone in the treatment of acute leukemia in adults. Scand J Haematol. 23:1-8; 1979.

88. Foon. KA; Naein, F; Yale, C; et al. Acute myelogenous leukemia: morphologic subclass and response to therapy. Leuk Res. 3:171-174; 1979.

89. Fourth International Workshop on Chromosomes in Leukemia. A perspective study of acute nonlymphocytic leukemia. Cancer Genet Cytogenet. 11:249-360; 1984.

90. Freeman, AI; Journey, LJ Ultrastructural studies on monocytic leukemia. Br J Haematol. 20:225-231; 1971.

91. Freireich, E; Thomas, LB; Frei, E; et al. A distinctive type of intracerebral hemorrhage associated with blast crisis in patients with leukemia. Cancer. 13:l46-154; 1960.

92. Glucksberg, H; Cheever, MA; Farewell, V.T.; et al. High-dose combination chemotherapy for acute nonlymphoblastic leukemia in adults. Cancer. 48:1073-1081; 1981.

93. Goh,.; Klemperer, MR. In vivo leukemic transformation: cytogenetic evidence of in vivo leukemic transformation of engrafted marrow cells. Am J Hematol. 2:283-290; 1977.

94. Golomb, H.M. Diagnostic and prognostic significance of chromosomal abnormalities in acute nonlymphocytic leukemia. Cancer Genet Cytogenet. 1:249; 1980.

95. Gorin, N.C. Autologous bone marrow transplantation: a review of recent advances in acute leukemia. In: Gale, R.P.; Champlin, R., eds. Progress in Bone Marrow Transplantation, UCLA Symposium Molecular and Cellular Biology, New Series, vol. 53. New York, NY: Alan R Liss Inc; 1987:676-684.

96. Greene, W.A. Psychological problems in leukemias and lymphomas. In: Weed, R.I., ed. Hematology for Internists. Boston, MA: Little Brown and Co; 1971.

97. Groopman, J.; Ellman, L. Acute promyelocytic leukemia. Am J Hematol. 7:395-408; 1979.

98. Halterman, R.H.; Leventhal, B.G.; Mann, D,L. An acute leukemia antigen: correlation with clinical status. N Engl J Med. 297:1272-1274; 1972.

99. Hanker, J.S.; Lazio, J.; Moore, J.O. The light microscopic demonstration of hydroperoxide-positive phi bodies and rods in leukocytes in acute myeloid leukemia. Histochemistry. 58:241-252; 1978.

100. Hansen, J.A.; Beatty, P.J.; Anasetti, C. et al. Treatment of leukemia by marrow transplantation from donors other than HLA genotypically identical siblings. In: Gale, R.P.; Champlin R., eds. Progess in Bone Marrow Transplantation, UCLA Symposium on Molecular and Cellular Biology, New Series, vol 53. New York, NY: Alan R Liss Inc; 667-675; 1987.

101. Herrmann, F.; Komischk, E.B.; Odenwald, E. et al. Use of monoclonal antibodies as a diagnostic tool in human leukemia: acute myeloid leukemia and acute phase of chronic myeloid leukemia. Blut. 47:157-167; 1983.

102. Hess, C.E.; Nichols, A.B.; Hunt, W.B.; et al. Pseudohypoxemia secondary to leukemia and thrombocytosis. N Engl J Med. 301:361-363; 1979.

103. Higby, D.J.; Burnett, D. Granulocyte transfusions: current status. Blood. 55:2-8; 1980.

104. Keating, M.J.; Smith, T.L.; McCredie, K.B.; et al. A 4-year experience with combination chemotherapy in 325 adults with acute leukemia. Cancer. 47:2779-2788; 1981.

105. Killmann, S.A. A hypothesis concerning the relationship between normal and leukemic hematopoiesis in acute myeloid leukemia. In: Stohlman, F., ed. Hematopoietic Cellular Proliferation. New York, NY: Grune & Stratton; 267-277; 1970.

106. Kirsch, I.R. Molecular biology of the leukemias. Pediatr Clin of North Am. 35:(4)693-722; 1988.

107. Krause, J.R. Granulocytic sarcoma preceding acute leukemia. Cancer. 44:1017-1021; 1979.

108. Levine, A.S.; Siegel, S.E.; Schreiber, A.D.; et al. Protected environments and prophylactic antibiotics. N Engl J Med. 288:477-483; 1973.

109. Lichtman, M.A. The myelogenous leukemias. In: Lichtman, M.A., ed. Hematology and Oncology. New York, NY: Grune & Stratton; 144-147; 1980.

109a. Lichtman, M.A.; Brennan, J.K. Hematopoiesis. In: Lichtman, M.A. ed. Hematology and Oncology. New York, NY: Grune & Stratton; 4-6; 1980.

110. Lichtman, M.A.; Kearney, E.A. Filterability of normal and leukemic leukocytes. Blood Cells. 2:491-506; 1976.

110a. Lichtman, M.A., Segel, G.B. The leukemias. In: Rubin, P. (ed).

Clinical Oncology: A Multi-disciplinary Approach (6th ed). New York, NY: American Cancer Society, Inc.; 1983.

111. Lichtman, M.A.; Weed, R.I. Peripheral cytoplasmic characteristics of leukemia in monocytic leukemia: relationships to clinical manifestations. Blood. 40:52-61; 1972.

112. Linman, J.W.; Saami, M.I. The preleukemic syndrome. Semin Hematol. 11:93-100; 1974.

113. Look, A.T. Cytogenetics of childhood leukemia: clinical and biologic implications. Pediatr Clin of North Am. 35:(4)723-902; 1988.

114. Machover, D; Rappaport, H.; Schwarzenberg, L.;*et al.* Treatment of acute myelogenous leukemia with a combination of intensive induction chemotherapy, early consolidation, splenectomy and long term maintenance chemotherapy. Cancer. 53:1644-1648; 1984.

114a. Mandelli, F.; Petti, M.C.; Ardia, A.; *et al.* A randomized clinical trial comparing idarubicin and cytarabine to daunorubicin and cytarabine in the treatment of acute non-lymphoid leukaemia. Eur J Cancer 27(6):750-755; 1991.

115. Marcus, R.E.; Catovsky, D.; Goldman, J.M.; *et al.* Maintenance and consolidation of chemotherapy in AML. Lancet. 1:686-689; 1984.

116. Mathe, G. Immunological approaches of leukaemia treatment. Ann Inst Pasteur. 122:855-881; 1972.

117. Mayer, R.J. Current chemotherapeutic treatment approaches to the management of previously untreated adult with *de novo* acute myelogenous leukemia. Semin Oncol. 14:(4)384-396; 1987.

118. McKee, L.C. Jr.; Collins, R.D. Intravascular leukocyte thrombi and aggregates as a cause of morbidity and mortality in leukemia. Medicine. 53:462-478; 1974.

119. McKenna, R.W.; Bloomfield, C.D.; Dick, F.; *et al.* Acute monoblastic leukemia: diagnosis and treatment of 10 cases. Blood. 46:481-494; 1975.

119a. McMillan, A.K.; Goldstone, A.H.; Linch, D.C.; *et al.* High-dose chemotherapy and autologous bone marrow transplantation in acute myeloid leukemia. Blood 76(3):480-488; 1990.

120. Mertelsman, R.; Thaler, H.T.; Tol, T.; *et al.* Morphological classification, response to therapy, and survival in 263 adult patients with acute nonlymphoblastic leukemia. Blood. 56:773-781; 1986.

121. Mir, M.A.; Brabin, N.; Tang, O.T. Hypokalemia in acute myeloid leukemia. Ann Intern Med. 82:54-57; 1975.

122. Muss, H.B.; Maloney, W.C. Chloroma and other myeloblastic tumors. Blood. 42:721-728; 1973.

122a. Ohno R, Tomonaga M, Kobayashi T et al. Effect of granu;ocyte colnt-stimulating factor after intensive induction therapy in relapsed or refractory acute leukemia. N Engl J Med. 323 (13): 871-877; 1990.

123. Omura, G.A.; Moffitt, S.M.; Vogler, W.R.; *et al.* Combination chemotherapy of adult ALL with randomized CNS prophylaxis. Blood. 55:199-204; 1980.

124. O'Regan, S.; Arson, S.; Chesney, R.W.;*et al.* Electrolyte and acid-base disturbances in the management of leukemia. Blood. 49:345-354; 1977.

125. Ottolander, G.J.D.;te Velde, J.; Brederoo, P.; *et al.* Megakaryoblastic leukemia (acute myelofibrosis): a report of 3 cases. Br J Haematol. 42:9-20; 1979.

126. Powells, R.L.; Morgenstern, G.; Clink, H.M.; *et al.* The place of bone marrow transplantation in acute myelogenous leukemia. Lancet. 1:1047-1051; 1980.

127. Preisler, H.D.; Brecher, M.; Browman, G.; *et al.* Treatment of acute myelocytic leukemia in patients 30 years of age and younger. Am J Hematol. 13:189-193; 1982.

128. Quattrin, N. Leucemies aigues a basophils. Nouv Rev Hematol. 13:745-754; 1973.

129. Rees, J.K.H.; Gray, R.G.; Swirsky, D.;*et al.* Principal results of the Medical Research Council's 8th Acute Myeloid Leukemia Trial. Lancet. i:1236-1239; 1986.

130. Rheingold, J.J.; Kaufman, R.; Adelson, E.;*et al.* Smouldering acute leukemia. N Engl J Med. 268:812-815; 1963.

131. Rowley, J.D. Chromosome changes in acute leukemia. Br J Haematol. 44:339-346; 1980.

132. Sakurai, M.; Sandberg, A.A. Chromosomes and causation of human cancer and leukemia. XIII. Findings in erythroleukemia. Cancer. 37:790-804; 1976.

133. Sandberg, A.A.; Cartwright, G.E.; Wintrobe, M.M. Studies in leukemia. 1. Uric acid excretion. Blood. 11:154-166; 1965.

133a. Santos, G.W.; Tutschka, P.J.; Brookmeyer, R.; *et al.* Marrow transplantation for acute nonlymphocytic leukemia after treatment with busulfan and cyclophosphamide. N Engl J Med. 309:1347;1983.

134. Sauter, C.; Berchtold, W.; Fopp, M. Acute myelogenous leukemia: maintenance chemotherapy after early consolidation treatments does not prolong survival. Lancet. 1:379-383; 1984.

135. Schiffer, C.A. Some aspects of recent advances in the use of blood cell components. Br J Haematol. 39:289-294; 1978.

136. Schimpff, S.C.; Young, V.M.; Greene, W.H.; *et al.* Origin of infections in acute nonlymphocytic leukemia. Ann Intern Med. 77:707-714; 1972.

137. Scott, R.B.; Ellison, R.R.; Ley, A.B. A clinical study of 20 cases of erythroid-leukemia (Di Guglielmo's syndrome). Am J Med. 37:162-171; 1964.

138. Second International Workshop on Chromosomes in Leukemia. Chromosomes in preleukemia. Cancer Genet Cytogenet. 2:108-113; 1979.

139. Sexauer, J.; Kass, L.; Schnitrer, B. Subacute myelomonocytic leukemia. Am J Med. 57:853-861; 1974.

140. Shaw, M.T. The distinctive features of acute myelocytic leukemia. Am J Hematol. 4:97-103; 1978.

141. Solberg, C.O.; Schreiner, A.; HelIium, K.B. Neutrophil granulocyte function in the early diagnosis of acute myeloblastic leukemia. Acta Med Scand. 197:147-151; 1975.

142. Southam, C.M. Immunotherapy of leukemia. In: Damashek, W.; Dutcher, R.M., eds. Perspectives in Leukemia. New York, NY: Grune & Stratton; 1968.

142a. Stone RM, Mayer RJ. The unique aspects of acute promyelotic leukemia. J Clin Oncol 8: 1913-1921, 1990.

143. Straus, D.J.; Mertelsmann, R.; Koziner, B;*et al.* The acute monocytic leukemias. Medicine. 59:409-425; 1980.

143a. Tallman, M.S.; Applebaum, F.R.; Amos, D.; *et al.* Evaluation of intensive postremission chemotherapy for adults with acute nonlymphocytic leukemia using high-dose cytosine arabinoside with l-asparaginase and amsacrine with etoposide. J Clin Oncol. 5:918;1987.

144. Thomas, E.D.; Buckner, C.D.; Banaji, M.; *et al.* One hundred patients with acute leukemia treated by chemotherapy, total body irradiation, and allogeneic marrow transplantation. Blood. 49:511-533; 1977.

145. Thomas, E.D.; Storb, R.; Clift, R.A.; *et al.* Bone marrow transplantation. N Engl J Med. 292:832-843; 1975.

146. Van Der Weyden, M.B.; Clancy, R.L.; Howard, M.A.; *et al.* Qualitative platelet defects with reduced life span in leukemia. Aust NZ J Med. 2:339-345; 1972.

147. Wainer, R.A.; Wiernik, P.H.; Thompson, W.L. Metabolic and therapeutic studies of a patient with acute leukemia and severe lactic acidosis of prolonged duration. Am J Med. 55:255-260; 1973.

147a. Warrell RP, Frankel SR, Miller WH, *et al.* Differentiation therapy of acute promyelocytic leukemia with tretinoin (All-Trans-Retinoic acid). N Engl J Med 324: 1385-1393, 1991.

148. Weinstein, H.J. Congenital leukemia and the neonatal myeloproliferative disorders associated with Down's syndrome. Clin Hematol. 7:147-154; 1978.

149. Weinstein, J.H.; May, R.J.; Rosenthal, D.S.; *et al.* Chemotherapy for acute myelogenous leukemia in children and adults, VAPA update. Blood. 62:315-319; 1983.

149a. Wiernik, P.H. Acute leukemias. In: DeVita, V.T., Jr., Hellman, S., Rosenberg, S.A. (eds). Cancer: Principles and Practice of Oncology, 3rd ed. Philadelphia, PA: JB Lippincott Co.; 1989; 1809-1835.

150. Wiernik, P.H.; Serpick, A.A. Granulocytic sarcoma (chloroma). Blood. 35:361-369; 1970.

151. Wiggans, R.G.; Jacobson, R.J.; Fialkow, P.J.;*et al.* Probable clonal origin of acute myeloblastic leukemia following radiation and chemotherapy of colon cancer. Blood. 52:659-663; 1978.

152. Yam, L.T.; Li, C.Y.; Necheles, T.F.; *et al.* Pseudoeosinophilia, eosinophilic endocarditis, eosinophilic leukemia. Am J Med. 53:193-202; 1972.

153. Yunis, J.J.; Bloomfield, C.D.; Ensrud, K. All patients with acute nonlymphocytic leukemia may have a chromosomal defect. N Engl J Med. 305:135-139; 1981.

154. Zittoun, R. Subacute and chronic myelomonocytic leukemia: a distinct haematological entity. Br J Haematol. 32:1-7; 1976.

Chronic Myelogenous Leukemia

155. Barton, J.C.; Conrad, M.E. Current status of blastic transformation in chronic myelogenous leukemia. Am J Hematol 4:281-291; 1978.
156. Bernstein, R. Cytogenetics of chronic myelogenous leukemia. Semin Hematol. 25:(1)20-34; 1988.
157. Boggs, D.R. Hematopoietic stem cell theory in relation to possible lymphoblastic conversion of chronic myeloid leukemia. Blood. 44:449-453; 1974.
157a. Bolin, R.W.; Robinson, W.A.; Sutherland, J.; Hamman, R.F. Busulphan versus hydroxyurea in long-term therapy of chronic myelogenous leukemia. Cancer. 50:1683;1982.
158. Boruncle, B.A.; Doan, C.A. Myelofibrosis: Clinical, hematologic, and pathologic study of 110 patients. Am J Med Sci. 243:697-715; 1962.
159. Brandt, L; Mitelman, F.; Panani, A.; et al. Extremely long duration of CML with Ph^1 negative and Ph^2 positive bone marrow cells. Scand J Haematol. 16:321-325; 1976.
160. Breazen, O.; Canaanid, (X.X.); Gayle, R.P. Molecular biology of chronic myelogenous leukemia. Semin Hematol. 25:(1)35-49; 1988.
160a. Buckner, C.D.; Clift, R.A.; Fefer, A.; et al. Treatment of blastic transformation of chronic granulocytic leukemia by high dose cyclophosphamide, total body irradiation and infusion of cryopreserved autologous marrow. Exp Hematol. 2:138;1974.
161. Burnstein, R. Cytogenetics of chronic myelogenous leukemia. Semin Hematol. 25:(1)20-34; 1988.
162. Catovsky, D. Ph^1-positive acute leukemia and chronic granulocytic leukemia: 1 or 2 diseases. Br J Haematol. 42:493-498; 1979.
162a. Cervantes, F.; Rozman, M.; Rosell, J.; et al. A study of prognostic factors in blast crisis of Philadelphia chromosome-positive chronic myelogenous leukaemia. Br J Haematol. 76(1):27-32; 1990.
163. Champlin, R.; Gale, R.P.; Foon, K.A.; et al. Chronic leukemias: oncogenes, chromosomes, and advances in therapy. Ann Intern Med. 104:671-688; 1986.
164. Champlin, R.; Ho, W.; Arenson, E.; et al. Allogeneic bone marrow transplantation with chronic myelogenous leukemia in chronic accelerated phase. Blood. 60:1038-1041; 1982.
165. Chervenik, P.A.; Ellis, L.D.; Pan, S.F.; et al. Human leukemic cells: in vitro growth of colonies containing the Philadelphia (Ph^1) chromosome. Science. 174:1135-1136; 1971.
165a. Clarkson, B.D. Chronic myelogenous leukemia: is aggressive treatment indicated? J Clin Oncol. 3:135;1985.
166. Clift, R.A.; Buckner, C.D.; Thomas, E.D.; et al. Treatment of chronic granulocytic leukemia in chronic phase by allogeneic marrow transplantation. Lancet. ii:61-62; 1982.
166'. Cunningham, I. Bone marrow transplantation for chronic myelogenous leukemia. Oncol (USA) 4(11):101-108; 1990.
166a. Cunningham, I.; Gee, T.; Dowling, M.; et al. Results of treatment with Ph^1 + chronic myelogenous leukemia with an intensive treatment regimen (L-5 protocol). Blood. 53:375;1979.
167. De Grouchy, J; DeNava, C.; Cantu, J-M.; et al. Models of clonal evolutions: a study of chronic myelogenous leukemia. Am J Hum Genet. 18:485-503;1966.
167a. Deisseroth, A.B.; Arlinghous, R.D. (eds). Chronic Myelogenous Leukemia—Molecular Approaches to Research and Therapy. New York, NY: Marcel Dekker, Inc; 1991.
168. Dreazan, O.; Canaani, E.; Gayle, R.P. Molecular biology of chronic myelogenous leukemia. Semin Hematol. 25(1):35-49;1988.
169. Ezdinli, E.Z.; Sokal, J.E.; Crosswhite, L.H.; et al. Philadelphia chromosome positive and negative chronic myelocytic leukemia. Ann Intern Med. 72:175-182; 1970.
170. Fialkow, P.J.; Denman, A.M.; Jacobson, R.; et al. Chronic myelocytic leukemia: origin of some lymphocytes from leukemic stem cells. J Clin Invest. 62:815-823; 1978.
170a. Fefer, A.; Cheever, M.A.; Greenberg, P.D.; et al. Treatment of chronic granulocytic leukemia with chemoradiotherapy and transplantation of marrow from identical twins. N Engl J Med. 306:63;1982.
170b. Fefer, A.; Cheever, M.A.; Thomas, E.D.; et al. Disappearance of Ph^1-positive cells in four patients with chronic granulocytic leukemia after chemotherapy, irradiation and marrow transplantation from an identical twin. New Engl J Med. 300:33;1979.
171. Fialkow, P.J.; Jacobson, R; Papayannopoubs, T. Chronic myelogenous leukemia: clonal origin in a stem cell common to the granulocyte, erythrocyte platelet, and monocyte/macrophage. Am J Med. 63:125-130;1977.
172. Finney, R.; McDonald, G.A.; Baikie, A.G.; et al. Chronic granulocytic leukemia with p negative cells in bone marrow and a 10-year remission after busulfan hypoplasia. Br J Haematol. 23:283-288; 1972.
173. Gallo, R.C. Terminal transferase and leukemia. N Engl J Med. 292:804-805; 1975.
174. Geary, C.G.; Catovsky, D.; Wiltshaw, E.; et al. Chronic myelomonocytic leukemia. Br J Haematol. 30:289-302; 1975.
175. Goh K-O; Anderson, F.W. Cytogenic studies in basophilic chronic myelocytic leukemia. Arch Pathol Lab Med. 103:288-290;1979.
176. Goh, K-O.; Swisher, S.M. Identical twins and chronic myelocytic leukemia. Arch Intern Med. 115:475-478; 1965.
177. Goldman, J.M.; Apperly, J.F.; Jones, L.; et al. Bone marrow transplantation for patients with chronic myelogenous leukemia. N Engl J Med. 314:202;1986.
178. Goldman, J.M.; Apperley, J.F.; Jones, L.; et al. Bone marrow transplantation for patients with chronic myelogenous leukemia. N Engl J Med. 314:202-207; 1986.
178a. Goldman, J.M.; Grosveld, G.; Baltimore, D.; et al. Chronic myelogenous leukemia—the unfolding saga. Leukemia 4(3):163-167; 1990.
179. Goldman, J.M.; Th'ng, K.H.; Park, D.S.; et al. Collection, cryopreservation and subsequent viability of hemopoietic stem cells intended for treatment of chronic granulocytic leukemia in blast cell transformation. Br J Haematol. 40:185-195; 1978.
180. Gomez, G.A.; Sokal, J.E.; Walsh, D. Prognostic features at diagnosis of chronic myelocytic leukemia. Cancer. 47:2470-2477; 1981.
181. Gralnick, H.R.; Harbor, J.; Vigel, C. Myelofibrosis in chronic granulocytic leukemia. Blood. 37:152-162; 1971.
182. Griner, P.F. Chronic myelogenous leukemia. In: Weed, R.I., ed. Hematology for Internists. Boston, MA: Little, Brown & Co.; 1971.
183. Groopman, J.E. The pathogenesis of myelofibrosis in myeloproliferative disorders. Ann Intern Med. 92:857-858;1980.
183a. Haines, M.E.; Goldman, J.M.; Worsley, A.M.; et al. Chemotherapy and autografting for chronic granulocytic leukemia in leukemia in transformation: probable prolongation of survival for some patients. Br J Haematol. 58:711;1984.
184. Ihde, D.C.; Canellos, G.A.; Schwartz, J.H.; et al. Splenectomy in the chronic phase of chronic granulocytic leukemia. Ann Intern Med. 84:17-21; 1976.
185. Janossy, G.; Greaves, M.F.; Revesz, T.; et al. Blast crisis of chronic myeloid leukemia. II. Cell surface marker analysis of "lymphoid" and myeloid cases. Br J Haematol. 34:179-192; 1976.
185a. Kantarjian, H.M.; Villekoop, L.; McCredie, B.; Keating, M.; et al. Intensive combination chemotherapy (ROAP 10) and splenectomy in the management of chronic myelogenous leukemia. J Clin Oncol. 3:192;1985.
186. Kattlove, H.E.; Williams, J.C.; Gaynor, E.; et al. Gaucher cells in chronic myelocytic leukemia: an acquired abnormality. Blood. 33:379-390; 1969.
187. Kauer, G.L.; Engle, R.L. Eosinophilic leukemia with Ph^1 positive cells. Lancet. ii:1340; 1964.
187a. Kennedy, B.J. Hydroxyurea therapy in chronic myelogenous leukemia. Cancer. 29:1052;1972.
188. Koettler, H.P.; Goldem, D.W. Chronic myelogenous leukemia: new concepts. N Engl J Med. 304:1201-1209;1269-1274;1981.
189. Kyle, R.A.; Pease, G. Basophilic leukemia. Arch Intern Med. 118:205-210; 1966.
190. LeBien, T.W.; Hozier, J.; Minowada, J.; et al. Origin of chronic myelocytic leukemia in a precursor of pre-B lymphocytes. N Engl J Med. 201:144-147; 1979.
191. Lichtman, M.A.; Heal, J.; Rowe, J.M. Hyperleukocytic leukemia: rheological and clinical features and management. Clin Hematol. 1:(3)725-746; 1987.
191a. MacKinnon, S.; Hows, J.M.; Goldman, J.M.; et al. Bone marrow transplantation for chronic myeloid leukemia: The use of histocompatible unrelated volunteer donors. Exp Hematol. 18(5):421-425; 1990.
192. Marks, S.M.; Baltimore, D.; McCattrey, R. Terminal transferase as a predictor of initial responsiveness to vincristine and prednisone in blastic chronic myelogenous leukemia. N Engl J Med. 298:812-814; 1978.

192a. McGlave, P.; Arthur, D.; Haake, R.; *et al.* Therapy of chronic myelogenous leukemia with allogeneic bone marrow transplantation. J Clin Oncol. 5:1033;1987.

192b. McGlave, P.B.; Arthur, D.C.; Weisdorf, D. Allogeneic bone marrow transplantation as treatment for accelerating chronic myelogenous leukemia. Blood. 63:219;1984.

192c. Medical Research Council Report. Chronic granulocytic leukemia: comparison on radiotherapy and busulfan therapy. Br Med J. 1:201-208; 1968.

193. Minot, G.R.; Buckman, T.E.; Isaacs, R. Chronic myelogenous leukemia: age, incidence, duration and benefit derived from irradiation. JAMA. 82:1489;1924.

194. Moore, M.S.; Ekert, H.; Fitzgerald, M.G.; *et al.* Evidence for the clonal origin of chronic myeloid leukemia from a sex chromosome mosaic. Blood. 43:15-22; 1974.

195. Nowell, P.C.; Hungerford, D.A. A minute chromosome in human chronic granulocytic leukemia. Science. 132:1497;1960.

195a. Preisler, H.D.; Raza, A.; Hibby, D.; *et al.* Treatment of myeloid blast crisis of chronic myelogenous leukemia. Cancer Treat Rep. 68:1351;1984.

196. Ratain, M.J.; Larson, R.A.; Hooperman, A.; *et al.* Study of recombinant beta interferon in chronic myelogenous leukemia. Blood. 72:(5)222A; 1988. Abstract.

196a. Reiffers, J.; Trouette, R.; Marit, G.; *et al.* Autologous blood stem cell transplantation for chronic granulocytic leukaemia in transformation: A report of 47 cases. Br J Haematol. 77(3): 339-345; 1991.

197. Rosenthal, S; Canellos, G.P.; DeVita, V.T.; *et al.* Characteristics of blast crisis in chronic granulocytic leukemia. Blood. 49:705-714; 1977.

198. Rosner, F.; Schreiber, Z.R.; Parise, F. Leukocyte alkaline phosphatase. Arch Intern Med. 130:892-894; 1972.

198a. Rushing, D.; Goldman, A.; Gibbs, G.; *et al.* Hydroxyurea versus busulphan in the treatment of chronic myelogenous leukemia. Cancer. 29:1052;1972.

199. Sandberg, A.A. The cytogenetics of chronic myelocytic leukemia (CML): chronic phase and blastic crisis. Cancer Genet Cytogenet. 1:217-228; 1980.

199a. Sharp, J.C.; Joyner, M.V.; Wayne, A.W.; *et al.* Karotype conversion in Ph-1 positive chronic myeloid leukemia with combination chemotherapy. Lancet. 1:1370;1979.

199b. Smalley, R.V.; Vogel, J.; Hugley, C.M.; Miller, D. Chronic granulocytic leukemia: Cytogenetic conversion of the bone marrow with cycle-specific chemotherapy. Blood. 50:107;1977.

200. Sokal, E.; Baccarani, M.; Russo, B.; *et al.* Staging and prognosis in chronic myelogenous leukemia. Semin Hematol. 25:(1)19-61; 1988.

200a. Speck, B.; Bortin, M.M.; Champlin, R.; *et al.* Allogeneic bone marrow transplantation for chronic myelogenous leukemia. Lancet. i:665;1984.

201. Strife, A.; Clarkson, B. Biology of chronic myelogenous leukemia: is discordant maturation the primary defect? Semin Hematol. 25:(1)1-19; 1988.

202. Talpaz, M.; Kantarjan, H.M.; Kurzrock, R.; *et al.* Therapy of chronic myelogenous leukemia: chemotherapy and interferons. Semin Hematol. 25:(1)62-73; 1988.

202a. Talpaz, M.; Kantarjian, H.M.; McCredie, K.; *et al.* Hematologic remission and cytogenetic improvement induced by recombinant human interferon alpha-A in chronic myelogenous leukemia. N Engl J Med. 314:1065;1986.

203. Tanaka, M.; Kaneda, T.; Hirota, Y.; *et al.* Terminal deoxynucleatidyl transferase in blastic phase of chronic myelogenous leukemia. Am J Hematol. 9:287-293; 1980.

204. Thomas, E.D.; Clift, R.A.; Fefer, A.; *et al.* Marrow transplantation for treatment of chronic myelogenous leukemia. Ann Intern Med. 104:155-163; 1986.

205. Vallejos, C.S.; McCredie, K.B.; Brittin G.M.; *et al.* Biological effects of repeated leukapheresis of patients with chronic myelogenous leukemia. Blood. 42:925-933; 1973.

206. Youman, J.D.; Taddeini, L.; Cooper, T. Histamine excess symptoms in granulocytic leukemia. Arch Intern Med. 131:560-562; 1973.

Acute Lymphocytic Leukemia

207. Albo, V.; Miller, D.R.; Leiken, S.; *et al.* Nine brain tumors as a late effect on children "cured" of acute lymphoblastic leukemia (ALL) from a single protocol. Proc Am Soc Clin Oncol. 4:172; 1985. Abstract.

208. Aur, R.J.A.; Simone, J.V.; Verzosa, M.S.; *et al.* Childhood acute lymphocytic leukemia. Study VIII. Cancer. 42:2123-2134; 1978.

209. Binger, C.M.; Ablin, A.R.; Feruerstein, R.C.; *et al.* Childhood leukemia: emotional impact on patient and family. N Engl J Med. 280:414-418; 1969.

210. Blatt, J.; Poplack, D.G.; Sherins, R.J. Testicular function in boys after chemotherapy for acute lymphoblastic leukemia. N Engl J Med. 304:1121-1123; 1981.

211. Bleyer, W.A.; Drake, J.C.; Chabner, B.A. Neurotoxicity and elevated cerebrospinal fluid methotrexate concentration in meningeal leukemia. N Engl J Med. 189:770-773; 1973.

212. Bohinjec, J. Acute lymphoblastic leukemia relapsing as acute myelomonocytic leukemia after a remission of 7 years. Br J Haematol. 46:495-497; 1980.

212a. Brochstein, J.A.; Kernan, N.A.; Groshen, S, *et al.* Allogeneic bone marrow transplantation after hyperfractionated total body irradiation and cyclophosphamide in children with acute leukemia. N Engl J Med. 317:1618;1987.

213. Chessells, J.M.; Hardisty, R.M.; Rapson, N.T.; *et al.* Acute lymphoblastic leukemia in children: classification and prognosis. Lancet. ii:1307-1309;1977.

214. Clark, M.A.; Creegan, W.J.; Stass, S.A.; *et al.* Pseudoleukemia. Arch Pathol Lab Med. 105:122-125; 1981.

215. Clarkson, B.; Ellis, S.; Little, C.; *et al.* Acute lymphoblastic leukemia in adults. Semin Oncol. 12:160-177; 1985.

216. Dritschilo, A.; Cassady, J.R.; Camitta, B.; *et al.* The role of irradiation in central nervous system treatment and prophylaxis for acute lymphoblastic leukemia. Cancer. 37:2729-2735; 1976.

216a. Esterhay, R.J.; Wiernik, P.H.; Grove, W.R.; *et al.* Moderate-dose methotrexate, vincristine, asparaginase and dexamethasone for treatment of adult acute lymphocytic leukemia. Blood. 59:334;1982.

217. Evans, A.E.; Craig, M. Central nervous system involvement in children with acute leukemia: a study of 921 patients. Cancer. 17:256-258; 1964.

218. Evans, A.E.; Gilbert, E.S.; Zandstra, R. The increasing incidence of central nervous system leukemia in children. Cancer. 26:404-409; 1970.

218a. Gaynon, P.S.; Bleyer, W.A.; Steinherz, P.G.; Finklestein, J.Z.; Littman, P.; Miller, D.R.; Reaman, G.; Sather, H.; Hammond, G.D. Day 7 marrow response and outcome for children with acute lymphoblastic leukemia and unfavorable presenting features. Med. Pediatr. Oncol. 18:273-279; 1990.

219. George, S.L.; Aur, R.J.A.; Mauer, A.M.; *et al.* A reappraisal of the results of stopping therapy in childhood leukemia. N Engl J Med. 300:269-273; 1979.

219a. Gingrich, R.D.; Burns, C.P.; Armitage, J.O.; *et al.* Long-term relapse-free survival in adult acute lymphoblastic leukemia. Cancer Treat Rep. 69:153;1984.

220. Henderson, E.S.; Scharlau, C.; Cooper, M.R.; *et al.* Combination chemotherapy and radiotherapy for acute lymphocytic leukemia in adults. Leuk Res. 3:395-407; 1979.

221. Hoelzer, D.; Thiel, E.; Loffler, H.; *et al.* Intensified therapy in acute lymphoblastic and acute undifferentiated leukemia in adults. Blood. 64:38-42; 1984.

221a. Horowitz, M.M.; Messerer, D.; Hoelzer, D.; *et al.* Chemotherapy compared with bone marrow transplantation for adults with acute lymphoblastic leukemia in first remission. Ann Int Med. 115(1): 13-18; 1991.

222. Hussein, K.K.; Dahlberg, S.; Head, D.; *et al.* Treatment of acute lymphoblastic leukemia in adults with intensive induction; consolidation and maintenance chemotherapy. Blood. 73:(1)57-63; 1989.

222a. Jackson, J.F.; Boyett, J.; Pullen, J.; *et al.* Favorable prognosis associated with hyperdiploidy in children with acute lymphocytic leukemia correlates with extra chromosome 6: A Pediatric Oncology Group Study. Cancer 66(6):1183-1189; 1990.

223. Kirsch, I.R. Molecular biology of the leukemias. Pediat Clin North Am. 35:(4)693-722; 1988.

224. Leventhal, B.G.; Levine, A.S.; Graw, R.G.; *et al.* Long-term second remissions in acute lymphatic leukemia. Cancer. 35:1136-1140; 1975.

224a. Linker, C.A.; Levitt, L.J.; O'Donnell, M.; *et al.* Improved results of treatment of adult acute lymphoblastic leukemia. Blood. 69:1242;1987.

225. Look, A.T. Cytogenetics of childhood leukemia: clinical and biologic implications. Pediat Clin North Am. 35:(4)723-741; 1988.

226. Miller, D.R. Childhood acute lymphoblastic leukemia: I. biological features and their use in predicting outcome of treatment. Am J Pediatr Hemat Oncol. 10:(2)163-173; 1988.

227. Miller, D.R. Childhood acute lymphoblastic leukemia: II. Strategies and innovation for producing more cures. Am J Pediatr Hemat Oncol. 10:(2)174-179; 1988.

227a. Miller, D.R.; Albo, V.; Leiken, S. et al. Brain Tumors and Survivors of Childhood Acute Lymphoblastic Leukemia. Internat Soc Pediatr Oncol Proc XVII Meeting, Belgrade, Yugoslavia: 1986.

228. Miller, D.R.; Leinkin, S.; Albo, V.; et al. Prognostic importance of morphology (FAB classification) in childhood acute lymphoblastic leukemia (ALL). Br J Haematol. 48:199-206; 1981.

229. Moss, H.A.; Nannis, E.D.; Poplack, D.G. The effects of prophylactic treatment of the central nervous system on intellectual function in children with acute lymphocytic leukemia. Am J Med. 71:47-52;1981.

229a. Mulhern, R.K.; Fairclough, D.; Ochs, J. Prospective comparison of neuropsychologic performance in children surviving leukemia who received 18-Gy, 24-Gy, no cranial irradiation. J Clin Oncol. 9:1348-1356; 1991.

230. Nies, B.A.; Bodey, G.P.; Thomas, L.B.; et al. Persistence of extramedullary leukemic infiltration during marrow remission of acute leukemia. Blood. 26:133141; 1965.

231. Pochedly, C. Neurologic manifestations in acute leukemia. NY State J Med. 75:575-580; 1975.

232. Poplack, D.G.; Reaman, G. Acute lymphoblastic leukemia in childhood. Pediatr Clin North Am. 35:(4)903-932; 1988.

232a. Pui, C.H.; Behm, F.G.; Sing, B.; et al. Heterogeneity of presenting features and their relation to treatment outcome in 120 children with T-cell acute lymphoblastic leukemia. Blood 75(1): 174-179; 1990.

232b. Pui, C.H.; Crist, W.M.; Look, A.T. Biology and clinical significance of cytogenetic abnormalities in childhood acute lymphoblastic leukemia. Blood 76(8):1449-1463; 1990.

233. Ravindranath, Y; Inoue, S; Considine, B; et al. New leukemia in the course of therapy of ALL. Am J Hematol. 5:211-223; 1978.

233a. Riehm, H.; Gadner, H.; Henze, G.; et al. Results and significance of six randomized trials in four consecutive ALL-BFM studies. Haematologie and Bluttransfusion 33(Suppl):439-450; 1990.

234. Sarovitz, H.I.; Gilchrist, G.S.; Smithson, W.A.; et al. Testicular relapse in childhood leukemia. Mayo Clin Proc. 53:212-216; 1978.

235. Schauer, P.; Arlin, Z.A.; Mertelsmann, R.; et al. Treatment of acute lymphoblastic leukemia in adults: results of the L-1OM protocols. J Clin Oncol. 1:462-466; 1983.

235a. Schuster, J.J.; Falletta, J.M.; Pullen, D.J.; et al. Prognostic factors in childhood T-cell acute lymphoblastic leukemia: A Pediatric Oncology Group Study. Blood 75(1):166-173; 1990.

236. Silverstein, M.N.; Kelly, P.J. Leukemia with osteoarticular symptoms and signs. Ann Intern Med. 59:637-645;1963.

237. Simone, J.V. The treatment of acute lymphoblastic leukemia. Br J Haematol. 45:1-4; 1980.

238. Simone, J.V.; Holland, E.; Johnson, W. Fatalities during remission of childhood leukemia. Blood. 39:759-770;1972.

239. Siris, E.S.; Leventhal, B.G.; Vaitukaitis, J.L. Effects of childhood leukemia and chemotherapy on puberty and reproductive function in girls. N Engl J Med. 294: 1143-1146; 1976.

240. Trigg, M.E. Bone marrow transplantation for treatment of leukemia in children. Pediatr Clin North Am. 35:(4)933-948; 1988.

241. Viana, M.B.; Maurer, H.S.; Ferenc, C. Subclassification of acute lymphoblastic leukemia in children. Br. J. Hematol. 44:383-388;1980.

242. Weisdorf, D.J.; Nesbit, M.E.; Ransay, N.K.C.; et al. Allogeneic bone marrow transplantation for acute lymphoblastic leukemia in remission: prolonged survival associated with acute graft-versus-host disease. J Clin Oncol. 5:1348;1987.

242a. Williams, J.M.; Davis, K.S. Central nervous system prophylactic treatment for childhood leukemia, neuropsychological outcome studies. Cancer Treat Rev. 13:113-127; 1986.

243. Zusman, J.; Brown, D.M.; Nesbit, M.E. Hyperphosphatemia, hyperphosphaturia, and hypocalcemia in acute lymphoblastic leukemia. N Engl J Med. 289:1335-1340; 1973.

Chronic and Other Lymphocytic Leukemias

244. Adler, S.; Stutzman, L.; Sokal, J.E.; et al. Splenectomy for hematologic depression in lymphocytic lymphoma and leukemia. Cancer. 35:521-528; 1975.

245. Aisenberg, A.C.; Wilkes, B. Lymphosarcoma cell leukemia: the contribution of cell surface study to diagnosis. Blood. 48:707-715; 1976.

246. Armitage, J.O.; Dick, F.R.; Cooper, M.P. Diffuse histiocytic lymphoma complicating chronic lymphocytic leukemia. Cancer. 41:2360-2372; 1978.

247. Bearman, R.M.; Pangalis, G.A.; Rappaport, H. Prolymphocytic leukemia. Cancer. 42:2360-2372; 1978.

247a. Bennett, J.; Rubin, P.; Begg, C.; Zagars, G. Comparison of the response and toxicity of total body irradiation vs chlorambucil and prednisone for remission induction of chronic lymphocytic leukemia (active): An ECOG study. Int J Radiat Oncol Biol Phys. 6:1351-1352; 1980.

248. Bentwich, Z.; Kunkel, H.G. Specific properties of B and T lymphocytes and alterations in disease. Transplant Rev. 16:29-50; 1973.

249. Bergsagel, D.E. The chronic leukemias. Cancer Med Assoc J. 96:1615-1620; 1967.

250. Boggs, D.R.; Sofferman, S.A.; Wintrobe, M.M.; et al. Factors influencing the duration of survival of patients with chronic lymphocytic leukemia. Am J Med. 40:243-254; 1966.

251. Brody, J.I.; Beizer, L.H. Immunologic incompetence of the neoplastic lymphocyte in chronic lymphocytic leukemia. Ann Intern Med. 64:1237-1245; 1966.

252. Brouet, J-C.; Flandrin, G.; Sasportes, M.; et al. Chronic lymphocytic leukemia of T-cell origin. Lancet. ii:890-893;1975.

253. Brouet, J-C.; Preud'Homme, J.L.; Seligmann, M.; et al. Blast cells with monoclonal surface immunoglobulin in 2 cases of acute blast crises supeNening on chronic lymphocytic leukemia. Br Med J. 4:23-24; 1973.

254. Brouet, J-C; Preud'Homme, J.L.; Seligmann, M. The use of B and T membrane markers in the classification of human leukemias with special reference to acute lymphoblastic leukemia. Blood Cells. 1:81-90; 1975.

255. Byhardt, R.W.; Brace, K.C.; Wiernik, P.H. The role of splenic irradiation in chronic lymphocytic leukemia. Cancer. 35 :1621-1625; 1975.

256. Carey, R.W.; McGinnis, A.; Jacobson, B.M.; et al. Idiopathic thrombocytopenic purpurla complicating chronic lymphocytic leukemia. Arch Intern Med. 136:62-66; 1976.

256a. Cassileth, P.A.; Cheuvart, G.; Spiers, A.S.; et al. Pentostatin induces durable remissions in hairy cell leukemia. J Clin Oncol 9(2):243-246; 1991.

257. Chanana, A.D.; Cronkite, E.P.; Rai, K.R. The role of extracorporeal irradiation of blood in the treatment of leukemia. Int J Radiat Oncol Biol Phys. 1:539-548; 1976.

258. Chandra, P.; Chanana, A.D.; Chikkappa, G.; et al. Chronic lymphocytic leukemia: concepts and observations. Blood Cells. 3:637-649; 1977.

259. Cherchi, M.; Catovsky, D. Mouse RBC rosettes in CLL: different expression in blood and tissues. Clin Exp Immunol. 39:411-415; 1980.

260. Cheson, B.D.; Martin, A. Clinical trials in hairy cell leukemia; current studies and future directions. Ann Intern Med. 106:871-878; 1987.

261. Christensen, B.E; Hansen, M.M.; Videbaek, A.A. Splenectomy in chronic lymphocytic leukemia. Scand J Hematol. 18:279-287;1977.

261a. Chun, H.G.; Leyland Jones, B.; Cheson, B.D. Fludarabine phosphate: A synthetic murine antimetabolite with significant activity against lymphoid malignancies. J. Clin. Oncol. 9:175-188; 1991.

262. Clark, C.; Rydell, R.E.; Kaplan, M.E. Frequent association of IgM with chrystalline inclusions in chronic lymphatic leukemic lymphocytes. N Engl J Med. 289:113-117; 1973.

263. Cooper, I.A.; Ding, J.C.; Adams, P.B.; et al. Intensive leukapheresis in the management of cytopenias in patients with chronic lymphocytic leukemia (CLL) and lymphocytic lymphoma. Am J Hematol. 6:387-398; 1979.

264. Douglas, S.D.; Cohnen. G.; Konig, E.; et al. Lymphocyte lysosomes and lysosomal enzymes in chronic lymphocytic leukemia. Blood. 41:511-518; 1973.

265. Ebbe, S.; Wittels, B.; Dameshek, W. Autoimmune thrombocyto-

penic purpura (ITP type) with chronic lymphocytic leukemia. Blood. 19:23-37; 1962.

266. Fiddes, P.; Penny, R.; Wells, J.V.; *et al.* Clinical correlations with immunoglobulin levels in chronic lymphatic leukemia. Aust N Z J Med. 4:346-350; 1972.

267. Fitzgerald, P.H.; Hamer, J.W. Third case of chronic lymphocytic leukemia in a carrier of the inherited Ch1 chromosome. Br Med J. 3:752-754; 1969.

268. Fraumeni, J.F.; Vogel, C.L.; DeVita, V.T. Familial chronic lymphocytic leukemia. Ann Intern Med. 71:279-284; 1969.

268a. French Cooperative Group on Chronic Lymphocytic Leukemia: A randomized clinical trial of chlorambucil versus COP in stage B chronic lymphocytic leukemia. Blood 75(7):1422-1425; 1990.

268b. French Cooperative Group on Chronic Lymphocytic Leukemia: Effects of chlorambucil and therapeutic decision in initial forms of chronic lymphocytic leukemia (stage A): Results of a randomized clinical trial on 612 patients. Blood 75(7):1414-1421; 1990.

269. Frenkel, E.P.; Ligler, F.S.; Graham, M.S.; *et al.* Acute lymphocytic leukemia transformation of chronic lymphocytic leukemia. Am J Hematol. 10:391-398; 1981.

270. Galton, D.A.G.; Goldman, J.M.; Wiltshaw, E.; *et al.* Prolymphocytic leukemia. Br J Haematol. 27:7-23; 1974.

271. Grever, M.R.; Leyby, J.M.; Kraut, E.H.; *et al.* Low dose deoxycoformycin in lymphoid malignancy. J Clin Oncol. 3:(9)1196-1201;1985.

272. Golde, D.W. Therapy of hairy cell leukemia. N Engl J Med. 307:495-496; 1982.

273. Golomb, H.M. The treatment of hairy cell leukemia. Blood. 69:979;1987.

273a. Golomb, H.M.; Catovsky, D.; Golde, D.W. Hairy cell leukemia. Ann Intern Med. 89:677-683; 1978.

273b. Golomb, H.M.; Fefer, A.; Colde, I.W.; *et al.* Sequential evaluation of alpha-2b interferon treatment in 128 patients with hairy cell leukemia. Semin Oncol. 14(suppl 2):13;1987.

273c. Golomb, H.M.; Vardiman, J.W. Response to splenectomy in 65 patients with hairy cell leukemia: an evaluation of spleen weight and bone marrow involvement. Blood. 61:349;1983.

274. Han, T.; Erdinli, E.Z.; Shimaoka, K.; *et al.* Chlorambucil vs. combined chlorambucil-corticosteroid therapy in chronic lymphocytic leukemia. Cancer. 31:502-508; 1973.

275. Hoppe, R.T.; Fuks, Z.; Bagshaw, M.A. Radiation therapy in the management of cutaneous T-cell lymphomas. Cancer Treat Rep. 63:625-632; 1979.

276. Jacobs, A.D.; Champlin, R.E.; Golde, W. Recombinant alpha-2 interferon for hairy cell leukemia. Blood. 65:1017-1020;1985.

277. Johnson, R.E. Total body irradiation of chronic lymphocytic leukemia: incidence and duration of remission. Cancer. 25:523-531; 1970.

278. John, R.E.; Ruhl, U. Treatment of chronic lymphocytic leukemia with emphasis on total body irradiation. Intl J Radiat Oncol Biol Phys. 1:387-397; 1976.

279. Junior, V.M.; Catovsky, D.; Galton, D.A.G. The relationship between chronic lymphocytic leukemia and prolymphocytic leukemia: 1. Clinical and laboratory features of 300 patients and characterization of an intermediate group. Br J Haematol. 63:377-387; 1986.

280. Junior, V.M.; Catovsky, D.; Gregory, W.M.; *et al.* Relationship between chronic lymphocytic leukemia and prolymphocytic leukemia: 4. Analysis of survival and prognostic features. Br J Haematol. 65:23-29;1987.

280a. Kantarjian, H.M.; Schnachner, J.; Keating, M.J. Fludarabine therapy in hairy cell leukemia. Cancer 67(5):1291-1293; 1991.

281. Katayama, L.; Li, C.Y.; Yam, L.T. Ultrastructural cytochemical demonstration of tartrate-resistant acid phosphatase isoenzyme activity in "hairy cells" of leukemic reticuloendotheliosis. Am J Pathol. 69:471-477; 1972.

281a. Keating, M.J.; Kantarjian, H.; Talpaz, M. *et al.* Fludarabine: A new agent with major activity against chronic lymphocytic leukaemia. Blood 74:19-25; 1989.

282. Keating, M.J.; Kantarjian, H.; Talpaz, M.; *et al.* Fludaradine-results of therapy in previously treated and untreated chronic lymphocytic leukemia. Blood. 72(5):207a; 1988. Abstract.

282a. Kraut, E.H.; Bournocle, B.A.; Grever, M.R. Low-dose deoxycoformycin in the treatment of hairy cell leukemia. Blood. 68:1119; 1986.

283. Kyle, R.A.; Maldonado, J.E.; Bayard, E.D. Plasma cell leukemia. Arch Intern Med. 133:813-818; 1974.

284. Lagos, M.D.; Friedlander, L.M.; Wallerstein, R.O.; *et al.* Atypical azurophilic crystals in chronic lymphocytic leukemia. Am J Clin Pathol. 62:342-349; 1974.

284a. Leong, A.S.Y.; Forbes, I.J.; Cowled, P.A.; *et al.* Surface marker studies in chronic lymphocytic leukemia and non-Hodgkin's lymphoma. Pathology. 11:461-471; 1979.

285. Long, J.C.; Aisenberg, A.C. Richter's syndrome. Am J Clin Pathol. 63:786795; 1975.

286. Lutzner, M.; Edelson, R.; Schein, P.; *et al.* Cutaneous T-cell lymphomas: the Sezary syndrome. Mycosis fungoides, and related disorders. Ann Intern Med. 83:534-552; 1975.

287. Miller, D.G.; Diamond, H.D.; Cravner, L.F. The clinical use of chlorambucil. N Engl J Med. 261:525-535; 1959.

288. Minna, J.D.; Roenigk, H.H.; Glatstein, E. Report of the committee on therapy for mycosis fungoides and Sezary syndrome. Cancer Treat Rep. 63:729-736; 1979.

289. Mittleman, A.; Lichtman, S.; Budman, D.; *et al.* Therapy of chronic lymphocytic leukemia (CLL) with fludaradine phosphate. Blood. 72:(5)250a; 1988. Abstract.

290. Morse, B.N.; Shattil, S.J. Metabolic complications of aggressive therapy of chronic lymphocytic leukemia. Am J Med Sci. 267:311-313; 1974.

291. Naido, J.M.; Norton, W.L. Chronic lymphocytosis with lymphocyte inclusions. Ann Intern Med. 76:265-268; 1972.

292. Nair, K.G.; Han, T.; Minowada, J. T-cell chronic lymphocytic leukemia. Cancer. 44:1652-1655; 1979.

293. O'Dwyer, P.J.; Spiers, A.S.D.; Marsoni, S. Association of severe and fatal infection and treatment with pentostatin. Cancer Treat Rep. 70:(9)1117-1120; 1986.

294. O'Dwyer, P.J.; Wagner, B; Legland-Jones, B.; *et al.* 2-deoxycoformycin (pentostatin) for lymphoid malignancies. Ann Intern Med. 108:(5)733-743;1988.

295. Oken, M.M.; Kaplan, M.E. Combination chemotherapy with cyclophosphamide; vincristine, and prednisone in the treatment of refractory chronic lymphocytic leukemia. Cancer Treat Rep. 63:441-447; 1979.

296. Pirofsky, B. Autoimmune hemolytic anemia and neoplasia of the reticuloendothelium. Ann Intern Med. 68 :109-119; 1968.

297. Prchal, J.T.; Lucuvero, G.; Carroll, A.I.; *et al.* A study of a patient with CLL which demonstrates that proliferation of the lymphocytic clone in CLL does not include T-lymphocyte. Clin Immunol Immunopathol. 13:231-236; 1979.

298. Quesada, J.R.; Hersh, E.M.; Manning; J.; *et al.* Treatment of hairy cell leukemia with recombinant alpha interferon. Blood. 68:493-496;1986.

299. Rai, K.R.; Sawitsky, A.; Cronkite, E.P.; *et al.* Clinical staging of chronic lymphocytic leukemia. Blood. 46:219-234; 1975.

300. Ratain, M.J.; Golomb, H.M.; Vardiman, J.W.; *et al.* Treatment of hairy cell leukemia with recombinant alpha 2 interferon. Blood. 65:644-648; 1985.

301. Richards, F.; Spurr, C.L.; Pajak, T.F.; *et al.* Thymic irradiation: an approach to chronic lymphocytic leukemia. Am J Med. 57:862-869; 1974.

302. Rubin, A.D.; Havemann, K.; Dameshek, W. Studies on chronic lymphocytic leukemia: further studies of the proliferative abnormality of the blood lymphocyte. Blood. 33:313-328; 1969.

302a. Rubin, P.; Bennett, J.M.; Begg, C. *et al.* The comparison of total body irradiation vs chloramucil and prednisone for remission induction of active chronic lymphocyte leukemia: An ECOG study. Part I: Total body irradiation: Response and toxicity. Int J Radiat Oncol Biol. 7(12):1623-1632; 1981.

303. Sawitsky, A.; Rai, K.R.; Glidewell, O.; *et al.* Cancer and leukemia group B: comparison of daily vs. intermittent chlorambucil and prednisone therapy in chronic lymphocytic leukemia. Blood. 50:1049-1059; 1970.

304. Scamps, K.A.; Streeter, A.M.; O'Neill, B.J. Immunoglobulin levels in chronic lymphocytic leukemia. Med J Aust. 1:535-536; 1971.

305. Schnitzer, B.; Loesel, L.S.; Reed, R.E. Lymphosarcoma cell leukemia. Cancer. 26:1082-1096; 1970.

306. Schmacher, H.R.; Maugel, T.K.; Davis, K.D. The lymphocyte of chronic lymphatic leukemia. I. Electron microscopy. Cancer. 26:895-903; 1970.

307. Silver, R.T. Treatment of chronic lymphocytic leukemia. Semin Hematol. 6:344-356; 1969.

308. Smith, M.J.; Browner, F.; Slungaard, A. The impaired responsiveness of chronic lymphatic leukemia lymphocytes to allogeneic lymphocytes. Blood. 41:505-509; 1973.

309. Spiers, A.S.D.; Moore, D.; Cassileth, P.A.; et al. Hairy cell leukemia: complete remission with pentostatin (2'deoxycoformycin). N Engl J Med. 316:825;1987.

310. Spiers, A.S.D.; Moore, D.; Cassileth, P.A. Remission in hairy cell leukemia with pentostatin (two-deoxycoformycin). N Engl J Med. 316(14):825-830; 1987.

311. Turner, A.; Kjeldsberg, C.R. Hairy cell leukemia: a review. Medicine. 57:477-499; 1978.

312. Uchiyama, T.; Yodoi, J; Sagawa, K.; et al. Adult T-cell leukemia. Blood. 50:481-492; 1977.

313. Van-Scoy-Mosher, M.B.; Bick, M.; Capostagno, V. A clinicopathologic analysis of chronic lymphocytic leukemia. Am J Hematol. 10:9-18; 1981.

314. Vilpo, J.A.; Klemi, P.; Lassila, O.; et al. Concomitant presentation of 2 chronic leukemias. Am J Hematol. 8:206-211; 1980.

314a. Weeks, J.C.; Tierney, M.R.; Weinstein, M.C. Cost effectiveness of prophylactic intravenous immune globulin in chronic lymphocytic leukemia. N Engl J Med 325(2):81-86; 1991.

314b. Wiernik, P.H.; Schwartz, B.; Dutcher, J.P.; Turman, N.; Adinolfi, C. Successful treatment of hairy cell leukemia with b-ser Interferon. Am. J. Hematol. 33:244-248; 1990.

315 . Wilson, J.D.; Nossal, G.J.V. Identification of human T and B lymphocytes in normal peripheral blood and in chronic lymphocytic leukemia. Lancet. ii:788-791; 1971.

316. Zacharski, L.R.; Linman, J. Chronic lymphocytic leukemia vs. chronic lymphosarcoma cell leukemia. Am J Med. 47:75-81; 1969.

317. Zarabbi, M.H.; Grunwald, H.W.; Rosener, F: Chronic lymphocytic leukemia terminating in acute leukemia. Arch Intern Med. 137:1059-1064; 1977.

318. Zawadzki, A.; Kapadia, S.; Bames, A.E. Leukemic myelomatosis (plasma cell leukemia). Am J Clin Pathol. 70:605-611; 1978.

319. Zucker-Franklin, D. Thymus-dependent lymphocytes in lymphoproliferative disorders of the skin (Sezary syndrome and mycosis fungoides). J Invest Dermatol. 67:412-418; 1976.

Randy N. Rosier, M.D., Ph.D., Orthopedic Oncology
Louis S. Constine III, M.D., Radiation Oncology

Chapter 25

SOFT TISSUE SARCOMA

For extreme diseases, extreme methods of cure.

Hippocrates (45)

PERSPECTIVE

Soft tissue sarcomas are a class of malignant tumors arising largely, though not exclusively, from mesenchymal connective tissues. Their distinction from carcinomas is based on their origin from connective rather than epithelial tissues. Some types of epithelium, however, arise from the mesoderm and tumors derived from these tissues are also considered to be sarcomas. Consequently, tumors classified as sarcomas are characterized by a common morphology and clinical behavior, and, as such, are dealt with as a group, as well as individually. Metastases tend to appear late and most commonly are pulmonary, although bone and lymphatic metastases also occur (3,5).

Soft tissue sarcomas are uncommon neoplasms that represent approximately 1% of all malignancies in men and 0.6% in women (68). Perhaps because of their rarity and tendency to evolve with few significant early symptoms, they often are observed too long and treated inadequately. Suspicious soft tissue masses should be biopsied immediately, especially if they have recently changed in size, or if they have become symptomatic.

Sarcomas typically grow centrifugally, at least initially, and induce a pseudoencapsule with a poorly defined zone of reactive tissue. It is clear that sarcomas require a therapeutic approach that establishes local control and thereby eliminates the potential of metastasis for patients with truly limited disease. Localized sarcomas are generally treated by surgery. Excision must be complete, with a wide margin of normal tissue, and along anatomic planes, or recurrence will almost certainly follow. Amputations are still occasionally required, although limb salvage procedures are being used increasingly, particularly in the context of multimodality therapy with irradiation and/or chemotherapy. Previously reported recurrence rates following surgery alone were high, ranging from 33-77% in different series (68). However, more recent reports indicate recurrence rates as low as 5% (24). Five-year survival after primary excision is approximately 60% and falls to 30% if re-excision of the sarcoma is required (68). Resection of recurrent lesions and even of solitary metastases is worthwhile and has resulted in long-term cures. Radiotherapy can be highly effective for improving local control and is used as adjuvant therapy, either preoperatively or postoperatively (59). Use of adjuvant irradiation allows for more conservative surgery without compromising local control, and therefore often may allow limb salvage where amputation might otherwise be necessary. Chemotherapy is still being evaluated for efficacy in eliminating micrometastatic disease. Both are occasionally palliatively for advanced, symptomatic, and incurable tumors.

EPIDEMIOLOGY AND ETIOLOGY

Epidemiology (89)

1. The sarcoma is a rare tumor, comprising 0.7% of all cancers, and has an annual age-adjusted incidence rate of two per 100,000. In the United States there are 5,600 new cases and 1,600 deaths from this cancer reported annually. It is more common in children than in adults, constituting 6.5% of all tumors, and ranking fifth as a cause of death in the age group below aged 15 years (88).
2. The relative incidence of the different varieties of sarcoma indicates that liposarcomas, rhabdomyosarcomas, fibrosarcomas, and synovial sarcomas are the most common types, along with the unclassified sarcomas. The diagnosis of malignant fibrous histiocytoma is appearing with increasing frequency in more recent literature, and many lesions previously classified as fibrosarcomas or undifferentiated spindle cell sarcomas are now classified in this category (61).

Etiology

1. The etiology of soft tissue sarcoma is unknown. Although sarcomas occasionally have developed in old scars, trauma has never been proven as a cause. Intensive irradiation for benign conditions, such as tuberculosis of the skin or thyroid disease, has given rise to fibrosarcomas.
2. Post-irradiation sarcomas also occur following high-dose treatment for other types of cancer, generally with a latent period from 5 to 15 years (66).
3. Long-standing lymphedema has been followed by lymphangiosarcomas, especially after radical mastectomy. Patients with von Recklinghausen's disease occasionally develop neurofibrosarcomas or malignant schwannomas.

Biology

1. *Genetics*: A variety of genetically linked diseases, such as multiple neurofibromatosis, tuberous sclerosis, Werner's

syndrome, intestinal polyposis and Gardner's syndrome, and basal cell nevus syndrome have been associated with soft tissue sarcomas (35,36,52,77).

2. *Tumor markers*: All of these tumors produce reticulin. Some immunohistochemical techniques also are useful for demonstration of specific marker proteins such as vimentin (characteristic of sarcomas) and S-100 protein (a marker for tumors of histiocytic and neural origin, [99]).

DETECTION AND DIAGNOSIS

Clinical Detection (Table 25-1) (41)

Local signs in typical presentations: Most sarcomas become evident as soft tissue masses that grow, become symptomatic, and often develop a hard consistency. Peripheral neuralgia, paralysis, or edema can occur because of pressure on nerves or vascular supply. Restriction of joint motion or an effusion can develop in an adjacent joint. Night pain may occur with larger lesions. The tumors also may interfere with visceral functions and may obstruct bowel, ureters, or mediastinal structures. Relatively rapid growth, fixation of a mass to subcutaneous tissue or skin, or underlying fascia or muscle, and presence of warmth or a distended local venous pattern are all clinical indications of a malignant lesion. Table 25-1 lists the common soft tissue sarcomas by age, sex, site, size, histologic pattern of growth, grade, stage, and 5-year survival.

Systemic effects: In addition to weight loss, fever, and general malaise, some sarcomas cause severe episodic hypoglycemia. Other endocrine disorders, including goiter or pituitary dysfunction, may also occur. Sarcomas that cause these paraneoplastic syndromes are generally large and retroperitoneal or extrapleural. Most are fibrosarcomas, but a variety of other histologic types have been reported (14). In general, systemic symptoms are unusual with extremity sarcomas.

Early detection: A high index of suspicion is invaluable. All unexplained soft tumor masses require early incisional or excisional biopsy. These tumors grow insidiously, are often in inaccessible sites, and have poor encapsulation. Additionally, most sarcomas are not painful at presentation.

Diagnostic Procedures

Radiographic studies (Table 25-2) (14a): There is a large variety of imaging modalities available. These are listed and their diagnostic and staging capability is briefly discussed.

1. Soft tissue techniques: Since most sarcomas are not apparent on inspection and palpation, radiography, including contrast studies or soft tissue techniques, may be required to demonstrate occult lesions in the retroperitoneal space or within large tissue masses. Soft tissue films may demonstrate the decreased radiodensity of liposarcomas or the fine stippled calcification of synovial sarcomas.

2. Computed tomography (CT): CT scans are invaluable for diagnosis and staging, and are widely used when the diagnosis is first considered. The ability of this technique to differentiate normal and abnormal tissue is not as good as magnetic resonance imaging (MRI), however.

3. Arteriograms may show characteristic irregular, bizarre capillaries, puddling, flush, or arteriovenous communi-

cation. Arteriography may be particularly useful in delineating the extent of these tumors, especially within the body cavities or in large muscle masses.

4. MRI: This modality has largely replaced CT scanning and arteriography in anatomic localization of soft tissue sarcomas. The relationship of the tumor to vessels, nerves, tendons, muscles and other structures can be delineated with a high degree of accuracy. Enhancing agents such as gadolinium can be used to gain even higher contrast between normal and abnormal tissues. However, while MRI enables unprecedented assessment of the anatomic extent of tumors, it has not been very successful in differentiating benign or infectious lesions from malignancies.

Biopsy: Any soft tissue mass suspicious for sarcoma should be biopsied at once. Because the mode of therapy is determined in large part by the histology of the tumor, ample tissue must be delivered to the pathologist. Pathologists experienced with needle biopsy and cytologic interpretation can diagnose these tumors with a minimally invasive needle biopsy. This is particularly true of high-grade lesions, and may obviate the need for a diagnostic surgical procedure and reduce the contamination of local tissue planes by the dissection and hematoma which may result from surgical biopsy. Diagnostic accuracy of 90% or better has been obtained with this technique (53,75). The needle tract should always be marked for later surgical removal with the tumor. In some cases such as low-grade or intermediate lesions, however, or lesions with extensive necrosis, inadequate tissue for definitive diagnosis may be obtained with needle biopsy. In these cases, incisional biopsy is necessary. Thoughtful consideration must be given to the incision used for biopsy, so that it will be removed during the en bloc dissection, and so that it will not interfere with the design of the needed flaps. In general, biopsy incisions on the extremities should always be longitudinal, and planes near major neurovascular structures should be strictly avoided so that any contaminated tissues can be removed at subsequent definitive surgery. As few compartments as possible should be violated during the biopsy procedure. Meticulous hemostasis always should be obtained to minimize postoperative hematoma formation, and if needed, a drain can be used as long placed near the incision and in line with it to facilitate subsequent excision of the drain tract with the biopsy incision. Frozen section at the time of biopsy helps to assure that adequate tissue has been obtained for definitive diagnosis.

Radioisotope studies: Radioisotope studies with gallium may help to localize the soft tissue mass, but rarely add information not obtained by other means. On the other hand, localized osseous uptake of technetium pyrophosphate is useful if bony invasion is suspected. Such a "hot" area, even in the presence of normal conventional radiographs, requires sacrifice of the involved bone (57a). Bone scans may also indicate presence of bony metastases, although this is unusual.

CLASSIFICATION AND STAGING (41)

Histopathology

According to the study of over 1,200 patients by a panel of pathologists led by Suit and Russell (93), the single most important factor in the outcome for soft tissue sarcoma

Table 25-1. Detection and Diagnosis of Soft Tissue Sarcoma

		Average Age	Sex Prevalence	Most Common Site	Most Common Presentation	Average Size (cm)	Histologic Pattern of Growth	Histologic Grade	Most Common Stage	Average 5-year Survival (%)
Malignant tumors of fibrous tissue	Malignant fibroblastic fibrous histiocytoma	45	Male	Trunk	Superficial	10	Arranged	Low	I	85
	Malignant histiocytic fibrous histiocytoma	50	Male	Knee	Deep	15	Epithelioid	--*	II	55
	Malignant pleomorphic fibrous histiocytoma	50	Male	Buttock and arm	Deep	5	Disarranged	--	III	50
	Desmoid tumor	25	Male	Arm and thigh	Deep	5	Spreading	Low	I	95
	Fibroblastic fibrosarcoma	45	Male	Thigh	Deep	10	Arranged	High	III	40
	Peleomorphic fibrosarcoma	50	Male	Thigh	Deep	15	Disarranged	High	III	35
Malignant tumors of tendosynovial tissue	Biphasic tendosynovial sarcoma	35	Male	Knee	Deep	10	Alveolar	--*	II	55
	Monophasic tendosynovial sarcoma	24	Male	Thigh	Deep	15	Spreading	High	III	30
	Epithelioid sarcoma	35	Male	Forearm	Superficial	2	Epithelioid	--	II	65
	Clear cell sarcoma	30	Male	Leg	Deep	5	Epithelioid	High	II	55
	Choroid sarcoma	40	Male	Hand	Deep	2	Lacy	Low	0	75
Malignant tumors of adipose tissue	Well-differentiated liposarcoma	55	Male	Trunk	--	5	Lacy	Low	I	95
	Myxoid liposarcoma	40	Male	Thigh	Deep	10	Lacy	Low	II	95
	Lipoblastic liposarcoma	45	Male	Thigh	Deep	10	Epithelioid	High	III	50
	Fibroblastic liposarcoma	45	Male	Thigh	Deep	10	Arranged	High	III	60
	Pleomorphic liposarcoma	55	Male	Thigh	Deep	20	Disarranged Spreading	High	III	45
Malignant tumors of muscle	Leiomyosarcoma	55	Female	Leg	--*	5	Epithelioid	--	II	60
	Leiomyoblastoma	50		--	Deep	5	Epithelioid	--	II	60
	Embryonal rhabdomyosarcoma	10	Female	Thigh	Deep	15	Epithelioid	High	III	65
	Rhabdomyosarcoma	20	Male	--	Deep	5	Disarranged	High	II	40
	Pleomorphic rhabdomyosarcoma	50	Male Male	Thigh	Deep	20		High	III	25
Malignant tumors of vessels	Hemangiosarcoma	45	Male	Trunk		5	Alveolar	High	III	30
	Hemangiopericytoma	40	Male	--	Deep	10	Alveolar	--	II	60
	Kaposi's sarcoma	55	Male	Leg	Superficial	2	Alveolar	Low	0	90
	Lymphangiosarcoma	50	Female	Arm	--	5	Alveolar	High	III	10
Malignant tumors of peripheral nerves	Malignant peripheral nerve tumor	40	Female	Thigh	Deep	15	Spreading	--	II	60
	Primitive neuroectodermal tumor	25	Male	Trunk	Deep	5	Epithelioid	High	III	30
Extraskeletal malignant bone tumors	Osteogenic sarcoma	50	Male	--*	Deep	15	Disarranged	High	III	15
	Chondrosarcoma	45	Male	Thigh	Deep	15	Lacy	--	II	60
	Ewing's sarcoma	20	Male	Thigh	Deep	5	Epithelioid	High	III	--
Miscellaneous malignant soft tissue tumors	Malignant granular cell tumor	45	Female	--	Superficial	5	Epithelioid	--	II	75
	Alveolar soft part sarcoma	35	Female	Thigh	Deep	15	Epithelioid	--	III	50
		--	--	Thigh	Deep	10	--	--	--	--
	Malignant lymphoma	20	Male	--	Deep	5	Epithelioid	High	III	5
		50	--	--	Deep	10	--	High	III	45
	Granulocytic sarcoma	45	--	--	Deep	10	--	--	--	--
	Plasmacytoma Malignant mesenchymoma	--	--	--	Deep	10	--	High	III	75
	Postirradiation sarcoma	--	--	--	Deep	--	--	High	--	--

* All blank spaces mean that no data are available.

From Hajdu (41), with permission.

Table 25-2. Imaging Modalities for Evaluation of Soft Tissue Sarcomas

METHOD	DIAGNOSIS AND STAGING CAPABILITY	RECOMMENDED FOR USE
Primary tumor and regional nodes		
CT	Useful to stage tumor locally for medullary and soft tissue extension as well as presence of matrix or cortical disruption	Yes; essential in planning limb conservation surgery and radiation portal shaping
MRI with gadolinium	Soft tissue extent. Main use with soft tissue rather than bone tumors.	Yes; essential in planning limb conservation surgery and radiation shaping fields
Conventional roentgeno-grams	High sensitivity and specificity for primary bone tumors: lower sensitivity and specificity for metastatic lesions in bone	Yes; metastases tend to involve medullary canal and must be > 1 cm to be detected
Angiography	Seldom useful except to serve as a vascular road map for surgery	No (yes, if considering limb salvage and clear margin from tumor not demonstrated by CT)
Metastatic evaluation		
Chest roent-genograms	Essential for all tumor types	Yes
CT of lungs	Use in high risk patient group where treatment decisions hinge upon presence or absence of lung metastases	Yes
Radionuclide bone scan	Essential to evaluate for presence of bone lesions	Yes

CT = computed tomography; MRI = magnetic resonance imaging.
Adapted from Bragg et al. (14a).

patients is the histologic grade of the primary tumor. There are currently two different classification and staging systems in use, the Musculoskeletal Tumor Society (MTS) Surgical Staging System and the American Joint Committee (AJC) (6,33) classification. Both of these systems stress histopathologic grade (G), rather than histopathologic types of sarcomas.

AJC	*MTS*
• G1 Well differentiated	• G1 Low-grade
• G2 Moderately differentiated	• G2 High-grade
• G3 Poorly differentiated	

Fig. 25-1 lists the common histopathologic types according to their grade on presentation.

Histopathologic Types

The grade of the sarcoma dominates the stage determination, not the anatomic extent of the tumor. Grade is based on, among other factors, the number of mitoses present, necrosis, degree of cellularity, nuclear pleomorphism, encapsulation, neovascularity, and vascular invasion. The presence of aneuploid nuclei and abnormal mitotic figures also indicates a higher-grade lesion. The degree of tumor invasion into surrounding normal tissues is also taken into consideration in grading.

Soft tissue sarcomas originate from primitive mesenchymal tissue that has the potential to develop into a large variety of stromal elements and connective tissues. The connective tissue component may resemble fibrous, adipose, or synovial tissue, smooth and striated muscle, and Schwann cells. The sarcomas are classified histologically and named according to the tissues they most resemble. Special staining, electron microscopy for ultrastructural features, and tissue cultures usually permit exact classification. Chromosome rearrangements and cytogenetic aberrations are of diagnostic value in establishing a definitive diagnosis in 25% of cases in which routine microscopy was in doubt as to tissue of origin of the

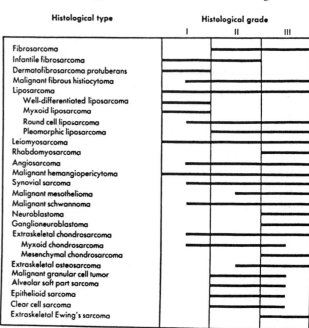

Fig. 25-1. Soft tissue sarcomas: Estimated range of degree of malignancy based on histologic type and grade. From Enzinger (3), with permission.

Table 25-3. Relative Incidence of Histologic Types of Soft Tissue Sarcomas

Type	Range of Incidence (%)	Average (%)
Unclassified	5.6-36.4*	11.2
Liposarcoma	11.5-33.9	19.2
Rhabdomyosarcoma	2.9-30.0	12.8
Synovialsarcoma	0.8-19.5	7.5
Neurofibrosarcoma	3.2-19.3*	5
Fibrosarcoma	3.6-44.0	22.6
Angiosarcoma	0.3-4.8*	1.6
Leiomyosarcoma	2.4-11.4*	4.9
Mesenchymoma	0.3-0.9*	0.1
Malignant fibrous histiocytoma	1.0-22.8*	8.5
Other	1.7-13.5*	6.3

*This "Range of Incidence" column is a composite of the incidence reported by several researchers. Total Number of cases: 4226. * signifies that at least one researcher found an incidence of 0%. In these cases the second lowest incidence reported is used in place of the lowest.
Adapted from Chang et al. (21b).

sarcoma (35a). The incidence according to histopathologic type is presented in Table 25-3 (21b) and the incidence of lesions to nodes according to tumor type is provided in Table 25-4 (102).

Anatomic Staging (Table 25-5, Fig. 25-2) (6)

Although the AJC staging system is more widely used by oncologists, orthopedic oncologists have favored the more recently introduced and simpler MTS (33) system because of its better predictive value and more direct relevance to the surgical aspects of treatment. Table 26-4 in "Bone Tumors" and Table 25-5 in this chapter present the features of the two staging systems. In the AJC system, the anatomic tumor (T) parameter depends on size or neurovascular invasion, whereas in the MTS system the parameter depends on whether the tumor is confined to a single compartment (T1) or involves more than one compartment (T2). The definition of compartments includes muscle groups bounded by a common fascial plane, bone, joint, skin and subcutaneous tissue, and major neurovascular structures. Nodal or other distant metastases are considered to be prognostically equivalent in the MTS system and define surgical stage III. The survival data of an interinstitutional analysis by the MTS as staged by the two systems demonstrates a clearer prognostic separation of the stages in the simpler MTS system (31). Regardless of the staging system used, a more advanced anatomic or histopathologic parameter and nodal or other metastases all correlate with a more advanced disease stage and consequently poorer prognosis. Lymph node metastases are unusual, but do occur with an increased incidence in certain histopathologic types of tumors such as synovial sarcomas, myxoid liposarcomas, and rhabdomyosarcomas (62,102).

Similarities of Staging Systems

The stage grouping is controlled by histopathologic grade of the sarcoma rather than anatomic extent of histopathologic type of sarcoma. The soft tissue sarcoma classification is relatively similar to previous editions with the major feature for T categories being size less (T1) or more (T2) than 5 cm. The node (N) category is simply absent (N0) or present (N1) and is an uncommon event for the group of malignancies. Surgical pathologic staging is critical because the grade and histopathology are essential elements, but clinical examination and imaging are also important.

Differences in Staging Systems

The major change is the elimination of T3, which indicates evidence of surrounding invasion into bone, major artery, or nerve. No reference or reason for this is given. The equivalence of N1 and metastases (M1) is another change. They are now clustered into the stage IV (A) and (B).

The soft tissue sarcoma grade is more important than histologic type in determining stage and prognosis. The anatomic extent is of secondary importance with a distinction only as to size independent of depth and compartmental invasion of bone or neurovascular structures. The presence of nodal involvement (N1) is equivalent to metastases and overrides grade in determining stage.

Table 25-4. Incidence of Lymph Node Metastases in Patients With Soft Tissue Sarcomas

Histology	No. Patients	Incidence of Lymph Node Metastases (%)
Liposarcoma	288	5.7
Fibrosarcoma	1083	5.1
Rhabdomyosarcoma	888	12.2
Synovial sarcoma	535	17.0
Unclassifiable	125	8.8
Neurofibrosarcoma	60	0.0

Adapted from Weingrad and Rosenberg (102).

Table 25-5. TNM Classification and Stage Grouping of Soft Tissue Sarcoma

TNM Classification		Stage Grouping				
T1	≤ 5 cm	Stage IA	G1	T1	N0	M0
T2	> 5 cm	Stage IB	G1	T2	N0	M0
		Stage IIA	G2	T1	N0	M0
N1	Regional	Stage IIB	G2	T2	N0	M0
		*Stage IIIA	G3-4	T1	N0	M0
G1	Well differentiated	*Stage IIIB	G3-4	T2	N0	M0
G2	Moderately differentiated	*Stage IVA	Any G	Any T	N1	M0
G3-4	Poorly differentiated/undifferentiated	Stage IVB	Any G	Any T	Any N	M1
* new category T = tumor; N = node; M = metastasis; G = grade. *From AJC (6), with permission.*						

Clinical radiographic evaluation of physical examination and imaging is less important than surgical pathologic assessment because tumor grade and histopathologic typing is key in this classification schema.

All of these tumors produce reticulin. Other helpful tumor markers in arriving at a specific diagnosis include vimentin and S-100 protein (99).

There are numerous pathologic classifications of soft tissue sarcomas. The commonly used systems differentiate between the soft tissue of origin and its malignant transformation.

In addition to benign varieties, there are borderline tumors that are locally invasive and have high recurrence rates. These tumors, however, such as desmoid tumors or aggressive fibromatosis, seldom metastasize. However, the treatment for such locally aggressive lesions is similar to that used for lower-grade sarcomas, and they are therefore treated as equivalent lesions. A typical system based on the putative cell of origin appears in Table 25-5.

Agreement among pathologists as to predominant cell type and grade is not as evident in the literature or in active practice, due to the great variation in subtypes of soft tissue sarcomas, as well as to the variable degree of expression of differentiated characteristics (76). In addition, reactive elements in the tissue, such as inflammatory cells and reactive fibrosis, can further complicate diagnosis. One of the factors in attempting to establish incidences of various types of sarcomas is the unclassifiable sarcoma. This diagnosis can account for from 5% to 35% of all patients, depending on the referenced series (Table 25-1). These differences may reflect the diagnostic criteria that the reporting pathologist uses.

Note that the classification of soft tissue sarcomas arbitrarily excludes growths associated with special organs, such as reticulum cell sarcomas or tumors of the alimentary tract, even though some of these tumors may arise from mesenchymal elements.

Staging Work-up

Recommended Procedures

Tumor extent must be assessed as precisely as possible to design therapeutic approaches accurately. The lesion must be carefully and gently palpated and measured, and regional draining lymphatic sites, though uncommonly involved, must carefully be evaluated. Careful neurologic and vascular examinations are necessary to assess any involvement of regional neurovascular structures. Pulmonary and abdominal examinations also may be important to rule out evidence of gross metastatic disease at presentation. Other useful tests, besides those generally ordered for routine admissions, include a variety of radiologic techniques.

1. CT scans (24,78) are much more useful than standard radiographs in delineating the extent of sarcomas and are strongly recommended, particularly if MRI is not available or feasible.

2. Arteriography is useful in all three phases. The early phase demonstrates the relationship to the large vessels; the midphase reveals the size of the tumor mass; and the late phase shows the major venous drainage that needs early control to limit embolization. Generally, arteriography is reserved for cases where a large bulky tumor may displace major vessels, such as intrapelvic lesions. Also, arteriography may permit preoperative embolization of lesions judged to be very vascular to decrease intraoperative blood loss.

3. MRI has become absolutely essential in the anatomic localization of the primary lesion (10,13). This modality is generally superior to CT scanning in all aspects of tumor imaging and the tumor's relationship to adjacent normal structures. In addition, subtle changes indica-

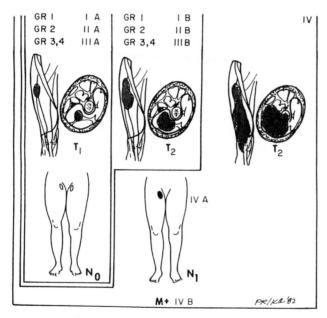

Fig. 25-2. Anatomic staging for soft tissue sarcoma. Adapted from AJC (6) (see Table 25-5).

tive of the reactive zone of the tumor, such as edema, can be better appreciated. MRI also assists the radiation oncologist in defining tissue planes and tumor compartmentalization for subsequent therapy (42). In most instances, MRI has replaced CT and arteriography. However, as previously mentioned, while MRI indicates the anatomic location and extent of the tumor precisely, its accuracy in differentiating benign from malignant lesions has been generally disappointing.

4. Radioisotope imaging of the bone with technetium-99 should be done if the sarcoma is close to the bone. Bone that is radiologically normal, may be hot by scan. However, a positive bone scan does not necessarily denote tumor invasion into bone, which is relatively uncommon, but may represent a periosteal reaction adjacent to the tumor. Nevertheless, tumor resection may require bone resection to meet the concept of an adequate radical resection. In addition, the bone scan can help rule out the presence of bone metastases, although these are quite unusual with soft tissue sarcomas.

5. Chest films to rule out pulmonary spread must be done routinely. Tomograms of both lungs have largely been supplanted by CT scans, which offer great accuracy in locating even small pulmonary metastases. In general, lung CT scanning should be carried out before surgery, as postoperative atelectasis can be misinterpreted as a false-positive scan. If sarcoma is not the anticipated diagnosis preoperatively and a chest CT is not done, waiting approximately 1 week after surgery generally allows any atelectasis to resolve prior to obtaining this study.

PRINCIPLES OF TREATMENT

General: Multidisciplinary Treatment Decisions

Optimal therapy for patients with ostensibly localized soft tissue sarcomas provides local control and eradicates micrometastatic disease, achieving these objectives with minimal functional disability (Table 25-6). While the ability to eliminate distant microscopic disease remains difficult, current strategies to obtain local control are effective, having evolved over the past 2 to 3 decades. In earlier years, patients were treated with local excisions of the tumor and its pseudocapsule. The high frequency of local recurrence caused surgeons to more aggressively excise tumors, often with

amputations. Although local control was thereby improved, functional and cosmetic deficits were substantial. As imaging modalities improved, and the efficacy of post-operative radiotherapy was confirmed, the potential for eliminating the primary tumor with less morbidity was provided. The addition of chemotherapy in some settings may further enhance the chance to cure patients. Thus, it is clear that a team approach to the treatment of patients with sarcomas is necessary.

Surgery (Table 25-7) (32a)

Resection of the primary: Soft tissue sarcomas usually spread by local extension along tissue planes, often far from palpable tumor. These tumors tend to respect anatomic boundaries, such as bony cortex or fascial planes, at least initially. They are among the most difficult tumors to control at their primary sites; they do not have a true capsule although they may appear at surgery to be encapsulated due to the compressed normal tissue and reactive inflammation and fibrosis around the lesion. This pseudocapsule, however, usually contains foci of malignant cells. Therefore these lesions must never be shelled out. Table 25-7 lists the surgical definitions of margins and associated surgical procedures. In general, wide or radical margins are mandated for high-grade lesions, while wide margins are adequate for lower-grade and smaller, more localized lesions. A radical margin encompasses all structures within every compartment involved by the tumor, while a wide margin encompasses the tumor, its reactive zone or pseudocapsule, and normal tissue in all directions around the lesion. With lesions confined to the skin and subcutaneous tissues, which are considered a single compartment, a radical resection is generally accepted as 5 cm in all directions around the lesion. Whether a wide or radical margin is used in a high-grade lesion may depend to some extent on whether the lesion is felt to be amenable to adjuvant therapy such as irradiation or chemotherapy, as well as the feasibility of obtaining a given margin in the context of preservation of vital structures such as major nerves or blood vessels. This is particularly true in areas such as the antecubital fossa, popliteal fossa, axilla, or inguinal areas, where separating fascial planes are absent (2,4)

Local recurrence rates in the past have been around 30% (68). This demonstrates that one out of every three tumors is inadequately excised. A local recurrence doubles the prob-

Table 25-6. Multidisciplinary Treatment Decisions: Soft Tissue Sarcomas   (3,4,73a,78,91a)

Stage	Surgery	Radiation Therapy		Chemotherapy
IA,B ($T_{1/2}$, G_1)	Conservative resection	If microresiduum, ART Postop 60 Gy		N R
IIA,B ($T_1 T_2$, G_2)	Conservative resection	ART Pre- or postop 50 or 60 Gy	and/or	SAC/MAC/IC II
IIIA,B (T_1, T_2, N_0, G_3)	Conservative resection	ART Pre- or postop 50 or 60-70 Gy	and/or	SAC/MAC/IC II
IVA (T_{any}, N_1, G_{any})	Amputation/ Lymphadenectomy	ART Pre- or postop 50 or 60-70 Gy PRT	and	SAC/MAC/IC II
B(T_{any}, N_{any}, $M+$, G_{any})	N R		and	MAC/IC II

RT = radiation therapy; ART = adjuvant; PRT = palliative; NR = not recommended; RCT = recommended chemotherapy; MAC = multiagent chemotherapy (investigational); SAC = single agent chemotherapy; IC II = investigational chemotherapy, phase I/II clinical trials.
PDQ: RCT - SAC = Adriamycin; MAC = Doxorubicin + Dacarbazine + Ifosfamide, or Adriamycin+ OTDTIC

Table 25-7. Surgical Procedures for Soft Tissue Extremity Sarcomas

Margin	How Margin Achieved		Plane of Dissection	Microscopic Appearance
	Limb-Salvage	Amputation		
Intracapsular	Intracapsular piecemeal excision	Intracapsular amputation	Within lesion	Tumor at margin
Marginal	Marginal en bloc excision	Marginal amputation	Within reactive zone-extracapsular	Reactive tissue ± microsatellites
Wide	Wide en bloc excision	Wide through-bone amputation	Beyond reactive zone through normal tissue within compartment	Normal tissue ± "skips"
Radical	Radical en bloc resection	Radical disarticulation	Normal tissue extracompartmental	Normal tissue

From Enneking (32a), with permission.

ability that the patient will die of the sarcoma. The Strong Memorial Hospital experience clearly shows that "performance of less than a radical operation in the hope of avoiding mutilation or loss of limb, accepts a high local recurrence rate and great risk that distant metastases will follow" (20). However, more recent studies involving use of aggressive surgery in conjunction with adjuvant radiation therapy and/or chemotherapy report substantially lower recurrence rates (28,50,81), which may approach 5%.

1. Treatment is determined by the tumor location and histology. If there is no evidence of distant spread, the excision must be wide or radical with frozen-section control to ensure total excision. The use of a tourniquet is strongly recommended for the resection of extremity sarcomas. This approach permits far more precise dissection with minimal blood loss and probably diminished tumor embolization. However, an elastic bandage should never be used to exsanguinate the limb as this may actually cause tumor embolization (32).

2. The excision of the sarcoma must be en bloc, through normal tissues on all sides and at least a 1 cm and preferably a 2 to 3 cm margin. There should be at least a 1 cm margin on all sides of the biopsy scar, and any needle biopsy tract or drain tract used for previous biopsy must be included with the resection. If adjuvant radiation therapy is a consideration, then the location of the scar should be oriented in anticipation of this treatment. Thus, for an extremity sarcoma, the scar should be vertical along the limb and lateral if possible, because the lymphatic drainage medially is generally richer. The resected specimen must include the entire musculoaponeurotic structures with contiguous neurovascular tissues, and, if possible, regional lymph nodes. Neurologic deficits resulting from resection of major nerves can often be managed effectively postoperatively with appropriate orthotic devices or braces, and if major blood vessels traverse the tumor or reactive zone in some cases they can be resected and grafts placed by a vascular surgeon. If skin and subcutaneous tissues are involved, they must be resected widely. Skin grafts are often needed to cover the defect, and for coverage of subcutaneous bones, free myocutaneous tissue transfers such as latissimus dorsi or rectus abdominus flaps can now be done. Any involved bone must be resected with a several centimeter margin, and skeletal continuity reestablished using bone grafts or allografts in conjunction with appropriate hardware for internal fixation. In cases involving resection of all or parts of joints, arthrodesis with segmental allografts or custom prosthetic joint replacements can be used. Of note is that radiotherapy can locally control unresected sarcomas in approximately 15% to 30% of patients, and thus is a consideration in selected settings (91).

3. Amputation of an involved limb may be indicated in the following cases:
   - the mass cannot be encompassed by wide excision, which would allow the use of adjuvant radiotherapy
   - surgery would leave a useless extremity without adequate vascular or neurologic supply
   - the mass is a recurrence of a previously excised primary tumor
   - soft tissue and skin defect following wide resection would be so large that soft tissue coverage over bones or joints is not feasible
   - tumor is impossible to palliate by medical measures because of bleeding, pain, or odor

   Amputations are subject to the same surgical definitions of margins as are other surgical resections. There is never any indication for an intralesional amputation, and even a marginal resection is a palliative procedure with high local recurrence risk. However, for a given tumor, either a wide or radical amputation may be appropriate. A wide level may preserve significantly more function with a prosthetic limb, and often will allow an acceptable recurrence risk if local adjuvant therapy can be used in conjunction with the surgical procedure. A radical amputation will by definition involve removal of the limb with inclusion of all bone to the next proximal joint and all muscle origins and insertions proximal to the tumor. For instance, a high-thigh amputation for a lesion in the distal thigh musculature or popliteal fossa would provide a wide margin, while a radical margin could be achieved only by a hip disarticulation.

4. Radical resections for sarcomas involving the trunk often require considerable ingenuity (60,82',86). Reference to the literature for such cases is essential.

5. Radical resection in an extremity frequently can be done without amputation, by complete compartmental resections (61a). Radical resection without amputation should not be undertaken without the realization by physician and patient that this approach requires a significantly longer rehabilitation time and more effort than amputation. Additionally the incidence of local complications such as skin sloughs and infection is fairly high in limb salvage procedures, and occasionally may lead to secondary amputation. This patient must also be apprised that intraoperative findings may force a change in plans and require amputation due to unresectability. This is now a relatively uncommon occurrence because the current use of bone scans and MRI precisely delineates tumor extent preoperatively.

Dissection of lymph nodes: Lymph node dissection generally is not indicated unless the lesion is contiguous to major node-bearing areas such as the axillary or inguinal areas, or adjacent regional nodes are clinically involved. Some advocate nodal dissection in those tumors with a higher propensity for lymphatic metastases, such as synovial sarcoma, rhabdomyosarcoma, myxoid liposarcoma, and epithelioid sarcoma. However, this is controversial due to lack of documented survival advantage and generally resection of only clinically involved nodes is the more accepted approach even with these tumors (37).

Resection of metastases: Solitary metastases should be removed. Solitary metastases in lung, for example, have a much better prognosis than do primary tumors of the lung (46). Such lesions have been excised with 5-year survival rates of up to 40% (12). The prognosis for survival improves with increasing time interval between initial therapy and the appearance of metastases (72).

Follow-up: The results of Simon et al. (88,89) provide an excellent review of the results attainable with appropriate radical surgery. Their local recurrence rate for all patients was 20%. Local recurrence is a function of location and size. Tumors in more central or relatively inaccessible sites such as pelvis, buttock, groin, and shoulder girdle recur more frequently than those in extremities (89). Once a tumor is greater than 10 cm in diameter, surgical removal may be problematic, depending on the anatomic location. Thirty-nine percent of the patients developed metastases, and three patients died of local recurrence without metastases. The probability of local recurrence diminished to zero 30 months after excision, and metastases occurred with a slowly decreasing frequency over the 48 months after surgery (31). This necessitates close periodic follow-up of patients after primary treatment. Assessment for local recurrence by clinical examination and MRI or CT scan should be done every 2 to 3 months for the first 2 years, and with decreasing frequency over the following 3 years. In cases where extensive metal implants have been used to allow limb salvage, CT scanning probably provides better imaging for follow-up studies, although both modalities are subject to artifact from the metal. Low-grade lesions probably should be followed for an even longer total period. Additionally, chest radiographs or CT scans should be performed with a similar frequency, to allow the option of early surgical treatment of pulmonary metastases, should these become apparent.

Radiation Therapy

The effective use of radiation therapy in the treatment of sarcomas was pioneered by Cade (17) during the 1940s and 1950s and Suit (93) at the M.D. Anderson Hospital in the 1960s (94). The objective of this work was to reduce the functional and cosmetic morbidity associated with radical surgical resection or amputation. The principles behind this approach are: (1) although radical surgery can provide local control, it often causes substantial disability (1); (2) conservative surgery alone is associated with a high frequency of local failure because of the presence of microscopic extension of tumor beyond palpable or radiographically demonstrable tumor; and (3) radiation therapy is capable of destroying tumor cells that constitute the microscopic extensions (95). Table 25-8 (91a) presents the results of the Massachusetts General Hospital series that demonstrate the efficacy of this approach. Radiation therapy is less effective when used as the sole treatment modality, but is used in selected patients who have inoperable tumors or advanced recurrent or metastatic disease. Local control in this setting is dependent primarily on the volume of the local tumor (97).

Techniques

1. Treatment volume: The tumor should be three-dimensionally defined by physical examination, imaging studies (including CT or, preferably, MRI), and clips if surgery is performed. The anatomic boundaries selected for irradiation are dependent on this information, the characteristics of the surgery, if performed,

Table 25-8. Local Control and Disease-Free Survival in 220 Patients With Soft Tissue Sarcoma Treated at Massachusetts General Hospital by Radiation and Surgery According to AJC Stage*

AJC Stage	No. of Patients	5-Year Actuarial Results	
		Local Control	Disease-free Survival
IA	17	1.00	1.00
IB	30	.93	.88
IIA	40	.88	.83
IIB	66	.85	.52
IIIA	33	.93	.87
IIIB	69	.79	.39
IVA	3	1.00	1.00
Total	258	.88	.66

*Excludes patients with distant metastases (stage IVB) and patients with sarcomas arising from thoracic, abdominal, pelvic, and retroperitoneal sites.

From Suit et al. (91a), with permission.

and the size and grade of the tumor. As previously described, sarcomas tend to spread along anatomic planes. In extremities, therefore, they generally grow longitudinally along fascial planes, and the deep margins are naturally limited, allowing a portion of the limb circumference to be spared from irradiation. In conjunction with a wide surgical resection, the volume chosen for irradiation traditionally has been the entire muscle compartment, as suggested by Simon *et al.* (89). However, if substantial surgical manipulation has been avoided, and extensive hematoma formation has not occurred, alternative guidelines can be considered: for histologic grade 1 sarcomas the proximal and distal margins are approximately 5 cm for small (< 5 cm) tumors and 10 cm for larger lesions; for histologic grade 3 tumors (high-grade lesions), the margins range from 7 to 14 cm for small and large tumors, respectively. Across the extremity, the margins are determined by suitable anatomic boundaries such as interosseus membranes and bones, or major fascial planes. Regional nodes generally are not treated unless determined by physical examination or radiographic studies to be involved with tumor (77,91b,98). This is uncommon, with an overall incidence of about 6% (0%, 2%, and 12% in histologic grade 1, 2, and 3 lesions, respectively, in a series by Mazeron and Suit [62]). However, for selected tumors with higher frequencies of nodal involvement such as synovial or epithelioid sarcomas, inclusion of regional clinically uninvolved nodes should be considered. If the surgical incision extends beyond the above-determined treatment volume, then the area to be irradiated is accordingly enlarged, although this is a matter of debate. Three-dimensional treatment planning should be used, resulting in complex field arrangements that often require wedges or tissue compensators. To effectively treat the designed volume, individualized, shaped blocks and excellent immobilization techniques are required.

2. Dose: When irradiation is combined with wide surgical resections, the total dose to the region of the tumor is usually in the range of 65 Gy. It is appropriate to shrink the field after 45 to 50 Gy to the initial volume, and at times two field reductions can be used. Recognition of sensitive structures (e.g., the Achilles tendon) or of areas at high risk for trauma (e.g., anterior surface of the tibia) should guide these field reductions. In the absence of a surgical resection, the total dose should be in the range of 70 to 80 Gy.

3. Beam Energy: Since soft tissue sarcomas usually involve superficial tissues, it is generally inappropriate to use energies greater than 6 MeV, and bolus is sometimes required. However, since the entire tumor volume is generally more than superficial, electron beams alone are usually inadequate; however, they can be used to chase scars that are extremely long or in treatment plans about the hands, feet, and face.

Strategies

1. Preoperative irradiation: This strategy has several potential advantages as well as disadvantages, but overall has been shown to be at least as effective as postoperative irradiation (11,77).

Advantages:
1. Patients who might have required amputation because of tumor abutting critical structures such as nerves or vessels may instead have a more conservative procedure. Although tumor regression is generally modest, it is nevertheless often sufficient to accomplish this goal. Histologic change is generally substantial. Additionally, the amount of preoperative tumor regression may allow some evaluation of tumor radiosensitivity.
2. Shrinkage of the tumor also may facilitate surgical resection by decreasing the vascularity and improving the delineation between the reactive zone and normal tissues.
3. Inactivation of malignant cells by irradiation may reduce the possibility of tumor embolization and implantation.
4. The lack of tissue hypoxia associated with postsurgical scarring allows maximal generation of free radicals and hence maximized effectiveness of the radiation dose delivered in terms of tumoricidal activity.
5. The volume of tissue requiring irradiation may be decreased because neither surgically manipulated tissues nor complicating factors (e.g., hematoma) are present.

Disadvantages:
1. Information from surgery regarding the exact extent of the tumor is not available. With CT and MRI imaging techniques, however, this is less of a problem than previously.
2. Difficulties with wound healing (dehiscence, infection, necrosis) are more likely in irradiated tissues, particularly in obese individuals and in certain locations such as the proximal thigh. Significant skin sloughs that ultimately result in the need for amputation occasionally occur (91b).
3. Theoretically the time between the initial period of irradiation and the boost dose (either following surgery or interstitially at the time of surgery) might decrease its efficacy; however, in practice this does not appear to be problematic.

Technique:
1. Using the previously stated guidelines for volume, machine energy, shielding etc., 50 Gy is administered in 5 weeks. After a 3-week rest, a conservative resection is performed, at which time 15 Gy is administered via an implant or after wound healing using teletherapy.
2. Postoperative irradiation: This approach is most commonly used because it involves immediate surgery providing an unirradiated histologic specimen and added information about tumor extent. Also, time is allowed for postoperative wound healing prior to initiation of radiotherapy, thus reducing wound complications. The technique and doses used are as previously stated.
3. Interstitial implantation: This technique, generally using iridium-192 or iodine-125, has been used as a primary treatment modality, or more commonly, in combination with external beam radiation therapy (88). Plastic tubes are generally sewn in place at the time of definitive surgery, and after loading of the catheters is accomplished a few days following the surgery. Detailed planning is necessary in this situation.
4. Intraoperative irradiation: This technique is under investigation and involves electron or orthovoltage irra-

diation of the tumor bed with 20 to 30 Gy in a single exposure, depending on the anatomic site, field size, and depth of penetration.

5. Irradiation alone: As previously stated, selected patients may be appropriate for this approach. Local control rates of 20% to 90% have been reported (90,97). Specifically, patients who are medically inoperable, have unresectable, inaccessible lesions, or recurrent or widely metastatic disease should be considered.

Chemotherapy

During the past decade, substantial advances have been made in the use of chemotherapy for soft tissue sarcomas in adults. Prior to the introduction of doxorubicin in the late 1960s, actinomycin D, cyclophosphamide, and vincristine were commonly used, either singly or in combination, with little clinical benefit for most patients (48). Treatment with doxorubicin increased response rates from 27% to 40%, but remissions were generally short-lived; the median survival was only 6 to 8 months (40). A recent report pooling 10-year results from three randomized cooperative group adjuvant studies (Eastern Cooperative Oncology Group (ECOG), Cancer and Leukemia Group B, and Southwest Oncology Group) of doxorubicin arm versus observation arm fail to show a difference between treatment groups with respect to survival (8a). There remains considerable controversy over the efficacy of adjuvant chemotherapy in adult soft tissue sarcoma. While fairly clear survival advantage has been demonstrated in some tumors such as malignant fibrous histiocytoma in bone (10), other randomized trials have suggested no benefit of chemotherapy when used in an adjuvant setting (15,30,58). A number of differing chemotherapeutic regimens currently are being used, but optimum regimens for specific tumors have not been firmly established (Tables 25-9 and 25-10) (21a,21b,102).

Doxorubicin and dacarbazine: In an attempt to improve results, doxorubicin was combined with other agents, the most effective being dacarbazine, an imidazole carboxamide derivative with alkylating properties. The rationale for this combination was:

- dacarbazine possesses antitumor activity against soft tissue sarcomas, with a response rate of 17%
- doxorubicin and dacarbazine are synergistic in animal tumors
- dose-limiting toxicities of each drug are less than additive, thereby allowing both drugs to be administered together in nearly full dosage
- doxorubicin and dacarbazine do not appear to be cross resistant. This combination has produced overall response rates from 42% to 47% of patients, with complete remissions (CRs) in 11%. More importantly, the survival of responding patients has increased to 15 months (35',105)

Four-drug program: CYVADIC yields responses in 50% of patients and CR in 17%. Median survival time for responders is 16 months (74,105). It is presently unclear whether CYVADIC is more effective than the doxorubicin/dacarbazine combination; the four-drug regimen is, however, more toxic. A large randomized study (716 patient) of the European Organization on Research and Treatment of Cancer (EORTC) Soft Tissue and Bone Sarcoma Group between CYVADIC versus doxorubicin (75 mgm/m²) versus doxoru-

Table 25-9. Response Rates According to Randomized Chemotherapy Trials for Soft Tissue Sarcoma

Regimen	% CR	% PR	Average
A	1-6	16-27	19
AD	3-14	18-44	28
ADCV	15-33	38-71	57
iM	2	18	
MAID	12	49	

A = doxorubicin ; AD = doxorubicin, dacarbazine;
ADCV = doxorubicin, dacarbazine,cisplatin,vincristine;
iM = ifosfamide methotrexate;
MAID = methotrexate,doxorubicin,ifosfamide,dacarbazine;
CR = complete response; RR = relapse rate.
Adapted from Chang et al. (21b) and Weingrad and Rosenbaum (102).

bicin + ifosfamide do not show any evidence of advantage to the combination versus single dose doxorubicin alone (82a). Despite this drawback, some patients have experienced long relapse-free remissions following intensive chemotherapy. An update of the M.D. Anderson experience (122 patients) favors CYVADIC over standard surgery and radiation therapy for local control, freedom from metastases and overall survival when the sarcoma is large (>10 cm) and high grade (G III) (i.e., 5- and 10-year local control rate of 89% and 81%, versus 68% for controls and 5- and 10-year overall survival of 72% and 58% versus 47% and 44%, respectively) (58a). The drugs methotrexate and cisplatin also possess antitumor activity; the introduction of additional active agents to these is clearly needed to continue building on these encouraging results (65a).

Some factors associated with poor responsiveness to chemotherapy and shortened survival time are (39):

- failure to respond to prior chemotherapy
- poor performance status
- significant weight loss
- large tumor burden
- primary lesions of the pelvis, trunk, and gastrointestinal tract (GI)
- metastatic involvement of liver, bone, and central nervous system (CNS)
- higher-grade tumors. Although all histologic subtypes show similar response rates to chemotherapy, higher-grade tumors are associated with a relatively poor prognosis
- Doxorubicin dose. This has been identified as an important factor, as patients who receive less than 50 mg/m² per course are less likely to achieve remissions (59).

Combined Modalities Approach

Limb salvage surgery: The efficacy of chemotherapy in advanced sarcomas has been well defined; its role in relatively early disease presently is unclear. For extremity sarcomas, drug administration by intra-arterial infusion (69), isolation-perfusion (63), or hyperthermic perfusion (54) has been combined with limb-sparing surgery and often with radiation therapy in an attempt to avoid amputation without increasing the risk of local recurrence (29). Such drugs as phenylalanine

Table 25-10. Randomized Chemotherapy Trials For Soft-Tissue Sarcoma

Group	Regimen	No. Patient	% CR	% RR	Comments
Studies Comparing the Addition of Dacarbazine					
GOG	A	80	6	16	Uterine sarcomas only
	AD	66	11	24	
ECOG	A	34	3	18	
	AD	32	3	44	Leiomyosarcomas only
ECOG	A q 3 wk	93	6	19	A 15 mg/m^2/wk
	A q wk	92	4	16	A 70 mg/m^2 q 3 wk
	AD	95	6	30	
SWOG	ACVD	221	14	52	
	ACVAd	224	12	40	
Studies Evaluating the Addition of Cyclophosphamide					
ECOG	A	66	6	27	A 70 mg/m^2
	ACV	70	4	19	A 50 mg/m^2
	CVAd	64	2	11	A 0 mg/m^2
SWOG	AD	79	14	32	
	ADC	95	13	35	
	ADAd	98	9	24	
GOG	A	50	1	19	
	AC	54	2	20	
Studies Evaluating Dose and Schedule					
SWOG	AD	135	7	19	Bolus
	AD	143	10	18	Continuous infusion
SWOG	ADCV	27	15	67	A 50 mg/m^2; C 500 mg/m^2
	ADCV	24	33	71	A 80 mg/m^2; C 800 mg/m^2
EORTC	ADCV	71	20	38	Full dose rate
	AD-CV	74	5	14	Half dose rate
Studies Evaluating Ifosfamide					
EORTC	I	68	3	18	5 g/m^2
	C	67	1	8	1.5 g/m^2

GOG = Gynecologic Oncology Group; ECOG = Eastern Cooperative Oncology Group; SWOG = Southwest Oncology Group; EORTC = European Organization for Research and Therapy of Cancer; A = doxorubicin; AD = doxorubicin/dacarbazine; ACVD = doxorubicin/cyclophosphamide/vincristine/dacarbazine; ACVAd = doxorubicin/cyclophosphamide/vincristine/actinomycin D; ADAd = doxorubicin/dacarbazine/actinomycin D; AC = doxorubicin/cyclophosphamide; ADCV = doxorubicin/dacarbazine/cyclophosphamide, vincristine; I = ifosfamide; CR = complete remission; RR = relapse rate.

mustard, nitrogen mustard, actinomycin D, and doxorubicin given intra-arterially may increase tumor responsiveness, but to date only isolation-perfusion has produced results similar to those achieved through postoperative irradiation (15% to 20% local recurrences) (54,57a,60,63); the isolation-perfusion approach has the potential to minimize systemic toxicity (25,43).

Chemotherapy, surgery, and irradiation: Impressive results have been obtained for multidisciplinary limb salvage using preoperative arterial doxorubicin (30 mg/d for 3 days) and radiation therapy (35 Gy in ten fractions, which is assumed to be equivalent to 48 Gy in 24 fractions). In a recent randomized study, Giuliano et al. (39) found no advantage between intravenous (IV) or intra-arterial (IA) route of administration, limb salvage was 100% verus 98%, respectively, with a median follow-up of 3 years. Surgery follows in 7 to 10 days with a radical en bloc resection of tumor with a 10 cm margin. Postoperative chemotherapy consists of vincristine and high-dose methotrexate and citrovorum rescue. Of 61 patients who had limb salvage, four had amputations because of major vessel, nerve, or bone involvement (103).

Adjuvant chemotherapy: Approximately 50% of patients already have micrometastatic disease at the time of diagnosis; therefore adjuvant chemotherapy is a conceptionally attrac-

tive approach. Preliminary data in two studies using historical and matched control groups suggest that survival is prolonged in patients treated with adjuvant therapy (8,70,79), but randomized, controlled trials failed to show any benefit for such patients (15,30,58). The proven effectiveness of combination chemotherapy in overt metastatic disease offers hope that adjuvant chemotherapy ultimately will prove beneficial in micrometastatic disease as well.

RESULTS AND PROGNOSIS

Results

1. *Surveillance, Epidemiology, and End Results Program Data*: The long-term 5- and 10-year observed survival rates for soft tissue sarcomas are 53% and 41%, respectively, with 89% of 5-year survivors reaching 10 years. In the pediatric age group, 5- and 10-year survival rates are somewhat better: 64% and 58%, respectively, with 90% of 5-year survivors reaching 10 years (98a).

2. *Survival by stage and histopathology* is detailed in Table 25-11 (36a). Survival rates are in the 40% to 55% range for the majority of common tumor types: fibrosarcomas, malignant fibrous histocytoma, liposarcoma, synovial sarcomas, and schwannomas. Stages I and II

Table 25-11. Five-year Survival Rates (%) By Histological Types and Stage

Histologic Type	All Stages		Stage I		Stage II		Stage III		Stage IV	
	No. of Cases	Rate	No. of Cases	Rate	No. of Cases	Rate	No. of Cases	Rate	No. of Cases	Rate
All types	1215	41	177	75	86	(55)	329	29	110	7
Fibrosarcoma	231	48	65	(73)	15	5/15	36	(43)	12	1/12
Malignant fibrohistiocytoma	128	46	15	11/13	29	(72)	45	(22)	7	1/7
Liposarcoma	221	55	57	(78)	18	10/17	48	(35)	13	0/12
Angiosarcoma	33	(24)	2	2/2	2	1/2	9	0/9	4	1/4
Synovial sarcoma	84	(43)	5	4/5	6	4/6	25	(16)	6	2/5
Rhabdomyosarcoma	234	23	1	0/1	0	0/0	97	(30)	35	0
Leiomyosarcoma	79	(32)	14	8/14	5	1/5	12	3/11	11	1/11
Malignant schwannoma	60	(45)	11	8/10	7	2/7	7	1/6	1	0/1
Unclassified	121	36	4	4/4	4	2/4	41	(31)	18	0/17

From Frederick et al. (36a), with permission.

resectable tumors do much better than advanced unresectable tumors.

3. *Survival by histopathologic grade* : According to Suit *et al.* (95) the tumor grade more than pathologic type determines anatomic staging. Thus metastases-free survival rates for all tumor types are 75% for grade I; 71% for grade II; and 41% for grade III.

4. *Surgery alone*: Simon *et al.* (89) definition of local recurrence rates is:
   * 100% following incisional biopsy
   * 805 to 100% following excisional biopsy
   * 50% following wide excision
   * 10% to 20% following radical resection
   * 5% following amputation

   Although *radical surgery* can achieve 80% local control rates with less radical procedures than amputations, rates tend to range closer to 50%, particularly with truncal or inaccessible sites, such as pelvis and head and neck (92,89).

5. *Radiation therapy*: (Table 25-12)
   a. *Preoperative irradiation:* This is currently preferred for larger lesions by Suit *et al.* (91b). Their Massachusetts General Hospital results are impressive, although the series is small. With doses of 50 Gy in 5 to 6 weeks, 24 of 25 patients were controlled. McNeer *et al.* report a 57% 5-year survival through either preoperative or postoperative irradiation (64).

   b. *Postoperative irradiation* (Table 25-12): Postoperative irradiation to dose levels of 63 to 70 Gy after local resection has achieved local control in 88% of patients (50,64). Of lesions in elbow-hand, knee-foot regions, 100% (46 of 46) local control has been achieved. Only 36% of lesions in proximal sites (upper arm and thigh) were successfully controlled. Metastasis-free survival was 58% for 2 to 10 years (64)

   M.D. Anderson Hospital's postoperative irradiation of 80 soft tissue sarcoma patients resulted in an 80% control rate, 80% of whom had a good functional result with minimal edema and a wide range of motion (57a).

   The Massachusetts General Hospital group has achieved 92% and 84% local control rates at 2 and 5 years, respectively. Local failures were likely in large and high-grade lesions. Tumor grade is an important determinant of outcome in this series (77,91b).

   The National Cancer Institute (NCI), in a study on soft tissue sarcomas in extremities, reported high rates of local control in both arms; there was a local control rate of 100% (15/15) for radical surgery versus 83% (20/24) for wide excision plus irradiation at a median follow-up of 4 months (79).

   c. *Interstitial Iridium Brachytherapy:* The use of interstitial brachytherapy and function-saving resections of

Table 25-12. Local Control and Survival of Soft Tissue Sarcomas with Preoperative, Postoperative Radiation and Radiation Alone

Author	Treatment	5-Year Local Control (%)	5-Year Survival (%)
Suit et al. (91b)	Preop. irradiation	86	62
Eilber et al. (29a)	Preop. irradiation and intra-arterial doxorubicin	97	-
Suit et al. (91b)	Postop. irradiation	84	73
Lindberg et al. (57a)	Postop. irradiation	78	61
Potter et al. (74a)	Postop. irradiation and chemotherapy	92	67
Lehti et al. (56a)	Preop. hyperthermic chemotherapy perfusion and postop irradiation	87	67
Shiu et al. (86,86a)	Postop. brachytherapy		
	Previously untreated	100	
	Recurrent	62	
Tepper and Suit (97,97a)	Radiation therapy alone	44	28
	<5 cm	88	
	5-10 cm	53	
	>10 cm	30	

STS of limbs yielding excellent local control has been illustrated in a number of recent articles. Using brachytherapy (60-70 Gy) in combination with wide excision for initially untreated limb soft tissue sarcomas results in long-term, 15-year local regional control and survival of 50-60% of patients as reported by Habrand *et al.* (40b). Necrosis, which usually heals, occurred in 35% of patients. For recurrent tumor and tumors exceeding 1 cm, the combined modality approach with chemotherapy and external irradiation is advised. In a review by Shiu *et al.* (84'), 88% local control was achieved and by postponing the loading of radioactive sources to the fifth postoperative day, they reduced wound healing complications from 48% in an early trial to 14%, subsequently.

6. *Combined irradiation and chemotherapy:*
   a. *Combined radiation therapy* with chemotherapy (cyclophosphamide and vincristine in six cycles over 1 year and maintenance cyclophosphamide for an additional 2 years) has yielded a high control rate (75%) in high-grade rhabdomyosarcoma and malignant synoviomas (93). Combined preoperative intra-arterial or IV doxorubicin and short course radiation therapy used by the University of California, Los Angeles (UCLA) group (83a) reports high local control rates of 90%, relapse-free survival and overall survival at 3 years of 63% and 83%, respectively, and limb and foot salvage with conservative surgery of approximately 90%.
   b. *Adjuvant chemotherapy* trials, often combining surgery and radiation therapy, have been used by a variety of groups such as ECOG, Mayo Clinic, EORTC, Scandinavian Group, Intergroup Sarcoma, UCLA, and NCI with a variety of combinations and most often doxorubicin alone in different regimens with no difference in overall survival, but some gain in disease-free survival (Table 25-13) (36 a). Some of the best results reported are by NCI investigators when the local control, 5-year disease-free survival was 100% and 94% for low grade tumors, respectively and 93% and 75% for high grade tumors, respectively. Stinson *et al.* (90a) in a retrospective review of 145 patients treated at NCI provide some of the answers to the conservative management of soft tissue sarcomas using combined modality limb sparing surgery. The focus of the review is the acute and chronic effects, which vary from 27% for acute skin reactions to 57% for late tissue induration to 32% for decrease in limb motion. Most severe changes were less than 10% for fracture, pain requiring narcotics, orthotic devices required, cane or crutch walking, or chronic infection. Only three amputations were performed in this series. High nominal standard dose (> 1760 rets) led to morbidity more than concomitant chemotherapy, which added to acute rather than late toxicity. The majority of patients (84%) were ambulating without severe complications or devicing.

Prognosis

There are a number of important prognostic factors to consider in assessing soft tissue sarcomas. Among these factors are size and anatomic site.

Clinical Investigations

1. *Autologous bone marrow transplantation (BMT) and High dose chemotherapy and total body irradiation (TBI):* Young *et al.* (106) reported on the treatment of chest wall sarcomas using very intensive chemotherapy, high-dose daily fractionated radiation treatment to the primary and nonpulmonary metastases plus TBI. Patients achieving CR received either a low-dose rate fractionated TBI or high-dose rate TBI plus an intensive cycle of chemotherapy followed by autologous BMT. This occurred successfully in 25 of 31 patients; the majority went into remission and remained so months to years later.
2. *Size:* The local recurrence rate increases dramatically once the tumor exceeds 10 cm in diameter. As the mass increases in size to exceed 20 cm, local control becomes virtually impossible.
3. *Anatomic location (Table 25-14) (84a):* Extremity tumors are detected earlier and are in favored sites because surgical resection is most often possible and full-dose irradiation with limb preservation can be achieved.

Table 25-13. Randomized Soft Tissue Sarcoma Adjuvant Chemotherapy Trials

Institution	Drugs	Observation DFS	Observation S(%)	Chemotherapy DFS(%)	Chemotherapy S(%)
EORTC	CVAD	52	94	67	79
MDA	VACAd	35	36	43	54
MAYO	VACAd	67	88	88	63
NCI	CAM	64	37	73	84
EORTC	A	65	81	65	81
MGH	A	81	81	90	90
ECOG	A	71	71	72	64
BOLOGNA	A	54	--	79	--
UCLA	A	52	70	56	80
SCAND	A	55	44	52	40
ISTSS	A	50	62	77	72

A:Adriamycin; Ad:actinomycin D; C:cytoxan; V:vincristine; M:methotrexate; D:DTIC; DFS:disease-free patients; S:living patients; MDA:M.D. Anderson; MAYO:Mayo Clinic; NCI:National Cancer Institute; EORTC:European Organization for Research and Treatment of Cancer; MGH: Massachusetts General Hospital; ECOG: Eastern Cooperative Oncology Group; BOLOGNA: Institute Rizzoli, Bologna, Italy; USLC: University of California, Los Angeles; SCAND: Scandinavian sarcoma trial; ISTSS: Intergroup soft tissue sarcoma study.
From Frederick et al. (36a), with permission.

Table 25-14. Site Correlated to Local Recurrence Rate

	Number of Patients	Percent Total	Number with Recurrence	Number without Recurrence	% Recurrence
Lower extremity (53)					
Intrapelvic	2	3	2	0	100
Buttock	8	11	3	5	38
Groin	7	10	1	6	14
Thigh	26	37	4	22	15
Knee	3	4	0	3	0
Below Knee	7	10	0	7	0
Upper extremity (17)					
Shoulder girdle	4	6	2	2	50
Arm	7	10	0	7	0
Below elbow	6	9	1	5	17

From Simon et al. (84a), with permission.

When tumors are axial in location, particularly the pelvis and abdomen, they are difficult to resect completely and become a major limitation in radiation dose delivery.

It is also difficult to resect and limit the radiation dose (i.e., < 50 Gy total dose) for neoplasms around the spinal cord, and therefore sarcomas in the paraspinal location in the chest and even neck are a challenge.

4. *Lymph node metastases*: As a general rule, lymph node metastases are uncommon. The incidence according to tumor type reflects locoregional invasive patterns (102). The overall incidence is 5% to 15%, with synovial sarcomas and rhabdomyosarcomas being more common problems than liposarcomas and fibro sarcomas.

SPECIFIC SOFT TISSUE SARCOMAS

The histopathologic type may be less important than the grade and stage of the sarcoma as major determinants of outcome (Table 25-1). However, the specific sarcoma type must be considered in planning treatment.

FIBROSARCOMA: (DESMOID TUMORS)

Fibrosarcomas, with all their variants, are the most common sarcomas. Seventy percent are seen in patients between the ages of 20 and 50 years, with a slight predominance in males. They may occur, however, in children and newborns. Lower-grade lesions must be differentiated from aggressive fibromatoses, and may occasionally arise in multiply resected and/or irradiated fibromatoses (73). A related tumor, malignant fibrous histiocytoma, comprises an increasing percentage of soft tissue sarcomas because many fibrosarcomas or previously unclassified sarcomas are now classified in this category. The behavior of these tumors is similar to high-grade fibrosarcomas, but histologically these tumors demonstrate a mixture of histiocytic cells and fibroblastic cells, often in a storiform pattern as opposed to the classic herringbone pattern of fibrosarcomas. Additionally, giant cells can often be seen in malignant fibrous histiocytoma. Further discussion of this tumor type is presented later. Although various types of fibrosarcoma have been reported as secondary malignancies following high-dose irradiation, in general etiology is unknown.

Principles of Treatment

Fibrosarcomas

Treatment consists of wide or radical excision. Fibrosarcomas have a high incidence of recurrence; 60% recur even when a wide excision has been performed. Postoperative irradiation is now strongly recommended (87a), and may markedly reduce the local recurrence rate (84). The importance of grading fibrosarcomas has been demonstrated; for poorly differentiated fibrosarcomas, radical compartmental resection or amputation is occasionally necessary, particularly with large tumors or multiple compartment involvement. Few fibrosarcomas have been controlled temporarily by definitive radiation therapy alone (83).

Desmoid Tumors

Surgery is the best approach for desmoid tumors and if a complete excision is obtained with clear margins, no radiation therapy is recommended, despite the risk of recurrence. For positive margins, an initial alternative to immediate irradiation is observation and frequent follow-up with CT/MRI. With recurrence and incomplete excision, or unresectable tumors, definitive radiation therapy is recommended. The radiation dose should be approximately 50 to 60 Gy, when given as 1.8 to 2 Gy fractions, five fractions per week, on the basis of evaluation of the available data. The dose would be raised to 60 to 65 Gy in at least two situations: recurrent desmoid and anatomic sites in which surgical salvage would not be feasible. The dose here refers to the final dose to the radiographically evident mass. Tissue suspected of subclinical disease should receive a dose in the range of 45 to 50 Gy (94).

Results and Prognosis

In spite of a recurrence rate of 42%, 5-year survivals of 96% have been reported in well-differentiated lesions. In contrast, poorly differentiated fibrosarcomas have a 75% recurrence rate and 50% mortality rate (96). There is a close relationship between histologic grade, recurrence rate, and failure to cure (92,90). Fibrosarcomas of the head and neck have a better prognosis than those of the extremities.

Dermatofibrosarcoma: This is a low-grade fibrosarcoma that occurs on the trunk or in the scalp in the third or fourth decade. It may remain stationary for many years as a purplish excrescence or keloid before rapid growth occurs. Thirty percent recur after simple excision, but they can usually be controlled by re-excision. Rare metastases have been reported.

Fibrosarcoma, grade 1, desmoid type: Desmoid tumor, or aggressive fibromatosis, is an infiltrative lesion with a high (50%) recurrence rate even after wide local resection, although it does not metastasize. However, multiple local recurrences can cause significant morbidity and disability, occasionally leading to amputations. The abdominal variants of this tumor have a somewhat better prognosis. These lesions were once thought to be radioresistant, but can be controlled by radiation therapy. Recent reports by Greenberger *et al.* (40a), Wara *et al.* (100), and Sherman *et al.* (83b) have demonstrated virtually complete control and regression with doses up to 50 to 60 Gy. Generally, however, radiation treatment is used for unresectable lesions or recurrent lesions. In some cases in which obtaining adequate margins may be technically difficult due to size or location of the tumor, definitive treatment primarily with both surgical resection and radiation therapy may be appropriate. Local control rates after irradiation postexcision are between 71% and 77% (83b,94).

Infantile fibrosarcoma: These rapidly growing fibrosarcomas with histologic features of high-grade malignancy are seen in infants and children less than 5 years of age. In spite of their frightening behavior and appearance, simple local excision appears to suffice for cure (47,101).

LIPOSARCOMA

Liposarcomas are the most frequent tumors after fibrosarcomas. They occur almost anywhere that fat is present and are usually malignant at inception. Only rarely do they arise from lipomas. They appear at all ages, but are most common between 40 and 60 years of age.

Distribution of the liposarcomas in Stout's and Lattes' series (91) of 262 patients was lower extremity, 118; head and neck, 17; abdominal cavity and retroperitoneum, 36; trunk, 36; upper extremity, 20; and miscellaneous, 35.

Grossly, the tumors are frequently large, with multiple convolutions; they may be yellowish and resemble fat, or may have a more myxoid appearance. There are often satellite nodules or multiple foci of origin. Microscopic examination may reveal well-differentiated adult fat cells or may show intense variation with bizarre giant cells. Specific fat staining may be useful, although identification of malignant lipoblasts is the key to diagnosis. Occasionally, distinction between well-differentiated myxoid liposarcoma and benign lipoma can be difficult. In such cases, the best course is complete marginal excision with careful follow-up consisting of periodic MRI scanning to detect any early recurrence.

Liposarcomas may attain tremendous proportions. In 1859, Delamater (22) reported a liposarcoma weighing 180 pounds; this tumor grew to about 250 pounds at the time of the patient's death.

Principles of Treatment

1. There is a predilection for pulmonary metastases, as with most soft tissue sarcomas. The myxoid variant of liposarcoma shows a higher incidence of regional nodal metastases, and any regional nodes suspicious either on physical examination or MRI or CT scanning should be removed surgically, although routine lymph node dissections are not recommended.

2. Treatment consists of wide surgical excision. For high-grade lesions, such as pleomorphic liposarcoma, a radical resection may be indicated.

3. Radiation therapy should be given postoperatively regardless of the completeness of resection. This tumor is among the most radioresponsive of the soft tissue sarcomatous types.

Results and Prognosis

The recurrence rate is high after surgical excision alone. In Anderson's (7) series of 100 cases, 60% recurred from one to ten times following radical local excision, although recurrences were sometimes delayed as much as 5, 10, or even 20 years. The recurrence rate is also related to size and histology; it is rare to have a recurrence of a well-differentiated small myxoid liposarcoma. Survival rates vary with differentiation: 10% if the tumor is nonmyxoid-pleomorphic, and 66% if it is myxoid. Overall 5-year survival is about 32%. With the use of adjuvant radiation treatment, the local recurrence rate is markedly improved (50). The role of adjuvant chemotherapy in this tumor is not as yet clearly defined, and it has not been routinely used. As with other soft tissue sarcomas, early resection of pulmonary metastases may be beneficial.

RHABDOMYOSARCOMA

The rhabdomyosarcomas are a group of common tumors of soft parts, divisible into three entities: adult pleomorphic type (13%), embryonal alveolar type (41%), and embryonal botryoid type (46%) (34).

Adult pleomorphic rhabdomyosarcoma: These tumors arise most frequently in the extremities, with special predilection for certain muscle groups: quadriceps, adductors, semimembranous muscles, biceps, and brachialis. They occur most commonly in the fourth to seventh decades and the typical patient tends to experience repeated local recurrences with ultimate metastases. A few, however, demonstrate explosive growth and early hematogenous and lymphatic spread. The tumor in these cases is hemorrhagic, cystic, and necrotic, with little apparent viable tumor.

Principles of Treatment

1. Wide excision remains the best treatment.

2. *Embryonal alveolar rhabdomyosarcoma:* This tumor occurs primarily in children and young adults, and is found chiefly in the extremities. The patient typically complains of severe intermittent or persistent pain in the area, sometimes months before a tumor mass becomes apparent. The tumor is grayish-white, almost cartilaginous, and has cystic areas. Although there is a pseudocapsule, adjacent tissues are almost always infiltrated.

3. Remarkable advances have been made in the treatment of embryonal rhabdomyosarcoma. Total excision remains the objective of surgery, but effective adjuvant therapy with radiotherapy and/or chemotherapy (actinomycin D, vincristine sulfate, cyclophosphamide, and doxorubicin) permits preservation of function and appearance where they previously had to be sacrificed.

4. *Embryonal botryoid rhabdomyosarcoma:* These tumors, named after their polypoid, grapelike appearance,

occur primarily in childhood. According to Anderson (7) 73% occurred in the first decade and 91% in the first 2 decades. They are more common in males. They are most common in the head and neck, the genitourinary tract, and especially the orbit and nasopharynx. The prognosis is grave.

Results and Prognosis

1. Reported local recurrence rates vary from 27% to 60% and 5-year survivals range from 37% down to 10% (23,52,55).
2. With embryonal rhabdomyosarcoma, cures of 80% to 90% without recurrence and even 20% survival with metastatic disease are not unusual (26), due to chemotherapy improvements.
3. In adults, the prognosis of rhabdomyosarcoma is poor, with only 10% to 15% 5-year survival, even with aggressive surgery, radiotherapy, and chemotherapy. In children, the prognosis is better, with 5-year survival rates of 20% to 80%, depending on stage and type (93).

Granular Cell Myoblastoma

These rare tumors are usually benign, but may be malignant or multiple in 10% of patients (23,56). Over half occur in the mouth; most of these arise in the tongue. Results of resection are good. The origin of these tumors continues to be disputed; they may arise from Schwann cells rather than from muscle.

Leiomyosarcoma

These tumors may be found along the distribution of smooth muscle. They may metastasize widely, most often to liver and lungs. They tend to be most common in the gastrointestinal, genitourinary, and vascular systems, or they may present as large masses in the retroperitoneal area. Smooth muscle tumors larger than 5 cm are almost always malignant.

Principles of Treatment

Radical resection or wide resection with adjuvant radiation offers the only hope of cure. The role of adjuvant chemotherapy is not currently defined.

SYNOVIAL SARCOMA

Synovial sarcoma is primarily a disease of children and young adults. Over 60% of cases were reported in patients under 40 years of age (23). Synovial sarcomas usually arise from primitive mesenchymal cells in the vicinity of ligaments, tendinous sheaths, bursae, and joints. They have the appearance of synovial tissues, but the tumors rarely involve the joint synovia, although they generally arise near major joints. Of these lesions, about 60% occur in the lower extremity in various series (16,23).

Many patients with synovial sarcoma have pain or tenderness for 1 to 18 months before a mass appears, but occasionally only the presence of a mass causes the patient to seek medical attention. Delay in seeking treatment is common, often about 12 months. The tumors vary greatly in rate of growth, and patients may present with pulmonary metastases.

Grossly, these sarcomas are firm and gray, with hemorrhage and often with foci of calcification; they are firmly fixed to underlying structures. There are two subtypes of synovial sarcoma, monophasic and biphasic. The biphasic types have adenomatous components as well as a sarcomatous spindle cell component, and have a somewhat better prognosis than the monophasic types (19). There is very little matrix in the monophasic types, and both forms demonstrate some glycoprotein matrix by periodic acid Schiff stain. Sparce collagenous material may be seen in the both types. The two subtypes of synovial sarcoma occur with approximately equal incidence. The microscopically evident calcifications can be seen by x-ray examination in about 30% of patients (18). Regional lymph nodes are involved in 10% to 15% of patients, and correlate to poor prognosis.

Principles of Treatment

Treatment consists of a wide or radical surgical excision. Surgical excision of any clinically or radiographically involved regional lymph nodes is also recommended. Amputations, including hip disarticulations, are often required. Radiation therapy has been reported to control these tumors and is strongly advocated postoperatively (21). Chemotherapy can play a significant role in the palliation of these tumors, but its role as an adjuvant form of primary treatment is unknown. Significant rates of local control have also been achieved with radiation therapy alone, particularly with smaller lesions

Results and Prognosis

Between 45% and 63% of patients have a recurrence within 20 months after excision. Published 5-year survival figures vary from 2% to 51%; with aggressive surgical management, 5-year survival rates on the order of 40% to 50% are probably realistic. The prognosis is better in children than in adults, and in more distal and smaller lesions (10,18,19).

SARCOMAS OF BLOOD VESSEL ORIGIN

Hemangioendothelioma and Angiosarcoma

Hemangioendothelioma is a tumor of low-grade malignancy, while angiosarcoma represents a high-grade tumor derived from vascular endothelial cells. These tumors are extremely rare, comprising less than 1% of sarcomas (34). Generally, the etiology of vascular sarcomas, like that of other sarcoma types, is unknown. The cutaneous form of angiosarcoma shows a predilection for exposed areas of skin, raising sun exposure as a possible etiologic agent.

Vascular sarcomas generally present with a mass that may be asymptomatic. With high-grade lesions, warmth, distended venous patterns in overlying skin, and occasionally a pulsatile nature of the mass may be present. The cutaneous form of angiosarcoma presents with one or more small reddish or purplish nodules which grow gradually.

Principles of Treatment

For angiosarcoma, the approach involves surgical resection according to the principles elaborated previously for other high-grade soft tissue sarcomas. More conservative surgery is generally indicated for hemangioendotheliomas, generally without adjuvant therapy. Although these tumors are not considered radiosensitive, they are managed in a fashion similar to that of other sarcomas with postoperative irradiation. Low-grade hemangioendotheliomas can respond particularly about the face and chest wall where progression is a relentless local spread pattern without metastasizing.

Results and Prognosis

These tumors are so rare that accurate statistical data are not readily available, but in general the prognosis for hemangioendothelioma with adequate treatment of the primary lesion is good, with reported metastatic rates of around 20% (34). The prognosis of angiosarcoma, however, is variable, depending on the type and histologic grade. High-grade angiosarcoma has a dismal prognosis, due to the propensity for early hematogenous metastases.

KAPOSI'S SARCOMA

Kaposi's sarcoma is a blood vessel sarcoma formerly seen in the United States primarily in Jewish and Italian men aged over 65 years. It is extremely common in equatorial Africa, where it occurs in all age groups and comprises 10% of all malignancies (82). However, since 1978, increasing numbers of cases of Kaposi's sarcoma have been reported in association with the acquired immunodeficiency syndrome (AIDS) caused by viral infection with human T-cell lymphotrophic virus type III (HIV). This has become by far the most common cause of Kaposi's sarcoma. The devastating effects of AIDS on the immune system, however, which usually lead to fatal complications, overshadow the effects of the sarcoma in most cases of the disease, and it is generally treated conservatively in these patients (49,67).

The lesion usually begins as a raised purplish nodule on the lower extremity. As the disease progresses, other nodules appear in both skin and viscera. Edema of the surrounding skin is a sign of advanced disease. The lesion is almost certainly multicentric in origin.

In AIDS patients, clinical diagnosis of the lesions may be sufficient, while in other patients biopsy of a skin lesion might be necessary to establish the diagnosis. Further diagnostic studies generally are not necessary, although any patient with Kaposi's sarcoma should be tested for HIV infection.

Principles of Treatment

Conservative local irradiation is used so that future nodules can also be treated, because this is generally considered a systemic disorder. Radiation therapy with modest doses is very effective for tumor regression, particularly for regionally advanced disease, i.e., multiple nodules in feet and in legs. Generous field to half-body radiation in modest to moderate doses result in complete regression in most cases. Regression requires 3 to 6 months to occur in classic Kaposi's, but the response is more rapid in AIDS-related lesions, particularly when associated with edema.

Results and Prognosis

There is a high associated incidence of lymphomas. Survival following diagnosis of Kaposi's sarcoma in the absence of AIDS is estimated to be about 8 years. Prognosis in the presence of AIDS is significantly worse, and the disease is essentially uniformly fatal within several years at most, although morbidity and mortality are generally secondary to the immunologic compromise and not the sarcoma itself.

LYMPHANGIOSARCOMA

Lymphangiosarcomas are multicentric tumors that arise in chronically edematous extremities. They are the most common complications of postmastectomy edema of the arm; however, they occur in less than 1% of patients with mastectomies (27,38,44). There seems to be an increased incidence of lymphangiosarcomas in patients who have undergone radiation therapy following their radical mastectomies. The average age of onset is 62 years and the average interval from mastectomy to tumor is 9 years, 7 months.

Principles of Treatment

Spread is rapid and hematogenous. Treatment, whether by radical amputation, irradiation, or chemotherapy, is generally ineffective.

Results and Prognosis

Mean survival after diagnosis is 19 months (27,38,44).

MALIGNANT FIBROUS HISTIOCYTOMA

These tumors arise from histiocytes and may arise in soft tissues of any part of the body. Benign fibrous histiocytomas generally occur in the skin and subcutaneous tissues, while the malignant lesions are usually found in deeper tissues. Since the original description of the lesion in 1963 (71), an increasing number of these tumors have been diagnosed, and it currently comprises the most common sarcoma in late adult life (61,65). This is an aggressive tumor which, like most soft tissue sarcomas, metastisizes hematogenously to the lungs. Malignant fibrous histiocytoma constitutes a significant proportion of postradiation therapy sarcomas, but aside from these cases the etiology is not known.

The histology of the tumor is variable, but generally includes both fibroblastic and histiocytic elements. Presence of giant cells, and a swirling cartwheel or storiform arrangement of the cells are common, as are bizarre aneuploid nuclear forms and pleomorphism. Several subtypes have been identified, including storiform/pleomorphic, myroid, giant cell, inflammatory (also called malignant xanthogranuloma), and angiomatoid (34). Except for the angiomatoid variant, which occurs in the dermis and subcutaneous tissues of children and young adults, these are tumors of older age groups.

Principles of Treatment

The route of spread is usually hematogenesis; rapidly disseminating metastases are the usual cause of treatment failure.

Treatment should consist of wide surgical excision followed by local radiation therapy, or radical local resection without irradiation. This will provide long-term control or cure, if metastases are not present. Pulmonary metastases may be amenable to resection when detected early. The tumors are often radiosensitive, responding to doses as low as 10 Gy. Radiation therapy is generally an extremely important treatment component, once the diagnosis is established. Most often, full doses of radiation therapy (50-60 Gy) are required for cure in conjunction with complete surgical excision as in most other sarcomas. There is evidence that adjuvant chemotherapy may significantly improve prognosis and decrease metastatic rate with this sarcoma (9, 79,81), and it is generally recommended in addition to treatment for the primary lesion in patients who are medically able to tolerate the drugs.

Results and Prognosis

According to one large series, 44% of patients develop a local recurrence and 42% metastases, which usually occur within 2 years of diagnosis (51). Metastases occur to the lung (82%), lymph node (32%), liver (15%), and bone (15%). Two-year survival with this disease is approximately 60%, but at least one third of patients surviving 2 years may develop later local recurrence or metastasis (104).

The size and depth of the tumor also correlate with prognosis. Only 10% of tumors confined to the subcutaneous tissue metastasize, while 27% which involve fascia and 43% of those which involve skeletal muscle will metastasize. More distal extremity lesions also have a somewhat better prognosis (105). However, given the more recent improved survival and decreased local recurrence rates obtained in a series of sarcomas using multimodality treatment, expected prognoses should improve significantly (8,12,36,38,44,103).

Recommended Reading

Enzinger and Weiss' book (3) is excellent for an overall understanding of soft tissue tumors. Section II of the Evarts' book (4) provides good surgical background and information. Rosenberg (78) focuses on adjuvant chemotherapy and gives an excellent summary of sarcomas of soft tissue and bone (80). Suit *et al.* deals with combination radiation therapy and surgery for soft tissue sarcomas (91a,91b).

REFERENCES

General References

1. Enneking WF. Limb Salvage in Musculoskeletal Oncology. New York, NY: Churchill Livingstone; 1987.
2. Enneking WF. Muskuloskeletal Tumor Surgery. New York, NY: Churchill Livingstone; 1983.
3. Enzinger FM, Weiss SW. Soft Tissue Tumors, 2nd edition. St. Louis, MO: C.V. Mosby; 1989.
4. Evarts CM, ed. Surgery of the Musculoskeletal System. 2nd ed. section 11: Bone and soft tissue tumors. New York, NY: Churchill Livingstone; 1989.
5. Lattes R. Tumors of the Soft Tissues, Armed Forces Institute of Pathology, fascicle 1, revised. Washington, D.C: AFIP; 1982.
5a. Lawrence, T.S.; Lichter, A.S. Soft tissue sarcomas (excluding retroperitoneum). In: Perez, C.A., Brady, L.W. (eds). Principles and practice of radiation oncology, Philadelphia, PA: JB Lippincott Co; 1992:1399-1412.

Specific References

6. American Joint Committee on Cancer. In: Manual for Staging of Cancer. Beahrs, OH: Myers MDH, eds. Philadelphia, PA: JB Lippincott; 1983.
7. Anderson WAD, ed. Pathology. St. Louis, MO: CV Mosby Co; 1971.
8. Antman K, Blum R, Corson J, et al. Effective adjuvant chemotherapy for localized soft tissue sarcoma. Proc Am Assoc Cancer Res. 21:141; 1980. Abstract.
8a. Antman K, Ryan L, Borden E, Wood W, Lerner H, Carson J, Carey R, Suit H, Balcerak S, Sherman M, Baker L. Pooled results from three randomized adjuvant studies of doxorubicin versus observation in soft tissue sarcoma: 10 year results. In: Salmon, S.E. (ed) Adjuvant therapy of cancer VI. Philadelphia, PA: WB Saunders Co; 1990.
9. Bacci G, Springfield D, Capanna R, Picci P, Bertoni F, Campanacci M. Adjuvant chemotherapy for malignant fibrous histiocytoma in the femur and tibia. J Bone Joint Surg. 67A:620-625; 1985.
10. Balzarini L, Ceglia E, Petrillo R, Tessoro-Tess JD, Reitano A, Musumeci R. MRI of lipomatous, fibrous and muscular tissue tumors. Radiol Med. 77(1-2):87-93, 1989.
11. Barkley H, Martin R, Romsdahl M, Lindberg R, Zagars G. Treatment of soft tissue sarcomas by preoperative irradiation and conservative surgical resection. Int J Radiat Oncol Biol Phys. 14:693-699; 1988 .
12. Belli L, Scholl S, Livartowski A, Ashby M, Palangie T, Levaseur P, Pouillart P. Resection of pulmonary metastases in osteosarcoma. A retrospective analysis of 44 patients. Cancer. 63(12):2546-2550; 1989.
13. Berquist TH. Magnetic resonance imaging of musculoskeletal neoplasms. Clin Orthop. 244:101-118; 1989.
14. Bertelsen CA, Eilbert FR. Paraneoplastic syndromes with soft-tissue sarcoma: a report of two unusual cases. J Surg Oncol. 24(3):170-172; 1983.
14a. Bragg DG, Rubin P, Youuker JE, eds. Oncologic Imaging. Elmsford, NY: Pergamon Press; 1985.
15. Bramwell VH, Crowther D, Deakin DP, Swindell R, Haris M. Combined modality management of local and disseminated adult soft tissue sarcomas. Br J Cancer. 51(3):301-318; 1985 .
16. Buck P, Mickelson MR, Bonfiglio M. Synovial sarcoma: A review of 33 cases. Clin Orthop. 156:211-215; 1981.
17. Cade S. Soft tissue tumors: their natural history and treatment. Proc R Soc Med. 19:19-36; 1951.
18. Cadman NL, Soule EH, Kelly P. Synovial sarcoma-an analysis of 134 tumors. Cancer. 18:613-627; 1965.
19. Cagle LA, Mirra JM, Storm FK, Roe DJ, Eilber FR. Histologic features relating to prognosis in synovial sarcoma. Cancer. 59:1810-1814; 1987.
20. Cantin J, McNeer GP, Chu FC, et al. The problem of local recurrence after Treatment of soft tissue sarcoma. Ann Surg. 168:47-53; 1968.
21. Carson JH, Harwood AR, Cummings BJ, Fornasier V, Langer F, Quirt I. The place of radiotherapy in the treatment of synovial sarcoma. Int J Radiat Oncol Biol Phys. 7:49-53; 1981 .
21a. Casali P, Di Pastorino U, Santoro A, Capri F, Viviani S, Azzarelli A, Bonadonna G. Full-dose eppirubicin, ifosfamide and dacorbazine (EID) combined with surgery in advanced soft tissue sarcomas. In: Proc Am Soc Clin Oncol. 9: 309; 1990. Abstract.
21b. Chang AE, Rosenberg SA, Gladstein FJ, Antman KH. Sarcomas of soft tissue. In: DeVita VT Jr, Hellman S, Rosenberg SA. Cancer Principles and Practice of Oncology. 3rd ed. Philadelphia, PA: JB Lippincott; 1989.
22. Delamater J. Mammoth tumor. Cleveland Medical Gazette. 1:31-41; 1859.
23. Delanay WE, Gross C, Nealon TF. The soft tissues. In: Nealon TF ed. Management of the Patient with Cancer. Philadelphia, PA: WB Saunders Co; 1976.
24. Demas BE, Heelan RT, Lane J, Marcove R, Hadju S, Brennan MF. Soft-tissue sarcomas of the extremities: comparison of MR and CT in determining the extent of disease. AJR. 150(3):615-620; 1988.
25. Didolkar MS, Kanter PM, Bart RR, et al. Comparison of regional vs. systemic chemotherapy with adriamycin. Ann Surg. 187:322-326; 1978.
26. Donaldson SS. Rhabdomyosarcoma: contemporary status and future directions. Arch Surg. 124:1015-1020; 1989.
27. Ebb CS, Brennan MJ, Fine G. Lymphangiosarcoma: a lethal complication of chronic lymphedema. Arch Surg. 94:223-230; 1967.
28. Eilber FR, Eckhardt J, Morton DL. Advances in the treatment of sarcomas of the extremity. Current status of limb salvage. Cancer. 54(suppl 11):2695-2701; 1984.
29. Eilber FR, Giuliano AE, Huth JF, Mirra J, Morton DL. High-grade soft-tissue sarcomas of the extremity: UCLA experience with limb salvage. Prog Clin Biol Res. 201:59-74; 1985.
29a. Eilber FR, Giuliano AE, Huth JF, Morton DL. A randomized prospective trial using postoperative adjuvant chemotherapy (Adriamycin) in high-grade extremity soft-tissue sarcoma. Am J Clin Oncol. 11:39-45;1988.
30. Elias AD, Antman KH. Adjuvant chemotherapy for soft tissue sarcoma: a critical appraisal. Semin. Surg Oncol. 4(1):59-65; 1988.
31. Enneking WF. Staging musculoskeletal tumors. In: Musculoskeletal Tumor Surgery. New York, NY: Churchill Livingstone; 69-88; 1983.
32. Enneking WF. Principles of musculoskeletal oncology. In: Surgery of the Musculoskeletal System. Evarts CM, ed. New York, NY: Churchill Livingstone. 47-69; 1983.
32a. Enneking WF. Staging of musculoskeletal neoplasms. In: Current Concepts of Diagnosis and Treatment of Bone and Soft Tissue Tumors. Heidelberg, Germany: Springer-Verlag; 1984.

33. Enneking W. A system of staging musculoskeletal neoplasms. Clin Orthop. 204:9-24; 1986.

34. Enzinger FM, Weiss SW. Soft Tissue Tumors. St. Louis, MO: CV Mosby Co; 1989.

35. Epstein CJ, Martin GM, Schultz AL, et al. Werner's syndrome. A review of its symptomatology, natural history, pathologic features, genetics, and relationship to the natural aging process. Medicine. 45:177-221; 1966.

35'. Essner R, Selch M, Eilber FR. Reirradiation for extremity soft tissue sarcomas. Cancer. 67(11):2813-2817; 1991

35a. Fletcher J, Morton C, Pavelka K, Weidner N, Pinkus G, Tepper R, Lage J, Kozakewich H, Carson J. Diagnostic relevance of chromosome rearrangements and genetic instability in malignant soft tissue (STT). Proc Am Soc Clin Oncol. 9: 310; 1990. Abstract.

36. Fraumeni JF Jr, Vogel CL, Easton JM. Sarcomas and multiple polyposis in a kindred. A genetic variety of hereditary polyposis? Arch Intern Med. 121:57-61; 1968.

36a. Frederick R, Eilber JF, Huth JM, Rosen G. Progress in the recognition and treatment of soft tissue sarcomas. Cancer. 65:660-666;1990.

37. Gaakeer HA, Albus Lutter Ch E, Gortzak E, Zoetmudder FAN. Regional lymph node metastases in patients with soft tissue sarcomas of the extremities, what are the therapeutic consequences?. Eur J Surg Oncol. 14(2):151-156; 1988.

38. Gajraj H, Barker SG, Burnand KG, Browse NL. Lymphangiosarcoma complicating chronic primary lymphoedema. Br J Surg. 74(12): 1180; 1987.

39. Giuliano AE, Juth JF, Weisenburger T, Eckardt J. Intravenus (IV) surgical excision for extremity soft tissue sarcomas: a randomized porspective trial. Proc Am Soc Clin Oncol. 9:309; March 1990. Abstract.

40. Gottlieb JA, Baker LH, O'Bryan RM, et al. Adriamycin (NSC123127) used alone and in combination for soft tissue and bony sarcomas. Cancer Chemother Rep. 6:271-282; 1975.

40a. Greenberger JS, Chatteh JT, Cassady JR: Radiation therapy in the treatment of aggressive fibromatosis. Int J Radiat Oncol Biol Phys. 7:305-310; 1981.

40b. Habrand JL, Gerbaulet A, Pejovic MH, et al. Twenty years experience of interstitial iridium brachytherapy in the management of soft tissue sarcomas. Int J Radiat Oncol Biol Phys. 20:405-412; 1991

41. Hajdu SI. Soft tissue sarcomas: classification and natural history. CA. 31:271-280; 1981.

42. Harle A, Reiser M, Erlemann R, Wuisman P. The value of MRI in staging bone and soft-tissue sarcomas. Orthopade. 18(1):34-40; 1989.

43. Haskell CM, Eber FR, Morton DL. Adriamycin (NSC-1 23127) by arterial infusion. Cancer Chemother Rep. 6:187-189; 1975.

44. Hermann JB. Lymphangiosarcoma of chronically edematous extremity. Surg Gynecol Obstet. 121:1107-1115;1965.

45. Hippocrates: The Theory and Practice of Medicine. Runes DD, Kiernan T eds. Secaucus, NJ: Citadel Press; 1964.

46. Huth JF, Holmes EC, Vernon SE, et al. Pulmonary resection for metastatic varcinoma. Am J Surg. 140:9-17; 1980.

47. Iwasaki H, Enjoji M. Infantile and adult fibrosarcomas of the soft tissues. Acta Pathol Jpn. 29:377-388; 1979.

48. Jacobs EM. Combination chemotherapy of metastatic testicular germinal cell tumors and soft part sarcomas. Cancer 25:324-332; 1970.

49. Jimenez Acosta F, Penneys NS. Treatment of cutaneous complications of AIDS. J Dermatol Treat. 1(2): 111-116;1989.

50. Karakousis CP, Emrich LJ, Rao U, Krishnamsetty RM. Feasibility of limb salvage and survival in soft tissue sarcomas. Cancer. 57(3):484-491; 1986.

51. Kearney MM, Soule EH, Ivins JC. Malignant fibrous histiocytoma: a retrospective study of 167 cases. Cancer. 45:167; 1980.

52. Keyhani A, Booher RJ. Pleomorphic rhabdomyosarcoma. Cancer. 22:956-957; 1968.

53. Kissin MW, Fisher C, Carter RL, Horton LW, Westbury G. Value of Tru-cut biopsy in the diagnosis of soft tissue tumours. Br J Surg. 73(9):742-4; 1986.

54. Krementz ET, Carter RD, Sutherland CM, et al. Chemotherapy of sarcomas of the limbs by regional pertusion. Ann Surg. 185:155-164;1977.

55. Lacey SR, Jewett TC Jr, Karp MP, Allen JE, Cooney DR. Advances in the treatment of rhabdomyosarcoma. Semin Surg Oncol. 2(3):139-146;1986.

56. Lattes R. Tumors of the Soft Tissues. Armed Forces Institute of Pathology, Fascicle 1. Washington DC: AFIP; 249; 1982.

56a. Lehti PM, Moseley HS, Janoff K, Stevens K, Fletcher WF. Improved survival for soft tissue sarcoma of the extremities by regional hyperthermia perfusion, local excision and radiation therapy. Surg Gynecol Obstet. 162:149-152;1986.

57. Lindberg RD, Martin RG, Romsdahl MM, Barkley HT Jr. Conservative surgery and postoperative radiotherapy in 300 adults with soft-tissue sarcomas. Cancer. 47:2391-2397;1981.

57a. Lindberg RD, Martin RG, Romsdahl MM. Surgery and postoperative radiotherapy in the treatment of soft tissue sarcomas in adults. Am J Roentgenol Radiol Ther Nucl Med. 123:123-129; 1975.

58. Lindberg RD, Murphy WK, Benjamin RS, et al. Adjuvant chemotherapy in the treatment of primary soft tissue sarcomas: a preliminary report. In: Clinical Conference on Cancer, 21st. M.D. Anderson Hospital and Tumor Institute, 1976. Management of Primary Bone and Sort Tissue Tumors. Chicago, IL: Year Book Medical Publishers. 343-352; 1977.

58a. Linke KA, Benjamin RS, Evans HL, Salem PA, Sherman NE, Pollack RE, Romsdahl MM. Proc Am Soc Clin Oncol. 9:314;1990. Abstract.

59. Lock S. Changes in treating soft tissue sarcomas. Br Med J. 2:562-563; 1979.

60. Lopez R, Didolkar MS, Karakousis C, et al. Problems in resection of chest wall sarcomas. Am Surg. 45:471-477; 1979.

61. Makepeace AR, Cannon SR. Malignant fibrous histiocytoma: the most common soft-tissue sarcoma. Br J Hosp Med. 39(2):122-127; 1988.

61a. Marcove RC. New limb sparing resections and results in the treatment of osteogenic sarcoma. Am Soc Clin Oncol. 9: 312; 1990. Abstract.

62. Mazeron JJ, Suit HD. Lymph nodes as sites of metastases from sarcomas of soft tissue. Cancer. 60(8):1800-1808; 1987.

63. McBride CM. Regional chemotherapy for soft tissue sarcomas. In: Clinical Conference on Cancer, 21st. M.D. Anderson Hospital and Tumor Institute, 1976. Management of Primary Bone and Soft Tissue Tumors. Chicago, IL: Year Book Medical Publishers. 353-360; 1977.

64. McNeer GP, Cantin J, Chu F, et al. Effectiveness of radiation therapy in the management of the soft somatic tissues. Cancer. 22:391-397; 1968.

65. Meister P. Malignant fibrous histiocytoma. History, histology, histogenesis. Pathol Res Pract. 183:1-7;1988.

65a. Meyers PA, Lane J, Marcove R, Healey J, Huros A, Rosen G. Osteogenic sarcoma (OS): experience at Memorial Sloan-Kettering Cancer Center (MSKCC). Proc Am Soc Clin Oncol. 9: 316;1990. Abstract.

66. Mindell E, Shah N, Webster J. Post-irradiation sarcoma of bone and soft tissue., Ortho Clin North Am. 8:821-834;1977.

67. Mitsuyasu RT. AIDS-related Kaposi's sarcoma: A review of its pathogenesis and treatment. Blood Rev. 2(4):222-231; 1988.

68. Mitts D, Gerhardt H, Armstrong D, et al. Chemotherapy for advanced soft tissue sarcomas: results of phase I and II cooperative studies. Tex Med. 75: 43-47; 1979.

69. Morton DL, Eilber FR, Townsend CM, et al. Limb salvage from a multidisciplinary treatment approach for skeletal and soft tissue sarcomas of the extremity. Ann Surg. 184:268-276; 1976.

70. National Institutes of Health. Consensus Development Conference Statement: limb-sparing treatment of adult soft tissue sarcomas and osteosarcomas. vol. 5. 1985.

71. Ozzello L, Stout AP, Murray MR. Cultural characteristics of malignant histiocytomas and fibrous xanthomas. Cancer. 16:331; 1963.

72. Pastorino U, Valente M, Gasparini M, Azzarelli A, Santoro A, Alloisio M, Ongari M, Tavecchio L, Ravasi G. Lung resection for metastatic sarcomas: total survival from primary treatment. J Surg Oncol. 40:275-280;1989.

73. Pettit VD, Chamness JT, Ackerman LV. Fibromatosis and fibrosarcoma following irradiation therapy. Cancer. 7:149; 1954.

74. Pinedo HM, Kenis Y. Chemotherapy of advanced soft tissue sarcomas in adults. Cancer Treat Rev. 4:67-86;1976.

74a. Potter DA, Kinsella T, Glatstein E, Wesley R, White EE, Seipp

CA, Chang AE, Lack EE, Costa J, Rosenberg SA. High-grade soft tissue sarcomas of the extremities. Cancer. 58:190-205;1986.

75. Presant CA, Russell WO, Alexander RW, Fu YS. Soft tissue and bone sarcoma histopathology peer review: the frequency of disagreement in diagnosis and the need for second pathology opinions. The Southeastern Cancer Study Group experience. J Clin Oncol. 4(11):1311-1319; 1986.

76. Rantakokko V, Ekfors, TO. Sarcomas of the soft tissue in the extremities and limb girdles. Acta Chir Scand. 125:385-394; 1979.

77. Risch M, Le Treut A, Dilhuydy MH, Coindre JM, Guibert JL, Bui NB. Adult soft tissue sarcomas. CT-scan initial findings and evaluation of response to neoadjuvant chemotherapy. Ann Radiol. 31(5):283-288; 1988.

78. Rosenberg SA. Adjuvant chemotherapy of adult patients with soft tissue sarcoma. Important Adv Oncol. 273-294; 1985.

79. Rosenberg SA, Suit H, Baker LH, et al. Sarcomas of the soft tissue and bone. In: DeVita VT, Hellman S, Rosenberg SA eds: Cancer: Principles and Practice of Oncology. Philadelphia, PA: JB Lippincott Co. 1036-1068; 1982.

80. Rosenberg SA, Kent H, Cost J, et al. Prospective randomized svaluation of the role of limb sparing surgery, radiation therapy, and adjuvant chemoimmunotherapy in the treatment of adult soft tissue sarcomas. Surgery. 84:62-69; 1978.

81. Rothman S. Remarks on sex, age, and racial distribution of Kaposi's sarcoma and on possible pathogenic factors. Acta: Unio Internationali Scontra Cancrum. 18:326-329; 1962.

82. Russell WO, Cohen J, Enzinger F, et al. A clinical and pathological staging system for soft tissue sarcomas. Cancer. 40:1562-1570; 1977.

82'. Rydholm A, Gustafson P, Rooser B, et al. Limb-sparing surgery without radiotherapy based on anatomic location of soft tissue sarcoma. J Clin Oncol 9:1757-1765; 1991.

82a. Santoro A, Rouesse DJ, Steward W, Mouridsen H, Verweif J, Somers R, Blackledge G, Buesa J, Sayer H, Tursz T, Thomas D, Sylevester R, Van Dosterom AT.. for EORTC Soft Tissue and bone Sarcoma Group. Proc Am Soc Clin Oncol. 9: 309;1990. Abstract.

83. Scott SM, Reiman HM, Pritchard DJ, Ilstrup DM. Soft tissue fibrosarcoma. A clinicopathologic study of 132 cases. Cancer. 64: 925-931; 1989.

83a. Selch MT, Kopald KH, Gerreiro GA, Mirra JM, Parker RG, Eilber FR. Limb salvage therapy for soft tissue sarcomas of the foot. Int J Radiat Oncol Biol Phys. 19:41-48;1990.85. Shiu M, Turnbull A, Nori D, Hajdu S, Hilaris B. Control of locally advanced extremity soft tissue sarcomas by function-saving resection and brachytherapy. Cancer. 53:1385-1398; 1984.

83b. Sherman NE, Romsdahl M, Evans H, Zagars G, Oswald MJ. Desmoid tumors: a 20-year radiotherapy experience. Int J Radiat Oncol Biol Phys. 19:37-40; 1990.

84. Shiu MH, Castro EB, Hajdu SI, et al. Surgical treatment of 297 soft tissue sarcomas of the lower extremity. Ann Surg. 182:597-602; 1975.

84'. Shiu MH, Hilaris BS, Harrison LB, Brennan MF. Brachytherapy and function-saving resection of soft tissue sarcoma arising in the limb. Int J Radiat Oncol Biol Phys. 21:1485-1492; 1991.

84a. Simon MA, Spanier SS, Enneking WF. Management of adult soft tissue sarcomas of the extremities. Surg Annu. 11:363-402; 1979.

85. Shiu M, Turnbull A, Nori D, Hajdu S, Hilaris B. Control of locally advanced extremity soft tissue sarcomas by function-saving resection and brachytherapy. Cancer. 53:1385-1398;1984.

86. Shiu MH, Collin C, Hilaris BS, Nori D, Manolatos S, Anderson LL, Hajdu SI, Lane JM, Hopfan S, Brennan MF. Limb preservation and tumor control in the treatment of popliteal and antecubital soft tissue sarcomas. Cancer. 57:1632-1639;1986.

86a. Shiu MH, Flancbaum L, Hajdu SL, et al. Malignant soft tissue tumors of the anterior abdominal wall. Arch Surg. 115:152-155; 1980.

87. Silverberg E: Cancer statistics, 1983. CA. 33:9-25; 1983.

88. Simon MA, Enneking WF. The management of soft tissue sarcomas of the extremities. J Bone Joint Surg. 58-A:317-327; 1976.

89. Simon MA, Spanier SS, Enneking WF. Management of adult soft tissue sarcomas of the extremities. Surg Annu. 11:363-402; 1979.

90. Slater J, McNeese M, Peters L. Radiation therapy for unresectable soft tissue sarcomas. Int J Radiat Oncol Biol Phys. 12: 1729-1734; 1986.

90a. Stinson SF, DeLaney TF, Greenberg J, et al. Acute and long-term effects on limb function of combined modality limb sparing therapy for extremity soft tissue sarcoma. Int J Radiat Oncol Biol Phys. 21:1493-1500; 1991.

91. Stout AP, Lattes R. Tumors of the soft tissues. Atlas of Tumor Pathology. 2nd Series. fascicle 1. Washington DC: Armed Forces Institute of Pathology; 1967.

91a. Suit HD, Mankin HJ, Willett G, et al. Limited surgery and external irradiation in soft tissue sarcomas. In: Recent Concepts in Sarcoma Treatment Proceedings of the International Symposium on Sarcomas. Tarpon Springs, FL.October 8-10, 1987. The Netherlands: Kluwer Academic Publishers; 1988.

91b. Suit HD, Mankin H, Wood W, Proppe K. Preoperative, intraoperative, and postoperative radiation in the treatment of primary soft tissue sarcoma. Cancer. 55:2659-2667; 1985.

92. Suit HD, Russell WO. Radiation therapy of soft tissue sarcomas. Cancer. 36:759-764; 1975.

93. Suit H, Russell W, Martin R. Sarcoma of soft tissue: clinical and histopathologic parameters and response to treatment. Cancer. 35:1478-1483; 1975.

94. Suit HD. Radiation dose and response of desmoid tumors. Int J Radiat Oncol Biol Phys. 19:225;1990.

95. Suit HD, Proppe KH, Mankin HJ, Wood WC. Preoperative radiation treatment for sarcoma of soft tissues. Cancer. 47:2269-2274. 1981.

96. Suit HD, Russell WO, Martin RG. Management of patients with sarcoma of soft tissue in an extremety. Cancer. 31 :1247-1255; 1973.

97. Tepper J, Suit H. Radiation therapy of soft tissue sarcomas. Cancer. 55:2273-2277, 1985.

97a. Tepper JE, Suit HD. Radiation therapy alone for sarcoma of soft tissue. Cancer. 56:475-479;1985.

97b. Tepper JE, Suite HD. Radiation therapy of soft tissue sarcomas. Cancer 55:2273-2277; 1985

98. Tepper J, Suit H. The role of radiation therapy in the treatment of sarcoma of soft tissue. Cancer Invest. 3:587-592; 1985.

98a. US Health and Human Services, Public Health Service Mortality Data, National Institute of Health, National Cancer Institute, Bethesda, MD; 1989.

99. Walker AN, Morton BD. Immunohistochemistry: a useful adjunct in the evaluation of malignant cutaneous spindle cell tumors. South Med J. 81(12): 1505-1508; 1988.

100. Wara WM, Phillips TL, Hill DR, et al. Desmoid tumors treatment and prognosis. Radiology. 124:225-226; 1977.

101. Wee A, Pho RWH, Ong LB. Infantile fibrosarcoma. Arch Pathol Lab Med. 103:236-238; 1979.

102. Weingrad DW, Rosenberg SA. Early lymphatic spread of osteogenic and soft tissue sarcomas. Surgery. 84:231-240;1978.

103. Weisenberger TH, Eilber FR, Grant TT, et al. Multidisciplinary "limb salvage" treatment for soft tissue and skeletal sarcomas. Int J Radiat Oncol Biol Phys. 7:1491-1499; 1981.

104. Weiss SW, Enzinger FM. Malignant fibrous histiocytoma: an analysis of 200 cases. Cancer. 41:2250;1978.

105. Yap BS, Baker LH, Sinkovic JG, et al. Cyclophosphamide, vincristine, Adriamycin, and DTIC (CYVADIC) combination chemotherapy for the treatment of advanced sarcomas. Cancer Treat Rep. 64:93-98; 1980.

106. Young MM, Kinsella TJ, Miser JS, Triche TJ, Glaubiger DL, Steinberg SM, Glatstein E. Treatment of sarcomas of the chest wall using intensive combined modality therapy. Int J Radiat Oncol Biol Phys. 16:49-58;1989.

Randy N. Rosier, M.D., Ph.D., Orthopaedic Oncology   Laszlo Boros, M.D., Medical Oncology
Andre Konski, M.D., Radiation Oncology

Chapter **26**

BONE TUMORS

Is this the poultice for my aching bones?

Romeo and Juliet II, v.65 (131a)

PERSPECTIVE

Nowhere is the value of the multidisciplinary approach to cancer management better exemplified than in the area of bone tumors. Improvements in multidisciplinary management and in diagnostic staging techniques have led to a rapid improvement in survival of patients with these traditionally devastating neoplasms. Primary malignant bone tumors are quite rare compared with other types of cancer (1-3,6,7). Diagnosis often depends on input from the orthopedist, pathologist, and radiologist.

Just as the diagnosis is based on the multidisciplinary process, so, too, are the treatment decisions. Chemotherapy has contributed substantially to the control of metastases and the management of bone tumors. Extremely aggressive drug combinations have been developed, particularly in the pediatric and young-adult age groups. Surgery and/or radiation therapy remain the mainstays of treatment of the primary tumor. Conservative limb-salvage procedures are firmly established as viable therapeutic methods to maintain function and cosmesis. Immunotherapy is still largely experimental, but has shown promise. Although previous data raised the question of changes in the natural history of certain tumors, e.g., osteosarcoma (134,135), subsequent studies indicate that improvements in survival with this tumor are more likely related to better staging technology and adjuvant therapy (36,78).

EPIDEMIOLOGY AND ETIOLOGY

Epidemiology

1. The incidence of bone tumors is highest during adolescence, with a rate of 3 per 100,000 (48). In spite of the high incidence at this age, bone tumors comprise only 3.2% of childhood malignancies that occur before the age of 15 years. The incidence falls to 0.2 per 100,000 at ages 30 to 35 years, and thereafter slowly rises until, at 60 years, the incidence rate equals that of adolescence (3,4).
2. Incidence of specific tumor types:
   a. Multiple myeloma, a nonosseous malignant tumor arising in the marrow of bone, should be considered a primary bone tumor. When it is included in such a classification, it becomes the most common malignant bone tumor comprising approximately 35% to 43% of such tumors (1,7). It is generally a tumor of middle-aged and older adults (peak incidence in 5th to 7th decades), and often must be differentiated clinically and radiographically from metastatic carcinoma.
   b. Osteosarcoma is the most common of the primary osseous malignant bone tumors; Dahlin (1) reported that it made up 28% of such tumors in his series. It is generally a tumor of adolescents and, occasionally, young adults. Secondary osteosarcomas can occur following radiation therapy for other tumors, in Paget's disease, and, rarely, in fibrous dysplasia in the older age group (150).
   c. The next most common type is chondrosarcoma which makes up approximately 13% of malignant bone tumors (61). Chondrosarcomas may be primary, but also occur as secondary malignancies developing in pre-existing benign lesions, such as the enchondroma or osteochondroma. In multiple forms of these lesions such as enchondromatosis (Ollier's disease) or hereditary multiple exostoses, the incidence of malignant transformation of one or more lesions can be as high as 15% to 25% (122).
   d. Fibrosarcoma primary in bone is rare less than 4% of primary malignant bone tumors (87). Malignant fibrous histiocytoma, a tumor similar in behavior to fibrosarcoma, is occasionally associated with bone infarctions or previous therapeutic irradiation to bone. It is rare as a primary sarcoma in bone, and is seen much more commonly as a soft tissue sarcoma (6,43).
   e. "Round cell tumors," which include primary lymphomas of bone, Ewing's sarcoma, and metastatic neuroblastoma, are discussed elswhere. Ewing's sarcoma, a relatively common primary bone tumor of childhood, comprises about 7% of all bone tumors (125).
   f. Giant cell tumors generally arise in the metaphysis or epiphysis of long bones in young adults, most commonly about the knee; they account for 4.5% of bone tumors. The majority of these lesions are classified as aggressive benign tumors, but a small percentage (about 7%) are malignant lesions. Malignant giant cell tumor is most commonly seen in the context of previous radiation treatment for a benign

giant cell tumor. It has been estimated that as many as 10% of irradiated benign giant cell tumors may ultimately demonstrate malignant transformation (6).

g. Most malignant lesions in bone (60% to 65%) are metastatic. Frequently, patients may present with a lesion in bone as the initial manifestation of carcinoma, and in some of such cases a primary site cannot be found (3). Metastatic carcinoma is encountered most frequently in the spine and pelvis; it becomes less frequent as the anatomic site becomes farther from the trunk. Metastatic bone lesions distal to the elbow or the knee are extremely rare, but are found more often in the foot than in the hand (7). In fact, the primary tumor associated most frequently with these distal or acral metastases is lung carcinoma (6). Other primary tumors commonly associated with bony metastases are breast, prostate, kidney, and thyroid (16).

Etiology

1. The observation of the high incidence in children supports the assumption that skeletal neoplasms arise in areas of rapid growth (1). In addition, the most common location of primary bone sarcomas is metaphyseal, near the growth plate. This is the region in the bone with the most intense cellular proliferation and remodeling activity during long-bone growth. The highest incidence is in the distal femur and proximal tibia, the two areas with the most active growth plates. Figure 26-1 (71) indicates the relative anatomic origins of the more common types of bone tumors.

2. Prolonged growth or overstimulated metabolism may blend imperceptibly with neoplasia. This may be seen in neoplasms arising in adult tissues affected by metabolic stimulation from long-standing Paget's disease (giant cell tumors or osteosarcomas), hyperparathyroidism (brown tumors), chronic osteomyelitis (squamous cell carcinomas and osteosarcomas), old bone infarcts (malignant fibrous histiocytoma), and fracture callus (3).

3. Certain developmental anomalies and benign tumors are prone to malignant transformation, as mentioned above for multiple exostoses and enchondromatosis.

4. Radiation has been linked to the formation of osteogenic sarcomas, chondrosarcomas, and fibrosarcomas as a result of both radiation treatment and internal bone-seeking radioisotopes from occupational and medicinal use (89a,119a).

5. The role of infectious agents, particularly in osteogenic sarcoma, has been suggested based on laboratory observations, i.e., induction of osteosarcomas in mice and chicks by extracts from human osteosarcomas (45). However, for most bone sarcomas it is generally felt that the cause may be multifactorial, that is, dependent on a combination of etiologic lesions for expression of neoplasia

6. A consistent cytogenic marker in Ewing's sarcoma of the bone is an 11:22 translocation (9b).

DETECTION AND DIAGNOSIS

Clinical Detection

1. Patients generally present with pain in the area of the lesion. The pain tends not to be activity-related, as with many types of musculoskeletal problems, and commonly may be worse at night. In more advanced lesions, patients may note a mass or swelling (generally only if there is significant periosteal reaction or the tumor has eroded through the bony cortex), and may occasionally

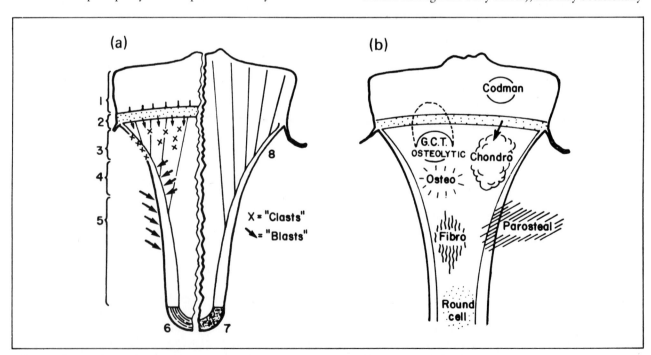

Fig. 26-1. The relationship of modeling processes to bone tumors. (A) Cross section of growing longbone illustrates the geographic distribution of osteoclasts and osteoblasts. Five zones of endochondral growth: epiphysis, growth plate/physics, subadjacet half of metaphysis, diaphyseal half of metaphysis, diaphysis. (B) Corresponding bone tumors in different sites to illustrate possible modeling aberrations. G.C.T. = Giant cell tumor; Codman = Codman's tumor. From Johnson (71), with permission.

present with a pathologic fracture. If the lesion is near a joint, a sympathetic effusion or stiffness of the joint also may occur. Occasionally, symptoms distant from the primary site may occur either by pain referral patterns (such as a hip lesion, which may present with pain referred to the knee), or by nerve compression that causes distal neurologic symptoms. Systemic or constitutional symptoms such as weight loss, fevers, malaise, or night sweats are quite uncommon with most bone sarcomas, but occur more commonly with Ewing's sarcoma, or in cases with multiple metastases at the time of presentation.

2. The history is extremely important for a number of reasons. A past history of carcinoma may suggest a metastatic etiology of a new bone lesion, while previous radiation treatment to an area may suggest a postradiotherapy sarcoma. Also, a long history (years) of symptoms from a bone lesion may indicate a benign nature, such as an osteoid osteoma, while symptoms that rapidly progress over weeks or a few months would signify a higher likelihood of a malignant process. In patients with known cartilaginous lesions, e.g., enchondroma or osteochondroma, occurrence of further growth in adulthood, or pain, may be an early indication of malignant transformation. Due to the possibility of sampling error in a biopsy of such a lesion, suspicious or symptomatic cartilage tumors should be treated by complete excision.

3. Early detection is extremely difficult; due to the rarity of primary bone tumors, presentation as an incidental finding on a diagnostic x-ray is unusual. Generally, the presence of pain initiates evaluation for a bone tumor, and pain is usually present early in the course of a malignant bone lesion. As most of these tumors progress rapidly, incidental discovery of these lesions is not common.

Diagnostic Procedures (Table 26-1)

1. Roentgenograms are the single most important diagnostic tool for diagnosis and prognosis of bone tumors. A number of roentgenographic parameters are considered in evaluation of a bone lesion, and influence the

Table 26-1. Imaging Modalities for Evaluation of Bone Cancer

METHOD	DIAGNOSIS AND STAGING CAPABILITY	RECOMMENDED FOR USE
Primary tumor and regional nodes		
CT	Useful to stage tumor locally for medullary and soft tissue extension as well as presence of matrix or cortical disruption	Yes; essential in planning limb conservation surgery
MRI	Applications at present are speculative. Main use with soft tissue rather than bone tumors	No
Conventional roentgenograms	High sensitivity and specificity for primary bone tumors; lower sensitivity and specificity for metastatic lesions in bone	Yes; metastases tend to involve medullary canal and must be > 1 cm to be detected
Angiography	Seldom useful except to serve as a vascular road map for surgery	No (yes, if considering limb salvage and clear margin from tumor not demonstrated by CT); essential if embolic or infusion therapy contemplated
Metastatic evaluation		
Chest roentgenograms	Essential for all tumor types	Yes
Film tomography	Useful to characterize questionable plain film findings	No
CT of lungs	Use in high-risk patient group where treatment decisions hinge on presence or absence of lung metastases	Yes
Radionuclide bone scan	Essential to determine if bone lesion is monostotic or polyostotic	Yes

CT = computed tomography; MRI = magnetic resonance imaging.

differential diagnosis. Radiographic patterns of bone destruction have been classified by Lodwick (5,79a), correlating with pathologic tumor aggressiveness.

  a. Lesions may be lytic (destroying bone) or blastic (either forming bone or inducing reactive bone formation). Osteosarcoma would be an example of a blastic, bone-forming tumor.

  b. With regard to lytic areas, a bone tumor may demonstrate several different patterns of bone destruction (5,70). Geographic lesions demonstrate a circumscribed area of bone destruction, without extension of the tumor beyond the radiographically evident lesion border. This implies a slower growth rate and typically would be seen with a lower-grade tumor such as a giant cell tumor, or a low-grade secondary chondrosarcoma.

  c. A "moth-eaten" pattern represents a more aggressive stage of bone involvement, with multiple lytic areas and, frequently, cortical destruction. The tumor extends within the bone beyond the radiographically evident lytic areas. This suggests an intermediate rate of growth.

  d. A permeative pattern implies extremely rapid and infiltrative growth, with diffuse areas of lytic destruction invading the bone. Permeative lesions are often associated with cortical disruption and extraosseous soft tissue mass.

  e. Periosteal reactions can be of several types (6). A "sunburst" periosteal reaction implies very proliferative malignant bone formation, and is characteristic of a classic osteosarcoma. Codman's triangle refers to the raised normal periosteum at the margin of a bone tumor associated with reactive periosteal new bone formation: it can be seen with a variety of malignant bone tumors. A lamellar periosteal reaction ("onion skin") implies rapid cyclic tumor growth, and is most classically associated with Ewing's sarcoma, although it is not specific for this tumor. Spiculated periosteal reactions also occur in aggressive, rapidly-growing tumors such as Ewing's sarcoma, and represent reactive periosteal bone being deposited along periosteal vessels as the expanding tumor stretches the periosteum.

2. Computed tomographic (CT) scans are extremely helpful in establishing the extent of the tumor within the bone, and in determining the presence of any extraosseus soft tissue mass. The CT can also help to delineate the three-dimensional anatomy of the lesion; this can be essential to planning either surgical biopsy or definitive treatment. One of the most important strengths of CT scanning compared to other modalities such as magnetic resonance imaging (MRI) scanning is the ability to assess even subtle degrees of cortical destruction quite accurately. This can be especially helpful in the case of secondary chondrosarcomas where focal cortical destruction may be key to differentiating a benign from a malignant lesion. Additionally, CT with contrast delineates very accurately the anatomic relationship between pelvic tumors and the bowel and ureters.

3. MRI is an alternative to CT scanning, and has replaced CT in many cases. Particularly in the case of highly malignant bone tumors with cortical destruction and a soft tissue mass, MRI shows with highly accurate detail the relationship between normal tissues and neurovascular structures and the tumor tissue. This is essential in planning surgical biopsy or treatment (16a). In addition, extent of the reactive zone of the tumor within the bone is also visualized with high sensitivity, as even edema of the marrow adjacent to tumor tissue is apparent. Newer techniques that use paramagnetic enhancing agents, such as gadolinium, also show promise in further delineating differences between normal and neoplastic tissue (146), but to date diagnostic specificity of MRI in differentiating benign from malignant lesions or indicating histogenic tumor type is limited.

4. Radionuclide imaging using technetium 99 (bone scan) has become an essential part of bone tumor evaluation. Although bone scans lack specificity for neoplasms, the studies are extremely sensitive, and can detect tumor foci in bone not visualized on standard radiographs. Thus, the extent of a tumor within a bone, including the reactive zone and the presence of skip metastases, can be demonstrated accurately. Also, although they are extremely uncommon, distant bony metastases can be identified. Bone scan results are frequently negative in multiple myeloma, however, and may underestimate the extent of disease with this particular tumor.

5. Angiography is no longer used as commonly in staging work-up due to the increasing use of CT with contrast or MRI, which accurately delineate the location of major vessels in their relationship to the primary tumor. However, in pelvic lesions, angiography is quite useful in defining the locations of the major vessels, and in neoplasms with excessive vascularity can facilitate embolization prior to biopsy or definitive surgical treatment to decrease intraoperative blood loss.

6. Laboratory studies have limited usefulness in bone sarcoma evaluation. Alkaline phosphatase concentration may be elevated, particularly in osteosarcoma, and is at extremely high levels in the secondary osteosarcoma of Paget's disease. Metastatic prostatic carcinoma can be excluded by lack of elevated levels of acid phosphatase or absence of prostatic specific antigen. Multiple myeloma can be diagnosed by serum protein electrophoresis if a significant level of abnormal immunoglobulin is present; serum immunoelectrophoresis is a more sensitivity test to detect a monoclonal gammopathy, and presence of light chains in the urine by Bence Jones testing or immunoelectrophoresis also can be helpful. The white blood cell count, differential, and sedimentation rate may be useful to exclude osteomyelitis, which can frequently mimic a primary bone tumor. The sedimentation rate may also be elevated in myeloma, Ewing's sarcoma, and bone, lymphomas, but generally not to the high levels seen in osteomyelitis. Hypercalcemia may suggest myeloma or disseminated metastatic disease, and can also be present in brown tumors of hyperparathyroidism, although with this lesion there is associated hypophosphatemia as well.

7. Biopsy obviously is essential in the diagnosis of any primary bone neoplasm. The biopsy should not be performed until staging studies such as CT, MRI, and bone scan evaluations of the local extent of the lesion have been completed (2). The accurate localization of

the lesion prior to biopsy facilitates placement of an appropriate biopsy site that will not subsequently interfere with resection of the tumor; compartmental contamination by the biopsy procedure also can be minimized. In general, biopsy sites should be placed so that major neurovascular structures are not encountered during the procedure. Any incision on the extremities should be longitudinal so that the biopsy tract or incision, along with at least 1 cm of skin and subcutaneous tissue on all sides, can be excised en bloc with the specimen during subsequent definitive surgery. The area of the tumor chosen for biopsy is also critical. The periphery of the lesion, where the interface between the tumor and normal tissues can be assessed, will generally provide the best assessment. This is because osteosarcomas and other bone sarcomas tend to demonstrate less differentiated characteristics peripherally, whereas central areas may contain more differentiated bone formation or necrosis. This procedure is also helpful in differentiating myositis ossificans from an osteosarcoma, which it can radiographically resemble in some cases. In myositis, the lesion tends to be most mature and differentiated at the periphery and more cellular and proliferative centrally (8). Additionally, if a bony defect exists in the cortex, biopsy should be performed at this site rather than making any additional surgical defect in the bone that could weaken it and predispose to pathologic fracture. Presence of a pathologic fracture in the extremities leads to contamination of multiple compartments and usually precludes limb-salvage procedures. Meticulous hemostasis always must be maintained after surgical biopsy to prevent hematoma from seeding additional tissue planes. Use of a drain tract placed in line with the biopsy incision and quite near it to facilitate its subsequent excision may also minimize hematoma formation. Another useful technique is packing of the biopsy defect in the bone with methyl methacrylate cement to stop any bleeding from the bone. Finally, a frozen section always should be obtained to be sure there is adequate

tissue for definitive diagnosis; however, permanent sections generally are needed for final diagnosis on which to base definitive therapy. Because of the reaction of normal bone and periosteal elements to the lesion, sampling error is a potential problem and can make diagnosis difficult. For this reason incisional biopsy is preferred by many, although needle biopsies are also effective and can achieve diagnostic accuracy of 70% to 90% at institutions with considerable experience with this technique (10,32).

CLASSIFICATION AND STAGING

Definitions

A primary bone cancer is any neoplasm that arises from the tissues or cells present within bone, and has the capability of producing metastases. As many types of cells are present within the medullary space of bone and adjacent to the bone surface, a number of histologic tumor types are possible, including tumors derived from osteoblasts, cartilage cells, fat, fibrous tissue, vascular elements, and hematopoietic and neural tissues. All these tumor types are referred to as sarcomas, a term that signifies a common derivation from mesenchymal tissues.

Bone sarcomas are named in relation to the predominant differentiated tissue type, although obviously multiple cellular elements may be present in any given tumor. Bone-forming tumors are referred to as osteosarcomas, cartilage tumors as chondrosarcomas, fibroblastic tumors as fibrosarcomas, fat-forming tumors as liposarcomas, and tumors derived from vascular elements as angiosarcomas. Table 26-2 (48a,89b) demonstrates the classification and incidence of various benign and malignant bone tumors in a large series from the Mayo Clinic (1).

Anatomic Staging

A anatomic staging system using the tumor, node, metastasis (TNM) parameters has not been formalized by the American Joint Committee on Cancer Staging and End-Results Reporting (AJC) as yet, although some TNM staging guidelines

---

Table 26-2. General Classification of Bone Tumors

Histologic Type*	(%)	Benign	Malignant
Hematopoietic	41.4		Myeloma
			Reticulum cell sarcoma
Chondrogenic	20.9	Osteochondroma	Primary chondrosarcoma
		Chondroma	Secondary chondrosarcoma
		Chondroblastoma	Dedifferentiated chondrosarcoma
		Chondromyxoid fibroma	Mesenchymal chondrosarcoma
Osteogenic	19.3	Osteoid osteoma	Osteosarcoma
		Benign osteoblastoma	Parosteal osteogenic sarcoma
Unknown origin	9.8	Giant cell tumor	Ewing's tumor
			Malignant giant cell tumor
			Adamantinoma
		(Fibrous) histiocytoma	(Fibrous) histiocytoma
Fibrogenic	3.8	Fibroma	Fibrosarcoma
		Desmoplastic fibroma	
Notochordal	3.1		Chordoma
Vascular	1.6	Hemangioma	Hemangioendothelioma, hemangiopericyoma
Lipogenic	<0.5	Lipoma	
Neurogenic	<0.5	Neurilemoma	

*Distribution based on Mayo Clinic experience.
From Fraumeni (48a) and Miller (89b), with permission.

have been suggested. Table 26-3 (2a) shows the suggested AJC guidelines for staging (Fig. 26-2). The Musculoskeletal Tumor Society (MTS) also has developed a surgical staging system for bone tumors that correlates very well with prognosis and is widely used by orthopedic oncologists. The MTS staging system is based on the concept of compartmental localization of the tumor (Table 26-4). Compartments are comprised of bone, musculofascial envelopes such as the muscular compartments of the extremities, joints, skin and subcutaneous tissues, and neurovascular sheaths (39). Involvement of more than one compartment leads to placement in a higher surgical stage and correlates with poorer prognosis. Thus, the anatomic (T) parameter is similar in both staging systems: T1 is within the bone (intracompartmental) and T2 indicates extension beyond the cortex of the bone. Spread of bone tumors to lymph nodes is rare; the usual pattern is hematogenous spread to pulmonary and other sites. In addition, distant metastases carry a similar poor prognosis whether the metastasis is to regional nodes or to the lung. Because of this, the MTS staging system does not differentiate N1 or M1, and nodal or other metastases place the patient in stage III. In this regard, the two staging systems differ. Finally, tumor grade is limited to G1 and G2 (low grade or high grade) in the MTS system, as opposed to G1 to G4 in the AJC system, due to frequent disagreement among pathologists on specific grading of tumors, particularly with intermediate-grade lesions (2,101). There is a good correlation with survival data for bone sarcomas versus the surgical stage, demonstrating the effectiveness of the MTS system for prognostication (2).

Staging Work-up

To place a patient in a given surgical stage of disease, a comprehensive evaluation for disease extent is necessary. This has important ramifications not only for prognosis, but also in evaluating treatment options.

1. Recommended procedures: (18a,34a,80a)
   a. Conventional radiographs of the involved bone are mandatory, and are the single most important diagnostic aid prior to biopsy. Oblique or magnification views may occasionally be needed, and tomograms may be helpful in selected cases, although these have been largely replaced by more sophisticated imaging techniques such as MRI and CT scanning.

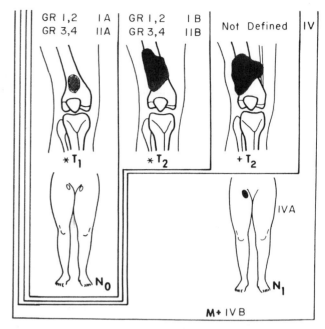

Fig. 26-2. Anatomic staging of bone cancer (see Table 26-3). G = grade; T = tumor; N = node; M = metastasis.

b. CT scanning demonstrates soft tissue extension of the lesion and is important in determining if the lesion is anatomically T1 or T2. In particular, CT is excellent in determining if there is any disruption of the bony cortex. However, assessment of extension into soft tissue planes or near major neurovascular structures is better accomplished with MRI scanning.

c. MRI scans demonstrate with great precision the exact anatomic extent of any soft tissue components and the relationship to other anatomic structures. This modality also demonstrates clearly the reactive zone of the tissue, as edema in the marrow or soft tissues is also evident (16a). Subtle marrow changes indicative of skip metastases can be readily visualized. The only shortcoming of MRI has been the inability to distinguish benign tumors from infec-

---

Table 26-3.   TNM Classification Summary and Stage Grouping for Bone Tumors

TNM Classification		Stage Grouping			
T1	Within cortex	**Stage IA**	G1,2	T1	N0	M0
T2	Beyond cortex	**Stage IB**	G1,2	T2	N0	M0
		Stage IIA	G3,4	T1	N0	M0
N1	Regional	**Stage IIB**	G3,4	T2	N0	M0
		Stage III	Not defined			
G1	Well differentiated	**Stage IVA**	Any G	Any T	N1	M0
G2	Moderately differentiated	**Stage IVB**	Any G	Any T	Any N	M1
G3	Poorly differentiated					
G4	Undifferentiated					

T = tumor; N = node; M = metastasis; G = grade.
From UICC (2a), with permission.

Table 26-4. Stages of Malignant Musculoskeletal Lesions

	IA	IB	IIA	IIB	IIIA	IIIB
Grade	G1	G1	G2	G2	G1-2	G1-2
Site	T1	T2	T1	T2	T1	T2
Metastasis	M0	M0	M0	M0	M1	M1
Clinical course	Symptomatic indolent growth	Symptomatic mass indolent growth	Symptomatic rapid growth	Symptomatic rapid growth fixed mass pathologic fracture	Systemic symptoms palpable nodes pulmonary symptoms	
Isotope scan	Increased uptake	Increased uptake	Increased uptake beyond radiographic limits	Increased uptake beyond radiographic limits	Pulmonary lesions no increased uptake	
Radiographic grade	II	II	III	III	III	
Angiogram	Modest neovascular reaction, involvement neurovascular bundle	Modest neovascular reaction, involvement of neurovascular bundle	Marked neovascular reaction - no involvement of neurovascular bundle	Marked neovascular reaction - involvement neurovascular bundle	Hypervascular lymph nodes	
CT	Irregular or broached capsule but intracompartmental	Extracompartmental extension or location	Broached (pseudo) capsule - intracompartmental	Broached (pseudo) capsule - extracompartmental	Pulmonary lesions or enlarged nodes	

CT = computed tomography; G = grade; T = tumor; M = metastasis.

tions or malignant lesions, or its lack of diagnostic specificity. However, increasing experience with this imaging modality, newer software techniques, and enhancing agents such as gadolinium (146) has not yet, but may, significantly improve diagnostic accuracy in the near future. In studies comparing MRI, CT, and radionuclide scan with proven histologic sections, MRI is consistently more accurate: 99%, 86%, and 56%, respectively. Soft tissue involvement can be overestimated secondary to hematoma, reactive edema and inflammatory response.

d. Arteriography has largely been replaced by MRI as a means of delineating the tumor location with respect to the major vessels. Arteriography is useful for pelvic lesions or for preoperative embolization of tumors judged to be highly vascular.

e. Radionuclide bone scanning is essential to further evaluate the extent of the lesion within the bone of origin, as well as to rule out skip metastases or distant bony metastases. This is particularly important with Ewing's sarcoma or lymphomas (133). If multiple myeloma is suspected, a skeletal survey of standard radiographs is indicated because this lesion is often not detected on the scan (123), but this is the only lesion in which the skeletal survey is routinely useful.

f. Chest x-ray is essential, and if positive should be followed up with a chest CT scan to detect any small metastases. If surgery is done (i.e., for biopsy), the chest CT should be obtained, preferably before surgery or otherwise at least 1 week after surgery, to allow resolution of any postsurgical atelectasis that might be misinterpreted as metastatic disease.

g. Laboratory studies should include complete blood cell count and, serum enzyme measurement, including alkaline phosphatase. Serum electrophoresis is included if myeloma is a possibility. Sedimentation rate may help to rule out an infectious process.

h. If sarcoma is suspected, it is essential to obtain consultations with the orthopedic radiologist, radiation oncologist, medical oncologist, and bone pathologist. The team approach to evaluation and treatment is extremely valuable in this group of diseases. The consultations should be done, whenever possible, before any surgery is undertaken, even for biopsy.

PRINCIPLES OF TREATMENT

Nonmalignant tumors are best removed surgically by the most direct route possible. Large defects in the bone are filled with suitable bone grafts, and occasionally protective internal fixation may be needed to prevent fracture or to stabilize a pathologic fracture. Intralesional resection (generally curettage), or, occasionally, marginal resection is generally adequate for treatment of these lesions. Marginal resection is preferred to curettage for more aggressive benign tumors such as chondromyxoid fibroma, juxtacortical chondroma, giant cell tumor, and aneurysmal bone cyst. Radiation treatment to benign tumors may eradicate the lesion but radiation doses to bone and cartilage have a high potential for late malignant change, both in the lesional tissue and in the normal surrounding bone (20). For this reason, radiotherapy to benign lesions in bone is limited to surgically inaccessible tumors or lesions that are responsive to very low doses of radiation, such as aneurysmal bone cysts in difficult surgical locations and eosinophilic granuloma (58,70,86,93).

Malignant tumors are managed best by a combination of surgery, radiotherapy, and chemotherapy (37,83,126,128), although this is strongly dependent on the tumor type (Table 26-5). Lower-grade sarcomas (MTS stage I) are almost always treated with definitive surgery alone, and results often depend largely on the adequacy of the resection margins. Such tumors include secondary chondrosarcomas arising in enchondromas or osteochondromas, and parosteal osteosarcomas. Central high-grade osteosarcoma is usually treated with surgery and adjuvant chemotherapy, while Ewing's sarcoma may be treated with irradiation and chemotherapy with surgery as the adjuvant treatment (120). In those tumors for which more limited data are available, the role of local radiation therapy and adjuvant chemotherapy is still controversial. A concise tabulation of multidisciplinary decisions in managing osteogenic sarcomas and Ewing's sarcoma is seen in Table 26-5.

Surgery

There is a shift from radical surgical amputation of a limb, which often included the joint above the tumor as well as the entire bone, to more conservative surgery. Limb-salvage surgery may allow better function and cosmesis without compromise of local control or survival (83,128). Improvements in imaging methods have allowed better preoperative assessment of disease extent, facilitating assessment of patient suitability for limb-sparing surgery. In addition, development of new techniques of limb reconstruction such as custom prosthetic implants, allograft, and free vascularized tissue transfers, along with advances in radiotherapy, have made limb salvage an increasingly available treatment option.

1. *Surgical definitions*: For consistency in evaluation of the surgical aspects of tumor treatment, some definitions have been proposed by the MTS (2,39). These definitions pertain to the anatomic extent and types of surgical procedures that are done, and provide a common ground for judging the efficacy of a given surgical treatment. Tumor resection margins are named similarly to the corresponding surgical procedure. An intralesional margin or surgical procedure means gross macroscopic tumor is left behind. This would generally be associated with incisional biopsy for diagnosis of a malignant lesion, or a curettage of a known benign lesion. A marginal resection or "marginal margin" indicates that the resection plane goes through the reactive zone of the tumor, allowing the possibility of residual microscopic disease within this zone. A wide resection or margin refers to removal of a tumor en bloc with normal tissue surrounding its reactive zone in all planes. The amount of normal tissue considered to constitute a wide margin varies greatly, depending on the location and tissue types. For instance, a resection through bone is generally considered to be wide if the resection level is 5 to 7 cm above the reactive zone of the lesion, whereas a layer of fascia from a muscular compartment might constitute a wide margin because of its efficacy as an anatomic barrier even though the tissue may be only a few millimeters thick. Finally, a radical surgical procedure (or margin) refers to a situation in which all structures in every compartment involved by the tumor are removed in their entirety. For a bone tumor this means, at the minimum, removal of the entire bone involved; any compartments with soft tissue extension would also have to be removed. Amputation nomenclature is identical, and therefore an amputation may be intralesional, marginal, wide, or radical depending on the level with regard to the above definitions. Figure 26-3 illustrates diagrammatically this scheme.

Table 26-5. Multidisciplinary Treatment Decisions for Bone Tumors   (2,6,96a,96b)

Stage	Surgery	Radiation Therapy	Chemotherapy
Multiple myeloma	NR	PRT 20-30 Gy	MAC*
Solitary myeloma	NR	CRT 50 Gy	NR
Osteogenic sarcoma	Conservation surgery or amputation	NR	MAC**
Ewing's sarcoma	Biopsy of soft tissue component Resection of tumor if possible or	CRT 50-60 Gy	MAC*** as VACA
Chondrosarcoma	amputation	If residuum postop	NR
	Biopsy	ART 60-70 Gy	
Histiocytic or NHL		DRT 45-50 Gy	and MAC**** as CHOP
	Resection if possible		NR
Giant cell tumor		DRT 50 Gy for central axial	
(malignant)	Conservative resection		NR
Parosteal osteosarcoma		NR	

RT = radiation therapy; ART = adjuvant; PRT = palliative; CRT = curative; DRT = definitive; NR = not recommended; MAC = multiagent chemotherapy.

PDQ: NR - MAC*   for MM - CYT + PRED

MAC**   for OS - high dose methotrexate, doxorubicin, bleomycin, cyclophosphamide, actinomycin D - CISPT,IFOS,VCR

MAC***   for Ewing's - VACA/IFOS + etoposide

MAC****   for NHL - CHOP

2. *Local control* can be achieved in 90% of patients with osteogenic sarcomas through careful selection of the level of amputation (144). While some authors have recommended radical disarticulation (2), a wide amputation is generally considered to be acceptable if careful preoperative evaluation discloses no evidence of skip metastases. Bone scans should be used to detect skip areas; a margin of at least 7 to 10 cm above the proximal extension of tumor is recommended. In addition, MRI may show subtle marrow abnormalities indicative of skip lesions, and should be included for preoperative assessment of the intraosseous extent of disease.

3. *Limb-sparing surgery* frequently may be an option but must fulfill certain requirements (Fig. 26-3). First, the level of function after surgical and adjuvant treatment must be considered, and the patient considered a candidate for limb salvage only if function of the extremity will equal or exceed function with a prosthetic limb after ablative surgery. In young children, limb salvage often is not an option because of the severe growth inhibition that results from the adjuvant radiation treatment, which renders the limb nonfunctional by the time of skeletal maturity. Preservation of major nerves and blood vessels must be feasible, and a wide margin (normal tissues or tissue planes removed in contiguity with the lesion in all directions) must be achievable. Finally, a relative factor is the availability of an effective adjuvant therapy for a given tumor type.

   a. Presurgical systemic chemotherapy leads to a high degree of tumor sterilization with some tumor types such as osteosarcoma (109,116,117). This may facilitate conservative surgery by shrinking a tumor mass away from major neurovascular structures; it also allows evaluation of the responsiveness of the tumor to the chemotherapeutic regimen and may therefore alter the subsequent protocol.

   b. Intra-arterial perfusion of chemotherapeutic agents, e.g., doxorubicin, and preoperative radiation treatment for radiosensitive tumors can also facilitate limb-sparing surgery (38,40,68).

4. *Reconstructive techniques* may allow replacement of large skeletal defects by any of several methods.

   a. Resection arthrodesis of a large joint such as the knee joint may be accomplished using sliding local bone or distant autogenous grafts with internal fixation devices (42). Similar procedures can be done for tumors about the hip or shoulder girdle.

   b. Cadaveric allografts are available in many situations; they can be used to replace all or part of a bone or joint, generally in combination with some form of internal fixation (40,54,81,82).

   c. Prosthetic bone and joint replacement with computer-designed custom metallic implants of titanium or stainless steel alloys provides another method of limb reconstruction. With the advent of porous ingrowth fixation systems, there has been decreased risk of long-term prosthetic loosening and failure. Consequently, these devices are being used increasingly in orthopedic oncology (40,74). Additionally, an expandable prosthesis has been developed for use in growing children, allowing sequential limb lengthening to simulate growth (54).

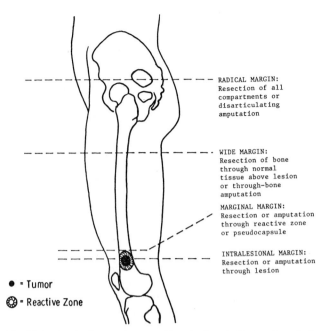

Fig. 26-3. Surgical procedures and terminology in the treatment of osteosarcoma: limb preservation.

5. *Contraindications to limb salvage* include invasion of major regional nerves or major blood vessels, or pathologic fractures (2), in which the resulting hematoma will contaminate many tissue planes and compartments.

6. *Internal hemipelvectomy* offers a method of resecting all or part of the hemipelvis while retaining a limb with some level of function, and may be applicable to many pelvic sarcomas. A number of reconstructive techniques can be used to enhance the function of the remaining extremity, including fusion of the femur to the remaining portion of the pelvis or sacrum, creation of a pseudarthrosis, or reconstruction with allografts and/or prosthetic devices (2,40,41,130).

7. *Surgical removal of pulmonary metastases* has been used with some success in some types of sarcoma (113).

Radiation Therapy

Historically, radiation therapy has not been the primary treatment modality in the treatment of most bone tumors. While radiation therapy is used almost exclusively for plasma cell tumors, metastatic tumors, and reticulum cell sarcomas, tumors such as osteogenic sarcoma, fibrosarcoma, and chondrosarcoma are relatively radioresistant. The amount of radiation and the size of the treatment portal necessary for treatment of bone tumors is dictated primarily by the histology of the tumor. Doses in the range of 10 to 40 Gy are required for adequate local control and palliation of tumors such as lymphomas, multiple myeloma, metastatic carcinomas, and leukemias, while osteogenic sarcomas, chondrosarcomas, Ewing's sarcoma, fibrosarcomas, and solitary plasmacytoma and reticulum cell sarcomas require higher doses (50 to 70 Gy) with prolonged fractionated-treatment schedules.

Limb preservation is an important aspect of radiation treatment. Radiation has been used alone, preoperatively, or postoperatively in the treatment of bone tumors, depending on the tumor histology. Multimodality treatment is used now because of new surgical techniques and chemotherapeutic agents available. The technical aspects of high-dose radiation therapy in the treatment of bone tumors are similar to those in the treatment of soft tissue sarcomas. Important points of limb preservation include sparing a strip of soft tissue to better preserve lymphatic drainage if possible, accurate delineation of the tumor volume with CT scans or MRI, and using shrinking field techniques to limit the high-dose treatment volume to as small a volume as possible. Management differs with each tumor type; therefore, discussion will be along histopathologic categories. The two major tumors, osteogenic sarcoma and Ewing's tumor, will be discussed as illustrations of a radioresistant and a radiosensitive tumor, respectively. The other tumor types will be presented under special considerations.

Osteogenic sarcoma: Osteogenic sarcoma is not a homogeneous pathologic entity but occurs in all age groups, at different locations in the bone, and in a number of anatomic sites. Osteogenic sarcoma in the mandible, for example, has a much better prognosis than if it presented in the femur (25,50). (This section will not deal with osteogenic sarcoma developing in patients with Paget's disease or in previously irradiated areas). Huvos *et al.* (63-65), have reviewed the Memorial Hospital for Cancer and Allied Diseases New York, New York experience with the former group of patients.

1. *Osteogenic sarcoma* is a relatively radioresistant tumor in which the exact mechanism of radiation resistance is unknown. Theories have been proposed to explain the relative radioresistance, ranging from the osteosarcoma possessing a broad shoulder on cell survival curves, to having a large capacity to repair sublethal damage, or having slow or inadequate reoxygenation of hypoxic compartments after irradiation (107,143,145). Phillips and Sheline (96), among others (139), as early as 1969 showed that doses in the order of 100 Gy are required for complete eradication of osteogenic sarcoma cells in pathologic specimens. Yanguas (151), however, found that osteogenic sarcoma is relatively radioresistant, with sterilization of pathologic specimens occurring when moderate doses of radiation are given in a short period or with higher doses if the time is prolonged longer than 40 days.

2. *Preoperative irradiation:* Surgical management along with chemotherapy has been the treatment of choice for osteogenic sarcoma, with radiation therapy given preoperatively or to patients unable to undergo definitive surgical resection because of medical contraindications to surgery or the location of the primary (9,21,31,47a,119,132). Pre-operative irradiation was used initially to shrink the primary tumor, followed by surgery 6 months later (9,21,31,121,132). This method of treatment was used to select for surgery those patients who did not develop pulmonary metastases (Cade technique) (22). Radiation doses used preoperatively ranged from 50 to 100 Gy (19). Five-year survival ranged from 23% to 60% (9,21,31,47a,119,121,132). Most series reported, however, are retrospective studies of patients treated over long periods with different treatment techniques. New reports have focused on combining infusional chemotherapy, doxorubicin or bromodeoxyuridine, with irradiation either pre-operatively or for inoperable tumors (34,55,85,144). Significant soft tissue toxicity has been reported in a number

of studies, forcing the investigators to modify the irradiation schedule.

3. *Dose:* Treatment with irradiation alone with doses ranging from 65 to 100 Gy has not been successful (16,19,31,75). Lee and Mackenzie (75) had 7 of 20 patients surviving at 5 years while Berg *et al.* (16), reported on 0 of 8 patients surviving at 5 years (78).

Ewing's sarcoma:

1. Volume considerations are essential for radiation treatment planning for Ewing's tumor. With the introduction of MRI and CT, excellent volumetric definition in three-dimension of bone and the large soft tissue component is possible, with careful field shaping and beam's eye view. The need to treat entire bones, particularly extremities, is being reassessed with exclusion of growth plates at the opposite end of the bone from eccentric lesions to lessen late effects of growth. Although generous margins are used, sparing of medial skin and lymphatic strips is important to maintain lymphatic flow.

2. The dose range has been 50 to 60 Gy with successive cone changes to the 60 Gy level. Dose modification will depend on the role of surgery or the inaccessibility of the tumor. The site modifies dose since centrally located masses in the pelvis, abdomen, and chest limit full-dose irradiation. Eventually this is reflected in better local control for peripheral versus control lesions, i.e., distal extremity, 90%; proximal extremity, 75%; central lesions, 65% (136).

Neutron and Charged Particle Therapy

Three institutions have reported on their experience with neutron therapy for bone tumors (28,33,94,105). Cohen *et al.* (28), reported that chondrosarcomas were more responsive than osteogenic sarcomas, 56% versus 22% respectively. Their review of the world literature found 60% of the bone tumors treated were locally controlled (28). Bone tumors are thought to be radioresistant because they contain a significant hypoxic fraction or they have a high capacity to repair radiation damage (107,143,145). For this reason high-linear energy transfer radiation has been investigated in the treatment of bone tumors.

Chemotherapy

Recently, several important developments in the treatment of osteosarcoma and Ewing's sarcoma have led to the use of improved chemotherapy regimens. Unfortunately, there are many problems in the interpretation of results of clinical trials that form the basis of these advances. Pathologic subtype, selection bias, location of the primary tumor, the presence or absence of metastases, time of treatment, use of a small sample size, reporting of premature results, CT for identifying pulmonary metastases, and a trend toward better survival because of earlier diagnosis are all important variables in evaluating treatment outcome.

1. *Osteogenic sarcoma*: The primary treatment for metastatic unresectable osteosarcoma is chemotherapy. (Table 26-6) (18b). The most effective single agents, with 30% to 40% response rates are doxorubicin (29), cisplatin (13), and high-dose methotrexate with leucovorin rescue (67). Effective combinations include the addition of other agents to high dose methotrexate with leucovorin rescue (100), BCD (90) (bleomycin, cyclo-

Table 26-6. OSTEOSARCOMA CHEMOTHERAPY RESPONSE RATES

SINGLE AGENTS		COMBINATION		
Drug	Response Rate (%)	Drugs		Response Rate (%)
Cyclophosphamide	15	ADIC		39
Actinomycin D	15	VADIC		23
Melphalan	15	CYVADIC I and II		24
Mitomycin C	13	CYVADACT		25
		BLEO/CPA/ACD		64
CTIC	14	VCR/HDMTX-CF/ADR		54
Methotrexate - high dose with folinic acid rescue	38-82 *	VCR/HDMTX-CF/CPA/ADR		37-77
		ADM	Doxorubicin	
Doxorubicin		VCR	Vincristine	
	26	ACD	Actinomycin D	
		HDMTX/CF	High-dose methotrexate with folinic acid rescue	

* Depends on schedule
Adapted from Bramwell & Piredo (18b).

phosphamide, dacatinomycin) and doxorubicin/dacarbazine (57), which give response rates of 25% to 62% (80). Responses tend to be partial and short-lived. Various combinations of these programs have failed to produce significant additional improvement in the response rates of patients with metastatic disease (Table 26-6).

a. Postoperative adjuvant intravenous (IV) chemotherapy: Observation of some effect with these drugs has led to evaluation of chemotherapy as an adjuvant to primary surgery in localized disease. Perhaps the most important result of investigations during the past 5 years is the clear demonstration that chemotherapy can significantly prolong disease-free survival (DFS) and overall survival in patients with osteosarcoma when used in the adjuvant setting.

Long-term survival of patients with localized primary osteogenic sarcoma treated with traditional surgical management is very poor—only 20% to 25% of patients alive at 3-year follow-up (120). The cause of death is metastatic disease; 60% to 80% of patients have metastases only in the lungs (120). A decade ago, considerable controversy developed over these figures when the Mayo Clinic published a retrospective report indicating improvements in survival that were not related to therapy. They noted that between 1963 and 1974, their 3-year survival was 25%; between 1972 and 1974, however, it had improved to 50% with no significant change in therapy (134). A follow-up report confirmed these earlier findings. In the more recently treated patients, there was improvement in duration of survival to death, survival to detection of metastases, and survival from occurrence of metastases to death. No significant differences were found between those patients treated with amputation alone and those also treated with chemotherapy or radiation therapy (135).

Having challenged the validity of historic controls in evaluating adjuvant therapy for osteosarcoma, these findings spawned a generation of studies comparing no treatment, control arms with adjuvant and neoadjuvant chemotherapy. In one of the first such studies, a surgery-alone control was compared with the study group treated with adjuvant vincristine and high-dose methotrexate with leucovorin rescue. There was no difference in the estimated 5-year survival, which was 52% in both groups (28). Such a high survival rate in the control arm suggested that the significant improvement in survival reported for patients with osteosarcoma was caused by changes in the natural history of the disease, not by improvements in chemotherapy.

In contrast, two more recently reported studies (36,78) showed contrary results. At University of California, Los Angeles, a prospective randomized comparison was made between patients who received postsurgical adjuvant chemotherapy and those who received no adjuvant treatment. Chemotherapy consisted of a 6-week course of vincristine/high-dose methotrexate/leucovorin rescue/doxorubicin and BCD repeated four times in a complex schedule over 7 months. At a median follow-up of 2 years, the chemotherapy arm had a greater DFS (55% versus 20%) and overall survival (80% versus 48%) compared with the no-chemotherapy arm. Further, their comparison showed no difference between these control patients and their historical controls who had a 15% survival at a median follow-up of 2 years (36).

A second prospective randomized study, the Multi-Institutional Osteosarcoma Study, showed similar results. Chemotherapy consisted of a complex four-regimen treatment using six drug combinations: bleomycin/cyclophosphamide/dactinomycin/high- dose methotrexate with leucovorin rescue/doxorubicin/cisplatin given over 1 year. At 2 years, actuarial relapse-free survival was 17% in the control group and 66% in the adjuvant chemotherapy group. Again, there was no difference between these control patients and historic controls from the same institutions (78).

Notwithstanding the Mayo Clinic reports, these two latter studies constitute compelling evidence for the benefit of adjuvant chemotherapy in localized osteosarcoma. Additional reasons for possible improvement in survival unrelated to chemotherapy include better diagnostic and staging tools (with the advent of CT and MRI scans), earlier diagnosis with more rapid access to skilled medical care, and the use of thoracotomy for pulmonary metastases (127). The best chemotherapeutic regimen has not been identified, but these and other treatment schedules suggest a fairly consistent benefit, with 40% to 50% DFS at 2 years (56,80). The next generation of studies will need to compare different schedules to find the least toxic and most effective combinations.

b. Preoperative IV chemotherapy: An exciting new approach to adjuvant chemotherapy (dubbed "neoadjuvant") has been advocated by Rosen et al. (114). They treated primary osteogenic sarcoma with high-dose methotrexate and leucovorin calcium rescue, doxorubicin, and BCD for 4 to 16 weeks prior to definitive surgery. The effect of the preoperative chemotherapy was assessed according to the percentage of tumor necrosis in the resected specimen. Postoperatively, the patients with greater than 90% necrosis were continued on the same chemotherapy program. Forty-eight of 49 (98%) of such patients were disease-free at 7 to 51 months (median, 31 months) of follow-up. Of those patients with less than 90% necrosis who remained on the same chemotherapy protocol postoperatively, ten of 15 (66%) had relapsed at 4 to 19 months' (median, 13 months) follow-up. In this same group (less than 90% necrosis) only two of 29 (7%) who had a change of chemotherapy postoperatively from high-dose methotrexate to cisplatin (78) with mannitol diuresis had relapsed; both patients relapsed at 14 months' follow-up. Twenty-seven of 29 (93%) patients were continually disease-free at 6 to 29 months' (median, 18 months) follow-up.

Neoadjuvant therapy avoids any delay in systemic therapy, which would otherwise be necessitated by the postoperative recovery period. In addition, the appearance of the tumor at the time of operation is used to plan further treatment. Advocates proposed that if there was tumor shrinkage as a result of chemotherapy, less extensive surgery would be possible. In addition, the drugs' effectiveness could be evaluated by histopathologic examination of the tumor for cell necrosis. This information in turn would help with the postoperative selection of chemotherapy. The results of Rosen et al. (114) suggested that those patients who had responsive tumors could be continued with the same chemotherapy postoperatively. Thus, neoadjuvant chemotherapy followed by histologic examination can be used to guide postoperative therapy (114).

Other studies have confirmed the discriminating value of this approach. Eighty-five patients with nonmetastatic high-grade osteosarcoma of the extremity received IV high-dose methotrexate (HDMTX)/leucovorin rescue and intra-arterial cisplatin (CPDD) followed by definitive surgical resection. Preoperative chemotherapy permitted limb-salvage surgery for some patients who would have had an amputation if surgery had been done first. Chemotherapy can shrink the tumor away from vital neurovascular structures, facilitating limb salvage. Postoperative chemotherapy was selected based on the histologic evidence or tumor response at the time of primary surgery. Nonresponders were no longer treated with the preoperative regimen, and instead received doxorubicin (DOX) and bleomycin/cyclophosphamide/dactinomycin (BCD) for 45 weeks. Patients with sensitive tumors continued the preoperative drugs and also received the additional regimen used in the resistant group. Overall survival in the entire group was 55% at 1 to 3 years' follow-up. Responders to neoadjuvant chemotherapy had an 80% to 89% DFS compared with 20% for those with resistant disease (12).

More recently, a series of studies by the Cooperative German/Austrian Study Group (148) called into question the overall benefit of the neoadjuvant approach. A nonrandomized early study (COSS-77) used DOX,HDMTX/leucovorin rescue/vincristine and cyclophosphamide as single sequential drugs for adjuvant postoperative chemotherapy. After almost 5 years of follow-up, there was a 56% DFS (148). Their neoadjuvant studies were compared to this initial result. The following study (COSS-80) compared the effect of neoadjuvant DOX,HDMTX/leucovorin/BCD with the neoadjuvant DOX,HDMTX/ leucovorin/CPDD. In both groups, the same chemotherapy was continued postoperatively regardless of histopathologic findings (147). At 5 year follow-up, the overall DFS was 68%, with no difference between the treatment arms. Histologically evaluated responders had an 84% DFS compared with 52% for those with resistant disease (149).

In the most recent study by the same group (COSS-82), histologic response was used to plan postoperative treatment with the same drug for responders or alternate drugs for nonresponders. In one arm, all patients received the same neoadjuvant chemotherapy with CPDD/DOX/and HCMTX/leucovorin rescue for two courses. Postoperatively, responders received an additional four courses of the same regimen. Nonresponders were treated with three courses of CPDD/IFO/BCD. In the second arm, the patients received neoadjuvant chemotherapy with BCD, HDMTX/leucovorin for two courses. Responders received four courses of the same regimen postoperatively. Nonresponders were treated with six courses of CPDD and DOX. The overall survival for both groups was 58% at 2 years. Nonresponders had a 44% DFS compared with 77% for responders (149).

The results in these studies suggest that response to neoadjuvant therapy can be used to identify those patients who will have an excellent prognosis. Thus, some investigators suggest that all patients should be treated preoperatively to identify that subset which needs only limited postoperative therapy (110). However, alterations in treatment based on histologic response have not resulted in better survival for the poorly responding group. As shown by the above results, the neoadjuvant approach has not had a significant impact on overall survival, but does identify the most highly responsive groups of patients. Additionally, it frequently allows salvage of extremities, when this might not otherwise be possible.

c. Preoperative intra-arterial chemotherapy: Preoperative intra-arterial chemotherapy for osteosarcoma has been advocated on the premise that tumor shrinkage prior to definitive surgery may alter the needed surgical procedure, allowing limb sparing and providing histologic assessment of tumor response as with IV neoadjuvant therapy. Although several abstracts have appeared describing results using this approach (15,52,97), only three articles (24,68,140) are available for full review.

In an early study, patients were randomized for treatment with intra-arterial high-dose methotrexate and intra-arterial cisplatin. Four of 15 in the methotrexate arm and nine of 15 in the cisplatin arm responded, but these results were not statistically different. Observed histologic response guided further therapy choices, but there was no significant difference in survival. There was no comment concerning changes in surgical procedure based on tumor response (68).

Continuous infusion of doxorubicin and intra-arterial cisplatin preoperatively in 40 other patients resulted in a meaningful change in surgical approach. Although only three of 40 patients met criteria for limb-sparing surgery preoperatively, 24 of 40 could undergo limb-sparing procedures after preoperative intra-arterial therapy (15).

The role of hyperthermic perfusion for the treatment of extremity osteosarcoma was evaluated in 76 patients. Hyperthermia alone, without surgery, led to only a 25% survival rate. When amputation was added to hyperthermia the survival rate increased to 51%. Adding the chemotherapy agents melphalan and dactinomycin to the arterial line of the circuit improved results, with a 5 year DFS of 67%. Some patients had limb-sparing surgery, rather than amputation, as a consequence of good local tumor response (24). More recently, intra-arterial cisplatin, systemic high-dose methotrexate, and hyperthermic chemotherapy have been combined with tolerable side effects (140). Survival information is not yet available from this latter study.

In summary, preoperative intra-arterial chemotherapy can be used to identify patients with responsive tumors. Some patients with tumors that require amputation may be treated with limb-sparing procedures if they exhibit a good response to preoperative intra-arterial therapy (11c). There are no studies available as yet to evaluate the survival benefit of this approach compared with systemic preoperative chemotherapy or standard amputation.

2. Ewing's tumor: Ewing's sarcoma is classically linked with a very poor prognosis. Overall, the 5-year survival following local treatment with surgery or radiation therapy is less than 15%. More than 75% of the patients who develop metastases do so within 2 years of treatment to the primary lesion (44). Therefore, a multidisciplinary approach is essential in the treatment of these patients (98). Chemotherapy has been shown to be effective in improving survival (Table 26-7) (89d). Single-agent treatment with cyclophosphamide, dactinomycin, doxorubicin, or vincristine has resulted in response rates of 40% to 60% (51). Complete remission with prolongation of survival is possible in patients with metastatic disease with the use of combination therapy (69,111,118).

Adjuvant chemotherapy for patients with localized disease has shown impressive improvement in DFS compared with patients who received treatment to the primary lesion alone.

a. Razek et al. (104) reported the results of the Intergroup Ewing's Sarcoma Study of 193 patients with localized disease. All patients received radiation therapy to the primary lesion, followed by chemotherapy with VAC or VACA or VAC + bilateral pulmonary irradiation. Continuous DFS was 58% at 172 weeks median to follow-up.

b. Rosen et al. (118) treated patients with adjuvant VACA. Fifteen of 20 patients had no evidence of

Table 26-7. Response Rates of Ewing's Sarcoma to Chemotherapy	
Drug	**Response Rate (%)**
Cyclophosphamide	47
Doxorubicin	42
Ifosfamide	32
Vincristine	40
Actinomycin D	19
Lomustine	33
5-FU	40
Etoposide	30
Cisplatin	7
Melphalan (high dose)	82
Ifosfamide/etoposide	84

From Miser et al. (89d), with permission.

recurrent disease at a median follow-up of 46 months. The actuarial 5-year DFS was 75%.

c. LeMevel *et al.* (76) described the 5-year results of the Intergroup European Ewing's Sarcoma Study. Twenty-three patients were treated with vincristine/cyclophosphamide/doxorubicin and procarbazine hydrochloride, or dactinomycin. The estimated DFS was 56% at 3 years.

d. More recent work (120) suggests that the prognosis for Ewing's sarcoma may be improved by addition of surgical resection as adjuvant treatment in conjunction with radiotherapy and chemotherapy as the primary modalities. Overall survival was 52% at 5 years, with 92% in the surgically treated group versus 37% in the nonsurgically treated group (120).

Immunotherapy

The role of immunotherapy in the treatment of bone tumors remains controversial. There is great promise, but the clinical application of knowledge about the immune response has been disappointingly inconclusive.

1. Interferon: Strander *et al.* (131) reported a comparison of 33 patients treated with a daily dose of 3 x 106 standard leukocyte interferon unit intramuscularly for 1 month, followed by the same dose three times a week for 17 months with 30 contemporary patients who did not receive adjuvant therapy. According to Life Table 26-Analysis, 58% of the study group would be free of disease at 3 years' follow-up, compared with 37% in the contemporary group. A recent update (92) showed a 58% 5-year survival rate in the study group.

Hidemoto *et al.* (62) used human leukocyte interferon and demonstrated partial regression of pulmonary metastases in two of three patients treated. In one of the two responders, an *in vitro* effect of interferon on cultured pleural fluid tumor cells also could be demonstrated.

2. *Transfer factor:* Levin *et al.* (77) studied 13 patients with osteogenic sarcoma who were treated with "tumor-specific transfer factor" that was derived from the blood of household contacts who had specific cell-mediated cytotoxicity against the tumor. Transfer factor was injected subcutaneously at a dose equivalent to ten leukocytes per dose until immunologic parameters increased by 20%. Five patients who were clinically tumor free at the initiation of immunotherapy had remained tumor free at 12 to 24 months' follow-up. Of seven patients with clinically advanced disease, one died at 7 weeks, two had stable disease, and four had increased size of metastases.

Ritts *et al.* (106) classified patients with osteogenic sarcoma as "convertors" or "nonconvertors," depending on changes in delayed cutaneous hypersensitivity after injection of transfer factor from donors who had been continuously disease free of their osteogenic sarcoma for at least 5 years. Convertors did not receive chemotherapy, while some nonconverters were treated with methotrexate, vincristine, and doxorubicin. At 24 months follow-up, 13 of 15 (87%) convertors were alive, while only seven of 15 (47%) nonconvertors lived.

A randomized study compared the effect of adjuvant combination chemotherapy with high-dose methotrexate, doxorubicin, and vincristine in 22 patients with adjuvant transfer

factor in 18 patients at the National Cancer Institute. Ten patients in the transfer factor group became convertors, and of those, five were alive and disease free at 14 to 25 months follow-up. There was no significant difference in survival between the two study arms.

Conclusion

For optimal management, patients with osteogenic sarcoma and Ewing's sarcoma must have a multidisciplinary approach to their disease. Every attempt should be made to enter each of these patients into randomized studies to further clarify and advance the role of chemotherapy. Patients with metastatic osteogenic sarcoma should be offered the potential benefit of combination chemotherapy. The role of adjuvant treatment is not yet established, but there is good reason to believe that DFS may be prolonged by combination chemotherapy. All patients with Ewing's sarcoma should have the benefit of chemotherapy, since complete responses are possible in advanced disease. Adjuvant chemotherapy has been shown to improve DFS and probably can cure many patients who would have otherwise died of their disease.

SPECIAL CONSIDERATIONS OF TREATMENT

The special challenges and the progress being made in managing malignant bone tumors is best illustrated by considering osteogenic sarcomas and Ewing's tumor. Each is representative of a specific genre of tumor—one is a radioresistant spindle cell sarcoma and the other is a radiosensitive small cell sarcoma. The progress in limb preservations, megavoltage radiation treatment with carefully shaped fields, and adjuvant multiagent neoadjuvant chemotherapy will be demonstrated in the pediatric setting, which also allows for a more aggressive approach, in particular, combination regimens.

OTHER TYPES OF TUMORS

Solitary Plasmacytoma: The diagnosis needs to exclude metastases or dissemination, i.e., multiple myeloma. These are rarely solitary lesions; despite local control, other foci appear, 5 to 10 years later in the majority of cases treated with 5,000 cGy, causing steady attrition of the solitary ranks. Although pain relief has been reported with doses ranging between 15 to 20 Gy for multiple myeloma (89), curative doses of 50 Gy are required for control of solitary plasmacytoma (89). Careful delineation of the tumor volume, including CT scans of the affected area, is required to encompass any soft tissue component of the disease. Forty-six cases of solitary plasmacytoma of bone, defined as solitary lytic bone lesions on skeletal survey, histologic confirmation of lesion and a bone marrow plasmacytosis of less than 10%, constitute the basis of a report by Frassica *et al.* (47). The 5- and 10- year survival is 43% and 25%, respectively, with 54% of patients developing multiple myeloma and 11% local recurrences. Interestingly, serum protein did not influence prognosis, even if elevated values persisted after appropriate therapy.

Chondrosarcoma of bone: Chondrosarcomas of bone are reported to be relatively radioresistant tumors. Studies reporting the results of irradiation used as a single modality consist of patients not suitable for surgery or who have surgically inaccessible lesions (60,72,88). Responses are, however, documented with doses in the range of 40 to 70 Gy (60,72,88). Surgical removal remains the treatment of choice, but one study quoted a 53-month survival of 65% with irradiation alone, which corresponds to the surgical studies (60). Radiosulfur has been used in the treatment of metastases (84).

Giant cell tumor of bone: Giant cell tumors of bone are generally aggressive benign tumors, although frankly malignant lesions do occur. These lesions are best treated surgically whenever possible, because of the risk of malignant transformation that has been reported to occur after radiation therapy. Radiation therapy is used, however, in the treatment of tumors that are surgically inaccessible (14,26,30,49,59,124). Controversy exists over the malignant transformation of these tumors after irradiation. Doses ranged from 30 to 40 Gy for post-operative treatment and 50 to 60 Gy for primary irradiation (14,26,30,49,59,124). Eighty percent local control has been reported (26).

Aneurysmal bone cysts: Aneurysmal bone cysts occur in all the bones of the body. Surgery is the treatment of choice with irradiation used for recurrent lesions or for surgically inaccessible lesions. Doses reported as achieving permanent local control range from 14 to 40 Gy (23,70,93).

Fibrosarcoma: As with other bone tumors, surgery is the treatment of choice with irradiation used for inoperable tumors, palliation, or for residual disease postoperatively (87).

Malignant fibrous histiocytoma of bone: Surgery is the treatment of choice for this tumor. Responses have been reported with radiation therapy in the histiocytic histology as opposed to the fibrocytic histology (129).

Reticulum cell sarcoma (non-Hodgkin's lymphoma): Irradiation alone with doses in the range of 45 to 50 Gy to the whole bone have been reported to give long-lasting local control to these tumors (11,66,91,99,141,142). No local recurrences were reported in one study when doses in this range were used (11).

Metastatic bone disease: Metastatic tumors of bone comprise the majority of bone tumors. A variety of fractionation schedules and total doses have been used with equal effectiveness (18,95,103,119b,138). Selection of a treatment schedule should consider the patient's overall condition, the biology and histology of the tumor, and machine availability. Hemibody irradiation has also been used with success in the treatment of metastatic disease (46,102,119b,121). Large lytic lesions in the femoral, humeral, and acetabular regions may need prophylactic pinning if judged to be at risk for fracture (27).

RESULTS AND PROGNOSIS (Fig. 26-4) (58)

The prognosis for patients with malignant bone tumors is not hopeless; these lesions are well worth aggressive treatment. Since most studies are small in patient number (<100) statistical percentages are unreliable and can be misleading. Each series of reported cases can include many unreported cell types, and comparison of case reports is difficult. Each patient must be treated as a separate entity based on a full study of the specific lesion. The site of a tumor greatly affects the patient's survival. Separation of tumors of the trunk from those of the extremities has rarely been done in statistical studies. A tumor of the pelvis is generally of a higher order of malignancy than one of the same type occurring in the hand. Both tumors may

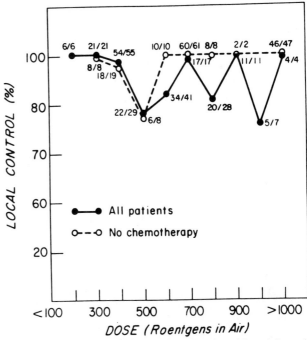

Fig. 26-4. Local control of bone lesions as function of dose delivered. Results are presented as percent of patients controlled (roentgenographic documented evidence of bone healing) after each designated dose of x-ray therapy. Doses are given in roentgens to standarize treatments to orthovoltage machines used in 1940-1960 period. From Greenberger *et al.* (58), with permission.

show similar histology, but the more centrally located tumors will metastasize earlier and more extensively. Localized tumors are limited to the bone of origin, although local skip metastases may be apparent within the bone, possibly indicating a worse prognosis (149a).

1. The results differ in accordance with the cell type, differentiation, and host response to chemoradiation therapy. According to the Surveillance, Epidemiology, and End Results data, 5-year survivals for bone tumors range from 46% to 49%, and at 10 years range from 38% to 44%. Patients who survive 5 years have an 88% chance to be alive at 10 years. These rates are somewhat less for soft tissue sarcomas.

2. Natural history changes (Mayo Clinic experiences): Taylor *et al.* (134,135) reported the Mayo Clinic experience with surgical management of osteogenic sarcoma from 1963 to 1974. They showed that the survival in the early years was typical of other reports—approximately 25%, but that by the years 1972 to 1974, the 3-year survival had become 50%. This change did not result from adjuvant chemotherapy or any basic change in the type of patients being treated. In light of this report, the validity of any study using historical controls is seriously questioned (Table 26-8).

3. The achievements of multidisciplinary treatment, particularly chemotherapy programs, are listed in the Principles of Treatment section, along with each regimen.

Table 26-8. Survival after Surgical Amputation for Osteogenic Sarcomas

Group	Time	No. Patients	2-yr Relapse-free Survival(%)	Overall Survival(%) 2-yr	Overall Survival(%) 5-yr	Ref
Memorial Sloan-Kettering Cancer Center	1949-1965	145	20		17*	84b
M.D. Anderson	1950-1973	106	16		9*	90a
Dana Farber Cancer Center	1950-1972	78	19	26	17	48b
Mayo Clinic	1963-1968	60	20	32	23	134
Mayo Clinic	1969-1974	68	20	65	55	135

* Number of survivors with no evaluable disease.

For both osteogenic sarcoma and Ewing's tumor, increasing response rates and survival are occurring. It is difficult to compare series because reported results vary due to short follow-up of many patients and changeability of chemotherapy. A brief description of results by each tumor type follows:

Osteogenic sarcoma: The natural history of osteogenic sarcomas has improved according to Mayo Clinic investigations without chemotherapy (Table 26-8) (134,135) but numerous investigators have reported an improvement in relapse-free survival from 40% to 60% with the aggressive use of chemotherapy (Table 26-9).

1. The Multi-Institutional Osteosarcoma Study (78) and the University of California, Los Angeles Study (34,36) are randomized clinical trials — both show better DFS: 64% versus 17% and 55% versus 20%, respectively (Table 26-9), but other randomized studies are less convincing.
2. Lung irradiation improved survival in Europe but has not been confirmed in the United States (Table 26-9).
3. In recently reported clinical trials, long-term responses and survival are reaching 75%, with conservation of limbs. The best results have been achieved by Rosen (108) with a 93% DFS.

Table 26-9. Reported Results of Representative Trials of Adjuvant Chemotherapy for Osteosarcoma

Adjuvant Regimen *	Investigators	% Relapse-free
HDMTX, VCR (Study I)	DFCI	42
HDMTC< VCR + BCG†	NCI	38
ADRIA	CALGB	39
ADRIA + HDMTX†	CALGB	50
ADRIA + HDMTX (Study II)	DFCI	59
ADRIA + VCR + (weekly) (Study III)	DFCI	60
ADRIA + VCR + (HDMTX or IDMTX)	CCSG	38
COMPADRI I (CTX, VCR, ADRIA, PAM, HDMTX)	SWOG	49
COMPADRI II (CTX, VCR, ADRIA, PAM, HDMTX)	SWOG	35
COMPADRI III (CTX, VCR, ADRIA, PAM, HDMTX)	SWOG	38
ADRIA + HDMTX + CTX	Stanford	47 (2 year) 13 (4 year)
ADRIA + HDMTX + CTX (OSTEO 72)	St.Jude	50
ADRIA + HDMTX + CTX (OSTEO 77)	St. Jude	51
ADRIA + CDDP	Roswell Park	64
HDMTX + VCR or no adjuvant therapy‡	Mayo Clinic	40 (chemotherapy) 44 (no chemotherapy)
BCG + HDMTX + ADRIA + CDDP or no adjuvant therapy	MIOS	64 (chemotherapy) 17 (no chemotherapy)
BCG + HDMTX + ADRIA + CDDP (+intra-arterial ADRIA + XRT)	UCLA	55 (chemotherapy) 20 (no chemotherapy)
Whole-lung irradiation 2000 rad or no adjuvant treatment	EORTC	43 (chemotherapy 28 (no chemotherapy)
Whole-lung irradiation (+ dactinomycin) or no adjuvant treatment	Mayo Clinic	40
HDMTX + VCR + ADRIA + CTX (T4 - T5 pooled)	MSKCC	48

HDMTX = high-dose methotrexate (5 g/m^2 or more) + leucovorin rescue; VCR = vincristine; BCG = bacillus Calmette-Guerin; ADRIA = Adriamycin; IDMTX = intermediate-dose methotrexate (750 mg/m^2) + leucovorin rescue; CTX = cyclophosphamide; PAM = phenylalanine mustard; CDDP = cisplatin; DFCI = Dana Farber Cancer Institute; NCI = Nation Cancer Institute; CALGB = Cancer and Leukemia Group B; CCSG = Children's Cancer Study Group; SWOG = Southwest Oncology Group MIOS - Multi-Institutional Osteosarcoma Study Group; UCLA = University of California, Los Angeles; EORTC = European Organization on Research and Treatment of Cancer; MSKCC = Memorial Sloan-Kettering Cancer Center.

In previously untreated osteogenic sarcoma patients, Memorial Sloan-Kettering Cancer Center investigators Marcove et al. (84a) and Meyers et al. (88a) confirm intensive chemotherapy prior to surgery achieves a 75% long-term survival, with limb-sparing surgery performed when feasible. There is a 5.5% local recurrence rate. The majority of cases do not develop pulmonary metastases (55%). Pulmonary resection of metastases can salvage one third of patients (56a).

A more aggressive three-drug neoadjuvant regimen (MTX, CDP, ADM) increased limb salvage, i.e., 87% versus 77%, good responders (>90% necrosis), i.e., 76% versus 52%, and 2-year DFS as compared with their two-drug schedule (CDP + MTX), i.e., 84% versus 59% (97a,119c).

Ewing's sarcoma (19a,22a,72a,90c'): The most dramatic improvement in survival with Ewing's sarcoma has occurred with chemoradiation programs that avoid limb resection. Without chemotherapy, 5-year survival has been dismal (8% to 10%) (Table 26-10) and surgery inevitably led to failure and loss of limbs. Current chemoradiation programs improved survival to 50% or more at 3 to 5 years, depending on drug program used (Table 26-11) and sites involved by tumor (Table 26-12); limb preservation is equally important.

Pelvic and sacral bone Ewing's sarcomas when managed by high dose multiagent chemotherapy (vincristine, cyclophosphamide, Adriamycin) and 55 Gy to the tumor bed have shown a survival advantage when comparing the different Inteagroup Ewing's Sarcoma Studies (IESS). At 5 years, the comparison between IESS-II versus IESS-I was 55% versus 23% for RFS and 63% versus 35% for S (42b). The importance of treating the whole bone was challenged by Arai et al. (9a), in applying limited volume radiotherapy and studying local failure patterns. Following induction chemotherapy, limited coverage of the tumor defined as initial bone involvement, and post-chemotherapy soft tissue extent (with 3 cm margins) was given a dose of 35 Gy-50 Gy, depending upon CR or PR chemotherapy response. Local control was 58%, and most local failures were infield not margin recurrences.

Table 26-10. Five-Year Survival of Patients with Ewing's Sarcoma Treated Without Chemotherapy

Series	No. Patients	No. Surviving at 5 Years (%)
Nesbit (90c)	374	36 (9.6)
Bacci (11a)	83	7 (8.4)
Dahlin (29a)	133	16 (12.0)
Wang (142a)	47	5 (10.6)
Total	637	64 (10.0)

Response to chemotherapy predicted response to irradiation, i.e., 62% versus 17%. The DFS at years is 59%—similar to local control rates. Utilizing multifractions (bid) daily, Marcus et al. (84c) produced better local control rates of approximately 80-90% with their radiation schedule—modified by the amount of tumor treated either with or without chemotherapy. The dose schedule consisted of 120 cGy twice a day to 50-60 Gy depending on micro or macrotumor residuum. Functional results were excellent with minimal late effects and no pathologic fractures.

CLINICAL INVESTIGATIONS

Because most malignant bone tumors metastasize so rapidly, the programs that have emerged are mainly directed at systemic multiagent chemotherapy at the time the primary is discovered.

Osteogenic Sarcoma

1. Conservative surgery is being studied in osteogenic sarcomas due to the effectiveness of chemotherapy.
2. Multiagent chemotherapy is yielding high response and control rates (69).
3. Biologic response modifier is being explored.

Table 26-11. Results of Therapy for Nonmetastatic Ewing's Sarcoma

Regimen	Outcome	Ref
	2-year RFS: 35%	90d
VCR, CTX, Dactine	2-year RFS: 74%	
VCR, CTX, Dactine, ADNA	2-year RFS: 58%	
VCR, CTX, Dactine, Pulmonary RT	N=62 pelvic tumors: 34% DFS at 5 yr	42a
As above	N=21 rib primaries: 11 (52%) disease-free at 18-64 mo	137
As above	All 12 patients alive NED at 10-37+ mo	112
T2	23 of 28 patients alive NED at 12-46+ mo	118
T6	N=67: 2-yr DFS: 79%	115
T2-9 CTX, ADRIA, MTX, VCR, BLEO	14/14 achieved CR, 12/14 disease-free at 9-41 +mos	60a
CTX, ADRIA	N=80: 31 (39%) disease-free at mean of 45 mo (21-96)	11b
VCR, ADRIA, CTX	N=124: 48% disease-free at median of 65 mo	11a
Same	N=21: 14 disease-free at median of 36 mo	118
VCR, ADRIA, CTX	N=28: 55% DFS at 3 yr	112
VCR, ADRIA, CTX	N=17: 49% survival at 3 yr (no beneficial effect of hemibody irradiation)	17
VCR, ADRIA, CTX	N=67 histologic responses: 41 good: 57% disease-free 26 bad: 9% disease-free	93a
	N=30: 6 yr DFS: 49%	152
VCR, ADRIA, CTX, Procarbazine	N=34: 53% RFS at yr	53a
VCR, ADRIA, CTX	N=24 high risk patients (pelvis, chest wall; 4 with metastasis): 25% DFS at 5 yrs	73
VCR, ADRIA, CTX	N=18: 70% DFS at 18 mo	89c
RFS = relapse-free survival; DFS = disease-free survival; NED = no evidence of disease; CR = complete remission.		

Table 26-12. Local Control and Disease-Free Survival in Ewing's Sarcoma

Site	Local Control (%)	Disease-free Survival (%)
Pelvis	85	47
Humerus	79	50
Femur	91	58
Tibia	89	59
Fibula	97	62
Ribs	94	58
Skull and spine	100	100
Sacrum	100	29
Ulna, radius, hand	80	80
Feet	75	75

Adapted from Perez et al. (95a).

Ewing's Sarcoma

1. Multiagent chemotherapy has been highly successful in controlling metastases (53).
2. Limb preservation with radiation dose reduction, particularly when doxorubicin and/or actinomycin D are used, depends on microresidual and macroresidual disease.
3. Elective central nervous system irradiation is being studied. Its value is debatable.

Recommended Reading

Tumors of Bone and Cartilage (7) and *Tumors and Tumorous Conditions of the Bone and Joint* (3) are good starting places for an understanding of bone tumor pathology and pathogenesis. *Bone Tumors: Diagnosis and Treatment* (6) provides an up-to-date and comprehensive review of the clinicopathologic features of bone tumors, and the section on musculoskeletal tumors in *Surgery of the Musculoskeletal System*, 2nd ed. (43) has a very thorough description of clinical features and treatment of bone tumors. Finally, *Musculoskeletal Tumor Surgery* (2) gives excellent detail on musculoskeletal tumor surgery and the rationale for surgical staging.

REFERENCES

General References

1. Dahlin, D.C. Bone tumors: general aspects and data on 6,221 cases. Springfield, IL.: Charles C Thomas; 1978.
2. Enneking, W.F. Musculoskeletal Tumor Surgery. New York, NY: Churchill Livingstone; 1983.
2a. International Union Against Cancer (UICC). TNM Classification of malignant tumors. 4th ed. New York, NY: Springer-Verlag; 1987:83-88.
3. Jaffe, H.L. Tumors and Tumorous Conditions of the Bones and Joints. Philadelphia, PA: Lea & Febiger; 1974.
4. Lichtenstein L. Bone tumors, 5th ed. St. Louis, MO: C V Mosby Co.; 1977.
5. Lodwick, G.S. The Bones and Joints. Chicago, IL: Year Book Medical Publishers; 1971.
6. Mirra, J.M. Bone tumors: Diagnosis and Treatment. Philadelphia, PA: JB Lippincott Co; 1989.
7. Spjut, H.J.; Dorfman, H.D.; Fechner, R.E.; Ackerman, L.V. Tumors of Bone and Cartilage. Washington, DC: Armed Forces Institute of Pathology; 1983.

Specific References

8. Ackerman, L.V. Extraosseous localized non-neoplastic bone and cartilage formation (so-called myositis ossificans). J. Bone Joint Surg. 40A:279; 1958.

9. Allen C.V., Stevens K.R. Preoperative irradiation for osteogenic sarcoma. Cancer. 31:1364-1366, 1973.
9a. Arai, Y.; Kun, L.E.; Brooks, M.T.; *et al.* Ewing's sarcoma: Local tumor control and patterns of failure following limited-volume radiation therapy. Int J Radiat Oncol Biol Phys. 1501-1508; 1991.
9b. Aurias, A.; Rimbaut, C.; Buffe, D.; *et al.* Chromosomal translocation in Ewing's sarcoma. N Engl J Med 309(8):496-497; 1983.
10. Ayala, A.G.; Zornosa, J. Primary bone tumors: percutaneous needle biopsy. Radiologic-pathologic study of 222 biopsies. Radiology. 149(3):675-679; 1983.
11. Bacci G., Jaffe N., Emmliani E., Van Horn J., Manfrini M., Picci B., Batoni F., Gherlinzoni F., Canpanacci M. Therapy for primary non Hodgkin's lymphoma of bone and a comparison of results with Ewing's sarcoma. Cancer. 57:1468-1472, 1986.
11a. Bacci, G.; Picci, P.; Gherlinzoni, F. *et al.* Localized Ewing's sarcoma of bone: ten years experience of the Istituto Ortopedico Rizzoli in 124 cases Tteated with multimodality therapy. Eur J Cancer Clin Oncol. 21:163-173;1985.
11b. Bacci, G.; Picci, P.; Gitelis; *et al.* The Treatment of localized Ewing's sarcoma. Cancer. 49:1561-1570;1982.
11c. Bacci, G.; Picci, P.; Ruggieri, P.; *et al.* Primary chemotherapy and delayed surgery (neoadjuvant chemotherapy) for osteosarcoma of the extremities: The Istituto Rizzoli experience in 127 patients treated preoperatively with intravenous methotrexate (high versus moderate doses) and intraarterial cisplatin. Cancer 65(11):2539-2553; 1990.
12. Bacci G., Springfield D., Capanna R.; *et al.* Neoadjuvant chemotherapy for osteosarcoma of the extremity. Clin. Orthop. 224:268-276;1987.
13. Baum E.S., Gaynon, P., Greenberg L.; *et al.* Phase II study of cis-dichlorodiammine platinum (II) in childhood osteosarcoma: Children's Cancer Study Group report. Cancer Treat. Rep. 63:9-10;1979
14. Bell R.S., Harwood A.R., Goodman S.B., Fornasier, V.L. Supervoltage radiotherapy in the treatment of difficult giant cell tumors of bone. Clin. Orthop. 174:208-216, 1983.
15. Benjamin R.S., Chawla S.P., Murray J.; *et al.* Response to preoperative chemotherapy of osteosarcoma improves disease-free survival and the chances of limb salvage. Proc. Am. Soc. Cancer. Res. 26:690, 1985. Abstract.
16. Berg N.O., Hahansson C.H., Lovdahl R., Persson B.M. Radiotherapy and surgery in 50 cases of osteosarcoma treated without adjuvant chemotherapy. Acta Orthop.Scand. 48:580-585; 1977.
16a. Berquist, T.H. Magnetic resonance imaging of musculoskeletal neoplasms. Clin. Orthop. 224:101-118; 1989.
17. Berry, M.P.; Jenkin, R.D.T.; Harwood, A.R.; *et al.* Ewing's sarcoma: a trial of adjuvant chemotherapy and sequential half-body irradiation. Int. J. Radiat. Oncol. Biol. Phys. 1:407-413;1976.
17a. Bertoli, R.J.; Brady, L.W. Bone. In: Perez, C.A., Brady, L.W. Principles and Practice of Radiation Oncology. Philadelphia, PA: JB Lippincott Co; 1992; 1382-1398.
18. Blitzer P.H. Reanalysis of the RTOG study of the palliation of symptomatic osseous metastasis. Cancer 55:1468-1472;1985.
18a. Bragg, D.G.; Rubin, P.; Youker, J.E., eds. Oncologic Imaging. Elmsford, NY: Pergamon Press; 1985.
18b. Bramwell, V.H.C.; Piredo, H.M. Treatment of metastatic bone and soft-tissue sarcomas In: Caster, S., Glasstein, E., Livingston, R.B., eds. Principle of Cancer Treatment. New York, NY: McGraw Hill; 1982.
19. Brennan J. Radiotherapy of osteogenic sarcoma. In: Osteosarcoma: New Trends in Diagnosis and Treatment. New York, NY: Alan R. Liss, Inc.; 1982:77-81.
19a. Burgert ED, Nesbit ME, Garnsey LA, *et al.* Multimodal therapy for the management of nonpelvic, localized Ewing's sarcoma of bone: Intergroup study IESS-II. J Clin Oncol 8(9):1514-1524; 1990.
20. Buschke F, Cantril SK. Roentgen therapy of benign giant cell tumor of bone. Cancer. 2:293-315;1949.
21. Caceres E., Zaharia M. Massive preoperative radiation therapy in the treatment of osteogenic sarcoma. Cancer. 30:634-638; 1972.
22. Cade S. Osteogenic sarcoma. A study based on 133 patients. J. Coll.Surg.Edinb. 1:79-111, 1955.
22a. Cangir A, Vietti TJ, Gehan EA, *et al.* Ewing's sarcoma metastatic at diagnosis: Results and comparisons of two intergroup Ewing's sarcoma studies. Cancer 66(5):887-893; 1990.

23. Cassady J.R. Radiation therapy in less common primary bone tumors. In: Jaffe, N, ed. Solid Tumors in Childhood. Boca Raton, FL: CRC, 1983:205-214.

24. Cavaliere R., Di Filippo F., Santori F.S.; et al. Role of hyperthermic perfusion in the treatment of limb osteosarcoma. Oncology (Basel). 44:1-5, 1987.

25. Chambers, R.G., Mahoney, W.D. Osteogenic sarcoma of the mandible: current management. Am. Surg. 36:463-467, 1970.

26. Chen Z.X., Zhoung G.U.D., Yu Z.H., Quin T.N., Huang Y.R., Hu Y.H., Gu X.Z. Radiation therapy of giant cell tumor of bone: analysis of 35 patients. Intl. J. Radiat. Oncol. Biol. Phys. 12:329-334;1986.

27. Cheng D.S., Seitz C.B., Eyre H.J. Nonoperative management of femoral, humeral, and acetabular metastases in patients with breast carcinoma. Cancer. 45:1533-1537, 1980.

28. Cohen L., Hendrickson F., Mansell J., Kurup P.D., Awschalon M., Rosenberg I., Tem Haken R.K. Response of sarcoma of bone and of soft tissue to neutron beam therapy. Intl.J. Radiat. Oncol. Biol. Phys. 10:821-824; 1984.

29. Cortes E.P., Holland J.F., Wang J.J.; et al. Doxorubicin in disseminated osteosarcoma. JAMA. 221:1132-1130, 1972.

29a. Dahlin, D.C.; Coventy, M.D.; Scanlon, P.W. Ewing's sarcoma: a Ccitical analysis of 165 cases. J. Bone Joint Surg. (Am). 43:185-192;1962.

30. Daugaard S., Johansen A.F., Barford G., Laustein G., Schiodt T., Lund B. Radiation treatment of giant-cell tumour of bone (osteoclastoma). Acta Oncol. 26:41-43, 1987.

31. de-Moor, N.G. Osteosarcoma a review of 72 cases treated by megavoltage radiation therapy, with or without surgery. S. Afr. J. Surg., 13(3):137-146, 1975.

32. Dollahite, H.A.; Tatum, L.; Moinuddin, S.M.; Carnesale, P.G. Aspiration biopsy of primary neoplasms of bone. J. Bone Joint Surg. 71A:1166-1169; 1989.

33. Duncan W., Arnott S.J., Jack W.J.L. The Edinburgh experience of treating sarcoma of soft tissues and bone with neutron irradiation. Clin. Radiol. 37:317-320; 1986.

34. Eckardt J.J.; Eilber F.R.; Grant T.T.; Mirra J.M.; Weisenberger T.H.; Dorey F.J. The UCLA experience in the management of stage IIB osteogenic sarcoma. In: Proc. NIH Consensus Development Conference on Limb-Sparing Treatment: Adult Soft Tissue and Osteogenic Sarcoma. Dec 3-5, 1987:61.

34a. Edeiken, J.; Karasick, D. Imaging in bone cancer. In: A.I. Holleb, ed. Imaging in Cancer. New York, NY: American Cancer Society Inc.; 1987:103-109.

35. Edmonson, J.H.; Green, S.J.; Ivins, J.C.; et al. A controlled pilot study of high-dose methotrexate with post surgical adjuvant treatment for primary osteosarcoma. J. Clin. Oncol. 2:152-156; 1984

36. Eilber, F.; Giuliano, A.; Eckhardt, J.; et al. Adjuvant chemotherapy for osteosarcoma: a randomized prospective trial. J. Clin. Oncol. 5:21-26; 1987.

37. Eilber, F.R., Eckhardt, J., Morton, D.L. Advances in the treatment of sarcomas of the extremity. Current status of limb salvage. Cancer. 54(11 suppl.):2695-2701, 1984.

38. Eilber, F.R., Morton, D.L., Eckhardt, J., Grant, T., Weisenberger, T. Limb salvage for skeletal and soft tissue sarcomas. Multidisciplinary preoperative therapy. Cancer. 53:2579-2584; 1984.

39. Enneking, W. A system of staging musculoskeletal neoplasms. Clin. Orthop. 204:9-24; 1986.

40. Enneking, W.F., ed. Limb Salvage in Musculoskeletal Oncology. New York, NY: Churchill Livingstone; 1987.

41. Enneking, W.F.; Dunham, W.K. Resection and reconstruction for primary neoplasms involving the innominate bone. J. Bone Joint Surg. 60A:731-746; 1978.

42. Enneking, W.F., Shirley, P.D. Resection-arthrodesis for malignant and potentially malignant lesions about the knee using an intramedullary rod and local bone grafts. J. Bone Joint Surg. 59A(2):223-236; 1977.

42a. Evans, R.; Nesbit, M.; Askin, F.B., et al. Local recurrence rate, sites of metastasis and time to relapse as a function of treatment regimen, size of primary, and surgical history in 62 patients presenting with non-metastatic Ewing's sarcoma of the pelvic bones. Int. J. Radiat. Oncol. Biol. Phys. 11(1):129-136; 1985.

42b. Evans, R.G.; Nesbit, M.E.; Gehan, E.A.; et al. Multimodal therapy for the management of localized Ewing's sarcoma of pelvic and

43. sacral bones: A report from the Second Intergroup Study. J Clin Oncol 9:1173-1180; 1991.

43. Evarts, C.M., ed. Surgery of the Musculoskeletal System, 2nd ed. Bone and soft tissue tumors, Vol. 5. New York, NY: Churchill Livingstone, New York; 1990:4595-5070.

44. Falk S.; Albert, M. Five-year survival of patients with Ewing's sarcoma. Surg. Gynecol. Obstet. 124:319-324; 1967.

45. Finkel, M.P.; Biskis, B.O.; Reilly, C.A., Jr. Interaction of FBJ osteosarcoma virus with Sr-90 and with Sr-90 osteosarcomas. In: Clark, R.L.; Cumley, R.W.; McCoy, J.E.; et al., eds. Oncology, 1970. vol. 1. Chicago, IL: Year Book Medical Publishers; 1971.

46. Fitzpatrick P.J., Rider W.D. Half-body radiotherapy. Intl. J. Radiat. Oncol. Biol. Phys. 1:197-207, 1976.

47. Frassica, D.A.; Frassica, F.J.; Schray, M.F.; Sim, F.H.; Kyle, R.A. Solitary plasmacytoma of bone: Mayo Clinic experience. Int. J. Radiat. Oncol. Biol. Phys. 16:43-48;1989.

47a. Flatman G.E. Osteosarcoma surgery, Radiotherapy and Chemotherapy. Radiography. 44(518):35-40; 1978.

48. Fraumeni, J.F., Jr. Bone cancer: epidemiologic and etiologic considerations. In: Vaeth, J.M., Jr., ed. Frontiers of Radiation Therapy and Oncology, vol. 10. Basel, Germany: S. Karger; 1975:17-27.

48a. Fraumeni, J.F.; Glass, A.G. Rarity of Ewing's sarcoma among US Negro children. Lancet. i:366-367;1970.

48b. Frei, E.; Jaffe, N.; Gero, M.; et al. Adjuvant Chemotherapy of osteogenic sarcoma: progress and perspectives. JNCI. 60:3;1978.

49. Friedman M., Pearlman A.W. Benign giant-cell tumor of bone, Radiation dosage for each type. Radiology. 91:1151-1158, 1968.

50. Garrington, G.E., Scofield, H.H., Cornyn, J., Hooker, S.P. Osteosarcoma of the jaws. Analysis of 56 cases. Cancer. 20:377-391, 1967.

51. Gasparini, M. Current Results with a Combined Treatment Approach to Localized Ewing's Sarcoma. Recent Results. Cancer Res. 68:45-51, 1979.

52. Gasparini M.; Azzarelli A.; Fossati-Bellani A.; et al. HD-MTX + VCR + CDDP as pre-operative intra-arterial therapy for osteogenic sarcoma. Intl. Soc. Pediatr. Oncol. 16:234; 1985.

53. Gasparini M, Fossati Bean F, Lattuada A, et al. Adjuvant Treatment with Adriamycin, Cytoxan, and Vincristine. In: Proc. Am. Soc. Clin. Oncol. 1977:77.Abstract 307.

53a. Gasparini, M.; Lombardi, F.; Gionni, C. et al. Localized Ewing's Sarcoma: Results of Integrated Therapy and Analysis of Failures. Eur. J. Cancer Clin. Oncol. 17:1205-1209; 1981.

54. Gitelis, S.; Heligman, D.; Quill, G.; Piasecki, P. The use of large allografts for tumor reconstruction and salvage of the failed total hip arthroplasty. Clin. Orthop. 231:62-70; 1988.

55. Goffinet D.R.; Kaplan S.H.; Donaldson S.S.; Bagshaw M.A.; Wilbury J.R. Combined radiosensitizer infusion and irradiation of osteogenic sarcomas. Radiology. 117:211-214; 1975.

56. Goorin A. M.; Perez-Atayde A.; Gebhart M.; et al. Weekly high-dose methotrexate and doxorubicin for osteosarcoma: the Dana Farber Cancer Institute/Children's Hospital-Study III. J. Clin. Oncol. 5:1178-1184, 1987.

56a. Goorin, A.M.; Shuster, J.J.; Baker, A.; et al. Changing pattern of pulmonary metastases with adjuvant chemotherapy in patients with osteosarcoma: Results from the multiinstitutional osteosarcoma study. J Clin Oncol 9(4):600-605; 1991.

57. Gottlieb J.A.; Baker L.H.; O'Bryan R. M.; et al. Adriamycin (NSC 123127) used alone and in combination for soft tissue and bony sarcoma, Cancer Chemother. Rep. 6 (part 3): 271-282, 1975

58. Greenberger, J.S.; Cassady, J.R.; Jaffe, N.; Vawter, G.; Crocker, A.C. Radiation therapy in patients with histiocytosis: management of diabetes insipidus and bone lesions. Intl. J. Radiat. Oncol. Biol. Phys. 5:1749-1755, 1979.

59. Harwood A.R., Fornasiez V.L., Rider W.D. Supervoltage irradiation in the management of giant cell tumor of bone. Radiology. 125:223-226, 1977.

60. Harwood A.R., Krajbeck J.I., Fornasiez V.L. Radiotherapy of chondrosarcoma of bone. Cancer. 45:2769-2777, 1980.

60a. Hayes, F.A.; Thompson, E.I.; Hustu, H.O.; et al. The response of Ewing's sarcoma to sequential cyclophosphamide and Adriamycin induction therapy. J Clin Oncol. 1:45-51;1983.

61. Henderson, E.D.; Dahlin, D.C. Chondrosarcoma of bone-a study of 288 cases. J. Bone Joint Surg. 45A:1450-145B; 1963.

62. Hidemoto, I.; Koichi, M.; Yanagawa, T.; et al. Effect of human

leukocyte interferon on the metastatic lung tumor of osteosarcoma. Cancer. 46:1 562-1565, 1980.

63. Huvos, A.G. Osteogenic sarcoma of bones and soft tissues in older persons. Cancer. 57:1442-1449; 1986.

64. Huvos, A.G.; Butler A., Bretsky S.S. Osteogenic sarcoma associated with Paget's disease of bone: a clinicopathologic study of 65 patients. Cancer. 52:1489-1495; 1983.

65. Huvos, A.G.; Woodard H.Q.; Cahan W.G. Postradiation osteogenic sarcoma of bone and soft tissues: a clinicopathologic study of 66 patients. Cancer. 55:1244-1255; 1985.

66. Jack, G.A. Radiotherapy of reticulum cell sarcoma of bone. Radiol. Clin. Biol. 40:230-242; 1979.

67. Jaffe N. Recent advances in the chemotherapy of metastatic osteogenic sarcoma, Cancer, 30:1627-1631;1972

68. Jaffe, N.,Robertson, R., Ayala, A., Wallace, S., Chuang, V., et al. Comparison of intra-arterial dis-diamminedichloroplatinum II with high-dose methotrexate and citrovorum factor rescue in the treatment of primary osteosarcoma. J. Clin. Oncol. 3:1101-1104; 1985.

69. Jaffe N, Traggis D, Salian S, et al. Improved outlook for Ewing's sarcoma with combination chemotherapy (vincristine, actinomycin D, cyclophosphamide) and radiation therapy. Cancer. 38:1925-1929; 1976.

70. Jereb B., Smith J. Giant aneurysmal bone cyst of the innominate bone treated with irradiation. Br. J. Radiol. 53:489-491, 1980.

71. Johnson, L.C. General theory of bone tumors. Bull. NY Acad. Med. 29: 164-171;1958.

72. King R.Y., Salten M.M., Brascho D.J. High-energy irradiation in the management of chondrosarcoma. South Med. J. 76(6):729-731, 1983.

72a. Kinsella, T.J.; Miser, J.S.; Waller, B.; et al. Long-term follow-up of Ewing's sarcoma of bone treated with combined modality therapy. Int J Radiat Oncol Biol Phys. 20(3):389-395; 1991.

73. Kuo, K.N.; Gitelis, S.; Sim, F.H.; et al. Segmental replacement of long bones using titanium fiber metal composite following tumor resection. Clin. Orthop. 176:108-114, 1983.

74. Lee E.S., Mackenzie D.H. Osteosarcoma; study of value of preoperative megavoltage radiotherapy. Br. J. Surg. 51:252-274; 1964.

75. LeMevel, B.P.; Hoerni, D.; Durant, O.; et al. EORTC/GTO Adjuvant Chemotherapy Program for primary Ewing's sarcoma: results at 5 years. Recent results. Cancer Res. 68:52-59; 1979.

76. Levin AS, Byers VS, Fudenberg, et al. Osteogenic sarcoma immunologic parameters before and during immunotherapy with tumor-specific transfer factor. J. Clin. Invest. 55:499, 1975.

77. Link, M.P.; Goorin, A.M.; Miser, A.W.; et al. The effect of adjuvant chemotherapy on relapse-free survival in patients with osteosarcoma of the extremity. N. Engl. J. Med. 314:1600-1606; 1986.

78. Lodwick, G.S. Solitary malignant tumors of bone. Semin. Roentgenol. 1:293-313; 1966.

79. Malawer M.M., Link, M.P.; Donaldson, S.S. Sarcomas of bone. In: DeVita, V.T., Jr., Hellman, S., Rosenberg, S. A., eds. Cancer: Principles and Practice, 3rd ed. Philadelphia, PA: JB Lippincott Co; 1989:1418-l468.

80. Manaster, B.J.; Ensign, M.F. The role of imaging in musculoskeletal tumors. In: Raymond, H.W., Zweibel, W.J., Harnsberger, H.R., eds. Seminars in Ultrasound CT and MR. Philadelphia, PA: WB Saunders Co. 10:498-517; 1989.

81. Mankin, H.J., Doppelt, S., Tomford, W. Clinical experience with allograft implantation. The first ten years. Clin. Orthop. 174:69-86; 1983.

82. Mankin, H.J., Doppelt, S.H., Sullivan, T.R., Tomford, W.W. Osteoarticular and intercalary allograft transplantation in the management of malignant tumors of bone. Cancer. 50:613, 1982.

83. Mankin, H.J., Gebhardt, M.C. Advances in the management of bone tumors. Clin. Orthop. 200:73-84, 1985.

84. Marcove R.C. The Surgery of Tumors of Bone and Cartilage. New York, NY: Grune & Stratton, 1981.

84a. Marcove, R.C.; Lane, J.M. New limb sparing resections and results in the treatment of osteogenic sarcoma. Proc. Am. Soc. Clin. Oncol. 9:1206;1990. Abstract.

84b. Marcove, R.C. En bloc resection of osteogenic sarcoma. Cancer Treat. Rep. 62:225; 1978.

84c. Marcus, Jr., R.B.; Cantor, A.; Heare, T.C.; et al. Local control and function after twice-a-day radiotherapy for Ewing's sarcoma of bone. Int J Radiat Oncol Biol Phys. 21:1509-1516; 1991.

85. Martinez A., Goffinet D.R., Donaldson S.S., Bagshaw M.A., Kaplan H.S. Intra-arterial infusion of radiosensitizer (BUdR) combined with hypofractionated irradiation and chemotherapy for primary treatment of osteogenic sarcoma. Intl. J. Radiat. Oncol. Biol. Phys. 11:123-128; 1985.

86. McCullough, C.J. Eosinophilic granuloma of bone. Acta. Orthop. Scand. 51:389-398, 1980.

87. McLeod, J.J.; Dahlin, D.C.; Ivins, J.C. Fibrosarcoma of bone. Am. J. Surg. 94:431-437; 1957.

88. McNaney D., Lindberg R.D., Ayala A.G., Barkley H.T., Hussey D.H. Fifteen year radiotherapy experience with chondrosarcoma of bone. Intl. J. Radiat. Oncol. Biol. Phys. 8:187-190; 1982.

88a. Meyers, P.A.; Heller, G.; Healy, J.; et al. Chemotherapy for nonmetastatic osteogenic sarcoma: The Memorial Sloan-Kettering experience. J Clin Oncol. 10:5-15; 1992.

89. Mill W.B., Griffith R. The role of radiation therapy in the management of plasma cell tumors. Cancer. 45:647-652, 1980.

89a. Miller, E.C.; Miller, J.A. Mechanisms of chemical carcinogenesis. Cancer. 47:1055-1064; 1981.

89b. Miller, R.W. Contrasting epidermiology of childhood osteosarcoma, Ewing's tumor and rhabdomyosarcoma. NCI Monogr. 56:9-14;1981.

89c. Miser, J.S.; Steis, R.; Longo, D.L. et al. Treatment of newly diagnosed high-risk sarcomas and primitive neuroectodermal tumors (PNET) in children and young adults. Proc of Am Soc Clin Oncol. 4:C-935;1985.Abstract.

89d. Miser, J.S.; Triche, T.J.; Pritchard, D.J.; Kinsella, T. Ewing's sarcoma and the non-rhabdomyosarcoma soft tissue sarcomas of childhood. In: Pizzo, P.A., Poplack, D.G. eds. Principles and Practice of Pediatric Oncology. Philadelphia, PA: JB Lippincott Co; 1988.

90. Mosende C., Gutierrez M, Caparros B.; et al. Combination chemotherapy with bleomycin, cyclophosphamide and dactinomycin for the treatment of osteogenic sarcoma. Cancer. 40:2779-2786, 1977.

90a. Murphy, W.K.; Benjamin, R.S.; Eyre, H.J. et al. Adjuvant chemotherapy in osteosarcoma of adults. In: Salmon, S.E., Jones, S.E., eds. Adjuvant Therapy of Cancer. Amsterdam, Netherlands: Elsevier/North-Holland Biomedical Press; 1977.

90b. Myers, J. In: Proceedings of the American Society of Clinical Oncology. Washington, D.C.: American Society of Clinical Oncology; 9: 1223; 1990.

90c. Nesbit, M.E.; Gehan, E.A.; Burgert, E.O.; et al. Multimodal therapy for the management of primary, nonmetastatic Ewing's sarcoma of bone: A long-term follow-up of the First Intergroup Study. J Clin Oncol. 8(10):1644-1674; 1990.

90c. Nesbit, M.E. Bone tumors in infants and children. Pediatrician. 1:273-287;1972-1973.

90d. Nesbit, M.E.; Perez, C.A.; Tefft, M.; et al. Multimodal therapy for the management of primary non-metastatic Ewing's sarcoma of bone: an Intergroup Study. NCI Monogr. 56:255-262;1981.

91. Newall, J., Friedman M. Reticulum-cell sarcoma: radiation dosage for each type. Radiology. 94:643-647, 1970.

92. Nilsonne U. The treatment of osteosarcoma with interferon and local tumor resection. J. Bone Joint Surg. 628:528-529;1980.

93. Nobler M.P., Higenbothan N.L., Phillips R.F. The cure of aneurysmal bone cyst. Irradiation superior to surgery in an analysis of 33 cases. Radiology. 90:1185-1192, 1968.

93a. Oberlin, O.; Patte, C.; Demeocq, F.; et al. The response to initial chemotherapy as a prognostic factor in localized Ewing's sarcoma. Eur J Cancer Clin Oncol. 21:463-467;1985.

94. Ornitz R., Hershavig A., Schell M., Fender F., Rogers C.C. Treatment experience: Locally advanced sarcomas with 15 MeV Fast neutrons. Cancer. 45:2712-2716, 1980.

95. Penn C.R.H. Single-dose and fractionated palliative irradiation for osseous metastases. Clin. Radiol. 27:405-408, 1976.

95a. Perez, C.A.; Tefft, M.; Nesbit, M.E.; et al. Radiation therapy in the multimodal managment of Ewing's sarcoma of bone: report of the Intergroup Ewing's Study. NCI Monogr. 56:262-271;1981.

96. Phillips T.L.; Sheline G.E. Radiation therapy of malignant bone tumors. Radiology. 92:1537-1545, 1969.

97. Picci P., Bacci G., Guerra A.; et al. Neoadjuvant chemotherapy for osteosarcoma: a study of 93 cases. Proc. Am. Soc. Clin. Oncol. 5:493, 1986.

97a. Picci, I.; Bacci, G.; Neff, J.R.; Capanna, R.; Baldini, N.; et al. The influence of preoperative chemotherapy (POC) in the surgical planning in patients (Pts) with osteosarcoma (OS). A histopathological study on 205 pts. Proc. Am. Soc. Clin. Oncol. Washington, DC: 9:1198;1990.

98. Pomeroy, C.T.; Johnson, R.E. Integrated therapy of Ewing's sarcoma. In: Vaeth, J.M., ed. Frontiers of Radiation Therapy and Oncology. vol. 10. Basel, Germany: S. Karger; 1975:152-166.

99. Potdar G.G. Primary reticulum-cell sarcoma of bone in Western India. Br.J.Cancer, 24(1):48-55, 1970.

100. Pratt C.B., Howarth C., Ransom J.L.; et al. High-dose methotrexate used alone and in combination for measurable primary or metastatic osteosarcoma. Cancer Treat. Rep. 64:11-20, 1980.

101. Presant, C.A., Russell, W.O., Alexander, R.W., Fu, Y.S. Soft-tissue and bone sarcoma histopathology per review: the frequency of disagreement in diagnosis and the need for second pathology opinions. The Southeastern Cancer Study Group experience. J. Clin. Oncol. 4(11):1658-1661, 1986.

102. Qasin M. Half-body irradiation (HBI) in metastatic carcinomas. Clin. Radiol. 32:215-219, 1981.

103. Qasin M. Single dose palliative irradiation for bone metastasis. Strahlenther. 153:154-532, 1977.

104. Razek A, Perez CA, Tefft M, et al. Intergroup Ewing's Sarcoma Study: local control related to radiation dose. volume and site of primary lesion of Ewing's sarcoma. Cancer. 46:516-521, 1980.

105. Reimers M., Castro J.R., Leinstadt D., Collier J.M., Henderson S., Hannigan J., Phillips T.L. Heavy charged particle therapy of bone and soft tissue sarcoma. Am. J. Clin. Oncol. 9(6):488-493, 1986.

106. Ritts, R.E. Jr; Prichard, D.J.; Taylor W.F.; et al. Comparison of transfer factor and combination chemotherapy as postsurgical adjuvants in osteogenic sarcoma: results of 3 years. In: Rainer, N., ed. Immunotherapy of Malignant Disease. New York, NY: Schattauer; 1978:343-352.

107. Rofstad E.K., Brustad T. Radiosensitizing effect of misonidazole in acute and fractionated irradiation of a human osteosarcoma xenograft. Intl. J. Radiat. Oncol. Biol. Phys. 6:1163-1167; 1980.

108. Rosen, G. The Medical Management of Osteogenic Sarcoma. In: American Society of Clinical Oncology Education Manual. Chicago, IL: 1990; 90-93.

109. Rosen, G. Malignant musculoskeletal tumors: the clinical investigative approach to combined therapy. In: Proceedings of the National Conference on the Care of the Child with Cancer. New York, NY: American Cancer Society; 1979:72-82.

110. Rosen G. The current management of malignant bone tumors: where do we go from here? Med. J. Aust. 148:373-378, 1988.

111. Rosen, G.; Caparros, B.; Mosende, C.; et al. Curability of Ewing's sarcoma and considerations for future therapeutic trials. Cancer. 41:868-899, 1973.

112. Rosen, G.; Carparros, B.; Nirenburg, A. et al. Ewing's sarcoma of bone: An Intergroup study. Natl Cancer Inst Monogr. 56:255-262;1981.

113. Rosen, G.; Huvos, A.G.; Mosende, C.; et al. Chemotherapy and thoracotomy for metastatic osteogenic sarcoma. A model for adjuvant chemotherapy and the rationale for the timing of thoracic surgery. Cancer. 41:841-849; 1978.

114. Rosen G., Huvos A.G., Nirenberg A.; et al. Osteogenic sarcoma: selection of adjuvant chemotherapy based upon the response of the primary tumor to preoperative chemotherapy. Proc. Am. Soc. Clin. Oncol. 1:429, 1981. Abstract C-378.

115. Rosen, G.; Juergens, H.; Caparros, B. et al. Combination chemotherapy (T6) in the multidisciplinary treatment of Ewing's sarcoma. NCI Monogr. 56:289-299;1981.

116. Rosen, G.; Marcove, R.C.; Caparros, B.; et al. Primary osteogenic sarcoma. The rationale for preoperative chemotherapy and delayed surgery. Cancer. 43:2163-2177; 1979.

117. Rosen G, Murphy ML, Huvos AG, et al. Chemotherapy, en bloc resection and prosthetic bone replacement in the treatment of osteogenic sarroma. Cancer. 37:1-11; 1976.

118. Rosen, G.; Wollner, N.; Tan, C.; et al. Disease-free survival in children with Ewing's sarcoma with radiation therapy and adjuvant 4-drug sequential chemotherapy. Cancer. 33:384-393, 1974.

119. Royster R.L., King R., Ebersole J., DeGiorgi L.S., Levitt S. High dose preoperative supervoltage irradiation for osteogenic sarcoma. Am. J. Roentgenol. Radium Ther. Nucl. Med. 114(3):536-43, 1972.

119a. Rubin, P.; Carter, S. Combination radiation therapy and chemotherapy: a logical basis for their clinical use. Cancer. 26:274-292; 1976.

119b. Rubin, P.; Salazar, O.; Zagar G.; Constine, L.S.; Keys, H.; Poulter, C.A.; Van Ess, J.D. Systemic hemibody irradiation for overt and occult metastases. Cancer. 55:2210-2221, 1985.

119c. Ruggieri, P.; Picci, P.; Marangolo, M.; Biagini, R.; Madon, E.; et al. Neoadjuvant chemotherapy for osteosarcoma of teh extremities (OE): preliminary results in 116 patients)(Pts) treated preoperatively wiith methotrexate (MTX) (IV), cisplatinum (CDP) (IA) and Adriamycin (ADM). Proc. Am. Soc. Clin. Oncol. 9:1199;1990. Abstract.

120. Sailer, S.L., Harmon, D.C., Mankin, H.J., Truman, J.T., Suit, H.D. Ewing's sarcoma: surgical resection as a prognostic factor. Intl. J. Radiat. Oncol. Biol. Phys. 15(1) :43-52, 1988.

121. Salazar O.M., Rubin P., Hendrickson F.R., Poulter C., Zagar G., Feldman M.J., Asbell S., Doss L. Single-dose half-body irradiation for the palliation of multiple bone metastases from solid tumors: a preliminary report. Intl. J. Radiat. Oncol. Biol. Phys. 7:773-781, 1981.

122. Schwartz, H.S.; Zimmerman, N.B.; Simon, M.A.; Wroble, R.R.; Millar, E.A.; Bonfiglio, M. The malignant potential of enchondromatosis. J. Bone Joint Surg. 69A:269-274; 1987.

123. Scutellari-P-N.; Spanedda-R.; Feggi-L-M.; Calzolari-F.; Cervi-P-M. Comparison between traditional skeletal radiography and total body bone scintigraphy in the diagnosis of multiple myeloma. Radiol-Med (Torino). 70(5):271-276; 1984.

124. Seider, M.J., Rich T.A., Ayala A.G., Murray J.A. Giant cell tumors of bone: treatment with radiation therapy. Radiology. 161:537-540, 1986.

125. Silverberg, E. Cancer statistics, 1989. CA. 39(1); 1989.

126. Sim, R.H. Musculoskeletal oncology: state of the art. Orthopedics. 10(12):1673-1684, 1987.

127. Simon, M.A. Current concepts review: causes of increased survival of patients with osteosarcoma: current controversies. J. Bone Joint Surg. 66A:306-310; 1984.

128. Simon, M.A., Nachman, J. The clinical utility of preoperative therapy for sarcomas. J. Bone Joint Surg. 68A:1458-1463, 1986.

129. Spanier SS, Enneking WF, Enriques P. Primary malignant fibrous histiocytoma of bone. Cancer. 36:2084-2089, 1975.

130. Steel, H.H. Partial or complete resection of the hemipelvis. An alternative to hindquarter amputation for periacetabular chondrosarcoma of the pelvis. J. Bone Joint Surg. 60A:719-730; 1978.

131. Strander H, Adamson U, Aparisi T, et al. Adjuvant interferon treatment of human osteosarcoma. Recent results. Cancer Res. 68:40-44, 1979.

131a. Strauss, M.B. Familiar Medical Quotations. Boston, MA: Little, Brown and Co; 1968.

132. Suit H.D. Radiotherapy in osteosarcoma. Clin. Orthop. 111:71-75, 1975.

133. Sweet, D.L.; Mass, D.P.; Simon, M.A.; Shapiro, C.M. Histiocytic lymphoma (reticulum-cell sarcoma) of bone. J. Bone Joint Surg. 63A:79-84; 1981.

134. Taylor, W.F., Ivins J.C., Dahlin D.C.; et al. Trends and variability in survival from osteosarcoma. Mayo Clin. Proc. 53:695-700; 1978.

135. Taylor, W.F., Ivins, J.C., Pritchard D.J.; et al. Trends and variability in survival among patients with osteosarcoma: a 7-year update. Mayo Clin. Proc. 60: 91-104; 1985.

136. Tepper, J.; Glaubiger, D.; Lichter, A.; Wackenhut, J.; Glatstein, E. Local control of Ewing's sarcoma of bone with radiotherapy and combination chemotherapy. Cancer. 46:1969-1973;1983.

137. Thomas, P.R.; Foulkes, M.A.; Gilula, L.A.; et al. Primary Ewing's sarcoma of the ribs. A report from the Intergroup Ewing's Sarcoma Study. Cancer. 51:1021-1027;1983.

138. Tong D., Gillick L., Hendrickson F.R. The palliation of symptomatic osseous metastases. Cancer. 50:893-899; 1982.

139. Urtasun R.C., McConnachie P., Merz T. Radiation damage to the periphery and center of human osteogenic sarcoma. Cancer. 31:1354-1358; 1973.

140. Vaglini M., Belli F., Santinami M. Isolation perfusion of the lower limb with platinum. World J. Surg. 12:307-309; 1988.

141. Wang C.C. Treatment of primary reticulum cell sarcoma of bone by irradiation. N. Engl. J. Med. 278(24):1331-1332; 1968.

142. Wang, C.C.; Fleischli, D.J. Primary reticulum cell sarcoma of bone: with emphasis on radiation therapy. Cancer. 22:994-998;1968.

142a. Wang, C.C.; Schultz, M.D. Ewing's sarcoma. N. Engl. J. Med. 248:571-576;1953.

143. Weichselbaum, R.; Little, J.B.; Nove, J. Response of human osteosarcoma *in vitro* to irradiation. Evidence for unusual cellular repair activity. Intl. J. Radiat. Biol. 31:295-299; 1977.

144. Weisenburger, T.N.; Eilber, F.R.; Grant, T.; *et al.* Multidisciplinary limb salvage treatment of soft tissue and skeletal sarcomas. Intl. J. Radiat. Oncol. Biol. Phys. 7:1495-1499; 1981.

145. Wheldon T.E. Optimal fractionation for the radiotherapy of tumor cells possessing wide-shouldered survival curves. Br. J. Radiol. 52:417-418; 1979.

146. Wikstrom, M G.; Moseley, M.E.; White, D L.; Dupon, J.W.; Winkelhake, J.L.; Kopplin, J.; Brasch, R.C. Contrast-enhanced MRI of tumors. Comparison of Gd-DTPA and a macromolecular agent. Invest. Radiol. 24(8):609-615; 1989.

147. Winkler K., Beron G., Kotz R.; *et al.* Neoadjuvant chemotherapy for osteogenic sarcoma: results of a cooperative German/Austrian study. J. Clin. Oncol. 2:617-624; 1984.

148. Winkler K., Beron G., Schellong G.; *et al.* Kooperative Osteosarkomstudie COSS-77 Ergebnisse nach über 4 Jaren. Klin. Padiatr. 194:251-256; 1982.

149. Winkler K., Oeron G., Delling G.; *et al.* Neoadjuvant chemotherapy of osteosarcoma: results of a randomized cooperative trial (COSS-02) with salvage chemotherapy based on histologic tumor response. J. Clin. Oncol. 6:329-337, 1988.

149a. Wuisman, P.; Enneking, W.F. Prognosis for patients who have osteosarcoma with skip metastasis. J Bone and Joint Surg. Am Vol 72-A(1):60-68; 1990.

150. Yabut, S.M. Jr.; Kenan, S.; Sissons, H.A.; Lewis, M.M. Malignant transformation of fibrous dysplasia. A case report and review of the literature. Clin. Orthop. 228:281-289; 1988.

151. Yanguas, M.G. A study of the response of osteogenic sarcoma and adjacent normal tissues to radiation. Intl. J. Radiat. Oncol. Biol. Phys. 7:593-595;1981.

152. Zucker, J.M.; Henry-Amar, M.; Sarrazin, D.; *et al.* Intensive systemic chemotherapy in localized Ewing's sarcoma in childhood. A historical trial. Cancer. 52:411-423;1983.

Alvin L. Ureles, M.D., Medical Oncology
Alex Yuang-Chi Chang, M.D., Medical Oncology

Louis S. Constine III, M.D., Radiation Oncology
Charles D. Sherman, Jr., M.D., Surgical Oncology

Chapter **27**

CANCER OF THE ENDOCRINE GLANDS:
THYROID, ADRENAL, AND PITUITARY

Heed the lesson of Lau Tsu, Aristotle, Leonardo and Darwin, who teach that the truth is less often attained by gaping at the grand than by scrutinizing the small.

Timothy Ferris (3)

THYROID CANCER

PERSPECTIVE

Thyroid cancers are generally characterized by slow growth, delayed symptoms, and low morbidity and mortality. Although they account for only 0.4% of all cancer deaths (60), they command our attention because they most often present as a thyroid nodule and thus must be identified from among the many other more common causes of thyroid nodules seen in 4% of our population (2,2a). Furthermore, although the clinical course is the most prolonged of all cancers (excluding anaplastic cancers), thyroid cancers do cause death in sufficient numbers to justify early diagnosis and treatment.

Controversy continues over the proper diagnosis and treatment of thyroid cancer. Most nodules are not cancerous. Some cancers are not nodules. Most thyroid cancers behave benignly for many years, even after local or distant metastases. Some thyroid cancers are very aggressive and cause severe morbidity and death. The combination of needle biopsy, improved radioisotope and ultrasound scanning, along with such biochemical markers as thyroglobulin and calcitonin have improved our diagnostic acumen. When feasible, surgery and radioactive iodine (RAI) have been the touchstones of therapy.

Cancers of the adrenal cortex are rare and highly malignant tumors that are usually diagnosed only after regional and/or distant metastatic spread. Cancer of the adrenal cortex presents either as a large, nonfunctioning mass that encroaches on neighboring structures, or as a functioning carcinoma that produces severe Cushing's syndrome, virilization, feminization, hypertension, or combinations of these clinical states (82). It has a mortality rate of less than 0.2% of all the cancer deaths combined. Computed tomography (CT) and magnetic resonance imaging (MRI) and improved ultrasound machines have made clinical detection and diagnosis easier.

However, generally early diagnosis still relies on clinical suspicion. The impact on survival of finding incidental tumors remains to be defined. Prolonged survival is attainable with aggressive surgical approach and adjuvant therapy in some patients.

The human pituitary gland, first described in 1524 by the Italian anatomist Berengario da Carpi (132), is of central importance by virtue of its endocrinologic functions and anatomic relationships. The hypothalamic-pituitary axis has a regulatory role in growth and development, as well as thyroid, adrenal, and gonadal function (172). The pituitary gland is strategically located near the optic chiasm, hypothalamus, third ventricle, and medial temporal lobes (136). The ability of pituitary tumors to elaborate hormones and depress their secretion, or to compress critical anatomic structures, heightens their clinical impact. Advances in neuroradiologic, pathologic, and endocrinologic diagnoses, and in surgical, radiation, and chemical therapies have greatly improved the prognosis for patients with these highly curable tumors.

General Definitions

1. *Goiter* is any enlargement of the thyroid, whether diffuse or nodular.
2. *A thyroid nodule* is any discrete lump in the gland; for clinical purposes, it is usually located on or near the gland surface and measures more than 1 cm in size. Quite often, a clinically single nodule is associated with other, smaller, nonpalpable nodules.
   a. *A functioning nodule* is usually an encapsulated neoplasm (adenoma), elaborating thyroxine (T4) and/or triiodothyronine (T3), and has a variable degree of autonomy from the pituitary thyroid-stimulating hormone (TSH) feedback mechanism. It is rarely malignant and is capable of suppressing the normal thyroid tissue, taking up significant amounts of RAI, and producing a clinical spectrum ranging from euthyroidism to hyperthyroidism.

b. *A nonfunctioning nodule* does not accumulate significant amounts of RAI, and is often composed of a cluster of enlarged colloid follicles with or without a capsule. It is often cystic, hemorrhagic, or calcified. Some are true encapsulated neoplasms (adenomas) of a primitive trabecular or tubular histologic type.

When a nodule is solitary, especially in a patient under 30 years of age or in a male, a malignant neoplasm should be suspected. The younger the patient, the greater the risk of malignancy (69).

c. *Metastatic nodules* to the thyroid from carcinoma of lung, breast, and kidney are rarely noted clinically.

d. Lymphoma, sarcoma, rare tumors, and granulomas can present as *nodules*.

e. *Chronic thyroiditis* of the lymphocytic form may present with varying degrees of nodularity, particularly in goiters, where fibrosis interlaces with large areas of cellular infiltrations.

EPIDEMIOLOGY AND ETIOLOGY

Epidemiology

Magnitude of the problem: There are an estimated 11,300 new cases annually of thyroid cancer, 8300 in women and 3000 in men, and a United States mortality of approximately 1025 deaths per year (64). The disparity between the incidence and mortality in thyroid carcinoma is a reflection of its low morbidity.

Surgical evidence: Prior to needle biopsy, a screened population had a 9% incidence of cancer in nodular goiters (24% in solitary nodules) (18). There is a 0.5% incidence of cancer reported in toxic nodular goiter (54).

Autopsy incidence in clinically normal thyroid glands ranges from 0.% to 2.0% (100 per million to 20,000 per million). Data vary with the care and number of sections studied (65). These cancers are predominantly occult papillary thyroid carcinomas that grow slowly and remain occult in most patients. They are significantly higher in Japanese population studies than in matched studies conducted in the western hemisphere (34). According to Surveillance, Epidemiology and End Result data, there had been a rising incidence of papillary and follicular thyroid cancer during the past decade (64).

Etiology

Prolonged TSH stimulus (6b,9): Thyroid cancer is experimentally produced in animals by severe iodine restriction, goitrogens (such as cabbage and rapeseed), subtotal gland resection, and RAI singly or in various combinations. There are case reports of thyroid cancer developing in the untreated hyperplastic glands in congenital cretins and those with congenital goiter (26). Recently, thyroid-stimulating immunoglobulins have been suspect as tumor-promoting agents in patients with Graves' disease (16a,32).

Radiation effects cause cell nuclear atypicality (46). There is a significant incidence of thyroid cancer in children and in young adults who received therapeutic head and neck or thymus irradiation as infants (29,59). The effect of this exposure is characterized by latency (5 to 30 years) and, usually, a slow-growing papillary follicular cancer (29a,58). All patients with suspected thyroid cancer should be questioned about a history of radiation therapy (i.e., Hodgkin's disease [37a]).

A significant number of adults exposed to the intensive radiation of the Hiroshima explosion have developed thyroid cancer (55). Iodine-131 therapy for hyperthyroidism is not associated with an increased incidence of thyroid cancer (40).

Less well-defined *etiologic factors* are:

- The relationship of long-standing nontoxic colloid goiter to papillary and anaplastic carcinoma
- The relationship of follicular adenoma as a premalignant lesion to follicular carcinoma
- The role of genetics and neural crest anlage in medullary carcinoma

Pregnancy has no apparent effect on the course of thyroid cancer (39).

DETECTION AND DIAGNOSIS

Clinical Detection (See Table 27-1 for Symptoms and Signs)

1. All *solitary nodules and multinodular goiters* that are changing in size and any nodule in a male, young adult, or infant should be suspected to be cancerous.
2. Twenty percent of patients have a *family history* of goiter (8).

Table 27-1. Clinical Symptoms and Signs in 106 Patients with Thyroid Carcinoma

Symptoms and Signs	66 Patients With Papillary Carcinoma (%)	33 Patients With Follicular Carcinoma (%)	7 Patients With Anaplastic Carcinoma (%)
Hoarseness	9	15	55
Dysphagia	11	12	28
Pain-pressure	8	6	28
Dyspnea	3	6	43
Increasing size	56	75	85
Solitary nodule	60	65	14
Multinodular	33	20	70
Found in routine examination	27	30	0

3. Occasionally, thyroid cancer presents as an *enlarged lymph node in the neck*, or a *lytic bone lesion* or *pulmonary infiltrate*, and no nodule or palpable enlargement is noted in the thyroid.

Diagnostic Procedures

Radioisotopic thyroid scanning (33) (rectilinear or gamma camera) has been useful in delineating the poorly functioning "cold" nodule from the "hot" hyperfunctioning mass. A cold nodule is suggestive of cancer, but is more commonly colloid cyst, hemorrhage, calcification, or solid thyroid adenoma. The "warm" nodule, which concentrates isotope equal to the adjacent thyroid tissue, may be troublesome diagnostically and may harbor a cancer. Normally functioning thyroid tissue surrounding a cold nodule may mask its hypofunction. A warm nodule that fails to suppress with exogenous thyroid is autonomous and, like the hot nodule, is unlikely to be cancerous.

The main choices for preoperative thyroid scanning are iodine-123 (43) and technetium-99m because of their short half-lives, low radiation doses, useful energy peaks, and physiologic behaviors of labeling functioning tissue but not cancer (12). Gallium-67 thyroid uptake appears to correlate to the degree of malignancy. It does not label differentiated thyroid cancer, but can identify highly malignant anaplastic cancer and lymphoma and therefore may prove to be a predictor of prognosis, although more studies are needed (38). Thallium-201 imaging may have a place in localizing thyroid metastases or recurrences in patients with a negative iodine-131 scan and abnormal levels of serum thyroglobulin, and may prove useful in its capacity to seek out tumor even in the presence of oral thyroid suppression in some patients (21,55a).

Finally, a number of promising recent studies have demonstrated significant visualization of thyroid medullary cancer, for example, using radiolabeled metaiodobenzylguanidine (11) and pertechnetate-labeled dimercaptosuccinic acid (52b,53). Their specificity and sensitivity will need further confirmation.

Needle biopsy (22a,37): Fine needle aspiration biopsy, large needle aspiration biopsy, and cutting needle biopsy have emerged as major diagnostic procedures for thyroid nodules in the past several years. Fine needle aspiration biopsy is the simplest and most widely used and has high specificity and sensitivity for thyroid malignancy. It requires good technique and an experienced cytologist. As in all other procedures, it fails to differentiate benign follicular adenoma from well-differentiated adenocarcinoma. When there is poor regression of a nodule treated with T4, repeat needle biopsy may be preferable to surgery.

Metastatic survey by plain radiographic screening (especially chest and bone films) is useful when using iodine-131, to identify the presence of local or remote nodal invasion, osteolytic bone lesions, or soft tissue infiltrates; it is most effective after all normal functioning tissue has been ablated and metastatic tissue has been stimulated by TSH (16).

Imaging of the neck (Table 27-2)
1. *Barium swallow* showing displacement and fixation of the trachea by goiter might add to one's suspicion of malignancy.
2. *Tracheal stenosis, when present*, is readily seen in regular chest films.
3. *Uniform, poorly marginated, fine, hazy calcifications* in streaked or nebular formation seen in special soft tissue x-rays of the thyroid (psammoma bodies) are noted in some papillary follicular carcinomas.
4. Medullary carcinomas of the thyroid often have characteristic *dense homogenous conglomerate calcifications* on one or both sides of the trachea. Involved nodes are also calcified.

Indirect laryngoscopy should be performed routinely. Unilateral or bilateral vocal cord paralysis is often an ominous sign of invasive thyroid carcinoma. The right-angle distal lens laryngoscope is particularly useful to view vocal cords.

Simple Transillumination might indicate a simple, fluid-filled, colloid cyst if it is very superficial; however, papillary carcinoma may be found in a degenerating cyst.

Thyroid *function tests*, aside from the radioisotopic scan, are of little value. Patients most often have normal radioimmunoassay T4, T3, free T4, T3 uptake, T4 binding, and antibody tests.

Elevated human thyroglobulin levels measured by radioimmunoassay are a valuable but not specific marker for well-differentiated thyroid cancer (56,56a). In totally thyroidecto-

METHOD	DIAGNOSIS AND STAGING CAPABILITY	RECOMMENDED FOR USE
Primary tumor and regional nodes		
CT	Extent of primary and regional nodal disease	Yes
MRI	Extent of primary and regional nodal disease for extensive lesions	Yes
Sonography	Detect primary, help determine nature of margins and extent	No
Radionuclide thyroid scan	Functioning v. nonfunctioning solitary thyroid nodule	Yes
Metastatic evaluation		
Radionuclide total body ^{131}I scan	For detecting functioning metastases after thyroid ablation	Yes
Radionuclide brain, bone, liver scan	For detecting metastases in symptomatic patients or advanced lesions	No

Table 27-2. Imaging Modalities for Evaluating Thyroid Tumors*

*Depending on histologic type and clinical or surgical estimate of extent of lesion.
CT = computed tomography; MRI = magnetic resonance imaging.

mized and iodine-131-ablated patients, persisting or recurrent elevations are highly correlated with active disease. Many patients are monitored with this assay as an alternate method of follow-up while still taking thyroid suppression therapy (see below). More data are needed (17).

Rare cases of hyperthyroidism with carcinoma *in situ* and functioning follicular carcinoma with extensive metastases will elevate all the above modalities (24). T3 might be the predominant hormone synthesized and released. Thyroid storm has been reported (23).

Ultrasound (19) evaluation of cystic versus solid thyroid nodules has improved rapidly over the past few years using high resolution probes with refined "B-mode" gray scale techniques. Ultrasound shows a high sensitivity for lesion detection; however, specificity is still low for malignancy. It is safe, fast, and an excellent localizing technique when combined with needle aspiration biopsy (70).

CT scanning and (MRI) scanning are the most recent imaging approaches to thyroid nodules diagnosis. Goiters and nodules greater than 0.5 cm are delineated and measured by both techniques but tissue signatures may be enhanced by high-field strength surface-coil MRI. Cost considerations are still major deterrents in selecting these modalities.

CLASSIFICATION AND STAGING

Histopathology (44) (Table 27-3)

Papillary carcinoma (with varying degrees of papillary and follicular formation), the most common type, comprises more than 50% of all adult and 80% of all childhood thyroid cancers (58). It tends to remain localized for years, and then spreads to local cervical nodes and later to mediastinal nodes and to lungs. At times, the primary focus is occult and requires careful serial section; often it is multifocal and bilateral. Papillary carcinoma becomes more aggressive in later life and metastasizes widely; death rarely occurs until past age 40 years(45,48a).

Follicular carcinoma represents about 25% of all thyroid cancer. It peaks in the third to fifth decades and can spread to nodes, but readily invades blood vessels and causes distant metastases, especially to bone. Types I and II well-differentiated follicular carcinoma with gradations of local infiltration are similar to papillary cancer in behavior. Type III (invasive follicular carcinoma) is more aggressive, often bilateral, tends to recur, and has a graver prognosis (68).

Medullary thyroid carcinoma (MTC) (75) constitutes 7% of thyroid malignancies. Derived from neural crest C cells rather than thyroid follicles, it is an aggressive tumor with

sporadic and familial forms. Secretory markers such as calcitonin allow for early discovery and cure in the familial form and serve as an index for recurrence (73). MTC frequently involves both thyroid upper lobes, with associated well-demarcated, hyalinized, fibrous, and amyloid-containing tumor. Additional, less common, biochemical markers secreted are histaminase, prostaglandin E2 and F2, corticotropin, vasoactive intestinal peptide, serotonin, lipotropin b, carcinoembryonic antigen, somatostatin, chromagranin A, and a novel neuroendocrine protein (28), some of which may have clinical expressions.

Three familial types of disease have been identified, all of which are autosomal dominant, have high penetrance, and exhibit variable expression. Multiple endocrine neoplasia (MEN) IIa is associated with hyperparathyroidism and bilateral pheochromocytoma. MEN IIb is also associated with pheochromocytoma and characteristic mucosal neuromata of lips and tongue, intestinal ganglioneuromatoses, marfanoid features, and skeletal deformities (62). Non-MEN familial disease has no extrathyroidal manifestations and, unlike its counterparts, is strikingly indolent.

The sporadic form of MTC is most common, often is only present in one thyroid lobe, and usually is detected in older age groups, which accounts for its poorer prognosis.

RAI therapy is useless and radiation therapy has little effect in MTC (57).

Anaplastic carcinoma appears as squamoid, giant or spindle cell cancer, and may arise out of long-standing, transforming, papillary cancers of Hürthle cell tumors (45a). These are highly lethal forms, not susceptible to therapy, with a median survival of 4 months (52a). A less virulent form, recently characterized as insular carcinoma, has been identified (41b).

Histologic Grading (4,5)

1. *Grade I*: Encapsulated, circumscribed neoplasms with only minimal invasion of adjacent gland or vessels.
2. *Grade II*: More extensive infiltration of surrounding gland, less differentiated, and greater cellular pleomorphism and mitoses.
3. *Grade III*: Extensive growth in gland, often with extraglandular invasion, dedifferentiated, pleomorphic with multinucleated cells, very mitotic.

Anatomic Staging

The American Joint Committee for Cancer Staging and End-Results Reporting (1) recommends the following classification to allow for the collection of data describing disease extent. It will undoubtedly be modified and refined (Table 27-4) (1,6). It is different from a clinical staging system proposed by the International Union Against Cancer (6).

1. *TNM (tumor, node, metastases) Classification* (Table 27-4).
   - *Primary tumor* (T)
   - *Nodal involvement* (N)
   - *Distant metastases* (M)
2. *Stage grouping*: *clinical staging* (using TNM system) (1) (Table 27-4, Fig. 27-1). Thyroid carcinoma evolves and can spread by (4):
   a. *Intraglandular pathways*:
   - Direct extension through true or pseudocapsule to invade normal parenchyma.
   - Multifocal seeding progressing to bilateral involvement via thyroidal lymphatics.

Table 27-3. Histologic Classification of Thyroid Tumors	
Tumor Type	**Incidence (%)**
Malignant	
Follicular carcinoma	25
Papillary carcinoma	60
Squamous cell carcinoma	
Undifferentiated (anaplastic) carcinoma	
Spindle cell type	
Giant cell type	15
Small cell type	
Medullary carcinoma	3

Table 27-4. TNM Classification and Stage Grouping for Cancer of the Thyroid

TNM Classification			Stage Grouping			
			Under 45 years	45 years and older		
T1	< 1 cm, limited to thyroid					
T2	> 1 cm, < 4 cm, limited to thyroid	ST I	T_{any}, N_{any}, M_0	Stage IA	T0	N0-3	M0
T3	> 4 cm, limited to thyroid	ST II	T_{any}, N_{any}, M_1	Stage IB	T1	N0-3	M0
T4	Extension beyond capsule			Stage II	T2	N0-3	M0
				Stage III	T3	N0-3	M0
N1$_a$	Ipsilateral cervical			Stage IV	T0-3	N0-3	M1
N1$_b$	Bilateral/midline/contralateral cervical/mediastinal						

T = tumor; N = node; M = metastasis.

Adapted from AJC/UICC (1,6).

b. *Extraglandular pathways*:
- Direct invasion of lobe capsule and isthmus into neighboring muscle, connective tissue, nerves, or trachea.
- Lymphatic spread to regional, cervical, mediastinal, or more distant nodes.
- Blood vessel invasion and metastases to distant sites.

Staging Work-up

Recommended Procedures

T work-up: Determine whether there is fixation to the trachea or invasion outside of the capsule into muscle. As noted in the classification, except for size, mobility is the important consideration.

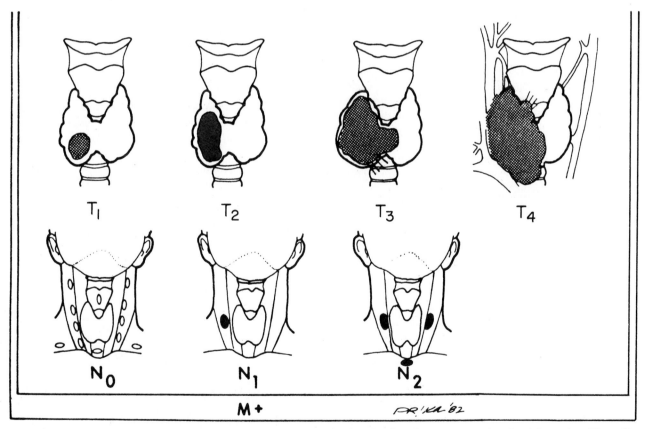

Fig. 27-1. Anatomic staging for thyroid cancer. Tumor *(T) classifications:* The size (less than or greater than 4 cm) determines T1a and b; fixation — partial versus complete — determines T2 versus T3. *Node (N) categories:* Since adenopathy is less ominous, all regional nodes are N1 if nodes are mobile. Thus, homolateral, contralateral, and bilateral are 1a, 1b, and 1c. If fixed, then nodes become N2. *Stage grouping:* None is recommended at the present time, but an example of clinical staging is shown in Table 27-3. *AJC versus UICC classification:* The UICC classification is entirely different and has 4 categories. It is based on single versus multiple nodules (T1 versus T2), homolateral versus bilateral (T2 versus T3), mobility versus fixation (T3 versus T4), and extension beyond capsule. *Pathologic (presurgical) stage (p)* TNM is totally different, and is based onsimilar features, but nodules less than 1 cm or greater than 1 cm in size are a critical distinction between pT1 and pT2. Modified from AJC (1) and UICC (6).

N work-up: Careful palpation of neck nodes is important. Chest films can be used to assess mediastinal widening. Barium swallow is also valuable.

M work-up: Chest films, skeletal survey, Sequential Multiple Analysis, RAI profiles, and body scans are important. In follicular and mixed follicular papillary cancer, it is essential to search for occult metastases with RAI after the primary is removed by surgical and iodine[131] ablation. Occasionally, metastases will pick up RAI in spite of a functioning thyroid gland.

PRINCIPLES OF TREATMENT

Treatment of thyroid carcinoma remains one of the pivotal controversies in clinical medicine. Early diagnosis and extirpation are essential before intraglandular and extraglandular invasion occurs or distant metastases take place. Because thyroid cancer is usually an indolent disease, the classical 5- and 10-year assessments are less meaningful than longer follow-up for morbidity, recurrence, and death. Host factors and biologic behavior of the tumor also may be more important than procedures. Clinicians who must treat these rare patients with advanced local or metastatic disease must ultimately decide if more aggressive treatment at an earlier stage would make a difference. There is need for a large, national, multicentered, standardized, therapeutic trial conducted over time to answer this question (48). A concise tabulation of recommended therapeutic approaches for common, well-differentiated thyroid cancer is shown in Table 27-5 (62).

Surgery (45)

For *papillary cancer*, (a solitary nodule), total lobectomy is done as an excision biopsy. If frozen section shows a papillary tumor, then the opposite lobe is removed, leaving a bit of posterior capsule and the adjacent superior parathyroid. All peritracheal lymph nodes and thymus are removed. If neck nodes are clinically involved, neck dissection is done (usually leaving the sternomastoid muscle to minimize deformity). This treatment plan is somewhat controversial. Occult carcinoma, which has been defined by Woolner *et al.* (76) as that less than 15 mm, is treated by unilateral lobectomy and node dissection.

For *follicular cancer* (types I and II), lobectomy and isthmectomy with local node excision are performed when indicated. For type III, treat as above for papillary cancer.

For *medullary cancer, aggressive* total thyroidectomy and node dissection is performed when possible (20). Progressive tracheal obstruction is common and palliative tracheotomy is usually indicated with resection of tumor lying anterior to the trachea, if possible.

Radiotherapy

The response of thyroid cancer to radiation therapy needs more evaluation. Smedal *et al.* (67) report encouraging results in patients with differentiated cancer who were given 2 MeV treatments postoperatively in place of radical neck dissection. Temporary, but gratifying, responses have been noted in bone metastases.

1. *Follicular* and *papillary cancers* are fairly radioresistant. If the deposit is small, the best chance for control of residual disease lies in postoperative external irradiation. Adequate doses, in the range of 5000 to 6000 cGy, require angled wedged fields with megavoltage photons or electrons. Large, inoperable neck masses can be partially reduced and growth can be temporarily halted, but rarely eradicated.

2. *Anaplastic small cell carcinomas* can be radiosensitive and deserve rigorous radiation treatment. Sometimes pathologic diagnosis is incorrect, and lymphoma is detected in the follow-up. Doses similar to those for papillary cancers are required.

3. *Anaplastic large cell carcinoma* is virtually radioresistant and rarely regresses even with full doses of irradiation to 6000 cGy. As noted (57), radiotherapy for medullary carcinoma has not been beneficial.

RAI Therapy

In spite of more than 40 years of RAI therapy, controversy continues over the specific indications and methodology, as well as the fundamental efficacy of this modality. Proponents (15,46) argue as follows:

> Of the more than 1000 patients dying each year from thyroid cancer, most have had differentiated malignancies that have metastasized. Aggressive treatment, early in their disease, would have resulted in a significant salvage rate. Thirty-nine percent of patients with metastatic cancer in the University of Michigan series were not detected by RAI tracer study at the time of surgery until after the normal competing residual tissue was totally ablated. Since we cannot predict

Table 27-5. Multidisciplinary Treatment Decisions for Well-Differentiated Thyroid Cancer (6a,55a)

Patient Age	Size of Lesion	Extrathyroidal Disease	Recommended Therapy
Any	≤ 2 cm	Absent	Thyroid lobectomy or NTT with suppression
< 45	2-4 cm	Absent	NTT/TT with suppression
≥ 45	2-4 cm	Absent	NTT/TT with suppression and ^{131}I ablation
Any	> 4 cm	Present with direct invasion	NTT/TT with suppression and ^{131}I ablation *
Any	Any	Distant metastases (bone on lung)	NTT/TT with suppression and ^{131}I ablation

NTT/TT = near total/total thyroidectomy; suppression = thyroxine to decrease thyroid stimulating hormone levels; [131]I = treatment with [131]I.

* One may consider additional local radiation therapy.

PDQ: NR.

Adapted from Norton et al. (6a).

who these patients will be, the proponents argue that all patients (except those with occult carcinoma) with proven thyroid cancer should have a bilateral lobectomy and isthmectomy followed by RAI ablation of the residual protective tissue. After a suitable period of induced hypothyroidism (6 weeks), a large RAI tracer is given to identify any stimulated metastatic disease and, if present, it is treated. Patients are then treated with suppressive oral thyroid. Treated metastases are followed yearly and rechallenged off thyroid therapy and treated until there is no longer uptake. Side effects are few. Subsequent fertility and birth histories are comparable with untreated populations. Patients whose distant metastases are adequately treated survive 2.2 to 3 times longer than patients not free of disease (14).

Our treatment protocol includes:

1. A 5 to 10 Mc iodine-131 tracer study 6 weeks after modified total thyroidectomy, after measurements of serum thyroglobulin and TSH are obtained in a nonpregnant, stable, iodine- restricted patient (74). Residual thyroid tissue and/or nodes are treated with 150 to175 Mc, extrathyroidal metastases are treated with 200 millicuries (47).
2. The tumor is suppressed with oral thyroxine.
3. Repeat steps 1 and 2 after 1 and 2 years until metastases do not take up RAI.
4. If there are no metastases, patients are maintained on oral suppression and followed with a yearly serum thyroglobulin and chest x-ray.

Thyroid Suppressive Therapy

1. Exogenous thyroid in high doses will suppress TSH and will probably induce regression in TSH-dependent tumors. Suppressive exogenous thyroid therapy should be given to all patients after appropriate primary therapy. It is possible to increase tolerance to large doses of exogenous T_4 by adding a ß-adrenergic blocker, such as propranolol.
2. Monitoring the effectiveness of suppression by TSH radioimmunoassay may prove useful. Recurrence on adequate suppressive therapy is uncommon.
3. There is a growing body of opinion that patients exposed to head and neck irradiation as infants should have regular clinical evaluation of their thyroid glands. The prophylactic use of exogenous thyroid therapy to suppress the gland at risk is still under study (13).
4. TSH receptors on cell membranes of papillary carcinoma have recently been identified and may prove useful in identifying tumor likely to suppress (41).
5. A surprising regression of metastatic tumor has been reported in medullary cancer treated with oral thyroid, a tumor type in which one would not expect to find TSH receptors; further clarification of this aspect of therapy is needed (31).

Chemotherapy

Numerous antineoplastic drugs have been administered for MTC that does not respond to conventional therapy. Doxorubicin to a dosage of 60 mg/m^2 appears to be the most promising. Responses were noted in tumors of all cell types (Table 27-6) (6a) (35,36). Combined modality treatment using immunotherapy (50), doxorubicin, and surgery in anaplastic disease may prove useful (22).

SPECIAL CONSIDERATIONS

Complications of Disease (25)

1. Patients dying of thyroid cancer most commonly have respiratory obstruction, pneumonia, hemorrhage, and thromboembolism.
2. Disability from metastatic bone disease is often painful and frequently presents with pathologic fracture.
3. Functioning follicular carcinoma may cause hyperthyroidism. Cases of thyroid storm have been reported (23).

Complications of Treatment

Surgery (61)

1. *Recurrent nerve paralysis* is rare in experienced hands.
2. *Hypothyroidism* is readily corrected and does not present a management problem.
3. *Hypoparathyroidism* is a more difficult problem to manage medically and when performing a total thyroidectomy, care must be taken to leave at least one parathyroid and its blood supply intact, even if it requires compromising the resection margins.

Iodine[131] Treatment (33)

1. Radiation sickness is usually mild or absent.
2. Sialoadenitis presenting as dry mouth or gland tenderness or swelling may last 3 weeks to more than 2 years (10).
3. Rare symptoms may be seen secondary to local posttherapy edema in metastases (27).
4. The radiation hazard of induced leukemia or malignancies does not appear to be a problem in the doses and intervals noted. Indeed, higher doses may be used without even using the blood dosimetry approach of Benua, Leeper et al. (71).

RESULTS AND PROGNOSIS

The personal experience of one of the authors (A. Ureles) is documented in Table 27-7 (7), Fig. 27-2. Note that the 10-year survival is excellent for stage I disease - approximately 90%. Survival decreases as a function of cancer invasion beyond the gland. Papillary and follicular cancers have long-term survival (Table 27-8), but anaplastic cancers are lethal and survival is short.

Table 27-6. Chemotherapy Response Rates for Thyroid Carcinoma		
Combination Chemotherapy	**Responders (%)**	**Complete Response (%)**
Doxorubicin	17-35	0
Doxorubicin + cisplatin	9-26	0-12
Doxorubicin+bleomycin+vincristine + melphalan	36	19
Doxorubicin+bleomycin+vincristine	64	0
From Norton et al. (6a), with permission.		

Survival Studies (29) (Fig. 27-2, Table 27-7)

1. *Long-term survival rates:* Approximately 20% of patients with thyroid cancer die of their disease (papillary 13%, follicular 22%, anaplastic 84%). Ten- and 20-year survival are similar for both papillary and follicular carcinomas — for papillary carcinomas 10-year survival is 90% and 20-year survival is 60% (Fig. 27-3a). Invasive follicular carcinoma has a poorer prognosis — 10-year survival is 60% and 20-year survival is 35% (52) (Fig. 27-3b).

   a. In a recent study of distant metastatic papillary cancer, patients under age 40 years often responded to iodine-131 treatment and their prognosis was good. Patients older than 40 years had a poor response and the disease was often lethal. However, 30% of distant metastatic follicular cancer patients responded at all ages and survival was significantly better than for those who were untreated (42).

   b. In another series of patients with more localized disease (72), death rates for thyroid ablated patients under 40 years old did not differ in those treated with surgery alone versus those treated with surgery plus iodine-131. Surgery plus iodine-131 treatment in patients over age 40 years, however, resulted in a significantly lower death rate.

2. Results of iodine-131 therapy on metastatic control by site: The best results and most cures are reported in patients with pulmonary metastases, although pulmonary fibrosis can be a serious complication of therapy with excessive doses. Bone metastases can be palliated, but successful control with complete remodeling and healing of the lesion is rare. Recent data suggest that pure follicular thyroid cancer, if extensive but localized to the neck, can be effectively treated with iodine-131 (77).

Table 27-7. Frequency and Survival in 1,006 Cases of Thyroid Cancer

Stage	Frequency (%)	10-Year Survival (%)	20-Year Survival (%)
IA	14	90	88
IB	55	89	82
II	15	54	42
III	10	29	16
IV	6	10	10

From Ureles (7), with permission.

Reasons for Failure

1. Failure to recognize intraglandular bilateral extension of the disease.
2. Failure to remove involved lymph nodes.
3. Failure to remove primary tumor before blood vessel invasion and distant metastases have occurred.
4. Failure to use the combination of total thyroidectomy, postoperative RAI, and thyroid hormone in patients with primary tumors greater than 1.5 cm in diameter (68).

Prognosis (66)

Nine prognostic factors, ranked by P value, for overall survival after treatment in papillary and follicular cancer have now been defined. Their order of importance is listed below:

1. Postoperative status, i.e., the presence or absence of residual gross or microscopic malignancy near the resected margin, postsurgery, is to be an important factor.
2. Age at diagnosis continues to be of major significance, with a worse prognosis after age 45 years and a second downward turn after age 60 years.
3. Extrathyroidal invasion into neighboring tissue remains a major negative finding.

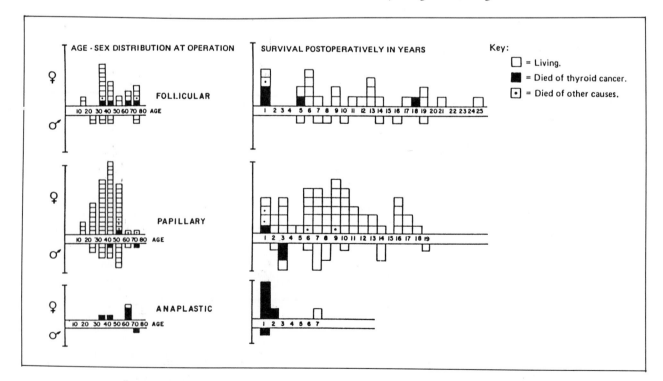

Fig. 27-2. Thyroid Cancer, 107 cases: Author's series. Courtesy of Ureles (7), with permission.

Table 27-8. Survival of Well-Differentiated Thyroid Carcinoma After Surgical Resection ± Ablation or Suppression, or Both

Group	5-Year Survival (%)	10-Year Survival (%)	20-Year Survival (%)
Papillary (41a,49,60a)	92–97	74–92	93
Follicular	73–96	43–94	
Schroader *et al.* (60a)			
Lang *et al.* (41b)			
Harness *et al.* (37a)			
Crile *et al.* (26a)			
Joensuu *et al.* (41a)			

4. Distant metastases is an especially important predictor in follicular cancer.
5. Nodal involvement is significant only if combined with the above factors.
6. The degree of differentiation is more significant for papillary-follicular than follicular cancer.
7. Males, in general, have a poorer survival than females, but sex has an overall low ranking.
8. Tumors more than 4 cm in diameter have a significantly poorer prognosis.
9. The characterization of follicular versus papillary-follicular cancer appears to be the lowest ranking prognostic factor.

CANCER OF THE ADRENAL CORTEX

EPIDEMIOLOGY AND ETIOLOGY

Epidemiology

Most of the literature consists of case studies reported singly or in small numbers. The best series are those of Lipsett and Wilson (110), and Hajjar *et al.* (101).

Magnitude of the problem: The incidence rate of adrenal cortex cancer is one to two cases per 1 million people. It is found in all decades, with a median age of 40 years at detection. Occurrence is not distinctive according to race or sex. The majority of tumors reported in small series and case studies are functioning cancer, i.e., virilism and Cushing's syndrome, and therefore are preponderantly in females. However, pathologic diagnosis reported in the large cancer registries offset this bias, because nonfunctioning tumors occur more frequently in male and older patients. Incidental finding of adrenal corticocarcinoma has increased in recent years in spite of lack of clinical suspicion (107,112). This may change the clinical picture and epidemiology.

Etiology

No etiologic factors have been elicited for adrenocortical malignancies. There does not appear to be a familial predisposition. Reports from Europe and throughout the United States do not suggest any particular geographic or climatic distribution.

Certain tumors may be sensitive to endogenous corticotropin and are, therefore, analogous to TSH-sensitive thyroid cancer (83). Carcinoma development in long-standing suppressible adrenal hyperplasia has been reported (88).

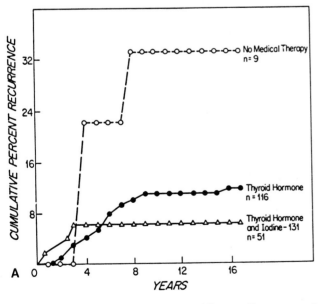 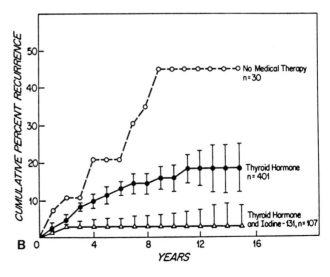

Fig. 27-3. Cumulative recurrence rates (A) according to type of postoperative therapy for papillary. From Mazzaferi *et al.* (49), with permission; (B) cumulative recurrence rates according to type of postoperative therapy for follicular carcinoma. From Young *et al.* (77), with permission.

DETECTION AND DIAGNOSIS

Clinical Detection

Typical Presentation

1. Frequently, local extension may displace, obstruct, or destroy the kidney and cause pain, hemorrhage, distention, and a large abdominal mass (44% in one study) (110). Weight loss, fatigue, anorexia, fever, and sweating are common, as in any advanced malignancy.
2. Widespread metastases to deep and to superficial nodes can appear as silent lymphadenopathy on chest x-ray or on physical examination. Metastatic lesions can erupt in any organ or system, causing symptoms. Bone metastases are unusual and can be lytic or blastic.
3. Lungs and liver are most commonly involved and occur in the course of most patients affected. Leg edema and distal myopathy are noted in 10% of cases. As in renal carcinoma, adrenal cancer tends to invade the veins locally producing thrombosis and occlusion. Embolic complications are not uncommon.

Hormonal Patterns

When the neoplasm involves functioning tissue, clinical endocrinopathies may or may not manifest. It is clear that adrenal cancer can excrete large amounts of 17-ketosteroids (17-KS) and 17-hydroxycorticoids (17-HOC) without clinical evidence of steroid excess. This has led to a confusion of terminology in the literature. The following are recognized types of endocrine syndromes:

1. Nonfunctioning: Steroid output is normal or low, and emanates from normal adrenal residue (95).
2. Functioning: Steroid production and excretion are increased with a normal or abnormal spectrum, but no syndrome is produced.
3. Syndrome-producing: Steroid production is excessive (94) and there is an abnormal spectrum producing homogeneous, or more commonly, mixed endocrinopathy or precocious puberty. These syndromes constitute about 50% of cases. The clinical manifestations are as follows:
   a. Feminization in males: Progressive loss of libido, impotence, gynecomastia, edema, and atrophic testes occurring variably over months or years (83,123). Young males may become sexually precocious.
   b. Virilization in females: Hypertrichosis, male pubic escutcheon, amenorrhea, voice deepening, oily skin, bitemporal hair recession, and enlarged clitoris (127).
   c. Cushing's syndrome: Often presents as an advanced clinical picture associated with hirsutism and is more often noted in females. Classical Cushing's syndrome may comprise up to 20% of syndrome-producing carcinomas (85,90,101). In a child, it is frequently due to adrenal cancer.
   d. Hypertension: Rarely, aldosteron-producing cancers have been reported (92). Hutter and Kayhoe (80) raise the question as to whether this is due, in some cases, to secondary renal artery compression. This is unlikely when patient's aldosterone level is markedly elevated, associated with profound hypokalemia, and there is a heterogenous adrenal mass (91).
   e. Mixed syndromes: One particular pattern often predominates, but underlying mixed syndromes are common. Shifting patterns evolving during the course of the disease also have been described.
   f. Inappropriate polypeptide hormones: Rarely, adrenal cancers produce gonadotropin (87) and a hypoglycemic substance that is presumably insulin-like. Walters *et al.* (128) have reported an unusual cortical cancer that appeared to produce catecholamines and presented as a pheocromocytoma. An antidiuretic hormone-like syndrome has been reported (96).

Diagnostic Procedures

A number of excellent imaging studies are available (Table 27-9) (78).

Imaging for Localization

Intravenous pyelography can give the first clue of a suprarenal mass displacing the kidney and nephrotomograms can give additional diagnostic support.

Suprarenal CT scan is the most commonly used single test to evaluate adrenal gland neoplasms. It is simple, effective, and noninvasive, and can evaluate bilateral adrenal glands and adjacent anatomic structures in one setting and detect neoplasms greater than 1 cm in size. Its use has eliminated the need for retroperitoneal pneumography, which was a standard test in evaluating adrenal glands and other retroperitoneal lesions. Both adrenal glands have been visualized and characterized in site and shape in 78% to 90% of normal persons (114) by CT scan. It was successfully localized in pheochromocytoma in 10 of 11 patients (57). In other reports, 11 of 13 patients with adrenal cortical adenoma and seven of seven with adrenal cortical carcinoma were identified by CT (105). The same group reported a false-negative

Table 27-9. Imaging of the Adrenal: Ability to Predict Histology	T_2 Image Adrenal Mass /Liver Ratio
Nonfunctioning or hyperfunctioning cortical adenomas	0.7 - 1.4
Metastases from other primary	1.2 - 2.8
Adrenal carcinoma	1.2 - 2.8
Pheochromocytoma	>3
From Doppman et al. (78), with permission.	

rate of 11% (3 of 26) that was due to the small size of the lesion (<0.5 cm in diameter) or lack of retroperitoneal fat. Tumor mass greater than 6 cm is highly suggestive of malignant carcinoma. Although a negative CT scan result does not rule out the possibility of adrenal cancer, it is the test of choice for screening the adrenal gland.

Real time ultrasonography of the retroperitoneum and upper abdomen is the most innocuous method for evaluating adrenal lesions (97). Its use is limited by individual skill and obesity of the patients. It often provides useful guidance for percutaneous skinny needle biopsy, which has less morbidity and mortality compared with open biopsy (115). In a prospective study (108) comparing adrenal cortical photoscanning using iodocholesterol I-131, adrenal arteriography, and ultrasound in 27 patients who underwent adrenal exploration, ultrasound examination was recommended as the first choice in localizing biochemically suspected adrenal lesion because it is rapid, noninvasive, inexpensive, and reasonably accurate. The predictive values of a positive result of ultrasound, photoscanning, and arteriography were 100%, 100%, and 83%, respectively, while a negative result gave 79%, 85%, and 64% predictive values. Sample and Sarti (119) prospectively compared CT scan and gray scale sonography in evaluation of adrenal lesions in 34 patients and found that results were comparable and complementary. The drawback of ultrasound examination is that the interpretation relies heavily on the performer's technique and experience. Therefore, CT scan remains as a preferred initial test.

MRI can demonstrate useful information regarding the size and extent of the adrenal tumor. It can also study the vasculature of adrenal, renal, and inferior vena cava to determine vessel invasion. MRI may help to make differential diagnosis, since adrenal metastasis, carcinoma, and pheochromocytoma may have different signal intensities in MRI from those of benign adrenal adenoma, lipoma or myelolipoma, although overlapping of signal intensities have been reported (98). However, the role of MRI in evaluating adrenal carcinoma is still in the early development stage.

Angiography can demonstrate an extensive vascular network in the adrenal neoplasm and differentiate adrenal gland from upper pole renal tumors. A more precise outline, however, can be obtained by the newer technique of adrenal venography, which is needed in cases of primary hyperaldosteronism (Conn's syndrome) for functional localization of the lesion.

Photoscanning, in the form of iodocholesterol I-131 or ^{131}I-6-beta-iodomethyl-19-norcholesterol (NP-59) for imaging adrenal tumors, is a pathophysiologic study of adrenal gland diseases. This technique can identify a hot tumor, that is synthesizing corticoids with contralateral suppression or a unilateral adrenal destruction from a non-functioning cancer (124-126). Its use in identifying metastases appears encouraging (129). The scanning is time-consuming and requires 48 hours to complete. Nonetheless, it remains a complementary test to CT scan, especially in a patient with Cushing's syndrome and a normal CT scan. More recently, Gross *et al.* (99) reported that functional NP-59 scanning in patients with euadrenal mass (nonfunctioning), adrenal mass shown on CT scan had high specificity and accuracy in distinguishing benign from malignant adrenal mass. If there is a concordant imaging result of NP-59 and CT scan, the adrenal mass is likely to be adenoma, otherwise it is more likely to be metastatic disease or primary adrenal carcinoma.

Laboratory Studies (93)

Urinary excretions of steroids are valuable. (Be wary of daily fluctuations [110].) Although 24-hour values are high, the actual efficiency of steroid production in the cancers per gram of tissue is low, hence the large growth before detection.

1. In functioning cancers, 17-KS evaluations are most common, either alone or in combination with other metabolites. An increase in the beta fraction indicates carcinoma. This has now been identified as predominantly increased dehydroepiandrosterone (DHEA).
2. Normal or moderately depressed steroid excretions can be found in nonfunctioning cancers.
3. Some cancers function as noted previously, but produce no apparent clinical syndrome.
4. Increased 17-HOC are also common, though not as striking as 17 KS. Failure to suppress production with dexamethasone 2 mg qid for 72 hours is suggestive of adrenocortical cancer.
5. Steroid patterns frequently include large amounts of intermediates. Complete and relative failures in 11 beta-hydroxylation are often noted (130). Increases in DHEA, pregnanetriol, androstenedione, deoxycorticosterone, testosterone, estrogens, aldosterone, and tetrahydro-S all have been reported. Increased compound S: compound F ratio in the urine may be useful in selected cases.

Biopsy

Biopsy of abnormal lymph nodes, suspicious skin, or subcutaneous lumps is indicated. Adrenal cancers metastasize widely.

CLASSIFICATION AND STAGING

Histopathology

1. Grossly, adrenal carcinomas are characteristically large bulky tumors whose cut surfaces are yellow, frequently hemorrhagic, cystic, and necrotic. They are partly encapsulated. There appears to be no site predilection for the right side or left side.
2. Early, they can be small, encapsulated tumors similar to adenomas; the first evidence of their malignancy is metastasis. They can grow into the adrenal vein or the vena cava and can extend into the lymphatics.
3. Histologically, they can appear either benign or widely malignant. Capsule invasion and metastasis clearly indicate the malignant nature of the tumor.
4. Aggregates of lipid-laden polygonal cells are easily confused with renal adenocarcinoma.
5. Pleomorphism, multinucleated cells, and spindle shapes compose the usual picture.
6. When functional, the metastatic areas or the recurrence maintain the same hormonal pattern of the parent lesion, although variations have been reported.

Anatomic and Clinical Staging

A staging system with prognostic significance has recently been presented by Bradley (Table 27-10) (85).

PRINCIPLES OF TREATMENT

Surgery

Curative surgery should be attempted in 18 of 38 patients (47%) in the National Institute of Health series, but usually in a somewhat lower percentage of patients in other series. Aggressive, surgical, en bloc dissection of the primary tumor, resection of adjacent organs for local invasion, and excision of resectable metastatic disease in the lung or liver are the basic principles of surgical therapy and remain the most effective means of producing long-term survival (87,122). It is now felt that attack on the primary tumor in spite of metastatic spread is worthwhile.

Radiotherapy

Preoperative and postoperative radiation therapy have been used in an attempt to eradicate local extension. However, radiotherapy's adjuvant role to surgery has not been finally established (113). However, radiation therapy can be useful in palliation of bone pain from metastasis (109).

Chemotherapy

Mitotane has been used in the treatment of adrenal cancer since 1960 (Table 27-11). Almost all published reports agree that there is an induced regression in tumor size, both primary and metastatic, and commensurate decreases in steroid output when present (111). Although protocols vary, 0.5 g tablets are usually given in doses of 1 g tid, increasing to a total dosage of 8 to 10 g/d. After ingestion, mitotane is about 40% absorbed and deposits in subcutaneous fat, liver, brain, and both normal and malignant adrenal tissues (116). Plasma levels of mitotane were measurable up to 8.5 months posttherapy (102). Therefore, full glucocorticoid and mineralocorticoid replacement are necessary in most cases to prevent adrenal insufficiency during and after therapy. High-dose mitotane may not be needed and careful monitoring of the patient by adrenal cortical function test is the key in management of those patients receiving mitotrane.

In steroid metabolism, both mitotane and aminoglutethimide favor the 6,8 hydroxy derivatives and, therefore, 24-hour urine 170 hydroxy steroid values can be misleading. Plasma cortisol levels can be more meaningful (120).

A few case reports and retrospective analyses have shown that alkylating agents (cyclophosphamide, carmustine), doxorubicin, cisplatin, may have some antitumor activity (100). Combination chemotherapy with 5-FU and methotrexate, cisplatin and doxorubicin, etoposide, streptozotocin and mitotane (89,106) has been reported to cause tumor regression and reduction of steroid production in a few patients. Adequate evaluation of each chemotherapeutic agent either singly or in combination is not available and multi-institutional cooperative studies are needed.

Aminoglutethimide produces a dramatic decrease in urinary steroid levels and, although it may relieve symptoms, has poor tumoricidal properties.

Complication of Disease and Treatment

1. Local recurrences of large masses encroach on bowel and retroperitoneal structures. Rarely, the primary tumor may rupture spontaneously and present a picture of acute abdomen (85).
2. In functioning cancers, there can be severe and complete contralateral atrophy requiring vigorous preoperative and postoperative substitution therapy is required.
3. Mitotrane drug toxicity is usually dose related and is reversible. Ninety percent of patients have one or more of the following untoward effects:
   - gastrointestinal (GI)   83%
   - neuromuscular   41%
   - skin rash   19%

Table 27-10. Proposed Clinical Staging System for Carcinoma of the Adrenal Cortex

T = Extent of primary tumor
    1 = < 5 cm and confined to adrenal gland
    2 = < 5 cm, but < 10 cm or adherence to kidney
    3 = > 10 cm or invasion of surrounding structures including renal vein
M = Presence and type of metastases
    0 = no demonstrable metastases
    1 = regional lymphatics
    2 = distant metastases, eg. liver, lung, bone
R = Tissue remaining after resection
    0 = tumor completely excised
    1 = tumor entered at operation
    2 = tumor tissue remaining after resection
D = Degree of histologic differentiation
    1 = differentiated, no capsular or vascular invasion
    2 = moderately undifferentiated, either capsular or vascular invasion
    3 = anaplastic, both capsular and vascular invasion
Stage 1 = 3 or fewer; eg, T1, M0, R0, D1
Stage 2 = 4 and 5; eg, T2, M0, R1, D2
Stage 3 = 6 amd 7; eg, T3, M1, R1, D2
Stage 4 = 8 or more; eg, T3, M2, R2, D3

From Bradley (85). By permission of Surgery, Gynecology & Obstetrics.

Table 27-11. Chemotherapy Response Rates for Adrenal Cortical Carcinoma

Drug	Dose	Frequency	No. Patients	Efficacy
Mitotane	1-12 g/d	bid or tid		33% PR* 0 CR
Cisplatin + etoposide	40 mg/m^2/d 100 mg/m^2/d	Daily x 3	2	2 PR 0 CR
Cyclophosphamide + doxorubicin + cisplatin	600 mg/m^2 40 mg/m^2 50 mg/m^2	q 3 wk	11	2 PR 0 CR
Cyclophosphamide + vincristine + semustine + bleomycin	Not given		2	1 PR 0 CR
Doxorubicin alone	40 mg/m^2	q 4 wk	8	1 PR 0 CR
Cyclophosphamide, melphalan, or peptichermio	Not given		12	2 CR 0 CR
Cisplatin	120 mg/m^2	q 4 wk	5	0 PR 0 CR
Cisplatin + etoposide + bleomycin	40 mg/m^2 100 mg/m^2 30 U	q 4 wk	4	1 CR 2 PR

PR = partial remission; CR = complete remission.
From Norton et al. (6a), with permission.

A recent study (112) of mitotrane in Cushing's disease combined the active agent with cellulose acetatephthalate. In a series of 62 patients, little GI discomfort was noted, even with doses of 8 to 12 g/d. The cellulose acetatephthalate prevents absorption of mitotrane from the stomach and may account for the marked decrease in GI side effects.

4. Roginski and Schick (118) reports a case of combined therapy (mitotane and 5-FU) inducing acute Addison's disease in a patient with hyperfunctioning adrenal carcinoma.

RESULTS AND PROGNOSIS

Results

Surgical: Total ablation of functioning cancers is usually accompanied by gradual regression of the clinical syndrome. Recurrence is common and often heralded by a recurring increase in steroid production.

Radiotherapy: Its value is questionable due to the lack of well-documented data. Most reports have been disappointing. However, a significant palliative response was recorded in 6 of 16 patients from Walter Reed Army Medical Center (109) without improvement of survival. Its value in the immediate postoperative period as an adjuvant therapy remains unknown.

Chemotherapy: Mitotrane therapy is warranted for inoperable patients with both functioning and nonfunctioning adrenal cancer (Table 27-11). A review of 138 patients by Hutter and Kayhoe (80) demonstrates a steroid response rate of 72% and a measurable disease response rate of 34% for a mean duration of 5 and 10 months, respectively. A more recent review by Lubits *et al.* (111) continues to support the earlier impressions. Becker and Schumacher (84) reports two inoperable patients treated with mitotrane with prolonged survival. Ostuni and Roginski (117) reports a 9-year survival on mitotrane combined with 5-FU for a patient who had widespread metastases.

Prognosis

Prognosis is poor. Well-controlled studies on survival in this group of carcinomas are not available (121). Lipsett and Wilson (110) found that 50% of the patients died within 2 years of onset of symptoms. Only 30% of the inoperable patients survived 2 years. Histopathologic characterization and staging are the two most important prognostic factors. Anaplastic carcinoma occurred more often in male patients, produced more frequent cutaneous metastasis associated with a lack of clinical or laboratory evidence of hormone production, and had a shorter median survival time (5 months). In contrast, differentiated carcinoma usually occurred in women, produced clinical and laboratory evidence of hormone excess, and a longer median survival time (40 months) (103). Hough *et al.* (104) analyzed the histologic patterns in 41 cases of adrenal cortical tumors after curative surgery. They found that clinical evidence associated with a poor prognosis and early metastasis included weight loss, broad fibrous bands traversing the tumor, a diffuse growth pattern, vascular invasion, and tumor cell necrosis.

PITUITARY TUMORS

EPIDEMIOLOGY AND ETIOLOGY

Epidemiology

1. *Clinical incidence*: Pituitary tumors comprise up to 10% of symptomatic intracranial neoplasms (131).
2. *Autopsy incidence*: Asymptomatic adenomas are found in 10% to 20% of presumably normal pituitary glands (134,144).
3. *Population characteristics*: Male: female ratios and age ranges vary depending on the clinical syndrome.

Etiology

1. Most tumors arise from epithelial cells of the anterior pituitary (131).

2. Pathogenesis is not known, but two theories predominate (131,163,172).
   a. Spontaneous development of the tumor in a clone of cells within the pituitary.
   b. Hypersecretion or abnormal elaboration of releasing factors by the hypothalamus, causing tumor development in the pituitary.

In fact, both of these events may participate. Pituitary adenomas are usually benign and localized, and incapable of metastasis. Although the component cells are clearly transformed, as yet unidentified cellular restraining factors presumably prevent the expression of a true malignancy. Through a process of initiation and promotion (see Chapter 3, "Pathology of Cancer"), the resulting transformed cell replicates and actively expresses the products of specific genes (Fig. 27-4). This is likely due to the presences of altered surface receptors to neurotransmitters and hypothalamic hormones (169). For example, the pathogenesis of prolactinomas may involve cell responsiveness to defective synthesis or release of hypothalamic dopamine or the excessive elaboration of some prolactin-releasing factor (169).

3. Oral contraceptives may be associated with the development of prolactin-secreting tumors. However, since the use of contraceptives in premenopausal women is high, this association may be coincidental.

DETECTION AND DIAGNOSIS

Clinical Detection

Pituitary tumors cause symptoms by secreting or depressing the secretion of hormones, or by mass-related effects.

1. The variety of functions (Table 27-12) (172) regulated by pituitary hormones accounts for the variety of syndromes caused by these tumors.
   a. *Acromegaly*: The earliest symptoms of excess growth hormone (GH) are often nonspecific and include fatigue or lethargy, paresthesia, and headache. Patients then exhibit acral enlargement, weight gain, or excessive perspiration (164).
   b. *Cushing's syndrome*: Sustained hypercorticoidism causes obesity, hypertension, hirsutism, glucose intolerance, easy bruising, striae, osteoporosis, and psychologic changes (136).
   c. *Nelson syndrome*: This may follow bilateral adrenalectomy for Cushing's disease with development of hyperpigmentation and visual field defects (170).
   d. *Prolactin-hypersecretion syndromes*: Females present with galactorrhea, amenorrhea, oligomenorrhea, or infertility. Males complain of decreased libido or impotence. Galactorrhea may also occur in male groups.

2. Mass-related symptoms are also manifold because of the many critical structures in the vicinity of the pituitary gland (131,136,166).
   a. *Optic nerve compression* with bilateral visual field loss that often begins in the superior temporal quadrants is the most common mass effect. Loss of visual acuity with optic disc atrophy may occur.
   b. *Cranial nerves III, IV, and VI may be compressed* by lateral tumor extension. Abnormalities in extraocular muscle function result. Cranial nerve V is rarely affected.
   c. *The hypothalamus may be involved by tumor extension* superiorly through the diaphragm sellae. Increased

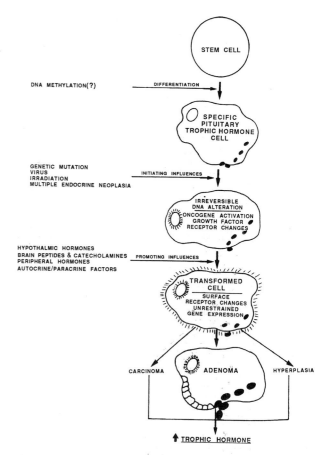

Fig. 27-4. Multistage model of pituitary tumor tumorigenesis. Reproduced with permission, from Melmed, S.; Braunstein, G.; Chang, R.; Becker, D. Pituitary tumors secreting growth hormone and prolactin. Ann. Intern. Med. 105:238-253; 1986.

appetite, diabetes insipidus, or changes in anterior pituitary hormone secretion may occur.
   d. Headache, increased intracranial pressure, seizures, or cerebrospinal fluid rhinorrhea (CSF) may all occur.
   e. *Hypopituitarism* may be caused by anterior pituitary compression or hypothalamic involvement. Sequential loss of hormone secretion usually begins with loss of growth hormone or the gonadotropins (luteinizing hormone [LH] and follicle-stimulating hormone [FSH]). Depressions of TSH and corticotropin may follow.

3. Although hormonally active tumors are usually detected before the occurrence of mass effects, exceptions can be expected (e.g., prolactin-secreting tumors in nonmenstruating women).

Diagnostic Procedures

1. *Endocrinologic testing*: All patients with suspected or documented pituitary tumors should be evaluated for gonadal, thyroid, and adrenal function including (136):
   a. Gonadal: LH, FSH, plasma estradiol in females, plasma testosterone in males.
   b. Thyroid: T4, T3, TSH.
   c. Adrenal: Basal plasma or urinary steroids. The ability of the pituitary-adrenal axis to respond to stress, trauma, or surgery should be assessed by testing cortisol response to insulin hypoglycemia and the plasma corticotropin response to metyrapone.

Table 27-12. Properties and Cellular Origin of Anterior Pituitary Hormones

Hormone	Pituitary Cell	Hormone Structure	Some Biologic Actions
Growth hormone	Acidophil	Peptide	Growth of bone, cartilage, muscle, connective tissue, viscera Elevates blood sugar
Prolactin	Acidophil	Peptide	Promotes lactation
Follicle-stimulating hormone	Basophil	Glycoprotein	Female: promotes maturation of ovarian follicles and formation of ovarian steroids Male: Promotes spermatogenesis
Luteinizing hormone	Basophil	Glycoprotein	Female: Promotes formation of corpus luteum and ovarian steroids Male: Stimulates testosterone formation by interstitial cells of testis
Thyoid-stimulating hormone	Basophil	Glycoprotein	Increases thyroid growth and synthesis of thyroid hormones
Adrenocorticotrophic	Basophil	Peptide	Promotes adrenocortical growth and steroidogenesis
Melanocyte stimulating hormone	Basophil	Peptide	Skin darkening

From Ontjes and Ney (172), with permission.

2. *Specific stimulation and suppression tests* for pituitary hormones (Table 27-13) (172) are performed in selected situations for tumor detection or response to treatment.
3. *Radiographic studies* determine the presence, size, and extent of the lesion (Table 27-14) (1a).
   a. *Plain radiographs* can demonstrate gross enlargement of the sella turcica with a rounded ballooned configuration or concavity of the anterior sellar wall (136).
   b. *CT* provides substantial three-dimensional information on tumor size and extension and may obviate the use of other procedures.
   c. *Sellar polytomography* provides better definition of sellar abnormalities, including unilateral sellar enlargement, sloping of the sellar floor, and focal sellar erosion.
   d. *Pneumoencephalography* reliably demonstrates suprasellar extension and excludes the empty sella syndrome.
   e. *Carotid arteriography* can assist in defining extrasellar (primarily lateral) tumor extension and exclude aneurysm as a cause for bony erosion.
4. Visual perimetry and other *neurophthalmologic and neurologic testing* is carefully performed.

Table 27-13. STIMULATION AND SUPPRESSION TESTS FOR PITUITARY HORMONES

Hormone	Diagnostic Agent	Site of Action	Normal Respons	Response with Tumor
Prolactin	Chlorpromazine	Hypothalamus	↑	→ or ↑ (high basal level)
	TRH	Pituitary	↑	Usually ↑
	L-dopa	Hypothalamus	↓	Usually ↓
Growth hormone	Insulin hypoglycemia (also arginine, L-dopa)	Hypothalamus	↑	→
	Hyperglycemia	Hypothalamus	↓	Usually →
LH and FSH	Clomiphene	Hypothalamus	↑	→
	LHRH	Pituitary	↑	↑ or →
TSH	TRH	Pituitary	↑	↑ or → (response may be delayed)
ACTH	Metyrapone	Adrenal-hypoth alamus	↑	→ in hypopituitarism ↑ in Cushing's disease
	Dexamethasone	Hypothalmus	↓	→ (low dose) Cushing's disease ↓ (high dose) Cushing's disease

↓= hormone secretion increased; ↑ = decreased secretion; → = no change in secretion; TRH=thyrotrophin releasing hormone; L-dopa=levo-dopamine; LHRH=luteinizing hormone-releasing hormone; LH=luteinizing hormone; FSH=follicle-stimulating hormone; TSH=thyroid-stimulating hormone; ACTH=adrenocorticotropic hormone.

From Ontjes and Ney (172), with permission.

Table 27-14. Imaging Modalities for Evaluating Pituitary Tumors

METHOD	DIAGNOSIS AND STAGING CAPABILITY	RECOMMENDED FOR USE
Primary tumor and regional nodes		
CT	Best test at present for detection, definition, and follow-up of sellar tumors.	Yes
MRI	Excellent for soft tissue extent of pituitary tumors. Excellent for patients allergic to iodine contrast agents.	Yes
Biopsy	Required for most CNS tumors. May be done very accurately in brain with CT stereotactic guidance.	Yes

CT = computed tomography; MRI = magnetic resonance imaging; CNS = central nervous system. *Adapted from Bragg (1a).*

CLASSIFICATION AND STAGING

Histopathology (Table 27-15) (135,139)

The traditional classification of pituitary tumors is based on the tinctorial staining properties of the cell cytoplasm viewed by light microscopy. The four commonly recognized types include chromophobe adenomas (53%), assumed to be endocrinologically inactive; acidophilic (eosinophilic) adenomas (8%), primarily associated with acromegaly; basophilic adenomas (27%), associated with Cushing's disease; and mixed types (13%) (Table 27-15).

The use of electron microscopy and specific immunohistochemical techniques revealed the limitations of conventional histopathology (139). Essentially all pituitary cells (except the follicular cells) have identifiable granules, including those considered to be chromophobic by classic techniques (176,182). Cells with a paucity of granules may in fact be secreting hormones so rapidly that accumulation is not observed or, alternatively, may be cells in a relative resting state.

The classical types of adenomas and hormones produced are summarized in Table 27-15 (139,172).

The demonstration of hormone-specific granules in tumor cells may not correlate to a clinical endocrinologic syndrome (184). The schemata most commonly used are thus based on the secretory characteristics of the cells (187). Such a schema with associated tumor frequency in 250 patients appears in Table 27-15.

Anatomic Staging

Because of the correlation of tumor growth characteristics and size with outcome, anatomical staging systems also are used in conjunction with the endocrinologic-based classifications. Hardy and Vezina (155) developed a system based on the extent of expansion and erosion of the sella (Table 27-16) (155):

- grade I: sella is of normal size but with asymmetry of the floor
- grade II: enlarged sella but with intact floor

Table 27-15.   Histopathology of Anterior Pituitary Cells

Classic Light Micro-scope	Classification Using Ultrastructure and Immunoperoxidase Stain	Hormones Produced	Secretory Granules
Acidophil	Somatotroph, well granulated	GH	Dense, 300-600nm
	Prolactin cell, well granulated	PRL	Dense, 200-1200 nm
Basophil	Corticotroph, well granulated	ACTH-MSH	Variable, 250-450 nm (halo)
	Thyrotroph, well granulated	TSH	Dense, 50-150 nm (halo)
	FSH gonadotroph, well granulated*	FSH	Dense, 250-300 nm, and variable, 400-450 nm
	LH gonadotroph, well granulated*	LH	Medium dense, 150-350 nm
Chromophobe †	Somatotroph, sparsely granulated	GH	Dense, 100-250 nm
Hormone-secreting	Prolactin cell, sparsely granulated	PRL	Dense, 130-50 nm
Nonhormone-secreting	Corticotroph, sparsely granulated	ACTH-MSH	
	Thyrotroph, sparsely granulated	TSH	
	FSH gonadotroph, sparsely granulated	FSH	
	LH gonadotroph, sparsely granulated	LH	Dense, 100-250 nm (halo)
	Acidophilic stem cell	GH and/or	Dense, 150-300 nm
	Undifferentiated cells (only in tumors)	PRL	
	Nononcocytic	None	
	Oncocytic (may be acidophilic)		

* Some investigators do not separate FSH and LH gonadotrophs, suggesting that one cell produces both hormones.
†When all available methods are used, there are no true chromophobes in the normal human pituitary.

GH = growth hormone; PRL = prolactin; ACTH = adrenocorticotrophic hormone; MSH = melanocyte-stimulating hormone; TSH = thyroid-stimulating hormone; FSH = follicle-stimulating hormone; LH = luteinizing hormone.
From Bloodworth et al. (139), with permission.

- grade III: localized erosion or destruction of the sellar floor
- grade IV: diffusely eroded floor

This system has been further modified to include a Grade V that equals tumor spread via the CSF or blood, and incorporates the criteria that the tumor is less than 10 mm in diameter in grade I, and greater than or equal to 10 mm in grade II (186). Patients with tumors with extrasellar extension are further subclassified into the following stages (based on modification by Wilson [186]):

- suprasellar extension
  - 0: none
  - A: tumor occupies the chiasmatic cistern
  - B: tumor obliterates recesses of the third ventricle
  - C: tumor grossly displaces the third ventricle
- parasellar extension
  - D: intracranial (intradural) extension
    anterior fossa = 1, middle fossa = 2, posterior fossa = 3
  - E: extension into or beneath the cavernous sinus (extradural)

Staging Work-up

1. Light microscopy shows small cells with large, round nuclei and scant cytoplasm lacking fibrils. Useful stains include Alcian blue and periodic acid-Schif orange G.
2. Electron microscopy demonstrates angulated polyhedral cells with granules than can be quantified by size.
3. Radioisotopic and fluorescent-labeled antibodies to the peptide hormones are used in the identification of endocrinologic types.

PRINCIPLES OF TREATMENT

Management begins with careful definition of the tumor extent and endocrinologic abnormalities. The principles of therapy are based on these factors and their clinical sequelae. Any direct effect of the mass (e.g., visual) must be addressed, and endocrinologic dysfunction must be corrected. Certain deficiencies, particularly corticosteroid, should immediately be corrected. Complications of therapy, most prominently hypopituitarism, and tumor recurrence can be manifested many years up to 30 years after therapy, and must be carefully and continuously considered (150).

The choice of treatment modality is determined by several factors (Table 27-17):

- need for immediate relief of mass effect or endocrinologic abnormalities
- potential for obtaining long-term control
- character and frequency of possible morbidities

Table 27-17 presents a concise summary of recommended therapeutic procedures using a multidisciplinary approach.

Surgery

The role of surgery in the management of pituitary adenomas includes histologic confirmation of the diagnosis, cyst evacuation, decompression of a hemorrhagic tumor, the optic chiasm or cranial nerves, reduction of obstructive hydrocephalus, complete excision of microadenomas and macroadenomas, and reduction of the tumor bulk of invasive adenomas. Either a transfrontal or trans-sphenoidal approach is used (Table 27-18).

1. The transfrontal approach via craniotomy provides added visualization of the tumor and surrounding structures. Indications include suprasellar or lateral tumor extension, dumbbell-shaped lesions, involvement of the chiasm or cranial nerves by tumor, and invasion of the surrounding vascular structures or pituitary apoplexy. Disadvantages of the transfrontal approach include the high morbidity and mortality that result from damage to vital structures, and the substantial incidence of postoperative hypopituitarism and diabetes insipidus (131,136).
2. The transsphenoidal technique involves entry into facial portion of the sphenoid sinus, thereby gaining access to the pituitary fossa. The binocular surgical microscope is coupled with fluoroscopic monitoring for direct visualization of the surgical field (187). The trans-sphenoidal approach offers the capability for tumor destruction by freezing, coagulation, or resection. Indications include removal of tumor confined to the sella turcica, tumors associated with CSF rhinorrhea, pituitary apoplexy, tumors with sphenoidal extension, and tumors with only modest suprasellar extension.

Contraindications to this approach include dumbbell-shaped tumors with constriction at the diaphragma sellae, massive suprasellar tumors, lateral suprasellar extension, and

---

Table 27-16. Staging System of Hardy-Vezina for Pituitary Tumors

Grade I: sella is of normal size but with asymmetry of the floor
Grade II: enlarged sella but with an intact floor
Grade III: localized erosion or destruction of the sellar floor
Grade IV: diffusely eroded floor

Suprasellar extension
0: None
A: Tumor occupies the chiasmatic cistern
B: Tumor obliterates recesses of the third ventricle
C: Tumor grossly displaces the third ventricle

Parasellar extension
D: Intracranial (intradural) extension
anterior fossa=1, middle fossa=2, posterior fossa=3
E: Extension into or beneath the cavernous sinus (extradural)

From Hardy and Vezina (155), with permission.

Table 27-17. Multidisciplinary Treatment Decisions Based on Tumor Type in Pituitary Adenomas (131,132a,135,135a)

Tumor Type and Characteristics	Surgery		Radiation Therapy		Chemotherapy
Nonsecreting adenoma					
Micro, no or limited suprasellar extension, minimal visual loss	TSS	or	CRT 45 - 50 GY		N R
Macro, severe visual loss, pituitary apoplexy	TSS	and	ART Postop 45-50 Gy		N R
GH-secreting adenoma					
Micro, well-defined	TSS	and	ART * Postop 45-50 Gy		Somatostatin
Prolactin-secreting adenoma	NR	or	ART * Postop 45-50 Gy	or	Bromocriptine
Micro					
Amenorrhea or infertility	TSS				
Macro	TSS	and	ART Postop 45-50 Gy	and/or	*Bromocriptine
Corticotropin-secreting adenoma					
Children	TSS	or	CRT 45-50 Gy		Mitotane
Adults	TSS	and	Postop RT *		N R

* If subtotal resection or continued hypersecretion; TSS = transsphenoidal surgery; RT = radiation therapy; CRT = curative; ART = adjuvant; N R = not recommended; GH = growth hormone.

incompletely pneumatized sphenoids (186). Morbidities include transient diabetes insipidus and, rarely, meningitis or persistent CSF rhinorrhea. When selective resection of an adenoma is possible, hypopituitarism is uncommon.

Radiation Therapy

Radiation therapy has been used extensively in the treatment of pituitary adenomas (141,151,173,181). External megavoltage photon therapy is generally used, although heavy particle photon or alpha -particle irradiation, and implantation of pellets containing radioactive isotopes (e.g., yttrium-90, gold-198) are alternative approaches (165).
1. Indications:
   a. Primary treatment of intrasellar adenomas.
   b. Adjunct to the surgical treatment of tumors with suprasellar extension or of large tumors presenting with mass effects.
   c. Adjunct to medical or surgical management of hormone-secreting adenomas in patients with a suboptimal response or inability to tolerate medical therapy.
   d. Primary therapy in patients whose tumors are inoperable or for invasive adenomas when surgical excision carries high risks.
   e. Primary therapy for selected patients with tumors have limited suprasellar extension.
2. Treatment techniques are variable, with the treatment volume tailored to the tumor volume and a minimum dose delivered to adjacent structures. Optimal techniques include bilateral coaxial wedge fields plus a vertex field, moving arc fields, and 360° rotational fields (181). The use of two bilateral opposed fields is occasionally necessary for large, asymmetric tumors, but is to be discouraged because of the increased dose delivered to the temporal lobes. Optimum doses are based on

evidence that doses under 40 Gy provide a lower probability of tumor control and doses above 50 Gy or fractions above 2 Gy/d are associated with higher complication rates, including injury to the optic nerves/chiasm and hypopituitarism. A dose of 50 Gy plus or minus 5 Gy is recommended. If the macrotumor is completely removed with microresiduum and the patient is young, 45 to 50 Gy is advisable, but if there is recurrent tumor, macroresiduum postresection, and suprasellar extension, a higher dose, 50 to 55 Gy depending on tumor bulk, is recommended (133).
3. The frequency of clinically significantly hypopituitarism is rare at these doses. GH secretion and gonadotropin abnormalities may occur after 40 to 50 Gy, but are either clinically well tolerated or medically manageable.
4. Disadvantages include the delay in therapeutic benefit for patients with hormonally active tumors, and the rare occurrence of radiation-induced malignancies.

Chemotherapy

Increased understanding of the hypothalamic control of pituitary function has led to the development of drugs to modulate pituitary hormone secretion (131,159).
1. Bromocriptine and other ergot derivatives with dopaminergic properties (e.g., pergolide mesylate).
   a. Bromocriptine effectively reduces elevated serum prolactin levels in most patients with prolactin-secreting pituitary adenomas (156,167,171). Bromocriptine therapy is thus indicated as primary treatment for microadenomas. Macroadenomas have also been successfully medically managed (167), although such management is generally used in this setting prior to definitive surgery or irradiation.

Table 27-18. Results of Treatment of Pituitary Tumors

Author	Type of Procedure	Type of Disease	No. Patient	No. Operation	Success (%)	Mortality (%)	Recurrence (%)	Visual Improvement
Ray	Transfrontal craniotomy	Chromophobe adenoma	63	68				
		Acromegaly	14	14				
		Cushing's syndrome	3	3				
		Total	80	85	100	0	8-10	75
Laws	Transseptal–transsphenoidal	Pituitary adenoma		408	99.02			
		Functioning	265					
		Nonfunctioning	135					
		Other	89	97				
		Total	489	505	98.61	1.39		95.3 (81 of 85 studied)
Wilson (186)	Transsphenoidal microsurgical	Cushing's disease						
		Basophilic adenoma	1					
		Chromophobe adenoma	10					
		Mixed	3					
		Insufficient tissue	3					
		Total						
		Hypophysectomy	1					
		No specimen	2					
		Total	20	20	100	0		
Hardy (153, 154)	Transsphenoidal	Pituitary adenoma						
		Chromophobe	8					
		Recurrent chromophobe	3					
		Mixed	4					
		Eosinophilic	1					
		Craniopharyngioma	2					
		Reticulosarcoma	1					
		Chondrosarcoma	1					
		Total	20	20	100	0		90

Ovulatory and menstrual cycles may resume in 75% to 80% of patients (143). Patients with macroadenomas who become pregnant are at risk for complications related to tumor growth. For these patients pregnancy should either be prevented by contraceptive methods, or definitive ablative therapy should be performed prior to pregnancy (169,175). Patients with intrasellar microadenomas are at a less than 10% risk for substantial tumor growth and associated complications (157). Bromocriptine should be discontinued when pregnancy is confirmed, although concerns regarding the teratogenicity of bromocriptine have not, to date, been substantiated (140).

b. Bromocriptine and pergolide also substantially decrease GH secretion in the majority of patients with acromegaly. Improved glucose tolerance and a reduction in acromegaly enlargement may occur (148), particularly for soft tissue component.

2. Cyproheptadine is a serotonin antagonist that significantly reduces corticotropin secretion in up to 60% of patients with Cushing's disease (161). Experience is nevertheless limited and hyperphagia is a side effect.

3. Somatostatin, the hypothalamic GH release inhibitory factor, and its analog SMS 201-995, reduce GH secretion when given parenterally or subcutaneously, respectively (131,162). Somatomedin-C, insulin secretion, and tumor mass decrease in some patients. The short half-life of somatostatin limits its usefulness. These drugs are, however, options in patients who do not benefit sufficiently from surgery or radiotherapy and do not respond to treatment with dopaminergic drugs.

Treatment Recommendations (Table 27-17)

Nonsecreting Adenomas

1. Radiation therapy (45 to 50 Gy) or transsphenoidal surgery are appropriate for small tumors with no or limited suprasellar extension and minimal vision loss.
2. Surgery with postoperative radiation therapy (50 Gy) is performed for patients with progressive or severe visual loss, large tumors, or pituitary apoplexy.
3. Selected patients with small, incidentally discovered adenomas may be carefully followed without immediate therapy.

GH-secreting Adenomas

1. Transsphenoidal surgery when the tumor is small and well defined.
2. Postoperative radiation therapy (50 to 55 Gy) for partially resected tumors or when GH levels remain elevated.

Prolactin-secreting Adenomas (Chromophobe Adenomas Mainly)

1. Selected patients with microadenomas may be carefully followed without treatment or given bromocriptine alone.
2. Because of the rapidity of response, transsphenoidal surgery is appropriate for patients who desire pregnancy. It effectively controls microadenomas but is less reliable for larger tumors. Bromocriptine therapy is an alternative approach for patients with microadenomas, or for selected patients with macroadenomas.

3. Radiation therapy (50 Gy + 5 Gy) is an appropriate consideration for patients with large, incompletely resected tumors. Patients who continue to have elevated prolactin values and amenorrhea following surgery may be treated with bromocriptine; if this medication is not tolerated or is ineffective, radiation therapy is administered. Although recent experience supports its efficacy as primary therapy for patients with prolactin-secreting adenomas (151), the effectiveness of the other modalities suggests that radiotherapy be reserved as stated above.

Corticotropin-secreting Tumors

1. Primary therapy for children is irradiation alone (40 to 45 Gy), or transsphenoidal surgery if a microadenoma can be identified.
2. Primary therapy for adults is generally transsphenoidal surgery, with radiotherapy (50 Gy) reserved for patients who are subtotally resected or remain hypersecretory.

RESULTS AND PROGNOSIS (Tables 27-18 and 27-19) (180)

Nonsecreting Adenomas (results cited are generally for chromophobe adenomas)

1. The strategy of observation only for patients with clinically evident but apparently inactive pituitary adenomas is inappropriate. Sheline (179) reported that 87% of such patients eventually required definitive

therapy and 50% developed permanent damage that might have been preventable with earlier therapy.
2. Depending on tumor size, 10-year recurrence-free survival is 80% or higher with radiation therapy alone or the combination of irradiation and surgery (133,136,147,151).
3. Visual improvement depends on the duration and extent of pretreatment visual loss but overall can be expected in 50% to 95% of patients, a broad range that reflects a variety of pretreatment variables (136,147,151,174,183).

GH-secreting Tumors (results cited are for patients with acromegaly) (Table 27-18)

1. The potential for tumor control is excellent with either radiotherapy or surgery. Ten-year recurrence-free survival is reported at 69% following radiotherapy, and is even higher for patients treated with 44 Gy or higher (151,160,173). Reduction in GH levels to less than 5 ng/mL with 10-year follow-up is also seen in 69% of patients after 40 to 50 Gy (145). Transsphenoidal surgery provides a remission in 78% of patients; the overall success of treatment is greater than 95% for grades I to III and 82% for grade IV (182). A similar percentage of patients will have GH levels reduced to less than 5 ng/mL(155).
2. Bromocriptine provides a return of GH to normal levels in 20% of patients and a response in 70% to 80% (184). The somatostatin analog SMS 201-995 was given to eight patients and the mean GH concentrations de-

---

Table 27-19. ACROMEGALY: Transsphenoidal Microsurgical Removal with Curative Intent as Initial Therapy at UCSF [*][†]

	Remission Rate (No. Remission /No. at Risk)	
Tumor classification		
Grade I	4/4	(100%)
Grade II	57/59	(97%)
Grade III	21/22	(96%)
Grade IV	14/17	(82%)
Total	96[c]/102	(94%)
Treated		
Surgery alone	80/102	(78%)[‡]
Surgery and irradiation	16/16 to	16/22[§]
Suprasellar extension of tumor		
None	51/51	(100%)
Into cistern	19/19	(100%)
3rd ventricle recesses obliterated	14/17	(82%)
3rd ventricle grossly displaced	12/15	(80%)
Surgical complications		
Hypopituitarism	4	(5%)
Meningitis	2	
False aneurysm	2	
Cerebrospinal fluid leak	1	
Nasal deformity	3	
Recurrence	3	

[*] A few others (number unspecified) had only biopsy followed by irradiation and are not included in this table.

[†] Mean follow-up: 35 months (range 6 wk-10 yr).

[‡] Four required a second surgical procedure before remission achieved.

[§] Radiation therapy given postresection for failure of surgery to achieve remission. Sixteen of between 16 and 22 (total number irradiated is not identifiable) reached remission after radiotherapy.

Adapted from Sheline et al. (180).

creased from an initial mean level of 57 ng/ml to 7.5 ng/mL, which suggests its usefulness for patients unresponsive to other measures (162).

Prolactin-secreting Tumors

1. The success of surgery is dependent on the size or grade of the adenoma and the pretreatment prolactin level. For patients with microadenomas, grades 1 to 2 tumors, or prolactin levels less than 500 ng/mL, clinical cures (normalization of prolactin levels and apparent complete tumor removal without recurrent hypersecretion or tumor growth) occur in 96% and 86% at 5 and 10 years, respectively (Table 27-19). However, in patients with macroadenomas, grades 3 to 4 tumors, or prolactin levels greater than 500, ng/mL clinical cures are seen in only 15% to 30% of patients (137,154,169,177,178).

2. Radiotherapy appears to provide better results than surgery; about 40% to 70% of patients are clinically cured surgically, but radiation therapy results are 90% to 100% in most series (137,149), although a recent report from Grigsby (133,155) shows a 10-year recurrence-free survival of 85% for both modalities combined.

3. Bromocriptine as a primary mode of therapy, or as an adjuvant following surgery or radiotherapy, is successful in lowering serum prolactin levels to normal in 90% of patients (167,185). Patients can be expected to show recurrence of hypersecretion following bromocriptine withdrawal, and isolated reports of tumor growth during bromocriptine therapy have been made (142).

Corticotropin-secreting Tumors

1. Transsphenoidal microsurgery is exceedingly effective treatment (Table 27-19). In a recent report of 221 patients, 78% could be treated with selective adenomectomy, 11% required total hypophysectomy, and the remainder had either a partial hypophysectomy or exploration only (168). Disease remission was achieved in 76%; success was relatively greater in patients with microadenomas or intrasellar adenomas than in patients with macroadenomas or extrasellar extension. Five patients were found to have an ectopic source of corticotropin secretion. Other series report similar results (153). Radiotherapy alone is less successful (50% to 60% in most series). Recurrence after complete clinical and biochemical remission is rare (136).

2. Primary radiation therapy is more effective in children, with up to 80% achieving a complete clinical remission (152).

Prognosis

Prognosis depends on the type of tumor and a combination of other factors, including (181):

- severity of the endocrinologic disturbance or mass-related symptoms and signs. The size and the extent of the tumor (as reflected in the staging systems) are also correlated to outcome, as indicated under "Results"
- success of therapy in reversing these abnormalities
- morbidities of therapy
- permanency of the therapeutic response

Although pituitary tumors are generally benign, the failure to provide adequate therapy can lead to severe functional deficits and death (181). Optimal therapy can vastly improve quality and duration of life.

Recommended Reading

For students who wish to peruse the subject of thyroid cancer in more detail we recommend the following: the 6th edition of *Werner and Ingbar's The Thyroid: A Fundamental and Clinical Text* (1b) and Falk's in-depth text *Thyroid Disease* (2a).

For more detailed information on adrenal cancer, we recommend: Hutter and Kayhoe (79); Lipsett *et al.* (81); King and Lock (109) on the natural course of the disease; Montagne *et al.* (114); Sample and Sorti (119) on diagnosis strategy by CT scan or ultrasound; Lubitz *et al.* (111); and Luton *et al.* (112) on the use of mitotrane in the treatment of adrenocortical carcinoma.

An overview of pituitary adenomas with particular attention to endocrinologic evaluation is given in Earp and Ney's chapter in *Cancer Medicine* (131) and Leavens *et al.* (163a). Comprehensive discussions on diagnosis (description of syndromes and physical, endocrinologic, and neuroradiographic examination), pathology, and therapy (surgical, radiation, and chemical) are presented in Gauger's chapter in Linfoot (132). Additional details on pathology are available in Kernohan and Sayre (134) and Bergland (138), and on surgery in Hardy and Vezina (155), Wilson and Dempsey (187), and Comtois *et al.* (141a). A recent article by Maroldo *et al.* (168a) gives information on advances in diagnostic techniques. Finally, a self-learning study text with insights into current literature is provided by Sheline (136).

REFERENCES

Thyroid Cancer

General References

1. American Joint Committee for Cancer Staging and End-Results Reporting. Manual for Staging of Cancer. 3rd ed. Philadelphia, PA: JB Lippincott Co; 1988.

1a. Bragg, D.G.; Rubin, P.; Youker, J.E., eds. Oncologic Imaging. New York, NY: Pergamon Press; 1985.

1b. Braverman, L.E.; Utiger, R.D. (eds). Werner and Ingbar's The Thyroid: A Fundamental and Clinical Text. 6th ed. Philadelphia, PA: JB Lippincott Co.; 1992.

2. DeGroot, L.J.; Stanbury, J.B. The thyroid and Its Diseases. 5th ed. New York, NY: John Wiley & Sons; 1984.

2a. Falk, S. Thyroid Disease. 1st ed. New York, NY: Raven Press; 1990.

3. Ferris, T. Galaxies. San Francisco, CA: Sierra Club Books; 1980:7.

3a. Greenfield, L.D.; Luk, K.H. Thyroid. In: Principles and practice of radiation oncology. 2nd ed. Perez, C.A., Brady, L.W. (eds). Philadelphia, PA: JB Lippincott C.; 1992: 1356-1381.

4. Hediger, C.E. Thyroid cancer. International Union Against Cancer (UICC) Monograph Series, vol. 12. New York, NY: Springer-Verlag; 1969.

5. International Histologic Classification of Tumors, nos.1-20. Geneva, Switzerland: World Health Organization; 1978.

6. International Union Against Cancer (UICC). Commission on clinical oncology. TNM Classification of Malignant Tumors. Geneva, Switzerland: UICC; 1968.

6a. Norton, J.A.; Doppman, J.L.; Jensen, R.T. Cancer of the endocrine system. In: DeVita, V.T. Jr.; Hellman, S.; Rosenberg, S.A., eds. Cancer Principles and Practice of Oncology. Philadelphia, PA: JB Lippincott Co.; 1989.

6b. Robbins, J.; Meriono, M.J.; Boice, Jr., J.D.; Ron, E.; Ain, K.B.; Alexander, H.R.; Norton, J.A.; Reynolds, J. Thyroid cancer: A Lethal endocrine neoplasm. Annals Int Med. 115:133-147;1991.

7. Ureles, A.L. Cancer of the endocrine glands: thyroid and adrenal. In: Rubin, P., ed. Clinical Oncology for Medical Students and

Physicians. 5th ed. New York, NY: American Cancer Society; 1978.

8. Werner, S.C. The thyroid: a Fundamental and Clinical Text. 5th ed. Philadelphia, PA: JB Lippincott Co; 1986.

9. Young, S.; Inman, P.R. Thyroid neoplasia. New York, NY: Academic Press; 1968.

Specific References

10. Allweiss, P.; Braunstein, G.D.; Katz, A.; *et al.* Sialadenitis following I-131 therapy for thyroid carcinoma: concise communication. J. Nucl. Med. 25:755-758; 1984.

11. Ansari, A.N.; Siegel, M.; DeQuattro, V.; *et al.* Imaging of medullary thyroid carcinoma and hyperfunctioning adrenal medulla using iodine-131 metaiodobenzylguanidine. J. Nucl. Med. 27:1858-1860; 1986.

12. Arnold, J.E.; Pinsky, S. Comparison of Tc-99m and I-123 for thyroid imaging. J. Nucl. Med. 17:261-267; 1976.

13. Beahrs, O.H.; Upton, A.C.; Land, C.E.; *et al.* Irradiation to the head and neck area and thyroid cancer. JAMA. 244:337-338; 1980.

14. Beierwaltes, W. Medical treatment of thyroid carcinoma. In: Santen, R.J.; Andrea, M., eds. Endocrine-Related Tumors. Hingham, MA: Martinus Nijoff; 1984:451-481.

15. Beierwaltes, W.; Nishiyama, R.H.; Thompson, N.W.; *et al.* Survival time and "cure" in papillary and follicular thyroid carcinoma with distant metastases: statistics following University of Michigan therapy. J. Nucl. Med. 23:561-568; 1982.

16. Beierwaltes, W.H. The treatment of thyroid carcinoma with radioactive iodine. Semin. Nucl. Med. 8:79-94; 1978.

16a. Belfiore, A.; Garofalo, M.R.; Giuffrida, D.; Runello, F.; Filetti, S.; Fiumara, A.; Ippolito, O.; Vigneri, R. Increased aggressiveness of thyroid cancer in patients with Graves' Disease J Clin Endocrine Metab. 70:830-835;1990.

17. Blahd, W.H.; Drickman, M.V.; Porter, C.W.; *et al.* Serum thyroglobulin, a monitor of differentiated thyroid carcinoma in patients receiving tyroid hormone suppression therapy: concise communication. J. Nucl. Med. 25:673-676; 1984.

18. Block, M.A. Management of carcinoma of the thyroid. Ann. Surg. 185:133-144; 1977.

19. Blum, M. Enhanced clinical diagnosis of thyroid disease using echography. Am. J. Med. 59:301-307; 1975.

20. Breaux, E.P., Jr.; Guillamondegui, O.M. Treatment of locally invasive carcinoma of the thyroid: how radical? Am. J. Surg. 140:514-517; 1980.

21. Brendel, A.J.; Guyot, M.; Jeandot, R.; *et al.* Thallium-201 imaging in the follow-up of differentiated thyroid carcinoma. J. Nucl. Med. 29:1515-1520; 1988.

22. Brun, J.; Barre, Y.; Barre, T.; *et al.* Response of undifferentiated thyroid carcinoma to combined modality treatment. World J. Surg. 3:517-522; 1979.

22a. Caruso, D.; Mazzaferri, E.L. Fine needle aspiration biopsy in the management of thyroid nodules. The endocrinologist. 1:194-202;1991.

23. Cerletty, J.M.; Listwan, W.J. Hyperthyroidism due to functioning metastatic thyroid carcinoma. JAMA. 242:269-270; 1979.

24. Chapman, C.N.; Sziklas, J.J.; Spencer, R.; *et al.* Hyperthyroidism with metastatic follicular carcinoma. J. Nucl. Med. 25:466-468; 1984.

25. Cline, R.E.; Shingleton, W.W. Long term results in the treatment of carcinoma of the thyroid. Am. J. Surg. 115:545-551; 1968.

26. Cooper, D.; Axelrod, L.; DeGroot, L.J.; *et al.* Congenital goiter and the development of metastatic follicular carcinoma with evidence for a leak of nonhormonal iodide. J. Clin. Endocrinol. Metab. 52:294-306; 1981.

26a. Crile, G.; Pontius, K.I.; Hawk, W.A. Factors influencing the survival of patients with follicular carcinoma of the thyroid gland. Surg Gunecol Obstet. 1985:409.

27. Datz, F. Cerebral edema following iodine-131 therapy for thyroid carcinoma metastatic to the brain. J. Nucl. Med. 27:637-640; 1986.

28. Deftos, L.J.; Woloszczuk, W.; Krisch, I.; *et al.* Medullary thyroid carcinomas express chromogranin A and a novel neuroendocrine protein recognized by monoclonal antibody HISL-19. Am. J. Med. 85:780-784; 1988.

29. DeGroot, L.J. Thyroid carcinoma. Med. Clin. North Am. 59:1241-1245; 1975.

29a. DeGroot, L.J.; Kaplan, E.L.; McCormick, M.; Straus, F.H. Natural history, treatment, and course of papillary thyroid carcinoma. J Clin Endocrinol Metab 71:414-424;1990.

30. DeGroot, L.J.; Reilly, M.; Pinnameni, K.; *et al.* Retrospective and prospective study of radiation-induced thyroid disease. Am. J. Med. 74:852-862; 1983.

31. Didolkar, M.S.; Moore, G.E. Hormone-dependent medullary carcinoma of thyroid. Am. J. Surg. 128:100-102; 1974.

32. Filetti, S.; Belfiore, A.; Amir, S.M.; *et al.* The role of thyroid stimulating antibodies of Graves' disease in differentiated thyroid cancer. New Engl. J. Med. 318:753-759; 1988.

33. Freitas, J.E.; Gross, M.D.; Ripley, S.; *et al.* Radionuclide diagnosis and therapy of thyroid cancer: current status report. Semin. Nucl. Med. 15:106-131; 1985.

34. Fukunaga, F.H.; Yatani, R. Geographic pathology of occult thyroid carcinomas. Cancer. 36:1095-1099; 1975.

35. Gottlieb, J.A.; Hills, C.S., Jr. Chemotherapy of thyroid cancer. Cancer. 30:848-853; 1972.

36. Gottlieb, J.A.; Hill, C.S., Jr. Chemotherapy of thyroid cancer with Adriamycin: experience with 30 patients. New Engl. J. Med. 290:193-197; 1974.

37. Hamburger, J. Consistency of sequential needle biopsy findings for thyroid nodules. Management implication. Arch. Intern. Med. 147:97-99; 1987.

37a. Hancock, S.L.; Cox, R.S.; McDougall, I.R. Thyroid diseases after treatment of Hodgkin's Disease. N Engl J Med 325:599-604;1991.

37b. Harness, J.K.; Thompson, N.W.; McLeod, M.K.; *et al.* Follicular carcinoma of the thyroid gland: trends and treatment. Surgery. 96:972;1984.

38. Higashi, T.; Watanabe, Y.; Yamaguchi, M.; *et al.* The relationship between the Ga-67 uptake and nuclear feulgen content in thyroid: concise cummunication. J. Nucl. Med. 23:988-992; 1982.

39. Hill, S.H. Jr.; Clark, R.L.; Wolf, M. Effect of subsequent pregnancy on patients with thyroid cancer. Surg. Gynecol. Obstet. 122:1219-1222; 1966.

40. Holm, L.; Dahlgvist, I.; Israelsson, A.; *et al.* Malignant thyroid tumors after iodine-131 therapy. New Engl. J. Med. 303:188-191; 1980.

41. Ichikawa, Y.; Saito, E.; Yoshigum, A.; *et al.* Presence of TSH receptor in thyroid neoplasms. J. Clin. Endocrinol. Metab. 42:395-398; 1976.

41a. Joensuu, H.; Klemi, P.F.; Paul, R., *et al.* Survival and prognostic factors in the thyroid carcinoma. Acta Radiol. 25:243;1986.

41b. Justin, e.P.; Seabold, J.E.; Robinson, R.A.; Walder, W.P.; Gurll, N.J.; Hawes, D.R. Insular carcinoma: A distinct thyroid carcinoma with associated Iodine-131 localization. J Nucl Med. 32:1358-1363;1991.

41b. Lang, W.; Choritz, H.; Hundeshage, H. Risk factors in follicular thyroid carcinomas. Am J Surg Pathol. 10(4):246;1986.

42. Leeper, R.D. The effect of I-131 therapy on survival of patients with metastatic papillary or follicular thyroid carcinoma. J. Clin. Endocrinol. Metab. 36:1143-1152; 1973.

43. Lip, C.J.M.; Vette, J.K.; Ruys, J.H.J.; *et al.* Visualization of "cold" thyroid nodules with nonradioactive iodine. New Engl. J. Med. 306:1491; 1982.

44. LiVolsi, V.A. Pathology of thyroid cancer. In: Greenfield, L., ed. Thyroid Cancer. West Palm Beach, FL: CRC Press Inc; 1978:85-141.

45. McConahey, W.M.; Hay, I.D.; Woolner, L.B.; *et al.* Papillary thyroid cancer treated at the Mayo Clinic 1946 through 1970: initial manifestations, pathologic findings, therapy, and outcome. Mayo Clin. Proc. 61:978-996; 1986.

45a. McDonald, R.J.; Wu, S.; Jensen, J.L.; Parker, L.N.; Lyons, K.P.; Moran, E.M.; Blahd, W.H. Malignant transformation of a Hurthle cell tumor: Case report and survey of the Literature. J Nucl Med 32:1266-1269;1991.

46. Maxon, H.R.; Saenger, E.L.; Thomas, S.R. Clinically important radiation-associated thyroid disease. JAMA. 244:1802-1806;1980.

47. Maxon, H.R.; Thomas, S.R.; Hertzberg, V.S.; et al Relation between effective radiation dose and outcome of radioiodine therapy for thyroid cancer. New Engl. J. Med. 309:937-941; 1983.

48. Mazzaferri, E.I. Papillary thyroid carcinoma: factors influencing prognosis and current therapy. Semin. Oncol. 14:315; 1987.

48a. Mazzaferri, E.L.; Young, R.L. Papillary thyroid carcinoma: 10-year follow-up report of the impact of therapy in 576 patients. Am. J. Med. 70:511-518; 1981.

49. Mazzaferi, E.L.; Young, R.L.; Oertel, J.E., *et al.* Papillary thyroid carcinoma: the impact of therapy in 576 patients. Medicine. 56:171;1977.

50. Melmed, S.; Harada, A.; Hershman, J.M.; *et al.* Neutralizing antibodies to bovine thyrotrophin in immunized patients with thyroid cancer. J. Clin. Endocrinol. Metab. 51:358-363; 1980.

51. Miller, J.M.; Kini, S.R.; Hamburger, J.I. Needle Biopsy of the Thyroid. New York, NY: Praeger Publishers; 1983.

52. Mustacchi, P.; Cutler, S.J. Survival of patients with cancer of the thyroid gland. JAMA. 173:1795-1798; 1960.

52a. Nel, C.J.; vanHeerden, J.A.; Goellner, J.R.; Gharib, H.; McConahey, W.M.; Taylor, W.F.; Grant, C.S. Anaplastic carcinoma of the thyroid: A clinicopathologic study of 82 cases. Mayo Clin Proc 60:51-58;1985.

52b. O'Driscoll, C.M.; Baker, F.; Casey, M.J.; Duffy, G.J. Localization of recurrent medullary thyroid carcinoma with Technetium-99m-Methoxyisobutylnitrile scintigraphy: A case report. J Nucl Med. 32:2281-2283:1991.

53. Ohta, H.; Yamamoto, K.; Endo, K.; *et al.* A new agent for medullary carcinoma of the thyroid. J. Nucl. Med. 25:323-325; 1984.

54. Olen, E.; Klinck, G.H. Hyperthyroidism and thyroid cancer. Arch. Pathol. 81:531-535; 1966.

55. Parker, L.N.; Blesky, J.L.; Yamamoto, T.; *et al.* Thyroid carcinoma after exposure to atomic radiation. Continuing survey of a fixed population. Hiroshima and Nagasaki 1958-1971. Ann. Intern. Med. 80:600-604; 1974.

55a. Ramanna, L.; Waxman, A.; Braunstein, G. Thallium-201 scintigraphy in differentiated thyroid cancer: Comparison with radioiodine scintigraphy and serum thyroglobulin determinations. J Nucl Med 32:441-446;1991.

56. Retetoff, S.; Lever, E.G. The value of serum thyroglobulin measurement in clinical practice. JAMA. 250:2352-2357; 1983.

56a. Ruiz-Garcia, J.; Ruiz de Almodovar, J.M.; Olea, N.; Pedraza, V. Thyroglobulin level as a predictive factor of tumoral recurrence in differentiated thyroid cancer. J Nucl Med. 32:395-398;1991.

57. Samaan, N.; Schultz, P.N.; Hickey, R.C. Medullary thyroid carcinoma: prognosis of familial versus sporadic disease and the role of radiotherapy. J. Clin. Endocrinol. Metab. 67:801-805; 1988.

58. Samaan, N.A.; Schultz, P.N.; Ordonez, N.G.; et al A comparison of thyroid carcinoma in those who have and have not had head and neck irradiation in childhood. J. Clin. Endocrinol. Metab. 64:219-224; 1987.

59. Schlumberger, M.; De Vathaire, F.; Travagli, J.P.; *et al.* Differentiated thyroid carcinoma in childhood: long term follow-up of 72 patients. J. Clin. Endocrinol. 65:1088-1094; 1987.

60. Schottenfeld, D.; Gershman, S. Epidemiology of thyroid cancer. CA. 28:66-86; 1978.

60a. Schroader, D.M.; Chambous, A.; France, C.J. Operative strategy for thyroid cancer: is total thyroidectomy worth the price? Cancer. 58:2320;1986.

61. Shanon, E. Total thyroidectomy: rationale, technique, and morbidity. Arch. Surg. 103:339-342; 1971.

62. Shimke, R.N.; Hartmann, W.H.; Prout, T.E.; et al Syndrome of bilateral pheochromocytoma, medullary thyroid carcinoma, and multiple neuromas. New Engl. J. Med. 279:1-18; 1968.

63. Silverberg, E. Cancer statistics, 1988. CA. 38(1):14-15; 1988.

64. Silverberg, E. Cancer statistics, 1989. CA. 39(1):3-20; 1989.

65. Silverberg, S.G.; Vidone, R.A. Carcinoma of the thyroid in surgical and postmortem material: analysis of 300 cases at autopsy and literature review. Ann. Surg. 164:291-295; 1966.

66. Simpson, W.J.; McKinney, S.E.; Carruthers, J.S.; Gospodarowicz, M.K.; et al Papillary and follicular thyroid cancer, prognostic factors in 1,578 patients. Am. J. Med. 83:479-488; 1987.

67. Smedal, M.I.; Salzman, F.A.; Meissner, W.A. The value of 2 MV roentgen-ray therapy in differentiated thyroid carcinoma. AJR. 99:352-364; 1967.

68. Thompson, N.W.; Nishiyama, R.H.; Harness, J.K. Thyroid carcinoma: current controversies. Curr. Probl. Surg. 15:1-67; 1978.

69. Vander, J.B.; Gaston E.A.; Dawber, T.R. Significance of nontoxic thyroid nodules: final report of 15-year study of incidence of thyroid malignancy. Ann. Intern. Med. 69:537-539; 1968.

70. VanHerle, A.J.; Rich, P.; Britt-Marie, E. The thyroid nodule. Ann. Intern. Med. 96:221-232; 1982.

71. Van Norstrand, D.; Neutze, J.; Atkins, F. Side effect of "rational dose" iodine-131 therapy for metastatic well-differentiated thyroid carcinoma. J. Nucl. Med. 27:1519-1527; 1986.

72. Varma, V.M.; Beierwaltes, W.H.; Mohammed, M.N.; *et al.* Treatment of thyroid cancer: death rates after surgery and after surgery followed by sodium iodide-131. JAMA. 214:1437-1442; 1970.

73. Vasen, H.F.A.; Kruseman, A.C.N.; Berkel, H.; *et al.* Multiple endocrine neoplasia syndrome type 2: the value of screening and central registration. Am. J. Med. 83:847-852; 1987.

74. Waxman, A.; Ramanna, L.; Chapman, D. The significance of I-131 scan dose in patients with thyroid cancer: determination of ablation. J. Nucl. Med. 22:861-865; 1981.

75. Wells, S.A.; Dilley, W.G.; Farndon, J.A.; *et al.* Early diagnosis and treatment of medullary thyroid carcinoma. Arch. Intern. Med. 145:1248-1252; 1985.

76. Woolner, L.B.; Lemmon, M.L.; Beahrs, O.H.; *et al.* Occult papillary carcinoma of the thyroid gland: a study of 140 cases observed in a 30 year period. J. Clin. Endocrinol. Metab. 20:89-105; 1960.

77. Young, R.L.; Mazzaferri, E.L.; Rahe, A.J.; *et al.* Pure follicular thyroid carcinoma: impact of therapy in 214 patients. J. Nucl. Med. 21:733-737; 1980.

Adrenal Cortex Cancer

General References

77a. Brady, L.W.; Calvo, F.A. Adrenal Gland In: Principles and practice of radiation oncology. 2nd ed. Perez, C.A., Brady, L.W. (eds). Philadelphia, PA: JB Lippincott Co.; 1992: 1302-1306.

78. Doppman, J.L.; Reinig, J.W.; Dwyer, A.J.; *et al.* Differentiation of adrenal masses by magnetic resonance imaging. Surgery. 102:1018; 1987.

79. Hutter, A.M.; Kayhoe, D.E. Adrenal cortical carcinoma: clinical features of 138 patients. Am. J. Med. 41:572-580; 1966.

80. Hutter, A.M.; Kayhoe, D.E. Adrenal cortical carcinoma, results of treatment with Op'-DDD in 138 patients. Am. J. Med. 41:581-592; 1966.

81. Lipsett, M.B.; Hertz, R.; Ross, G.T. Clinical and pathophysiological aspects of adrenal cortical carcinoma. Am. J. Med. 35:374-383; 1963.

81a. Norton, J.A.; Doppman, J.L.; Jensen, R.T. Cancer of the endocrine system. In: DeVita, V.T., Hellman, S., Rosenberg, S.A.Cancer: Principles and practice of oncology. Philadelphia, PA: JB Lippincott Co; 1989: 1269-1344.

82. Samaan, N.A.; Hickey, R.D. Adrenal cortical carcinoma. Semin. Oncol. 14:292-296; 1987.

Specific References

83. Axelrod, L.R.; Goldzieher, J.W.; Woodhead, D.M.. Steroid biosynthesis in feminizing adrenal carcinoma. J. Clin. Endocrinol. Metab. 29:1481-1488; 1969.

84. Becker, D.; Schumacher, O.P. Op'-DDD therapy in invasive adrenocortical carcinoma. Ann. Intern. Med. 82:677-679; 1975.

85. Bradley, E.L. Primary and adjunctive therapy in carcinoma of the adrenal cortex. Surg. Gynecol. Obstet. 141:507-511; 1975.

86. Chambers, W.L. Adrenal cortical carcinoma in a male with excess gonadotropin in the urine. J. Clin. Endocrinol. 9:451; 1949.

87. Cohn, K.; Gottesman, L.; Brennan, M. Adrenocortical carcinoma. Surgery. 100:1170-1177; 1986.

88. Dluhy, R.G.; Barlow, J.J.; Mahoney, E.M.; *et al.* Profile and possible origin of an adrenocortical carcinoma. J. Clin. Endocrinol. Metab. 33:312-317; 1971.

89. Erikson, B.; Oberg, K.; Curstedt, T.; *et al.* Treatment of hormone-producing adrenocortical cancer with QP'DDD and streptozotocin. Cancer 59:1398-1403; 1987.

90. Eymontt, M.J.; Gwinup, G.; Kruger, F.A.; *et al.* Cushing's syndrome with hypoglycemia caused by adrenocortical carinoma. J. Clin. Endocrinol. 25:46-52; 1965.

91. Farge, D.; Chatellier, G.; Pagny, J-Y; Jeunemaitre, X.; Plouin, P-F.; Carvol, P. Isolated clinical syndrome of primary aldosteronism in four patients with adrenocortical carcinoma. Am. J. Med. 83:635-640; 1987.

92. Filipecki, S.; Feltynowski, T.; Polawska, W.; *et al.* Carcinoma of the adrenal cortex with hyperaldosteronism. J. Clin. Endocrinol. Metab. 35:225-229; 1972.

93. Fishman, L.M.; Liddle, G.W.; Island, P.; *et al.* The effects of

amino-glutethimide on adrenal function in man. J. Clin. Endocrinol. 27:481-490; 1967.

94. Fukushima, D.K.; Bradlow, H.L.; Hellman, L.; Gallagher, T.F. Origin of pregnanetriol in a patient with adrenal carcinoma. J. Clin. Endocrinol. 22:765-772; 1962.

95. Fukushima, D.K.; Gallagher, T.F. Steroid production in "nonfunctioning" adrenal cortical tumor. J. Clin. Endocrinol. 23:923; 1963.

96. Fulchuk, K.R. Case report: inappropriate antidiuretic hormone-like syndrome associated with an adrenal carcinoma. Am. J. Med. Sci. 266:393-395; 1973.

97. Ghorashi, B.; Holmes, J.H. Gray scale sonographic appearance of an adrenal mass: a case report. J. Clin. Ultrasound 4:121; 1976.

98. Glazer, G.M.; Woolsey, E.J.; Borrello, J.; et al. Adrenal tissue characterization using MR imaging. Radiology 158:73-79; 1986.

99. Gross, M.D.; Shapiro, B.; Bouffard, A.; et al. Distinguishing benign from malignant enadrenal masses. Ann. Intern. Med. 109:613-618; 1988.

100. Hag, M.M.; Legha, S.S.; Samaan, N.A.; et al. Cytotoxic chemotherapy in adrenal cortical carcinoma. Cancer Treat. Rep. 64:909-913; 1980.

101. Hajjar, R.A.; Hickey, R.C.; Samaan, N.A. Adrenal cortical carcinoma: a study of 32 patients. Cancer. 35:549-554; 1975.

102. Hogan, T.F.; Citrin, D.L.; Johnson, B.M.; et al. Op'-DDD (Mitotane) therapy of adrenal cortical carcinoma. Cancer. 42:2177; 1978.

103. Hogan, T.F.; Gilchrist, K.W.; Wesring, D.W.; et al. A clinical and pathological study of adrenocortical carcinoma. Cancer. 45:2880-2883; 1980.

104. Hough, A.J.; Hollifield, J.W.; Page, D.L.; et al. Prognostic factors in adrenal cortical tumor. A mathematical analysis of clinical and morphological data. Am. J. Clin. Pathol. 73:390-399; 1979.

105. Javadpour, N.; Woltering, E.A.; Brennan, M.F. Adrenal neoplasms. Curr. Probl. Surg. 17:16-27; 1980.

106. Johnson, D.H.; Greco, F.A. Treatment of metastatic adrenal cortical carcinoma with cisplatin and etoposide. Cancer. 58:2198-2202; 1986.

107. Katz, R.L.; Shukhoda, A. Diagnostic approach to incidental adrenal nodules in the cancer patient. Cancer 55:1995-2000; 1985.

108. Kehlet, H.; Blicher-Toft, M.; Hancke, S.; et al. Comparative study of ultrasound, iodine-131-19-iodocholesterol scintigraphy, and aortography in localizing adrenal lesions. Br. J. Med. 2:665-667; 1976.

109. King, D.R.; Lock, E.E. Adrenal cortical carcinoma. A clinical and pathological study of 49 cases. Cancer. 44:239-244; 1979.

110. Lipsett, M.B.; Wilson, H. Adrenocortical cancer: steroid biosynthesis and metabolism evaluated by urinary metabolites. J. Clin. Endocrinol. 22:906-915; 1962.

111. Lubitz, J.A.; Freeman, L.; Okun, R. Mitotane use in inoperable adrenal cortical carcinoma. JAMA. 223:1109-1112; 1973.

112. Luton, J.P.; Mahondeau, J.A.; Bouchard, P.H.; et al. Treatment of Cushing's disease by Op'-DDD. New Engl. J. Med. 300:459-464; 1979.

113. Magee, B.J.; Gattamaneni, H.R.; Pearson, D. Adrenal cortical carcinoma: survival after radiotherapy. Clin. Radiol. 38:557-558; 1987.

114. Montagne, J.P.; Kressel, H.Y.; Korobkin, M.; et al. Computed tomography of the normal adrenal glands. AJR. 130:963-966; 1978.

115. Montali, G.; Solbiati, L.; Bossi, M.C.; Pra, L.D.; Donna, A.D.; Ravetto, C. Sonographically guided fine-needle aspiration biopsy of adrenal masses. AJR. 143:1081-1084; 1984.

116. Moy, R.H. Studies of the pharmacology of Op'-DDD in man. J. Lab. Clin. Med. 58:296-304; 1961.

117. Ostuni, J.A.; Roginsky, M.S. Metastatic adrenal cortical carcinoma — documented cure with combined chemotherapy. Arch. Intern. Med. 135:1257-1258; 1975.

118. Roginsky, M.S.; Schick, M. Addison's disease following combined chemotherapy for hyperfunctioning adrenocortical carcinoma. Arch. Intern. Med. 117:673-676; 1966.

119. Sample, W.F.; Sarti, D.A. Combined tomography and grey scale ultrasonography of the adrenal gland. A comparative study. Radiology. 128:377-383; 1978.

120. Schein, P.S. Chemotherapeutic management of the hormone-secreting endocrine malignancies. Cancer. 30:1616-1626; 1973.

121. Schick, M. Survival with adrenal carcinoma. JAMA. 224:1763; 1973.

122. Schteingart, D.E.; Motazedi, A.; Noonan, R.A.; et al. Treatment of adrenal carcinomas. Arch. Surg. 117:1142-1146; 1982.

123. Solomon, S.S.; Swersie, S.P.; Paulsen, C.A.; et al. Feminizing adrenocortical carcinoma with hypertension. J. Clin. Endocrinol. 20:608-612; 1968.

124. Sturman, M.F.; Beierwaltes, W.H.; Ice, R. Imaging of functional nodules of the adrenal glands in relatively asymptomatic individuals. Abstract. J. Nucl. Med. 14:458; 1973.

125. Thompson, N.W.; Cheung, P.S.Y. Diagnosis and treatment of functioning and nonfunctioning adrenocortical neoplasms including indicentalomas. Surg. Clin. North Am. 67:423-436; 1987.

126. Thrall, J.H.; Freitas, J.E.; Beierwaltes, W.H. Adrenal scintigraphy. Semin. Nucl. Med. 8:23-41; 1978.

127. Vilee, D.B.; Rotner, H.; Kliman, B.; et al. Androgen synthesis in a patient with virilizing adrenocortical carcinoma. J. Clin. Endocrinol. Metab. 27:1112-1122; 1967.

128. Walters, G.; Wyatt, G.B.; Kelleher, J. Carcinoma of the adrenal cortex presenting as a pheochromocytoma. Report of a case. J. Clin. Endocrinol. Metab. 22:575-580; 1962.

129. Watanabe, K.; Kamoi, I.; Nakayama, C.; et al. Scintigraphic detection of a hepatic metastases with iodine-131-labeled steroid in recurrent adrenal carcinoma: case report. J. Nucl. Med. 17:904-906; 1976.

130. West, C.D.; Kumagai, L.F.; simons, E.L.; et al. Adrenocortical carcinoma with feminization and hypertension associated with a defect in 11-beta-hydroxylation. J. Clin. Endocrinol. 24:567-579; 1964.

Pituitary Tumors

General References

131. Earp, H.S.; Ney, R.L. Pituitary tumors. In: Holland, J.F.; Frei, E., eds. Cancer medicine. 2nd ed. Philadelphia, PA: Lea & Febiger; 1982:1634-1647.

132. Gauger, G.E. Anatomy of the pituitary and hypothalamus. In: Linfoot, J.A., ed. Recent Advances in the Diagnosis and Treatment of Pituitary Tumors. New York, NY: Raven Press; 1979:5-16.

132a. Grigsby, P.W.; Sheline, G.E. Pituitary. In: Principles and practice of radiation oncology. Perez, C.A., Brady, L.W. (eds). Philadelphia, PA: JB Lippincott Co; 1992:564-582.

133. Grigsby, P.W.; Simpson, J.R.; Emami, B.N.; Fineberg, B.B.; Schwartz, H.G. Prognostic factors and results of surgery and postoperative irradiation in the management of pituitary adenomas. Int. J. Radiat. Oncol. Biol. Phys. 16: 1411-1418; 1990.

134. Kernohan, J.W.; Sayre, G.P. Tumors of the pituitary gland and infundibulum. section 10,fasc. 36. Armed Forces Institute of Pathology, Washington D.C: AFIP; 1956:7-57.

135. Levin, V.A.; Sheline, G.E.; Gutin, P.H. Neoplasms of the central nervous system. In: DeVita, V.T.; Hellman, S.; Rosenberg, S.A., eds. Cancer: Principles and Practice of Oncology. 3rd ed. Philadelphia, PA: JB Lippincott Co; 1989:1557-1611.

136. Sheline, G.E. Oncologic: Multidisciplinary Decisions in Oncology: Pituitary adenomas. New York, NY: Pergamon Press; 1981.

Specific References

137. Antunes, J.; Houseplan, E.; Frantz, A.; et al. Prolactin-secreting pituitary tumors. Ann. Neurol. 2:148-153; 1977.

138. Bergland, R.M. Pathologic considerations in pituitary tumors. Prog. Neurol. Surg. 6:62-94; 1975.

139. Bloodworth, J.M.B.; Kalman, K.; Horvath, E. Light and electron microscopy of pituitary tumors. In: Linfoot, J.A., ed. Recent Advances in the Diagnosis and Treatment of Pituitary Tumors. New York, NY: Raven Press; 1979:141-159.

140. Canales, E.; Garcia, I.; Ruiz, J.; Zarate, A. Bromocriptine as prophylactic therapy in prolactinoma during pregnancy. Fertil. Steril. 36:524-526; 1981.

141. Chun, M.; Masko, G.; Hetelekidis, S. Radiotherapy in the treatment of pituitary adenomas. Intl. J. Radiat. Oncol. Biol. Phys. 15:305-309; 1988.

141a. Comtois, R.; Beauregard, H.; Somma, M.; Serri, O.; Aris-Jilwan, N.; Hardy, J. The clinical and endocrine outcome to transsphenoidal microsurgery of nonsecreting pituitary adenomas. Cancer 68:860-866; 1991.

142. Crosignani, P.; Mattei, A.; Ferrari, C.; et al. Enlargement of a prolactin-secreting pituitary microadenoma during bromocriptine

treatment — case report. Br. J. Obstet. Gynaecol. 89:169-170; 1982.

143. Crosignani, P.; Ferrari, C.; Scarduelli, C.; Picciotti, M.; Caldara, R.; Malinverni, A. Spontaneous and induced pregnancies in hyperprolactinemic women. Obstet. Gynecol. 58:708-713; 1981.

144. Earl, K.M.; Dillar, S.H. Pathology of adenomas of the pituitary gland. In: Kohler, P.O.; Ross, G.T., eds. Diagnosis and Treatment of Pituitary Tumors. Amsterdam, Excerpta Medica; New York, NY: American Elsevier; 1973:3.

145. Eastman, R.; Gorden, P.; Roth, J. Conventional supervoltage irradiation is an effective treatment for acromegaly. J. Clin. Endocrinol. Metab. 48:931; 1979.

146. Edmonds, M.; Simpton, W.; Meakin, J. External irradiation of the hypophysis for Cushing's disease. Calif. Med. 107:860; 1972.

147. Erlichman, C.; Meakin, J.W.; Simpson, W.T. Review of 154 patients with nonfunctioning pituitary tumors. Intl. J. Radiat. Oncol. Biol. Phys. 5:1981-1986; 1979.

148. Goldfine, I.D. Pharmacologic treatment of acromegaly. In: Linfoot, J.A., ed. Recent Advances in the Diagnosis and Treatment of Pituitary tTmors. New York, NY: Raven Press; 1979:341-346.

149. Gomez, F.; Reyes, F.; Faiman, C. Nonpuerperal galactorrhea and hyperprolactinemia. Am. J. Med. 62:648; 1977.

150. Grigsby, P.; Simpson, J.; Fineberg, B. Late regrowth of pituitary adenomas after irradiation and/or surgery: hazard function analysis. Cancer. 63:1308-1312; 1989.

151. Grigsby, P.; Stokes, S.; Mards, J.; Simpson, J. Prognostic factors and results of radiotherapy alone in the management of pituitary adenomas. Intl. J. Radiat. Oncol. Biol. Phys. 15:1103-1110; 1988.

152. Grigsby, P.; Thomas, P.; Simpson, J.; Fineberg, B. Long-term results of radiotherapy in the treatment of pituitary adenomas in children and adolescents. Am. J. Clin. Oncol. 11:607-611; 1988.

153. Hardy, J. Trans-sphenoidal surgery for hypersecreting adenomas. In: Kohler, P.O.; Ross, G.T., eds. Diagnosis and Treatment of Pituitary Tumors. Amsterdam, Excerpta Medica; New York, NY: American Elsevier; 1973:179-194.

154. Hardy, J.; Beauregard, H.; Robert, F. Prolactin-secreting pituitary adenomas: transsphenoidal microsurgical treatment. In: Robyn, C.; Harter, M., eds. Progress in Prolactin Physiology and Pathology. Amsterdam, Netherlands: Elsevier/North Holland Biomedical Press; 1978:361-370.

155. Hardy, J.; Vezina, J.L. Trans-sphenoidal neurosurgery of intracranial neoplasm. In: Thompson, R.A.; Green, J.R. eds. Advances in Neurology, vol. 15. New York, NY: Raven Press; 1976:261-274.

156. Imura, A. Hyperprolactinemia. In: Linfoot, J.A., ed. Recent Advances in the Diagnosis and Treatment of Pituitary Tumors. New York, NY: Raven Press; 1979:189-206.

157. Jewelewicz, R.; Bande Wiele, R. Clinical course and outcome of pregnancy in twenty-five patients with pituitary microadenomas. Am. J. Obstet. Gynecol. 136:339-343; 1980.

158. Joplan, G.F.; Banks, L.; Cassar, J.; et al. Implantation of yttrium-90 or gold-198 seeds. In: Linfoot, J.A., ed. Recent Advances in the Diagnosis and Treatment of Pituitary Tumors. New York, NY: Raven Press; 1979:331-336.

159. Kleinberg, D.; Boyd, A.; Wardlaw, S.; et al. Pergolide for the treatment of pituitary tumors secreting prolactin or growth hormone. New Engl. J. Med. 309:704-709; 1983.

160. Kramer, S. Indications for, and results of, treatment of pituitary tumors by external radiation. In: Kohler, P.O.; Ross, G.T., eds. Diagnosis and Treatment of Pituitary Tumors. Amsterdam, Excerpta Medica New York, NY: American Elsivier; 1973:271.

161. Krieger, D.T. Pharmacologic therapy of Cushing's disease and Nelson's syndrome. In: Linfoot, J.A., ed. Recent Advances in the Diagnosis and Treatment of Pituitary Tumors. New York, NY: Raven Press; 1979:337-340.

162. Lamberts, S.; Uitterlinden, P.; Vershoor, L.; Dongen, K.; Pozo, E. Long-term treatment of acromegaly with the somatostatin analogue SMS 201-995. New Engl. J. Med. 313:1576-1580; 1985.

163. Lawrence, A.M.; Wilbur, J.F.; Hage, T.C. The pituitary and primary hypothyroidism. Enlargement and unusual growth hormone secretory responses. Arch. Intern. Med. 132:327-333; 1973.

163a. Leavens, M.E.; McCutchen, I.F.; Samann, N.A.. Management of pituitary adenomas. Oncology (June):69; 1992.

164. Levin, S. Manifestations and treatment of acromegaly. Calif. Med. 116:57-64; 1972.

165. Linfoot, J.A. Heavy ion therapy: Particle therapy of pituitary tumors. In: Linfoot, J.A., ed. Recent Advances in the Diagnosis and Treatment of Pituitary Tumors. New York, NY: Raven Press; 1979:245-268.

166. Linfoot, J.A. Neuro-ophthalmological considerations in pituitary tumors. In: Linfoot, J.A., ed. Recent Advances in the Diagnosis and Treatment of Pituitary Tumors. New York, NY: Raven Press; 1979:131-139.

167. Liuzzi, A.; Dallabonzana, D.; Oppizzi, G., et al. Low doses of dopamine agonists in the long-term treatment of macroprolactinomas. New Engl. J. Med. 313:656-659; 1985.

168. Mampalam, T.; Tyrrell, B.; Wilson, C. Transsphenoidal microsurgery for Cushing's disease. Ann. Intern. Med. 109:487-493; 1988.

168a. Maroldo, T.V.; Dillon, W.P.; Wilson, C.B. Advances in diagnostic techniques of pituitary tumors and prolactinomas. Curr. Opinion in Oncol. 4:105-115; 1992.

169. Melmed, S.; Braunstein, G.; Chang, R.; Becker, D. Pituitary tumors secreting growth hormone and prolactin. Ann. Intern. Med. 105:238-253; 1986.

170. Moore, T.J.; Dluhy, R.G.; Gordon, H.W.; et al. Nelson's syndrome: frequency prognosis, and effect of prior pituitary irradiation. Ann. Intern. Med. 85:731-734; 1976.

171. Mori, H.; Mori, S.; Saitoh, Y.; et al. Effects of bromocriptine on prolactin-secreting pituitary adenomas. Mechanism of reduction in tumor size evaluated by light and electron microscopic, immunohistochemical and morphometric analysis. Cancer. 56:230-238; 1985.

172. Ontjes, D.A.; Ney, R.L. Pituitary tumors. CA. 26:330-350; 1976.

173. Pistenma, D.A.; Goffinet, D.R.; Bagshaw, M.A.; et al. Treatment of acromegaly with megavoltage radiation therapy. Intl. J. Radiat. Oncol. Biol. Phys. 1:885; 1976.

174. Pistenma, D.A.; Goffinet, D.R.; Bagshaw, M.A.; et al. Treatment of chromophobe adenomas with megavoltage irradiation. Cancer. 35:1574-1582; 1975.

175. Randall, S.; Laing, I.; Chapman, A.; et al. Pregnancies in women with hyperprolactinaemia: obstetric and endocrinological management of 50 pregnancies in 37 women. Br. J. Obstet. Gynaecol. 89:20-23; 1982.

176. Randall, R.; Scheithauer, B.; Laws, E.; Abboud, C.; Ebersold, M.; Kao, P. Pituitary adenomas associated with hyperprolactinemia: a clinical and immunohistochemical study of 97 patients operated on transsphenoidally. Mayo Clin. Proc. 60:753-762; 1985.

177. Rodman, E.; Molitch, M.; Post, K.; Biller, B.; Reichlin, S. Long-term follow-up of transsphenoidal selective adenomectomy for prolactinoma. JAMA. 252:921-924; 1984.

178. Serri, O.; Rasio, E.; Beauregard, H.; et al. Recurrence of hyperprolactinoma after selective transsphenoidal adenomectomy in women with prolactinoma. New Engl. J. Med. 309:280-283; 1983.

179. Sheline, G.E. Untreated and recurrent chromophobe adenomas of the pituitary. Am. J. Roentgenol. Radium Ther. Nucl. Med. 112:768-773; 1971.

180. Sheline, G.E.; Goldberg, M.V.; Feldman, R. Pituitary irradiation for acromegaly. Radiology. 76:70-75,82;1961.

181. Sheline, G.; Tyrrell, J. Pituitary tumors. In: Perez, C.; Brady, L., eds. Principles and Practice of Radiation Oncology. Philadelphia, PA: JB Lippincott Co; 1987:1108-1125.

182. Sheline, G.; Tyrrell, J. Pituitary adenomas. In: Phillips, T.; Pistemma, D., eds. Radiation oncology annual. New York, NY: Raven Press; 1983:1-35.

183. Urdaneta, N.; Chessen, H.; Fischer, J.J. Pituitary tumors and craniopharyngioma; analyses of 99 cases treated with radiation therapy. Intl. J. Radiat. Oncol. Biol. Phys. 1:895-902; 1976.

184. Wass, J.A.H.; Thorner, M.O.; Morris, D.V.; et al. Long-term treatment of acromegaly with bromocriptine. Br. Med. J. 1:875-878; 1977.

185. Werder, K.; Fahlbusch, R.; Landgraf, R.; et al. Treatment of patients with prolactinomas. J. Endocrinol. Invest. 1:47-59; 1978.

186. Wilson, C. Neurosurgical management of large and invasive pituitary tumors. In: Tindall, G.; Collins, W., eds. Clinical Management of Pituitary Disorders. New York, NY: Raven Press; 1979:335-352.

187. Wilson, C.B.; Dempsey, L.S. Trans-sphenoidal microsurgical removal of 250 pituitary adenomas. J. Neurosurg. 48:13-22; 1978.

James L. Peacock, M.D., Surgical Oncology
James W. Keller, M.D., Radiation Oncology

Robert F. Asbury, M.D., Medical Oncology

Chapter **28**

ALIMENTARY CANCER

"I hav finally kum to the konklusion that a good reliable sett ov bowels iz wurthmore tu a man, than enny quantity ov brains".

Henry Wheeler Shaw (10)

PERSPECTIVE

Cancer occurring in the alimentary tract continues to be a common health problem. Almost 200,000 new cases of gastrointestinal malignancy will be diagnosed in the United States this year. Most of these will be colorectal tumors, but cancer of the esophagus and stomach continue to occur with calculated regularity and very high mortality. Although hereditary factors may play some role in the etiology of gastrointestinal cancer, increasing evidence implicates environmental toxins as causative agents. The surface area of the alimentary tract is the largest barrier of the body between the environment and the internal milieu. Logically the exposure to mutagenic agents in food and liquids is important to the development of cancer in this organ system.

The problems common to all alimentary tract cancers relate to delay in clinical presentation. Pain or palpation of a mass, signs which give early warning to other types of cancer, do not occur early. Instead, most patients present with symptoms of obstruction or gross hemorrhage, which invariably are associated with large primary tumors, high risk of spread, and lower chance of cure. All physicians must search for earlier signs of gastrointestinal cancer, and educate their patients likewise to be aware of certain symptoms in order to make earlier diagnoses. In general, these early warning signs include vague abdominal discomforts, unexplained weight loss, change in bowel habits, or new onset anemia. Routine sigmoidoscopy and stool testing for occult blood are recommended screening procedures. Other tests such as routine contrast radiography, upper endoscopy, or cytology analysis have yet to demonstrate cost effectiveness. Eventually, however, these screening procedures may apply to high risk populations.

Surgery remains the primary mode of treatment for cure of gastrointestinal malignancies. Surgery alone, however, has been unable to change survival rates over the last decade. Adjuvant and neo-adjuvant utilization of radiation and chemotherapy offer the best prospect of improving cure rates. A great deal of investigational studies are being pointed appropriately towards this strategy.

Radiation therapy has been capable of producing responses in gastrointestinal malignancies adequate to down-stage large primary masses prior to surgery. Both pre-operative and/or post-operative irradiation have been used as effective adjuvants from the esophagus to the rectum with modest gains.

Intraoperative and intracavitary modes of delivering radiation are on the horizon for increasing response rates. In addition, effective palliation can be accomplished with radiation therapy.

Chemotherapy for malignancy of alimentary tract is plagued by the lack of a single effective agent. 5 Fluorouracil (5-FU) has been the historic standard. Response rates with this drug, however, continue to be poor. Addition of leucovorin recently has increased optimism for treatment of these malignancies with 5-FU. In the adjuvant setting, the addition of levamisole to 5-FU has increased survival significantly for Stage C subsets of colon cancer patients.

Conquering cancer of the gastrointestinal tract will ultimately require multimodality therapy. For the most part combination treatments are experimental, and are not currently considered standard treatment. Emphasis on enrolling patients in clinical trials of this nature will help develop effective treatment strategies in the future. The most impressive success story for chemoradiation has been in anal cancers where moderate dose irradiation combined with simultaneous infusions of 5-FU, mitomycin C, and/or cisplatin have yielded high response rates, improved survival and have allowed for anal sphincter preservation avoiding the use of abdomino-perineal resections.

ESOPHAGUS

EPIDEMIOLOGY AND ETIOLOGY

Epidemiology (1b)

Incidence

Esophageal cancer accounts for approximately 5% of all gastrointestinal malignancies. 11,100 new cases will occur in the United States in 1992, with an overall incidence of 3.5 per 100,000 persons. The incidence is higher among males (3:1) and blacks (3.5:1). Worldwide, northern China, Japan, Finland, and Iran have the highest incidence.

Death Rate

Esophageal cancer will lead to an estimated 10,000 deaths in the United States this year. This figure approximates the actual incidence of the disease, and forebodes the poor prognosis that most patients have. One study defines a lower mortality for women compared to men, though the reasons for this are unclear (66).

Age

This disease is most common in elderly males over age 60, yet it may appear at a younger age in association with achalasia or hiatal hernia, although cancer is not associated frequently with either of these entities.

Etiology (15,61)

Direct causative factors for esophageal cancer have not been established. However, numerous associative conditions have been defined and subsequently assigned as risk factors.

1. Woman with Plummer-Vinson syndrome, (sideropenic anemia, glossitis, esophagitis) have a 10% incidence of esophageal cancer, particularly common in Sweden.
2. Chronic consumption of hot or heavily seasoned foods and liquids have been associated with this disease especially in regions of east and south Africa.
3. Heavy alcohol and tobacco use are independent risk factors for developing esophageal cancer. Combination of these two factors multiplies the risk even more.
4. Esophageal strictures secondary to Lye injuries are at risk for development of carcinoma. These malignancies tend to be less aggressive than esophageal cancer from other causes (13).
5. Long standing achalasia is accompanied with a 5% incidence of esophageal cancer. Interestingly, performing a myotomy to relieve achalasia does not decrease this risk.
6. The only hereditary transmission of esophageal cancer is among patients with tylosis, an autosomal dominant disorder characterized by hyperkeratosis of the palms and soles. 37% of these patients will develop squamous cell carcinoma of the esophagus (21).
7. Barrett's esophagus, a condition of gastric columnar epithelium extending more than 3cm into the distal esophagus, is commonly associated with occurrence of adenocarcinoma. While most adenocarcinomas of the distal esophagus arise from Barrett's esophagus, the incidence of this cancer developing in patients followed with Barrett's epithelium is low, approximately 1 in 175-441 patient years. This is the same risk as developing lung cancer after smoking one pack of cigarettes per day for 20 years. Anti-reflux therapy, medical or surgical, does not reduce this risk which is almost 30 times the normal risk of developing carcinoma of the esophagus. Close follow-up of these patients is essential (16,41,63).
8. Linxian is in Honan Province in northern China and has an extraordinary high incidence of human esophageal cancer, but also in domestic chickens (60). Nitrosamines in the food or water are the probable culprit.

DETECTION AND DIAGNOSIS

Clinical Detection (59a)

Dysphagia and *weight loss* are the most common symptoms at presentation, occurring in 90% of patients. *Hematemesis* is an uncommon occurrence and can herald a rapid fatal outcome due to aortic wall penetration by the cancer.

Early symptoms may include chest pain or *odynophagia*, but usually are not severe enough to stimulate medical attention. Signs of invasion of adjacent organs are late and include hoarseness (related to recurrent laryngeal nerve), superior vena cava syndrome, cough related to tracheal- or bronchial-esophageal fistula, Horner's syndrome (sympathetic nerves), paralyzed diaphragm (phrenic nerve), malignant pleural effusion, or massive hematemesis related to aorto-esophageal fistula which is ominous.

Screening procedures such as endoscopy and cytology brushings, are common in the Orient but have not been cost effective in the United States.

Diagnostic Procedures (44,49,50,68) (Table 28-1)

Fluoroscopy and barium swallow: Irregular filling defects or ulcerative strictures are characteristic findings of carcinoma. Deviation or angulation of the barium column is another sign of malignancy. Double contrast with air and barium should be used to find smaller lesions. Barium swallow is used to determine the length of the lesion and the extent of circumferential involvement. Degree of obstruction can also be assessed.

Esophagoscopy: Flexible endoscopes with biopsy and cytology capabilities have improved the diagnosis of esophageal cancer. The combination of cytology brushings and perimeter biopsies of a mass will make the diagnosis of cancer with 90% accuracy.

Ultrasound: Ultrasound with endoscopy is a relatively new mode of assessment which shows promise in determining depth of penetration through wall and into surrounding structures (52,69).

CT scan evaluates the presence of nodal involvement, invasion of adjacent structures, as well as metastatic spread to lung, liver, or celiac nodes (35).

MR is less valuable to assess esophageal cancers due to cardiac and aortic motion. If corrected for motion artifacts, it is highly competitive with CT for estimation of esophageal and mediastinal invasion but less accurate for nodal assessments.

Bronchoscopy to rule out invasion of the left mainstem bronchus is especially important for lesions in the middle third of the esophagus. Assessment of vocal cord function is also performed with this procedure (35).

Exploratory laparotomy and biopsy of celiac lymph nodes and or other sites of distant spread are important maneuvers for clinical staging which if positive would contraindicate radical surgery.

If metastatic disease is suspected depending upon symptoms and signs, CT scan of liver and/or radioisotope bone scans are recommended.

Generally less helpful studies include mediastinoscopy, scalene node biopsies, and skeletal surveys (35).

CLASSIFICATION AND STAGING

Histopathology (Table 28-2)

Squamous cell carcinomas: The majority of esophageal cancers (60%) are squamous in nature, and no attempt is made to grade these tumors. Approximately 15% occur in the cervical subsite, 45% in the upper and mid thoracic areas and 40% in the lower.

Table 28-1. Diagnostic Procedures for Esophageal Cancer (1a)

METHOD	DIAGNOSIS AND STAGING CAPABILITY	RECOMMENDED FOR USE
Primary tumor and regional nodes		
CT	Most useful of all modalities for determining local invasion and regional nodes.	Yes
Double-contrast esophagogram	Useful to detect and define primary lesion, occasionally to demonstrate second tumor	Yes
Percutaneous biopsy guided by imaging technique, usually CT	Invasive but very accurate for squamous cell; will rarely be used in chest, has been used in neck and abdomen.	No, only in selected cases.
MetastaticTumors		
Chest films	Good for detecting metastases and second primary. Controversial local invasion.	Yes
Ultrasound	Useful for evaluating clinically suspected abdominal metastases. CT as good or better than ultrasound.	No
Bone films	Useful only to confirm metastatases.	No
Radionuclide studies liver-spleen, brain and bone scans	Useful in evaluation of clinically suspected metastases. CT better than RN scans for liver brain.	No

Adenocarcinomas (40%) of the esophagus comprise anywhere from 20%-40% of modern series and the increase appears to be real (29,63). It has been questioned whether these are true esophageal cancers or gastric cancers that have invaded the esophagus. Some insist on their esophageal origin and argue that adenocarcinomas of the lower esophagus or cardia behave the same as their squamous counterpart (25). The origin of these adenocarcinomas is debated to arise in : (1) esophageal mucosa or submucosal glands, (2) heterotopic gastric mucosa that has failed squamous differentiation, or (3) metaplastic gastric mucosa (Barrett's esophagus) (19). The most convincing pathologic differences between these adenocarcinomas and gastric adenocarcinomas is the presence of Barrett's epithelium in the esophageal site (63). Other unusual malignancies of the esophagus include adenosquamous variants, oat cell carcinoma, carcinosarcomas and melanoma.

Table 28-2. Histologic Classification of Espohageal Tumors

MALIGNANT	% INCIDENCE
1. Squamous cell carcinoma	90
2. Adenocarcinoma	10
3. Adenoid cystic carcinoma	
4. Mucoepidermoid carcinoma	
5. Adenosquamous carcinoma	<1
6. Undifferentiated carcinoma	

TNM Classification

Anatomy

It is important to appreciate the various divisions of the esophagus.

1. Cervical — from the bottom of the cricoid cartilage (C6) to the suprasternal notch which spans 15 to 18 cm from the incisors. Areas of extension — trachea.
2. Upper Thoracic — from the suprasternal notch to the carina (T4 or T5); 18 to 24 cm from incisors. Areas of extension — aorta and trachea.
3. Mid-thoracic — from tracheal bifurcation to esophagogastric junction; 24 to 32 cm. Areas of possible extension — aorta, pericardium, and left main stem bronchus.
4. Lower thoracic — approximately 8 cm in length which includes the abdominal esophagus; 32 to 40 cm from the incisors. Areas of extension — diaphragm, prevertebral fascia or thoracic vertebrae.

The current AJCC (3rd) (1) and UICC (4th) (11) editions of the classification of cancer are the same in context but differ from previous editions.

Similarities

For most of the gastrointestinal tract (GIT), a hollow viscus, the classification is based upon depth of invasion through the 4-layered wall for all sites. The T1 lesion is confined to the mucosa or invades lamina propia and submucosa, T2 invades the muscularis propria, T3 invades to the adventitia or serosa and T4 invades surrounding structures. The staging process is surgical/pathologic rather than clinical radiographic with size, surface spread, mobility being excluded in criteria but presumably related to depth of invasion. The exception is the anus.

Differences

The nodal categories and stage grouping have been rearranged at most sites and is more confusing than before. There is no consistency as to nodal categories or stage grouping, which makes it necessary to refer to tables. Generally T3 is equivalent to N1 and N1 is equivalent to M1. A brief review of differences for the staging of esophagus from previous editions follows:

Size (>5cm) has been omitted, degree of obstruction and different categories of N stage. Invasion of adjacent structures was classified as T3 previously, now it is T4. The lymph node categories have been reduced to N0 and N1 since N1 carries so poor a prognosis that state of advancement to N2, N3 designation has been eliminated. The stage grouping is rearranged and unfortunately confusing. There are four instead of three T categories.

Clinical Staging (Table 28-3, Fig. 28-1)

Clinical staging is based on the anatomical extent of the primary tumor as determined by pretreatment studies. These studies include esophagoscopy, contrast radiography, and other examinations listed above. Most cancers occur in the middle or distal thirds of the esophagus. Fifteen percent occur in the upper third of the esophagus and by their critical location are associated with a worse prognosis and a different mode of treatment.

Staging Work-Up

Both CT and MR are highly accurate in staging cancer of the mediastinal esophagus with sensitivities and specificities of over 90% tumor invasion but lower (33%) sensitivity for involved lymph nodes. Computerized tomography and MR can detect mass effect, invasion and thickening of esophageal wall, invasions into fat, and can be used to predict aortic (CT>MR) and pericardial invasion (MR>CT), with a sensitivity of 92%-99% and a specificity of 96%.

Pathologic Staging (Fig. 28-2)

Pathologic staging is based on surgical exploration and histologic examination of the resected specimen and regional lymph nodes. For purposes of prognosis, the depth of invasion, involvement of lymph nodes, and visceral metastatic spread are the most important and independent variables affecting survival. Other features which have relative significance include: site of origin along the esophagus, vascular invasion, submucosal extension, histologic type, lymphocyte response to tumor, and presence of tumor necrosis (24,65).

Lymph node involvement is depicted in Fig. 28-2 and distribution in the mediastinum is a function of tumor location.

PRINCIPLES OF TREATMENT (Table 28-4)

At the time of presentation, only 40% of T1 patients have localized disease, 25% have disease outside the esophagus, and 35% are metastatic. For T2 lesions, only 10% are localized, 15% are outside the esophagus, and 75% are metastatic. Frequent sites of local disease outside the esophagus at autopsy include trachea (54%), mediastinum (13%), lung (16%), pleura (7%), aorta (6%), and heart (5%) (22). Patterns of failure at autopsy include 83% with local + regional + distant spread, 53% liver, 35% lung, 11% bone, 8% adrenals, and 4% brain (25). Hence, esophageal cancer is a disease that is rarely localized at diagnosis and characterized by high incidence of local/regional and distant spread at death. Any successful treatment strategy must address these issues.

Cure rates average 5% at 5 years. Despite this pessimistic outlook, the approach to therapy is still tempered towards cure. In most cases a therapeutic goal of cure eventuates the best palliation. Unfortunately, treatment of esophageal cancer is largely palliative. A multidisciplinary approach is essential to achieve desirable outcomes and is presented in Table 28-4.

Table 28-3. TNM Classification for Esophagus Cancer

TNM Classification		Clinical Classification	
		Cervical and Intrathoracic	
T1	Lamina propria/submucosa	T1	≤ 5 cm/no obstruction
T2	Muscularis propria	T2	> 5 cm/obstriction/whole circumference
T3	Adventitia	T3	Extension outside esophagus
T4	Adjacent structures		
N1	Regional lymphnodes	**Cervical**	
		N1	Supraclavicular, cervical nodes

Stage Grouping		
		Intrathoracic
Stage I	$T_1 N_0 M_0$	
Stage IIA	$T_{2,3} N_0 M_0$	N1 Mediastinal, perigastric (incl. celiac)
Stage IIB	$T_{1,2} N_1 M_0$	M1 Nodes not considered regional
Stage III	$T_3 N_1$ or $T_4 N_0 N_1$	
Stage IV	$T_{any} N_{any} M_1$	

T = tumor; N = node; M = metastases.
Modified from AJC (11).

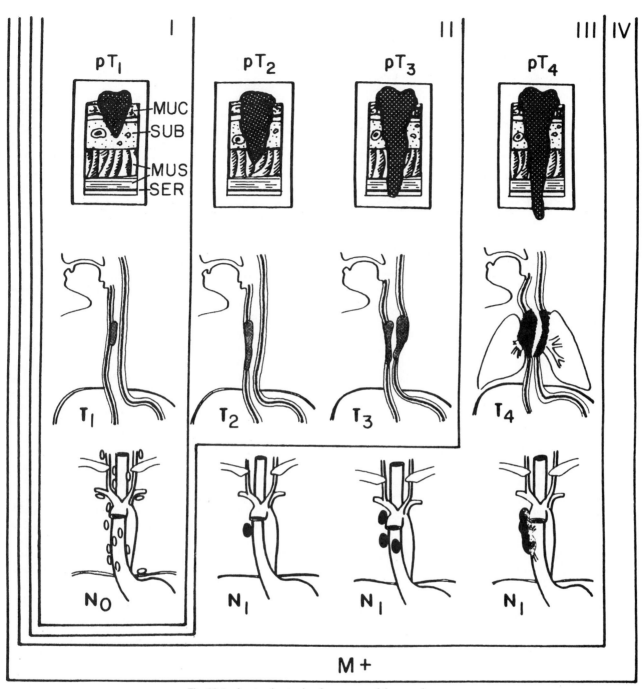

Fig. 28-1. Anatomic staging for cancer of the esophagus.

Surgery

Surgery is the standard treatment for Stage I and II carcinoma of the esophagus in patients capable of withstanding a major operation. Operative mortality ranges from 5%-20% depending on patient selection. Over all, 5-year survival following esophagectomy is less than 10%. When considering "curative" resections alone, however, survival is as high as 21% (21,23,49).

Despite low overall survival rates, surgical resection offers good palliation of dysphagia. In one study over 50% of patients after esophagectomy had no recurrence of dysphagia and most patients with recurrent dysphagia were eating satisfactorily nonetheless (39).

The principles of surgical treatments for esophageal cancer include extended longitudinal margins of resection because of the proclivity for submucosal spread. Over 40% of patients will have involvement of the submucosa 5cm above the gross margin of the tumor (45). Many authors recommend total esophagectomy as minimal treatment. The most widely used approach is a midline laparotomy to mobilize the stomach and rule out metastatic disease. This is followed by a right thoracotomy for esophagectomy. Subsequent reconstruction of the gastrointestinal tract is usually obtained by esophagogastrostomy with the stomach drawn through the resection bed and posterior mediastinum. Depending on the location of the primary tumor anastomosis may be at the

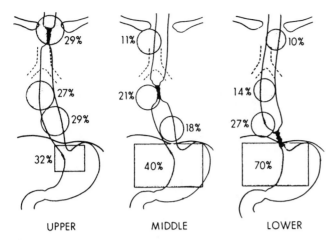

UPPER   MIDDLE   LOWER

Fig. 28-2. The percentage of positive lymph nodes found at surgery for esophageal carcinoma in the upper, middle, and lower esophagus.

level of the azygos vein or in the neck through a separate cervical incision. Other alternatives include interposition with colon or jejunal segments (20). Many surgeons have converted to esophagectomy without thoracotomy (transhiatal esophagectomy). Esophagogastrostomy is performed in the neck. Comparative studies have shown reduced morbidity with this procedure and no differences in tumor recurrence (54a).

Radiotherapy (13b,27,28,56)

1. Esophageal epidermoid carcinoma is radioresponsive, and local tumor eradication is frequently attainable. Irradiation is favored for lesions above the aortic arch since surgical mortality rates rise for higher esophageal lesions without improvement in surgical outcome. The results in terms of survival are probably better than with surgery (51).
2. Radiation therapy has also been successful in palliating pain and improving dysphagia in 65%-80% of cases.

Unfortunately the palliation dose is close to the definitive dose, generally 50-60 Gy in 1.8 Gy fractions. Another frequent schedule is 25 Gy in 10 fractions over 14 days, followed by a 2-4 week rest, then repeat of the same (29,58,59).

3. Supervoltage irradiation and a very long radiation field are commonly utilized. Since the disease spreads longitudinally, a margin of 5-8 cm above and below the lesion is desirable, if possible. The tumoricidal dose for the major area of involvement is 5,000cGy/5 weeks. Care is taken to keep the maximum dose to the spinal to 4500 cGy by using oblique fields. The fields are reduced in size as therapy progresses so that the boost dose of 1,000-2,000 cGy is given to the tumor plus a 2 cm margin. Total accumulated doses range between 6000 and 7000 cGy.

4. Endocurietherapy, which uses intracavitary sources of irradiation like iridium-192 (n) to supplement and increase the dose to selected sites, is having a resurgence of interest because of high activity radioactive sources with safe after-loading systems (33,33a,55).

5. Radiation Tolerance of Esophagus and Surrounding Structures: The esophagus is quite tolerant to radiation and "curative doses" have been in the 60-70 Gy range. In order to treat to this high dose, it is necessary to avoid exceeding tolerance to the spinal cord, heart and lungs. The patient is usually treated with a combination of AP/PA ports followed by posterior oblique fields with the patient in the prone position to take advantage of the esophagus falling anteriorly away from the spinal cord. It is doubtful that treatment of the celiac and/or supraclavicular nodes improves local control and survival results. Side effects of radiation are mainly dysphagia which has its onset after 20-30 Gy and regresses within 1-2 weeks of completion. Because of this development, and knowing the marginal nutritional status of many of these patients, one must be prepared for alimentation in the form of percutaneous gastric-tubes or percutaneous

Table 28-4. Multidisciplinary Treatment Decisions: Esophagus   (18a,31a,60b)

Stage	Surgery		Radiation Therapy		Chemotherapy
I T_1, N_0, M_0	Esophagectomy anastomosis	or/and	DRT 60-70 Gy for lesions above aortic arch		NR
II $T_{1,2}, N_1, M_0$ T_3, N_0	If good response to RT, then resection attempted		ART preop 40-50 Gy	and/or	CCR
III T_3, N_1, M_0 T_4, N_0, N_1	Bypass procedure if obstruction is severe		DRT 60-70 Gy	and	CCR
IV $T_{any} N_{any}, M_+$	Bypass procedure if obstruction is severe		PRT 50 Gy		CCR IC II

RT = radiation therapy; DRT = definitive; ART = adjuvant; PRT = palliative; NR = not recommended; RCT = recommended chemotherapy;

CCR = concurrent chemotherapy and radiation; IC II = investigational chemotherapy, phase I/II clinical trials.

PDQ: RCT - CCR - 5-FU + mitoC or Cispt with DRT

endoscopic gastrostomy (PEG) tubes. Although radiation has been implicated as a cause of esophageal stricture, all too often the stricture is found to be related to recurrent disease. Fistulae: tracheo-, bronchio-, or aortoesophageal, depending on the location of the cancer and adjacent structures, may develop during the treatment as the tumor regresses and is often disastrous. Aortic perforation leads to sudden hemoptysis and exsanguination within hours to a day. Myelitis as a complication should be rare nowadays given knowledge of spinal cord tolerance, CT treatment planning and oblique fields. Pericarditis is rare as is significant radiation pneumonitis.

Chemotherapy (Table 28-5)

Single agent chemotherapy for metastatic or localized esophageal cancer has been associated with low response rates of < 20% of short duration of 2-5 months.

There are sporadic reports of good palliation with chemotherapy (38). The drugs most studied have been Bleomycin, Methotrexate, Cisplatin, Mitomycin C, Adriamycin, 5-FU, CCNU, Vindesine, and VP-16. These studies were performed in patients with advanced disease, and complete responders were rare. It was natural to study combination chemotherapy, and indeed responses have been higher in the 40%-50% range. Most combinations consisted of Cisplatin plus one of the above agents and duration of response has been approximately 7 months (26). Neoadjuvant chemotherapy has produced high response rates but impact on survival is modest. Consistently, response rates for combination chemotherapy, cisplatinum containing, for local regional disease are 30%-50% (Table 28-5a) and have been higher than response rates with more extensive metastatic cancer with rates of 20%-30%.

Adenocarcinoma of the esophagus may respond to 5-fluorouracil (5-FU), mitomycin C, and doxorubicin (Adriamycin) in a manner similar to that of gastric carcinoma.

Combined Modality Therapy

Attempts to improve response rates in this disease have resulted in combined modality approaches.

Pre-operative Radiation

Pre-operative radiation has theoretical advantages such as reduction of tumor bulk to improve surgical resectability, reduction in transplantable tumor cells by the surgery, curative effect on disease in the para-esophageal region, and sterilization of occult foci in lymph nodes. A variety of studies have been reported using accelerated schemes (20 Gy in 5 days, to 30-45 Gy in 8-12 days), conventional fractions with moderate doses (40-50 Gy in 4-5 weeks) to high doses (50-66 Gy in 6-7 weeks). Unfortunately, pre-operative irradiation goals were not realized and there was no improvement in survival. Indeed the accelerated and high doses were disadvantageous due to increased complications (27,28,40,65).

Post-operative Radiation

Post-operative radiation should ideally allow one to select the most suitable patients for adjuvant therapy. Disadvantages of this strategy include the presence of hypoxic tissue and the intolerance of the stomach or colon to "curative" doses of radiation. Doses should not exceed 50 Gy, but again survival has not been improved with this strategy (28,40).

Pre-operative Chemotherapy

Chemotherapy has been added to pre-operative irradiation and more surgical specimens have been free of disease. However, only those patients with a complete response benefit. Series are non-randomized but the follow-up is short and it is doubtful that this strategy will be curative without concurrent drugs (26,32,49).

Chemo-radiation Therapy (Table 28-6)

Investigators at Wayne State were the first to report on a combined modality approach for squamous cell carcinoma of the esophagus using pre-op chemo-radiation. Surgical specimens were totally free of disease in 5/15 (33%) (43). Although the patient survival was longer, all of these five patients died of recurrent disease (42). A larger, non-randomized study performed by SWOG started with 106 evaluable patients and 71 went on to surgery. The pathology specimens were free of disease in 18/71 (25%) and complete responders had a longer survival (57). RTOG reported on a similar trial with similar results (62). Toxicity was significant and surgical mortality

Table 28-5a.	Response to Chemotherapy Combinations		
		% RESPONSE	MED SURVIVAL
	DDP-/BLEO	17-24	4 mo
	+MTX	26-50	5-7.5 mo
	+VIND	29-33	4 mo

Table 28-5b.	Pre-Op Chemotherapy			
Combination	OPERATION(%)	PR (%)	CR (%)‡	Median Survival
DDP-Bleo	(79)	6 (14)	0	10.0 mo
DDP-Bleo-Vind	(77)	28 (63)	1 (2)	16.2 mo
DDP-Vind-MGBG	(74)	8 (42)	1 (5)	8.5 mo
DDP-Vind-MGBG	(100)	6 (55)	1 (9)	14.0 mo
DDP-5-FU	(35)	13 (76)	0	17.6 mo
DDP-5-FU	(92)	14 (58)	1 (4)	

DDP = cisplatin; Bleo = bleomycin; Vind = vindesine; MGBG = mitoguazone; 5-FU = 5-fluoroacil
‡ Pathologic CR.

Modified from Rosenberg et al. (59a).

Table 28-6. Treatment of Carcinoma of Esophagus With CCIC* and RT

No. of Patients	Treatment	Complete Response Rate (%)	Two-year Survival (%)	Reference
55	3000 cGy/3 wk 5-FU infusion mitomycin or cisplatin bolus (preop)	25	60	43a
140	3000 cGy/3 wk + 5-FU infusion+ cisplatin bolus	22	60	43a
35	6000 cGy x 6 wk 5-FU infusion + mitomycin bolus	48	28	36a
30	6000 cGy 5-FU infusion mitomycin bolus	-	Median 24 mo	17a
21	3000-5040 cGy /3.5-5.5 wk,5-FU infusion mitocycin bolus alternating with cisplatin	77	Median 15 mo	35b

*CCIC = Concomitant Continuous Infusion Chemotherapy.

was increased. The role of surgery came into question from the above studies, so various investigators decided to proceed with chemo-radiation alone (Table 28-7). Again these are small series, non-randomized and presumably selected cases (17,18,19,42). Most of these reports show improvement over historical controls with complete response rates of 25%-75%. There are better 2-year survival rates of 30%-40% with occasional patients surviving at 5 years; however it is doubtful that long-term survival will be improved. An Intergroup study of patients with localized, squamous cell carcinoma of the esophagus was recently reported. Patients were randomized between concurrent radiation (5000cGy) and chemotherapy (5-FU and Cisplatin), followed by two courses of the same chemotherapy or to radiation alone (6400 cGy). Survival in the radiation alone group at 12 and 24 months was 33% and 10%, respectively, while the radiation, chemotherapy arm was 50% and 38%, respectively; a highly significant difference (30). As Tannock (67) stated in a recent review on combined modality therapy, chemotherapy should be used only in a clinical trial and not be considered the standard therapy, however, the above results are challenging.

Treatment According to Clinical Stage

Stages I and II

Surgery and reconstruction is the primary mode of treatment. Preoperative radiation can be used but has not been demonstrated in randomized studies to effect survival or local recurrence. Postoperative adjuvant treatment may be applicable depending on pathologic stage.

Stage III

Irradiation alone is advised for palliation of these patients. Few selected patients may be candidates for palliative resection depending on performance status and location of the primary tumor. Most of these patients will require parenteral or enteral hyperalimentation. Smaller boosting radiation fields are used to deliver maximum doses that are often required.

Stage IV

Radical surgery or radiation therapy is contraindicated in this group of patients with disseminated disease. Effective palliation without major morbidity and mortality is difficult. Silas-

Table 28-7. Nonsurgical Treatment of Locoregional Esophageal Cancer

Reference	Treatment Plan	No. of Patients	Survival Median (mo)	1 Year (%)	2 Year (%)
Leichman et al. (42)	Cisplatin 100 mg/m² + 5-FU 1,000 mg/m² x 96 h x 2 cycles + RT 3000 cGy, mitomycin + bleomycin + RT 2000 cGy	20	22	—	—
Coia et al. (17b)	Mitomycin 10 mg/m² day 1 + 5-FU 1,000 mg/m²/d x 96 h days 2 + 29 + RT 6000 cGy	57	18	—	—
Lokich et al. (44a')	5-FU 300 mg/m² CI weeks 1-6, 5-FU + RT weeks 6-10	13	16	—	—
Herskovic et al. (30)	Cisplatin 75 mg/m² + 5-FU 1,000 mg/m²/d x 96 h weeks 1, 5, 8, 11 + RT 5000 cGy	61	12.5*	50*	38*
	v				
	RT 6400 cGy	60	8.9	33	10

Abbreviations: RT, radiotherapy; CI, continuous infusion.
*Difference statistically significant.
From Forastiere (25a), with permission.

tic tubes can be used to bypass obstructive lesions. Laser therapy offers hope for better palliation of this group.

SPECIAL CONSIDERATIONS OF TREATMENT

Surgical Complications

Esophagectomy and reconstruction is an extensive surgical endeavor with considerable morbidity and significant mortality. Early complications include anastomotic leak and respiratory failure. Later complications which occur are anastomotic strictures, reflux esophagitis and motility disorders (12,64).

Radiation Complications

The untoward reaction to irradiation depends upon normal tissue tolerance and varies with type of tissue, volume irradiated, total dosage, and rate of administration. The type of complicator depends upon the structure involved.

Esophagus: Early during therapy, perforation or hemorrhage may occur due to rapid tumor dissolution. A later effect is stricture.

Lung: Early, there may be radiation pneumonitis during the post therapy period and late, radiation fibrosis. This is an infrequent complication, occurs in a small volume and fortunately a small percentage of patients. Other structures such as heart and spinal cord are rarely involved due to appropriate shielding.

Transverse myelitis is reported after doses greater than 5,000 rad to spinal cord, but should be avoidable with modern shielding techniques.

Chemotherapy Complications

There are a wide range of toxicities that depend upon the drugs used. Using chemotherapeutic agents requires careful considerations because of their limited palliative gains.

Palliation

Local invasion of vital structures, presence of distant metastases, or severe debilitation renders 60% of patients with esophageal cancer unresectable. The alternatives for palliative care are:

Substernal gastric bypass: This is a procedure that leaves the esophagus in place and creates a bypass conduit using the stomach placed through the anterior mediastinum. This procedure recently has become unfavorable due to significant morbidity and mortality (26%), with survival no greater than 5 months (46,54).

Radiation Therapy: External irradiation is 50%-60% successful for palliation of dysphagia. Intracavitary treatment with radioactive Iridium may improve this figure (33,55).

Dilatation and Intubation: Placement of prosthetic tubes to stent malignant obstructions of the esophagus has been used for many years. These devices are probably no more successful at palliation than dilatation alone with Bougie or Maloney dilators. Morbidity from aspiration pneumonia and migration of the prosthetic tubes is high (14,71).

Laser therapy: Endoscopic ND:YAG and Argon Laser treatments, with or without photodynamic dyes, are the most resent advance in palliation of the unresectable carcinoma. Generally, three to five sessions of laser therapy are required in conjunction with dilation to establish patency in most obstructing tumors. Bleeding perforation and fistula formation have been reported but symptoms are improved in 80 90% of patients (47,53).

Gastrostomy and Cervical Esophagostomy: These procedures rarely provide good palliation and are discouraged except for rare situations in which a debilitated patient is receiving neoadjuvant treatment with the hope of undergoing subsequent resection. Feeding jejunostomy would be preferable in these cases to preserve later use of the stomach for reconstruction.

RESULTS AND PROGNOSIS (Table 28-8)

It has been stated that of 100 consecutive patients with esophageal cancer 20% have distant metastases at presentation, 20% have a medical contraindication for surgery, and 60% will be explored. Of the 60 patients explored, 40 are resectable (66%) and of these 40, 13 die in the hospital and 26 are eventually discharged (<50%). Of those discharged, 18 live 1 year, 9 live 2 years, and 4 are alive at 5 years (6%) (23). Hence, treatment of esophageal cancer is largely palliative.

Treatment Results by Stage (Table 28-8)

Stages I and II

Surgery remains the primary strategy in these patients. Surgical treatment for resectable esophageal cancers results in 5-

Table 28-8.	Definitive Radiation for Esophageal Cancer					
Author	Patients Treated	Dose	Median Survival	2 Years Survival (%)	5 Years Survival (%)	Ref
Beatty	146	4000-6000	9	20	6	13b
Cedarquist	388	4500-7000	8	11	4	16a
Hussey	69	5500-6500	10	16	10	34a
Lewinsky	85	5000-6000	8	11	4	43a
Lowe	244	Not stated	5	7	1	44b
Newaisky	444	5000-5500	12	18	9	53a
Pearson	388	5000	12	28	20	52a
Schuchmann	77	4500	10	-	0	61a
Van Andle	115	6000-6600	-	4	1	69a
Van Houtte	81	6000-7500	8	9	3	69b
Wara	103	5000-6000	7	8	1	70a
Wei-Bo Yin	1212	6000-7000	-	11 (3 yr)	7	71a
TOTAL	3352	4000-7000	8.9	13	4.6%	

year survival rates of 5–20%. This is associated with a 7% operative mortality rate (37b). One can expect greater than 50% 5-year survival for the rare T1, NO stages. For T2NO and T1N1 stage, 5-year survival is 10%-15% with an operative mortality of 7-18% (34). Radiation is also given for these stages of disease with 2-year results usually less than 20% and 5-year results generally < 10% with one exception (56) (Table 28-7). The better results reflect better patients as Pearson had the opportunity to treat resectable early stage patients. Generally patients irradiated are older, with poor performance status, and poor surgical candidates. Perhaps the most optimistic results have come from combined modality therapy for this disease, but this remains investigational.

Pre-op RT: There are no randomized studies but in this group of operable patients utilizing a variety of doses (20-70 Gy) there are suggestive but not consistent gains in survival of 20%-30% at 2 years and 10%-25% at 5 years (Table 28-9a).

Post-op RT: Two randomized studies by Kasai (36) show a dramatic increase in survival in node negative patients at 5 years, i.e., 87% versus 17% at 5 years, respectively, but no difference for node positive patients which are the majority i.e., 11% versus 18%. Overall survival showed a benefit for irradiated patients, i.e., 35% versus 20% (Table 28-9b). This study is the exception, however.

Combined chemoradiation: A number of Phase II pilot studies report a 30%-40% 2-year survival for 5-FU + mitomycin or cisplatin which is an improvement. Preoperative neoadjuvant chemotherapy has relapse rates of 15%-75% clinically but

pathologic complete remissions are very few, i.e., < 1%. (Table 28-5b) (Table 28-10). One series of radiation therapy and chemotherapy from Fox Chase with 5-FU and mitomycin produced a 75% local control rate alleviating dysphagia and a 30% actuarial disease-free survival (18% overall survival) at 5 years for stage I and stage II patients (18a). An intergroup randomized trial of chemotherapy and radiation therapy versus radiation therapy alone resulted in an improvement in 2-year survival for the combined modality group (42% versus 10%) (30a).

Stage III

Radiation alone is used for palliation of these cases. Some undergo palliative resection depending on performance status and location of the tumor. A recent intergroup study has shown a survival advantage to definitive irradiation combined with 5-FU and Cisplatin.

Stage IV

There is no standard therapy for this stage disease. Some patients are treated with combination chemotherapy, and others, depending on the symptoms, may receive radiation, e.g., to relieve pain or obstruction. Celiac block will frequently relieve pain from metastases to this area. Other palliative strategies were listed above.

CLINICAL INVESTIGATIONS

Screening of high risk populations with endoscopy and cytology brushings is an important area of investigation.

Table 28-9a. Studies of Preoperative Radiation Therapy for Esophageal Cancer

Preoperative Dose (cGy)	Operative Mortality	2-year Survival (%)	5-year Survival (%)	Reference
5000-6000	21	32	25	13a
5000-6000	33	12	5	22a
3300	25	25	10	27a
2000-4500	12	10	5	37a
4000	20	20	10	41a
3000-7000	9	70	60	44a
4500	18	23	14	47a
2000-3000	6	-	13	35a
4500	19	15	10	55a
2500-3000	6	28	17	65a
4000	21	-	14	69a

Table 28-9b. Survival After Postoperative Irradiation for Esophageal Carcinoma   (36)

Mediastinal Nodes	1 Year	2 Years	5 Years
Negative (39)			
Radiation (20)	19/10 (95%)	17/18 (94.4%)	7/8 (87.5%)
No radiation (19)	10/19 (53%)	8/17 (47%)	3/11 (17%)
Positive (72)			
Radiation (32)	20/32 (63%)	11/30 (37%)	2/18 (11%)
No radiation (40)	21/40 (51%)	9/36 (24%)	4/22 (18%)
Overall Survival			
* Radiation		58%	35%
No radiation		30%	20%

* Not actuarial. Follow-up is 1 to 6 years.

Table 28-10. Preoperative Chemoradiotherapy

Reference	No. of Patients	Preoperative Treatment	Pathologic CR Rate (%)	Median Survival (mo)
Steiger et al. (65')	30	Mitomycin/5-FU/RT 3000 cGy	6/23 (26)	12
Leichman et al. (43)	21	Cisplatin/5-FU/RT 3000 cGy	5/19 (26)	18
Poplin et al. (57)	113	Cisplatin/5-FU/RT 3000 cGy	18/71 (25)	12
Seydel et al. (62)	41	Cisplatin/5-FU/RT 3000 cGy	8/27 (29)	13*
Forastiere et al. (26a)	43†	Cisplatin/5-FU/vinblastine/RT 3750-4500 cGy	10/41 (24)	29

Abbreviation: RT = radiotherapy.
*Mean survival.
†Adenocarcinoma and squamous cell carcinoma.
From Forastiere (25a), with permission.

Oriental investigators have proven that earlier detection of carcinoma of the esophagus will lead to higher cure rates.

Research continues for radiation sensitizing agents which will improve the effectiveness of radiotherapy in both preoperative and palliative phases.

Laser modalities are being investigated to reduce the morbidity and increase the effectiveness of this form of treatment.

STOMACH

EPIDEMIOLOGY AND ETIOLOGY

Epidemiology (1b)

Gastric carcinoma is the 7th leading cause of cancer death in the United States. For unknown reasons the frequency of gastric cancer has been steadily decreasing over the past 50 years. The death rate from this disease was 5 times greater in the 1930s. The estimated new cases for 1992 in the United States is 24,400; 15,000 will be males and approximately 9,400 will be females.

The death rate remains high in other countries especially Chili, Costa Rica, Japan and the Soviet Union where the rates >45/10⁵ population. The expected deaths from gastric carcinoma in 1992 for the US are 13,300 for an incidence to death ratio of 1.7. Deaths occur mostly in the 50 to 59 year age group.

Social and ethnic trends: Low socio economic groups have a higher incidence of gastric cancer. White populations more frequently have proximal lesions where as pyloric and antral lesions are more common among blacks.

Etiology (78)

Diet: The high incidence of gastric cancer in Japan is attributed partly to a diet high in pickled, highly salted and smoked foods. This theory is substantiated by the observation that Japanese persons who migrate to the western world develop a lower incidence of this disease. Nitrosamines and nitrosamides are known gastric carcinogens. Some evidence suggests that food containing ascorbic acid antagonizes these mutagenic chemicals.

Environment: Occupational risks for developing gastric cancer are inherent with the following: coal mining, nickel refining, rubber workers, and asbestos exposure. Infection with Helicobacter pylori is associated with increased risk of gastric cancer (104a).

Alcohol and Tobacco use have not been associated with gastric cancer in a statistically meaningful study.

Historically blood group A individuals where thought to carry an elevated risk of gastric cancer. Subsequent epidemiologic studies, however, have not confirmed this finding. If any, the risk is extremely small.

The transformation of a benign gastric ulcer into a cancer is rare. Conversely, however, gastric carcinomas frequently are ulcerative and misdiagnosed as benign ulcers. For this reason a gastric ulcer which fails to heal is always suspect for malignancy.

Gastric polyps are not precancerous unless villous changes are found on histology. Villous adenomas of the stomach have a definite association with malignancy. In general, all gastric polyps should be biopsied; and all polyps greater than 2 cm in size should be excised.

The risk of developing gastric carcinoma is 2.4 times greater in individuals who have previously had resection for ulcer disease. These cancers occur anywhere from 15 to 40 years after the initial resection.

DETECTION AND DIAGNOSIS

Clinical Detection (91,95)

Vague epigastric discomfort is the most frequent symptom associated with gastric cancer and 90% of patients experience epigastric pain. Weight loss occurs in 80% of patients, early satiety in 65%, anorexia in 60%, and 50% of patients experience dysphagia and vomiting. Only 1% of patients are asymptomatic.

Physical findings: The physical signs of gastric cancer are invariably related to metastatic or unresectable disease. One-third of patients will have signs of metastatic disease, i.e., palpable epigastric mass, ascites, jaundice, supraclavicular adenopathy (Virchow's node), left axillary adenopathy (Irish's node), hepatomegaly, rectal shelf (Blumer's), generalized cachexia, on their initial presentation.

Laboratory findings indicated that 85% of patients are afflicted with anemia and 50% have guaiac positive stools. Hypoalbuminemia is also common as well as elevated CEA levels which occur in 50% of gastric cancers.

DIAGNOSTIC PROCEDURES (95,112) (Table 28-11)

1. *Stool exam* for occult blood.
2. *Upper GI series* is an accurate method for detecting malignant gastric lesions. Ten percent of malignant gastric lesions may be missed unless a double contrast technique is used. Lesions with smooth, sharply defined borders and rugal folds which radiate from the ulcer are usually benign. Malignant lesions generally have

Table 28-11. Diagnostic Procedures for Gastric Cancer (1a)

METHOD	DIAGNOSIS AND STAGING CAPABILITY	RECOMMENDED FOR USE
Primary tumor and regional nodes		
CT	Most valuable of all modalities for determining local invasion and distant metastases	Yes
MRI	Of limited value with massive disease	No
Double-contrast upper GI studies	Very useful in detecting early gastric CA	Yes-should be performed along with single-contrast
Single-contrast upper GI studies	Useful in detecting and defining primary advanced lesions in stomach	Yes-should be performed along with double-contrast
Gastroscopy	Very accurate modality for detecting and defining primary lesions	Yes. If use to confirm lesion detected in UGI series to screen high risk patients
Ultrasound	May be able to detect primary lesions appearing as abdominal masses. May also be able to detect abdominal metastases	No
MetastaticTumors		
Chest films	Good for detecting metastases	Yes
Bone films	Useful only for confirming metastases	No
Radionuclide studies liver-spleen, brain, and bone scans	Useful in evaluation of clinically suspected metastases. CT is better than RN scans for liver and brain	No

elevated irregular margins and rugal folds that do not radiate from the ulcer. Duodenal invasion carries a poorer prognosis (92').

3. *Endoscopy*: Flexible gastroscopy allows visualization and biopsies of most gastric lesions. Generous biopsies of all gastric ulcers should be performed. Infiltrative lesions are the type least likely to be biopsied accurately.

4. *CT scan* is a technique most helpful for detecting evidence of metastatic spread to liver, ovaries, and peritoneal surfaces. Obliterations of the lesser sac might indicate unresectability of the primary tumor. Newer studies with CT scanning are improving the ability to stage the primary (103) lesion. CT has not been successful in the determinations of local invasion into gastric wall and even less for gastric lymph node involvement with a 61% specificity and 67% sensitivity. Determination of pancreatic invasion was accurate in only 27% of instances. Magnetic resonance has similar limitations to CT.

5. At present *laparotomy* is the primary procedure for staging and assessment of resectability. Studies have shown that using laparotomy for staging does not increase mortality rates, and provides the best information for effecting cure or palliation (92).

6. *Exfoliative cytology* using abrasive balloon or chymotrypsin lavage is highly accurate when positive. However, it is time consuming and requires skilled personnel (88).

7. *Molecular genetics:* Two recent studies, one of fractional allelic chromosomal loss and another of allelic deletions of the gene nm23 have both demonstrated a significant association between loss of putative tumor suppressor gene function and the eventual development of distant metastases in patients with initially localized colorectal cancer (76a).

CLASSIFICATION AND STAGING

Histopathology (79) (Table 28-12)

Adenocarcinoma is the most common malignant tumor of the stomach, comprising 95% of these lesions. Among the remaining gastric malignancies, 60% are lymphomas. Leiomyosarcomas are third in frequency. Leiomyosarcomas and undifferentiated cancers comprise 1%-2%.

Leiomyomas are the most common benign tumors of the stomach. They are very frequent in autopsy series but are usually asymptomatic.

Four histologic subtypes of adenocarcinomas have been described and include (1) intestinal — because it resembles intestinal mucosa, (2) pylorocardial — because it resembles glands of the gastric antrum, (3) signet ring cells, and (4) anaplastic.

The gross appearance of gastric adenocarcinomas is characterized by four different types of presentation which are important for their varied prognosis.

1. Ulcerative carcinoma is the most common and is the reason all gastric ulcers should be biopsied.
2. Polypoid cancers or fungating are also common, and all polypoid lesions should be surgically excised.
3. Scirrhous carcinoma has the worst prognosis. These lesions infiltrate the gastric wall producing a thickened,

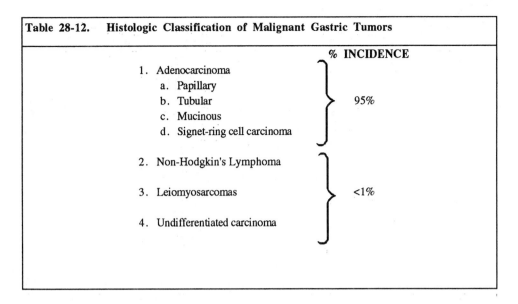

Table 28-12.   Histologic Classification of Malignant Gastric Tumors

		% INCIDENCE
1. Adenocarcinoma		
a. Papillary		
b. Tubular		95%
c. Mucinous		
d. Signet-ring cell carcinoma		
2. Non-Hodgkin's Lymphoma		
3. Leiomyosarcomas		<1%
4. Undifferentiated carcinoma		

nodular, foreshortened stomach which is referred to as linitis plastica.

4. Superficial gastric cancer is an uncommon variety which is characterized by sheet-like collections of cancer cells replacing the normal mucosa.

TNM Classification (Table 28-13 and Fig. 28-3)

The current AJCC (4th) (1) and UICC (4th) (11) editions of the classification of cancer are the same in context but differ from previous editions. The T4 category has been simplified and is divided into an a and b categories; the N category was reduced from 5 to 4. Many abdominal lymph nodes which were considered regional nodes are now metastatic and include periaortic, hepato-duodenal, retropancreatic and mesenteric. Stage grouping is splintered into A and B for

early stages and requires reference to a schema to be appreciated. Unlike most other stage grouping, advanced adenopathy does not advance stage and is confusing.

Stage Grouping (Table 28-13)

Stage classification depends on anatomic extent of the disease. This is most reliably assessed at the time of surgical exploration. Some clinical studies such as CT scanning, gastroscopy, and contrast radiography are helpful in separating patients with advanced local disease and metastases which would obviate the need for surgical exploration.

Changes which have occurred in the staging system include subdivision of stages I and III into two groups each. Extra regional lymph nodes, previously designated N3, are now considered M1. Biologic typing of tumor by DNA

Table 28-13. TNM Classification for Stomach Cancer

	TNM Classifcation		**Pathologic Classification**	
T1	Invades Lamina propria or submucosa		T1/pT1	Mucosa or submucosa only
T2	Muscularis propria or subserosa		T2	Deep invasion $\leq 1/2$ region
T3	Penetrates serosa		pT2	Extension to serosa
T4	Invades adjacent structures		T3	Deep invasion > 1/2 region
			pT3	Extension through serosa
N1	Perigastric lymphnodes <3 cm of tumor		T4/pT4	Extension outside stomach
N2	Perigastric lymphnodes >3 cm of tumor		N1/2	Regional (operable) nodes

p = Pathologic (postsurgical) stage.

Stage Grouping

IA	$T_1 N_0$
IB	$T_1 N_1 T_2 N_0$
II	$T_1 N_2 T_2 N_1 T_3 N_0$
IIIA	$T_2 N_2 T_3 N_1 T_4 N_0$
IIIB	$T_3 N_2 T_4 N_1$
IV	$T_4 N_2 T_{any} N_{any} M_1$

T = tumor; N = node; M = metastases.
Modified from AJC (11).

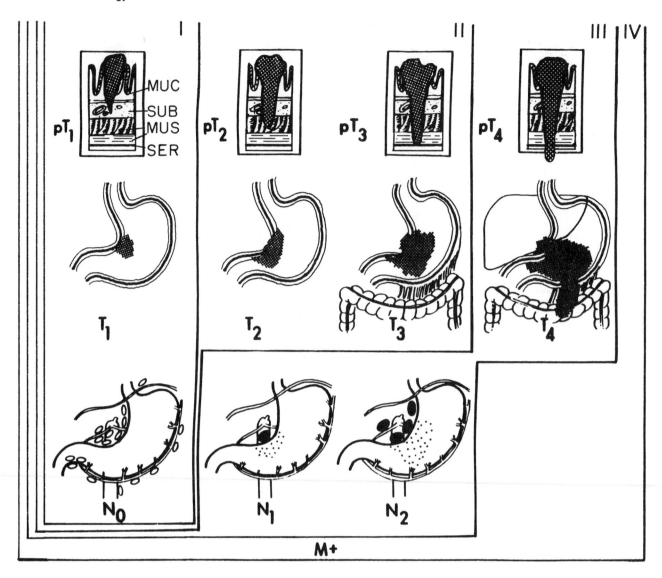

Fig. 28-3. Anatomic staging for cancer of the stomach.

content (ploidy) and cell proliferation characteristics by flow cytometry have identified a favorable (diploid, low proliferation) and unfavorable group (aneuploid and high proliferation) (111c).

PRINCIPLES OF TREATMENT (Table 28-14)

All methods of treating gastric cancers suffer from the predominance of advanced stage disease at the time of presentation. The stage of disease is the most important predictor of outcome for any treatment modality. Most patients who present with gastric cancer have disease outside the stomach at diagnosis, but this is not known without surgical staging. Generally about 20%-30% will be considered inoperable at diagnosis because of metastatic disease or medical contraindications. The remaining will undergo surgery, which at this time is the only treatment modality that influences survival. Of the 75 patients who undergo surgery, 20 will be found to be unresectable, 25 have non-curative resections (palliative) and 30 will have "curative" resections (43%). These figures will undoubtedly vary with institutions by 5-15%. Local/regional recurrence and liver metastases, however, will be the

patterns of failure in most surgical series (87). A multidisciplinary approach is essential to managing gastric cancers and a concise summary is offered in Table 28-14.

Surgery

Surgery is the only modality capable of curing gastric cancer. Results however continue to be poor overall. The goals of surgery are to provide safe removal of all tumor, palliate symptoms such as bleeding and obstruction, and third produce the least mortality and morbidity (84,106).

The extent of resection is governed by the location of the primary tumor. Total gastrectomy should be reserved for removal of large lesions in the body of the stomach. Radical subtotal gastrectomy is the most standard operation. This entails removal of a large part of the stomach *en bloc* with greater and lesser omenta, and occasionally splenectomy and distal pancreatectomy. Direct extension into contiguous organs such as liver and transverse colon is treated by excision of involved areas. Reconstruction is generally accomplished with a gastrojejunostomy. Cancer of the cardia can be resected with a more limited esophagogastrectomy and reconstruction with an esophagogastrostomy in the chest (81,86,107,108).

Table 28-14.   Multidisciplinary Treatment Decisions: Stomach   (82a,104b,111b)

Stage	Surgery	Radiation Therapy	Chemotherapy
I $T_1 N_0 M_0$ $T_1 N_1, T_2 N_0$	Radical subtotal gastrectomy and regional lymph nodes	NR	NR
II $T_2 T_3, N_0, M_0$ $T_1 N_2 T_2 N_1$ $T_3 N_1$	Radical subtotal gastrectomy and regional lymph nodes	NR	NR
III $T_3 N_{1-3}, M_0$	Radical subtotal gastrectomy and regional lymph nodes	ART postop 45-50 Gy	MAC IC II
IV $T_4 N_3 M_0$ $T_4 N_3 M_1$	Radical subtotal gastrectomy and regional lymph nodes and resection of contiguous organs involved if possible	ART postop 45-50 Gy PRT for selected sites 45-50 Gy PRT if feasible	MAC IC II
V (Relapse and recurrence)	Palliative if feasible		MAC IC II

RT = radiation therapy; ART = adjuvant; PRT = palliative; NR = not recommended; RCT = recommended chemotherapy; MAC = multiagent chemotherapy; IC II = investigational chemotherapy, phase I/II clinical trials.

PDQ: RCT - MAC = FAM = 5-Flourouacil, doxorubicin, and mitomycin-c, also, FAP, FAB, EAP

Wide lymph node dissection has been associated with improved survival in Stage I, II, and III lesions. These regions include greater curvature, lesser curvature, splenic, celiac and hepatic lymph nodes. Splenectomy and distal pancreatectomy may be indicated to facilitate a wide lymphadenectomy (74,104).

Palliation is best accomplished by resection. Bypass procedures which leave the primary tumor *in situ* are not recommended. Palliative resection reduces the occurrence of perforation, bleeding, or obstruction; as well as improving the results of chemotherapy (80,90).

Radiation Therapy

As a rule, radiation therapy is ineffective in offering palliation in advanced gastric cancer for either obstruction or hemorrhage. The unfavorable therapeutic ratio limits doses with conventional radiation so that the only possible role for radiation therapy is as an adjuvant. Unfortunately, there is no evidence for suggesting that it has improved survival with one exception — intraoperative irradiation (72).

1. Based upon a careful analysis of failure patterns in a reoperation series of patients, including elective second look procedures, a high local and regional recurrence rate of 50-80% was found by Gunderson and Sosin (87).
2. 4,500 rad is recommended by Gunderson for a newly designed radiation field based upon a careful anatomical mapping of recurrences (87).
3. Intraoperative radiation therapy for gastric cancer has demonstrated improvement of survival in stage II and III disease by several Japanese cooperative group studies (72). A randomized trial at the National Cancer Institute failed to show any difference in disease free or overall survival, and this modality remains investigational (110).

Chemotherapy (96) (Table 28-15)

Chemotherapy for gastric cancer in general is more successful than in colorectal cancers. Single agents that are most active include 5-FU, nitrosoureas, doxorubicin, and Mitomycin C with response rates that range from 18%-30% (76,77,105). Response rates with these combinations are almost invariably partial and in the 30%-40% range. Current interest is focused on the combination of Etoposide, Adriamycin, and Platinum (EAP) which has been reported to produce complete responses in about 20% of patients and a total response rate of 64% (105,111). The regimen has significant side effects.

Surgery and Chemotherapy

This has been attempted in a number of large randomized studies (82,83,84,92,94). None of these studies, except the GITSG's study has shown a survival advantage associated with treatment. Results of that study are in conflict with a large ECOG study using the same drugs (82). At the present time adjuvant postoperative chemotherapy in patients with gastric cancer is not beneficial. Recently, the same authors who have reported success with EAP for advanced disease have used this combination (neoadjuvantly) in patients with locally advanced, unresectable gastric cancer. Following chemotherapy a second look operation was performed. Of 33 patients entered on this study 7/33 (21%) had a CR and 16/33 (48%) a PR. At the time of the second look, five patients with clinical complete remission were noted to be pathologically free of disease and 10 patients with PR's were converted to CR. The same chemotherapy was administered to responders after the second surgery. Four patients are disease-free >36 months (111). These results are encouraging.

Table 28-15. Combination Chemotherapy for Gastric Cancer		
Drug Combination	% Response (Range)	Med Survival (mos)
5-FU, Mito-C	24 (14-32)	4-6
5-FU, BCNU	26 (11-41)	3-8
FAM (original)	33 (17-55)	6-8
intensified	32	7-9
variants	26	6-9
FAB	43	6-8
FAP	36	6-13
FAMtx	43	8
EAP	56	9-18
ELF	52	11

F = 5-FU; M = Mitomycin-C; A = Doxorubicin; B = carmustine; P = cisplatin;
Mtx = methotrexate; E = etoposide; L = leucovorin.
Modified from MacDonald (99a) and Wilke (111a).

Radiation and Chemotherapy

Combinations of concurrent irradiation (35-40Gy) plus 5-FU given on the first 3 days at doses of 15 mg/kg/day to patients with inoperable gastric carcinoma significantly increased survival over that of radiotherapy alone in a prospective, randomized, double blind study from the Mayo Clinic (102). The median survival improved, but overall survival was unchanged for both groups. Although other studies show a gain with this combination over 5-FU alone, analysis of an ECOG trial did not confirm the true benefit of this combined program compared with 5-FU alone in a maintenance regimen (99). Response rates range from 30%-77%, but rarely include complete remissions of lasting duration.

Treatment According to Clinical Stage

Stages I and II

Total surgical resection of adenocarcinoma as a radical subtotal gastrectomy (see surgery for details) with reconstruction with gastrojejunostomy. Neither single agent chemotherapy or radiotherapy is recommended except in the clinical trial setting.

Stage III

In locally unresectable gastric cancer combination of radiation and 5-FU or combination chemotherapy can be utilized. Clinical trials are encouraged.

Stage IV

In metastatic cancer chemotherapy combinations are applicable. Radiation therapy can be used for painful local metastatic lesions but is otherwise not indicated.

SPECIAL CONSIDERATIONS AND TREATMENT

Malignant Lymphoma

The gastrointestinal tract is the most common extranodal site for non-Hodgkin's lymphoma with the highest incidence of primary disease in the Western world arising in the stomach (89). The Ann Arbor staging system is utilized to stage these patients, however, the degree of gastric wall penetration, and histology do have prognostic significance (98,109). The standard approach to gastric lymphoma has been surgical resection which was therapeutic and served to pathologically stage the disease. Some have argued that better diagnostic (endoscopy and biopsy) and staging tests (CT, lymphangiography, etc.) may obviate the need for surgical staging. There has always been concern that chemotherapy and radiation could lead to rapid tumor lysis and gastric hemorrhage and perforation. This concept has recently been challenged by Maor *et al.* (101), who treated a group of patients primarily with combined chemotherapy and radiation and obtained favorable results without increased morbidity. Suffice it to say that the optimal staging-treatment strategy of surgery, radiation, chemotherapy is still in a state of debate for patients with IE and IIE disease (75,85,89,100).

Gastric Leiomyosarcoma

Resection is effective for leiomyosarcoma and may be less radical than with carcinoma. These lesions rarely metastasize to lymph nodes and do not require en bloc node removal (97).

RESULTS AND PROGNOSIS

Overall Survival

Despite decreasing incidence and overall mortality of this disease success with treatment has improved only slightly in the past 30 years. Overall 5-year survival is 16%, compared to 10% in 1960. Survival in localized disease is reported as high as 57%; with metastatic disease 0%-8% 5 year survival is expected (9).

  1. SEER Data: Pooled data from 18,767 gastric cancer patients revealed survival rates between 4.7% and 16.9%. Only 10%-20% of patients who present with gastric cancer will have disease capable of curative resection. For this subgroup, however, survival rates of 30%-50% over 5 years are commonly reported. Five-year survival rates adjusted for stage are presented in Table 28-14 and Fig. 28-4 for surgical procedures. In log scale, one notes the limited survival for subtotal gastrectomy which ranges from 10%-20% which is superior to total gastrec-

RESULTS

Gastric Carcinoma: Survival by procedure

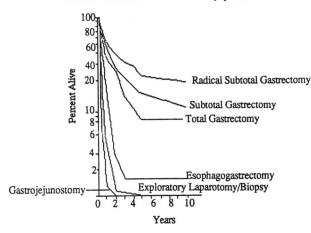

Fig. 28-4. Results: Gastric carcinoma: Survival by procedure.

tomy (<10%). Esophago-gastrectomy is very poor — less than 2%—and reflects more advanced stages.

2. Prognostic Factors: As with other alimentary tract cancers the two most prognostic features are depth of invasion and lymph node involvement. In Table 28-16a, the 5-year survival is shown by depth of invasion on T stage (50%-80%) and nodal involvement which reduces survival dramatically (<20%). The other features which are associated with worse prognosis are: duration of symptoms less than 6 months indicating rapid onset of disease; size of primary tumor greater than 4 cm; location: proximal tumors have worse prognosis; histological: diffuse, undifferentiated and signet ring cell types; DNA ploidy using flow cytometry correlates to survival.

Survival by Combination Chemotherapy (CCT):

1. Adjuvant chemotherapy programs are more hopeful than therapeutic applications. The strategy of CCT is reserved for patients with residual or unresectable local-regional disease. One of the best results are with FAM plus irradiation, which had 41% 2-year actuarial survival in a study from Massachusetts General Hospital. Randomized trials are yet to be completed. The GITSG surgical adjuvant chemotherapy trial using 5-FU and Methyl CCU is the only study which showed a survival benefit (59% versus 44% survival at 4 years) (84). Four other cooperative group studies show no real gain, i.e., 40%-65% 5-year survival (5) (Table 28-17). The overall survival of patients with gastric cancer is about 12%.

2. Enthusiasm is expressed for EAP (Etoposide, Adriamycin, Platinum) in the adjuvant and advanced setting, but confirmatory studies are needed.

3. A randomized series of patients treated with adjuvant mitomycin-C has shown a survival advantage but needs further confirmation (82a).

Survival by Stage

Stage 0

Experience in Japan, where Stage 0 is diagnosed frequently, indicated 90% of patients treated by gastrectomy with lymphadenectomy will survive beyond 5 years (104b).

Stage I and II

Total surgical resection of the cancer as a radical subtotal gastrectomy with reconstruction with gastrojejunostomy (Fig. 28-4). Neither single agent chemotherapy or radiotherapy is recommended adjuvantly except in clinical trials. Expected 5-year survival rates for Stage I is 50%-85% and Stage II < 20%. Intraoperative irradiation of gastric cancer has shown a modest improvement in results by Japanese investigators (Table 28-16b) (72a) for Stage II (22%) and for Stage III (8%).

Stage III

In locally unresectable gastric cancer combination of radiation and 5-FU or combination chemotherapy can be utilized. Expected 5-year survival is 10%-20%.

Table 28-16a. Surgery: Five Year Survival and Initial Stage of Gastric Cancer		
Extent of Disease	5-Year Survival (%)	(92a)
Lymph nodes (-)		
Mucosa only	85	
Mucosa and gastric wall	52	
Through gastric wall	47	
Lymph nodes (+)		
Extent of lymph node involvement		
Regional only	17	
Other areas	5	

Table 28-16b. Intraoperative Irradiation of Gastric Cancer		(72a)
Stage	5-Year survival	
	Surgery alone	Surgery plus IORT
I	93% (43)	88% (20)
II	55% (11)	77% (18)
III	37% (38)	45% (19)
IV	0% (18)	20% (27)

Numbers in the parenthesis indicate the total number of patients treated.

Table 28-17. Surgical Adjuvant Chemotherapy of Gastric Cancer - Randomized Studies

Group	Treatment	5-year Survival		Ref
		Treated	Control	
VASOG	Thiotepa vs. control	25.5%	33.7%	78a
	FudR vs. control	23.9%	21.3%	107a
	5-FU + methyl-CCNU vs. control	37.8% *	38.9% *	92
GITSG	5-FU + methyl-CCNU vs. control	59%	44%	84
			(p<0.03)	
ECOG	5-FU + methyl-CCNU vs. control	44%	47%	82
			(p<0.03)	
NCCTG	5-FU + doxorubicin vs. conrol	52%	51%	94a
Cancer Institue of Tokyo	Mitomycin C + Ara-C +5-FU	68%		103a
	vs.		51%	
	Mitomycin-C + Ftorafur Ara-C	63%		
	vs.			
	Control	* 4 Year Survival		

Stage IV

In metastatic cancer chemotherapy combinations are applicable. Radiation can be used for painful local metastatic lesions. The exception is to have any survivors at 5 years.

CLINICAL INVESTIGATIONS

Screening tests (i.e., brush cytology) for high risk subgroups are being developed. These populations might include patients with pernicious anemia, chronic atrophic gastritis and previous gastrectomy for ulcer disease. Earlier diagnosis is essential to improving cure rates.

Innovative combination chemotherapy trials are underway. Response rates must be correlated to survival as these new treatment programs are evaluated. Only durable responses are clinically meaningful.

Radiation dose modifiers and sensitizers are being investigated. These agents could reduce the toxicity and improve the efficacy of radiation therapy.

Intraperitoneal administration of adjuvant chemotherapy is being tested in some centers (110a).

SMALL INTESTINE

EPIDEMIOLOGY AND ETIOLOGY

Although 90% of the mucosal surface of the alimentary tract is small bowel, less than 5% of GI tumors or carcinomas occur in this organ (115). Three thousand four hundred cases of small bowel cancer are estimated this year, proportionally split between men and women. The death rate in this country is approximately 900 patients per year, the mean age of onset is 59 years (1b).

The most common benign tumors are leiomyomas and adenomatous polyps (118). The most common malignant tumor is adenocarcinoma in the proximal small bowel and carcinoid in the distal bowel. Lymphomas and sarcomas are less frequent malignancies of small bowel. A typical distribution of small bowel tumors is outlined in Table 28-18.

Several factors contribute to the low rate of mutagenesis in the small bowel (113,117,118):

1. Neutralization of acids by pancreatic and small bowel secretions protects against carcinogenic effects of nitrosamines, which usually require the presence of acid for activity (113,118).
2. Rapid peristalsis decreases exposure of mucosal surfaces to intraluminal carcinogens.
3. High concentrations of IgA and abundant lymphoid tissue are immunologic factors which probably help protect the small bowel from the development of cancer.

One of the most important etiologies of small bowel cancer is inherited disorders. These include familial polyposis, Gardner syndrome, Peutz-Jegher syndrome, and Crohn's disease.

DETECTION AND DIAGNOSIS

Clinical Detection

Clinical detection of small bowel tumors can be very difficult and requires special attention to various signs and symptoms. Frequently, the symptoms of these lesions are insidious and non-specific. Over a third of patients have symptoms for 6 to 12 months before diagnosis is made (113).

Table 28-18. Distribution of Malignant Neoplasms in the Small Intestine (118)

Type of Neoplasm	Number and Percentage by Region						Total	
	Duodenum		Jejunum		Ileum			
Adenocarcinoma	427	(40%)	408	(38%)	241	(22%)	1076	(46%)
Sarcoma	46	(10%)	162	(36%)	239	(54%)	447	(19%)
Lymphoma	4	(16%)	9	(36%)	12	(48%)	25	(1%)
Carcinoid	48	(6%)	78	(10%)	682	(84%)	808	(34%)
TOTAL	525	(22%)	660	(28%)	1171	(50%)	2356	(100%)

Symptoms

Abdominal pain is usually cramping in nature and related to obstruction. A benign small bowel tumor is the most common cause of intussusception in adults (117). Carcinomas are more likely to cause a napkin ring obstruction. Lymphomas generally obstruct by extrinsic compression and dysmotility through nerve invasion.

Hemorrhage is usually slow and chronic. Hemangiomas, on the other hand, are the exception which can bleed massively. Carcinoid tumors rarely bleed.

Weight loss occurs in 50% of patients and is especially associated with lymphoma.

Signs (118)

1. An abdominal mass is palpable in nearly 25% of patients that is usually moveable
2. Jaundice is a particular finding in duodenal tumors which involve the ampulla;
3. Occult or gross blood per rectum can be an early sign of a small bowel neoplasm.

Syndromes

Syndromes that are associated with small bowel tumors help the clinician diagnose small bowel cancers that might otherwise be silent. Examples include the following:

Carcinoid syndrome: Carcinoid tumors have the capacity to produce serotonin, histamine, and bradykinin. These compounds cause a clinical syndrome manifested by attacks of watery diarrhea, cutaneous flushing, and asthmatic-type respiratory distress. Lesions of tricuspid and pulmonic valves also occur. This syndrome does not occur in all instances of carcinoid tumor. The syndrome is most frequently associated with carcinoids of the ileum or extensive hepatic metastases. Carcinoids most commonly occur on the appendix, but rarely produce carcinoid syndrome from this site (116).

Peutz-Jegher's syndrome is a genetically determined syndrome transmitted in a dominant sex-linked pattern of inheritance. Hamartomas appear along the small bowel with malignant transformation being rare. The syndrome includes pigmented lesions of the skin and mucous membranes at an early age (118).

Gardner's syndrome is a familial syndrome of small and large intestinal polyps. These polyps are true adenomas. Associated anomalies are desmoid tumors, osteomas, and abnormalities of teeth. Periampullary carcinomas are increased in these patients.

Diagnostic Procedures

The small bowel is difficult to evaluate by radiographic methods. An upper GI series with small bowel follow through can characterize some lesions, although the redundancy of the small bowel frequently obscures the ability of this examination to detect small lesions. Enteroclysis is a radiographic method of examining the small bowel by passing a nasoenteral tube instilling contrast with pressure to delineate smaller lesions in the intestine. A barium enema can be used to visualize the terminal ileum if reflux is obtained through the ileocecal valve.

Other radiographic methods for evaluating small bowel cancers include angiography through the superior mesenteric artery. This test is helpful for cases of acute hemorrhage. Also, CT scan may be helpful to evaluate metastatic disease. MR is of no value due to bowel motion.

Pertinent laboratory studies in patients who are thought to have small bowel tumors include a CBC to detect anemia and liver function tests with particular interest in bilirubin and amylase. In cases of carcinoid tumors, a 5 hydroxyindole acetic acid (5 HSAA) level is indicated.

Abdominal exploration is frequently the best diagnostic test and is usually required when a specific diagnosis or site of bleeding cannot be determined. Unfortunately, explorations for small bowel tumors are usually unproductive when preoperative X rays are negative and the patient does not have acute obstruction or hemorrhage.

CLASSIFICATION AND STAGING

Classification of small bowel tumors correlates to their histopathologic type. Table 28-18 is a compilation of these tumors.

PRINCIPLES OF TREATMENT

Surgery

Surgery is standard treatment for all small bowel tumors. Mortality is very low. A wide mesenteric resection is used for carcinomas. Primary resection is justified for metastatic lesions also to prevent obstruction.

Villous adenomas of the duodenum frequently require pancreaticoduodenectomy (119). Fifty percent of these lesions are malignant if their size is greater than 5 cm.

Wide resection of lymphomas is indicated, although follow-up radiation and chemotherapy is also necessary (89).

Carcinoid tumors usually occur in the distal ileum, and therefore, require right hemicolectomy in most cases. Surgical debulking of liver metastases is indicated for control of carcinoid syndrome (114,118).

Radiotherapy

Most carcinomas of the small bowel are insensitive to radiation therapy. Whole abdominal field irradiation is used, however, for carcinoid and lymphomas of the small intestine involving peritoneal cavity. Adjuvant radiotherapy can be considered following resection of leiomyosarcoma of small bowel but is not often used.

Chemotherapy

5-fluorouracil and nitrosoureas have been used with very little benefit in most small bowel cancers. Lymphomas have shown responds to common chemotherapeutic programs as outlined in Chapter 18. Streptozotocin and 5-FU are standard systemic agents for unresectable carcinoid tumors. Carcinoid syndrome is treated with antiserotonin agents and somatostatin analog as outlined in Chapter 29.

RESULTS AND PROGNOSIS

General Survival

The 5-year survival results are shown by site in the small intestine in Table 28-19 and have similar 5-year mean survivals of 20%-30%.

Survival by Tumor Type

Adenocarcinoma most frequently occurs in the duodenum and five-year survival rates following resection are approximately 20%.

Table 28-19. Clinical Series of Carcinoma of the Duodenum, Jejunum, and Ileum (47)

	Year	No. of Patients	Resection Rate (%)	Operative Mortality (%)	5-Year Survival (%)* (Resected Group) (%)
Duodenum	1963-1985	213	44-100 69 Mean	0-40	0-37 22 Mean
Jejunum	1959-1985	100	44-100 77 Mean		6-50 27 Mean
Ileum	1959-1985	57	68-100 75 Mean		0-38 19 Mean

Sarcomas have an overall better prognosis with 5-year survival rate of almost 50%.

Lymphomas which can be resected have 40%-50% survival rate if radiation is added (118). Unresectable lymphomas have a prognosis of 25% survival.

Carcinoids: Survival of carcinoid tumor also depends on resectability. Generally, however, these tumors are slow growing and have relatively longer survival rates. Even metastatic carcinoid disease has a 60%-70% 5-year survival if the metastatic tumors can be resected. A 40% 5-year survival rate is reported in those instances where the carcinoid tumors are unresectable.

COLON AND RECTUM

EPIDEMIOLOGY AND ETIOLOGY

Epidemiology

Incidence: Colorectal cancer will afflict 156,000 Americans in 1992, representing almost 15% of all newly diagnosed cancers. The incidence is equal among men and women. Japan and Finland, countries with a high incidence of esophageal and gastric cancer, have distinctly low rates of colorectal cancer. The American Cancer Society estimates that there will be 45,000 new cases of rectal carcinoma diagnosed in 1992 which amounts to approximately 30% of all cases included under the rubric "colon and rectum" (1b,9).

Death rate: Overall, 58,000 deaths are anticipated in 1992: 51,000 from cancer of the colon and 7,300 from rectal cancers. These results are second only to lung cancer in terms of nationwide mortality. Overall, the 5-year survival of colorectal cancer is approximately 50%. Disease which is localized at the time of presentation generally has greater than 80% 5-year survival. However, disseminated disease has an expectancy of less than 35% 5-year survival (1b).

Age: Most patients are over 50 years of age. Subgroups of patients including familial polyposis or ulcerative colitis can develop colorectal cancer at a much earlier age. Rectal carcinoma is uncommon below 20 years of age; median age is approximately 60 years old.

Location: Several series have reported a trend of higher occurrence of colorectal cancer in the right side of the large bowel, as opposed to more distal lesions (177,202). This may be secondary to wider use of sigmoidoscopy and polypec-

tomy, which have decreased the relative incidence of rectal cancers. Approximately 50% of colorectal cancers are now found beyond the range of the rigid 25 cm. sigmoidoscope. A typical distribution of cancers in the large bowel is the following: ascending, 24%; transverse, 16%; descending, 7%; sigmoid, 38%; rectum, 15% (177).

Etiology (183,193,201,209)

Environmental factors: The prevalence of colorectal cancer in the Western world is attributed to a diet high in animal fat and low in fiber. Supportive epidemiologic data are derived from immigrants from Japan who develop colorectal cancer with a 2.5 times greater frequency than native Japanese. In rural Africa where fiber and cellulose are more commonly consumed, colon cancer is rare.

Dietary fat stimulates the production of bile acids which influences proliferation of gut epithelium. Fiber increases fecal bulk, lowers transit time, and decreases fecal pH; all of these are factors which reduce the impact of intraluminal carcinogens.

Alcohol may be a co-carcinogen, but is not statistically associated with colon cancer in epidemiologic studies.

Genetic causes: Familial polyposis syndrome is an hereditary disease with autosome dominant transmission which is characterized by pancolonic adenomatous polyps. If not treated, most patients die before age 60 (125).

Gardner's syndrome includes desmoid tumors, osteomas, and fibromas in addition to colorectal adenomas. The risk for developing adenocarcinoma is similar to those patients with familial polyposis syndrome.

Recently, nonpolyposis familial cancer syndromes have been described. These patients are typically young, have multiple colonic lesions, and have higher incidences of other intra-abdominal malignancies (127).

Age is a risk factor for developing colon cancer. Incidence begins to rise after age 40 and peaks between the ages of 55 and 65.

Colon polyps are mucosal tumors which may be pedunculated on a stalk or sessile. Polyps have variable degrees of malignant potential. Hyperplastic polyps are most common, and do not progress to adenomas or carcinomas. Adenomatous polyps, however, have a higher chance of malignant change. Histologically they may be tubular or villous, with variable degrees of mixture. Factors of risk for malignancy include size greater than 2 cm, villous features, and amount of dysplasia.

Most polyps can be removed by colonoscopic polypectomy. The finding of carcinoma in a polyp does not necessarily mandate colon resection. The following conditions in a polyp would mitigate in favor of resection versus observation following endoscopic polypectomy: poorly differentiated histology, positive margins, lymphatic invasion, and sessile lesion.

Inflammatory bowel disease: Chronic ulcerative colitis is associated with increased risk of colorectal cancer. The risk correlates to the duration of ulcerative colitis and the degree of colon involvement. Patients with a pancolitis for more than 7 years have increased risk of cancer. After 30 years the incidence of cancer reaches 35%. At any time during the process of ulcerative colitis the finding of dysplasia in the colonic mucosa confers a 50% chance of developing carcinoma (140).

Crohn's disease of the colon has a slight increase in colon cancer, but much less than ulcerative colitis.

Previous history of colon cancer is associated with the 5% risk of a new primary malignant lesion in the colon.

Diverticulosis and cancer may be found together but there is no evidence that diverticula are important in the development of cancer.

DETECTION AND DIAGNOSIS

Clinical Detection (156,208) (Table 28-20)

History

History and physical examination can alert the physician to colorectal cancer. A change in bowel habit, whether constipation or diarrhea, in a patient over 40 years old may be a harbinger of this disease. Other symptoms depend largely on the location of the tumor in the large bowel.

Right Colon: Microcytic anemia, occult blood in stool, palpable mass in right lower quadrant.

Left Colon: Hematochezia (usually red blood mixed with stool), obstructive symptoms and small caliber stools.

Rectum: Lesions of the rectum often present with rectal bleeding (65%-90%), pain (10%-25%), change in bowel habits (45%-80%) and stool caliber and later with tenesmus. It is not uncommon for the bleeding to be ascribed to hemorrhoids and the lesions to go uninvestigated for long periods of time. Most cancers in this area can be detected by a simple digital examination (65%-80%); once discovered proctosigmoidoscopy should follow with appropriate biopsies to establish the diagnosis (170).

Metastatic disease: hepatomegaly.

Laboratory Studies

Electrolytes: Villous adenomas are known to secrete potassium and can cause profound hypokalemia.

Serum carcinoembryonic antigen (CEA) is an oncofetal antigen which frequently is expressed by colorectal tumors. CEA should be used only after a diagnoses of adenocarcinoma has been made. It is not useful as a screening test due to numerous benign conditions which may also elevate CEA levels (196).

Screening Tests

Cost effective screening for colorectal cancer varies depending on the population at risk (122,207).

Average risk population: Digital rectal exam and occult blood testing should be performed annually after age 40. Sigmoidoscopy should be done every 3-5 years.

Population with positive family history for colorectal cancer. The same screening as in a. except to begin at age 35. Add air contrast barium enema every 3-5 years.

Patients with ulcerative colitis for 10 years duration should have an elective colectomy or annual colonoscopy with biopsies.

Patients with familial polyposis should have an elective colectomy with either rectal mucosectomy or preservation of the rectum and follow-up proctoscopy every 6 months.

Mass screening of the average risk population with fecal occult blood testing will produce between 2% and 6% positive findings. One third of these will be benign adenomas; 5%-10% will be carcinoma (142).

Diagnostic Procedures (122,197) (Tables 28-20 and 28-21)

Similar diagnostic procedures are used for both the colon and the rectum. The sensitivity for cancers and polyps as well as cost benefit and patient discomfort are tabulated in Table 28-20.

Rectal exam should be a part of every physical exam on patients over age 40 regardless of symptoms or physical condition.

Sigmoidoscopy is indicated for screening and should be performed on any patient with lower GI symptoms or positive occult blood test. Flexible sigmoidoscopy (60-65 cm) is the best yielding for the cost and discomfort involved. (Table 28-18).

Table 28-20. Qualitative Analysis of Screening Options for Colorectal Cancer (129a)				
Technique	Sensitivity for Cancer	Sensitivity for Polyps	Cost	Patient Discomfort
Digital rectal examination	+	1/2+	1/2+	+
Fecal occult blood	++	+	1/2+	1/2+
Rigid sigmoidoscopy	++	++	++	++
Flexible sigmoidoscopy (60-65 cm)	+++	+++	++	+
Single column barium enema	++	+	++	++
Air contrast barium enema	+++	+++	++	+++
Colonoscopy	++++	++++	++++	+++

Table 28-21. Diagnostic Procedures for Colorectal Cancer (1a)

METHOD	DIAGNOSIS AND STAGING CAPABILITY	RECOMMENDED FOR USE
Primary tumor and regional nodes		
CT	Most valuable of all modalities for determining local invasion and distant metastases	Yes
MRI	Of limited value with massive disease	No
Double contrast Barium enema	Very useful in detecting and defining primary lesion s in the colon.	Yes
Single contrast Barium enema	Less sensitive than double-contrast study in detecting polyps	No. Should be used in patients unable to cooperate in double-contrast study
Colonoscopy	Very accurate modality for detecting and defining primary lesions	Yes. If used to confirm lesion detected on BE or to screen high risk patients

Colonoscopy is not a screening device, but is reserved for patients with evidence of gastrointestinal bleeding or follow-up of high risk patients.

Barium enema is indicated for unexplained iron deficient anemia. Air contrast technique is required to detect mucosal polyps and should always be done (134,157). This exam is especially important for patients who have suboptimal colonoscopy (Table 28-20).

Endorectal ultrasound (US) is a promising technique for local spread into the rectal wall and occasionally perirectal node detection (123).

CLASSIFICATION AND STAGING

Histopathology (197) (Table 28-22)

The vast majority of cancers are adenocarcinoma (>90%) and, to a lesser degree, carcinoid tumors, leiomyosarcomas, and lymphoma. The grading system used refers to the Broder's system and concludes with the degree of differentiation and anaplasticity.

Anatomic Staging (Table 28-23, Figs. 28-5 and 28-6)

The new attempt to achieve compatibility with Duke's classification is more successful. The T categories of T1, T2 superficial and muscular invasion are the same as Duke's A

Table 28-22. Histologic Classification of Colorectal Tumors

MALIGNANT	% INICIDENCE
1. Adenocarcinoma	90-95%
2. Mucinous adenocarcinoma	10%
3. Signet-ring carcinoma	4%
4. Squamous cell carcinoma	
5. Adenosquamous carcinoma	
6. Undifferentiated carcinoma	<1%
7. Unclassified carcinoma	

and T3,T4 categories of transerosal are equivalent to Duke's B with nodal disease Duke's C. The T categories are reduced to 4 rather than 5 and the N categories are expanded from N1,N2, and N3 depending on the number of nodes and regional and jutaregional categories.

Stage Grouping (Table 28-23)

Duke's Classification: The Duke's classification depends on depth of wall invasion and presence or absence of nodal metastasis. The simplified version is: A) mucosa, B) muscularis, C) node involvement, D) metastatic disease.

This classification has been modified by several groups and presents difficulty in comparing institutional results. The AJCC classification is based upon surgical-pathologic evaluation. Most large bowel cancer studies have adopted this classification system and staging shown in Table 28-21 and Figs. 28-5 and 28-6.

Metastatic Spread

Spread to regional lymph nodes generally correlates to depth of invasion by the primary tumor and the grade of differentiation. Nodal spread occurs in 10%-20% of tumors confined to the bowel wall. Overall, low grade tumors have a 30% chance of nodal spread, while high grade lesions have positive nodes in 80% of cases.

Hematogenous spread is usually to the liver via portal venous transmission. One study found a 32% incidence of tumor cells in the mesenteric vein during colon resection.

Staging Work-up (Table 28-21)

The colon and rectum are evaluated by available clinical diagnostic procedures as to spread and extension, but require surgical and pathologic evaluation in the new AJCC schema, which is designed to be compatible with the Duke's classification.

The recommended procedures are:
1. Barium enema with air contrast and/or colonoscopy. (Obviously barium enema can not be performed with obstruction. Proximal bowel should be examined at the time of surgery).

Table 28- 23. TNM Classification for Colon Cancer

AJC	TNM Classification	DUKES	UICC		AJCC
T1	Submucosa				
		A	T1/pT1	Mucosa or submucosa only	T1
T2	Muscularis		T2/pT2	Muscle or serosa	T2
			T3a/pT3a	Extension to contiguous structures	T3
T3	Subserosa/Nonperitonealized			No fistula	
	pericolic or perirectal tissues		T3b/pT3b	With fistula	T4
		B	T4/pT4	Extension beyond contiguous structures	T5
T4	Perforates visceral peritoneum				
	Directly invades other organis			No regional node involvement	
			N0	Regional	N0
N1	1-3 pericolic / perirectal		N1		N1
	lymphnode				
		C			
N2	≥4				
N3	Vascular trunk				
M1		D			

T = tumor; N = node; M = metastases.

Modified from UICC (7) / AJC (11).

2. Colonoscopy (Favored preoperatively, if possible, to identify synchronous carcinomas and adenomas).
3. Cystoscopy for low sigmoid and rectal lesions
4. Chest film
5. Laboratory tests including CBC with differential and platelet count, liver enzymes, PT, PTT, BUN, Creatinine, and CEA. CEA levels should be done pre- and postoperatively. Post-operative CEA levels which fail to drop to normal range are suggestive of metastatic disease.
6. CT scan for rectal cancers is helpful to define the local extent into vital structures or pelvic bones. Also CT is useful for liver metastases detection.
7. CT and MR (Table 28-21) are both of some limited value in determining primary tumor extent and lymph node involvement. For colon, CT and MR are limited in their ability to determine transmural spread in the colon and are not efficacious in determining involved lymphadenopathy. CT accuracy of 48%-74% is reported for primary staging and ranging from 25%-73% for lymph nodes. For rectum, MR may be superior to CT since perirectal fat invasion may be easier to identify. However, neither mode discriminated stage A (T1) from stage B (T2) accurately or consistently, nor could stage C (node positive) lymphadenopathy be distinguished.
8. Because of the low incidence of bone and brain metastases, scans of these areas are not indicated.

PRINCIPLES OF TREATMENT FOR COLON CANCER (Table 28-24)

The staging of colon cancer is based on surgical finding and as such is pathologic. The colon measures approximately 1.5.

meters (about 5 feet). The terminal 12 cm is the rectum which is defined by the pelvic peritoneum; since different treatment strategies are used for the rectum and "proximal" colon, the rectum will be discussed separately in the following section. The colon is an intra-abdominal structure but the peritoneal covering varies with location. The transverse and sigmoid portions have a complete encircling mesentery and are mobile, while the ascending and descending colon posteriorly do not have a mesentery and therefore are fixed retroperitoneally. This anatomy suggests the potential for more peritoneal seeding in the former and more posterior invasion in the latter sites. The patterns of spread of colon cancer are: hematogenous (generally to the liver), lymphatic, transperitoneally and by direct extension. Obviously direct extension through the serosa and peritoneum can be the harbinger of transperitoneal seeding. Generally cancers in the colon tend to extend circumferentially rather than longitudinally, and hence proximal and distal surgical margins are easily obtained, but this does not ensure against anastomotic and local recurrences since submucosal lymphatic channels run longitudinally.

At the time of presentation representative stages of colon cancer include: stage A - 8%, B- 39%, C - 28%, D - 25% (179). After surgical resection for cure (stages A,B,C) local/regional recurrence with or without distant metastases is found in 20% of patients, distant metastases alone in 11%, and local/regional plus distant in 30% of cases. The liver is the prime organ for metastatic disease (65%); extra-abdominal metastases in lung (25%), and bone and brain (10%) are much less common. Most recurrences appear within 2 years (about 70%) and almost all (90%) within 5 years. Local recurrences are related to stage with a 7% risk in patients with Astler-Coller stage A,B1,B2,C1, and 40% for B3,C2,C3

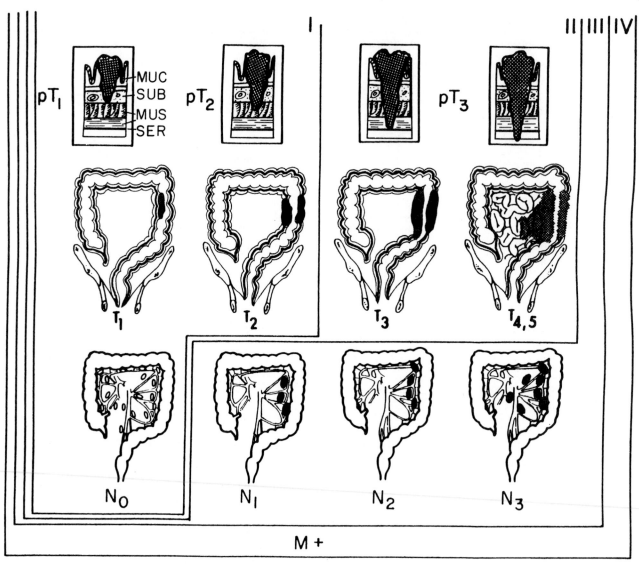

Fig. 28-5. Anatomic staging for cancer of the colon.

Table 28-24.   Multidisciplinary Treatment Decisions: Colon   (129b,129c,180c

Stage	Surgery	Radiation Therapy	Chemotherapy
I $T_{1/2}N_0M_0$ Duke A	Wide segmental resection and regional nodes in mesentery and primary anastomosis	NR	NR
II $T_{3/4},N_0,M_0$ Duke B	Wide segmental resection and regional nodes in mesentery and primary anastomosis	NR	IC III
III $T_{any}N_{1/2/3}M_0$ Duke C	Wide surgical resection if feasible and anastomosis	NR	MAC
IV T_4,N_1,M_0 Duke D	By-pass colostomy or Palliative resection	PRT 40-50 Gy	IC II

RT = radiation therapy; ART = adjuvant; PRT = palliative; NR = not recommended; RCT = recommended chemotherapy; MAC = multiagent chemotherapy; IC II = investigational chemotherapy, phase I/II clinical trials; IC III = investigational chemotherapy, phase II/III clinical trials.

PDQ: RCT - MAC = 5-FU Levamisole

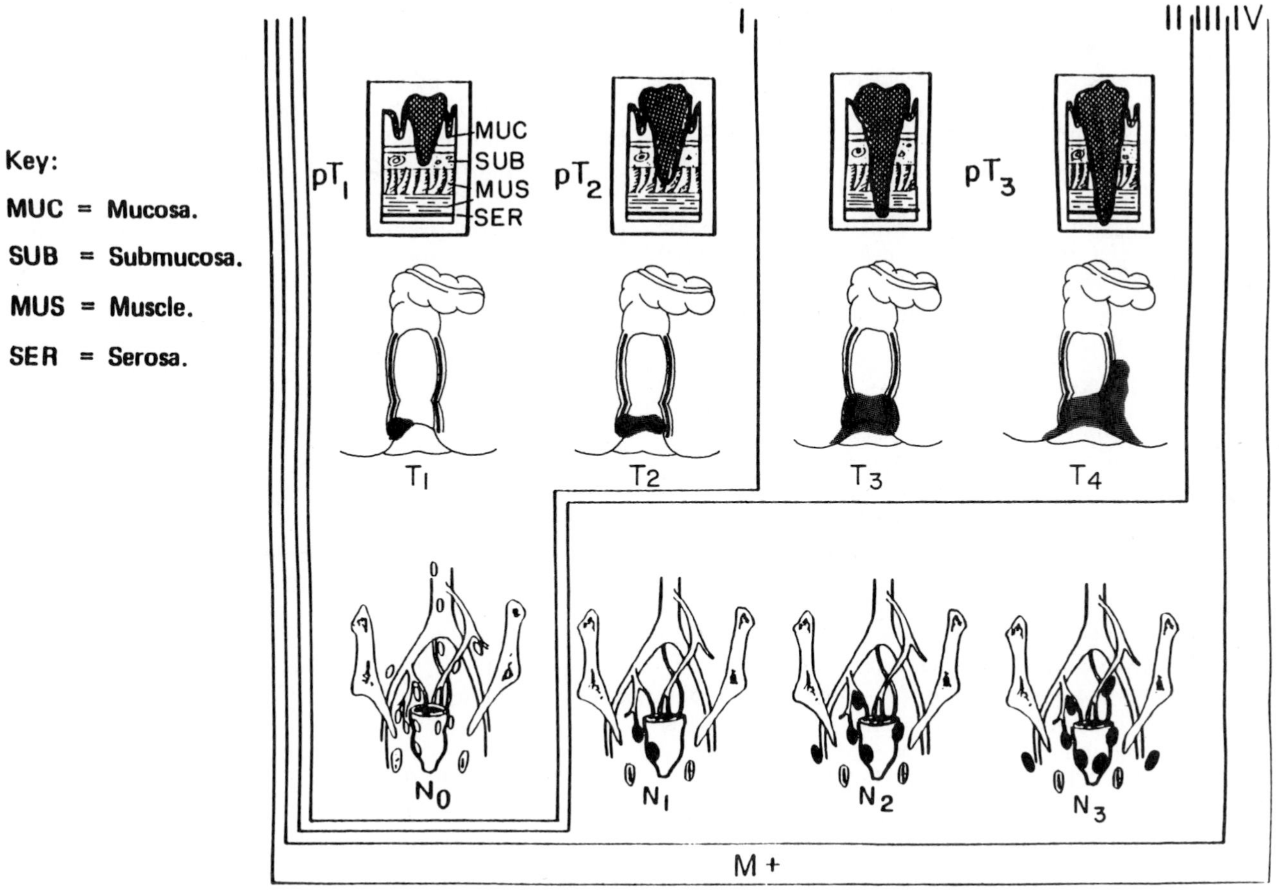

Fig. 28-6. Anatomic staging for cancer of the rectum.

(203). Adhesion or invasion of the primary tumor to local structures, as well as perforation of the bowel, are factors associated with significantly earlier recurrence (143a).

A multidisciplinary approach is essential and is summarized in Table 28-24.

Surgery (122,130,149,171)

1. Polyps or polypoid masses should be removed endoscopically if possible, or at least biopsied. Polyps which are greater than 1 cm in size should be removed surgically if colonoscopic polypectomy is unsuccessful. The finding of invasive cancer on a polyp mandates laparotomy and resection of the involved segment. Exceptions for this treatment include small, low grade carcinomas meeting the criteria listed earlier.
2. *Carcinoma*: Surgery is the primary mode of therapy for colon and rectal cancer. The principles of surgical therapy are:
   a. laparotomy for staging
   b. wide *en bloc* resection of the primary tumor
   c. lymphadenectomy for staging as well as possible therapeutic benefit (137)

Good evidence exists to indicate that implantation of tumor cells onto the suture line during resection contributes to local recurrence. Although randomized trials of the "no touch" technique have failed to confirm a significant difference in survival, reasonable efforts should be made intraoperatively to prevent intraluminal and intraperitoneal spread of tumor cells (200). Primary reconstruction of the colon after resection is almost always feasible.

Synchronous metastatic disease to the ovaries is reported in almost 8% of colorectal cancers. This occurrence justifies simultaneous oophorectomy in women being treated for colorectal cancer; a slight survival benefit has been observed (5,124a,131).

3. *Metastases:* Resection of metastases can prolong survival in stage D patients with disease confined to the liver (195b).

Radiation Therapy

There is no well-defined role for radiation therapy as primary treatment in colon cancer, nor as adjuvant therapy. The basis for consideration of adjuvant radiation is the high incidence of local recurrence in certain stages. These data have been accumulated by a number of institutions from second-look surgery in asymptomatic and symptomatic patients as well as autopsy series (128,143,152,173,190,203).

The radiation oncologists have investigated the role of both preoperative and postoperative radiation using small local fields, extended fields and even whole abdominal fields. They have generally selected patients with stages B2,C2,C3 for treatment, sometimes concentrating on the cecum, sigmoid or ascending/descending portions of the colon (160,194,198,204). These studies have been non-randomized, selected, generally small (< 80 patients), and from single institutions. Most have concluded that local control and survival have been improved compared to historical controls. However, this adjuvant treatment strategy has never been tested in randomized studies, is not widely used clinically and currently there is more enthusiasm for adjuvant chemotherapy than radiotherapy.

Chemotherapy

After many years and many negative trials, adjuvant therapy with 5-FU and levamisole has been shown to increase survival in patients with Duke's C colon cancers. The response rates to chemotherapy in recurrent and metastatic cancer remain poor and are of limited duration.

Advanced and Metastatic Disease

Chemotherapy for palliation, usually for liver or lung metastases, produced responses in approximately 10%-20% of patients treated with 5-FU (174). Despite this relatively low response rate, it has been shown that 5-FU responders have a prolonged median survival (18 months) compared to non-responders (< 6 months) (174). A wide variety of other agents have been studied with only mitomycin-C and the nitrosoureas showing over 10% response rates (174). Combinations of 5-FU and MeCCNU with or without vincristine were initially reported to have response rates of 32%-43% (139,176,182). Subsequently, a larger experience at the Mayo Clinic has shown a reduction in response rates: 5-FU + MeCCNU + vincristine, 27% of 137 patients; and 5-Fu + MeCCNU, 16% of 61 patients (174). The combinations produce no response or survival advantage over treatment with 5-FU alone as shown by a recent report of a series of 1314 patients by the Eastern Cooperative Oncology Group (ECOG) (165).

Postoperative Adjuvant Chemotherapy (Table 28-25, Fig. 28-7)

After innumerable unsuccessful trials finally two recent studies (163,175) have found that combination of 5-FU and levamisole given to patients with Duke's Stage C colon cancer dramatically reduced cancer recurrence and significantly improved survival. 5-FU was given at a dose of 450 mg/

m²/day intravenously for 5 days and then beginning at day 28 at a dose of 450 mg/m² weekly for 1 year. Levamisole dose was 150 mg/day for 3 days every 2 weeks for 1 year. Levamisole is a fascinating drug whose only previous proven efficacy has been as an antihelmintic agent. In this capacity it has had genuine importance in areas where such infections in humans and livestock pose an importance public health problem. Combination of levamisole and 5-FU has reduced the risk of dying from recurrent colon cancer at 5 years by 17% (178a).

There is no evidence that intravenous or intra-arterial standard chemotherapy with or without resection of liver metastases has improved the survival of patients with colon cancer, although useful palliation may be seen in certain patients. However, some evidence suggests that survival may be enhanced in some patients if resection results in no measurable tumor being left behind (191a,195b). Regional adjuvant therapy directed at reducing liver metastasis has been tested using both portal vein infusion of 5-FU and hepatic radiation, and an early trial by Taylor showed promising results. The preliminary results of confirmatory trials from the NSABP and the Mayo Clinic, however, have failed to demonstrate a significant benefit for hepatic-directed adjuvant therapy in the reduction of liver recurrences (122a,207b).

Combination Therapy

Disillusionment with combination therapy has led to a search for more innovative ways of using existing agents. Currently studies using folinic acid to potentiate 5-FU are in progress. Folates bind to thymidylate synthetase and tighten the binding of 5-FU to this enzyme (155). This has been shown to increase the tumor cell kill *in vitro* (158). It appears that the biochemical modulation occurs in normal as well as tumor cells since toxicity, especially diarrhea, has been much greater than that seen with 5-FU. There are now several randomized studies which have shown response rates significantly different from 5FU alone, and a few demonstrated improved survival too (136,138,145,181).

Table 28-25. Colon Cancer Adjuvant Therapy Trials					(129a)
Study	Chemo-therapy	Immunio-therapy	Chemoim-munotherapy	Results	Ref.
VASOG	5-FU, methyl/CCNU			MF results in survival benefit for Dukes' C1	152a
GITSG	5-FU, methyl/CCNU	BCG-MER intradermally	MF + BCG-MER	Apparent overall improved survival compared to historical controls	144a
NSABP	MR, same as GITSG + VCR	BCG		MOF resutls in 67% 5-year survival, vs. 58% for control	207a / 180a
SWOG	5-FU, methyl/CCNU		MF + BCG (6 x 10 organisms PO) every other wk for 26 wk	Superior disease-free survival benefit for MT + BCG	163a
NCCTG	5-FU	Levamisole		5-FU + levamisole results in increase recurrence-free interval in Dukes C colon Carcinoma	175
NCCTG UPDATE 1990	5-FU	Levamisole		5-Fu + levamisole results in increased recurrence-free interval in Dukes C colon (see figure)	

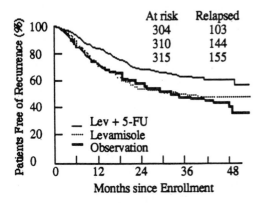

RESULTS

LEVAMISOLE AND FLOUROURACIL DUKES STAGE C COLON CARCINOMA

	At risk	Relapsed
	304	103
	310	144
	315	155

— Lev + 5-FU
······ Levamisole
— Observation

Recurrence-freee Interval, According to Study Arm. Lev+ 5-FU denotes combination therapy with levamisole and flourouracil.

Fig. 28-7. Results: Levamisole and Flourouracil Duke's stage C colon carcinoma.

Chemotherapeutic Agents

The search for new chemotherapeutic agents has been in progress for thirty years. A list of all agents tested would be long, but of little use. Unfortunately, although some drugs have produced an occasional response, none has had activity approaching 5-FU and most have been more toxic. Although this is a discouraging legacy, it is essential to pursue all avenues including new drug testing for a disease which is such an important public health issue.

BiologicResponse Modifiers

Biologic response modifiers, primarily the interferons and interleukin-2 (IL-2) have been used in patients with colon cancer. At the present time it does not appear that they will play an important role, at least as single agents, in management of these patients (187). This is obviously a rapidly developing field with research currently in progress which may point to new treatment possibilities (180b,200a).

PRINCIPLES OF TREATMENT FOR RECTUM (Table 28-26)

The rectum comprises the penultimate 15 cm of the alimentary tract with the anus being the terminal 3-4 cm. It is important to separate these lesions from the colon and not lump them together as "colorectal cancer," because the local failure pattern and treatment strategies are different.

The rectum is divided into thirds: upper 12-16 cm above the anal verge, middle 7.5-12 cm above the verge and lower 3.5-7.5. cm from the verge. The upper third is covered by the

Table 28-26a. Multidisciplinary Treatment Decisions: Rectum (162,180a,180d,201a)

Stage/Dukes	Surgery	Radiation Therapy	Chemotherapy
I (A)	Abdominoperineal or low anterior resection and regional nodes	Contact therapy for selected cases CRT 30 Gy x 3 = 90 Gy	NR
II (B)	Abdominoperineal or anterior resection and regional nodes	ART postop 50 Gy	CCR
III (C)	If unresectable, colostomy	ART preop 20-50 Gy with surgical reassessment ART postop 50-60 Gy and/or PRT 50-60 Gy	CCR
IV (D)	If unresectable, colostomy		IC II

RT = radiation therapy; CRT = curative; ART = adjuvant; PRT = palliative; NR = not recommended; RCT = recommended chemotherapy; CCR = concurrent chemotherapy and radiation; IC II = investigational chemotherapy, phase I/II clinical trials.

PDQ: RCT - CCR: 5-FU + DRT 50 Gy

Table 28-26b. Multidisciplinary Treatment Decisions: Anus (218b)

Stage/Dukes	Surgery	Radiation Therapy	Chemotherapy
I-III	N R*	CRT 50-60 Gy	CCR
I V	N R	PRT 50 GY	CCR

* N R--unless chemoradiation response is less than CR

CRT = curative radiation therapy; PRT = palliative radiation therapy; NR = not recommended; RCT = recommended chemotherapy; CCR = concurrent chemotherapy and radiation.

PDQ: RCT - CCR: 5-FU + Mito C

peritoneal reflection posteriorly, but most of it is within the free peritoneal cavity. The middle third is covered by peritoneum anteriorly only. The lower third has no peritoneal coverage.

The venous drainage of the upper rectum is to the inferior mesenteric vein then to the portal system, while the lower portion is to the internal iliac veins and inferior vena cava; hence one may see pulmonary metastases with lesions in the lower segments, without liver metastases.

Similarly, lymphatic drainage is along the inferior mesenteric vein in upper lesions, while middle and lower third drainage is to internal iliac and presacral nodes. Direct invasion by cancer of the rectum can involve the bladder, prostate, seminal vesicles, urethra, ureters, vagina, small intestines, sacrum, and surrounding nerves and vessels. Inguinal lymph nodes are not at risk for metastases unless the lesion extends to the dentate line and anus.

There has always been an emphasis on adequate proximal and distal surgical margins in alimentary tract cancers, but we are increasingly aware of radial or lateral margins as a cause of local failure. These margins are difficult for the surgeon to obtain in the cramped pelvic quarters and for the pathologist to adequately identify. Local failure in the pelvis after surgery occurs in 25-40% of B2,B3,C1 cases and 40%-65% of C2,C3 (180,206) and is important not only because it portends an almost uniformly poor outcome, but also because of the local pain symptoms, bladder dysfunction and sepsis; hence the emphasis on adjuvant therapy.

Surgery (171,186,188,206)

Surgery remains the mainstay of treatment for all T1-4, Nx, MO (Duke's A,B,C) lesions; other modalities are adjunctive. The principles of surgical therapy are (1) laparotomy for staging, (2) wide *en bloc* resection of the primary tumor and (3) lymphadenectomy for staging as well as possible therapeutic benefit. The traditional operations have been either an abdominoperineal resection (APR) which implies a permanent colostomy, or a low anterior resection (LAR) in which bowel continuity is restored after resection of the involved segment of bowel. The abdominoperineal resection, which is also called the Miles procedures, involves a separate abdominal and perineal incision in order to radically excise the entire rectum, most of the sigmoid colon and mesocolon with its regional lymphatic drainage, anal sphincter, and canal, the levator ani muscles and ischiorectal fat. Lesions within 5 cm of the anal verge usually require APR, while the other are treated with LAR (133,188). New techniques are emerging to preserve the anal sphincter and gastrointestinal continuity, and these are being tested to determine if adequate tumor control is obtained (176a). These operations include combined abdominal transsacral resection, transsacral resection (Kraske procedure), abdominal transphincteric resection and various pull-through procedures (133). The circular, intraluminal stapling device has been of great technical help. Operative mortality for APR is on average 5%, but varies between 1%-12% depending on the surgical series. Complications related to surgery in this site include fistulae (vesicovaginal, vesicoperineal, ureteroperineal), abscess, hemorrhage, stomal problems, and small bowel obstruction (186).

Conservative local therapies have been used for early rectal cancer and as palliation to avoid obstruction: electrocoalgulation, local excision, cryosurgery, laser vaporization and contact radiotherapy, all of which have their proponents (133). Colostomy without some form of local therapy is rarely palliative for incurable rectal lesions. The procedure may be done, however, in preparation for pre-operative radiation therapy to be followed by APR or other multimodal treatment. With the trend toward adjuvant postoperative radiation therapy, there has been emphasis on pelvic reconstruction to decrease the amount of small intestine in the radiation field. This may take the form of reperitonealization of the pelvic floor, use of omental slings or pedicle flaps, absorbable polyglycolic acid mesh (135) or temporary pelvic prosthetic devices.

Radiotherapy

The role of radiotherapy in rectal carcinoma is several:
1. Primary treatment if the patient is considered medically inoperable;
2. Primary treatment in some early, Duke's A lesions (exophytic, < 4 cm in size and well differentiated histology) using contact radiotherapy (Pappillon technique), depending upon the experience and expertise of the radiation oncologist, (164,195);
3. palliative treatment for pain or bleeding;
4. treatment for recurrent disease;
5. adjuvant therapy after primary resection (B2 and C) for patients with complete resection as well as those with microscopic and macroscopic disease remaining.

Primary radiation treatment is not recommended for rectal carcinoma, except for patients who refuse surgery or are medically inoperable (132,166).

It is the adjunctive setting, where no residual disease is suspected, that radiation has been utilized most frequently to reduce the incidence of local recurrence. Meta-analyses of various studies have substantiated the role of radiation in reducing local recurrences, however, this has not been translated into improved survival (126,199). The importance of local control cannot be over-emphasized, however, since pelvic recurrences lead to significant problems of pelvic pain. The proponents of preoperative radiation stress reduction in tumor cell viability at time of surgery and thus dissemination, better tissue oxygenation, smaller treatment volume with less risk of small bowel injury, no need to treat the perineum and conversion of some inoperable lesions into operable. Postoperative advocates stress better patient selection for adjuvant therapy (Duke's A and D would avoid irradiation), surgical measures to exclude small bowel from the field (see above), placement of surgical clips to delineate areas of special interest, and histologic confirmation of pre-op staging.

Preoperative radiation doses have varied from a single dose of 500 cGy to 4500 cGy in 25 fractions. Surgery is usually performed anywhere from 1 week after radiation for the short, higher fraction courses to 5-7 weeks for the more conventional treatment course (148,153,159,184,192). The randomized studies (148,153,192) did not demonstrate any improvement in survival; the recently completed European Organization for Research and Treatment of Cancer (EORTC) study did find reduced local recurrence in the radiation arm (192). Several recent non-randomized studies reported improved local control and overall survival in the irradiated group compared to historical surgical controls (159,184).

Postoperative irradiation alone in at least three randomized studies did not demonstrate any survival benefit (121,141,146,147).

Complications of pelvic radiation in this setting include cystitis, proctitis if the sphincter has been retained, perineal skin reactivity if an APR has been performed since inclusion of the scar is recommended. Small bowel injury with late complications of obstruction, possibly requiring surgery occurs in < 5% (150). Technical factors include use of megavoltage linear accelerators, standard fractionation treatment (180-200 cGy), use of multiple fields, and displacement of small bowel from the field are believed important in delivering the radiation therapy (151).

Chemotherapy

The role of chemotherapy in this disease has been studied either as an adjuvant or as a palliative modality. The use of single agents or combinations of drugs used are similar to those for colon cancer because there is no evidence to suggest that the response to rectum will be different than colon. 5-Fluorouracil has long been the "standard" with only 20% response rates. Various combinations 5-FU + MeCCNU, 5FU + MeCCNU + VCR, etc.) have been used, but none have been better than 5-FU alone. Recently, there has been enthusiasm for the combination of 5-FU and levamisole in Stage C colon cancer. Patients with rectal carcinomas were not included in these studies (163,175). Chemotherapy as a surgical adjuvant has not demonstrated any survival advantage in general (180). The recent NSABP study did demonstrate an improved survival in the chemotherapy arm (methyl CCNU, vincristine, 5-FU) as compared to surgery alone, but only in men < 65 years (141). According to Marsh *et al.* (167a), the combination of methotrexate (MTX) with leucovorin (LV) rescue and fluorouracil (5-FU) is an active regimen in advanced colorectal cancer; its efficacy is increased in colon, but not rectal cancer, when the interval between MTX and 5-FU is long (24 hours) rather than short (1 hour).

Combined Modality Therapy

The search for improved local control and survival, especially Stages B2 and C, has naturally progressed to studies of all three modalities. There have now been two randomized studies that have demonstrated improved overall survival and better local control for patients treated with postoperative radiation and chemotherapy. The now classic study performed by the Gastrointestinal Study Group (GITSG) randomized patients with post-operative Duke stages B2 or C to one of four arms: (1) observation alone, (2) pelvic radiation to a dose of 40-48 Gy, (3) chemotherapy with bolus 5-FU nd MeCCNU, or (4) radiation and chemotherapy with the two given concomitantly initially. After a period of 7 years it was found that the survival in the adjunctive radiation/chemotherapy arm was 58% and only 34% in the surgery plus observation group (146,147). A more recent study by the North Central Cancer Treatment Group, the Mayo Clinic and Duke University (162) in which patients with predominantly B-2 and C disease were randomized between post-op radiation alone (50Gy) or post-op radiation plus chemotherapy with bolus 5-FU and methyl CCNU corroborates the GITSG study and demonstrates improved disease-free and overall survival as well as reduced local recurrence and distant metastases in the combined arm. Thus, at this time a combined modality approach appears to be the most rational, especially the concomitant administration of 5-FU and radiation to take advantage of the radiosensitizing effects of the 5-FU (180',201a). Studies currently in progress are testing radiation with 5-FU alone, 5-FU + levamisole, 5-FU + low dose leucovorin and 5-FU + levamisole + leucovorin. Preoperative combined modality therapy is also being investigated.

SPECIAL CONSIDERATIONS OF TREATMENT

Familial Polyposis: Patients with familial polyposis syndromes should have total colectomy before age 40. If the rectum is preserved a 7%-13% incidence of carcinoma is reported. These patients should have proctoscopy every 6 months or undergo rectal mucosectomy with ilioanal anastomosis.

Aggressive surgical resection of advanced local disease without metastasis is warranted. This approach may require *en bloc* removal of adjacent organs, or in the case of rectal cancer, total pelvic exenteration. These heroic measures have been associated with improved survival (205).

A persistent or recurrent sinus in the perineum after abdominal perineal resection suggests residual or recurrent tumor in the pelvis. Likewise, persistent pelvic or perineal pain is a sign of recurrence.

Circumferential carcinoma of the descending and sigmoid colon may present with obstruction or perforation. This situation requires a two-stage surgical approach with formation of a diverting colostomy. More proximal lesions can be treated safely with a one-step procedure in spite of these complications.

Patients who are unsuitable for surgery may have palliation of obstruction by endoscopic laser therapy (138a).

RESULTS AND PROGNOSIS

Overall Survival

Based on SEER data for patients diagnosed between 1973-1975, the overall 5 and 10 year survival rates for colon cancer were 38% and 26% respectively. During the same period the rectal cancer rates were 37% and 25%, respectively. Disease specific survival is higher by 10%-20% which agrees with the frequently quoted survival of 50% at 5 years. Once 5-year survival is achieved the chances of 10-year survival are excellent with 85%-90% of the survivors reaching the tenth year free of disease (178).

Colon Cancer

By Stage there is no major difference in survival as the invasion increases from Duke's Stage A-B or as the disease progresses from T1 to T3 (Table 28-27). With very high 5-year survivals for submucosal extensions in the 90% range, and with minimal penetration into the muscularis, it decreases but is still relatively high at 70%-80%. However, once nodal invasion occurs (Duke's C) the survival drops to half, approximately 40%, and will be somewhat higher or lower depending on degree of nodal involvement. From Table 28-26 with 1 to 4 nodes the 5-year survival is 56% versus 26% for more than four nodes.

By Grade: The 5-year survival reflects the degree of differentiation of the adenocarcinoma (Table 28-28). Grade I cancers tend to be more superficial and the majority of

Table 28-27.	Percent Five Year Survival Rates for Colorectal Cancer by Stage (163a,180a,203,137b, 171a,195a)				
Stage	**COLON**		**Stage**	**RECTUM**	
	N -	N +		N -	N +
T1	97		Dukes A	88-93	
T2	89-90	74			
T3	78-80	48	Dukes B	71-79	
T4	63	38			
Dukes' C		40	Dukes C		29-41
Dukes' C (1-4 nodes)		56			
Dukes' C (>4 nodes)		26			

patients survive with a 60%-90% outcome in contrast to totally differentiated tumors Grade 3 where the survival is under 50% and can be as low as 10% when the depth of invasion and nodal involvement becomes a prominent feature.

Adjuvant Biologic Response Modifiers and Immunomodulators: The most dramatic recent study which has been established in two large controlled clinical trials has been the utilization of levamisole and Fluoraroucil for Duke's Stage C colon cancer (Fig. 28-7). The RFS has improved by 15-20% at 5 years (163,175). With confirmation of NCCTG trial (784852) (163) by INTERGROUP trials (0035) (175), the conclusions seem firm. However, in Stage B, the results are less impressive and 40%-50% of patients DFS is possible with surgery alone.

RECTAL CANCER

By stage, survival for rectal cancer is similar to colon. The 5 year survival for stage A averages about 85% (range 75%-100%), and B 65% (range 40%-80%). Stage C 5 year survival is approximately 40% with a range of 15%-60% depending upon stage subset and histology. Local relapses after surgery are <10%, 5%-40%, and 40%-60%, respectively, for the same stages, and specifically 25%-40% for B2, B3, and C1, and 40%-65% for C2,C3 (125,180). The need for adjuvant therapy in stages B2 and C disease is apparent.

Radiation Therapy: There is little doubt that radiation given either pre- or postoperatively reduces local recurrences, however, overall survival was not improved significantly in randomized studies. At a mean follow-up of 6 years, the local failure rate was 21% in the patients receiving postoperative therapy versus 12% in the preoperative radiotherapy group (p = 0.02). No difference was seen in the rate of distant metastases, cancer-specific or overall survival (195c). Control of local disease is important, however, since it improves the quality of life. Tobin *et al.* (197a) deal with the preservation of the anal-rectal sphincter in relatively advanced rectal cancers using preoperative irradiation (176a).

Combined Modality Therapy: The most significant advance in rectal cancer has been the demonstration now in two

Table 28-28. Percent 5-Year Survival Colorectal Cancer By Histologic Grade	
Grade	**% Survival**
1	59-93
2	33-75
3	11-56
(Refs 172a,184a,182a)	

independent studies that post-operative treatment with chemotherapy and radiation improves survival. The most recent study is positive for reduction in local recurrence and distant metastases, as well as overall and disease-free survival (162). Indeed this study is so striking that a recently held NIH consensus conference concluded that this should be the standard treatment for stage B2 and C rectal cancer, until other investigative approaches are completed.

Prognosis: Many clinical factors have relative influence on prognosis of colorectal cancer (172,173).

1. *Sex:* Women tend to have a higher survival rate than men (5).
2. *Symptoms:* Asymptomatic patients have better prognosis. Those patients with a very short duration of symptoms tend to have a worse prognosis (185).
3. *Obstruction or Perforation:* These complications increase operative mortality and uniformly decrease overall survival to approximately 20% (191).
4. *Rectal bleeding* is generally associated with a tumor which presents early and has better prognosis.
5. *Transfusion:* Multivariate analysis have shown that increased amount of blood transfusion perioperatively is inversely related to survival. The mechanisms for this finding are not entirely known (124).
6. *Adjacent organ involvement:* T4 lesions (Duke's B3 or C3) are tumors which are associated with higher local recurrence and lower survival. Aggressive surgical treatment is warranted (185).
7. *Blood vessel invasion:* This histopathologic finding is associated with three times greater incidence of liver metastasis (161).

The detection and treatment of asymptomatic recurrences can have an impact on survival and quality of life. This requires a plan of regular follow-up and specific diagnosis tests.

Patients should be examined each 3-4 months for the first 3 years after initial treatment. Rectal exam and occult blood tests should be done on each visit. Colonoscopy should be done each 6 months for 3 years. Chest x-ray and Barium enema should be done yearly. CEA levels can detect recurrent disease by a rising serum titer. Two thirds of colorectal cancer recurrences will be heralded by a rising CEA as the first indication. This test should be performed each 2-3 months after surgery. Several studies justify re-exploration based on a rising CEA as the only sign of recurrent disease (120,168,169).

CLINICAL INVESTIGATIONS

1. Numerous biological response modifiers are being tested for their effect on colorectal cancer. These include:

alpha-interferon, levamisole, interleukin-2 and lymphokine activated killer cells, and monoclonal antibodies.

2. Bone marrow transplantation allows more potent combinations of chemotherapy. A 50% complete response rate has been reported, but durations of response have been short.

3. Laser surgery is beginning to make a place in colorectal surgery also. Excision of polyps may be more precise with this modality and allow more accurate determination of invasion.

4. The treatment of rectal cancer and locally advanced colon cancers may be effective by the use of interoperative radiation therapy. This modality has been proven to be feasible. Clinical trials have yet to show a significant survival benefit (202a).

ANAL CARCINOMA

EPIDEMIOLOGY AND ETIOLOGY

Anal carcinomas are relatively rare with about 1500 cases expected in the United States in 1992 (1b). In most series, females predominate over males, but male/female ratios in different series varies from 1:1.5 to 1:6. Good statistics for anal carcinomas are lacking because they are often included with rectal cancers, and the anatomical nomenclature used varies (e.g., definition of anal margin cancers) with the report. The average age for most series is between 60-65 years, with a broad range of ages between 30-85 years (1b,220).

The cause of anal carcinoma is unknown. It has been associated with a variety of chronic anorectal conditions, such as, condylomata (human papilloma virus), fistulae, fissures, leucoplakia, Bowen's Disease, and prior radiation. More recently, it has been seen in the homosexual population and the incidence is higher in patients with renal transplants; this suggests immunodeficiency may play a role (213,216).

DETECTION AND DIAGNOSIS

Clinical Detection

The following symptoms may lead to the detection of anal carcinoma: GI bleeding (50%); rectal pain (20%-40%); palpable mass (25%); pressure sensation; change in bowel habits; rectal discharge; tenesmus (210,216).

Diagnostic Procedures

1. Physical examination is recommended, with special emphasis for the presence of *hepatomegaly* and *enlarged inguinal nodes*, signs of metastatic disease.

2. Anoscopic examination and biopsy will confirm the diagnosis and clinically stage the disease. Rectal examination will confirm the presence of an abnormality which will require further investigation.

   It is reasonable to proceed with sigmoidoscopy to exclude a second lesion located superiorly.

3. Barium enema is optional if colonoscopy has been performed.

4. CT scan provides evidence for or against local extension into prostate, bladder, vaginal, and/or nodes, as well as liver metastases.

5. Transrectal ultrasound does not have the value that it does when performed in the rectum.

6. The role of MRI has not yet been defined.

CLASSIFICATION AND STAGING

Histopathology (Table 28-29)

There are two predominant histologic types of anal carcinomas both of which are variants of squamous cell carcinoma: squamous cell (epidermoid), and basaloid (cloacogenic, transitional). Other much less common varieties include mucoepidermoid, adenocarcinoma, and undifferentiated. In most series the squamous variety predominates (>70%) with the basaloid comprising most of the rest. Of the squamous types >70% are moderately or poorly differentiated. The basaloid

Table 28-29. Histologic Classification of Anal Carcinoma	
Type	**% of Patients**
Squamous cell carcinoma	63
Transitional (cloacogenic) carcinoma	23
Adenocarcinoma	7
Paget's disease	2
Basal cell carcinoma	2
Melanoma	2

Modified from Peters (218a).

variety occur most commonly in the upper portion of the anus originating from the rectal column area. Adenocarcinomas and mucoepidermoidal arise from the anal crypts which have mucus-filled goblet cells and also occur in the upper anus. The squamous types arise predominantly from the pecten line area. Malignant melanomas may also occur as a primary malignancy in the anus being the third most common site after eye and skin. Other rare varieties are sarcomas which may arise from the soft tissue and invade the anus and lymphomas. Perianal tumors other than squamous variety include adnexal tumors, extramammary Paget's, Bowen's disease and basal cell carcinomas (211,216).

TNM Classification

Since there has been some controversy as to just what constitutes the anus canal and the perianal skin; a description and some definitions follow (212):

1. Anal margin — perianal region: the skin within 5 cm radius of the anal verge. Lesions located here are skin cancers.
2. Anal verge: the edge of the anal orifice leading into the anal canal.
3. Anal canal: extends from the rectum to the perianal skin (junction with hair-bearing skin), and measures about 3-4 cm in length. It is lined by the mucous membrane overlying the internal sphincter, including the transitional epithelium and dentate line.
4. Pecten or dentate line: located 1 cm above the anal verge and identified as a visible groove, or depression.
5. Upper margin of anus — palpable border of the anal sphincter and puborectalis muscles, at the level of the apex of the prostate in men. This is an area of transition from rectum to anus in which the epithelium more closely resembles transitional cells of the bladder, and anatomically consists of vertical folds (the rectal columns of Morgagni) which are then united at their lower border into the anal valves.

This is a new classification and T categories are based on size using 2 and 5 cm as critical sizes for T1,T2,T3 with T4 representing invasion of surrounding viscera. N categories relate distance from primary and whether nodes are unilateral or bilateral.

Staging Work-Up

1. Blood tests: CBC, platelets, differential, SMA-12 (or bilirubin, alkaline phosphatase, AST, BUN, and Creatinine).
2. Chest x-ray.

3. Careful rectal/vaginal examination and proctosigmoidoscopy (under EUA, if necessary) with appropriate biopsies. Palpable inguinal nodes: some investigators first perform a fine needle aspirate and only biopsy if this is negative, others do a bilateral groin dissection at the tme of or just after definitive surgery.
4. Barium enema. This is useful for extensions into rectum.
5. CT scan of abdomen and pelvic searching for metastatic pelvic nodes and liver metastases.

PRINCIPLES OF TREATMENT

Surgery (210,219)

Surgery has been the traditional treatment for anal cancers especially of the canal, usually in the form of an abdominal perineal resection and permanent colostomy; local excision has been utilized more frequently for margin cancers. Failures with this approach are believed related to the profuse blood supply and dense lymphatics in this area, and the limited amount of tissue around the rectum for safe surgical removal. Beneath the thick mucous membrane of the rectal columns lies the dilated and tortuous tributaries of the superior and inferior hemorrhoidal veins. Cancers may spread hematogenously into the portal system via the inferio-mesenteric vein or into the systemic circulation via the internal iliac veins. Similarly, the lymphatic drainage may be due to the inguinal nodes or the internal iliac chain.

Sphincter sparing is more widely accepted and considered in view of gains due to chemoradiation.

Radiotherapy versus Chemoradiation Therapy (Tables 28-30 and 28-31)

Definitive radiation for anal cancers was initially rejected because the perianal skin and mucocutaneous juncture were sensitive to radiation and associated with severe reactions. However, in 1974, Nigro *et al.* (218) reported on three patients who were treated with intermediate doses of radiation (30-35 Gy) and concomitant 5-FU infusion and a single bolus of Mitomycin C. Two of the patients subsequently underwent an APR with no tumor being found and the third refused surgery and was clinically NED at 14 months. He subsequently updated his series in 1984 combining 44 cases from his institution with 60 from surgeons in the US who followed his regimen. At 2 years of follow-up, 60 patients were NED with chemoradiation alone and another 22 NED with chemoradiation followed by APR, two were alive with disease, and 20 had died, seven of unrelated causes. Two

Table 28-30. Anal Carcinoma: External Radiation				
Dose (cGY)	**Complications (%)**	**5-Year Survival %**	**Local Control**	**Ref**
5000-7000	8	51	67	219b
6000-6500	14	72 (T1,2)	91	215a
		35 (T3,4)	76	
6500	13	79	80	211a
4500-6000	12	72	60	211c

Table 28-31. Selected Concomitant Radiation/5-Fluorouracil/Mitomycin Protocols

Reference	Radiation (cGy)	Primary Tumor Control %	Survival
Leichman et al. (215b')	3000	86	80%, 5-yr crude
Sischy et al. (221)	4080	71	73%, 3-yr actuarial
Flam et al. (215a')	4500	90	Not stated
Papillon and Montbarbon (218')	4200 + 2000 implant	81	Not stated
Cummings et al. (211c')	5000	88	75%, 5-yr actuarial
Cummings et al. (211c')	4800-5000	87	65%, 5-yr actuarial
Nigro (217)	3000	89	80%, 5-yr crude

From Cummings (211b'), with permission.

startling findings were: (1) 97/104 (93%) had no gross tumor remaining after the chemoradiation was completed and (2) 22/31 (70%) who had APR had no tumor seen in the specimen (217). Other authors have since presented their data confirming the good results with 82% (153/216) of surgical specimens (APR or local excision) free of cancer (214). As more experience was gained with chemoradiation, APR was less often performed, local excision was used to document response and the sphincter was retained. Currently radical surgery no longer plays a role in the initial management of these patients except for groin dissection of clinically involved nodes and colostomy in case of anal obstruction. A counterpoint to this development which coincides with a better understanding of radiation techniques and megavoltage equipment, has been the use of radiation alone. Doggett *et al.* (215) have reported on 35 selected patients (lesions < 5 cm) treated with definitive radiation alone with excellent results. There were eight local failures in this group of which five were salvaged with APR (anal continence - 80%) and one with local excision. The patients were treated between 1973-1986, and only two have died of disease. Schlienger *et al.* (220) have recently reported on 193 patients treated only with radiation.

RESULTS AND PROGNOSIS

Surgery versus Radiation Therapy

Results for anal carcinoma have improved dramatically in recent years with improved survival with anal sphincter preservation through the use of chemoradiation. It is also been true for the use of irradiation alone and needs to be compared to surgery which has been the traditional mode of treatment. The general survival for anal cancers all stages treated surgically, requiring an abdominal perineal resection with colostomy, has been in the range of 50% 5 years (range 35%-68%). With the introduction of full dose radiation therapy and attempt at anal preservation figures have improved so that the overall 5-year survival ranges from 50%-75% with doses of 60-70 Gy as a rule (Table 28-29). The complication rate has a range from 10%-15% with anal strictures and soft tissue necrosis. Percentage of local control, however, is high; it ranges from 60%-90%. Anal sphincter preservation occurs in 80% of survivors.

Chemoradiation

Chemoradiation has been used with increasing success initially introduced by Nigro and then developed in clinical trials by Sichy (221) both for the RTOG and ECOG. Generally, 5-Fu and Mitomycin C and/or cisplatinum have been utilized with radiation therapy simultaneously. There has been some radiation dose modification so that 30-40 Gy are used. With survival rates being reported ranging from 75%-85% at 5 years and the majority of patients showing complete response, approximately 90%-95% strive for anal preservation (Table 28-31). Some series have exceeded 90% 5-year survival, but most series have 5-year survival in excess of 70% with low levels of acute and resifual toxicity (211b,222). The experience of searching for the optimal timing and sequencing of radiation therapy and concommitant chemotherapy in anal cancers is presented by Cummings *et al.* (211c'), reviewing the treatment of 192 patients based on eight consecutive protocols over a span of three decades. It begins with the use of irradiation alone followed by simultaneous use of 5-FU (FUR) and Mito-C (FUMIR). The primary tumor control rate was 68% at 5-year, and for each of the arms — RT, FUR, FUMIR — the rates were 58%, 60%, and 86%, respectively; the overall survival was 69%, and for each of the arms, 69%, 64%, and 76%, respectively. Anal preservation occurred in 88% of patients whose primary was controlled, and 64% overall. Complications, both acute and late, were greater with FUMIR, as was improved local regional control leading to split-course irradiation and lowering the daily functional dose to 2 Gy.

REFERENCES

General References

1. Beahrs, O.H., Henson, D.E., Hutter, R.V.P., Myers, M.H. eds. Manual for Staging of Cancer, 4th ed. New York, NY: JB Lippincott Co; 1992.
1a. Bragg, D.G., Rubin, P., Youker, J.E. eds. Oncologic Imaging. Elmsford, NY: Pergamon Press; 1985.
1b. Boring, C.C.; Squires, B.A.; Tony, T. Cancer Statistics, 1992 Ca. 42:19-38;1992.
2. Boros, L. Gastrointestinal Cancers. In: Rosenthal, S.N., Bennett, J.M. eds. Practical Cancer Chemotherapy. Garden City, NJ: Med. Exam. Publ. Co; 1981; pp 226-262.
3. Carter, S.K., Glatstein, E., Livingstone, R.B. eds. Principles of Cancer Treatment. New York, NY: McGraw-Hill; 1982.
4. del Regato, J.A., Spjut, H.J., Cox, J.D. Cancer, Diagnosis, Treatment, and Prognosis, 6th ed. St. Louis, MO: C.V. Mosby; 1985.
5. DeVita, V.T., Hellman, S., Rosenberg, S.A. eds. Cancer, Principles and Practice of Oncology, 3rd ed. Philadelphia, PA: J.B. Lippincott Co; 1989.
6. International Histologic Classification of Tumors, Nos. 1-20. Geneva, Switzerland: World Health Organization; 1978.
7. Monfardini, S., Bnunner, K., Crowther, D. *et al.* Gastrointestinal Tumors. In: Monfardini S, Bnunner K, Crowther D *et al.* eds. Manual of Cancer Chemotherapy, 3rd ed. UICC Technical Report Series. Geneva, Switzerland: International Union Against Cancer (UICC); 1981:115-121.
8. Rubin, P. ed. Current Concepts in Cancer: Multidisciplinary Views. Chicago, IL: American Medical Association; 1974.
9. Silverberg, E.; Boring, C.C.; Squires, T.S. Cancer Statistics. CA 40: 9-26; 1990.
10. Strauss, M.B. Familiar Medical Quotations. Boston, MA: Little, Brown and Co; 1968.

11. TNM Classification of Malignant Tumors (Hermanek P, Sobin LH), 4th ed.New York, NY: Springer-Verlag;1987.

Specific References

Esophagus

12. Abe, S.; Tachibana, M.; Shimokawa, T. *et al.* Surgical treatment of advanced carcinoma of the esophagus. Surg. Gynecol Obstet. 168: 115-20; 1989.

13. Appelquist, P.; Salmo M. Lye corrosion carcinoma of the esophagus. Cancer 45:2655-2658; 1980.

13a. Akakura, I.; Nakamura, Y.; Kakegawa, T. *et al.* Surgery for carcinoma of the esophagus with preoperative irradiation. Chest 57:47; 1970.

13b. Beatty, J.D.; DoBoer, G.; Rider, W.D. Carcinoma of the esophagus-pretreatment assessment, correlation of radiation treatment parameters with survival and identification and management of radiation treatment failure. Cancer 43:2254;1979.

14. Boyce, H.W. Palliation of advanced esophageal cancer. Semin. Oncol. 11:186-95; 1984.

15. Broitman, S.A.; Vitale, J.J.; Gottlief, L.S. Ethanolic beverage consumption, cigarette smoking, nutritional status and digestive tract cancers. Semin. Oncol. 10: 322-29; 1983.

16. Camerson, A.J.; Oh, B.J.; Payne, W.S. The incidence of adenocarcinoma in columnar-lined (Barrett's) esophagus. N. Eng. J. Med. 313: 857-59; 1985.

16a. Cedraquist, C.; Nielsen, J.; Bertheelsen, A. *et al.* Cancer of the esophagus II. Therapy and outcome. Acta Chir. Scand. 144:223;1979.

17. Chan, A.; Wong, A.; Arthur, K. Concomitant 5-Fluorouracil infusion, Mitomycin C, and radiation therapy in esophageal squamous cell carcinoma of the esophagus: An RTOG study. Int. J. Radiat. Oncol. Biol. Phys.16: 59-65; 1989.

17a. Coia, L.R. Esophageal cancer. Is esophagectomy necessary? Oncology 3:101-110;1989.

17b. Coia LR, Engstrom PF, Paul AR, *et al.* Long-term results of infusional 5-FU, mitomycin-C, and radiation as primary management of esophageal carcinoma. Int J Radiat Oncol Biol Phys 20:29-36; 1991.

18. Coia, L.R.; Engstrom, P.F.; Paul, A. Nonsurgical management of esophageal cancer: Report of a study of combined radiotherapy and chemotherapy. J Clin Oncol 5:1783-90; 1987.

18a. Coia LR, Engstrom PF, Paul AR, *et al.* Long-term results of infusional 5-FU, mitomycin-C, and radiation as primary management of esophageal carcinoma. Int J Radiat Oncol Biol Phys. 20(1):29-36; 1991.

19. Coia LR, Plaul AR, Engstrom PF. Combined radiation and chemotherapy as primary management of adenocarcinoma of the esophagus and gastroesophageal junction. Cancer 61:643-49; 1988.

20. DeMeester, T.R. Carcinoma of the esophagus (Part I & II). Curr. Prob. Surg. 25: 477-605; 1988.

21. DeMeester, T.R.; Barlow, A.P. Surgery and current management for cancer of the esophagus and cardia. Curr. Prob. in Cancer 12: 243-327; 1988.

22. Demeester, T.R.; Lafontaine, E.R. Surgical Therapy. In: Demeester, T.R., Levin, B. eds. Cancer of the Esophagus. New York, NY: Grune and Stratton; 1985: 141-197.

22a. Doggett, R.L.S.; Guernsey, J.M.; Bagshaw, M.A. Combined radiation and surgical treatment of carcinoma of the thoracic esophagus. Front. Radiat. Ther. Oncol. 5:147;1970.

23. Earlam, R.; Cunha, Melo, J.R. Oesophageal squamous cell carcinoma: I. A critical review of surgery. Brit. J. Surg. 67: 381-90; 1980.

24. Edwards, J.W.; Hellier, V.F.; Lawson, R.A. Squamous carcinoma of the esophagus: Histological criteria and their prognostic significance. Brit. J. Cancer 59: 429-33; 1989.

24a. Fisher, .SA., Brady, L.W. Esophagus. In: Preez, C.A., Bardy, L.W. (eds). Principles and Practice of Radiation Oncology (2nd ed). Philadelphia, PA: JB Lippincott Co; 1992, pp 853-870.

25. Flores, A.D.; Nelems, B.; Evans, K.; Hay, J.H.; Stoller, J.; Jackson, S.M. Impact of new radiotherapy modalities on the surgical management of cancer of the esophagus and cardia. Int. J. Radiat. Oncol. Biol. Phys. 17:482-87; 1986.

25a. Forastiere, A.A. Treatment of locoregional esophageal cancer. Semin Oncol 19(4) (Suppl 11):57-63; 1992.

26. Forastiere, A.A.; Gennis, M.; Orringer, M.B.; Agha, F.P. Cisplatin, Vinblastine, and Mitoguazone chemotherapy for epidermoid and adenocarcinoma of the esophagus. J Clin Oncol 5:1143-49; 1987.

26a. Forastiere, A.A.; Orringer, M.B.; Perez-Tamayo, C.; *et al.* Concurrent chemotherapy and radiation therapy followed by transhiatal esophagectomy for local-regional cancer of the esophagus. J Clin Oncol 8:119-127; 1990.

27. Gignoux, M.; Roussel, A.; Paillot ,B.; Gillet ,M.; Schlag, P.; Dalesio, O.; Buyse, M.; Duez, N. The value of preoperative radiotherapy in esophageal cancer : Results of a study by the EORTC. Recent Results in Cancer Research 110:1-13; 1988.

27a. Gignoux, M.; Roussel, A.; Pallot, B. *et al.* The value of preoperative radiotherapy in esophageal cancer. Results of a study of the EORTC. World J. Surg. 11:426;1987.

28. Hancock, S.F.; Glatstein, E. Radiation therapy of esophageal cancer. Semin. Oncol. 11: 144-158; 1984.

29. Hankins, J.R.; Cole, F.N.; Ward, A. *et al.* Carcinoma of the esophagus. The philosophy for palliation. Ann. Thorac. Surg. 14:189-197; 1972.

30. Herskovic, A.; Martz, K.; Al-Sarraf, M. *et al.* Combined chemotherapy and radiotherapy compared with radiotherapy alone in patients with cancer of the esophagus. N Engl J Med 326:1593-1598; 1992.

30a. Herskovic, A.; Martz, K.; Al-Sarraf, M.; *et al.* Intergroup esophageal study: Comparison of radiotherapy (RT) to radio-chemotherapy combination: A phase III trial. Proc Am Soc Clin Oncol 10:A-407,135; 1991.

31. Hesketh, P.J.; Clapp, R.W.; Doos, W.G.; Spechler, S.J. The increasing frequency of adenocarcinoma of the esophagus. Cancer 64:526-530; 1989.

32. Hilgenberg, A.D.; Carey, R.W;, Wilkins, E.W.; Choi, N.C.; Mathisen, D.J.; Grillo, H.C. Pre-operative chemotherapy, surgical resection and selective post-operative therapy for squamous cell carcinoma of the esopohagus. Ann. Thorac. Surg. 45:357-63; 1988.

33. Hishikawa, Y.; Kamikonya, N.; Tanaka, S.; Miura, T. Radiotherapy of esophageal carcinoma: Role of high-dose-rate intracavitary irradiation. Radiotherapy and Oncology. 9: 13-20; 1987.

33a. Hishikawa Y, Kurisu K, Taniguchi M, *et al.* High-dose-rate intraluminal brachytherapy (HDRIBT) for esophageal cancer. Int J Radiat Oncol Biol Phys 21:1133-1136; 1991.

34. Hurt, R.L. Historical Survey of Surgical Treatment. In: Hurt, R.L. ed. Management of Oesaphageal Carcinoma. London, UK: Springer-Verlag; 1989:1-19.

34a. Hussey, D.H.; Barkley, H.T. Jr.; Bloedron, F.G. Carcinoma of the Esophagus. In: Fletcher, G.H. ed. Textbook of Radiotherapy. Philadelphia, PA: Lea & Febiger; 1980:688-703.

35. Inculet ,T.I.; Keller, S.M.; Dwyer, A.; Roth, J.A. Evaluation of noninvasive tests for the preoperative staging of carcinoma of the esophagus: A preoperative study. Ann. Thorac. Surg. 40: 561-651; 1985.

35a. Isono, K.; Onoda, S.; Ishikawa, T. *et al.* Studies on the causes of deaths from esophageal carcinoma. Cancer 49:173;1982.

35b. John, M.J.; Flam, M.S.; Mowry, P.A. *et al.* Radiotherapy alone and chemoradiation for nonmetastatic esophageal carcinoma. Cancer 63:2397-2403;1989.

36. Kasai, M.; Moris, Watanabe, T. Follow-up results after the resection of esophageal carcinoma. World J. Surg. 2: 543;1980.

36a. Keane, T.J.; Harwood, A.R.; Rider, W.D. *et al.* Concomitant radiation and chemotherapy for squamous cell carcinoma of esophagus (Abstract). Int. J. Radiat. Oncol. Biol. Phys. 10:89;1984.

37. Kelsen, D. Neoadjuvent therapy of esophageal cancer. Canc. J. Surg. 32:410-14; 1989.

37a. Kelsen, D.P.; Ahuja, R.; Hopfan, S. *et al.* Combined modality therapy of esophageal carcinoma. Cancer 48:31;1981.

37b. Kelsen, D.P; Bains, M.; Burt, M. Neoadjuvant chemotherapy and surgery of cancer of the esophagus. Semin Surg Oncol 6(5):268-273; 1990.

38. Kelser, D. Chemotherapy of esophageal cancer. Semin. Oncol. 11:159-168; 1984.

39. King, R.M.; Pairolero, P.C.; Trastek, V.F. *et al.* Ivor Lewis Esophagogastrectomy for carcinoma of the esophagus: Early and late functional results. Ann. Thorac. Surg. 44: 119-122;1987.

40. Kinzie, J.J. Radiation Therapy. In: Demeester, T.R.; Levin, B. Cancer of the Esophagus. New York, NY: Grune & Stratton; 1985: 247-57.

41. Kuster, G.G.; Foroozan, P. Early diagnosis of adenocarcinoma developing in Barrett's esophagus. Arch. Surg. 124: 925-27; 1989.

41a. Launois, B.; DeLaRue, D.; Campion, J.P. *et al.* Preoperative radiotherapy for carcinoma of the esophagus. Surg. Gynecol. Obstet. 153:690;1981.

42. Leichman, L.; Herskovic, A.; Leichman, C.G.; Lattin, P.B.; Steiger, Z.; Tapazolglou, E.; Rosenberg, J.C.; Arbulu, A.; Asfaw, I.; Kinzie, J. Nonoperative therapy for squamous cell cancer of the esophagus. J. Clin. Oncol. 5:365-370; 1987.

43. Leichman, L.; Steiger, Z.; Seydel, H.G.; Dindogru, A.; Kinzie, J.; Toben, S.; Mackenzie, G.; Shell, J. Preoperative chemotherapy and radiation therapy for patients with cancer of the esophagus: A potentially curative approach. J. Clin. Oncol. 2:75-79; 1984.

43a. Leichman, L.; Steiger, Z.; Sydel, H.G.; Vaitkevicus, V.K. Combined preoperative chemotherapy and radiation therapy for cancer of the esophagus. The Wayne State University Southwest Oncology Group and Radiation Therapy Oncology Group experience. Semin. Oncol. 11:178-195;1984.

43b. Lewinsky, B.S.; Annes, G.P.; Mann, S.G. *et al.* Carcinoma of the esophagus: An analysis of results and of treatment techniques. Radiol. Clin. North Am. 44:192;1975.

44. Lightdale, D.J.; Winawe, S.J. Screening diagnosis and staging of esophageal cancer. Semin. Oncol. 11: 101-112; 1984.

44a'. Lokich, J.; Shea, M.; Chaffey, J. Sequential infusional 5-fluorouracil followed by concomitant radiation for tumors of the esophagus and the gastroesophageal junction. Cancer 60:275-279; 1987.

44a. Liu, G.; Huang, Z.; Rong, T. *et al.* Measure for improving therapeutic results of esophageal carcinoma in Stage III: Preoperative radiotherapy. J. Surg. Oncol. 32:248;1986.

44b. Lowe, W.C. Survival with carcinoma of the esophagus. Ann. Intern. Med. 77:915;1972.

45. Maillet, P.; Bauliewx, J.; Bouley *et al.* Carcinoma of the thoracic esophagus: Results of one-stage surgery (271 cases). Am.J. Surg. 143: 629; 1982.

46. Mannell, A.; Becker, P.J.; Nissenbaum, M. Bypass surgery for unresectable esophageal cancer: Early and late results in 124 cases. Br. J. Surg. 75: 283-86; 1988.

47. Manyak, M.H.; Russo, A.; Smith, P.D.; Glatstein, E. Photodynamic therapy. J. Clin. Oncol. 6:380-91; 1988.

47a. Marks, R.D. Jr.; Scruggs, H.J.; Wallace, K.M. Preoperative radiation therapy for carcinoma of the esophagus. Cancer 38:84; 1976.

48. Matthewson, K. Laser Therapy. In: Hurt, R.L. ed. Management of Oesophageal Carcinoma. London,UK: Springer-Verlag: 251-266.

49. McFarlane, S.D., Ilver, R. Carcinoma of the Esophagus. In: Hill, L., Kozarek,R., McCallum, R., Mercer,C.D. eds. The Esophagus, Medical and Surgical Management. Philadelphia,PA: WB Saunders Co; 1988: 237-256.

50. McLean, A.M., Reznek, R.H. Radiologic Diagnosis and Assessment. In: Hurt, R.L. ed. Management of Oesophageal Carcinoma. London,UK: Springer-Verlag; 1989: 69-101.

51. Mendenhall, W.M. Carcinoma of the Cervical Esophagus. In: Million, R.R., Cassissi, N.J. eds. Management of Head and Neck Cancer, A Multidisciplinary Approach. Philadelphia, PA: JB Lippincott Co; 1984: 393-405.

52. Murata, Y.; Muroi, M.; Yoshida, M. *et al.* Endoscopic ultrasound in the diagnosis of esophageal carcinoma. Surg. Endos. 1:11;1986.

53. Murray, F.E.; Bowers, G.J.; Birkett, D.H. *et al.* Palliative laser therapy for advanced esophageal carcinoma: An alternative perspective. Am. J. Gastroent. 83: 816-819; 1988.

53a. Newaishy, G.A.; Read, G.A.; Duncan, W. *et al.* Results of radical radiotherapy of squamous cell carcinoma of the esophagus. Clin. Radio. 33:347;1982.

54. Orringer, M.B. Substernal gastric bypass of the excluded esophagus—results of an ill advised operation. Surgery 96:467; 1984.

54a. Orringer, M.B. Surgical therapy for esophageal carcinoma. In: Sawyers, J.L., Williams, L.F. eds. Difficult Problems in General Surgery. Chicago, Year Book Medical Publishers, Inc. 1989:21-42.

55. Pagliero, K.M. Brachytherapy (Intracacitary Irradiation). In: Hurt, R.L. ed. Management of Oesophageal Carcinoma. London,UK: Springer-Verlag;1989: 243-250.

55a. Parker, E.F.; Gregorie, H.B.; Prioleau, W.H., Jr. *et al.* Carcinoma of the esophagus — observations of 40 years. Ann.Surg. 195:618;1982.

56. Pearson, J.G. The value of radiotherapy in the management of esophageal cancer. Am.J. Roentgenol. 105:500-513; 1969.

56a. Pearson, J.G. The present status and future potential of radiotherapy in the management of esophageal cancer. Cancer 39:82; 1977.

57. Poplin, E.; Fleming, T.; Leichamn, L.; Seydel, H.G.; Steiger, Z., Taylor, S., Vance, R.; Stuckey, W.J.; Rivkin, S.E. Combined therapies for squamous-cell carcinoma of the esophagus: A Southwest Oncology Group Study (SWOG-8037). J. Clin. Oncol. 5:622-628; 1987.

58. Pringle, R.; Winsey, H.S. The palliation of esophageal carcinoma. J. R. Coll. Surg. Edinb. 18:188-190; 1973.

59. Rider, WD.; Diaz Mendoza, R. Some opinions on the treatment of cancer of the esophagus. Am. J. Roentgenol. 105:514-517; 1969.

59a. Rosenberg, J.C.; Lichter, A.S., Leichman, L.P. Cancer of the Esophagus. In: De Vita, V.T., Jr., Hellman, S., Rosenberg, S.A. eds. Cancer, Principles and Practice of Oncology. Philadelphia, PA: JB Lippincott Co; 1989.

59b. Rotman, M.; Aziz, H. Concomitant continuous infusion chemotherapy and radiation. Cancer 65:823-835;1990.

60. Rubio, C.A.; Fu-Sheng, L. Spontaneous squamous carcinoma of the esophagus in chickens. Cancer 64: 2511-14; 1989.

61. Schottenfeld, D. Epidemiology of cancer of the esophagus. Semin. Oncol. 11: 92-100; 1984.

61a. Schumann, G.F.; Heydorn, W.H.; Hall, R.V. *et al.* Treatment of esophageal carcinoma. J. Thorac. Cardiovasc. Surg. 79:67;1980.

62. Seydel,H.G.; Leichamn, L.; Byhnardt ,T.; Cooper, J.; Herdkovic, A.; Libnock J.; Pazdur, R.; Speyer, J.; Tschan, J. Preoperative radiation and chemotherapy for localized squamous cell carcinoma of the esophagus: An RTOG study. Int. J. Radiat. Oncol. Biol. Phys. 14:33-35; 1988.

63. Sjogren, R.W.; Johnson, L.F. Barrett's esophagus: A review. Am. J. Med. 74:313-321; 1983.

64. Skinner, D.B. Surgical treatment for esophageal carcinoma. Semin. Oncol. 11: 136-143; 1984.

65. Skinner, D.B.; Ferguson, M.K.; Sariano, A. *et al.* Selection of operation for esophageal cancer based on staging. Annals Surg. 204: 391-401; 1986.

65'. Steiger Z, Franklin R, Wilson RF, *et al.* Eradication and palliation of squamous cell carcinoma of the esophagus with chemotherapy, radiotherapy, and surgical therapy. J Thorac Cardiovasc Surg 82:713-719; 1981.

65a. Sugimachi, K.; Matsufuji, H.; Kai, H. *et al.* Preoperative irradiation for carcinoma of the esophagus. Surg. Gynecol. Obstet. 172:174;1986.

66. Sugimachi, K.; Matsuoka, H.; Matsufuji, H. *et al.* Survival rates of women with carcinoma of the esophagus exceed those of men. Surg. Gynecol. Obstet. 164: 541-544; 1987.

67. Tannock, I.F. Combined modality treatment with radiotherapy and chemotherapy. Radiotherapy and Oncology 16:83-101; 1989.

68. Thompson, W.M. Esophageal Cancer. In: Bragg, D.G., Rubin, P., Youker,J.E. eds. Oncologic Imaging. Elmsford, NY: Pergamon Press; 1985: 207-242.

69. Tio, T.L.; Cohen, P.; Coene, P.P. *et al.* Endosonography and computed tomography of esophageal carcinoma: Pre-operative classification comparted to new (1987) TNM system. Gastroenterology 96:1478-86; 1989.

69a. Van Andel, J.G.; Dees, J.; Diskhuis, C.M. *et al.* Carcinoma of the esophagus - results of treatment. Ann. Surg. 190:684; 1979.

69b. Van Houtte, P. Radiotherapie du cancer l'oesophage. Acta Gastroenterol. Beig. 40:121;1977.

70. Wang, H.H.; Antonioli, D.A.; Goldman, H. Comparative features of esophageal and gastric adenocarcinomas. Human Path. 17: 482-487; 1986.

70a. Wara, W.M.; Mauch, P.M.; Thomas, A.N.; Phillips, T.L. Palliation for carcinoma of the esophagus. Radiology 121:717;1976.

71. Watson, A. Palliative Therapy. In: Hurt,R.L. ed. Management of Oesophagealcarcinoma. London,UK: Springer-Verlag;1989:211-222.

71a. Yin, W.; Zhang, I.J.; Miao, Y. *et al.* The results of high-energy electron therapy in carcinoma of the esophagus compared with telecobalt therapy. Clin. Radiol. 34:113;1983.

Stomach

72. Abe, M.; Takahashi, M.;Ono, K.;Tobe, T.; Inamoto, T. Japan

gastric trials in the intraoperative radiation therapy. Int. J. Radiat. Oncol. Biol. Phys. 15:1431-1433; 1988.

72a. Abe, M.; Takahashi, M. Intraoperative radiotherapy: The Japanese experience. Int. J. Radiat.Oncol. Biol. Phys. 7:863-868;1981.

73. Baker, L.H.; Talley, R.W.; Matter, R. *et al*. Phase III comparison of the treatment of advanced gastrointestinal cancer with bolus weekly 5-FU vs. methyl-CCNU plus bolus weekly 5-FU. A Southwest Oncology Group study. Cancer 38:1-7;1976.

74. Baker, T.; Nakane, Y.; Okusa, T. *et al*. Strategy for lymphadenectomy of gastric cancer. Surgery 105:585-592; 1989.

75. Burgers, J.M.V.; Taal, B.G.; van Heerde, P.; Somers, R.; den Hartog, Jager, F.C.A.; Hart, A.A.M. Treatment results of primary stage I and II non-Hodgkin's lymphoma of the stomach. Radiotherapy and Oncology 11:319-326; 1988.

76. Carter, S.K.; Comis, R.L. Gastric cancer: Current status of treatment. J. Natl. Cancer Inst. 58:567-578; 1977.

76a. Cohn KH, Wang F, DeSota-LaPaix F, *et al*. Association of *nm*23-H1 allelic deletions with distant metastases in colorectal carcinoma. Lancet 338:722; 1991.

77. Comis, R.L.; Carter, S.K. A review of chemotherapy in gastric cancer. Cancer 34:1576-1586; 1974.

78. Correa, P. Clinical implications of recent developments in gastric cancer pathology and epidemiology. Semin. Oncol. 12:2-10; 1985.

78a. Dixon WJ, Longmire WP, Holden, WD. Use of triethylenethiophosphoramide as an adjuvant to the surgical treatment of gastric and colorectal carcinoma: Ten-year follow-up. Ann Surg 173:16; 1971.

79. Douglass, H.O.; Nava, H.R. Gastric adenocarcinoma — management of the primary disease. Semin. Oncol. 12:32-45; 1985.

80. Dupont, J.B.; Cohn, I. Gastric aenocarcinoma. Curr. Probl. Cancer 4:25; 1980.

81. Ellis, F.H.; Gibb, S.B.; Watkins, E. Limited esophagogastrectomy for carcinoma of the cardia. Ann. Surg. 208:354-361; 1988.

82. Engstrom, P.; Lavin, P. Post-operative adjuvant therapy for gastric cancer patients. Proc. Am. Soc. Clin. Oncol. 2:114; 1983.

82a. Estape J, Grau JJ, Lcobendas F, *et al*. Mitomycin C as an adjuvant treatment to resected gastric cancer: A 10-year follow-up. Ann Surg 213(3):219-221; 1991.

83. Galiano, R.; McCracken, J.D.; Chen, T. Adjuvant chemotherapy with 5-Fluorouracil, Adriamycin, and Mitomycin (FAM) in gastric cancer. Proc. Am. Soc. Clin. Oncol. 2:114; 1983.

84. The Gastrointestinal Tumor Study Group : Controlled trial of adjuvant chemotherapy following curative resection for gastric cancer. Cancer 49: 1116-1122; 1982.

85. Gospodarowicz, M.K.; Bush, R.S.; Brown, T.C.; Chua, T. Curability of gastrointestinal lymphoma with combined surgery and radiation. Int. J. Radiati. Oncol. Biol. Phys. 9:3-9; 1983.

86. Gouzi, J.L.; Huguier, M.; Gagniez, P.L. et al Total versus subtotal gastrectomy for adenocarcinoma of the gastric antrum. A French prospective controlled study. Ann. Surg. 209:162-166; 1989.

87. Gunderson, L.L.; Sosin, H. Adenocarcinoma of the stomach: Areas of failure in a reoperation series (second or symptomatic look) clinicopathologic correlation and implications for adjuvant therapy. Int. J. Radiat. Oncol. Biol. Phys. 8:1-12; 1982.

88. Gupta, J.P.; Jain, A.L.; Agrawal ,B.K.; Gupta, S. Gastroscopic cytology and biopsies in diagnosis of gastric malignancies. J. Surg. Oncol. 22: 62-64; 1983.

89. Haber, D.A.; Mayer, R.J. Primary gastrointestinal lymphoma. Semin. Oncol. 15:1154-1169; 1988.

90. Hallissey, M.T.; Allum, W.H.; Roginski, C.; Fielding, J.W.L. Pallative surgery for gastric cancer. Cancer 62: 440-444; 1988.

91. Hendricks, J.C. Malignant tumors of the stomach. Surg Clin N Am 66:683-693; 1986.

92. Higgins, G.A.; Amadeo, J.H.; Smith, D.E.; Humphrey, E.W.; Keehn, R.J. Efficacy of prolonged intermittent therapy with combined 5-FU and Methyl-CCNU following resection for gastric carcinoma. Cancer 52:1105; 1983.

92'. Kakehi Y.; Tsujitani S.; Baba H.; *et al*. Clinicopathologic features and prognostic significance of duodenal invasion in patients with distal gastric carcinoma. Cancer 68(2):380-384; 1991.

92a. Kennedy, B.J. TNM classification for stomach cancer. Cancer 6:971;1970.

93. Klarfield, J.; Resnick, G. Gastric remnant carcinoma. Cancer 44:1129-1133; 1979.

94. Koyama, Y.; Kimura, T. Controlled clinical trials of chemo-

therapy as an adjuvant to surgery in gastric surgery. Proc. II Int. Cancer Congr., Buenos Aires,Argentina: A978: 1-21.

94a. Krook, J.E.; O'Connell, M.J.; Wieland, H.S. *et al*. Adjuvant therapy of gastric cancer with doxorubicin and 5-Flourouracil. Proc. Am. Soc. Clin. Onco. 7:93;1988.

95. Kurtz, R.C.; Sherlock, P. The diagnosis of gastric cancer. Semin. Oncol. 12: 11-18; 1985.

96. Lechebalier, T.; Smith, F.P.; Harter, W.K.;Schein, P.S. Chemotherapy and combined modality therapy for locally advanced and metastatic gastric carcinoma. Semin. Oncol. 12: 46-53; 1985.

97. Licht,J.D.; Weissmann, L.B.; Antman, K. Gastrointestinal sarcomas. Semin Oncol 15:181-88; 1988.

98. List AF, Greer JP, Cousar JC, *et al*. Non-hodgkin's lymphoma of the gastrointestinal tract: An analysis of clinical and pathologic features affecting outcome. J Clin Oncol 6:1125-1133; 1988.

99. MacDonald, J.S.; Schein, P.S.; Wooley. P.V. *et al*. 5-fluorouracil, doxorubicin and mitomycin C (FAM) combination chemotherapy for advanced gastric cancer. Ann. Intern. Med. 93:533-536; 1980.

99a. MacDonald, J.S.; Steele, G.S.; Gunderson, L.L. Cancer of the Stomach. In: DeVita, V.T. Jr., Hellman, S., Rosenberg, S.A. Cancer, Principles and Practice of Oncology. Philadelphia, PA: J.B. Lippincott Co; 1989, pp 765-799.

100. Maor, M.H.; Maddux, B.; Osborne,B.M.; Fuller, L.M.; Sullivan, J.A.; Nelson, R.S.; Martin, R.G.; Libshitz, H.I.; Valasquez, W.S.; Bennett, R.W. Stage IE and IIE non-Hodgkin's lymphomas of the stomach. Comparison of treatment modalities. Cancer 54:2330-2337; 1984.

101. Maor, M.H.; Velasquez, W.S.; Fuller, L.M.; Silvermintz, K.B. Stomach conservation in stage IE and IIE gastric non-Hodgkin's lymphoma. J. Clin. Oncol. 8:266-271; 1990.

102. Moertel, C.G.; Childs, D.S.; Colby, M.Y. *et al*. Combined 5-FU and supervoltage radiation therapy of locally unresectable gastrointestinal cancer. Lancet 2:865-867; 1969.

103. Moss, A.A.; Schnyder, P.; Marks, W. *et al*. Gastric adenocarcinoma: A comparison of the accuracy and economics of staging by computed tomography and surgery. Gastroenterology 80: 45-90; 1981.

103a. Nakajima, T.; Takahashi, T.; Takagi, K. Comparison of 5-FU with Fltorafus in adjuvant chemotherapies with combined inductive and maintenance therapies for gastric cancer. J. Clin. Oncol. 2:1366-1371;1984.

104. Okamura, T.; Tsujitan, S.; Korenaga, O. *et al*. Lymphadenectomy for cure in patients with early gastric cancer and lymph node metastasis. Am. J. Surg. 155:476-480; 1988.

104a. Parsonnet, J.; Friedman, G.D.; Vandersteen, D.P. *et al*. Helicobacter pylori infection and the risk of gastric carcinoma. NEJM. 325:1127-1136;1991.

104b. Physicians' Data Query. Stomach Cancer. National Cancer Institute, Bethesda, MD: January 1992.

105. Preusser, P.; Achterrath, W.; Wilke, H.; Lenaz, L.; Junk, W.; Heineke, A.; Meyer, J.; Buente, H. Chemotherapy of gastric cancer. Canc. Treat. Reviews 15:257-277; 1988.

106. ReMine, W.H. Preoperative Assessment and Palliative Surgery. In: Fielding, J.W.L., Newman, C.E., Ford, C.H.J., Jones, B.G. eds. Gastric Cancer: Advances in the Biosciences, vol.32. Oxford, UK: Pergamon Press; 1981: 123-138.

107. Salo, J.A.; Saario, I.; Kimilankao, E.O. *et al*. Near total gastrectomy for gastric cancer. Am. J. Surg. 155:486-489; 1988.

107a. Serlin, O; Wolkoff, J.S.; Armadeo, J.M. *et al*. Use of 5-flurodeoxyuridine (FudR) as an adjuvant to the surgical management of carcinoma of the stomach. Cancer 24:23;1969.

108. Shiu, M.H.; Moore, E.; Sanders, M. *et al*. Influence of the extent of resection on survival of the curative treatment of gastric carcinoma. Arch. Surg. 122:1347-1351; 1987.

109. Shiu, M.H.; Nisce, L.Z.; Pinna, A.; Straus, D.J., Tome, M.; Filippa, D.A.; Lee, B.J. Recent results of multimodal therapy of gastric lymphoma. Cancer 58:1389-1399; 1986.

110. Sindelar, W.F. Intraoperative radiotherapy in carcinoma of the stomach and pancreas. Recent Results in Cancer Research 110:226-243; 1988.

110'. Smalley S.R., Gunderson L.L. Stomach. In: Perez CA, Brady LW (eds). Principles and Practice of Oncology (2nd ed). Philadelphia, PA: JB Lippincott Co; 1992; pp 970-984.

110a. Sugarbaker, P.H. Early postoperative intraperitoneal adriamycin as an adjuvant treatment for advanced gastric cancer with lymph node or serosal invasion. In: Sugarbaker PH (ed.) Management of Gastric Cancer. Boston, MA: Kluwer Academic Publishers; 1991; pp 277-284.

111. Wilke H, Preusser P, Fink U, *et al.* Preoperative chemotherapy in locally advanced and nonresectable gastric cancer: A phase II study with Etoposide, Doxorubicin, and Cisplatin. J Clin Oncol 7:1318-1326; 1989.

111a. Wilke H, Preusser P, Fink U, *et al.* New developments in the treatment of gastric carcinoma. Seminars in Oncology 17:1(S2), 61-70; 1990.

111b. Wils JA, Klein HO, Wagener DJ Th, *et al.* Sequential high-dose methotrexate and fluorouracil combined with doxorubicin — A step ahead in the treatment of advanced gastric cancer: A trial of the European Organization for Research and Treatment of Cancer Gastrointestinal Tract Cooperative Group. J Clin Oncol 9:827-831; 1991.

111c. Witzig TE, Loprinzi CL, Gonchoroff NJ, *et al.* DNA ploidy and cell kinetic measurements as predictors of recurrence and survival in stages B₂ and C colorectal adenocarcinoma. Cancer 68:879; 1991.

112. Wong, W.S.; Goldberg, H.I. Gastric Small Bowel and Colorectal Cancer. In: Oncologic Imaging. Bragg, D.G.; Rubin, P.; Youker, J.E. eds.New York, NY: Pergamon Press; 1985.

Small Intestine

113. Ashley, S.W., Wills, Jr, S.A. Tumor of the Small Intestine. Semin. Oncol. 15(2): 116-128; 1989.

114. Dial, P., Cohn, Jr, I. Tumors of the Jejunum and Ileum. In: Scott, Jr, H.W., Sawyers, J.L. eds. Surgery of the Stomach, Duodenum and Small Intestine. Boston,MA: Blackwell Scientific Publications; 937-951: 1987.

115. Garvin, P.J.; Herrman, V.; Kaminski, D.L. *et al.* Benign and malignant tumors of the small intestine. Curr. Publ. Cancer 3(3): 1-46; 1979.

116. Marks, C. Carcinoid tumors. A clinicopathologic study. Boston,MA: GK Hall;1979: 1-154.

117. River, L.; Silverstein,J.; Tope, J.W. Collective review. Benign neoplasms of the small intestine. Critical comprehensive review with reports of 20 new cases. Intl. Abstr. Surg. 102:1-38; 1956.

118. Sidelar, W.F. Cancer of the Small Intestine. In: DeVita ,Jr ,V.T., Hellman ,S., Rosenberg,S.A. eds. Cancer, Principles and Practice of Oncology, 3rd edition, Philadelphia,PA: JB Lippincott Co; 1989: 875-894.

119. Tarayi, R.Y.; Hermann, R.E.; Vogt, O.P. *et al.* Results of surgical treatment of periampullary tumor: A thirty-five year experience. Surgery 100: 716-722; 1986.

Colorectal Cancer

120. Atliych, F.F.; Stearns, M.W. Second-look laparotomy based on CEA elevation in colorectal cancer. Cancer 47: 2119-2125;1981.

121. Balslev, I.; Pedersen, M.; Teglbjaerg, P. *et al.* Postoperative radiotherapy in Dukes' B and C carcinoma of the rectum and rectosigmoid. Cancer 58:22-28; 1986.

122. Beahrs, O.H., Higgins, G.A., Weinstein, J.J. Colorectal Tumors. Philadelphia,PA: JB Lippincott Co; 1986.

122a. Beart RW, Moertel CG, Wieand HS, *et al.* Adjuvant therapy for resectable colorectal carcinoma with fluorouracil administered by portal vein infusion. A study of the Mayo Clinic and the North Central Cancer Treatment Group. Arch Surg 125(7):897-901; 1990.

123. Beynon, J. An evaluation of the role of rectal endosonography in rectal cancer. Ann. R. Coll. Surg. Engl. 71: 131-139; 1989.

124. Blumberg, N. *et al.* Association between transfusion of whole blood and recurrence of cancer. Br. J. Med. 293: 530-533; 1986.

124a. Burt CA. Carcinoma of the ovaries secondary to cancer of the colon and rectum. Dis Colon Rectum 3:352-357; 1960.

125. Bussey, H.J.R. Familial Polyposis Coli. Family Studies, Histopathology, Differential Diagnosis, and Results of Treatment. Baltimore, MD: Johns Hopkins Univ Press; 1975.

126. Buyse, M.; Zeleniuch-Jacquotte, A.; Chalmers, T.C. Adjuvant therapy of colorectal cancer. Why we still don't know. JAMA 259: 3571-3578; 1988.

127. Cannon-Albright, L.A.; Skolnick, M.H.; Bishop, D.T.; Lee, R.G.; Burt, R.D. Common inheritance of susceptibility to colonic adenomatous polyps and associated colorectal cancers. N.Eng. J. Med. 319: 533-537; 1988.

128. Cass, A.W.; Million, R.R.; Pfaff, W.W. Patterns of recurrence following surgery alone for adenocarcinoma of the colon and rectum. Cancer 37: 2861-2865; 1976.

129. Chlebowski, R.T.; Nystrom, S.; Reynolds, R. *et al.* Long-term survival following Levamisole or placebo adjuvant treatment of colorectal cancer. Oncology 45:141-143; 1988.

129a. Cohen, M., Shank, B., Friedman, M.A. Colerectal Cancer. In: DeVita VT, Hellman S, Rosenberg SA (eds). Principles and Practice of Oncology. Philadelphia, PA: JB Lippincott Co; 1989; pp 895-964.

129b. Colorectal Cancer. Part I. Kane MJ (ed). Semin Oncol 18(4); 1991.

129c. Colorectal Cancer. Part II. Kane MJ (ed). Semin Oncol 18(5); 1991.

130. Corman ML: Colon and Rectal Surgery (2nd ed). Philadelphia, PA: JB Lippincott; 1989, pp 387-468.

131. Cotait, R., Lesser, M.C., Enker, W.E. Prophylactic Oophorectomy in surgery for large bowel cancer. Dis Colon Rectum 26: 6-11; 1983.

132. Cummings, B.J. Radiation therapy and rectal carcinoma: The Princess Margaret Hospital experience. Br. J. Surg. 72 (suppl): 64-65; 1985.

133. Curley, S.A.; Roh, M.S.; Rich, T.A. Surgical therapy of early rectal carcinoma. Hematol. Oncol. Clin. North Am. 3: 87-102; 1989.

134. Dent, T.L.; Kukora, J.S.; Buinewicz, B.R. Endoscopic screening and surveillance for gastrointestinal malignancy. Surg. Clin. N. Am. 69:1205-1225; 1989.

135. Devereux, D.F.; Eisenstat, T.; Zinkin, L. The safe and effective use of postoperative radiation therapy in modified Astler Coller stage C3 rectal cancer. Cancer 63: 2393-2396; 1989.

136. Einhorn, L.H. Improvement in Fluorouracil chemotherapy. J. Clin. Oncol. 7:1377-1379; 1989.

137. Enker, W.E.; Laffer, V.T.; Block, G.E. Enhanced survival of patients with colon and rectal cancer is based upon wide anatomic resection. Ann. Surg. 190:350-360;1979.

137a. Eisenberg, B.; DeCosse, J.J.; Harford, F. *et al.* Carcinoma of the colon and rectum: The natural history reviewed in 1704 patients. Cancer 49:1131-1134;1982.

138. Erlichman, C.; Fine, S.; Wong, A. *et al.* A randomized trial of Fluorouracil and folinic acid in patients with metastatic colorectal carcinoma. J. Clin. Oncol. 6:469-475; 1988.

138a. Escudero-Fabre, A.; Sack, J. Endoscopic laser therapy for neoplastic lesions of the colorectum. Am Journal Surg. 163:260-262;1992.

139. Falkson, G.; Falkson, H.C. 5-FU, Methyl CCNU, and Vincristine in cancer of the colon. Cancer 38:1368-1470; 1976.

140. Fenoglio-Preiser, C.M.; Hutter, R.V.P. Colorectal polyps: Pathologic diagnosis and clinical significance. CA 35: 322-344; 1985.

141. Fisher, B.; Wolmark, N.; Rockette *et al.* Postoperative adjuvant chemotherapy or radiation therapy for rectal cancer: Results from NSABP protocol R-01. JNCI 80: 21-29; 1988.

142. Fleischer, D.E.; Goldberg, S.B.; Browning, T.H. *et al.* Detection and surveillance of colorectal cancer. JAMA 261: 580-586;1989.

143. Flody, C.E.; Conley, R.G.; Cohen, I. Local recurrence of carcinoma of the colon and rectum. Am. J. Surg. 109:153; 1965.

143a. Galandiuk, S.; Wieand, H.S.; Moertel, C.G. *et al.* Patterns of recurrence after curative resection of carcinoma of the colon and recum. Surg. Gyn and Obstet. 174:27-32;1992.

144. Gastrointestinal Tumor Study Group: Adjuvant therapy of colon cancer: Results of a prospectively ranodmized trial. N. Engl. J. Med. 310:737-743;1984.

145. Gastrointestinal Tumor Study Group: The Modulation of 5-Fluorouracil with folinic acid (Leucokvorin) in metastatic colorectal carcinoma: A prospective randomized phase III trial. J. Clin. Oncol. 7:1419-426; 1989.

146. Gastrointestinal Tumor Study Group: Prolongation of the disease-free interval in surgically treated rectal carcinoma. N. Engl. J. Med. 312: 1465-1472; 1985.

147. Gastrointestinal Tumor Study Group: Survival after postoperative combination treatment for rectal cancer. N. Engl. J. Med. 314: 1294-1295; 1986.

148. Gerard, A.; Buyse, M.; Nordlinger, B.; Loygue, J. *et al.* Preopoerative radiotherapy as adjuvant treatment in rectal cancer. Ann. Surg. 208: 606-614; 1988.

149. Goldberg SM, Nivatvongs, Rothenberger DA. Colon, rectum and anus. In: Schwartz SI, Shires GT, Spenser FC (eds). Principles of

Surgery, ed 5. New York, NY: McGraw-Hill; 1989; pp 1225-1314.

150. Gunderson, L.L. Combined-treatment approaches in the management of rectal cancer. Recent Results in Cancer Res. 110:119-129; 1988.

151. Gunderson, L.L.; Russell, A.H.; Llewellyn, H.J.; Doppke, K.P.; Tepper, J.E. Treatment planning for colorectal cancer: Radiation and surgical techniques and value of small-bowel films. Int. J. Radiat. Oncol. Biol. Phys. 11:1379-1393; 1985.

152. Gunderson, L.L.; Sosin, H.; Levitt, S. Extrapelvic Colon - Areas of failure in a reoperation series: Implications for Adjuvant Therapy. Int. J. Radiat. Oncol. Biol. Phys. 11: 731-741; 1985.

152a. Higgins, G.A.; Amadeo, J.H.; McElhinney, J. et al. Efficacy of prolonged intermittent therapy with combined 5-fluorouracil and me-CCNU following resection for carcinoma of the large bowel. Cancer 53:1-8;1984.

153. Higgins, G.A.; Humphrey, E.W.; Dwight, R.W.; Roswit, B. et al. Preoperative radiation and surgery for cancer of the rectum: Veterans Administration Surgical Oncology Group trial II. Cancer 58:352-359; 1986.

154. Higgins, G.A. Jr ; Humphrey, E.; Juler, G.L. et al. Adjuvant chemotherapy in the surgical treatment of large bowel cancer. Cancer 38:1461-1467; 1976.

155. Houghton, J.A.; Maroda, S.J.; Phillips, J.O. et al. Biochemical determination of responsiveness to 5-Fluorouracil and its derivatives in xenographs of human colorectal adenocarcinoma in mice. Cancer Res. 41:144-149; 1981.

156. Kaufman, S.K.; Deckers, P.J., Gunderson, L.L, Cancer of the Colon and Rectum. In: Cancer: A Manual for Practitioners, ed. 5, Boston, MA: American Cancer Society; 1978:183-191.

157. Kelvin ,G.M. Radiologic approach to the detection of colorectal neoplasia. Radiol. Clin. N. Am. 20:743-759; 1982.

158. Keyomarsi, K.; Moran, R.G. Folinic acid augmentation of the effects of fluoropyrimidines on murine and human leukemic cells. Cancer Res. 46:5229-5235; 1986.

159. Kodner, I.J.; Shemash, E.I.; Fry, R.D.; Walz, B.J. et al. Preoperative irradiation for rectal cancer. Ann. Surg. 209:194-199; 1989.

160. Kopelson, G. Adjuvant postoperative radiaion therapy for colorectal carcinoama above the peritoneal reflection. I. Sigmoid colon. Cancer 51:1593-1598; 1983.

161. Krasna, M.J.; Glancbaum, L.; Cody, R.P.; Shneibaum, S.; Ari, G.B. Vascular and neural Invasion in colorectal carcinoma. Incidence and prognostic significance. Cancer 61:1018-1023; 1988.

162. Krook, J.; Moertel, C.; Gunderson, L.L. et al. Effective surgical adjuvant therapy for high-risk rectal carcinoma. N. Engl. J. Med. 324:709-715; 1991.

163. Laurie, J.A.; Moertel, C.G.; Fleming, T.R.; Wieand, H.S.; Leigh, J.E.; Rubin, J.; McCormich, G.W.; Gerstner, J.B.; KrkookJ.E.; Malliard, J.; Twito, D.I.; Morton, R.F.; Tschetter, L.K.; Barlow, J.F. Surgical adjuvant therapy of large-bowel carcinoma: An evaluation of Levamisole and the combination of Levamisole and Fluorouracil: the North Central Cancer Treatment Group and the Mayo Clinic. J. Clin. Oncol. 7: 1447-1456; 1989.

163a. Laurie, J.; Moertel, C.; Flemming, T. et al. Surgical adjuvant therapy of poor prognosis colorectal cancer with Levamisole alone or combined Levamisole and 5-Fluorouracil: A North Central Cancer Treatment Group and Mayo Clinic Study (Abstract). Proc. Am. Soc. Clin. Oncol. 5:81;1986.

164. Lavery, I.C.; Jones, I.T.; Weakley, F.L.; Saxton, J.P. et al. Definitive management of rectal cancer by contact (endocavitary) irradiation. Dis. Colon Rectum 30:835-838; 1987.

165. Lavin, P.; Mittelman, A.; Douglas, H. et al. Survival and response to chemotherapy for advanced colorectal carcinoma. An Eastern Cooperative Oncology Group report. Cancer 46:1536-1543;1980.

166. Leaming, R. Radiation Therapy in the Clinical Management of Neoplasm of the Colon, Rectum and Anus. In: Stearns, M.W. ed. Neoplasms of the Colon, Rectum and Anus. New York, NY: John Wiley and Sons:143-153.

167. Li ,M.C.; Ross, S.T. Chemoprophylaxis for patients with colorectal cancer. Prospective study with 5-year follow-up. J. Am. Med. Assoc. 235:2825-2828; 1976.

167a. Marsh, J.C.; Bertino, J.R.; Katz, K.H.; et al. Influence of drug interval on the effect of methotrexate and fluorouracil in the treatment of advanced colorectal cancer. J Clin Oncol 9:371-380; 1991.

167b. Martenson, J.A. Jr; Gunderson, L.L. Colon and rectum. In: Perez C.A., Brady L.W. (eds). Principles and Practice of Radiation Oncology (2nd ed). Philadelphia, PA: JB Lippincott Co; 1992; pp 1000-1014.

168. Martin, E.W.; Cooperman, M.; Carey, L.C. et al. A retrospective and prospective study of several CEA determinations in early detection of recurrent colorectal cancer. Am. J. Surg. 137: 167-169; 1979.

169. Martin, E.W.; Minton, J.P.; Carey, L.C. CEA-directed second-look surgery in the asymnptomatic patient after primary resection of colorectal carcinoma. Ann. Surg. 202: 310-317; 1985.

170. McDermott, F.T. Carcinoma of the Colon. In: Hughes, E., Cuthbertson, A.M., Killingback, M.K. eds. Colorectal Surgery. New York, NY: Churchill Livingstone; 1983:382-412.

171. McDermott, F.T. Carcinoma of the Rectum. In: Hughes, E., Cuthbertson, A.M., Killingback, M.K. eds. Colorectal Surgery. New York, NY: Churchill Livingston;1983: 347-381.

171a. McDermott, F.T.; Hughes, E.S.R.; Paihl, E. et al. Prognosis in relation to symptom duration in colon cancer. Br. J. Surg. 68:846-849;1981.

172. Minsky, C.D. et al. Potentially curative surgery of colon cancer: The influence of blood vessel invasion. J. Clin. Oncol. 6:119-127;1988.

172a. Minsky, B.D.; Mies, C.; Rich, T.A. et al. Colloid carcinoma of the colon and rectum. Cancer. 60:3103-3112;1987.

173. Minsky, B.D.; Mies, C.; Rich, T.A.; Techt, A.; Chaffey, J.T. Potentially curative surgery of colon cancer: Patterns of failure and survival. J. Clin. Oncol. 6: 106-118; 1988.

174. Moertel, C.G. Chemotherapy of gastrointestinal cancer. N. Engl. J. Med. 299:1049-1059; 1978.

175. Moertel, C.G.; Fleming, T.R.; MacDonald, J.S.; Haller, D.G.; Laurie, J.A.; Goodman, P.J.; Ungerleider, J.S.; Emerson, W.A.; Tormey, D.C.; Glick J.H.; Veeder, M.H.; Mailliard, J.A. Levamisole and Fluoracil for adjuvant therapy of resected colon cancer. N. Engl. J. Med. 322:352-358; 1990.

176. Moertel, C.G.; Schutt, A.J.; Hahn, R.G. et al. Therapy of advanced colorectal cancer with a combination of 5-FU, Methyl-CCNU, and Vincristine. J. Natl. Cancer Inst. 54:69-71; 1975.

176a. Mohiuddin M, Marks G. High dose preoperative irradiation for cancer of the rectum, 1976-1988. Int J Radiat Oncol Biol Phys 20(1):37-43; 1991.

177. Morgenstern, L.; Lee, S.E. Spatial distribution of colonic carcinoma. Arch. Surg. 113: 1142-1143; 1978.

178. Myers, M.H.; Ries, L.A.G. Cancer patient survival rates: SEER program results for 10 years of follow-up. CA 39: 21-32;1989.

178a. National Institutes of Health: NIH Consensus Conference: Adjuvant therapy for patients with colon and rectal cancer. JAMA 264(11):1444-1450; 1990.

179. Newland, R.C.; Chapuis, P.H.; Smythig, E.J. The prognostic value of substaging colorectal carcinoma. A prospective study of 1117 cases with standardized pathology. Cancer 60:852-857; 1987.

180. O'Connell, M.J.; Gunderson, L.L.; Fleming, T.R. Surgical adjuvant therapy of rectal cancer. Semin. Oncol. 15:138-145; 1988.

180'. O'Connell M, Wieand H, Krook J, et al. Lack of value for methyl-CCNU (MeCCNU) as a component of effective rectal cancer surgical adjuvant therapy: Interim analysis of intergroup protocol 86-47-51. Proc ASCO 10:A-403,134; 1991.

180a. Panettiere, F.J.; Chen, T.T. The SWOG large bowel study benefits from therapy (Abstract). Proc. Am. Soc. Clin. Oncol. 4:76;1985.

180b. Pazdur R, Ajani JA, Patt YZ, et al. Phase II study of fluorouracil and recombinant interferon alfa-2a in the treatment of colorectal carcinoma. Semin Oncol 17(1, suppl 1):16-21; 1990.

180c. Physicians Data Query. Colon cancer. National Cancer Institute, Bethesda, MD: January 1992.

180d. Physicians Data Query. Rectal cancer. National Cancer Institute, Bethesda, MD: January 1992.

181. Poon, M.A.; O'Connell, M.J.; Moertel, C.G. et al. Biochemical modulation of Flourouracil: Evidence of significant improvement of survival and quality of life in advanced colorectal carcinoma. J. Clin. Oncol. 7:1407-1418; 1989.

182. Posey, L.E.; Morgan, L.R. Methyl-CCNU vs. Methyl-CCNU and 5-FU in carcinoma of the large bowel. Cancer Treat. Rep. 61:1453-1458; 1977.

182a. Rao, A.R.; Kagan, A.R.; Chan, P.M. *et al.* Patterns of recurrence following curative resection alone for adenocarcinoma of the rectum and sigmoid colon. Cancer. 48:1492-1495;1981.

183. Rawson, R.W. Colonic polyps: antecedent or associated lesions of large bowel cancer. Semin. Oncol. 3:361-367;1976.

184. Reed, W.P.; Garb, J.L.; Park, W.C.; Stark, A.J. *et al.* Long-term results and complications of preoperative radiation in the treatment of rectal cancer. Surgery 103:161-167; 1988.

184a. Riboli, E.B.; Secco, G.B.; Lapertosa, G. *et al.* Colorectal cancer: Relationship of histologic grading to disease prognosis. Tumori. 69:581-584;1983.

185. Rosemungy, A.S.; Block, G.E.; Shihab, F. Surgical treatment of carcinoma of the abdominal colon. Surg. Gynecol. Obstet. 167:399-405; 1988.

186. Rosen, L.; Veidenheimer, M.C.; Coller, J.A.; Corman ,M.L. Mortality, morbidity and patterns of recurrence after abdomino-perineal resection for cancer of the rectum. Dis. Colon Rectum 25: 202-208;1982.

187. Rosenberg, S.A.; Lotze, M.T.; Yang, J.C.; Aebersold, P.M.; Linehan, W.M.; Seipp, C.A.; White, D.E. Experience with the use of high-dose Interleukin-2 in the treatment of 652 cancer patients. Ann. Surg. 210: 474-84; 1989.

188. Rothenberger, D.A.; Wong, W.D. Rectal cancer — adequacy of surgical management. Surg. Ann. 17:309-331; 1985.

189. Rousselot, L.M.; Cole, D.R.; Grossi, C.E. *et al.* Adjuvant chemotherapy with 5-Fluorouracil in surgery for colorectal cancer: 8-year progress report. Dis. Colon Rectum 15:169-174; 1972.

190. Russel, A.H.; Tong, D.; Dawson, L.E.; Wisbeck, W. Adenocarcinoma of the proximal colon. Sites of initial dissemination and patterns of recurrence following surgery alone. Cancer 53: 360-657; 1984.

191. Saadia, R.; Schain, M. Local treatment of carcinoma of the rectum. Surg. Gynecol. Obstet. 166:481-486; 1988.

191a. Scheele J, Stangl R, Altendorf-Hofmann A, *et al.* Indicators of prognosis after hepatic resection for colorectal secondaries. Surg 110(1):13-29; 1991.

192. Second Report of an MRC Working Party. The evaluation of low dose preoperative X-ray therapy in the management of operable rectal cancer; results of a randomly controlled trial. Br. J. Surg. 71:21-25; 1984.

193. Seitz, H.K., Simanowski, U.A., Wright, N.A. eds. Colorectal Cancer: From Pathogenesis to Prevention? New York, NY: Springer-Verlag; 1989.

194. Shehata, W.M.; Meyer, R.L.; Jazy, F.K.; Cormier, W.J.; Welling, R.E. Regional adjuvant irradiation for adenocarcinoma of the cecum. Int. J. Radiat. Oncol. Biol. Phys. 13: 843-846; 1987.

195. Sischy, B.; Graney, M.J.; Hinson, E.J. Endocavitary irradiation for adenocarcinoma of the rectum. CA 34:333-339; 1984.

195a. Slanetz, C.A. Jr.; Herter, F.P.; Grinnell, R.S. Anterior resection versus abdominoperineal resection for cancer of the rectum and rectosigmoid. Am. J. Surg. 123:110-117;1972.

195b. Steele, G.; Bleday, R.; Mayer, R.J. *et al.* A prospective evaluation of hepatic resection for colorectal carcinoma metastases to the liver: Gastrointestinal Tumor Study Group Protocol 6584. J. Clin. Oncol. 9:1105-1112;1991.

195c. Stockholm Rectal Cancer Study Group. Preoperative short-term radiation therapy in operable rectal carcinoma. Cancer 66:49; 1990.

196. Sugarbaker, P.H. Role of carcinoembryonic antigen assay in the management of cancer. Adv. Immunity Cancer Therapy 1: 167-193; 1985.

197. Sugarbaker, P.H.; Gunderson, L.L.; Wittes, R.E. Colorectal Cancer. In: DeVita, V.T., Hellman, S., Rosenberg, S.A. eds. Cancer, Principles and Practice of Oncology. Philadelphia, PA: JB Lippincott Co; 1985: 795-884.

197a. Tobin RL, Mohiuddin M, Marks G. Preoperative irradiation for cancer of the rectum with extrarectal fixation. Int J Radiat Oncol Biol Phys 21:1127-1132; 1991.

198. Turner, S.S.; Vieira, E.F.; Ager, P.J.; Alpert, S.; Efron, G.; Ragins, H.; Weil, P.; Ghossein, N.A. Elective postoperative radiotherapy for locally advanced colorectal cancer. A preliminary report. Cancer 40: 105-108; 1977.

199. Twomey, P.; Burchell, M.; Strawn, D.; Guernsey, J. Local control in rectal cancer. A clinical review and meta-analysis. Arch. Surg. 124:1174-1179; 1989.

200. Umpleby, H.C.; Williamson, R.C.W. Anatomic recurrence in large bowel cancer. Br. J. Surg. 74:873-878; 1987.

200a. Wadler, S.; Lembersky, B.; Atkins, M.; *et al.* Phase II trial of fluorouracil and recombinant interferonalfa-2a in patients with advanced colorectal carcinoma: An Eastern Cooperative Oncology Group study. 9(10):1806-1810; 1991.

201. Walker, A.R.P.; Burkitt, D.P. Colon cancer: epidemiology. Semin. Oncol. 3:341-350; 1976.

201a. Weaver D, Lindblad AS. Radiation therapy and 5-fluorouracil (5-FU) with or without MeCCNU for the treatment of patients with surgically adjuvant adenocarcinoma of the rectum. Proc ASCO 9:A-409, 106; 1990.

202. Welch, C.E.; Giddings, W.P. Carcinoma of colon and rectum. Observations on Massachusetts General Hospital Cases. N. Engl. J. Med. 244:859-867; 1951.

202a. Willett CG, Shellito PC, Tepper JE, *et al.* Intraoperative electron beam radiation therapy for primary locally advanced rectal and rectosigmoid carcinoma. J Clin Oncol 9:843-849; 1991.

203. Willett, C.G.; Tepper, J.E.; Cohen, A.M.; Orlow, E.; Welch, C.E. Failure patterns following curative resection of colonic carcinoma. Ann. Surg. 200:685-690; 1984.

204. Willett, C.G.; Tepper, J.E.; Skates, S.J. *et al.* Adjuvant postoperative radiation therapy for colonic carcinoma. Ann. Surg. 206: 694; 1987.

205. Williams, L.F.; Huddleston, C.B.; Sawyers, J.L. *et al.* Is total pelvic exenteration reasonable primary treatment for rectal carcinoma? Ann. Surg. 207:670-678; 1988.

206. Williams, N.S. Changing patterns in the treatment of rectal cancer. Br. J. Surg. 76:5-6; 1989.

207. Winawer, S.J.; Miller, D.G.; Sherlock, P. Risk and screening for colorectal cancer. Adv. Int. Med. 30: 471-496; 1984.

207a. Wollmark, N.; Fisher, B.; Rockette, H. Adjuvant Therapy in Carcinoma of the Colon: Five Year Results of NSABP Protocol C-01. In: Salmon, S.E. ed. Adjuvant Therapy of Cancer. New York, NY: Grune & Stratton; 1987: 531-536.

207b. Wollmark N, Rockette H, Wckerman DL, *et al.* Adjuvant therapy of Dukes' A, B, and C adenocarcinoma of the colon with portal-vein fluorouracil hepatic infusion: Preliminary results of National Surgical Adjuvant Breast and Bowel Project Protocol C-02. J Clin Oncol 8(9):1466-1475; 1990.

208. Wooley, P.V. Clinical manifestations of cancer of the colon and rectum. Semin. Oncol. 3: 373-376; 1976.

209. Wynder, E.L.; Reddy, B.S. Dietary fat and liver and colon cancer. Semin. Oncol. 10:264-272; 1983.

Anal Cancer

210. Beahrs, O.H. Management of cancer of the anus. Am. J. Roent 133:791-795; 1979.

211. Boman, B.M.; Moertel, C.G.; O'Connell *et al.* Carcinoma of the anal canal. A clinical and pathologic study of 188 cases. Cancer 54:144-125; 1984.

211'. Cummings, B.J. Anal canal. In: Perez, C.A.; Brady, L.W. (eds). Principles and Practice of Radiation Oncology, 2nd ed. Philadelphia, PA: JB Lippincott Co; 1992:1015-1024.

211a. Cantril, S.T.; Green, J.P.; Schall, G.L. *et al.* Primary radiation therapy in the treatment of anal carcinoma. Int. J. Radiat. Oncol. Biol. Phys. 9:1271-1278;1983.

211b'. Cummings, B.J. Concomitant radiotherapy and chemotherapy for anal cancer. Semin. Oncol. 19(4) (Suppl 11):102-108; 1992.

211b. Cummings BJ. Anal cancer. Int J Radiat Oncol Biol Phys 19(5):1309-1315; 1990.

211c. Cummings, B.; Keane, T.; Thomas, G. *et al.* Results and toxicity of treatment of anal carcinoma by radiation therapy or radiation therapy and chemotherapy. Cancer. 54:2062-2068;1984.

211c'. Cummings BJ, Keane TJ, O'Sullivan B, *et al.* Epidermoid anal cancer: Treatment by radiation alone or by radiation and 5-fluorouracil with and without mitomycin C. Int J Radiat Oncol Bio Phys 21:1115-1126; 1991.

211d. Cummings, B.J.; Harwood, A.R.; Keane, R.J. Anal canal carcinoma: Improving the therapeutic ratio with combined radiation and chemotherapy. Int. J. Radiat. Oncol. Biol. Phys. 9:11;1983.

212. Cummings, B.J. The treatment of anal cancer. Int. J. Radiat. Oncol. Biol. Phys. 17:1359-1361; 1989.

213. Daling, J.R.; Weiss, N.S.; Hislop, T.G. *et al.*: Sexual practices,

sexually tranmitted diseases and the incidence of anal cancer. N. Engl. J. Med. 317: 973-977; 1987.

214. Denecke, H.; Roloff, R. Preoperative radio-chemotherapy in anal carcinoma. Recent Results in Cancer Res. 110: 134-139; 1988.

215. Doggett, S.W.; Green, J.P.; Cantril, S.T. Efficacy of radiation therapy alone for limited squamous cell carcimoma of the anal canal. Int. J. Radiat. Oncol. Biol. Phys. 15: 1069-1072; 1988.

215a. Eschwege, F.; Lasser, P.; Chavy, A. *et al.* Squamous cell carcinoma of the anal canal. Treatment by external beam irradiation. Radiother. Oncol. 3:145-150; 1985.

215a'. Flam MS, John MJ, Mowry PA, *et al.* Definitive combined modality therapy of carcinoma of the anus. Dis Colon Rectum 30:495-502; 1987.

215b. John, M; Flam, M.; Lovalva, L. *et al.* Feasibility of nonsurgical definitive management of anal canal carcinoma. Int. J. Radiat. Oncol. Biol. Phys. 13:299-303;1987.

215b'. Leichman L, Nigro N, Vaitkevicius VK, *et al.* Cancer of the anal canal: Model for preoperative adjuvant combined modality therapy. Am J Med 76:211-215; 1985.

215c. Michaelson, R.; Magell, G.; Quan, S. *et al.* Preoperative chemotherapy and radiation therapy in the management of anal canal epidermoid carcinoma. Cancer. 51:390-395;1983.

216. Mitchell EP: Carcimoma of the anal region. Semin. Oncol. 15: 146-153; 1988.

217. Nigro, N.D. An evaluation of combined therapy for squamous cell cancer of the anal canal. Dis. Col. Rect. 27:763-766; 1984.

218. Nigro, N.D.; Vaitkevicus, V.K.; Considine, B. Combined therapy for cancer of the anal canal: A preliminary report. Dis. Col. Rect. 17: 354-356; 1974.

218'. Papillon J, Montbarbon J. Epidermoid carcinoma of the anal canal. A series of 276 cases. Dis Colon Rectum 30:324-333; 1987.

218a. Peters, R.K.; Mack, T.M. Patterns of anal carcinoma by gender and marital status in Los Angeles County. Br. J. Cancer. 48:629-636;1982.

218b. Physicians Data Query. Anal cancer. National Cancer Institute, Bethesda, MD: January 1992.

219. Pyper, P.C.; Parks, T.G. The results of surgery for epidermoid carcinoma of the anus. Br. J. Surg. 72:712-714; 1985.

219a. Rotman, M.; Hassan, A. Concomitant continuous infusion chemotherapy and radiation. Cancer. 65:823-825;1990.

219b. Salmon, R.J.; Fenton, J.; Asselain, B. *et al.* Treatment of epidermoid anal cancer. Am. J. Surg. 147:43-48;1984.

220. Schlienger, M.; Krzisch, C.; Pene, F. *et al.* Epidermoid carcinoma of the anal canal: Treatment results and prognostic variables in a series of 242 cases. Int. J. Radiat. Oncol. Biol. Phys. 17:1141-1151; 1989.

220'. Shank, B.; Cohen, A.M.; Kelsen, D. Cancer of the anal region. In: DeVita VT, Hellman S, Rosenberg SA (eds). Principles and Practice of Oncology (3rd ed). Philadelphia, PA: JB Lippincott Co; 1989; pp 965-978.

220a. Sischy, B. The use of radiation therapy combined with chemotherapy in the management of squamous cell carcinoma of the anus and marginally resectable adenocarcinoma of the rectum. Int. J. Radiat. Oncol. Biol. Phys. 11:1587-1593;1985.

221. Sischy, B.; Doggett, R.L.; Krall, J.M. *et al.* Definitive irradiation and chemotherapy for radiosensitzation in management of anal carcinoma: Interim report on Radiation Therapy Oncology Group study No. 8314. J. Natl Cancer Inst. 81: 850-856; 1989.

222. Zucali, R.; Doci, R.; Bombelli, L. Combined chemotherapy-radiotherapy of anal cancer. Int J Radiat Oncol Biol Phys. 19(5):1221-1223; 1990.

James W. Keller, M.D., Radiation Oncology
James L. Peacock, M.D., Surgical Oncology

Julia L. Smith, M.D., Medical Oncology

Chapter **29**

CANCER OF THE MAJOR DIGESTIVE GLANDS:
PANCREAS, LIVER, BILE DUCTS, GALLBLADDER

"It usually requires a considerable time to determine with certainty the virtues of a new method of treatment and usually still longer to ascertain the harmful effects."

Alfred Black (7)

PERSPECTIVE

Cancer of the pancreas is the most common cancer of the major digestive glands in the United States, the other sites are affected much less frequently. They have in common a propensity for advanced stage at presentation. Our ability to image these tumors has been refined and improved over the past decade, as has the technique for histopathologic diagnosis using fine needle aspirates. Epidemiologic studies have not been clinically useful in identifying high-risk groups for close surveillance, except in hepatic cancer, and new markers for these cancers have not been found. Recent treatment strategies have included combined modality therapy, but in most cases a significant survival advantage has not been realized. Thus our ability to diagnose early has not occurred, our treatment has not improved, and overall prognosis has remained gloomy.

PANCREATIC CANCER

Epidemiology (11a)

In the United States it is projected that 28,300 new cases of pancreatic carcinoma will be diagnosed in 1992 or about 10 cases per 10,000 population, with an almost equal sex distribution. The incidence has gradually risen, and currently this cancer is the fourth leading cause of cancer deaths in this country; in 1992 25,000 deaths are expected. The incidence:death ratio is almost equal and relates to its almost uniform fatal outcome. It is rare before aged 40 years and the majority of cases occur between aged 60 and 80 years.

Etiology (9,11,17,39)

There is no known cause for this disease, and in pancreatic cancer there are few clues. No particular chemical carcinogens have been implicated. Smokers have a higher than expected incidence of this cancer, but it does not approach that of lung cancer. A questionable association with coffee drinking has been made (26). Alcohol, diabetes mellitus, tea, and pancreatitis are not associated.

Clinical Detection (10)

Unfortunately this cancer is invariably diagnosed when it is advanced because of the lack of specific symptoms or signs. The insidious onset of abdominal or back pain, anorexia, early satiety, weight loss, dyspepsia, weakness, fatigue, bloating, nausea, and vomiting are the most common symptoms. New-onset hyperglycemia without a family history of diabetes mellitus could be a clue. Back pain that characteristically worsens when lying flat or stretching the back occurs in about 25% of cases and is related to the retroperitoneal location of the gland; this occurs more with lesions in the body of the gland. If the cancer is located in the head of the pancreas, signs of obstructive jaundice will predominate. If the periampullary region or duodenum is involved, gastrointestinal (GI) bleeding may be noted. Lesions in the tail of the gland often go undiagnosed until there are advanced locoregional extensions or distant metastases. Less common presentations include psychiatric disturbances (e.g., depression) and migratory thrombophlebitis or thromboembolic phenomenon.

Physical signs of pancreatic cancer may include weight loss, jaundice, abdominal mass, epigastric tenderness, palpable gallbladder, and hepatomegaly; at least half of the patients have no physical findings. Metastatic signs include supraclavicular adenopathy (Virchow's nodule), umbilical nodule (Sister Joseph's Node), or peritoneal shelf on rectal exam (Blumer's shelf).

Diagnostic Procedures (Table 29-1) (1a)

Diagnosis requires a biopsy of the pancreas or peripancreatic area demonstrating a carcinoma of ductal origin. Frequently, however, the diagnosis is made indirectly by a biopsy of a metastatic site that reveals a histology compatible with pancreatic origin, and a constellation of other findings that includes: (a) appropriate presentation for pancreatic carcinoma; (b) a mass in the pancreas detected on ultrasound, computed tomography (CT), magnetic resonance imaging (MRI), or endoscopic retrograde cholangiopancreatography (ERCP) (Table 29-1); and (c) absence of another primary.

Table 29-1. Imaging Modalities for Evaluating Carcinoma of the Pancreas

METHOD	DIAGNOSIS AND STAGING CAPABILITY	RECOMMENDED FOR USE
Primary tumor and regional nodes		
CT	Most useful and beneficial of all imaging modalities in determining local invasion and distant metastases.	Yes
MRI	Morphological imaging of pancreas and peripancreatic tissues for local as well as distant metastases. Additional diagnostic information may be present with tissue-specific MRI variables.	Yes
ERCP/PTC	Very accurate in defining deformity of bile and pancreatic duct and localizing site of obstruction. May be useful in the jaundiced patient or the patient with diagnostic uncertainty or questionable diagnosis.	No
Barium - upper gastrointestinal	Useful to define effect on stomach and duodenum. Helpful to rule out other causes of upper gastrointestinal symptoms such as ulcer disease.	Yes
Upper abdominal ultrasound	Useful for evaluating suspected abdominal metastases, especially hepatic metastases. May be helpful in defining the primary tumor as well as evaluating for dilated bile ducts and ascites.	Yes
Metastatic Tumors		
Chest roentgenograms	Good for detecting pulmonary parenchymal metastases, which are generally late and usually seen only terminally.	Yes
Bone roentgenograms	Useful to confirm the uncommon bone metastasis.	No
Radionuclide studies (liver spleen scan)	May be useful in evaluating clinically suspected hepatic metastasis.	No (selected cases only)

CT = computed tomography; MRI = magnetic resonance imaging; ERCP /PTC = endoscopic retrograde cholangiopancreatography/transhepatic cholangiography.
From Bragg et al. (1a), with permission.

Tissue or cells for cytology for diagnosis are obtained from duodenal drainage, ERCP or fine needle aspirates under ultrasound or CT guidance. It is of interest that from 1% to 57% of cases in some series do not have histologic proof of cancer (22). The reasons for this are varied, but surgeons have been reluctant to perform operative pancreatic wedge or needle biopsies of the pancreas directly for fear of triggering pancreatitis, intraabdominal hemorrhage, spreading cancer cells, or producing a pancreatic fistula, abscess, or pseudocyst. Operative biopsies are generally reliable in diagnosing carcinoma and complications are low; however, biopsy complications are higher in patients with inflammatory disease. Transduodenal biopsies for lesions of the head of the pancreas are popular and fine needle aspirates are considered safe (8,46).

A variety of diagnostic procedures have been used to diagnose pancreatic cancers; their multiplicity belies the difficulty. However, this has changed recently. Flat films of the abdomen, pancreatic function tests, upper GI series, hypotonic duodenography, and currently available nuclear scans currently are seldom used, nowadays. Ultrasound and CT scans are essentially the gold standards at the moment (43).

Ultrasound

This test is almost invariably used for initial screening of anyone presenting with jaundice, because of its low cost and ready availability. It is 95% accurate in diagnosing obstructive jaundice. However, its accuracy in detecting the site of obstruction falls to 60% to 90%. The presence of abdominal gas limits its accuracy as do residual barium in the bowel, obesity, ascites, and hemoclips. Liver metastases can be detected with this modality.

Computerized Tomography (CT)

This test is the current test of choice for pancreatic carcinoma, and the initial test for suspected carcinoma of the body or tail of the pancreas. It is more reliable (85% to 95% accuracy) than ultrasound in detecting a mass in the gland and in determining the level of obstruction, and is also helpful in determining local and nodal extension and liver metastases. CT-guided fine needle aspirate biopsies can also be performed for histologic confirmation.

The combined use of ultrasound and CT has reduced the percentage of unnecessary laparotomies in this disease in some centers from 28% to 5% and has increased the resectability rate from 5% to 20% (30,44).

Once pancreatic carcinoma is highly suspected, it is usually the surgeon's preference whether percutaneous confirmation will be needed before exploration, and if the tumor is considered operable, whether an angiogram to help delineate the blood supply and anatomy should be done.

Endoscopic Retrograde Cholangiopancreatography (ERCP)

If the patient is jaundiced, and the site of obstruction is not defined, this test is extremely helpful. It allows visualization (and biopsy) of the duodenum and Vater's ampulla, as well as visualization (and cytology) of both the pancreatic and bile duct ,which could be important for resection.

MRI

The role of this modality is yet to be defined.

Laparoscopy

This procedure has been used in some centers to determine resectability, but it has not been popular in the United States (39).

Laparotomy

This strategy is used frequently (approximately 80% of cases) if the patient is considered resectable and a diagnosis has not been established. If resectability is not possible, then bilioenteric and gastroenteric bypass is often performed.

CLASSIFICATION AND STAGING

Histopathology (5,12,39) (Table 29-2)

The most common pancreatic carcinoma is the solid adenocarcinoma that arises from the ductal epithelial cells. Other exocrine varieties are rare and include acinar cell adenocarcinomas, cystadenocarcinomas, anaplastic, and squamous cell carcinomas. Cancers of the pancreas may also arise from endocrine or islet cell components of the gland (see below).

The cancer is situated in the head of the gland approximately 50% to 60% of the time and the remaining are distributed evenly in the body and tail or some combination of sites. Lesions of the head average 5 cm in diameter at diagnosis, while tail and body lesions are 10 cm; which speaks to the latter's worse prognosis. Unfortunately more than 80% of cases are found to have extension outside the gland at diagnosis. Direct extension to the duodenum, stomach, retroperitoneum (especially body and tail), and portal vein is

Table 29-2. Histological Classification of Carcinoma of the Pancreas	
Malignant	**Incidence (%)**
Adenocarcinoma	80
Squamous cell carcinoma	4
Cystadenocarcinoma	4
Acinar cell carcinoma	4
Undifferentiated carcinoma	4

common, as is local lymph node and para-aortic nodal metastases. Liver metastases are also frequent. Distant metastases to lung, brain, bone, and other sites occur; indeed there are few distant sites where it has not been described.

Staging Work-up (Table 29-3, Fig. 29-1)

Physical examination is essential with emphasis on sites of metastases or local extension: abdominal mass, hepatomegaly, palpable gallbladder, supraclavicular adenopathy, rectal shelf, and umbilical nodule.

Laboratory tests must include complete blood cell counts (CBC) with differential, and platelet count, liver enzyme tests, creatinine and blood urea nitrogen (BUN), glucose, as are coagulation tests, calcium and electrolytes measurements. These tests determine if the patient has any medical contraindications for surgery and evaluate for paraneoplastic manifestation. There are no good markers for pancreatic cancer.

Special Tests: As mentioned above, ultrasound and CT are performed on almost all patients. Other specialized tests, including fine needle aspirate biopsy of the pancreas or metastatic sites. ERCP and angiography are performed depending on the clinical presentation, possibility of resection, and judgment of the surgeon. Chest x-ray is indicated.

Surgical exploration is performed in 80% of cases to either establish the diagnosis, define disease extent, or perform bypass surgery or definitive resection (22).

Table 29-3. TN Classification and Stage Grouping for Carcinoma of the Pancreas		
TN Classification		
EXOCRINE PANCREAS		**AMPULLA OF VATER**
T1 Tumor limited to the pancreas	**T1**	Tumor limited to ampulla of Vater
T1a Tumor 2 cm or less in greatest dimension	**T2**	Tumor invades duodenal wall
T1b Tumor more than 2 cm in greatest dimension	**T3**	Tumor invades 2 cm or less into pancreas
T2 Tumor extends directly to the duodenum, bile duct, or peripancreatic tissues	**T4**	Tumor invades more than 2.0 cm into pancreas and/or into other adjacent organs
T3 Tumor extends directly to the stomach, spleen, colon, or adjacent large vessels		
N1 Regional lymph node metastasis	**N1**	Regional lymph node metastasis

STAGE GROUPING FOR CARCINOMA OF THE PANCREAS

Stage I	T1, N0, M0
	T2, N0, M0
Stage II	T3, N0, M0
Stage III	Any T, N1, M0
Stage IV	Any T, Any N, M1

T = tumor; N = node; M = metastasis.

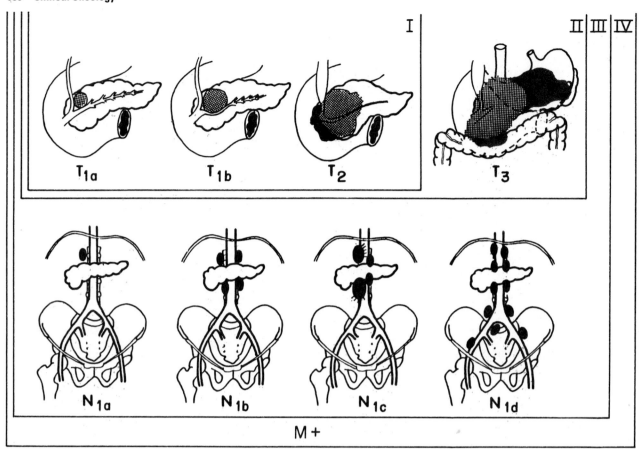

Fig. 29-1. Anatomic staging for cancer of the pancreas.

PRINCIPLES OF TREATMENT (Table 29-4)

A multidisciplinary approach is essential. Table 29-4 summarizes treatment options.

Surgery

Surgery is the only known curative modality, but even with surgery cure is very infrequent. The percentage of cases resectable for cure and resectable technically with minor local extension is about 5% to 15% depending on the experience and enthusiasms of the surgeon. A large retrospective analysis of approximately 2,300 patients found only 92 survivors, and four of these did not have surgery (22). In general, 20% of patients will be inoperable at presentation, and another 25% will have a laparotomy with biopsy only. Approximately 40% will be explored and undergo some type of palliative bypass procedure, and only 15% will be resected for cure.

The standard operation for lesions in the tail of body or the gland is a partial pancreatectomy. For lesions in the head a pancreaticoduodenostomy or Whipple procedure is standard (47). This operation consists of en bloc removal of the duodenum, head of pancreas, distal portion of the common duct, and distal stomach with the pylorus. The gastric pouch

Table 29- 4. Multidisciplinary Treatment Decisions: Pancreas   (3,6,36a)

Stage	Surgery		Radiation Therapy	Chemotherapy
Localized T_1, T_2, N_1	Whipple procedure	or	DRT 65 Gy	N R
Advanced T_3, T_4 N_1	Unresectable		DRT 65 Gy Intraoperative RT High-dose rate brachy therapy	IC II
T_{any} N_{any}, M_+	N R		PRT	IC II

RT = radiation therapy; DRT = definitive; PRT = palliative; N R = not recommended;

IC II = investigational chemotherapy, phase I/II clinical trials.

PDQ: NR

is reanastomosed to the jejunum and the common duct and pancreatic duct are joined to the jejunum proximal to the gastrojejunostomy. The operative mortality with this procedure depends much on the experience of the surgeon and support staff and can be between 5% to 20%. Complications of surgery include hemorrhage, sepsis, and anastomotic leaks. Recent reports, however, document improvements in morbidity and survival (8). Some surgeons prefer a total pancreatectomy for a lesion anywhere in the gland, because it avoids pancreaticojejunal anastomotic problems. Pyloric sparing, if possible, avoids a vagotomy and gastric resection, reduces operating time, and avoids some of the nutritional problems (27). Palliation procedures include biliary-enteric bypass to relieve the jaundice, a gastroenteric bypass if duodenal obstruction exists or likelihood of this happening is high, and celiac axis alcohol or phenol block for pain relief, which is effective in 80% cases. Clips can also be placed around the tumor area for identification, if post-operative radiation therapy is planned (9,10,22).

Radiotherapy

Potentially, radiation therapy could be used in several postoperative settings: (1) adjuvantly when there is no residual disease, but still a high incidence of recurrence; (2) when microscopic or macroscopic disease has been left behind; and (3) when the disease is considered locally unresectable, and there is no evidence of distant metastases. As in other cancers that originate in the abdominal cavity, definitive radiation is made difficult by the tolerance of surrounding normal tissues, such as spinal cord, stomach, liver, small bowel, and kidney. To overcome this problem, external radiation has been combined with intraoperative or interstitial radiation and radiosensitizers (42) and chemotherapy for radiopotentiation.

Randomized studies have been performed in patients with surgically unresectable disease who lack distant metastases. Split course radiation was compared with this same radiation and bolus 5-FU. These studies demonstrated improved survival in the combined modality arm, with medial survival of 37 to 42 weeks versus 23 weeks in the radiation alone arm. A similar study comparing radiation with 5-FU or doxorubicin demonstrated no difference in survival: almost all the patients had died at the time of the report (21,33,34). Postoperative external irradiation, or external and intraoperative or interstitial radiation for unresectable pancreatic carcinoma is not curative, and has not impacted on survival although local control is considered better (14,29,35,37,41). The major problems are locoregional and distant failures (especially the liver). Frequently survival is 40% to 50% at 1 year and 20% at 2 years, and occasionally there are survivors over 5 years.

The Gastrointestinal Study Group performed a study of patients who underwent curative resection and were then randomized between no further therapy versus two courses of 20 Gy split-course irradiation and bolus 5-FU. Of the patients who had curative surgery, essentially 95% of lesions were located in the head of the pancreas (as might be expected), approximately 33% had disease confined to the gland, 40% had contiguous invasion, and 30% had adjacent nodal involvement. Surgery consisted of a Whipple procedure or total pancreatectomy. Median survival was 10.9 months in the control group, and 21 months in the treated group. Two-year survival was 46% for the treated and 18% for the no-further-treatment group (20,28).

Chemotherapy (Table 29-5) (11b)

For adenocarcinoma of the pancreas, a small percentage of patients may have temporary palliation with chemotherapy. Drugs with known activity include 5-FU (26% response), mitomycin (27%), streptozotocin (11%), lomustine (15%), and doxorubicin(8%) (23).

There has been limited success in improving either response rates or survival by use of combination chemotherapy. FAM has yielded response rates as high as 40%, although a confirmatory trial yielded only a 9% response. Combinations of streptozotocin + mitomycin + 5-FU, FAM + streptozotocin, and 5-FU + doxorubicin + cisplatin also give rates ranging from 14% to 43%. Survival is about 5 months in responding patients. Clearly, there is a need for new agents to treat this cancer (23).

Trimodality Therapy

The use of aggressive trimodality therapy in pancreatic cancer has many advocates and shows some promise. Whittington et al. (47a), using 45–48 Gy with 5-FU, present their evidence for favoring infusion over bolus and the use of chemoradiation as an adjuvant to surgery in a consecutive series of patients over a decade. The local control rates for surgery (S) alone, S + 5-FU bolus, and S + 5-FU infusion are 85%, 55%, and 25%, respectively; and 2-year survival rates are 35%, 30%, and 43%, respectively, improved to 41%, 33%, and 59% if surgical resection margins are negative.

Table 29-5. Selected Combination Chemotherapy for Carcinoma of the Pancreas

Common Regimen	Range of Response Rates (%)	Range of Median Survival (wk)
FAM	13-40	12-24
SMF	14-43	13-24
FAC	21	16
FAM-chlorozotocin	13	25
FAM-streptozotocin	18-48	18-22
FAMMe	22	

F = 5-fluorouracil, A = doxorubicin, M = mitomycin-C, S = streptozotocin, Me = semustine, C = cisplatin.
Adapted from Brennan et al. (11b), with permission.

Palliation

As mentioned above, at the time of surgery, biliary enteric or gastroenteric bypass are often performed to relieve obstructive jaundice and actual or imminent duodenal obstruction. Pain has been managed by analgesic pharmacotherapy and celiac plexus blocks are quite effective. Radiation therapy has also helped relieve pain and frequently used for symptomatic metastatic disease (38).

RESULTS

1. Overall 5-year survival is 2 to 5%, with a median survival of 6 months (Tables 29-6 and 29-7) (11b,35a) (Fig. 29-2).
2. Best Results: Approximately 40% of patients whose tumors are confined to the head of the pancreas may be alive at two years, particularly those with T1, N0 tumors (11c).

CLINICAL TRIALS

Clinical trials are evaluating modulated fluorouracil, new anticancer agents, or biologicals (phase I and II) (11d,28a).

ISLET CELL TUMORS

Other tumors of the pancreas include the infrequent islet cell or neuroendocrine tumors. These tumors generally have been recognized by their autonomous secretion of various hormones that originate in the pancreas. However, 15% to 25% are nonfunctioning or have as yet no detectable hormone abnormality (19,45). Fifty percent to 70% of these tumors are considered malignant, based not on their histo-

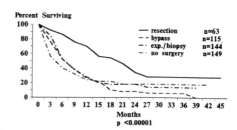

Fig. 29-2. Survival for adenocarcinoma of the pancreas, Memorial Sloan-Kettering Cancer Center, 1983–1987. From Brennan *et al.* (11b), with permission.

logic features, but on metastases outside the pancreas (especially abdominal lymph nodes and liver) (16). Many are associated with an inherited disorder termed multiple endocrine neoplasia syndrome (MEN I) in which in addition to an islet cell tumor there are parathyroid and/or pituitary (especially prolactin) abnormalities. The islet cell tumors most often associated with MEN I are gastrinoma (30%) and insulinoma (20%) (16,25). The tumors for the most part are characterized as slowly progressive.

The number of hormones secreted by these tumors continues to grow and includes: insulin, gastrin, glucagon, somatostatin, pancreatic polypeptide, neurotensin, serotonin, corticotropin, corticotropin-releasing factor, growth hormone, growth hormone releasing hormone (GHRH), thyrocalcitonin, parathyroid hormone, melanocyte stimulating hormone and vasoactive intestinal peptide (45). The most common types include: (1) insulinoma, (2) gastrinoma (Zollinger-Ellison syndrome), (3) nonfunctioning types, (4) watery diarrhea hypokalemia achlorhydria (WDHA, VIPoma, Verner-Morrison syndrome, pancreatic diarrhea), (5) glucagonoma, and (6) somatostatinoma (16,19,25,36).

There is no staging system for these tumors and the treatment is frequently symptomatic, occasionally surgical (especially for insulinomas, but also for tumors localized to the pancreas), and chemotherapy for symptomatic, metastatic disease. In 1989 the Food and Drug Administration approved the drug, octreoide, an analogue of somatostatin which is effective in controlling some of the symptoms of the hormonal excess, e.g., hypoglycemia, diarrhea and nausea

Table 29-6. Results of Pancreatic Resection for Cure of Exocrine Cancer			
Year	No. Patients	Operative Mortality (%)	Mean Survival (mo)
1958-1975	605	5-44	6-23
1976-1982	1502	8-19	9-23
Adapted from Morrow et al. (35a).			

Table 29-7. Selected Two-Drug Combination Chemotherapy in Randomized Trials for Pancreatic Cancer			
Treatment	Number	Objective Response Rate (± 95% CI)*	Median Survival (wk)
5-FU + BCNU†	30	10 (33 ± 9%)	24
5-FU	31	5 (16 ± 7%)	26
BCNU	21	0 (0%)	22
5-FU + streptozotocin	42	5 (12 ± 5%)	16
Streptozotocin - cyclophosphamide	51	6 (12 ± 5%)	9
5-FU + spironolactone	89		18
5-FU + streptozotocin ± spironolactone	87		16
5-FU + mitomycin C	45	10 (22 ± 6%)	19
5-FU + methyl-CCNU	43	2 (5 ± 3%)	17

* 95% confidence interval.
† 5-FU = 5-flourouracil; BCNU = carmustine; methyl-CCNU = semustine.
From Boring, et al. (11a), with permission.

(31,32). The chemotherapy agents used, mainly in some combination, include steptozotocin, doxorubicin, and 5-FU; interferon has also been used (15,32). A discussion of the individual pathophysiology, diagnosis and treatment is beyond the scope of this chapter, and interested readers are referred to the above references.

PRIMARY LIVER (HEPATOCELLULAR) CANCER

Epidemiology

In the United States, about 3000 cases of liver cancer are diagnosed annually (13,40). Most cases occur between the ages of 45 and 60 years, it is uncommon before age 20 in the United States, but not in areas with high incidence. Men are more likely to contract the disease than women. The incidence in the United States has declined by about 50% over the past 50 years but the death rate has remained constant (40,57).

Hepatocellular cancer is the most common cancer among males world wide. In both Nationalist and Communist China, Korea, and Africa below the Sahara, there is a particularly high rate (13,59).

Etiology

There is extensive evidence that hepatitis B surface antigen (HBsAG) plays a role for the majority of cases (13,48,51,59). There is 100 times the carrier rate of HBsAG in sub-Saharan Africa as in the United States. The cancer is more likely to develop in carriers than in noncarriers and middle-aged carriers have a 0.5% incidence of hepatocellular cancer per year (13).

Hepatitis B viral antigens and nucleic acids can be recovered from tissue of hepatocellular carcinoma (68).

In the United States, the correlation is not as close with HBsAG but there is a close correlation with cirrhosis. At autopsy 20% to 40% of cirrhotics have foci of hepatocellular carcinoma and the combination of HBsAG and cirrhosis is synergistic with higher rates of the cancer than either alone

(13). Idiopathic hemochromatosis and other chronic liver diseases have also been linked to this cancer (13,51).

Other etiologic factors include aflatoxins, which are derived from the fungus *Asperigillus flavus* in poorly stored grain crops. The radio-contrast agent Thorotrast is associated with hepatocellular carcinoma and Thorotrast, vinyl chloride, and arsenic are associated with angiosarcomas of the liver (55).

Anabolic steroids have also been associated with hepatocellular cancer (13,51). Oral contraceptives, although known to promote benign adenomas are not convincingly related to hepatocellular cancer (52).

Efforts are under way in parts of China to reduce or eliminate hepatocellular carcinoma by aggressive programs to vaccinate newborns against hepatitis B (13).

DETECTION AND DIAGNOSIS (Table 29-8)

At diagnosis the majority of patients have advanced disease. The presenting symptoms relate to effects of hepatomegaly and ascites and include pain, anorexia, weight loss, malaise, occasionally abdominal mass, and, rarely jaundice. Patients with cirrhosis may have unexplained changes in liver enzymes, clinical deterioration, pain, or fever.

On physical examination there is usually hepatomegaly, right upper quadrant tenderness, occasionally an audible bruit, ascites, and portal hypertension with associated esophageal varices and splenomegaly.

Using a radioimmunoassay technique, 50–70% of American patients with hepatocellular carcinoma have elevated alpha-fetoprotein levels. However, patients with other malignancies (germ cell carcinoma, and rarely pancreatic and gastric carcinoma) also demonstrate elevated serum levels of alpha-fetoprotein (64a). Other prognostic variables include performance status and liver functions (67a).

Imaging studies with ultrasound are highly sensitive for detecting the disease and directing percutaneous fine needle aspirate biopsies. These tumors are hypervascular and biopsy can be associated with bleeding even with normal

Table 29-8. Clinical Features of Hepatocellular Carcinoma in High- and Low-Incidence Areas

Variables	High Incidence	Low Incidence
Geographic location	Asia, Africa	North America, Europe
Race	Asians, blacks	Whites
Median age	Asians, 40-50 yr	50-60 yr
	Blacks, 20-30 yr	
Duration of symptoms	Usually short, especially in young blacks	Can be indolent
Abdominal pain or discomfort	70-90%	50-70%
Anorexia and weight loss	Common	Common
Hemorrhage secondary to ruptured tumor	10-20%	<10%
Cirrhosis	60-80%	60-80%
Cirrhosis evolving to hepatocellar carcinoma	50% or more	5-10%
Type of cirrhosis	Mostly macronodular	Mostly micronodular
Etiology of cirrhosis	HBV probably most important	Often alcohol and HBV
Hepatocellular carcinoma associated with hepatitis B	80% or more	30-50%
Hepatitis B antigen	70-90%	15-40%
Possible exposure to aflatoxin	High	Most unlikely
AFP> 400 ng/ml (radioimmunoassay)	70-85%	30-65%

HBV = hepatitis B virus; AFP = α-fetoprotein.

Table 29-9. Histologic Classification of Malignant Tumors of the Liver

Type of Tumor	% Incidence
Hepatocellular carcinoma (liver cell carcinoma)	70-90
Cholangiocarcinoma (intrahepatic bile duct carcinoma)	5-30
Bile duct cystadenocarcinoma	
Combined hepatocellular and cholangiocarcinoma	<1
Hepatoclastoma	
Undifferentiated carcinoma	

coagulation studies (55). Using alpha-fetoprotein and ultrasound is a sensitive screening system for in high-risk populations (50,66).

Once the diagnosis is suspected, further diagnostic workup is necessary to determine resectability. CT, MRI, and arteriography may be used.

Associated paraneoplastic syndromes include hypoglycemia, erythrocytosis from an erythropoietin-like substance secreted by the tumor, hypercalcemia, and hypercholesterolemia (51).

Histopathology (55)

Cancers of the liver may arise in the parenchymal cells (hepatocellular cancers), or from the intrahepatic bile ducts (cholangiocarcinomas). The bulk of these cancers (70% to 95%) originate in the liver cells, and eight histologic varieties have been described: hepatic, pleomorphic, adenoid or acinar, clear cell, sclerosing, giant cell, fibrolamellar, and mixed (Table 29-9). The remaining cancers (5% to 30%) that arise from the bile duct are adenocarcinomas and they differ from hepatocellular cancers in that sex incidence is equal, patients are usually older than those with hepatocellular cancer, cirrhosis is much less common, and alpha fetoprotein is usually normal. Malignant hemangioendothelioma (angiosarcoma or Kupffer cell sarcoma) is a rare liver malignancy but is an important variant because of its strong association with Thorotrast, arsenic, and vinyl chloride.

Metastatic Spread

Spread occurs by direct extension within the liver and to adjacent organs. It can also spread by lymphatic and vascular invasion to lungs, bone, adrenals, and brain (67).

CLASSIFICATION AND STAGING (Table 29-10, Fig. 29-3)

Anatomic Staging (24)

This system applies to primary hepatocellular and intrahepatic bile duct carcinoma of the liver.

PRINCIPLES OF TREATMENT (Table 29-11)

A multidisciplinary approach is essential. Treatment options are summarized in Table 29-11.

Surgery

Excision of the tumor is the only curative therapy. Concomitant cirrhosis generally precludes surgery because of associated high operative mortality. The noncirrhotic patient must be free of jaundice and ascites and the lesion must be solitary or localized to a single lobe of the liver; there must be no nodal or distant spread (60). The expected 5-year survival is 10%.

Total hepatic lobectomy should be performed. There is an operative mortality of 10% to 20%. The role of liver transplantation in this disease is evolving and fibrolamellar histol-

Table 29-10. TN Classification and Stage Grouping for Carcinoma of Liver

TN Classification		Stage Grouping			
T1	Solitary, ≤ 2 cm, without vascular invasion	Stage I	T1	N0	M0
T2	Solitary, ≤ 2 cm, with vascular invasion	Stage II	T2	N0	M0
	Multiple, one lobe, ≤ 2 cm, without vascular invasion	Stage III	T1	N1	M0
	Solitary, > 2 cm, without vascular invasion		T2	N1	M0
T3	Solitary, > 2 cm, with vascular invasion		T3	N0,N1	M0
	Multiple, one lobe, ≤ 2 cm, with vascular invasion	Stage IVA	T4	Any N	M0
	Multiple, one lobe, > 2 cm, with or without vascular invasion	Stage IVB	Any T	Any N	M1
	Multiple, > one lobe				
T4	Invasion of major branch of portal or hepatic veins				
N1	Regional nodes				
	Solitary, ≤ 2 cm, with vascular invasion				

T = tumor; N = node; M = metastasis.
From AJC (1). with permission.

Table 29-11. Multidisciplinary Treatment Decisions: Liver   (58a*,58b,67)

Stage	Surgery	Radiation Therapy		Chemotherapy
T_{1-3}, N_0	Resection	N R		N R
T_4, N_{any}	Unresectable	External RT Radiolabeled antibodies	and/or	IC I

Multidisciplinary Treatment Decisions: Gallbladder

Stage	Surgery	Radiation Therapy	Chemotherapy
$T_{1,2} N_0$	Resection	N R	N R
$T_3 N_0$	Palliative resection	DRT, intraluminal BRT	IC I
T_4, N_{any}	Unresectable	DRT, intraluminal BRT	

RT = radiation therapy; BRT = brachy; DRT = definitive; N R = not recommended; IC I = investigational chemotherapy, phase I clinical trial.

PDQ: NR

ogy does better (53). Hepatic ligation for palliation is not recommended (49). Cryosurgery may become a useful modality for ablating liver tumors in the near future (58b).

Radiotherapy

The liver does not tolerate so-called definitive doses of external irradiation. The tolerance dose generally accepted is 30 to 35 Gy given in 1.8 to 2.0 Gy fractions; at higher fractions the chance of significant radiation hepatitis in-creases. The radiation injury site is the hepatic venules thus producing a clinical picture similar to the Budd-Chiari syndrome. Hepatic tolerance may be reduced when chemotherapy also is used (63). Thus, it is obvious that external irradiation alone or with chemotherapy plays little role in this disease. Order et al. (58a) at Johns Hopkins have developed protocols combining external radiation, chemotherapy (5-FU and doxorubicin), and radiolabelled antibodies. Iodine-131 or yttrium-90 antiferritin has been used for hepatocellu-

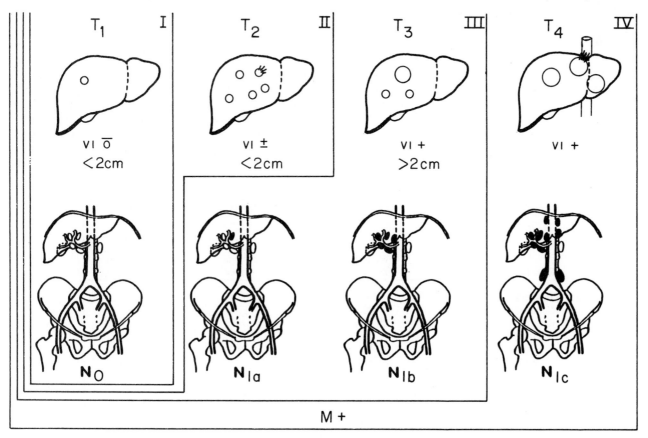

Fig. 29-3. Anatomic staging for cancer of the liver.

Table 29-12.   Liver Cancer Combination Chemotherapy Responses

	Range of Response (%)	(%) Average	Mean Survival (mo)
5-FU combinations*	0-40	8.8	2.6
Doxorubicin combinations†	8-44	19	3
Total (570 patients)			

* cytarabine, carmustine, semustine,mitomycin-C, streptozotocin, cyclophosphamide, vincristine
† Prednisone, 5-FU, semustine, streptozoticin, bleomycin, Mitomycin-C
Adapted from Wanebo et al. (67).

lar carcinomas and iodine-131 anti-carcinoembryonic antigen has been used for cholangiocarcinomas. This strategy is most interesting; several unresectable lesions have become resectable with this technique and a few long-term survivors have been observed (58a,62,64). In a randomized trial comparing radiolabelled polyclonal antiferritin to chemotherapy alone, no significant improvement occurred in median survival, but 30% achieved a response to antiferritin therapy and some (40%) appear to have been made resectable (58').

Chemotherapy

There have been efforts to treat unresectable hepatocellular cancer with both systemic and intrahepatic artery chemotherapy. In a small percentage of cases there is shrinkage of the tumor but the effect is temporary and of no advantage to patient survival compared with untreated patients.

Doxorubicin, etoposide, 5-FU, and its analog floxuridine have been used (56,67) (Table 29-12). The patients who are entered onto chemotherapy trials represent a subset of patients with good performance status and more localized disease. The overall group of patients often have poor hepatic function, are generally quite ill, and may tolerate chemotherapy poorly. Older studies with standard agents have demonstrated responses in 15–30% in patients receiving regional chemotherapy with external beam radiation therapy (51').

RESULTS

The overall survival in this disease is 2% to 6% at 5 years (Table 29-13) (56a,57a). Favorable prognostic factors include the lack of cirrhosis, female sex, and resectability (Fig. 29-4) (65). Only about 10% to 20% of cases are surgically resectable and of these probably 20% to 30% are cured. Although hepatocellular cancer is rapidly fatal in the advanced, unresectable stages with an average life expectancy of 6 months, the growth rate of hepatocellular cancer is actually comparatively slow. Using serial ultrasound, it has been shown that average doubling time is 4 months (61).

When the tumor is Stages III or IV the 5-year survival is less than 1% (67).

CLINICAL INVESTIGATIONS (18)

Radioisotope therapy systemically administered in conjugated biologic combinations as radiolabeled tumor antibodies for hepatocellular cancer is being actively explored by Order (58). Radioisotope therapy deserves careful consideration by academic radiation oncologists in terms of collaborative training with other disciplines such as nuclear medicine and pathology, but there is also a need to foster more laboratory research and clinical investigational protocols.

Table 29-13.   Summary of Resection Experience with Primary Hepatic Malignancies

Resection Data	Clinical Cancers		Japan National Study	Small or "Minute" Cancers Found by Screening in High-Risk Groups Requiring Limited Resections
	Western Experience	Eastern Experience		
Total patients	~2000	4983	5496	147
No. of resections	482	969	1186	110
Resectability rate	20-25%	19%	21.5%	73%
(range)		(7-46%)		(54-76%)
With cirrhosis, mean	17%	68%	~80%	90%
(range)	(0-43%)	(40-90%)		
Hospital mortality after resection	15%	18%		0-5%
Overall survival (yr)				
1	81%	48%	55%	73%
3	48%	24%	30%	66%
5	30%	14.5%		33-70%

Adapted from Nagorney and Adson (56a) and Okuda (57a).Courtesy of Marcel Dekker Inc.

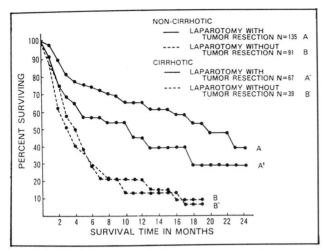

Fig. 29-4. Survival curves for the laparotomized cases in Japanese national study (1980-1981). Reprinted from Ref. 57a, pp. 219-238 by courtesy of Marcel Dekker Inc.

The major paradox is the effectiveness of the low doses achieved in treating hepatocellular carcinomas with 30 to 150 mCi of [131]antiferritin with doses of only 1100 to 1200cGy. The introduction of tumor volumetrics to measure objectively the response rates has clearly demonstrated that partial remissions are possible and when combined with other standard modalities of external beam irradiation and chemotherapy, unresectable tumors have been made resectable. In the Radiation Therapy Oncology Group experience, 11 patients converted to resectability by the use of radioisotope therapy and 80% are alive more than 3 years. The radiobiological basis for the current usefulness of low-dose radioisotope therapy is postulated by Fowler (51a). Low dose rates in the range of 10 to 300 cGy/h might allow cells to progress into the radiosensitive G_2M phase and allow for their destruction. Radioisotope therapy at 15 cGy/h with an effective half-life of 4 days would deliver a total dose of 2100 cGy to a tumor and account for two to three logs of cell kill. Radioisotope therapy could be an effective boost dose and therefore needs to be used with other modalities such as surgery, radiation therapy, and chemotherapy.

EXTRAHEPATIC BILE DUCT CANCER

Epidemiology (40,82)

Bile duct cancers, or cholangiocarcinoma, are uncommon cancers, and the least common of those categorized as liver and biliary passage cancers. The annual incidence in the United States is approximately 2500 cases and the annual death rate approaches the incidence. Men predominate over women and it usually has its onset between 50 to 70 years of age, with a mean of 65 years.

Etiology (71,75,82)

The cause of this cancer is unknown. Gallstones are found in only 30% of cases, unlike gallbladder cancer. There is some suggestion that chronic inflammation and cholestasis may be contributory. Patients with inflammatory bowel disease (especially ulcerative colitis, and to a lesser degree, Crohn's disease) may have associated sclerosing cholangitis and with this there is an increased incidence of cholangiocarcinoma.

Biliary passage parasites, especially the liver fluke, *Clonorchis sinensis*, are also associated with this cancer in a higher than expected ratio. There is also an increased incidence in patients with choledochal cysts.

DETECTION AND DIAGNOSIS

Clinical Detection (74,82)

The majority of patients present with cholestatic (obstructive) jaundice, defined as jaundice (mostly direct hyperbilirubinemia) associated with an aspartate aminotransferase of less than 300 and a serum alkaline phosphatase more than 3 times the upper limit of normal. This presentation is not specific for this type of cancer and can be found in a number of other conditions causing bile duct obstruction: cholecystitis, sclerosing cholangitis, primary biliary cirrhosis, cholestatic hepatitis (frequently drug related), intrahepatic cholestasis, and alcoholic hepatitis.

Symptoms of obstructive jaundice include nausea, vomiting, epigastric pain, weight loss (frequently secondary to malabsorption) and pruritus. The pruritus itself can be severely debilitating. Dark urine, light-colored stools, steatorrhea, and hepatomegaly are common. The gallbladder is palpable in about one third of cases (Courvoisier's sign). A palpable gallbladder is tantamount to bile duct obstruction; bile calculi rarely lead to a palpable gallbladder. Signs of liver failure are a late manifestation. Laboratory tests invariably demonstrate the liver pattern mentioned above, but also elevated prothrombin time (corrected by administration of vitamin K) and frequently anemia.

Diagnostic Procedures (80,82-84)

The best tests for patients with obstructive jaundice, if no clues are forthcoming from the history and physical examination, are among cholangiography, ultrasound, and CT scan. (Table 29-14). The major question asked of these tests include: (1) site and possible cause of the obstruction; (2) extent of disease locally; and (3) evidence of metastatic disease. Despite advances in this area, frequently surgical exploration is necessary to define resectability or need for bilioenteric bypass.

Ultrasound: This test is performed early because it is associated with few complications, is readily available, and is cost-effective. It is 85% to 90% accurate in detecting bile duct dilatation, but its accuracy in detecting the site of obstruction (27% to 86%) or cause of obstruction (23% to 52%) is much less. Ultrasound will also help detect nodal enlargement and hepatic metastases.

CT scan is about 90% to 95% accurate in detecting dilated bile ducts, and is better than ultrasound in determining the level of obstruction (88%) and the cause (70%). CT scan is also used to determine local extent of disease and liver metastases. This test is undoubtedly our best single noninvasive test, but it is more expensive and requires oral and intravenous contrast media and therefore, a small, but definite allergic risk.

Cholangiography: Direct cholangiography may be either from above (percutaneous transhepatic cholangiography [PTC]) or below (endoscopic retrograde cholangiopancreatography [ERCP]). These tests are associated with more complications, therefore, they usually are performed after ultrasound or CT scans. Complications include sepsis,

Table 29-14.   Imaging Modalities for Gallbladder Tumors

METHOD	CAPABILITY	BENEFIT/COST RATIO	RECOMMENDED FOR USE
Primary tumor and regional nodes			
CT	Minimally invasive with intravenous contrast, which is strongly recommended for optimal scanning technique. Most useful of all imaging modalities for determining local invasion, extent of tumor, defining site of biliary ductal obstruction and evaluating for distant metastases.	High	Yes
MRI	May be useful in staging and evaluating primary spread of tumor as well as distant metastases.	?	?
Barium contrast upper gastrointestinal roentgenograms	May be used to define mass affect on the stomach or duodenum secondary to metastatic disease.	Moderate	No (selected cases only)
Oral cholecystogram	Not useful because biliary system usually does not opacity	Low	No
Radionuclide liver/spleen and hepatobiliary scans	May be useful in evaluating for hepatic metastases. Biliary radionuclide scanning may demonstrate level of obstruction.	High	No (selected cases only)
Hepatobiliary sonography	Excellent for evaluating metastatic disease of the liver and for evaluating the biliary tract. Even when the primary tumor is not seen dilated bile ducts may be visualized.	High	Yes
ERCP/PTC	Extremely accurate in localizing the site of obstruction, and evaluating the type of obstruction.	High	Yes
Percutaneous biopsy guided by imaging technique	Accurate in confirming malignant nature of identified mass. Usually peripheral mass in the liver is biopsied. Biopsy of the gallbladder should not be performed percutaneously. Cholangiocarcinoma may demonstrate no mass.	High	No (selected cases only)

CT = computed tomography; MRI = magnetic resonance imaging; ERCP/PTC = endoscopic retrograde cholangiopancreatography/transhepatic cholangiography.

bile duct leakage, hemorrhage, perforation, and pancreatitis. The cost of these tests is higher than CT scans. Exfoliative cytology from brush biopsies is useful in establishing a diagnosis. However, choleangiographies remain the gold standards for sensitivity, specificity, and accuracy in the diagnosis or exclusion of bile duct obstruction. Some investigators would argue that the noninvasive tests are not reliable enough and that the "last test should be done first."

Histopathology (71,75,82)

Almost all of these cancers are adenocarcinomas; only a few (1% to 2%) are anaplastic or squamous. (Table 29-15) Microscopically they have been divided into sclerosing, nodular, and papillary. They are frequently considered multicentric and significant submucosal spread is not unusual.

Anatomically these cancers have been divided into three locations. The upper third is the area from the main right and left hepatic ducts, to the confluence, the common hepatic duct to the level of the cystic duct. The middle third encompasses from the entrance of the cystic duct down to the intrapancreatic part of the common bile duct. The lower third is that portion of the common duct that runs through the pancreas and wall of the duodenum. The common bile duct unites with the pancreatic duct in the duodenum to form a common opening termed the Vater's ampulla.

Over half the cases of bile duct cancers are found in the upper one third of the duct. Those found at the bifurcation of the hepatic duct within the porta hepatis have been called Klatskin tumors, after the clinician who stressed their small size, their tendency to remain localized, and need for cholangiography to establish the site of obstruction (78). About one fourth are found in the middle third and the other fourth in the distal third. Distant metastases are rare: most patients die from hepatic failure or infections. Direct extension to liver,

Table 29-15. Histologic Classification for Gallbladder and Bile Ducts

Type	% Incidence
Adenocarcinomas	60 -90%
Undifferentiated carcinomas	3 - 10%
Squamous cell carcinomas	3 - 6%
Mixed carcinomas or acanthomas	± 8%

portal vein, or pancreas occurs in 70% of patients, and local node metastases (choledochal, pancreaticoduodenal, hepatic artery) are found in 50%. Peritoneal seeding is rare.

Staging-Workup

The staging of bile duct cancers is surgical/pathologic (Table 29-16). Noninvasive and invasive tests as mentioned above are used to determine the site of obstruction, possible cause of obstruction, and evidence of local/regional or metastatic spread. Work-ups include:

- CBC, differential, platelet count, bilirubin, and liver enzymes, prothrombin time, BUN, creatinine, glucose, and electrolytes
- chest x-ray
- ultrasound and CT scan as mentioned above
- possible PTC or ERCP
- Exploratory laparotomy: in the past most of these cancers required surgical exploration for diagnosis, operability, and evaluation for bypass. Currently, diagnosis (ultrasound or CT-directed biopsies or cholangiograms brushings) and extent of disease (ultrasound and CT) and nonsurgical bypass (percutaneous or endoscopi-

cally) can be established in some patients and surgery avoided.

PRINCIPLES OF TREATMENT

Surgery (69,70-72,82)

Surgery is the only known curative modality. Its aim is resection of the tumor and reanastomosis of bile drainage to the bowel. Unfortunately only 20% to 40% are resectable for cure and local/regional recurrences are the norm (60% to 80%). The type of surgery performed is related to the location of the carcinomatous obstruction, status of the common bile duct, and the extent of disease.

Resectable disease in the distal duct is best managed with a pancreaticoduodenal resection (Whipple procedure), with or without pylorus preservation (27,47). Approximately 40% of cancers in this area are resectable. Those that involve the Vater's ampulla have a more favorable prognosis than patients with cancer of the head of the pancreas, because these lesions are more frequently localized.

Resectable lesions in the mid common bile duct are rare because of involvement of the portal vein and hepatic artery

Table 29-16. TNM Classification and Stage Grouping for Gallbladder and Bile Ducts

TNM Classification		Stage Grouping	
Primary Tumor			
T0	No evidence of primary tumor	Stage I	T1, N0, M0
T1A	Invasion of mucosa only	Stage II	T2, N0, M0
T1B	Invasion of muscle layer	Stage III	T1, N1, M0
T2	Invasion of perimuscular connective tissue		T2, N1, M0
T3	Invasion of adjacent structures (liver, pancreas, duodenum, gallbladder, colon, stomach)		
		Stage IVA	T3, any N, M0
Node Involvement		Stage IVB	Any T, any N, M1
N0	No regional lymph nodes involved		
N1A	Cystic duct or hepatoduodenal nodes involved		
N1B	Peripancreatic, periduodenal, celiac or superior mesenteric nodes involved		
Distant Metastases			
M0	No known metastases		
M1	Distant metastases		

T = tumor; N = node; M = metastasis.

and are usually treated with block resection of the gallbladder, common hepatic and common bile ducts, and surrounding lymph nodes. The hepatic ducts are then anastomosed to a defunctionalized portion of the jejunum (Roux-Y-hepaticojejunostomy) to reduce the incidence of cholangitis. Many surgeons prefer to perform a Whipple procedure.

Lesions in the common hepatic duct or right or left hepatic ducts are frequently unresectable (50% to 70%). When resection is undertaken, in addition to the structures removed for mid duct lesions, the confluence of ducts and partial hepatectomy is added with Roux-Y- intrahepatic cholangiojejunostomy. Some 5-year survivors are reported (71). An understanding of the vascular and ductal anatomy of the liver has increased the number of hepatic duct bifurcation tumors (Klatskin tumors) that can be resected (61a).

Complications of this surgery are primarily anastomotic leaks and infections.

For situations where resection is not possible, palliative procedures include biliary enteric bypass, or transtumoral or paratumor bypass intubation.

Radiotherapy (77,79,80)

The techniques available to the radiation oncologist for treatment of this include: (1) external irradiation with high energy machines, with field size reduction for boost, (2) intraoperative irradiation using orthovoltage equipment or electrons, and (3) intracavitary irradiation using a 192-iridium ribbon in a cholangiogram decompression tube primarily for boost. As in other areas of the abdomen, normal surrounding structures (liver, kidney, small bowel, and spinal cord) limit the external dose; hence the rationale for intracavitary or intraoperative irradiation.

In general, the use of external irradiation alone as adjuvant therapy for gross or microscopic residual disease after palliative resection or as definitive treatment in cases of unresectable disease has produced reasonable (>80%) palliation (relief of jaundice, pruritus, and pain) in small series from single institutions (71,79). To obtain higher doses and avoid exceeding tolerance to normal tissue, brachytherapy, and intraoperative techniques have come into use.

Recently Fields and Emami (73) and Hayes et al. (76) retrospectively reviewed their experience with 17 and 24 patients, respectively. Many of these patients were treated with combined external and transcatheter irradiation. In general this approach has not been curative, but survival may be prolonged over external irradiation alone; however, randomized studies have not been performed and enthusiasm varies (81); side effects, including infections and GI bleeding, are not insignificant. It is not clear how much these complications are related to the long-term presence of percutaneous catheters. Intracavitary hyperthermia using microwave antennae and iridium ribbons have also been used to take advantage of the synergism between photon irradiation and heat (85).

Chemotherapy (80,82)

Due to the rarity of this type of cancer, there are no large studies of chemotherapy. Responses have been seen with 5-FU, mitomycin C, and FAM and combined doxorubicin, carmustine, and Ftorafur in patients with advanced disease (Table 29-17). Responses were seen in 30% of cases with duration from 8.5 to 18 months. Because of the low response rates, adjuvant chemotherapy has not been investigated.

Palliation

Biliary enteric bypass may be accomplished surgically or with stents placed through or around the tumor at the time of surgery. Catheter can also be placed percutaneously or endoscopically for external or internal decompression. Basically this is based on many factors including medical condition of the patient, his or her performance status, prospect for curative resection, and patient preferences (71,72,80).

RESULTS

Overall survival is less than 5% at 5 years.

Survival for distal lesions where radical pancreaticoduodenectomy is possible ranges from 16-68% at 5 years with an average of 42%.

Midduct cancer for the most part is much less common and generally unresectable; 5-year survival is less than 5%.

Carcinomas of the proximal ducts are resectable in only 30% to 40% of cases. There are some reported 5-year survivors; mean survival is 30 months (71,79).

Table 29-17. Chemotherapeutic Responses of Biliary Cancer		
Drug	**Response (%)**	**References**
5-Flourouracil	4/1/7 (24)	Haskell (1980)
	3/23 (13)	Davis et al. (1980)
Mitomycin C	7/15 (42)	Crooke and Bradner (1976)
	0/10 (0)	Von Dyben et al. (1980)
BCNU	2/2 (100)	Haskell (1980)
Doxorubicin	1 (anecdotal)	Adolphson and Carpenter (1981)
Neocarzinostatin	Anecdotal response	Bodey et al. (1981)
m-AMSA	2/23 (9)	Bukowski et al. (1983)
FAM	4/14 (31)	Harvey et al. (1984)
Ftorafur, doxorubicin and BCNU	3/7 (43)	Hall et al. (1979)
Doxorubicin and bleomycin	1/5	Ravey and Hester (1979)
5-Flourouracil and mitomycin C via hepatic artery	9/13 (69)	Misra et al. (1977)

BCNU = carmustine; m-AMSA = Amsacrine; FAM = 5-flourouracil, doxorubicin; mitomycin.
From Andrews and Smith (86a), with permission.

GALLBLADDER CARCINOMA

Epidemiology (40,82)

Cancer of the gallbladder is a rare form of cancer but the most common cancer of the liver and biliary passages. Approximately 6000 cases are diagnosed in the United States each year and the annual death rate is almost comparable. The incidence is between 2.5 and 4.0 per 100,000. It is rare in patients less than aged 50 years, with the peak incidence between 50 and 70 years. The female to male ratio is 3:1 which is similar to the incidence of cholelithiasis.

Etiology (96,101)

The cause of this disease is unknown but several associations have been noted.

Most patients with gallbladder cancer have associated gallstones, but there is no conclusive evidence that this is a cause-and-effect relationship. American Indians from the Southwest, who have a high rate of gallstones, also have a high rate of gallbladder cancer at an early age. The general incidence of this cancer in patients with cholelithiasis is less than 1%. Given this low incidence, and considering the operative morbidity/mortality, prophylactic cholecystectomy cannot be recommended for patients with gallstones, perhaps with one exception. Patients with the so-called "porcelain" or calcified gallbladder have a 25% risk of cancer and accordingly once detected selective cholecystectomy is suggested (100,102).

There is some evidence to suggest that an anomalous pancreaticobiliary union with associated reflux of pancreatic secretion may have an etiologic relationship. In those patients with an anomalous union as judged by a cholangiopancreatography, gallbladder cancer was found to be significantly increased (92,93).

Clinical Detection (82)

The most common symptoms reported by patients with this disease include: pain (75%), jaundice (45%), nausea, vomiting, anorexia, and weight loss (40%). Symptoms of right upper quadrant pain and nausea and vomiting are similar to patients with cholelithiasis and cholecystitis. Jaundice implies extension to produce common duct obstruction or, less frequently, metastases to the liver. Malaise, anorexia, fever and weight loss all suggest advanced disease. Hepatomegaly suggests liver metastases as does elevated alkaline phosphatase with hyperbilirubinemia; the gallbladder may be palpably enlarged.

Diagnostic Procedures (80,82,94)

Since fewer than 5% of patients are diagnosed preoperatively, the surgeon/pathologist makes the diagnosis in the majority of cases.

Ultrasound: This procedure is capable of diagnosing the disease early by detecting polypoid, solid masses, if the patient is seen early (87).

However, there are many shortcomings to this test (91). Bile duct obstruction, gallstones, regionally enlarged nodes, and hepatic metastases can also be detected with this procedure.

CT Scan: This modality is capable of detecting wall thickness, masses, and liver, nodal, and duodenal extension, and complements ultrasound.

Oral cholecystogram, angiography, CT scans, and ERCP are much less useful.

Histopathology

Adenocarcinoma comprises 85% of these cancers, with squamous, anaplastic, and adenocanthoma accounting for the remainder (Table 29-15). Three growth patterns have been identified: papillary, nodular, and infiltrative. As in most adenocarcinomas, these cancers are graded as well, moderately, and poorly differentiated. From a prognostic viewpoint the papillary and well- differentiated types fare best (89,99).

As with most intra-abdominal cancers, the pattern of spread may be hematogenous, lymphatic, direct extension, and peritoneal seeding; the last is uncommon. The predominant pattern of spread, as determined from surgery and post mortem examination, is by direct extension: (l) gallbladder fossa of the liver, 60% to 83%; (2) extrahepatic bile ducts, 57%; (3) duodenum or transverse colon, 40%; (4) portal vein or hepatic artery, 15%; and (5) pancreas, 23%. Regional cystic, choledochal or pancreaticoduodenal nodes occurs in 42% to 70%, and para-aortic nodes in 25%. Frequent sites of hematogenous spread include the liver (64%), lung (24%), and bone (12%) (82,86,101,103). For staging, see Table 29-16.

PRINCIPLES OF TREATMENT

Surgery (Table 29-18) (104)

Surgery is the only know curative modality. However, this cancer is rarely detected early. Indeed, only about 10% of cases will have disease confined to the gallbladder and another 10% to 20% will involve associated local spread that is resectable. The patients who do best are those where the disease is found incidentally. One prominent surgeon has been quoted as saying that if the diagnosis is made preoperatively, you can avoid the surgery (101). The other 75% are inoperable for cure but bypass for obstruction is frequently performed. The standard surgery is a cholecystectomy for patients with stages I, II, and III disease (98). More radical procedures have been performed, including resection of the gallbladder fossa of the liver, regional nodes, and the gall bladder, for stage III disease; however, enhanced survival has not been documented (82,97).

Radiotherapy

It was often stated in the past that this tumor was radioresistant, however, relief of jaundice and osseous pain suggest that this may not be so. The limiting feature of irradiation is the tolerance of surrounding structures. Numerous small series have been reported but without improvement in survival. Some investigators have suggested postoperative irradiation for patients with high risk of residual microscopic disease, e.g., transmural penetration and/or regional nodes. The usual doses recommended are 45 to 50 Gy to include the tumor bed and regional lymphatic drainage. Data, however, are too sparse to recommend this routinely (73,79,80).

Chemotherapy

Currently, chemotherapy for this disease is investigational. A number of agents have been tried and not found to be active. These include 5-FU, mitomycin C, streptozotocin, and lomustine either alone or in combination (80,82,88).

Table 29-18. Five-Year Survival After Resection of Gallbladder Cancer in Collected Staged Series

Stage	Extent of Invasion	Survival (%)
I	Mucosa	Stage I-II
		18/33 (55)
II	Muscularis	Stage I-III
		27/106 (26)
III	Subserosal	
IV	Cystic LN+	1/24 (4.2)
VA	Extension to liver or adjacent organ (resectable)	1/123 (8)
VB	Regionally advanced or metastatic (unresectable)	
Total series	(microstaged)	28/398 (7)

LN = lymph node
Adapted from Wanebo (104). Courtesy of Marcel Dekker Inc.

Palliation

Biliary-enteric bypass is reasonable if biliary obstruction is present. The decision for operative, percutaneous catheter decompression or use of an endoprosthesis is often debated, but final decisions are often individualized, based on risk of surgery, extent of disease, clinical status of the patient, and patient preference (90,95). Radiotherapy can be used to palliate symptomatic metastatic disease.

Results

Overall survival is less than 5%; average survival after diagnosis is approximately 9 months. Five-year survival for patients with stage I and II disease is 70–80%. Most of these patients were probably found to have gallbladder cancer incidently at the time of cholecystectomy for other reasons. Survival for stage III at 5 years is 15%, and for stage IV is less than 1%.

Recommended Reading

There are a number of sources on all aspects of pancreatic cancer. *Tumors of the Pancreas*, edited by Moosa (6), deals with experimental and clinical pathology, diagnostic radiologic studies and treatment principles. *Pancreatic Cancer*, edited by Cohn (3), a supplement to *Cancer* (2), and a recent Medical Progress article by Warshaw and Fernandez-Castillo (7a) review epidemiologic and diagnostic approaches. Clinical features and treatment are well covered in issues of *Seminars in Oncology* (8,11) devoted entirely to pancreatic cancer, in an article by Wils (47b), and again in the Medical Progress article noted above (7a). The increase in the number of articles on pancreatic cancer, however, is not reflected in an increase in long-term survival.

The student can also use del Regato and Spjut as a general reference (4a). Islet cell tumors are reviewed by Moertel (33) and in the articles in the September 1987 issue of *Seminars in Oncology*. The NIH conference (51) and the Wanebo *et al.* chapter (67) on hepatocellular cancer are good. Biliary obstruction is reviewed by Lokich *et al.* (80). See article by Nagorney and McPherson (82) for gallbladder and extrahepatic bile duct carcinomas.

REFERENCES

General References

1. American Joint Committee for Cancer Staging and End-results Reporting. Manual for Staging Cancer. 3rd Ed. Philadelphia, PA: JB Lippincott Co; 1988.
1a. Bragg DG, Rubin P, Youker JE, eds. Oncologic Imaging. Elmsford, NY: Pergamon Press; 1985.
2. Cancer of the Pancreas Task Force. Staging of Cancer of the Pancreas. Cancer 47:1631-1637; 1981.
3. Cohn I Jr, ed. Pancreatic Cancer: New Directions In Therapeutic Management. New York, NY: Masson Publishing; 1980.
4. Del Regato JA, Spjut HJ. Cancer of the digestive tract. In: Del Regato JA, Spjut HJ (eds). Ackerman and Del Regato's Cancer: Diagnosis, Treatment, and Prognosis. 5th Ed. St. Louis, MO: CV Mosby, Co; 1977:572-611 .
4a. Del Regato JA, Spjet HJ, Cox JD (eds). Ackerman and del Regato's Cancer: Diagnosis, Treatment and Prognosis. 6th ed. St. Louis: MO; C.V. Mosby; 1985.
5. International Histologic Classification of Tumors, Nos. 1-20. Geneva, Switzerland; World Health Organization; 1978.
6. Moosa AR, ed. Tumors of the Pancreas. Baltimore, MD: Williams & Wilkins; 1980.
7. Strauss MB. Familiar Medical Quotations. Boston, MA: Little Brown and Co; 1968.

Specific References

Pancreatic Cancer

7a. Warshaw AL, Fernandex-Castillo C. Pancreatic carcinoma. N Engl J Med 326:455-465; 1992.
8. Beazley RM. Percutaneous Needle Biopsy for Diagnosis of Pancreatic Cancer. Semin. Oncol. 6:344-46, 1979.
9. Beazley RM, Cohn I. Decisions In Pancreatic Carcinoma. Seminars Oncol. 7:435-443, 1980.
10. Beazley RM, Cohn I: Update On Pancreatic Cancer. Cancer. 38:310-319, 1988.
11. Berg JW, Connelly RR. Updating the Epidemiologic Data On Pancreatic Cancer. Semin. Oncol. 6:275-289, 1979.
11a. Boring CC, Squires TS, Tong T. Cancer Statistics, 1992. CA 42:19-38; 1992.
11b. Brennan MF, Kinsella T, Friedman M. Cancer of the Pancreas. In: Devita VT Jr, Hellman S, Rosenberg SA, eds. Cancer, Principles and Practice of Oncology. Philadelphia, PA: JB Lippincott; 1989, p 830.
11c. Cameron JL, Crist DW, Sitzmann JV, et al. Factors influencing survival after pancreaticoduodenectomy for pancreatic cancer. Am J Surg 161(1):120-125; 1991.
11d. Crown J, Casper ES, Botet J, et al. Lack of efficacy of high-dose

leucovorin and fluororacil in patients with advanced pancreatic adenocarcinoma. J Clin Oncol 9(9):1682-1686; 1991.

12. Cubilla AL, Fitzgerald PJ. Cancer of the Pancreas (nonendocrine): A Suggested Morphologic Classification. Semin Oncol. 6:285-297, 1979.

13. Dibisceglie AM, Hoofnagle, JH. Hepatitis B Virus Infection and Hepatocellular Carcinoma Etiologic Relationship and Clinical Implicatioins. Updates of Cancer: Principles and Practice of Oncology. 1 (10):1-10; 1987.

14. Dobelbower RR, Howard JM, Bagne FR, Eltake A, Merrick HW: Treatment of Cancer of the Pancreas By Precision High Dose (PHD) External Photon Beam and Intraoperative Electron Beam Therapy (IOEBT). Int J Radiat Oncol Biol Phys. 16:205-209, 1989.

15. Eriksson B, Skogseid B, Lundqvist G, Wide L, Wilander E, Oberg K: Medical Treatment and Long-term Survival In A Prospective Study of 84 Patients With Endocrine Pancreatic Tumors. Cancer. 65: 1883-1890, 1990.

16. Fajans SS, Vinik AI. Insulin-producing Islet Cell Tumors. Endocrinol Metab Clin North Am. 18:45-74, 1989.

17. Fonthan ETH, Correa P. Epidemiology of Pancreatic Cancer. Surg Clin North Am. 69:55-67; 1989.

18. Fowler, JF. Radiobiological Aspects of Low Dose Rates In Radioimmunotherapy. Int J Radiat Oncol Biol Phys. 18(5):1261-1269; 1990.

19. Friesen SR: Update of the Diagnosis and Treatment of Rare Neuroendocrine Tumors. Surg Clin North Am. 67:379-393, 1987.

20. Gastronintestinal Tumor Study Group. Further Evidence of Effective Adjuvant Combined Radiation and Chemotherapy Following Curative Resection of Pancreatic Cancer. Cancer. 59:2006-2010; 1987.

21. Gastrointestinal Tumor Study Group. Radiation Therapy Combined With Adriamycin Or 5-fluorouracil for Treatment of Locally Unresectable Pancreatic Carcinoma. Cancer. 56:2563-268; 1985.

21a. Gunderson LL, Willett CG. Pancreas and hepatobiliary tract. In: Perez CA, Brady LW (eds). Principles and Practice of Radiation Oncology. 2nd ed. Philadelphia, PA: J.B. Lippincott Co., 1992; pp 985-999.

22. Gudjonsson B. Cancer of the Pancreas: 50 Years of Surgery. Cancer 60:2284-2303, 1987.

23. Haller DG. Chemotherapy In Gastrointestinal Malignancies. Semin Oncol. 15 (suppl 4): 50-64; 1988.

24. Hermanek P, Sobin LH, eds. TNM Classification of Malignant Tumours. Ed 4. New York,NY: Springer-Verlag; 1987

25. Howard TJ, Passaro E. Gastrinoma. New Medical and Surgical Approaches. Surg Clin North Am. 69:667-81, 1989.

26. Hsieh CC, Macmahon B, Yen S, Trichopolos D, Walrren K, Nardi G. Coffee and Pancreatic Cancer (chapter 2). New Engl J Med. 315:587-589, 1986.

27. Itani KMF, Coleman RE, Akwari WC. Pylorous-preserving Pancreatoduodenectomy. A clinical and physiologic appraisal. Ann Surg. 204:655-664, 1986.

28. Kalser MH, Ellenberg SS: Pancreatic cancer. Adjuvant combined radiation and chemotherapy following curative resection. Arch Surg. 120:899-903, 1985.

28a. Kelsen D, Hudis C, Niedzwiecki D, et al. A phase III comparison trial of streptozotocin, mitomycin, and 5-fluorouracil with cisplatin, cytosine arabinoside, and caffeine in patients with advanced pancreatic carcinoma. Cancer 68(5):965-969; 1991.

29. Komacki R, Wilson JF, Cox JD, Line RW. Carcinoma of the Pancreas: Results of Irradiation for Unresectable Lesions. Int J Radiat Oncol Biol Phys 6:209-212, 1980.

30. Kummerle F, Ruckert K. Surgical Treatment of Pancreatic Cancer. World J Surg. 8:889-894, 1984.

31. Kvols LK, Buck M, Moertel CG, et al. Treatment of metastatic islet cell carcinoma with a somatostatin analogue (SMS 210-995). Ann Intern Med. 107:162-168,1987.

32. Moertel CG: An odyssey on the land of small tumors. J Clin Oncol. 5:150322, 1987.

33. Moertel CG, Childs DS, Reitemeier RJ, Colby MY, Holbrook MA. Combined 5-fluorouracil and supervoltage radiation therapy of locally unresectable gastrointestinal cancer. Lancet. Ii:865-867, 1969.

34. Moertel CG, Frytak S, Hahn Rg, et al. Therapy of locally

unresectable pancreatic carcinoma: A randomized comparison of high dose (6000 Rads) radiation alone, moderate dose radiation (4000 Rads + 5-fluorouracil), and high dose radiation + 5-fluorouracil. Cancer. 48:1705-1710; 1981.

35. Mohiuddin M, Cantor RJ, Biermann W, Weiss SM, Barbot D, Rosato FE: Combined modality treatment of localized unresectable adenocarcinoma of the pancreas. Int J Radiat Oncol Biol Phys. 14:79-84, 1988.

35a. Morrow M, Hilaris B, Brennan MF. Comparison of conventional surgical resection, radioactive implantation, and bypass procedures for exocrine carcinoma of the pancreas, 1975-1980. Ann Surg. 199:1-5; 1984.

36. O'dorisio TM, Mekhjian HS, Gaginella TS. Medical therapy of vipomas. Endocrinol Metab Clin North Am. 18:545-556, 1989.

36a. Physician's Data Query. Pancreatic Cancer. National Cancer Institute, Bethesda, MD; January 1992.

37. Roldan GE, Gunderson LL, Nagorney DM, Martin JK, Ilstrukp DM, Holbrook MA, Kvols LK, Mcilrath DC: External beam versus intraoperative and external beam irradiation for locally advanced pancreatic cancer. Cancer. 61:1110-1116, 1988.

38. Saltzbury D, Foley KM: Management of pain In pancreatic cancer. Surg Clin North Am. 69:629-649, 1989.

39. Sarner M. Cancer of the Pancreas. In: Gazet, JC, ed. Carcinoma of the Liver, Biliary Tract and Pancreas. London, UK: Edward Arnold; 1983;152-190.

40. Silverberg E, Boring CC, Squires TS. Cancer Statistics, 1990. Ca. 40:9-26, 1990.

41. Syed AMN, Puthawala AA, Neblett DL. Interstitial Iodine-125 implant: In the management of unresectable pancreatic carcinoma. Cancer. 52:808-813, 1983.

42. Tepper JE, Shipley WU, Warshaw AL, Nardi GL, Wood WC, Orlow El. The role of misonidazole combined with intraoperative radiation therapy in the treatment of pancreatic carcinoma. J Clin Oncol. 5:579-584, 1987

43. Thompson WM:.Imaging Strategies for Tumors of the gastrointestinal system. Cancer. 37:165-185, 1987.

44. Trede M. The surgical treatment of pancreatic carcinoma surgery. 97:28-35; 1985.

45. Vinik AI, Moattari Ar. Treatment of Endocrine Tumors of the Pancreas. Endocrinol Metab Clin North Am. 18:483-518, 1989.

45a. Warshaw AL, Fernandez-del Castillo C. Pancreatic carcinoma. N Engl J Med. 455-465; 1992.

46. Weiss SM, Skibber J, Dobelbower RR, Whittington R, Rosato FE: Operative Pancreatic Biopsy. Ten-year Review of Accuracy and Complications. Am Surg. 48:214-216, 1982.

47. Whipple AO. Present Day Surgery of the Pancreas. N Eng J Med. 226:515-526;1942.

47a. Whittington R, Bryer MP, Haller DG, et al. Adjuvant therapy of resected adenocarcinoma of the pancreas. Int J Radiat Oncol Biol Phys 21:1137-1144; 1991.

47b. Wils JA. Treatment of pancreatic carcinoma: Therapeutic nihilism? Recent Results in Cancer Research 110:87-94; 1988.

Primary Liver (Hepatocellular) Cancer

48. Beasley RP, Hwaang LY, Lin CC, Chien, CS. Hepatocellular Carcinoma and Hepatitis B Virus. A Prospective Study Of 22707 Men In Taiwan. Lancet. 2:1129-1133; 1981.

49. Bengmark S, Jeppsson B: Status of Ischemic Therapy for Hepatic Tumors. Surg Clin North Am. 69:411-418; 1989.

50. Chen DS, Sung JL, Shen JC, Lai MY, How SW, Hsu HC, Lee CS, Wei TC. Serum Alpha-fetoprotein In the Early Stage of Human Hepatocellular Carcinoma. Gastroenterology. 86:1404-1409,1984.

51. Dibisceglie AM, Rustgi VK, Hoofnagle JH, Dusheiko GM, Lotze MT. NIh Conference: Hepatocellular Carcinoma. Ann Int Med. 108:390-401; 1988.

51'. Epstein B, Ettinger D, Leichner PK, et al. Multimodality cisplatin treatment in nonresectable alpha-fetoprotein-positive hepatoma. Cancer 67(4):896-900; 1991.

51a. Fowler JF. Radiobiological aspects of low dose rates In radioimmunotherapy. Int J Rad Oncol Biol Phys. 18:1261-1270; 1990.

52. Ishak KG. Hepatic neoplasms associated with contraceptive and anabolic steroids. Recent results Cancer Res. 66:73-128, 1979.

53. Jenkins RL, Fairchild Rb. The role of transplantation in liver disease. Surg Clin North Am. 69:371-382; 1989.

54. Jones DB, Koorey Dj. Screening studies and markers. Gastroenterol Clin North Am. 16:563-573; 1987.

55. Murray-lyon IM. Primary and Secondary Cancer of the Liver, In Gazet JC (ed): Carcinoma of the Liver, Biliary Tract and Pancreas. London, UK: Edward Arnold; 1983;1-81.

56. Nerenstone S, Friedman M. Medical Treatment of Hepatocellular Carcinoma. Gastroenterol Clin North Am 16:603-612; 1987.

56a. Nagorney, D.M.; Adson, M.A. Major Hepatic resections for Hepatoma In the West. In: HJ Wanebo Ed. Hepatic and Biliary Cancer. New York, NY: Marcel Dekker; 1987;167-185.

57. Oberfield RA, Steele G, Gollan JL, Sherman D. Liver Cancer. Ca. 39:206-218; 1989.

57a. Okuda K, Ryu M, Tobe T. Surgical Management of Hepatoma, the Japanese Experience In: Wanabo HJ, Ed. Hepatic and Biliary Cancer. New York, NY: Marcel Dekker; 1987; 219-238.

58. Order SE. Presidential Address: Systemic Radiotherapy — the New Frontier. Int J Radiat Oncol Biol Phys. 18:979-980; 1990.

58'. Order S, Pajak T, Leibel S, et al. A randomized prospective trial comparing full dose chemotherapy to 121I antiferritin: An RTOG study. Int J Radiat Oncol Biol Phys 20(5):953-963; 1991.

58a. Order S, Stillwagon G, Klein J et al: Iodine 131 Antiferritin, A New Treatment Modality In Hepatoma: A Radiation Therapy Oncology Group Study. J Clin Oncol. 3:1573-1582, 1985.

58a*. Physician's Data Query. Liver Cancer. National Cancer Institute, Bethesda, MD; January 1992.

58b. Ravikumar, T.S.; Steele, G.; Kane, R.; King. V. Experimental and Clinical Observations On Hepatic Cryosurgery for Colorectal Metastases. Cancer Res. 51:6323-6327; 1991.

59. Rustgi VK: Epidemiology of Hepatocellular Carcinoma. Gastroenterol Clin North Am. 16.545-551, 1987.

60. Schwartz SI: Liver, In: Schwartz SI, Ed: Principles of Surgery, 5th Ed. New York, NY: Mcgraw-hill; 1989;1327-1380.

61. Sheu JC, Sung JL, Chen DS, Yang PM, Lai, MY, Lee CS, Hsu HC, Chuang CN, Yang PC, Wang TH, Lin JT, Lee CZ: Growth Rate of Asymptomatic Hepatocellular Carcinoma and Its Clinical Implications. Gastroenterology. 89:259-266; 1985.

61a. Shutze WP, Sack J, Aldrete JS. Long-term follow-up of 24 patients undergoing radical resection for ampullary carcinoma, 1953 to 1988. Cancer 66(8):1717-1720; 1990.

62. Sitzmann JV, Order SE, Klein JL, Leichner PK, Fishman EK, Smith GW: Conversion By New Treatment Modalities of Nonresectable To Resectable Hepatocellular Cancer. J Clin Oncol. 5:1566-1573, 1987.

63. Stevens KR. The Liver and Biliary System. In: Moss WT, Cox JD, Eds: Radiation Oncology. Rationale. Technioues. Results. Baltimore, MD: Cv Mosby Co; 1989;381-387.

64. Stillwagon GB, Order SE, Guse C, Klein JL, Leichner PK, Leibel SA, Fishman EK. 194 Hepatocellular Cancers Treated By Radiation and Chemotherapy Combinations: Toxicity and Response: A Radiation Therapy Oncology Group Study. Int J Radiat Oncol Biol Phys. 17:1223-1229; 1989.

64a. Stillwagon GB, Order SE, Guse C, et al. Prognostic factors in unresectable hepatocellular cancer: Radiation Therapy Oncology Group study 83-01. Int J Radiat Oncol Biol Phys 20(10):65-71; 1991.

65. Sutton FM, Russell NC, Guinee VF, Alpert E. Factors Affecting the Prognosis of Primary Liver Carcinoma. J Clin Oncol 6:321-328; 1988.

66. Takashima T, Matsui O, Suzuki M, et al. Diagnosis and Screening of Small Hepatocellular Carcinomas. Radiology. 145:635-638; 1982.

67. Wanebo HJ, Falkson G, Order SE. Cancer of the Hepatobiliary System. In: Devita VT, Hellman S, Rosenberg SA, Eds. Cancer Principles and Practice of Oncology, 3rd Ed. Philadelphia, PA: JB Lippincott Co; 198;9; 836-856.

67a. Yamashita Y, Takahashi M, Koga Y, et al. Prognostic factors in the embolization and arterial infusion. Cancer 67(2):385-391; 1991.

68. Zhou XD, Detolla L, Custer RP, London WT: Iron, Ferritin, Hepatitis B Surface and Core Antigens In the Liver of Chinese Patients With Hepatocellular Carcinoma. Cancer. 59:1430-1437; 1987.

Extrahepatic Bile Duct Cancer

69. Adkins RB, Dunbar LL, Mcknight WG, Farringer JL. An Aggressive Surgical Approach To Bile Duct Cancer. Am Surg. 52:134-139; 1986.

70. Beazley RM, Blumgart LH: Malignant Stricture At the Confluence of the Biliary Tree Diagnosis and Management. Surg Ann 17125-141; 1985.

71. Bengmark S. Biliary Duct Cancer: Therapeutic Nihilism Or Prospect. Recent Results In Cancer Research 110:74-78; 1988.

72. Dawson SL, Mueller PR. Non-operative management of biliary obstruction. Ann Rev Med. 36:1-11; 1985.

73. Fields JN, Emami B: Carcinoma of the extrahepatic biliary system results of primary and adjuvant radiotherapy. Int J Radiation Oncology Biol Phys. 13:331-38; 1987.

74. Fry DE. Obstructive Jaundice. Causes and Surgical Interventions. Postgrad Med. 84:217-230; 1988.

75. George P. Cancer of the Bile Ducts. In: Gazet JC, Ed. Carcinoma of the Liver, Biliary Tract and Pancreas. London, UK: Edward Arnold; 1983;104-151.

76. Hayes JK, Sapozink D, Miller FJ. Definitive Radiation Therapy In Bile Duct Carcinoma. Int J Radiat Oncol Biol Phys. 15:735-744; 1988.

77. Johnson DW, Safai C, Goffinet DR. Malignant Obstructive Jaundice: Treatment With External-beam and Intracavitary Radiotherapy. Int J Radiat Oncol Biol Phys. 11:411-416; 1985.

78. Klatskin G. Adenocarcinoma of the Hepatic Duct At Its Bifurcation Within the Porta Hepatis. An Unusual Tumor With Distinctive Clinical and Pathologic Features. Am J Med. 38:241-256, 1965.

79. Kopelson G, Harisiadis L, Tretter P, Chang CH. The Role of Radiation Therapy In Cancer of the Extrabiliary System: An Analysis of Thirteen Patients and Review of the Literature of the Effectiveness of Surgery, Chemotherapy and Radiotherapy. Int J Radiat Oncol Biol Phys. 2:883-894; 1977.

80. Lokich JJ, Kane RA, Harrison DA, Mcdermott WV: Biliary Tract Obstruction Secondary To Cancer: Management Guidelines and Selected Literature Review. J Clin Oncol. 5:969-981; 1987.

81. Molt P, Hopfan S, Watson RC, Botet JF, Brennan F. Intraluminal Radiation Therapy In the Management of Malignant Biliary Obstruction. Cancer. 57:536-544; 1986.

82. Nagorney DM, Mcpherson GAD. Carcinoma of the Gallbladder and Extrahepatic Bile Ducts. Semin Oncol. 15:106-116; 1988.

83. Thompson WM. Imaging Strategies for Tumors of the Gastrointestinal System. Ca. 37:165-185; 1987.

84. Wolcott JK, Chem PS. Radiologic Evaluation of the Jaundiced Patient. Diagnostic and Therapeutic Role of Current Procedures. Postgrad Med. 84:233-246; 1988.

85. Wong JYC, Vora NL, Chou CK, et al. Intracavitary Hyperthermia and Iridium192 Radiotherapy In the Treatment of Bile Duct Carcinoma. Int J Radiat Oncol Biol Phys. 14:353-359; 1988.

Gallbladder Carcinoma

86. Adson M. Carcinoma of the Gallbladder. Surg Clin North Am. 53:1203;1973.

86a. Andrews W, Smith F. Chemotherapy for cholangiocarcinoma and gallbladder cancer. In: Wanebo HD (ed). Hepatic and biliary cancer. New York, NY: Marcel Dekker; 1987, pp 453-457.

87. Elvin A, Erwald R, Muren C, Mare K. Gallbladder Carcinoma. Diagnostic Procedures With Emphasis On Ultrasound Diagnosis. Ann Radiol (Paris). 32:282-287; 1989.

88. Falkson G, Macintyre JM, Moertel CG. Eastern Cooperative Group Experience With Chemotherapy for Inoperable Gallbladder and Bile Duct Cancer. Cancer. 54:965-969; 1984.

89. Friedman RB, Anderson RE, Gilchrist KW, Carbone PP. Prognostic Factors In Invasive Gallbladder Carcinoma. J Surg Oncol. 23:189-194; 1983.

90. Hall RI, Denyer ME, Chapman AH. Percutaneous-endoscopic Placement of Endoprothesis for Relief of Jaundice Caused By Inoperable Bile Duct Strictures. Surgery 107:224-227; 1990.

91. Hederstrom E, Forsberg L: Ultrasonography In Carcinoma of the Gallbladder. Diagnostic Difficulties and Pitfalls, Acta Radiol 28:711-714; 1987.

92. Kato O, Hattori K, Skuzukki T, Tachino F, Ylkuasa T. Clinical Significance of Anomalous Pancreaticobiliary Union. Gastroinest Endosc. 29:94-98; 1983.

93. Kimura K, Ohto M, Saisho H, et al. Association of Gallbladder Carcinoma and Anomalous Pancreaticobiliary Ductal Union. Gastroenterology. 89:582; 1985

94. Lawson TL, Berland LL, Foley WD. Malignant Neoplasms of the Pancreas, Liver and Biliary Tract. In: Bragg DG, Rubin P, Youker

JE, Eds. Oncologic Imaging. New York, NY: Pergamon Press; 1985; 287-342.

95. Malangoni MA, Mccoy DM, Richardson JD, Flint LM. Effective Palliation of Malignant Biliary Duct Obstruction. Ann Surg. 201:554-55; 1985.

96. Maringhini A, Moreau JA, Melton LJ, Hench VS, Zinsmeister AR, Demagno EP: Gallstone, Gallbladder Cancer, and Other Gastrointestinal Malignancies. An Epidemiologic Study In Rochester, Minnesota. Ann Intern Med. 107:30-35; 1987.

97. Muir IM, Morris DL. Carcinoma of the Gallbladder. Br J Hosp Med. 36:278-280; 1986.

98. Nivin JE, Moran TJ, Kay S, *et al.* Carcinoma of the Gallbladder: Staging, Treatment and Prognosis. Cancer. 37:141-148;1976.

99. Ouchi K, Owada Y, Matsukno S, Sata T. Prognostic Factors In the Surgical Treatment of Gallbladder Carcinoma. Surgery. 101:731-737; 1987.

100. Peterson H. Carcinoma of the Gallbladder. A Review of 158 Cases. Acta Radiol Diag. 15:225-236;1974.

101. Piehler JM, Crichlow RW. Primary Carcinoma of the Gallbladder. Surg Gyn Obstet. 147:929-942;1978.

102. Polk HC. Carcinoma In the Calcified Gallbladder. Gastroenterology. 50:582; 1966.

103. Sons HU, Borchard F, Joel BS. Carcinoma of the Gallbladder: Autopsy Findings In 287 Cases and Review of the Literature. J Surg Oncol. 28:199-206; 1985.

104. Wanebo, H.J. Carcinoma of the Gallbladder. In: HJ Wanebo, Ed. Hepatic and Biliary Cancer. New York, NY: Marcel Dekker; 1987, pp 431-445.

105. Wanebo HJ, Falkson G, Order SE. Cancer of the hepatobiliary system. In: DeVita VT Jr., Hellman S, Rosenberg SA (eds). Cancer: Principles and Practice of Oncology. 3rd ed. Philadelphia, PA: JB Lippincott; 1989, pp 836-874.

Diana F. Nelson, M.D., Radiation Oncology
Joseph V. McDonald, M.D., Surgical Oncology
Lowell W. Lapham, M.D., Neuropathology

Raman Qazi, M.D., F.A.C.P., Medical Oncology
Philip Rubin, M.D., Radiation Oncology

Chapter 30

CENTRAL NERVOUS SYSTEM TUMORS

Keep unshak'd that temple thy fair mind.

William Shakespeare (3)

PERSPECTIVE

Any growth within the cranial vault can cause symptoms by compressing the brain against the rigid bony calvarium. In addition, if the growth happens to block a midline ventricle, it can block the flow of cerebral spinal fluid (CSF), thereby creating hydrocephalus with its associated symptoms of increased intracranial pressure. Because of the rigid, bony encasement of the brain and spinal cord, even a benign tumor can produce significant symptoms and possibly death, as a brain or upper cervical spinal cord neoplasm. Additional symptoms can be produced by direct invasion and destruction of brain parenchyma. The specific symptoms produced depend on the location of tumor in the brain (Table 30-1).

Without surgical intervention, malignant tumors do not usually disseminate beyond the central nervous system (CNS). Low-grade benign tumors tend to grow slowly and some of them may be cured by surgery with or without radiation therapy. The malignant, or high-grade, tumors grow more rapidly and are associated with a shorter survival. Some of the malignant tumors have a tendency to disseminate throughout the CNS. Some of these highly lethal tumors, such as medulloblastoma and ependymoblastoma, otherwise known as primitive neuroectodermal tumors (PNET), tend to occur in children. They are potentially curable by either surgery or radiotherapy in combination with chemotherapy or by surgery and radiotherapy alone (21c).

A better prognosis is associated with a younger age, with possibly the exception of young children less than 4 years of age, whose brains are still developing and whose therapy is modified to minimize the adverse effects of radiation therapy and chemotherapy. This is evident in the Surveillance, Epidemiology and End Results program data in which the overall 5- and 10-year survival rates for patients of all ages with brain tumors are 16% and 12%, respectively, compared with 43.3% and 38.6% for children less than 5 years old, 50.8% and 44.3% for children 5 to 9 years old, 57.6% and 49.3% for children aged 10 to 14 years 58.2% and 51.9% for children aged 15 to 19 years of age, and 52.8% and 39.8% for young adults aged 20-24 years (19). Compare these figures to a zero 5-year survival for patients older than 60 years of age regardless of histology; those with glioblastoma multiform (GBM) have a median survival of 6 months (79); those with anaplastic astrocytoma a median survival of 9 months (79); and those with primary non-Hodgkin's lymphoma of the brain a median survival of 7 months (80a). Low-grade glio-

mas are rarely observed in elderly patients and when they are the survival rate is no better than that for malignant gliomas (personal observation). Whether there truly are low-grade gliomas in the elderly, or whether the diagnosis of low-grade astrocytoma results from a sampling error, remains to be determined. The important point is that age is a significant prognostic variable in addition to histopathology (79-80b). The Karnofsky performance status (KPS) is also a significant prognostic variable in adult malignant glioma (79,80) and CNS lymphoma (80a). Analysis of patterns of care of brain tumor patients in the United States has been recently completed (15a).

EPIDEMIOLOGY AND ETIOLOGY

Epidemiology

Currently, 15,000 new cases of primary brain tumors and a little more than 4,000 new spinal cord tumors occur each year. Approximately 2% of all cancer deaths are caused by brain tumors; these account for 11,000 deaths annually (5b).

CNS tumors comprise 2% to 5% of all tumors. Eighty percent involve the brain and 20% involve the spinal cord. Twenty percent to 40% of brain tumors are metastatic lesions from lung, breast, kidney, melanoma, and the gastrointestinal (GI) tract. In one study, 70% of cases had multiple deposits (5b).

In children, brain tumors are second only to leukemia as a cause of death — 1,600 children and young adults die annually (5b). In contrast to adult tumors, they are largely infratentorial rather than supratentorial, and involve cerebellum, midbrain, pons, and medulla.

Tumors of Adults

1. Gliomas comprise 50% of all primary brain tumors and glioblastomas comprise over 50% of all gliomas (15). They occur most commonly in the cerebrum and most frequently between the ages of 40 to 74 years (19).
2. Meningioma is the most common of the nongliomatous tumors. It constitutes 15% of primary intracranial neoplasms. The average age of patients is about 50 years (159). The parasaggital area and the anterior part of the base of the skull are common sites. Rarely, there are more aggressive changes evidenced by more rapid growth and local invasiveness.

617

Table 30-1.   Brain Tumor Localization Chart

	Frontal	Parietal	Temporal	Occipital
Symptoms	Often asymptomatic until late Symptoms of increased ICP Bradyphrenia Personality changes Libido changes Impetuous behavior Excessive jocularity Defective memory Urinary incontinence Seizures (generalized, becoming focal) Gait disorders Weakness Loss of smell Speech disorder Tonic spasms of fingers/toes	Symptomatic earlier than frontal lobes Symptoms of increased ICP Loss of vision Spatial disorientation Tingling sensation Dressing apraxia Loss of memory Seizures (focal sensory epilepsy) Weakness (anterior extension)	Speech disorders (left hemisphere dominant, not only for right-handed but for most left-handed persons) Loss of smell (superior lesion) Disturbance in hearing, tinnitus, etc Speech disturbance Uncinate fits Seizures with vocal phenomena in aura, including speech arrest Hallucinations, Dreams, Deja vu Space perception disturbances Dysarthrisa Dysnomia Disturbance of comprehension	Seizures, relatively less common, but with auras including flashing lights and unformed hallucinations Loss of vision Tingling (early) Weakness (late)
Specific cerebral functions	Behavioral problems (anterior location) Labile personality Mental lethargy Defective memory Motor aphasia	Anosognosia Autotopagnosia Visual agnosia Graphesthesia (X) Loss of memory Proprioceptive agnosia	Dysarthria Sensory asphasia Defective hearing Defective memory	Visual agnosia Visual impulses
Cranial nerve functions	Anosmia (inferior lesion) Nerve VI palsy with increased ICP Papilledema with increased ICP Foster Kennedy's syndrome Proptosis	Hemianopsia Papilledema (with increased ICP)	Superior quadrantanopsia (X), could be homonymous hemianopsia with tumor extension Central weakness of the cranial nerve VI Papilledema with increased ICP	Macular sparing hemianopsia Horizontal nystagmus
Motor system	Contralateral weakness (late) Paresis (flaccid spastic) Disturbed gait (midline lesion) Automatism Persistence of induced movement (Kral's phenomenon) Diagonal rigidity [arm (X); leg (-)] Loss of skilled movement (X) Urinary incontinence (superior lesion)	Weakness Atrophy Clumsiness Dysdiadochokinesia Independent movements (unrecognized by patient)	Dysdiadochokinesia (early) Drigt, secondary in later stages, involving arm more than leg	Motor signs appear late manifested by drift or dysdiadochokinesia
Sensory functions	Rarely involved initially unless invasion of sensory area (posterior lesion)	Dysesthesias (tingling) (X) Pallesthesia (loss of vibratory sense) (X) Loss of touch, press, and position sense (X), but pain and temperative usually unaffected	Initially minimal	Somatosensory disturbances earlier than motor changes, as adjacent structures are involved Visual phenomena, such as persisting images, unformed hallucinations, aura.
Reflex changes	Tonic plantar reflex Hoffmann's sign Grasp reflex Babinski's sign	Babinski's sign Hoffmann's sign	May occur contralateral to tumor	Not affected in early stages

ICP = Intracranial pressure, (X) = Contralateral,   (-) = Ipsilateral

3. Pituitary adenomas comprise 12% to 18% of intracranial neoplasms, the majority of which are chromophobic (6). They are almost never malignant.
4. Neurilemoma (schwannoma) is chiefly a tumor of adults, and is usually benign.

Tumors of Childhood (103-112)

1. About 60% of childhood brain tumors are infratentorial and 75% or more are midline (6). Forty-five percent are astrocytomas (5c), 25% involve the cerebellum, and 10% the brain stem (6). Astrocytomas of varying degrees of malignancy also occur in the brain stem in children (32). They are all malignant. A few are cystic or exophytic and are amenable to surgery, although they cannot be excised completely. X-ray therapy and chemotherapy are used for these tumors.
2. *Optic pathway gliomas* are usually well-differentiated astrocytomas with slowly growing progressive extensions along the optic nerve and ultimate intracranial extension. These comprise 5% of childhood intracranial tumors (6). Enlargement of the optic foramen is present in a majority of cases. Optic pathway gliomas can be cured surgically if they are confined to one optic nerve. If they involve the optic chiasm alone or more posteriorly, they are treated with radiation therapy. They are usually well-differentiated astrocytomas with slow-growing, progressive extensions (109,147-155).
3. *Medulloblastomas* comprise 20% of primary brain tumors and are the most common posterior fossa tumor (4,5c,113-119,121-129). Ten percent of childhood brain tumors are *ependymomas* (5c, 130-135).
4. *Craniopharyngiomas* constitute 5% to 10% of all intracranial tumors in children. Eighty percent of craniopharyngiomas occur before aged 30 years. Symptoms and signs produced by enlargement of the cystic tumor are increased intracranial pressure (ICP), visual defects, endocrine dysfunction, and hypothalamic dysfunction. Symptoms can simulate those of pituitary adenomas. Suprasellar calcification is a characteristic x-ray finding (6). These tumors are benign but are difficult to remove completely because they often involve the hypothalamus and the third ventricle, the circle of Willis, and/or the optic nerve (140,143,146).
5. *Pineal tumors* constitute only about 1% to 2% of childhood brain tumors (5c). They classically present with paralysis of upward gaze (Parinaud's syndrome). Pineal tumors consist of a variety of tumors, including teratomas, pineoblastomas, and germinomas (6). Pineoblastoma have a high dissemination rate of 10% to 30% in different series. Teratomas with mixed elements may yield markers such as alpha-fetoprotein and choriogonadotrophic hormones (182-189).

Tumors of the Spinal Cord (13,15)

1. The majority of spinal axis tumors are extradural. They are predominantly metastatic carcinomas, lymphomas, or sarcomas, with only a rare chordoma.
2. Most primary spinal axis tumors are intradural: the extramedullary meningiomas and neurilemomas are more common (26% and 29%, respectively) than the intramedullary ependymomas (13%) and astrocytomas (7%) (15), although the 60% of ependymomas that occur in the lumbosacral region (filum terminale and conus medullaris) are not truly intramedullary (13).

Etiology

There are increasing data documenting a genetic basis, or at least a genetic association with some brain tumors. In some instances specific chromosomes and/or gene locations have been identified. An association of brain tumors with certain chemicals/drugs and irradiation has been reported.

Genetic (12,15)

1. Bilateral retinoblastoma and chemodectoma have an autosomal dominant pattern of inheritance in certain instances and are associated with specific gene deletions. A familial occurrence of glioma has been described in association with breast cancer and soft tissue sarcomas. In children, there appears to be a family association of gliomas and lymphomas/leukemia (12,15).
2. *Phakomatoses* are associated with certain CNS neoplasms with an autosomal dominant pattern (15).
   a. Tuberous clerosis is associated with astrocytoma, glioblastoma, ependymoma, and ganglioneuroma.
   b. Von Recklinghausen's neurofibromatosis, especially the central form that has multiple schwannomas of the cranial and spinal nerve roots, is associated with multiple meningiomas, multiple ependymomas, and optic gliomas.
   c. Von Hippel-Lindau disease is associated with hemangioblastoma, particularly in the cerebellum, renal carcinoma, and pheochromocytoma.
   d. Nevoid basal cell carcinoma syndrome is associated with medulloblastoma and ovarian tumors.
   e. In Turcot syndrome, brain tumors are associated with polyposis coli.
3. In addition, meningiomas appear to be associated with breast cancer and this association may be genetic and/or hormonally linked. Meningiomas are also associated with 22 chromosome abnormalities (8).

Chemical and Viral (8,15,23)

An increased risk of brain tumors has been reported in the rubber manufacturing industries and in workers exposed to vinyl chloride. In rat studies, brain tumors have been associated with polyaromatic hydrocarbons exposure, N-vitroso compounds, and ovarian sarcoma virus.

Immunosuppression

Renal transplant patients have an increased incidence of primary non-Hodgkin's lymphoma of the brain. Patients with malignant gliomas are immunologically compromised; whether this is cause or effect remains to be determined.

Radiation Treatment (12)

Prior irradiation to the head has been reported in association with brain tumors in approximately 100 patients, with 70% meningiomas, 11% astrocytomas, 6% sarcomas, and 10% miscellaneous histologies (12).

DETECTION AND DIAGNOSIS

Clinical Detection (11)

Brain tumors cause generalized, or nonlocalizing, symptoms and signs by increasing the pressure within the skull, and cause localized symptoms and signs by direct compression, invasion, or irritation of the brain (Table 30-1).

1. Increased ICP is due to rapidly increasing tumor mass and/or associated edema, and, less commonly, hemorrhage or infarction within the tumor. A rapid increase in the tumor's mass or associated surrounding edema can cause such early symptoms as headache, nausea and vomiting, and later depression of the state of consciousness. On the other hand, slowly growing tumors, such as meningiomas or low-grade gliomas, may be present for many years and become large before symptoms are caused by increased pressure within the skull. Tumors that obstruct the flow of CSF through the ventricles can also cause a rapid and severe rise in ICP. Examples include thalamic gliomas, colloid cysts of the third ventricle, ependymomas, or cerebellar tumors blocking the fourth ventricle.

2. Localizing signs:. Involvement of specific regions(s) of the brain give rise to specific symptoms and signs that permit tumor localization.

   a. Epileptic seizures in an adult who has never had them before should alert the doctor to the possibility of a tumor. Magnetic resonance (MRI) scan of the brain should be done if a computerized tomography (CT) scan is negative.

   b. Headache is a common symptom. It is often diffuse, but can localize to the involved side of the tumor. Suboccipital tenderness is common with posterior fossa tumors.

Diagnostic Procedures

1. *Physical and neurologic examinations* are indicated in the presence of seizures, inappropriate affect, somnolence, lethargy, disorientation, subtle degrees of aphasia or apraxia, asymmetry of cranial nerve function, incoordination, musculature weakness, or loss of sensation in extremities. A thorough neurologic examination is indicated, testing for cerebral and cerebellar function, cranial nerves, sensory dermatoses, reflexes, and muscle strength and coordination (1).

2. *Funduscopic examination* should be routine. If the room is darkened, this can usually be done without mydriatics. These drugs should be avoided, if possible, because they can obscure or suggest nerve involvement to later observers.

3. *Visual field examination* is often forgotten or slighted, yet it can give precise information about the location of a tumor above the tentorium, because there are different places between the retina and the occipital cortex in which the optic fibers can be compromised, and the visual field alterations at each of these sites are different.

4. *MRI* is a noninvasive, safe, painless, highly sensitive, and efficient technique (Table 30-2) (5a). It can be done on an outpatient basis. MRI scans can be performed with or without contrast. MRI done with contrast agents such as gadolinium can identify regions of the tumor where the blood-brain barrier is altered. MRI of the brain has become the screening procedure of choice for diagnosing and localizing tumors in the brain stem, posterior fossa, and spinal cord, and for defining the extent of low-grade gliomas. It can be used to differentiate between intrinsic and extrinsic spinal cord problems, and metastatic disease versus disc problems. This technique can provide three-dimensional tumor imaging. The capabilities of this technique are still being explored (10).

5. *CT scanning can be performed to complement the i*nformation available from MRI (Table 30-2). CT can detect intracranial calcifications and separate them from acute hemorrhage. In contrast, MRI cannot detect calcifications and can only demonstrate acute hemorrhage with

METHOD	DIAGNOSIS AND STAGING CAPABILITY	RECOMMENDED FOR USE
Table 30-2. Imaging Modalities for Evaluating Brain and Spinal Cord		
Primary tumor and regional nodes		
CT	Best test at present for detection, definition and follow-up of brain tumors. Limited use in cord tumors	Yes
MRI	Excellent for low-grade gliomas, posterior fossa tumors, tumors of the cerebellopontine angle, brain stem & spinal cord evaluation. Excellent for patients allergic to iodine contrast agents. Will replace myelogram as an initial procedure for evaluating spinal cord tumors and discs	Yes
Nuclear medicine scan	Will detect most brain tumors. Best for detection of bone metastases from non-CNS neoplasms	Brain - No Spine - Yes
Angiography	Aids differentiating tumors from AV malformation. Aids in planning surgical approach. Rarely used for either detection or follow-up	No
Myelography	Best test at present for small epidermal and nerve root lesions, whether primary or secondary	Yes, if MRI unavailable or negative despite a positive clinical picture
Biopsy	Required for most CNS tumors. May be done very accurately in brain with CT stereotactic guidance	Yes

CT = computed tomography; MRI = magnetic resonance imaging; CNS = central nervous system; AV = arterovenous.
Adapted from Bragg et al. (5a)

special techniques. CT performed with contrast demonstrates blood-brain alterations, as does MRI when contrast agents are injected intravenously (IV).

6. *Skull roentgenograms* are no longer routinely done. Skull roentgenograms will show some abnormality in about 30% of patients with brain tumors (27). Roughly three quarters of craniopharyngiomas are calcified. Meningiomas can also be calcified and, not infrequently, cause a thickening of the calvaria of the sphenoidal ridge at their point of attachment. Generalized ICP can cause erosion of the posterior clinoid processes of the sella turcica, or can cause a "beaten silver" or hammered effect in the inner table of the skull in the very young. A calcified pineal body or habenular commissure can be pushed away from the midline by a cerebral tumor confined to one hemisphere.

7. *Electroencephalography* has been of some value in screening suspected brain tumor. It is abnormal in about 75% of cases, but well localized in only 40% (20). Because it is imprecise and not specific for brain tumors, its use in the diagnosis of brain tumors is limited. CT and MRI have minimized the usefulness of electroencephalography in the diagnosis and localization of brain tumors.

8. Technetium pertechnetate brain scanning (technetium-99m) is no longer widely used in spite of a positive rate — 75% to 86% for meningiomas, glioblastomas, and large metastatic tumors.

9. *Cerebral angiography* of the intracranial vessels is used by surgeons who desire information about the intrinsic vasculature of the tumor and its relationship to adjacent blood vessels — important matters in planning surgery.

10. Air study *pneumoencephalography, and ventriculography* are no longer done.

11. *Lumbar puncture* is avoided when there is obvious evidence of increased ICP. There is a definite risk of herniation when this procedure is used under such circumstances. When the CSF is withdrawn or continues to leak through the hole made by the puncture in the leptomeninges, there can be a shift of the intracranial contents, which will cause or aggravate a medial temporal or cerebellar herniation.

A lumbar puncture can be useful to determine whether ICP is elevated. It is most helpful in differentiating patients with meningitis or subarachnoid hemorrhage from those with suspected tumors, although MRI or unenhanced CT scan should demonstrate hemorrhage.

12. *CSF examination* is valuable because the CSF protein is elevated approximately one third of the time in the presence of intracranial tumor and almost always in the presence of a spinal cord tumor. CSF glucose may be low in the presence of highly malignant tumors or metastatic meningeal deposits. CSF cytology is positive in meningeal carcinomatosis and in tumors that involve the meninges or are situated in a subependymal location. Cerebral spinal fluid cytology should be evaluated in PNET tumors and primary non-Hodgkin's lymphoma. A positive cytology obtained within 1 week to 10 days of surgery can be falsely positive and should be repeated after 2 weeks postsurgery.

Histopathology (Table 30-3) (62)

Reliance on a pathologic classification of brain tumors is a requisite to understanding their clinical behavior, prognosis, and treatment. In fact, histopathology is more important than anatomic staging in determining the clinical behavior and prognosis of brain tumors. Histopathology is also more important than staging in determining treatment. Although our present knowledge is too limited to provide a fully satisfactory classification of brain tumors, the following is empirically useful and provides the basis for therapeutic procedures. Pathologic diagnosis is required for understanding the biologic behavior of brain tumors and their prognoses.

Intrinsic Tumors

1. *Astrocytomas*: Historically there have been two grading systems: the Kernohan system (27,28) consisting of four grades, and the three-grade system of Bailey-Cushing that was presented by Russell and Rubinstein (34) and Burger and Vogel (25) and later substantiated by the Radiation Therapy Oncology Group (30,66,79,80,80b) and the Brain Tumor Study Group studies (24,73,90,91). The Kernohan system distinguished four groups using the criteria of cellularity, degree and frequency of anaplasia, presence or absence of mitotic figures, presence or absence of giant cells and necrosis, number of blood vessels, and degree of endothelial and adventitial proliferation (27,28). These four grades have been too difficult to use reproducibly. Therefore, the grades were grouped into low-grade or benign gliomas (grades I and II), and high-grade or malignant gliomas (grades III and IV). When Kernohan's Mayo Clinic cases were updated and expanded to include subsequent cases in a recent evaluation of the Mayo Clinic low-grade gliomas, Shaw *et al.* (100a) found the curves for grades I and II to be superimposable. Nelson *et al.* (30) demonstrated that grades III and IV had no prognostic significance in RTOG 7401 - Eastern Cooperative Oncology Group (ECOG) 1374, but the presence or absence of tumor necrosis did have prognostic significance and this has

Table 30-3. Histologic Classification: Incidence of Different Brain Tumor Types

	Percent of Brain Tumors
Gliomas	43.0
Glioblastoma multiforme	23.0
Astrocytoma	13.0
Ependymoma	1.8
Oligodendroglioma	1.6
Mixed and other	1.9
Medulloblastoma	1.5
Meningioma	16.0
Pituitary adenoma	8.2
Neurilemoma	5.7
Craniopharyngioma	2.8
Sarcoma	2.5
Hemangioblastoma	2.7
Pineal tumor	1.1
Metastastic	13.0
Other	6.0

Number of brain tumors studied = 17,580.

From Walker (62), with permission.

been further substantiated by later RTOG studies (66,79,80,80b). This three-tier classification divides gliomas into astrocytomas that are low grade or benign, anaplastic astrocytoma (also called astrocytoma with foci of anaplasia (AAF)), and GBM, which has the worst prognosis. This classification is essentially that used by the World Health Organization (WHO) classification (36).

The low-grade tumors are characterized by a degree of cellularity that is only slightly greater than that seen in reactive hyperplasia. The nuclei may show slight to moderate pleomorphism. The WHO classification further divides low-grade gliomas into a favorable group that includes pilocystic astrocytomas (including juvenile pilocystic astrocytomas and microcystic cerebellar astrocytomas), subependymal giant cell astrocytomas, and pleomorphic xanthoastrocytomas; and an unfavorable group that includes ordinary astrocytomas (including fibrillary, protoplasmic, gemistocytic, and mixed), oligoastrocytomas, and oligodendrogliomas (36). The *AAF is an intermediate grade* that is malignant. In this grade, cellularity is increased, and there may be rare mitotic figures. Pleomorphism may be more pronounced, and there may be slight endothelial hyperplasia (30). In the *highest grade gliomas*, the most important feature is necrosis. In addition, marked cellularity is a prominent characteristic. There may be marked pleomorphism, marked endothelial hyperplasia and abundant mitotic figures. Giant cells sometimes are present. No feature is as important as necrosis (30).

There is an approximate correlation between survival rate (with or without treatment) and tumor grade. Patients with supratentorial low-grade gliomas have a 5-year survival rate of 28% to 76% following surgery plus radiotherapy and 0% to 34% for surgery alone (92,94-96,100-102), whereas patients with completely excised cerebellar astrocytomas may survive 20 or more years (100a). Those patients with AAF usually survive 2 to 5 years (median 28 to 36 months) (66,80,80b). GBM, on the other hand, carries a grave prognosis with survival of no more than 12 months and a median of 8 to 10 months (66,80,80b). Because of their infiltrative character and lack of encapsulation, all astrocytomas can be regarded as malignant lesions, as they ultimately usually are fatal. There are occasional exceptions to this when the tumor can be totally removed, as in cerebellar astrocytomas in childhood.

2. *Medulloblastomas* (113-129) are classified by some as primitive, undifferentiated cells (33), and by others as primitive neuronal tumors PNET (31). These are almost exclusively tumors of the vermis of the cerebellum in childhood. They are rapidly growing, infiltrative neoplasms with a marked tendency to spread throughout the subarachnoid space and to produce disseminated meningeal foci. Histologically, the cells are small and closely packed, with scanty cytoplasm. The tumors have similar features from one case to another, in contrast to the broad range of histologic appearance among the astrocytomas. The theory of origin of medulloblastomas contrasts with the current concept of origin of other tumors such as the gliomas that are thought to arise from dedifferentiation of adult cells.

Tumors of the Supporting Structures of the Nervous System (25)

1. *Meningiomas* (156-159,161-165) arise from cells in the pia-arachnoid, whereas neurilemomas develop from Schwann cells of cranial nerves or nerve roots. Meningiomas have a predilection for growth in certain localities so that characteristic clinical syndromes have come to be associated with meningiomas in specific areas.

2. *Intracranial neurilemomas* most commonly arise from the eighth nerve and, therefore, are most often found in the cerebellopontine angle, where compression of the eighth nerve, the adjacent brain stem, and the overlying cerebellum constitutes the anatomic basis for the ensuing clinical phenomena. Meningiomas and neurilemomas are also important tumors of the spinal canal that cause compression of the spinal cord and spinal roots.

Microscopically, many of the cells in meningiomas resemble arachnoidal lining cells, forming islands and sheets in which whorls and psammoma bodies frequently are found; others are elongated cells with a fibroblastic appearance of palisading. Neurilemomas can also display a looser structure with a more stellate type of cell predominating (25).

Developmental Tumors

Developmental tumors, a third category of tumor, presumably arise from cells that have developed abnormally and that have persisted throughout postnatal growth.

1. *Hemangioblastoma* is a tumor of blood vessels, generally appearing in adult life. It is slow-growing, frequently cystic, and occurs primarily in the cerebellum.

2. Other tumors of this group are craniopharyngiomas (136-146), epidermoid and dermoid cysts, colloid cysts of the third ventricle, and the rare chordomas. The neoplastic aspects of some of these lesions are readily established; in others (e.g., colloid cysts of the third ventricle and epidermoid or dermoid cysts) these aspects are equivocal. They gradually increase in size whether by proliferation of cells or by accumulation of desquamated or secreted materials and reactive connective tissue elements. Their clinical behavior, therefore, is that of an expanding lesion.

3. *Pituitary tumors* (hormonally active and inactive) (12,123,173-176) comprise a fourth major group of tumors. Although they are not true tumors of the CNS, they often cause neurologic signs and symptoms as a major complication resulting from pressure upon the optic chiasm, hypothalamus, third ventricle, and medial temporal lobe. Eventually, increased ICP can occur. These tumors are benign, slow-growing, and encapsulated lesions (15,25). There can be evidence of decreased pituitary activity, as in hypopituitarism, or increased activity, as seen in acromegaly and Cushing's syndrome. There also can be prolactin secretion by the tumor.

4. *Metastatic cancer* (single or multiple) is the fifth tumor category. Carcinomas are much more common than sarcomas, and lung and breast are by far the most frequent primary sources. Carcinomas from the pancreas, colon/rectum, and kidney, as well as malignant melanomas are also important sources of secondary

brain tumors. A metastatic lesion to the brain is a highly invasive and destructive growth, with a well-defined margin at the periphery of the lesion. Edema is often present in the surrounding white matter, which in some cases extends a considerable distance from the tumor. Occasionally, metastases give rise to diffuse carcinomatosis of the leptomeninges with multiple cranial nerve and spinal root involvement.

Edema deserves emphasis as a frequent and important secondary complication of any type of intracranial growth, whether intrinsic or extrinsic, benign or malignant. The mechanism of edema formation is not well understood, but it often contributes significantly to the clinical problem, as well as to the morbid anatomy. Edema is readily detected and visualized by either MRI or CT scans. It is treated with corticosteroids.

CLASSIFICATION

Anatomic Staging

Anatomic staging has not been widely used in supratentorial tumors. The only criteria that have been applied in selecting treatment have been the size (> 5 or < 6 cm) and noncentral location of lesions considered for brachytherapy (radioactive brain implant). The predominant factor in staging is tumor grade rather than tumor size (Table 30-4) (2).

For infratentorial tumors with a propensity to seed the CSF, as in medulloblastoma and empendymoblastoma, staging has some use in determining treatment and comparing treatment results. Tumor, node, and metastasis stage are given in Table 30-5 (2) and Fig. 30-1. This staging system has been used by the cooperative groups. It has more prognostic significance and is more useful for making treatment decisions than the American Joint Commission on Staging, which classifies all M positive categories in one.

Staging Work-up

The major purpose of the staging work-up is to determine tumor location, extent, size, and juxtaposition to ventricular cavities for the likelihood of subarachnoid seeding. Nodal and distant metastases are extremely uncommon. The major concern is the probability of spinal cord seeding in certain tumors, specifically medulloblastoma and ependymoblastoma (high-grade infratentorial ependymoma) and pineoblastoma.

Recommended Procedures (in sequence, depending on location of tumor) (5a, 10a, 10b)

1. *MRI* is the best noninvasive procedure. It also is an excellent method for evaluating tumor response or recurrence after surgery and irradiation.
   a. MRI has replaced CT as the principal imagery modality for detection and diagnosis of primary brain

Table 30-4.   TN Classification and Stage Grouping Suprtentorial Tumors and Malignant Gliomas

	TN Classification
T1	Diameter < 5 cm; confined to 1 side
T2	Diameter > 5 cm; confined to 1 side
T3	Diameter may be < 5 cm; invades or encroaches ventricular system
T4	Crosses midline, invades opposite hemisphere, extends infratentorially
N	Does not apply in this site

STAGE GROUPING

		Grade	Tumor	Metastases
Stage I				
	IA	G1	T1	M0
	IB	G1	T2,3	M0
Stage II				
	IIA	G2	T1	M0
	IIB	G2	T2,3	M0
Stage III				
	IIIA	G3	T1	M0
	IIIB	G3	T2,3	M0
Stage IV				
		G4	T1-4	M0
		G1-3	T4	M0
		Any G	Any T	Any M

T = tumor; N = node; M = metastasis; G = grade
Adapted from AJC (2).

Table 30-5. TNM Staging System for Infratentorial Tumors and Malignant Gliomas

T1	Tumor <3 cm in diameter and limited to the classic midline postion in the vermis, the roof of the fourth ventricle, and less frequently to the cerebellar hemisphere
T2	Tumor ≥3 cm in diameter, further invading one adjacent structure or partially filling the fourth ventricle
T3-A	Tumor further invading two adjacent structures or completely filling the fourth ventricle with extension into the aqueduct of Sylvius, foramen of Magendie, or foramen of Luschka, thus producing marked interal hydrocephalus
T3-B	Tumor arising from the floor of the fourth ventricle of brain stem and filling the fourth ventricle
T4	Tumor further spreading through the aqueduct of Sylvius to involve the third ventricle or midbrain, or tumor extending to the upper cervical cord
N	Does not apply to this site
M0	No evidence of gross subarachnoid or hematogenous metastasis
M1	Microscopic tumor cells found in cerebrospinal fluid
M2	Gross nodular seedings demonstrated in the cerebellar, cerebral subarachnoid space, or in the third or lateral ventricles
M3	Gross nodular seeding in spinal subarachnoid space
M4	Metastasis outside the cerebrospinal axis

T = tumor; N = node; M = metastasis
Adapted from AJC (2).

tumors and metastatic foci due to its ability to detect neoplasia smaller than 1 cm.

  b. MR has the following advantages over CT:
  • three-dimensional multiplanar imaging
  • no need for iodinated contrast
  • absence of bone artifacts allows posterior fossa to be better evaluated
  c. The high sensitivity but low specificity of MRI is overcome by stereotactic biopsy to determine pathology.
  d. MRI identifies by hyperintense lesions as T1 which on T2 does not discriminate tumor from edema or intracellular versus extracellular water.
  e. Gadolinium-pentetic acid, an IV contrast agent for MRI, is similar to iodinated contrast enhancement for CT and better distinguishes tumor from vasogenic edema on T1 weight sequence.

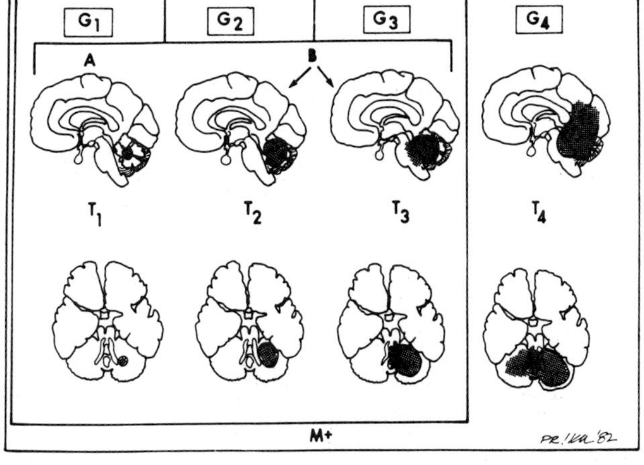

  f. MRI with gadolinium is exquisitely sensitive to detection of surface seeding in subarachnoid space and ventricular surface.
  g. MRI and contrast-enhancement sensitive tools detecting recurrent tumor but may not distinguish recurrence from treatment-related change. MRI can detect radiation demyelination or white signal on T2 weighted images.
2. *CT* scanning can complement MRI in the diagnostic work-up by confirming the presence of calcification or hemorrhage within a tumor when it is suspected by MRI. CT is also more economical in following the progress of patients in the postoperative period.
3. *Arteriogram* is helpful prior to surgery to determine tumor vascularity.
4. *CSF* analysis for cells can be helpful, particularly for determining the spread of medulloblastoma, ependymoma, GBM, and pinealoma. Myelogram and/or MRI of the spinal cord should be done for medulloblastoma and ependymoblastoma.
5. *Posterior-anterior and lateral chest films* can assist in the evaluation of suspected cerebral metastases from a primary malignancy outside the CNS.

Optional and Investigative Procedures

1. Bone scan and skeletal survey are recommended if bone metastases are suspected or if there is continual, unexplained back pain.
2. Neck node biopsy is indicated if there are suspicious nodes in neck; this is a very rare occurrence.

Fig. 30-1. Anatomic staging for infratentorial central nervous system tumors. G = grade; T = tumor; M = metastasis.

PRINCIPLES OF TREATMENT

Multidisciplinary Decisions

The challenges of managing malignant brain tumors is evident in the often life-threatening nature of the presentation. A multidisciplinary approach is essential both for diagnostic purposes and correct therapeutic decision making. Emergency imaging is often required, particularly if there is increased ICP or progressive neurologic changes. Corticosteroids allow for medical lowering of increased ICP and time for consultation by all disciplines. In both adult and pediatric brain tumors, the poor results for aggressive malignancies require careful consideration for new combined-modality approaches in investigative clinical trials. A summary of a trimodality standard management decision is shown by histopathologic type in Table 30-6.

Surgery (55,82,83,85,89)

Mortality and morbidity rates for intracranial tumor surgery have decreased steadily during the past 20 years, from the range of 20% to 40%, to less than 2% to 3%. There are multiple reasons for this. Earlier and more precise diagnosis using CT and MRI must be credited. It is now uncommon to see patients with marked papilledema as a sign of advanced ICP, or stupor or coma secondary to it. Tumor identification and localization with CT and MRI is simpler, quicker, safer, and noninvasive. Corticosteroid therapy to control edema around a brain tumor provides dramatic relief of symptoms (44,57,58), often within a day, and makes it easier to prepare patients for surgery. Much improved anesthetic techniques that avoid increased ICP prior to, during, and after surgery have made tumor exposure and dissection much more benign.

The surgeon has been helped personally by the use of magnified vision and micro-instrumentation provided by the dissecting microscope. The use of the ultrasonic tumor aspirator to morcellate and remove tumor tissue has minimized the need for retraction of the surrounding brain and thereby minimized the transmission of mechanical deformity to the brain. The carbon dioxide laser has permitted vapor-

ization of tumor deposits in relatively inaccessible areas. Ultrasonic devices, CT scanning, and stereotactic localization allow for biopsy of deeply seated lesions with greater accuracy and safety (39,42,51-53,55).

Working with a unique computer-guided stereotactic coupled laser system, neurosurgeons been able to eradicate a large number of varying types of cortical tumors. The patients have had relatively benign postoperative courses. Unfortunately, when the tumors have been malignant, recurrence of the tumor has not been prevented, even when it appeared to have been completely destroyed radiologically.

Initial treatment for all intracranial tumors is surgical excision (11,18,62). Removal is limited by the tumor location and invasiveness of the particular lesion, or, in the case of some benign lesions, by technical problems at the time of operation.

Meningiomas are almost always histologically benign (11,15). Usually, they can be removed completely. Sometimes only partial removal is possible, but even this will provide symptomatic relief. Since meningiomas can grow slowly, recurrent symptoms may not be a problem for years, although they may occur within a year or two. If there is postoperative residual disease, radiation therapy is recommended. Postoperative radiation therapy decreases the recurrence rate from 60% to 75% to 29% to 32% and increases the median survival from 66 to 125 months (15,156,157,159,161).

Malignant brain tumors can be cured only rarely in adults, although in children, as total an excision as possible plus radiation therapy can produce cures. Generally, by the time they are discovered, invasion of deep-seated areas of the brain has already occurred; this prevents their complete removal. In such cases, the surgeon usually attempts to perform an internal decompression, removing as much of the tumor as

Table 30-6. Multidisciplinary Treatment Decisions For Various Brain Tumors (12,52a,82,103a,107a)

Tumor	Surgery		Radiation Therapy	Chemotherapy
Low-grade glioma	Complete resection if possible	and/or	For residual and recurrent tumor ART/CRT 50-60 Gy	N R
Malignant glioma (AAF + GBM)	Partial resection Decompression	and/or	DRT High doses are used: 60-80 Gy with implants 100-120 Gy	CCR/IC* III
Medulloblastoma ependymoblastoma	Complete resection if feasible		CRT 45-55 Gy, depending on age	CCR/IC III
Meningioma	Complete resection if feasible	and/or	For residual and recurrent tumor: ART/CRT 60 Gy	N R
Pituitary adenoma	Complete resection if possible	and/or	ART/CRT 45-55 Gy	Bromocriptine is used to lower prolactin level N R
Craniopharyngioma	Complete resection		ART/CRT 55-60 Gy	N R
Pinealomas	Stereotactic only	and/or	CRT 50 Gy	N R
Midbrain and brain stem	Stereotactic biopsy at most, unless exophytic		DRT 50-60 Gy	

RT = radiation therapy; ART = adjuvant; CRT = curative; DRT = definitive; N R = not recommended; RCT = recommended chemotherapy; AAF = astrocytoma with foci of anaplasia; GBM = glioblastoma multiforme; CCR = concurrent chemotherapy and radiation; IC III = investigational chemotherapy, phase II/III clinical trials.
PDQ: RCT - *CCR=BCNU + RT for glioblastoma

possible to relieve the pressure on the brain. This generally restores function temporarily.

Astrocytomas are of varying degrees of malignancy and may occur anywhere in the brain, including the optic nerves. The more slowly growing cystic astrocytomas are more amenable to surgery and can sometimes be removed completely. Those located in the cerebellum in children can almost always be excised successfully (11,93). Malignant astrocytomas tend to recur rapidly, and about 80% of the patients who undergo surgery alone for AAF or GBM die within 6 months (11).

The ideal therapy is complete surgical excision, but this is rarely possible except for an occasional tumor isolated to an optic nerve or to a polar location in the brain such as the anterior frontal, temporal, or occipital lobe. Those patients treated with wide surgical excision generally do better, even if the tumor is malignant. Their symptoms are relieved because of decompression of adjacent viable areas of the brain. Surgery decreases the remaining tumor bulk for irradiation and chemotherapy (52,53,55,82,83,85,89). However, for tumors that are in or near the midline, involve both hemispheres, or lie very deep within the cerebrum only biopsy is done, as an attempt at surgical eradication would likely cause severe neurologic deficit that obviously would not improve the patient's status. A biopsy may be done under local or general anesthesia using various methods such as CT, ultrasonic or stereotactic guidance (39,42,51,67). The ability to diagnose an astrocytoma with such methods is better than 90%. However, because of the small sample of tissue taken and the variability of the histologic picture throughout such a tumor, sometimes a false impression may be gained as to the degree of malignancy. When wide surgical excision can be done, much more tissue is available to the pathologist for diagnosis. Then, the worst looking areas are taken as a measure of the tumor's actual degree of malignancy.

When *astrocytomas, oligodendrogliomas,* and other malignancies in the brain recur, therapeutic options are limited. Sometimes symptoms are caused by a necrotic mass within the tumor that has developed secondary to treatment with irradiation or chemotherapeutic agents. Resection of these necrotic areas and the tumor around them can be useful, especially if the patient's symptoms are primarily from increased ICP. Reresection of localized gliomas in favorable locations such as the frontal pole, temporal tip, occipital pole, or posterior parietal region is done occasionally. Interstitial irradiation by brachytherapy has also been used during the past 10 years for lesions less than 6 cm in diameter that do not involve the deep or midline structures. It was used 20 or 30 years ago, but can be controlled much more precisely now with CT guidance. Complications such as radionecrosis of the tumor region and adjacent brain do arise and sometimes can be treated with surgical excision. While some reports are encouraging, it is uncertain as to the exact value of these measures for recurrent tumors. In individual cases, they are occasionally gratifying, producing even a 5-year cure in some patients with GBM (74,75). Brain implants are also being evaluated as primary therapy in select cases of malignant glioma that meet the criteria of size and location.

Radiotherapy (12,15,22,50,81)

Most malignant brain tumors respond to external irradiation. Radiation therapy is the most important treatment modality; it produces cures in certain tumors and prolonged survival in others. It can also allay symptoms when tumors recur.

Radiotherapy is generally indicated when the tumor:

1. Is malignant (e.g., malignant gliomas AAF, GBM, and gliosarcoma (64-92); meningiosarcoma (50,156,157, 163,165); medulloblastoma (113-119,121-129); ependymoma and ependymoblastoma (130-135); pinealoma, pineoblastoma, and germinomas (182-189)].
2. Is a low-grade tumor that is incompletely excised (see below under 3).
3. Is centrally located and involves critical structures so that surgical intervention is not possible without a great deal of morbidity and/or mortality, such as tumor involving midbrain, third ventricle, and brain stem. Some of these tumors may not even be able to be safely biopsied.
4. Is a metastatic deposit (11,15). (Although clinically only one site may be suspected, there are usually multiple sites.)
5. Is a pituitary tumor (11,15,173-176).

Postoperative x-ray therapy is advocated for the following tumor types, if tumor removal has been incomplete:

- low-grade gliomas (92c-102) including optic glioma (147-155)
- oligodendroglioma (166-172)
- ependymoma (130-135)
- meningioma (156-165)
- craniopharyngioma (136-146)
- chordoma (177-181)
- neurilemoma

Radiation treatment dose is determined by the tumor's histologic type, radioresponsiveness, anatomic site, and level of tolerance. Treatment fields are determined by the anatomic extent of the tumor and the potential areas of spread. Elective irradiation of the spinal cord is advocated for neoplasms with high potential for meningeal seeding such as medulloblastomas, high-grade ependymomas, pineoblastomas, and malignant gliomas of the posterior fossa with positive CSF cytology.

In general, total tumor doses range from 5,000 to 7,000 cGy in 6 to 8 weeks with daily fractions of 150 to 200 cGy each. Doses in excess of 7,000 cGy have not resulted in curability of GBM. Coned-down fields are advised when doses to the whole brain, or large field, reach 3,500 to 4,000 cGy in children and 4,500 to 5,000 cGy in adults.

The total dose is limited by normal tissue tolerance. When normal tissue tolerance is exceeded in the brain, *radiation necrosis* develops (9,14,16,21b,47,48). The risk of brain necrosis, balanced against the risk from tumor progression, determines the dose that can be given. In adults with malignant tumors, such as GBM, where survival is usually measured in months, the risk of rapid tumor recurrence is high enough that a higher risk of necrosis (as high as 20%) is accepted and doses of 6,000 cGy in 30 to 35 fractions are routinely used. For adults with astrocytomas, that is, low-grade gliomas, whose survival is measured in years, an incidence of less 5% or less is generally accepted. Doses of 5,400 cGy delivered in 180 cGy fractions are frequently used. In patients with pituitary adenomas where survival is long, because of the potential risk of blindness the total dose is usually restricted to 5,000 cGy in 25 to 28 fractions (9,48,50).

There is one exception to the avoidance of necrosis when radioactive implant is considered for a relatively small tumor. If the tumor is located in a relatively silent region of the brain where necrosis can be excised without producing significant deficit, then total doses of 10,000 to 12,000 cGy can be delivered by external beam irradiation and implant. The use of an implant after external beam irradiation has resulted in a 5-year cure in some patients with GBM (74,75).

In children with malignant tumors, further dose modification is required. The developing brain is more sensitive to radiation therapy. Treatment in children less than aged 4 years is avoided, if possible. Very young children (< 4 years of age) are given chemotherapy or are simply followed after surgical resection until either tumor progression requires the use of radiation therapy or until the patient reaches 4 years of age, at which time the brain growth and development is virtually complete. Because the young brain is more sensitive to irradiation, with postradiation learning difficulties becoming a particularly severe problem at ages up to 6 years, doses are modified. For a child older than 4 years, posterior fossa tumors are usually treated to 5,400 cGy. Whole brain irradiation is usually limited to 3,500 to 4,000 cGy and spinal axis irradiation is given to 2,500 to 4,000 cGy, the lower doses being used for potential microscopic disease. The trend is to evaluate lower doses in clinical trials of various diseases.

Clinical radiation symptoms (9,14,15,48,50):

1. *Acute effects of irradiation* are usually minimal when daily doses of 180 to 200 cGy per fraction are used 5 days a week up to doses of 6,000 cGy. However, there are some patients who develop increased ICP or an exacerbation of their symptoms and/or signs associated with the lesion being treated. These are probably due to edema and usually respond to simple corticosteroid therapy, e.g., dexamethasone 2 to 4 mg bid to qid. Occasionally a patient with a large tumor mass develops a rapid deterioration that sometimes can be reversed or improved by the addition of IV mannitol and/or glycerol.

   With doses of 2,000 to 4,000 cGy delivered in 2 to 4 weeks, patients will experience temporary hair loss approximately 10 days to 2 weeks into treatment. It will take approximately 2 to 3 months after completion of irradiation for the hair to begin to regrow. However, if the dose to a region of the scalp is more than 4,000 cGy, then the loss is usually permanent. *Erythema* of the scalp, *tanning*, and dry desquamation will occur. *Moist desquamation* can occur behind the ears, particularly if the patient wears glasses and there is some rubbing by the glasses.

2. *Delayed acute reactions* or *early delayed reactions* (15,50) usually occur between 2 and 6 weeks following completion of irradiation and may continue for up to 3 months. Symptoms are usually somnolence and lethargy that can manifest as simply going to bed sooner, and/or taking a nap, up to the extreme of sleeping 20 hours a day or more. These symptoms may be associated with worsening of the original symptoms or the development of new symptoms. Such symptoms can be dysarthria, dysphagia, cerebral ataxia, and decreased mental status. These delayed acute reactions are thought to be associated with patchy demyelinization with petechial hemorrhages. The symptoms spontaneously improve without change in therapy or with simple increase in dexamethasone. The importance of recognizing the early delayed reaction is to reassure the patient that symptoms occurring during this time do not necessarily indicate tumor recurrence or the need to change therapy, although for patients over 60 years of age with a malignant glioma, deterioration is more apt to represent tumor progression.

3. Late (delayed) *radiation reactions* occur several months to years later. They are usually irreversible and progressive. Symptoms depend on the location of the lesion in the brain. Minor delayed reactions can occur with white matter loss producing cerebral atrophy on CT scan and possible difficulty in short-term memory. The most severe late delayed reaction is radiation necrosis discussed above. Radiation cataracts are possible. However, if the eyes are shielded or kept out of the beam, this usually can be avoided.

Radiation treatment volume: With the advent of CT scanning and MRI, we are now better able to localize and define tumor extent (10,77a). The contrast-enhancing lesion is generally considered to constitute the gross tumor volume and tumor edema in the white matter is considered to represent microscopic extension. Tumor cells have been documented in white matter edema. Therefore, the region of edema is usually treated with a margin to a dose which is used for microscopic disease. The gross tumor plus a 2.5 cm margin for malignant tumors and a 1.0-2.0 cm margin for benign tumors is treated to the total tumor dose.

Patterns of failure — local recurrence: Hochberg and Pruit (77a) reviewed serial CT scans in 42 patients with GBM before death and noted that 90% of recurrences were located within a 2 cm margin of the primary tumor. In 35 patients who had CT scan within 2 months of autopsy, gross and microscopic tumor were found to be within the volume identified on CT scan in 29 of 35 patients. An additional two patients who had multifocal disease identified on CT scan had additional nodules identified on postmortem examination that were not identified on CT scan. If the whole brain is treated in patients with multiple lesions, 90% of patients with solitary lesions treated with local field would have had tumor relapse within 2 cm of the contrast-enhancing lesion. Only 4% to 6% of patients with malignant glioma have multifocal disease and are not candidates for local radiotherapy (77a). In a report by Walner *et al.* (92) from Memorial Sloan-Kettering Cancer Center, 78% of 32 patients with unifocal tumors had recurrence within 2 cm of the presurgical initial tumor margin as defined on the enhancing edge of the tumor by CT scan.

Cranial spinal irradiation is given to tumors that have a high propensity to seed the subarachnoid space, such as the PNET, which include medulloblastoma. With cranial spinal irradiation, the patient is treated prone. Lateral fields are used to treat the whole brain. These lateral fields are gapped with the posterior field, which treats the spinal cord. Extremely technical maneuvers are used to match the divergence of the radiation beam so that there is no overlap. To make certain there are no significant hot spots or cold spots, edges of the fields are feathered; that is, the gap, or match line, is shifted 1 cm every thousand cGy so that the gap is located at three different levels or more to allow for smudging of the dose. An example of this is given in Fig. 30-2.

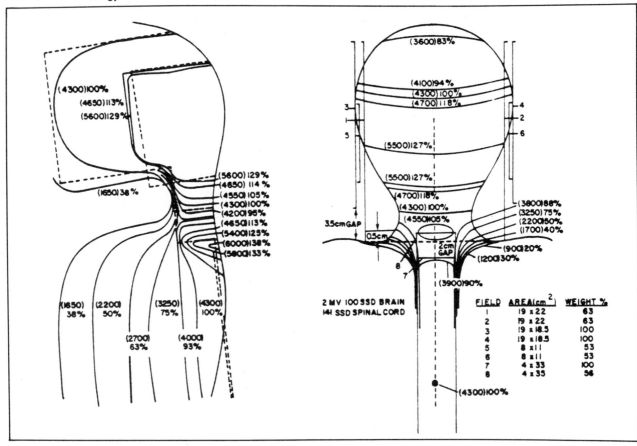

Fig. 30-2. Radiation therapy technique: matching fields. When the entire central nervous system is to be irradiated, such as in medulloblastoma with high potential of meningeal seeding, there is a need to avoid a gap or "cold spot" between the cranial field and the spinal cord field. More important is the need to avoid an overlap, creating a "hot spot" that would lead to exceeding the radiation tolerance dose in that area, and eventually result in necrosis and spinal cord transection. A shifting field arrangement in which the spinal field is move to three different levels, allows for the creation of a relatively uniform dose, avoiding cold or hot spots in this important area. The isodose curves indicate equal doses at specified levels. SSD = source-surface distance.

Local control remains the challenge: Even with doses of 7,000 or 8,000 cGy, local recurrence or tumor persistence remains the problem with malignant glioma and many other brain tumors. Malignant gliomas can be considered to be related to sarcomas, which are more radioresistant than carcinomas. GBM also contains areas of necrosis, and therefore, hypoxia. Hypoxia is a major reason for local failure of radiation therapy. Attempts to overcome this hypoxia have consisted of using: (1) hyperbaric oxygen; (2) high linear energy transfer radiation such as neutrons (21,65,70) and heavy particles, stripped nuclei (56), or negative pi-mesons; (3) electron effinic hypoxic cell radiation sensitizers such as misonidazole or metronidazole (7,64,69,80,81,87,88); and (4) the use of small individual fraction size with hyper-fractionation (twice daily treatments), in order to minimize the oxygen effect (69,81).

An additional factor that may contribute to the failure to control so many brain tumors, particularly malignant gliomas, may be the immunologic status of the patient. Many patients with malignant gliomas have an impaired immunologic status. In addition, there are no lymphatics within the brain, and the absence of lymphatics, along with the presence of the blood-brain barrier, may prevent killer T cells and

phagocytes from eliminating the last remaining tumor cells after treatment with radiation therapy, surgery, and/or chemotherapy.

Increasing the dose or total effective dose is another means of attempting to increase local control. Such attempts have included: (1) focused heavy particle beams (49,56); (2) hyperfractionation (twice daily treatments with two smaller than usual individual doses separated by 4 to 8 hours to allow for repair of radiation damage, which minimizes late radiation effects and permits delivery of a higher total dose) (81); (3) radiosurgery or gamma knife therapy (61,63); and (4) brachytherapy, a radioactive implant that delivers a high dose to the tumor with rapid fall-off to the normal brain (49a,74,75). Adding heat (hyperthermia) to radiation therapy may also increase the effectiveness of tumor cell killing (45,54).

Chemotherapy (4,15,17,37,40,41,46,59,66,69, 71-73,76,77,79,84,86,90,91)

Progress in this field has been slow because: a) Compared with breast and colorectal cancer, incidence of these tumors is low and only a limited number of patients are available for clinical trials; b) the inaccessibility of CNS tumors makes objective tumor response measurement hard to obtain;

c) most studies have used survival as a measurement of response. Because of the lack of a control group in most studies and the heterogeneity of important prognostic variables like tumor grade, histologic type, patient age, and KPS, the significance of several months' extension of survival is difficult to assess; d) at present there is no demonstrated benefit from chemotherapy for newly diagnosed low-grade gliomas or for brain stem gliomas; and e) the multi drug resistance gene expression was found in the vast majority of glioma samples studied by Feun et al. (41a) and may explain the intrinsic resistance of this tumor to chemotherapeutic agents, which is associated with median duration of response.

For malignant brain tumors, chemotherapeutic options remain somewhat limited. Lipid-soluble drugs such as the nitrosoureas lomustine, carmustine, and semustine, procarbazine, and vincristine remain the mainstays of treatment. Other investigated cytotoxic drugs include teniposide (a podophylotoxin derivative), dacarbazine, bleomycin, cisplatin, and carboplatinum (86).

Cortiosteroids have proven to be of considerable benefit to patients with metastatic brain tumors (44,57,58). The response of increased ICP secondary to primary brain tumors also has been equally impressive. The mechanism of action of corticosteroids is probably secondary to the effect of the amelioration of cerebral edema. There is some evidence that there is a specific antitumor effect of corticosteroids. This has been demonstrated in experimental animal work by Shapiro and Posner (58) in a study in mice with intracerebral ependymoblastomas. The most favored corticosteroid has been dexamethasone, although this is being replaced by methylprednisolone. The usual daily dose of dexamethasone is 16 mg, but some patients have received as much as 96 mg before maximal improvement has been noted. The general complications of this treatment are similar to those of corticosteroids used for other conditions. The incidence of GI bleeding appears to be less than 5% (58).

Chemotherapy for Recurrence

Carmustine has been used widely to treat malignant brain tumors. Responses are obtained in about half of the patients treated. Duration of response can vary from 3 to 12 months. Lomustine is also an active agent, although as a single agent it appears to be somewhat inferior to carmustine. Procarbazine has been useful in combination with other agents. Higher response rates have been obtained with carmustine and 5-FU or carmustine, 5-FU hydroxyurea and 6 mercaptomurine combinations. Effective single agents for recurrent malignant gliomas are listed in Table 30-7A. Ineffective agents with response rates less than 30% and/or durations less than 35 weeks are listed in Table 30-7A. Effective multiagent chemotherapy for recurrent gliomas also are listed in Table 30-7B.

Adjuvant Chemotherapy of Malignant Gliomas (66,69,71,71a,73,79,86,90,91)

Adjuvant chemotherapy seems to benefit some patients with malignant gliomas. Although there are a number of studies showing no survival advantage for adjuvant chemotherapy, the sample sizes of many of these studies have been small so that all but large improvement in survival would be missed. Large cooperative groups like the Brain Tumor Study Group (BTSG), RTOG, and ECOG have randomized several hundred patients and found modest beneficial effect of adjuvant chemotherapy in certain subsets of patients by way of prolongation of survival. Table 30-8 summarizes the results of the major chemotherapy trials. Patients between the ages of 40 and 60 years and those less than aged 40 years with GBM have demonstrated the most benefit. Patients over aged 60 years have shown no improvement in survival and have had worse toxicity unless chemotherapy doses were initially lowered.

Chemotherapy/Radiation Therapy Reactions (16,38,40,92a)

White matter necrosis or demyelination occurs with some chemotherapeutic agents, and is more apt to occur when

---

Table 30-7. Response Rates to Single Agent Chemotherapy in Recurrent or Malignant Gliomas

Single Agent Regimens		Multiagent Regimens	
Drug	Response rate (%)	Drug	Response Rate (%)
Effective Therapy			
Procarbazine	27-50	Carmustine + vincristine	25-41
Teniposide	63	Carmustine + 5-FU	31-39
Carmustine	48-51	Procarbazine, lomustine, vincristine	60
Lomustine	43-47	Teniposide+ lomustine	18-75
Semustine	56	Teniposide, lomustine, doxorubicin	72
		Methotrexate, lomustine, vincristine	36-40
Ineffective Therapy (Response rate < 30%, Duration < 35 wk)		Cyclophosphamide, lomustine, vincristine	38
Doxorubicin			
AZQ			
Chlorozotacin			
Cisplatin			
DDP			
Hydroxyurea			
Imidazole			
Carboxamide			
Methotrexate			
Mithramycin			
Thiotepa			
Triazinate			

Table 30-8. Randomized Trials of Chemotherapy in the Treatment of Gliomas

TREATMENT	SURVIVAL			
	Median no. months	18 mo (%)	24 mo (%)	Reference
BTSG Trial 6901				90
Support	39.	0	0	
Carmustine	5.8	4	0	
RT	8.7	4	1	
RT + carmustine	9.4	19	5	
BTSG Trial 7201				91
Semustine	5.5	10	8	
RT	11.8	15	10	
RT + carmustine	11.8	27	15	
RT + semustine	9.7	23	12	
BTSG Trial 7501				73
RT + carmustine	11.5	24	16	
RT + methylprednisolone*	9.2	15	6	
RT + procarbazine	10.9	29	23	
RT + carmustine + methylprednisolone	9.5	23	18	
BTSG Trial 7702				69
RT† + carmustine	9.9	16	10	
Hyperfraction RT-carmustine	10.4	25	16	
RT† + streptozotocin + carmustine	9.2	17	9	
RT† streptozotocin	9.9	24	19	
RTOG 7401 / ECOG 1374				79
< 60 Gy	9.3	18	14	
< 70 Gy	8.2	24	16	
60 Gy + carmustine	9.7	28	20	
60 Gy + semustine - dacarbazine/imidazole/carboxamide	10.1	17	21	
EORTC BTG '78				71
RT + lomustine postop	9.9			
RT postop lomustine at relapse	14.3			
EORTC BTG '81				71a
RT + teniposide + lomustine postop	12.7			
RT postop teniposide + lomustine at relapse	14.1			

BTSG = Brain Tumor Study Group; RT = radiation therapy; ECOG = Eastern Cooperative Oncology Group; RTOG = Radiation Therapy Oncology Group; EORTC - BTG = European Organization on Research and Treatment of Cancer Brain Tumor Group
* VSG = valid study group;
† RT = 55-60 Gy + 1.1 Gy bid to 66 Gy ++ grades III and IV

chemotherapy is combined with irradiation either simultaneously or sequentially. This is well illustrated by the late effects seen with methotrexate in survivors with acute lymphocytic leukemia. When high-dose methotrexate is given after brain irradiation there is an increased risk of leukoencephalopathy. This has been attributed to radiation-induced alterations in the blood-brain barrier, resulting in increased penetration of drugs across the blood-brain barrier after irradiation, and consequent increased drug concentrations in the brain. A diffuse demyelination process occurs, which is different from the distribution of radiation lesions, which tend to be perivascular. A whole series of acute and late

encephalopathies have been reported, particularly in children (38). Although drug delivery prior to irradiation minimizes the risk of late CNS toxicity, there is still some increased risk. The best example is again methotrexate, which when given to children prior to 4,000 cGy whole brain irradiation, has produced leukoencephalopathy in several cases (D'Angio, G.J., M.D., personal communication, 1987).

Pulmonary toxicity is a late effect of carmustine that can be fatal, reported by Mahaley *et al.* (16) and Weinstein *et al.* (92a) in long-term survivors maintained on carmustine. A dose-response curve indicates accumulated levels of above 903 mg/m² can be lethal. There is about a 10% incidence of pulmonary toxicity at total doses of 1,200 to 1,400 mg/m^2, and an almost 50% incidence at 2,000 mg/m^2.

Investigational Approaches

Interferon, intra-arterial infusional chemotherapy, and carmustine-soaked wafers implanted directly into the tumor, hyperosmolar attempts to disrupt the blood-brain barrier, interleukin 2-lymphocyte-activated killer cells, and high-dose chemotherapy with autologous bone marrow transplantation are new options being studied (41,60,77,92b).

SPECIAL CONSIDERATIONS OF TREATMENT MALIGNANT ADULT ASTROCYTOMAS

High-grade Astrocytomas

Anaplastic astrocytomas and GBM tumors can rarely be totally resected. Radiation therapy is commonly used if the patient is able to tolerate a full course of therapy. Large-field irradiation encompassing the tumor and edema plus a 2 cm margin is used to doses of 4,500 to 5,000 cGy, with a boost to the primary tumor plus a 2.5 cm margin to bring the total dose to 6,000 to 6,500 cGy. Despite radiation doses of 7,000 to 8,000 cGy to brain tumors, local control has not been achieved with photon irradiation. For this reason, a variety of clinical trials have been completed and a number of studies are in progress.

Chemotherapy: As noted in the previous sections on radiation therapy and chemotherapy (Table 30-8), a wide variety of combinations have been used. The combination of carmustine and radiation therapy appears to offer the longest median survival and is considered the standard treatment in clinical trial settings. The increase in median survival is associated with hematologic toxicity and depression in 30% to 40% of patients (66,79,90,91). Various drug combinations have been explored, but none have led to an overall increase in cure. Intra-arterial carmustine or intra-arterial platinum have been and are being evaluated. However, CNS toxicities, including blindness, have remained problems. High-dose (lethal) carmustine 300 mg/m^2/d x 3 followed by autologous bone marrow transplant and 6,120 cGy in 180 cGy fractions is being studied by the ECOG (protocol P-C387). Hydroxyurea, a cell cycle synchronizer, and bromodeoxyuridine, a radiosensitizing agent, are being explored by Levin *et al.* (78a,78b) with radiotherapy and PCV; their results demonstrated an increase in median survival.

Hypoxic cell radiosensitizers: Misonidazole, a hypoxic cell sensitizer, was expected to be effective in treating malignant tumors of the brain. This has been used alone as well as in combination with carmustine. The enhancement ratio predicted was between 1.3 and 1.7, which implies that for a given dose of irradiation, there would be a 30% to 70% increase in effectiveness with misonidazole compared with irradiation alone (88). In the first randomized study of cerebral GBM treated by postoperative irradiation with and without the sensitizer metronidazole, there was an initial significant gain in survival that was of brief duration (87). However, prognosis and survival beyond 12 months were not altered and the total radiation dose was low. More recent studies from the RTOG (80) and the Cambridge glioblastoma study (64), and the BTSG (69) have shown no overall advantage to misonidazole added to radiation therapy. In addition, the RTOG and BTCG have both observed a worse survival for

patients with anaplastic astrocytoma treated with misonidazole. This is either due to radiation damage/necrosis or added independent CNS toxicity, as misonidazole is known to produce CNS toxicity. Presently the halogens bromodeoxyuridine and idoxuridine are being evaluated. Incorporation of these halogens into pyrimidines increases the radiosensitivity of DNA three fold.

Heavy particle therapy: Heavy particle beams consisting of neutrons, pi mesons, and stripped nuclei possess certain biologic advantages that may achieve greater local control of more radioresistant tumors (78b'). The London neutron therapy trial (65) compared 6 MeV irradiation with doses of 5,000 cGy to neutron dose of 1.400 cGy. The encouraging finding was the pathologic evidence of nearly complete tumor eradication in 69% of neutron-treated patients versus 14% for photon-treated patients. The latter sterilization rate is similar to rates reported in other series in the literature, such as that of BTSG, which reports only 4% with a dose of 6,000 cGy. There was no improved survival with neutron beam therapy because the greater biologic effect of neutrons on the normal brain produced increasing radiation-induced degenerative changes in the cerebral white matter, leading to progressive dementia (65). A similar experience reported from Seattle showed no advantage for neutron versus megavoltage irradiation (21). For neutron therapy, there does not appear to be a therapeutic window that permits eradication of tumor without eradication of brain function (85a).

Immunotherapy: Efforts have been made to increase host immunity by nonspecific measures such as bacillus Calmette-Guerin or levamisole administration, but there is no convincing evidence that such maneuvers have prolonged survival in patients with malignant gliomas (60). A randomized clinical trial at the Royal Marsden Hospital (5) attempted to increase host resistance by injecting irradiated autologous brain tumor tissue subcutaneously and postoperatively. It failed to improve the results for patients who received irradiation alone; in fact, in 2.5 years, all patients treated with autologous tumor cells were dead, whereas 20% of the control group were still alive. Intratumor infusions of autologous leukocytes have been cited as improving clinical response, but no lasting effects have been noted (92b).

Hyperfractionation: With RTOG protocol 8302, hyperfractionation 120 cGy bid (separated by a 4 to 8 hour interval) was evaluated to total doses of 6,480 cGy, 7,200 cGy, 7,680 cGy, and 8,160 Gy in a phase II randomized trial. This study is presently closed and preliminary evaluation reveals no significant difference between hyperfractionation plus carmustine in this study versus historical control, that is, control arm of 7918 (radiotherapy plus carmustine). There is a suggestion that the 7,680 Gy arm is doing better. However, a phase III randomized trial needs to be conducted to evaluate this hypothesis (78d). Fulton *et al.* (72a) have reported that hyperfractionation using fractions of 89 cGy tid to a total dose of 6,140 cGy, with or without misonidazole, compared with 193 cGy/d to a total dose of 5,800 cGy demonstrates significant increase in survival for hyperfractionation with a median survival of 45 and 50 weeks for tid fractionation compared with 29 weeks for conventional fractionation. This is an example in which worse survival in a control group makes the experimental arm look better, that is, statistically significant. However, the control groups of other randomized trials with standard therapy are closer to the 45 to 50 weeks observed with the hyperfractionation arm (72a). The BTSG also evaluated hyperfractionation treating 110 cGy bid to 6,660 cGy in 60 fractions plus carmustine compared with conventional radiotherapy 6,000 cGy in 30 to 35 fractions plus carmustine in a randomized phase III trial. There was no statistical difference in survival. Median survival was 10.4 months for hyperfractionation versus 9.9 months for conventional fractionation. Eighteen months' survival was minimally better with hyperfractionation: 24.9% versus 16.1%. Similarly, 24-month survival was 15.6% compared with 10.4% (69). Although the initial radiation biology estimates were that hyperfractionation would permit an increase of 10% in total dose, this study proves that such an increase neither increased the complication rate nor the survival rate. With the RTOG hyperfractionation study, there is no dose response for toxicity and the best arm appears to be the total dose of 76.8 cGy. Marcial-Vega *et al.* (78c) have reported on an accelerated course of radiation therapy in a nonrandomized retrospective series of 73 patients with grade III or IV supertentorial gliomas who were treated with accelerated fractionation 300 cGy/d to 3,000 cGy in 2 weeks, followed by a 2 week rest and an additional 2,100 cGy in seven fractions to a total dose of 5,100 cGy in 17 fractions over 36 days. The overall median survival was 12.5 months, with 52% surviving 1 year, 23% alive in 2 years, and 10% surviving 5 years. The median survival for grade III histologies was 22.5 months and for the grade IV it was 10 months. These results are not statistically significant from other series of conventional radiation therapy, although it is a nonrandomized series in which case selection might influence outcome. Combining hyperfractionation with misonidazole was no more successful than irradiation alone in a recent BTSG Study (69). Lindstadt *et al.* (78b) have demonstrated excellent tolerance to brain stem for hyperfractionated irradiation with high control and survival rates.

Stereotactic interstitial brachytherapy: The use of interstitial implants in combination with external irradiation has resulted in minimum doses of 8,000 cGy and approximately half the patients receiving doses to as high as 12,000 cGy (75a). The survival for anaplastic astrocytomas was 46% and 28% at 18 months and 36 months, respectively; in contrast, survival for GBM was only 22% and 8% for the same time periods. Of special interest are the associated high rate of tumor necrosis that occurred in 49% of survivors and that excision or removal of the necrotic zone led to higher survival. Although 67% remain steroid-dependent, the majority of long-term (72 years) survivors remain stable as measured by KPS (49a).

Stereotactic radiotherapy: Stereotactic radiosurgery promises the delivery of high radiation doses to a well-defined target volume and is shifting its direction from treating benign arterio-venous malformations to defining its role in the management of malignant intracranial neoplasms—primary, recurrent, and metastatic tumors (78c'). The 3-D technique is well explained and illustrated by Kooy *et al.* (78') using a BRW localizing frame combined with CT (optimally MR and angiography) to provide the required accuracy and volumetric analyses. This is an investigational technique for boosting residual central focus of malignant gliomas after a course of external irradiation is completed.

RESULTS AND PROGNOSIS

Due to the wide spectrum of neoplasms with varied aggressiveness, long-term survival may occur in some subgroups. This should not necessarily be attributed to the effects of surgery, and/or radiotherapy, and/or chemotherapy. The tumor's natural history must be considered (27,34). The 5-year survival figures are of value in expressing long-term results of low-grade tumors and some malignant tumors (Table 30-9, Fig. 30-3) (6). However, in malignant gliomas, the 2-year survival rate and median survival are often used because survival is so short. Two recent excellent reviews of malignant gliomas have been reported by Davis (68) and Sheline (86a); they report management based on achievements in cooperative group clinical trial research and provide data on overall survival.

High-grade Astrocytomas (Anaplastic Astrocytoma and GBM)

More than 50% of patients with GBM will be dead within 9 months, with 5% to 12% surviving 2 years and virtually all dead in 3 years. There are a few exceptional 5-year survivors who are young adults (< 40 years of age). For patients with anaplastic astrocytoma, the survival is better, and a number of series report survivals of 20% to 35% at 5 years, depending upon treatment and distribution of prognostic variables. For malignant gliomas, the median survival improves with increasing dose from 5,000 to 7,000 cGy. There is a gain in 2-year survival, but this disappears by 3 years. Performance status improves after surgery and radiation therapy; 34% of patients return to work, 24% have moderately good function, and 42% stay at poor functional improvement (28%) in performance status after therapy (30). Another study examined posttherapy KPS. Forty-four percent had an improved KPS, 34% a stable status, and 22% a worse status. When neurologic function was scored on a scale of 4, 34% improved, 56% were stable, and 10% were worse (79).

Treatment Results

Survival rates in clinical trials: In a randomized, prospective trial in 1980, the BTSG reported a significant increase in survival when radiation therapy, or radiation therapy and carmustine was added to surgery. The median survival was 35

Table 30-9. Five and Ten-Year Survival Rates for Brain Tumors

	% Survival	
	5-year	10-year
Astrocytoma		
Grade I (cerebellar)	90-100	85-100
Grade I (all sites)	50-60	30-40
Grade II	16-46	8-15
Grade III	10-30	0-10
Grade IV	1-10	0-1
Medulloblastoma	40-50	20-30
Ependymoma	40-55	35-45
Oligodendroglioma	50-80	20-30
Brain stem	20-30	0-10
Third ventricle and midbrain	25-35	5-10
Pinealoma	50-90	55-65
Pituitary adenoma	80-95	70-90
Craniopharyngioma	80-90	65-80
Optic	75-100	70-85
Meningiomas	70-80	50-60

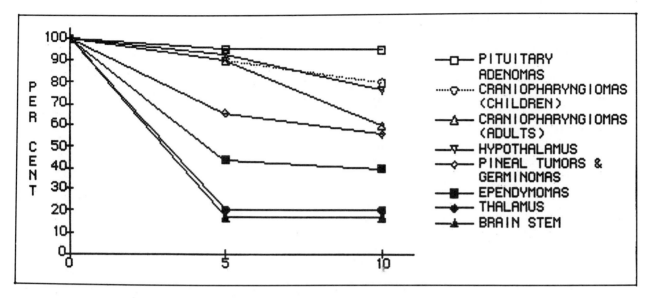

Fig. 30-3. Survival curves. This figure is a compilation of results in the literature illustrating that many of the childhood tumors carry a good to excellent prognosis with approximately 50% survival or better. Highly malignant thalamus and brain stem tumors as well as grade III-IV glioblastomas have a lower survival, but much better than adults. Numbers in graph are percent survival at 5 and 10 years. From Bloom (5), with permission.

weeks compared with 14 weeks for surgery with supportive care only, or 19 weeks for surgery plus carmustine. The 18-month survival rate for surgery with supportive care was zero; for surgery plus carmustine, 4%; for radiation therapy, 4%; and for radiation therapy plus carmustine, 19% (90). When the BTSG analyzed data from 621 patients treated between 1966 and 1975 with 180 to 200 cGy per fraction to doses of 5,500 to 6,000 cGy, a dose response was observed and median survival times were 28 weeks, 36 weeks, and 42 weeks respectively, which was statistically significant (p = 0.004). The distribution of prognostic variables between treatment groups was comparable (91a).

Importance of dose: The RTOG and ECOG evaluated 6,000 cGy whole brain versus 6,000 cGy whole brain plus 1,000 cGy boost to the tumor volume without significant increase in survival, although the patients less than aged 40 years treated to 70 cGy had a median survival of 47 months compared with those treated to 60 cGy, who had a median survival of 21.3 months. However, the number of patients was too small to be significant. For the AAF patients there was no real difference between 60 and 70 cGy, although those AAF patients less than aged 40 years treated to 70 cGy had a 72% 48-month survival, compared with a 30% 48-month survival for those who were treated to 60 cGy. However, the total number of patients for each group is only 7 and 12. Total dose did not affect survival for AAF patients aged 40 years or older. Their 48-month survival was approximately 18% to 20%, and their median survival was 6 months. When their median survival is compared with that of AAF patients younger than 40 years, the magnitude of the prognostic factor of age is evident. The median survival for AAF patients younger than aged 40 years treated with 70 cGy had not yet been reached with follow-up of more than 5 years, and the median survival for those treated with 60 cGy was 36 months. Age made a greater impact on survival than did treatment (79).

Prognostic factors: The difference in survival due to the prognostic factors of age, histology, and KPS has proven to

be more significant than therapy in most randomized trials with large numbers of patients. Because of the impact of prognostic factors on survival, the reader of the malignant glioma literature needs to have a healthy skepticism of any series that has less than 100, if not 150, patients per arm. If one considers all age groups and histologies together, small or modest differences in therapy may be masked.

1. *Histopathology:* When Nelson *et al.* (30) reviewed an RTOG trial to evaluate pathology criteria for grading, they found no difference in median survival for Kernohan grade 3 (median survival of 238 patients was 10 months) and Kernohan grade 4 (median survival of 220 patients was 9 months). When the same patients were reclassified on the basis of the presence of necrosis, there was a significant difference in survival (P < .0001). The median survival when necrosis was present (i.e., for GBM), was 8 months and when necrosis was absent (i.e., for AAF), 28 months. The respective 18-month survival rates were 15% and 62%. Although AAF only constitutes 15% to 20% of RTOG and BTCG protocol patients, their improved survival has been repeatedly confirmed (79,80,80b).

2. *Age:* Prognosis is inversely related to age; the older the patient, the worse is the prognosis. Prognosis is especially poor for patients older than 60 years of age. Overall, for malignant gliomas those aged 18 to 44 survive twice as long as those aged 45 to 55 years and three times as long as those aged over 55 years (80). For patients with GBM, the median survival for patients 60 to 70 years old is 6 months; for 40 to 59 year olds, 9 months; and for 18 to 39 year olds, 17 months. For patients with AAF, the median survival for those 60 to 70 years old is 9 months; for 40 to 59 years, 26 months; and for 18 to 39 years, 48 months (80a).

3. *Karnofsky performance status:* KPS has been repeatedly confirmed as a prognostic variable. Patients with KPS of 80 to 100 have a survival that is approximately twice that for patients with a KPS of 40 to 70 (80). For patients

with AAF histology, the survival difference is even greater with a median survival of 46.8 months for those with a KPS of 80 to 100 compared with a median survival of 9.5 months for those with a KPS of 40 to 70. The respective 1-year survival rates were 89% versus 49% and 3-year survival rates were 25% and 62% (80a,93a)

Low-Grade Astrocytomas (92c-102) (Table 30-10a)

Prognosis for low-grade cerebellar astrocytomas is extremely favorable. Usually cystic, they have a high curability of 90% at 5 years and 85% at 10 years (93). Children with cerebral gliomas also have a good survival: 46% at 5 years and 43% at 10 years. However, this is not as good as those with gliomas in the cerebellar location (98). In children, gliomas located at the third ventricle and hypothalamus yield a survival of 74% and 60%, respectively, indicating a more favorable trend than for adults (5). Using the new WHO histologic classification, these would be included in the pilocytic astrocytomas which include juvenile pilocytic and microcystic cerebellar astrocytomas. Laws reports 85% 5-year survival and 79% 10-year survival for 41 patients with pilocytic astrocytoma. For ten patients treated by gross total or radical subtotal resection, the 5- and 10-year survival rates were 100% compared with 22 patients who underwent subtotal resection who had 95% 5-year survival and 84% 10-year survival rates. This is compared with a 44% 5- and 10-year survival rate for nine patients who had biopsy only. The addition of postoperative irradiation only improved survival for those patients who had subtotal resection or biopsy only of the tumor. Survival for ordinary astrocytomas (fibrillary, protoplasmic, gemistocytic) and mixed oligoastrocytomas was 51% at 5 years and 23% at 10 years. Survival was not affected by the extent of surgery. In this group of ordinary astrocytomas, the addition of high-dose radiation therapy ($\geq 5{,}800$ cGy) made a statistically significant difference in survival; 68% at 5 years and 39% at 10 years compared with 47% at 5 years and 21% at 10 years for those treated with low-dose radiation therapy ($< 5{,}300$ cGy), and 32% at 5 years and 11% at 10 years for those who underwent surgery alone (100a). A review of the literature indicates that, when treated with surgery alone, ordinary low-grade gliomas have 5-year survival rates of 19% to 34% (Table 30-10a), and 10-year survival rates of 11% to 32% (94,97). The addition of postoperative radiotherapy in non-randomized series has increased the 5-year survival rate to 42% to 54% (Table 30-10a) and the 10-year rate to 35% and 26% (94,97). CT and MRI scanning have permitted identification of small, low-grade gliomas earlier in the natural history of the disease than did nuclear medicine isotope scans and electroencephalograms. Consequently, and because of the possibility of late radiation CNS toxicity affecting the quality of life, the question has been raised as to the optimal time to irradiate low-grade gliomas. This is being studied by two randomized trials; one conducted by the European Organization on Research and Treatment of Cancer in Europe, and one intergroup study conducted by the BTSG with the participation of the RTOG and Southwest Oncology Group (SWOG).

Oligodendrogliomas (Table 30-10b)

Approximately 5% of intracerebral gliomas are oligodendrogliomas, about three-quarters of which are calcified. Histologically, many of them actually are mixed tumors with a significant component of astrocytic tumor. Once thought to be more benign than other gliomas, their natural history is much like that of astrocytomas of the same grade. At surgery,

Table 30-10. 5 Year Survival Rates Following Surgery(s) and Surgery Plus Radiation Therapy (S + RT) in Retrospective Series

Low-Grade Astrocytoma

S		S + RT		
No. Patients	5 yr survival (%)	No. Patients	5 yr survival (%)	Ref
42	26	105	49	92b
17	20	28	42	102
37	19	71	46	101
23	32	45	54	94
6	0	10	50	100
167	34	74	49	96
23	21	57	50	95
10	32	35	68 High Dose RT	100a
		67	45 Low Dose RT	

Oligodendroglioma

S		S + RT		
No. Patients	Survival (%)	No. Patients	Survival (%)	Ref
A. Median Survival in Years				
208	2.9		3.8	169
34	4.5	37	5.2	166
58	2.2	106	3.2	168
B. 5 Year Survival				
11	82%	24	100%	167
58	27%	106	36%	168
11	18%	34	56%	172

they are usually a bit easier to differentiate from surrounding normal brain tissue because they have a gelatinous appearance and often a gritty texture, but microscopically tumor cells extend beyond the apparently clear surgical borders in most cases. A four-tier grading system (A-D) has been introduced by Smith *et al.* (35). Stage A has a very favorable prognosis, a median survival of 94 months, and a 71% 5-year survival rate; stage D has a grim prognosis with a median survival of 17 months and a zero 5-year survival rate (the maximum survival was about 40 months); and stage B and C have intermediate prognoses with median survivals of 51 months and 45 months and 5-year survival rates of 45% and 43%, respectively (29). Review of the literature of retrospective series reveals median survival ranges between 2.2 and 4.5 years for patients treated with surgery, and between 3.2 and 5.2 years for those patients treated with surgery and radiation therapy (Table 30-10b). The corresponding 5-year survival rates range between 18% and 82% for surgery, and 36% and 100% for surgery and radiation therapy.

Meningiomas (156-165)

These tumors commonly lie over the convexity of the cerebral hemispheres, especially in the frontal and central areas, as well as in the parasaggital regions on or near the superior longitudinal sinus or the falx cerebri. Substantial numbers also lie beneath the brain along the lesser sphenoidal ridge as well as on the tuberculum sellae, the olfactory groove anterior to it, and the parasellar region. There, they often distort or envelop the carotid arteries and the optic nerves. Other less common sites are the tentorium cerebelli, the cerebellopontine angle, and the clivus. Occasionally, meningiomas are aggressive, as evidenced by rapid growth and local invasiveness.

Almost invariably histologically benign, meningiomas are considered one of the most favorable intracranial tumors for surgical removal. This usually can be accomplished successfully over the convexity of the brain and when the tumors are attached to the falx cerebri or tentorium.

The tumors often become very large before patients become symptomatic. While it is less common since the use of MRI and CT scan diagnosis, it is not rare to see such tumors 6 cm or more in diameter.

Meningiomas may be multiple and more than one craniotomy may be necessary for the excision of all the tumors. Sometimes there are so many that some, which appear indolent and are not causing symptoms, are allowed to remain and are followed with serial scans at intervals of 6-12 months.

In the same way, small, asymptomatic meningiomas may be seen on scans, usually in older patients. When the tumors are not symptomatic, they may be followed with serial scans. If they appear to be enlarging, they may be irradiated or excised.

Meningiomas often are involved in the superior longitudinal sinus. In its posterior two thirds, this structure cannot be ligated unless it is already occluded by tumor. This may also require leaving some tumor along its wall at the time of surgery. Meningiomas of the clivus can almost never be removed completely.

When they rise along the base of the skull, meningiomas may be much more difficult to remove completely because their involvement with the internal carotid arteries, the nerves entering the cavernous sinus, or the optic nerves. Often the bulk of the tumor can be excised, but a small portion meshing these vital structures must be allowed to remain rather than destroy their function. Any residual tumor is best irradiated postoperatively while the tumor volume is microscopic.

Recurrence rate after total excision of meningiomas varies between 0% and 13% and 22% (32,163,165), whereas recurrence rates after partial surgical excision have ranged between 7% and 74% (163,165). When postoperative radiotherapy has been added to subtotal resection, the recurrence rates have been between 9% and 28% with a median of 21% (157,159,165). The Royal Marsden Hospital (5) reported 73% 5-year survival after partial removal of the tumor followed by postoperative radiotherapy versus 78% after total removal, with 10-year survival rates of 60% and 61%, respectively. This indicates that radiation therapy is effective in this group of tumors. The use of radiotherapy at time of recurrence, as opposed to postoperatively, has been associated with a much higher recurrence rate: 50% versus 9% in one series (157). In another series of recurrent tumors, 44% had objective responses to irradiation, with two thirds of the patients stabilizing without further recurrence for long periods. Women with meningioma have been reported to develop symptoms suggestive of rapid tumor growth during pregnancy and the luteal phase of the menstrual cycle; therefore SWOG has been evaluating the use of tamoxifen in unresectable and refractory meningiomas.

Pituitary Adenomas

Pituitary adenomas comprise 12% to 18% of intracranial neoplasms. The majority are prolactinomas. Many pituitary adenomas are small and asymptomatic. Only a tiny percentage are malignant. Pituitary adenomas are generally benign and carry a low mortality rate. Curability is 80% to 95% at 5 years with surgery and postoperative irradiation. Recurrences occur in less than 20% of the patients following modern megavoltage therapy alone, and cystic degeneration and hemorrhage during treatment are uncommon events (5% to 10%) (14). In the majority of cases, vision remains excellent and/or improved following the combined surgery/radiation therapy approach (120). Endocrine failure resulting from both pressure atrophy of the pituitary and irradiation is an uncommon late event in adults (172a).

Chordoma

Chordoma is an uncommon tumor that arises at the basisphenoid at the base of the skull just behind the sella turcica. Such tumors usually erode the bone of the base and involve multiple cranial nerves. Surgical resection can be done, but does not lead to a cure even though it may palliate symptoms. Local irradiation and brachytherapy are also used. Irradiation with heavy particles has produced encouraging results, with some prolonged cures.

Neurilemoma (Schwannoma)

Neurilemoma (schwannoma) is chiefly a tumor of adults. Intracranially it usually originates from the vestibular portion of the 8th cranial nerve, where it is not malignant (43). Much less commonly, it may originate from the 5th nerve and very rarely from the glossal, pharyngeal, or vagus nerves.

CNS Lymphoma (189a,190-197)

Primary lymphoma of the brain is relatively uncommon. It is usually cerebral and presents much like a glioma. Biopsy, and/or surgical excision, if the tumor is located favorably, followed by irradiation and chemotherapy is recommended. When the whole brain and meninges were treated to 4,000 cGy and the tumor plus a 2 cm margin boosted to another 2,000 cGy to a total of 6,000 cGy the RTOG found a median survival of 11.6 months (48% 1-year survival and 28% 2-year survival rate (80a). These results are no better than the survival reported in retrospective series where doses generally used were less and the whole meninges were not necessarily treated. In many of the retrospective series, at least some patients were staged without CT or MRI. The range of median survival of prior studies was 19.5 - 42 months with a median survival of 18 months. Even with treatment of the gross tumor to a high dose, and the whole brain and meninges to a dose for microscopic disease, local recurrence remained the major failure pattern in the RTOG study; 83% of the failures were local only and 9% were local plus distant. Most were in the region of full dose, suggesting the need for an additional treatment modality. Age and KPS were observed to be significant prognostic factors — patients less than 60 years of age had a median survival of 23.1 months compared to 7.6 months for patients 60 years or older. Similarly, patients with a KPS of 70 to 100 had a median survival of 21.1 months compared with 5.6 months for patients with KPS of 40 to 60. Clinical trials evaluating chemotherapy followed by radiotherapy are in progress to determine whether survival can be improved in this disease.

Metastases

Metastases to the brain are seen frequently. The most common sources are the lung, breast, and gut, but they may come from any malignant tumor in the body. Usually they are associated with a large amount of edema that responds well to treatment with corticosteroids. If the metastasis is solitary and is in a favorable location, such as the anterior frontal region, surgical excision usually is advisable. If, as is usually the case, there are metastases, surgery is not indicated unless the tumors are all in the same relatively small area of the brain. In any case, irradiation is usually advisable to retard growth and relieve symptoms, with continued use of corticosteriods to control edema. The median survival of lung cancer patients with brain metastases is 11 weeks, and for breast cancer patients with brain metastases it is 22 weeks. Obviously, the length of palliative radiotherapy should be kept short (~ 2 weeks) for most patients with brain metastases unless the patient meets strict criteria that suggest he or she has a more favorable prognosis.

Spinal Cord Tumors

Intramedullary tumors of the spinal cord are relatively favorable because they usually are of a low order of malignancy. High-grade astrocytoma (GBM) is infrequent. The ependymomas often have an associated intramedullary cyst. These tumors can be exposed through a longitudinal myelotomy and can sometimes be removed completely. Postoperative radiotherapy is recommended in most cases.

Extramedullary intraspinal tumors are almost invariably benign meningiomas or neurilemomas. Even in the face of very severe neurologic deficits, these usually can be removed satisfactorily with marked recovery in the patient's signs and symptoms. They are more common than the intramedullary tumors.

Unfortunately, metastatic tumor to the spine is frequent, usually at multiple sites. Sometimes the patient's spinal cord can be decompressed if it becomes symptomatic. Back pain, or pain that radiates anteriorly in the chest or abdomen and inferiorly to the legs should arouse suspicion of epidural metastases and appropriate work-up should be done. In a patient with a known malignancy one should not wait until the patient cannot walk and has lost bladder and bowel control before doing MRI of the spine or a myelogram. The best therapeutic results occur when spinal cord compression is diagnosed early, at which time radiation therapy and/or surgical decompression have the best chance of preserving leg, bladder, and bowel function. If the patient has lost all motor strength in the lower extremities, including loss of use of ankle and toe muscles, the chances of regaining function are slim.

Long-term survival: Spinal cord tumors generally do well; 10-year survival figures are as high as 90% for low-grade astrocytomas and ependymomas (192a).

Tumors of Childhood (Fig. 30-4) (103a)

The gold standard in pediatric brain tumors can be found in the recent and last update of results from Bloom *et al.* at the Royal Marsden Hospital (103a,111a). These achievements are noted in each special category of brain tumors. Long-term psychologic and late effects of chemoradiation are well studied (111a).

Medulloblastomas (103,106,108,111,113-119,121-129)

Medulloblastomas are common malignant tumors in the cerebellum (Fig. 30-4). Seeding often occurs in the subarachnoid space; therefore, irradiation is applied to the entire craniospinal axis. Although there is controversy about the dose of elective CNS and spinal cord irradiation, it is standard practice. The whole brain is irradiated to 4,500 cGy, the primary tumor in the cerebellum receives an additional 1,000 cGy boost, and the spinal cord is treated with 3,500 to 4,500 cGy, although there are data suggesting that doses of 2,500 cGy may be sufficient (118).

Medulloblastomas are rarely cured by surgery alone. A combined modality of surgery and radiation therapy is recommended for early-stage lesions and chemotherapy, radiation therapy, and surgery for advanced disease. The extent of surgical resection does make a difference in survival. At the University of Pennsylvania, the use of the dissecting microscope and preoperative CT scan to identify tumor extent increased relapse-free survival at 4 years from 38% to 84% in a historical comparison of treatment groups (108). Local control is additionally determined by dose to the posterior fossa with local control rates of 79% and 80%, and survival rates of 50% to 80% achieved with doses of 5,000 cGy or more, compared with local control rates of 20% to 50% and 5-year survival rates of 30% to 40% for doses less than 5,000 cGy (113,118,121,123). Local recurrences are the main pattern of failure, often associated with half of this group having spinal cord seeding. Distant metastases outside the CNS can also occur. Adjuvant chemotherapy initially had conflicting results. However, the International Society of Paediatric Oncology (SIOP) undertook a randomized trial in 1975 that demonstrated a gain of survival at 2, 3, and 4 years that was

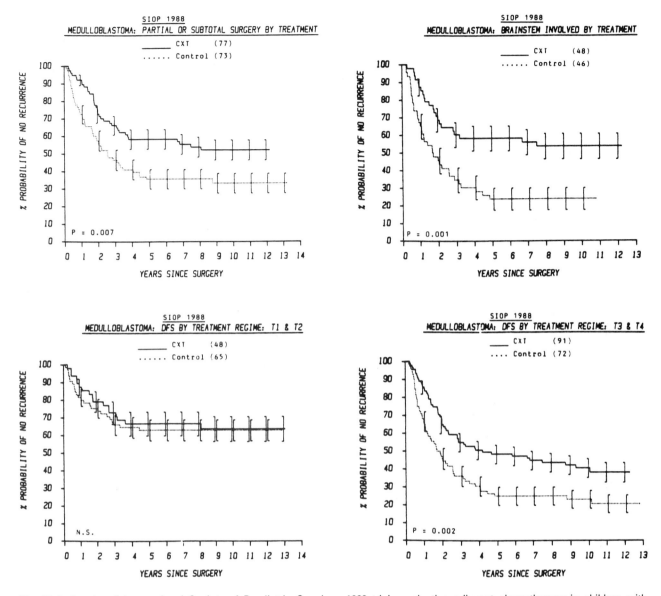

Fig. 30-4. Results of International Society of Paediatric Oncology 1988 trials evaluating adjuvant chemotherapy in children with medulloblastoma. Figures indicate that adjuvant chemotherapy may substantially improve the survival of children in certain high risk groups. From Bloom *et al.* (103a), with permission.

statistically significant (P = .03) (117). The Children's Cancer Study Group also conducted a Phase III randomized trial that demonstrated improved disease-free survival at 54 months — 59% with chemotherapy of lomustine, vincristine, and prednisone used in combination in addition to surgery and radiotherapy, versus 49% for surgery and radiotherapy (P < .05). However, when one does subset analysis, it is obvious that those patients with early-stage disease (i.e., T1 M0 or T2 M0) have disease-free survival at 5 years of 65% to 70% and do not benefit from chemotherapy. Those patients with intermediate stage diseases (T3,M0 and T4,M0) show a nonstatistically significant trend of improved survival with the addition of chemotherapy. Those patients with advanced disease, (T3-4,M1-3) have a significant improvement with chemotherapy: a 45% 5-year relapse-free survival compared with zero relapse-free survival at 3 years without chemotherapy (103,106). Other high-risk subgroups are age less than 3 years, subtotal

removal, and brain stem invasion, that benefited from adjuvant chemotherapy (103a).

Ependymomas (103a)

Ependymomas are another variety of intracerebral tumor that may occur at any age. About 9% of children's brain tumors are ependymomas. They may occur in any of the cerebral ventricles and are especially common in the fourth ventricle in children. They also can present as subcortical cerebral tumors, often lying near a ventricular wall. High-grade ependymomas (also known as anaplastic ependymomas, or ependymoblastomas) that are infratentorial are prone to spread via subarachnoid and intraventricular fluid pathways. As shown in Table 30-11, the risk of seeding depends on the location and histologic grading. Because of the rarity of this tumor and the propensity to seed, there is no complete consensus on how to treat these tumors. Even when treat-

Table 30-11. Ependymoma Rate of Intraspinal Metastases by Location and Grade in 163 Cases From 5 Series *

	Low Grade	High Grade
Supratentorial	0/35†	1/31 (3.2%)
Infratentorial	8/62† (13.1%)	15/36 (41.7%)

* See references 129a, 130, 132, 134,135.
† includes 3 cases that had infratentorial and supratentorial disease.

ment is limited to the whole brain, however, there have been significant neurologic sequelae such as speech and writing problems and difficulty in spatial orientation in 61% (132). (Only one quarter of the schoolchildren are at a normal academic level.) Since local recurrence in the treatment field appears to be the greatest problem for low-grade ependymomas (135), local field irradiation is recommended. The Mayo Clinic found no difference in spinal cord metastases between those infratentorial low-grade ependymomas treated with involved field only (1/7 = 14% spinal metastases) and those treated with craniospinal irradiation technique (1/2 = 8% spinal metastases). The craniospinal technique has been described in the medulloblastoma section. However, with a 13% to 15% rate of spinal cord metastases there are some recommendations for craniospinal irradiation for low-grade ependymomas. One possible compromise is posterior fossa and spinal irradiation, which would at least spare the cognitive brain. In supratentorial low-grade ependymomas, there appears to be no reason to treat more than local field to the disease plus a margin, especially with CT and MRI scanning with and without contrast. For supratentorial high-grade ependymomas, treatment to the whole brain with a boost to the gross disease is recommended (132,134). In the five series summarized in Table 30-11, there was only a 3.2% incidence of spinal cord metastases in supratentorial malignant ependymomas. Of course, the use of local therapy for tumors with the capability of seeding the CSF requires close attention to staging, particularly to adequate evaluation of CSF cytology.

Treatment of malignant ependymomas is least controversial, with a consensus in the literature to treat with craniospinal irradiation. However, since local failure at the site of the original primary is the major failure pattern, it may be that supratentorial irradiation may be able to be decreased, or even eliminated, especially if chemotherapy is used also.

The overall 5-year survival rate for patients with ependymomas is 62% according to Shaw *et al.* (134), 39% according to Pierre-Kahn *et al.* (132) for the entire series, but 51% when postoperative mortality is excluded, and 67% according to Wollner *et al.* (135). Grade and age are significant prognostic factors, with low-grade ependymomas having a 71% 5-year survival compared with 29% for high-grade ependymomas in the Mayo Clinic series. The University of California series (135) had only 4/20 patients with high-grade ependymomas. Adjuvant chemotherapy had improved survival for 2 to 5 years compared with historical controls. However, the improvement in survival has not been maintained in the long-term, with survival the same at 5 to 7 years. In the SIOP trial,

this subgroup has shown no gain compared with the medulloblastoma series.

Craniopharyngiomas (103a,136,146)

Craniopharyngiomas are congenital tumors which present usually in childhood or in the later decades of life. They are usually suprasellar in location, very commonly calcified, and often contain multiloculated cysts. In this location, they may cause compression of the optic nerve and invaginate and block the third ventricle, thereby causing hydrocephalus or deformation of the pituitary stalk. They are histologically benign and the ideal treatment is complete surgical excision if this can be accomplished without unacceptable sequelae. However, the price of aggressive surgical removal may be severe, i.e., permanent neurologic deficit with a poor prognosis. Even when the surgeon feels that there has been complete excision, the recurrence rate is 21.5% for 144 patients included in 10 series (145), because minute amounts of tumor have not been excised. Sometimes total surgical removal cannot be done because craniopharyngiomas are densely adherent to adjacent structures such as the carotid artery, optic nerves, or brain stem. When there has been only partial tumor removal, the overall recurrence rate for 88 patients included in 8 series was 71% to 76% (145). When postoperative irradiation was added to partial resection, the recurrence rate was 25.9% for 232 cases included in 14 series from the literature (145). The addition of postoperative irradiation has yielded survival results that approximate those of grade I cerebellar astrocytomas. The 10-year results reported initially by Kramer *et al.* (142) and updated by Bloom *et al.* (5,103a) using modern megavoltage irradiation are 80% in children and 60% in adults, with greater than 90% survival at 5 years and longer. Intracavitary irradiation of the cyst with radioactive phosphorus and local irradiation have both been shown to be valuable in the management of these tumors.

Optic Gliomas (109,147-155)

With precise tumor imaging using CT scanning and computerized radiation therapy treatment planning, 78% of patients with optic glioma retain their vision and between 75% and 100% of patients are long-term survivors (148). Optic nerve gliomas involving only the chiasm have a 100% 5-year survival rate and 90% 10-year survival rate, whereas optic gliomas involving the chiasm and hypothalamus have a 71% 5-year survival rate and 66% 10-year survival rate (148). Chiasmal gliomas treated with radiotherapy had better 10- and 15-year survivals than those not treated with radiation therapy at the University of California, San Francisco. Dose did make a difference in disease-free survival: 100% survived after doses equivalent to a normal standard dose greater than 1.385 versus 40% surviving after doses equivalent to normal standard doses of less than or equal to 1.385 (155).

Pineal Tumors and Suprasellar Germinomas (93a,182-189)

Pineal tumors have an excellent prognosis and a high rate of cure with radiotherapy, with a 5-year survival rate of 50% to 90%. The major problem is high operative mortality (30% to 60%) because of the location. To avoid biopsy, Bloom (5) advocated a trial of radiation therapy and CT scanning. If the tumor regressed markedly at 2,000 cGy, the assumption was made that it was a pinealoma. However, with the availability of CT scan and stereotactic brain biopsy techniques, a directed biopsy is almost always possible.

Ganglioglioma

An unusual cerebral tumor, more often seen in children than in adults, is the ganglioglioma. It is relatively amenable to treatment. Often the patient has a history of focal seizures followed by symptoms of ICP. When found, the tumors usually are large and can be excised completely. This should be done as aggressively as possible, since these tumors grow slowly and are of a low order of malignancy, but may become highly malignant at a later date. Microscopically, they are composed of abnormal neurons in a background of low-grade astrocytoma cells.

Recommended Reading

The following literature is highly recommended: *Principles and Practice of Radiation Oncology*, edited by Perez and Brady, specifically chapters entitled "Brain" (13) and "Spinal Canal" (8a) and "Brain Tumors in Children" (14a); *Cancer: Principles and Practice of Oncology*, edited by DeVita, Hellman, and Rosenberg, *"Neoplasms of the Central Nervous System"* (15); *Brain Tumor Therapy* (21a); "Malignant Astrocytic Neoplasms: Classification, Pathologic Anatomy, and Response to Treatment" (24); "Radiation Therapy for Neoplasms of the Brain" (50); "Resection and Reoperation in Neuro-oncology: Rationale and Approach" (55); *Oncology of the Nervous System* (82); "Controversies in the Management of Low-Grade Supratentorial Astrocytomas — Defining the Role of Postoperative Radiation Therapy" (100a); "Childhood Brain Tumors: Current Status of Clinical Trials in Newly Diagnosed and Recurrent Disease" (103); four journal articles by Finlay on brain tumors in children (105-108); and "Definitive Radiation Therapy in the Treatment of Primary non-Hodgkin's Lymphoma of the Central Nervous System, non-AIDS Related: Report of the RTOG Study 8315" by (80a). Two recent excellent reviews of malignant gliomas and their management are based on achievements in cooperative group clinical trials (69,86a). The gold standard in pediatric and adult brain tumors can be found in the April 1990 issue of the International Journal of Radiation Oncology Biology Physics, dedicated to Bloom's life's work (103a,117a).

REFERENCES

General References

1. Adams, R.D.; Victor, M. Principles of Neurology. New York, NY: McGraw-Hill; 1977.
2. American Joint Committee on Cancer Staging and End-Results Reporting. Manual for Staging of Cancer, 3rd ed. Philadelphia, PA: J.B. Lippincott, Co.; 1988.
3. Bartlett, J. Familiar Quotations. Boston, MA: Little, Brown and Co.; 1955.
4. Bennen, J.M.; Rosenthal, S.N., eds. Practical Cancer Chemotherapy. New York, NY: Med. Exam. Publishing Co.; 1981.
5. Bloom, H.J.G. Intracranial tumors response and persistence to therapeutic endeavors, 1970-1980. Intl. J. Radiat. Oncol. Biol. Phys. 8:1083-1113; 1982.
5a. Bragg, D.G.; Rubin, P.; Youker, J.E. Oncologic Imaging. Elmsford, NY: Pergamon Press; 1985.
5b. Cancer facts and figures. New York, NY: American Cancer Society, Inc.; 1990.
5c. Cohen, M.E.; Dugger, P.K. Brain Tumors in Children. Principles of Diagnosis and Treatment. New York, NY: Raven Press; 1984.
6. Chutorian, A.M.; Ganti, S.R. Diagnosis of intracranial tumors in infants and children. In: Chang, C.H.; Houspian, E.M., eds. Tumors of the Central Nervous System: Modern Radiotherapy in Multidisciplinary Management. New York, NY: Masson Publishing USA, Inc.; 1982:83-105.

7. Conference on chemical modification radiation and cytotoxic drugs, September 17-21 1981. Key Biscayne, FL. Intl. J. Radiat. Oncol. Biol. Phys. 8:323-815; 1982.
8. Copeland, D.D.; Bigner, D.D. Glial mesenchymal tropism of *in vivo* Avian sarcoma virus neuro-oncogenesis in rats. Acta Neuropathol. 41:23-25; 1978.
8a. Garcia, D.M.; Karlsson, U.L. Spinal Canal. In: Perez, C.A.; Brady, L.W. (eds). Principles and Practice of Radiation Oncology. Philadelphia, PA: JB Lippincott Co; 1992:583-594.
9. Gilbert, H.A.; Kagah, A.R., eds. Radiation Damage to the Nervous System. A Delayed Therapeutic Hazard. New York, NY: Raven Press; 1980.
10. Graif, M.; Bydder, G.M.; Steiner, R.E.; Niendorf, P.; Thomas, D.G.T.; Young, I.R. Contrast-enhanced MR imaging of malignant brain tumors. AJNR 6:855-862; 1985.
10a. Harnsberger, H.R.; Dillon, W.P. Imaging Tumors of the Central Nervous System and Extracranial Head and Neck. In: Imaging in Cancer. Holleb, A.I. ed. Syracuse, NY: American Cancer Society, New York State Div., Inc.: 1987; 89-102.
10b. Harnsberger, H.R.; Dillon, W.P. The Radiologic Role in Diagnosis, Staging, and Follow-up of Neoplasia of the Brain, Spine, and Head and Neck. In: Seminars in Ultrasound CT and Mr. Raymond, H.W.; Zwiebel, W.J.; Harnsberger, H.R., eds. Vol. 10 (6): 431-452; 1989.
11. Kahn, E.A.; Taren, J.A.; Schneider, R.C.; *et al.* Correlative Neurosurgery. Springfield, IL: Charles C. Thomas, Publisher; 1969.
12. Karlsson, U.L.; Brady, L.W. Primary intracranial neoplasms. In: Perez, C.A.; Brady, L.W., eds. Principles and practice of radiation oncology. Philadelphia, PA: J.B. Lippincott Co.; 1987:408-436.
13. Karlsson, U.L.; Leibel, S.A.; Wallner, K.; *et al.* Brain. In: Perez, C.A.; Brady, L.W., eds. Principles and practice of radition oncology. Philadelphia, PA: J.B. Lippincott Co.; 1992:515-563.
14. Kramer, S.; Southard, M.E.; Mansfield, C.M. Radiation effects and Tolerance of the Central Nervous System. In: Vaeth J, ed. Frontiers of Radiation Therapy and Oncology, Vol. 6. Baltimore, MD: University Park Press, 1972.
14a. Kun, L.E. Brain tumors in children. In: Perez, C.A., Brady, L.W. (eds). Principles and Practice of Radiation Oncology. Philadelphia, PA: JB Lippincott Co; 1992:1417-1441.
15. Levin, V.A.; Sheline, G.E.; Gutin, P.H. Neoplasms of the central nervous system. In: DeVita, V.T., Jr.; Hellman, S.; Rosenberg, S.A., eds. Cancer: principles and practice of oncology, 3rd ed. Philadelphia: J.B. Lippincott Co.; 1989:1557-1611.
15a. Mahaley, M.S., Jr.; Mettlin, C.; Natarajan, N.; Laws, E.R., Jr., *et al.* Analysis of patterns of care of brain tumor patients in the United States; a study of the Brain Tumor Section of the AANS and the CNS and the Commission on Cancer of the ACS. Clin. Neurosurg. 36:347-352; 1990.
16. Mahaley, M.S.; Vogel, F.S.; Burger, P. Neuropathology of Tissues from Patients Treated by the Brain Tumor Study Group. NCI Monogr. 46:7782, 1977.
17. Monfardini, E.S.; Brunner, K.; Crowther, D.; *et al.* Manual of Cancer Chemotherapy, 3rd ed. UICC Technical Report Series, Vol. 56. Geneva, Switzerland: UICC; 1981:165.
18. Mullan, S. Essentials of Neurosurgery for Students and Practitioners. New York, NY: Springer Publishing; 1961.
19. Myers, M.H.; Gloeckler Ries, L.A. Cancer patient survival rates: SEER program results for 10 years of follow-up. CA Cancer J. Clin. 39:21-32; 1989.
20. Northfield, D.W.C.; Russell, D.S. Intracranial Tumors. In: Felling, A., ed. Modern Trends in Neurology. New York, NY: Paul B. Hoeber, Inc.; 1951:291-362.
21. Parker, R.G.; Berry, H.C.; Caderao, J,B.; *et al.* Preliminary Clinical Results from US Fast Neutron Teletherapy Studies. Intl. J. Radiat. Oncol. Biol. Phys. 3:261; 1977.
21a. Rosenblum, M.L.; Wilson, C.B., eds. Brain tumor therapy. Basel, Germany: S. Karger; 1984.
21b. Rubin, P.; Cooper, R, Jr. Radiation biology and radiation pathology syllabus, vol. RT-1. Chicago, IL: American College of Radiology; 1975.
21c. Shapiro, W.R., ed. Brain tumors. Seminars in oncology. 13; 1986.
22. Sheline, G.E. Radiation therapy of primary brain tumors. Semin. Oncol. 2:29 - 42; 1975.
22a. Vick, N.A.; Bigner, D.d., eds. Symposium on neuro-oncology. Neruology clinics, vol. 3, no. 4. Philadelphia: W.B. Saunders Co.; 1985.

23. Wechsler, W.; Kleihues, P.; Matsumoto, S.; *et al.* Pathology of Experimental Neurogenic Tumors Chemically Induced during Prenatal and Postnatal Life. Ann .NY Acad. Sci. 159:360-408; 1969.

Specific References

Pathology

24. Burger, P.C. Malignant astrocytic neoplasms: classification, pathologic anatomy, and response to treatment. Semin. Oncol. 13:16-26; 1986.
25. Burger, P.C.; Vogel, F.S. Surgical pathology of the nervous System and Its Coverings. New York, NY: John Wiley & Sons; 1976.
26. Burger, P.C.; Vollmer, R.T. Histologic factors of prognostic significance in the glioblastoma multiforme. Cancer 46:1179-1186; 1980.
27. Kernohan, J.W.; Sayre, C.P. Tumors of the Central Nervous System. Washington DC: Armed Forces Institute of Pathology; 1952.
28. Kernohan, J.W.; Uihlein, A. Sarcomas of the Brain. Springfield, IL: Charles C. Thomas, Publisher; 1962.
29. Ludwig, C.L.; Smith, M.T.; Godfrey, A.D.; Armbrustmacher, V.W. A clinicopathological study of 323 patients with oligodendrogliomas. Ann. Neurol. 19:15-21; 1986.
30. Nelson, J.S.; Tsukada, Y.; Schoenfeld, D.; Fulling, K.; Lamarche, J.; Peress, N. Necrosis as aprognostic criterion in malignant supratentorial, astrocytic gliomas. Cancer 52:550-554; 1983.
31. Rorke, L.B. The cerebellar medulloblastoma and its relationship to primitive neuroectodermal tumors. J. Neuropathol. Experimental Neurol. 42:1-15; 1983.
32. Rubinstein, L.J. Embryonal central neuroepithelial tumors and their differentiating potential: a cytogenetic view of a complex neuro-oncological problem. J. Neurosurg. 62:795-805; 1985.
33. Rubinstein, W. Tumors of the central nervous system (2nd series). Washington, D.C.: Armed Forces Instititue of Pathology; 1972.
34. Russell, D.S.; Rubinstein, W. Pathology of tumors of the nervous system, 4th ed. Baltimore, MD: Williams & Wilkins Co.; 1977.
35. Smith, M.T.; Ludwig, C.L.; Godrey, A.D.; Armbrustmacher, V.W. Grading of oligodendrogliomas. Cancer 52:2107-2114; 1983.
36. Zuich, K.J. Principles of the new World Health Organization (WHO) classification of brain tumors. Neuroradiology 19:59-66; 1980.

Treatment

37. Blasberg, R.G.; Groothuis, D.R. Chemotherapy of brain tumors: physiological and pharmacokinetic considerations. Semin. Oncol. 13:70-82; 1986.
38. Bloom, H.J.G. Combined modality therapy for intracranial tumours. Cancer 35:111-120; 1975.
39. Bullard, D.E. Role of stereotaxic biopsy in the management of patients with intracranial lesions. Neurol. Clin. 3:817-830; 1985.
40. Burger, P.C.; Kamenar, E.; Schold, S.C.; Fay, J.W.; Phillips, G.L.; Herzig, G.P. Encephalomyelopathy following high-dose BCNU therapy. Cancer 48:1318-1327; 1981.
41. Feun, L.G.; Lee, Y.Y.; Wallace, S.; Charnsangavej, C.; Savaraj, N.; Carrasco, C.H.; Gianturco, C.; Yung, W-K.A. New drugs and new delivery techniques. Prog. Exp. Tumor Res. 29:131-139; 1985.
41a. Feun, L.; Savaraj, J.; Landy, H.J.; Lu, K.; Green, B.; Page, Li; Rosomoff, H.; Lampidis, T. Molecular Biology of the Primary Brain Tumor. Abstract. Proc Am Soc Clin Oncol 9:96;1990.
42. Goldstein, S.; Gumerlock, M.; Neuwelt, E. Comparison of CT guided and stereotaxic cranial diagnostic needle biopsies. J. Neurosurg. 67:341-348; 1987.
43. Hamer, S.; Ebersold, M. Management of acoustic neuromas. J. Neurosurg. 63:175-179; 1985.
44. Henaudin, J.; Fewer, D.; Wilson, C.B.; *et al.* Dose Dependency of Decadron in Patients with Partially Excised Brain Tumors. J. Neurosurg. 39:302-305; 1973.
45. Hill, S.A.; Denekamp, J. The Response of 6 Mouse Tumours to Combined Heat and X-rays: Implications for Therapy. Br. J. Radiol. 52:209-218; 1979.
46. Katz, M.E.; Glick, J.H. Nitrosoureas: a reappraisal of clinical trials. Cancer Clin. Trials 2:297-316; 1979.

47. Kjellberg, R.N.; Hanamura, T.; Davis, K.R.; Lyons, S.L.; Adams, R.D. Bragg-peak proton-beam therapy for arteriovenious malformations of the brain. New Engl. J. Med. 309:269-274; 1983.
48. Kramer, S. The Hazards of Therapeutic Irradiation of the Central Nervous System. Clin. Neurosurg. 15:301-318; 1967.
49. Kumar, P.; Good, R.; Skultety, M.; *et al.* Radiation induced neoplasms of the brain. Cancer 59:1274-1282; 1987.
49a. Leibel, S.A.; Gutin, P.H.; Wara, W.M.; Silver, P.S.; Larson, D.A.; Edwards, M.S.B.; Lamb, S.A.; arn, B.; Weaver, K.A.; Barnett, C.; Phillips, T.L. Int. J. Radiat. Oncol. Biol. Phys. 17:1129-1140; 1989.
50. Leibel, S.A.; Sheline, G.E. Radiation therapy for neoplasms of the brain. J. Neurosurg. 6:1-22; 1987.
51. Lunsford, D.; Martinez, A.J. Stereotactic exploration of the brain in the era of computed tomography. Surg. Neurol 22:222-230; 1984.
52. McKeever, P.E. Scanning Electron Microscopy in the Evaluation of Neurosurgical Neopiasms: A Review of New Approaches. Neurosurgery 4:343-352; 1979.
53. Rekate, H.L.; Ruch, T.; Nulsen, F.E.; *et al.* Needle Biopsy of Tumors in the region Of the Third Ventricle. J. Neurosurg. 54:338-341; 1981.
54. Salazar, O.M.; Samaras, G.M.; Eddy, H.A.; Amin, P.P.; Sewchand, W.; Drzymala, R.E.; Bajaj, K.G. Neurobrachytherapy: a new frontier. Endocurietherapy/Hyperthermia Oncol. 2:S-3 - S15; 1986.
55. Salcman, M. Resection and reoperation in neuro-oncology. Rationale and approach. Neurol. Clin. 3:831-842; 1985.
56. Saunders, W.M.; Chen, G.T.Y.; Austin-Seymour, M.; Castro, J.R.; Collier, J.M.; Gauger, G.; Gutin, P.; Phillips, T.L.; Pitluck, Walton, R.E.; Zink S.R. Precision, high dose radiotherapy. II. Helium ion treatment of tumors adjacent to critical central nervous system structures. Intl. J. Radiat. Oncol. Biol. Phys. 1:1339-1347; 1985.
57. Selker, R.G. Corticosteroids: their effect on primary and metastatic brain tumors. In: Walker, M.D., ed. Oncology of the nervous sytem. Boston, MA: Martinus Nijhoff Publishers; 1983:167-191.
58. Shapiro, W.R.; Posner, J.E. Corticosteroid hormones: effects in an experimental brain tumor. Arch. Neurol. 30:217-221; 1974.
59. Shapiro, W.R.; Shapiro, J.R. Principles of brain tumor chemotherapy. Semin. Oncol. 13:56-69; 1986.
60. Takahura, K.; Sano, K. Role of immunopotentiators in brain tumour therapy. In: Paoletti, P.; Walker, M.D.; Butti, G.; *et al.*, eds. Multidisciplinary aspects of brain tumour therapy. Amsterdam, the Netherlands: Elsevier North-Holland; 1979:223-234.
61. Valentino, V. Radiosurgery in cerebral tumors and AVM. Acta Neurochirurgia. 42(suppl.):193-197; 1988.
62. Walker, M.D. Brain and Peripheral Nervous System Tumors. In: Holland, J.F.; Frei, E., eds. Cancer Medicine. Philadelphia: Lea & Febiger; 1973:1385-1417.
63. Winston, K.R.; Lutz, W. Linear accelerator as a neurosurgical tool for stereotactic radiosurgery. Neurosurgery 22:454-464; 1988.

High-Grade Astrocytomas/Malignant Gliomas

64. Bleehan, N.M. The Cambridge Glioma Trial and Radiation Therapy with Associated Studies. Cancer Clin. Trials 3:267-273; 1980.
65. Caterall, M.; Bloom, H.J.G.; Ash, D.V.; *et al.* Fast neutrons compared with megavoltage x rays in the treatment of patients with supratentorial glioblastoma: a controlled pilot study. Intl. J. Radiat. Oncol. Biol. Phys. 6:261-266; 1980.
66. Chang, C.H.; Horton, J.; Schoenfeld, D.; Salazar, O.; Perez-Tamayo, R.; Kramer, S.; Weinstein, A.; Nelson, J.S.; Tsukada, Y. Comparison of postoperative radiotherapy and combined postoperative radiotherapy and chemotherapy in the multidisciplinary management of malignant gliomas: a joint Radiation Therapy Oncology Group and Eastern Cooperative Oncology Group study. Cancer 52:997-1007; 1983.
67. Coffey, R.J.; Lunsford, L.D.; Taylor, F.H. Survival after stereotactic biopsy of malignant gliomas. Neurosurgery 22:465-473; 1988.
68. Davis, L.W. Presidential Address: Malignant glioma - a nemesis which requires clinical and basic investiation in radiation oncology. Int. J. Radiat. Oncol. Biol. Phys. 16:1355-1366; 1989.
69. Deutsch, M.; Green, S.B.; Strike, T.A. Burger, P.C.; Rogertson,

J.T.; Selker, R.G.; Shapiro, W.R.; Mealey, J., Jr.; Ransohoff, J., II; Paoletti, P.; Smith, K.R.; Odom, G.L.; Hunt, W.E.; Young, B.; Alexander, E., Jr.; Walker, M.D.; Pistenmaa, D.A. Results of a randomized trial comparing BCNU plus radiotherapy, streptozotocin plus radiotherapy, BCNU plus hyperfractionated radiotherapy, and BCNU following misonidazole plus radiotherapy in the postoperative treatment of malignant glioma. Intl J. Radiat. Oncol. Biol. Phys. 16:1389-1396; 1989.

70. Duncan, W.; McLelland, J.; Davey, P.; Jack, W.J.L.; Arnott, S.J.; Gordon, A.; Kerr, G.R.; Williams, J.R. A phase I study of mixed (neutron and photon) irradiation using two fractions per day in the treatment of high-grade astrocytomas. Br. J. Radiol. 59:441-444; 1986.

71. EORTC Brain Tumor Group. Effect of CCNU on survival rate of objective remission and duration of free interval in patients with malignant brain glioma—final evaluation. Eur. J. Cancer 14:851-856; 1978.

71a. EORTC Brain Tumor Group. Evaluation of CCNU, VM-26 plus CCNU and procarbazine in supratentorial brain gliomas. J. Neurosurg. 55:27-31; 1981.

72. Evans, A.E.; Anderson, J.; Chang, C.; et al. Adjuvant Chemotherapy for Medulloblastomas and Ependymoma. In: Paoleni, P.; Walker, M.D.; Butte, G.; et al., eds. Multidisciplinary Aspects of Brain Tumor Therapy. Amsterdam, the Netherlands: Elsevier, North Holland; 1979:219-222.

72a. Fulton, D.S.; Urtasun, R.C.; Shin, K.H.; et al. Misonidazole combined with hyperfractionation in the management of malignant glioma. Intl. J. Radiat. Oncol. Biol. phys. 10:1709-1712; 1984.

73. Green, S.B.; Byar, D.P.; Walker, M.D.; Pistenmaa, D.A.; Alexander, E., Jr.; Batzdorf, U.; Brooks, W.H.; Hunt, W.E.; Mealey, J., Jr.; Odom, G.L.; Paoletti, P.; Ransohoff, J., II; Robertson, J.T.; Selker, R.G.; Shapiro, W.R.; Smith, K.R.; Wilson, C.B.; Strike, T.A. Comparisons of carmustine, procarbazine, and high-dose methylprednisone as additions to surgery and radiotherapy for the treatment of malignant glioma. Cancer Treat. Rep. 67:121-132; 1983.

74. Gutin, P.H.; Leibel, S.A.; Wara, W.M.; Choucair, A.; Levin, V.A.; Philips, T.L.; Silver, P.; Da Silva, V.; Edwards, M.S.B.; Davis, R.L.; Weaver, K.A.; Lamb, S. Recurrent malignant gliomas: survival following interstitial brachytherapy with high-activity iodine-125 sources. J. Neurosurg. 67:864-873; 1987.

75. Gutin, P.H.; Phillips, T.L.; Hosobuchi, Y.; et al. Permanent and Removable Implants for the Brachytherapy of Brain Tumors. Intl. J. Radiat. Oncol. Biol. Phys. 7:1371-1381; 1981.

75a. Gutin, P.H.; Prados, M.D.; Phillips, T.L.; et al. External irradiation followed by an interstitial high activity iodine-125 implant "boost" in the initial treatment of malignant gliomas: NCOG study 6G-82-2. Int J Radiat Oncol Biol Phys. 21:601-606; 1991.

76. Hildebrand, J. Radiotherapy and chemotherapy of malignant brain gliomas. Drugs Exptl. Clin. Res. XII:167-175; 1986.

77. Hochberg, F.H.; Parker, L.M.; Takvorian, T.; et al. High-dose BCNU with Autologous Bone-marrow Rescue for Recurrent Glioblastoma Multiforme. J. Neurosurg. 54:455-460; 1981.

77a. Hochberg, F.A.; Pruit, A. Assumptions from the radiotherapy of glioblastoma. Neurology. 30:907-911; 1980.

78. Hoshino, T.; Barker, M.; Wilson, C.B.; et al. Cell Kinetics of Human Gliomas. J. Neurosurg. 37:15-26; 1972.

78'. Kooy, H.M.; Nedzi, J.S.; Loeffler, J.S.; et al. Treatment planning for stereotactic radiosurgery of intracranial lesions. Int J Radiat Oncol Biol Phys. 21:683-694; 1991.

78a. Levin, V.A.; Silver, P.; Hannigan, J.; Wara, W.M.; Gutin, P.H.; Davis, R.L.; Wilson, C.B. Superiority of Post-Radiotherapy Adjuvant Chemotherapy with CCNU, Procarbazine, and Vincristine (PCV) Over BCNU for Anaplastic Gliomas: NCOG 6G61 Final Report. Int. J. Rad. Oncol. Biol. Phys. is:321;324;1990.

78b. Levin, V.A.; Wara, W.M.; Gutin, P.H.; Wilson, C.B.; Phillips, T.; Prados, M.; Flam, M.S.; Ahn, D.K. Initial analysis of NCOG 6G82-1: bromodeoxyuridine (BUdR) during irradiation followed by CCNU, procarbazine, and vincristine (PCV) chemotherapy for malignant gliomas. Abstract. In: Proceedings of the American Society of Clinical Oncology. Sem. Clin. Oncol. 9:91;1990.

78b*. Lindstadt, D.E.; Edwards, M.S.B.; Prados, M.; et al. Hyperfractionated irradiation for adults with brainstem gliomas. Int J Radiat Oncol Biol Phys. 20:757-760; 1991.

78b'. Lindstadt, D.E.; Castro, J.R.; Phillips, T.L. Neon ion radio-

therapy: Results of the phase I/II clinical trial. Int J Radiat Oncol Biol Phys. 20:761-769; 1991.

78c. Marcial-Vega, V.A.; Waram, M.D.; Leibel, S.; Clark, A.; Sweig, R.; Order, S.E. Treatment of supratentorial high-grade gliomas with split course high fractional dose post-operative radiation therapy. Intl. J. Radiat. Oncol. Biol. Phys. 16:1419-1424; 1989.

78c'. Nedzi, L.A.; Kooy, H.; Alexander III, E.; et al. Variables associated with the development of complications from radiosurgery of intracranial tumors. Int J Radiat Oncol Biol Phys. 21:591-600; 1991.

78d. Nelson, D.F.; Curran, W.J.; Nelson, J.S.; Weinstein, A.S.; Martz, K.L.; Ahmad, K.; Keller, J.W.; Murray, K.; Hanks, G.E. Hyperfractionation in malignant glioma. Report on a dose searching Phase I/II protocol of the Radiation Therapy Oncology Group. Abstract. In: Proceedings of the American Society of Clinical Oncology. Semin. Clin. Oncol. 9:90; 1990.

79. Nelson, D.F.; Diener-West, M.; Horton, J.; Chang, C.H.; Shoenfeld, D.; Nelson, J.S. Combined modality approach to treatment of malignnat gliomas. Reevaluation of RTOG 7401/ECOG 1374 with long-term follow-up: a joint Radiation Therapy Oncology Group and Eastern Cooperative Oncology Group study. NCI Monogr. 6:279-284; 1988.

80. Nelson, D.F.; Diener-West, M.; Weinstein, A.S.; Schoenfeld, D.; Nelson, J.S.; Sause, W.T.; Chang, C.H.; Goodman, R.; Carabell, S. A randomized comparison of misonidazole sensitized radiotherapy plus BCNU and radiotherapy plus BCNU for treatment of malignant glioma after surgery: final report of an RTOG study. Intl. J. Radiat. Oncol. Biol. Phys. 12:1793-1800; 1986.

80a. Nelson, D.F.; Martz, K.L.; Bonner, H.; Nelson, J.; Newell, J.; Kerman, H.D.; Thomason, J.W.; Murray, K. Definitive radiation therapy in the treatment of primary non-Hodgkin's lymphoma of the central nervous systme, non-AIDS related: report of RTOG study 8515. J. Neurosurg. (In press).

80b. Nelson, D.F.; Nelson, J.S.; Davis, D.R.; Chang, C.H.; Griffin, T.W.; Pajak, T.F. Survival and prognosis of patients with astrocytoma with atypical or anaplastic features. J. Neuro-oncol. 3:99-103; 1985.

81. Nelson, D.F.; Urtasun, R.C.; Saunders, W.M.; Gutin, P.H.; Sheline, G.E. Recent and current investigations of radiation therapy of malignant gliomas. Semin. Oncol. 13:46-55; 1986.

82. Ransohoff, J. The role of intracranial surgery for the treatment of malignant gliomas. In: Walker, M.D., ed. Oncology of the nervous system. Boston, MA: Martinus Nijhoff Publishers; 1983:101-115.

83. Ransohoff, J.; Kelly, P.; Laws, E. The role of intracranial surgery for the treatment of malignant gliomas. Semin. Oncol. 13:27-37; 1986.

84. Robertson, J.T.; Rogers, E.S.; Banks, W.L.; Young, H.F. Metabolic therapy of malignant gliomas. In: Walker, M.D., ed. Oncology of the nervous system. Boston, MA: Martinus Nijhoff Publishers; 1983:273-284.

85. Rossi, G.R.; Feoli, F.; Fernandez, E.; et al. The Role of Surgery in the Treatment Supratentorial Brain Gliomas. In: Paoleni, P.; Walker, M.D.; Buni, G.; et al., eds. Multidisciplinary Aspects of Brain Tumor Therapy. Amsterdam, the Netherlands: Elsevier-North Holland Publishing Co.; 1979:155-163.

85a. Saroja, K.R.; Mansell, J.; Hendrickson, F.R.; Cohen, L.; Lennox, A. Failure of accelerated neutron therapy to control high grade astrocytomas. Int. J. Radiat. Oncol. Biol. Phys. 17:1295-1298; 1989.

86. Shapiro, W.R. Therapy of adult malignant brain tumors: what have the clinical trials taught us? Semin. Oncol. 13:38-45; 1986.

86a. Sheline, G.E. Radiotherapy for high grade gliomas. Int. J. Radiat. Oncol. Biol. Phys. 18:793-804; 1990.

87. Urtasun, R.; Band, P.; Chapman, J.D.; et al. Radiation and High-dose Metronidazole in Supratentorial Glioblastoma. New Engl. J. Med. 294:1354-1367; 1976.

88. Urtasun, R.C.; Miller, J.D.R.; Frunchak, V.; et al. Radiotherapy Pilot Trials with Sensitizers of Hypoxic Cells: Metronidazole in Supratentorial Glioblastoma. Br. J. Radiol. 50:602-603; 1977.

89. Walker, M.D. Malignant glioma. In: Wilson, C.B.; Hoff, J.T., eds. Current surgical management of neurologic disease. New York, NY: Churchill Livingstone; 1980:72-78.

90. Walker, M.D.; Alexander, E. Jr.; Hunt, W.E.; et al. Evaluation of BCNU and/or Radiotherapy in the Treatment of Anaplastic Gliomas. A Cooperative Clinical Trial. J. Neurosurg. 49:333-343; 1978.

91. Walker, M.D.; Green, S.B.; Byar, D.P.; Alexander, E., Jr.; Batzdorf, U.; Brooks, W.H.; Hunt, W.E.; MacCarty, C.S.; Mahaley, M.S., Jr.; Mealey, J., Jr.; Owens, G.; Ransohoff, J. II; Robertson, J.T.; Shapiro, W.r.; Smith, K.R., Jr.; Wison, C.B.; Strike, T.A. Randomized comparisons of radiotherapy and nitrosoureas for the treatment of malignant glioma after surgery. New Engl. J. Med. 303:1323-1329; 1980.

91a. Walker, M.D.; Strike, T.A.; Sheline, G.E. An analysis of dose effect relationship in the radiotherapy of malignant gllomas. Intl. j. Radiat. Oncol. Biol. Phys. 5;1725-1731; 1979.

92. Walner, K.E.; Galichih, J.H.; Krol, G.; Aribit, E.; Malkin, N.G. Patterns of failure following treatment of glioblastoma multiforme and anaplastic astrocytoma. Intl. J. Radiat. Biol. Oncol. Phys. 16:1405-1409; 1989.

92a. Weinstein, A.S.; Nelson, D.F.; Pakuris, E.; Pajak, T. Pulmonary toxicity in patients with malignant glioma treated with BCNU and radiotherapy with or without misonidazole. An RTOG Study. Cancer Treatment Reports 70:947-956; 1986.

92b. Young, G.; Kaplan, A.; Regelson, W. Immunotherapy with autologous white cell infusions ("lymphocytes") in the treatment of recurrent glioblastoma multiforme. Cancer 40:1037-1044; 1977.

Low-Grade Astrocytomas

92c. Bouchard, J. Effects of irradiation in treatment of intracranial gliomas — treatment results by histologic groups. In: Bouchard, J., ed. Radiation therapy of tumors and diseases of the nervous system. Philadelphia, PA: Lea & Febiger; 1966:78-118.

93. Bucy, P.C.; Thieman, P.W. Cerebellar astrocytoma, long-term follow-up. Arch. Neurol. 18:14,1968.

93a. Dearnaley, D.P.; A'Hern, R.P.; Whittaker, S.; Bloom, H.J.G. Pineal and CNS germ cell tumors: Royal Marsden Hospital Experience 1962-1987. Int. J. Radiat. Oncol. Biol. Phys. 18:773-782; 1990.

94. Fazekas, J.T. Treatment of Grades I and II Brain Astrocytomas. The Role of Radiotherapy. Intl. J. Radiat. Oncol. Biol. Phys. 2:661-666; 1977.

95. Garcia, D.M.; Fulling, K.H.; Marks, J.E. The value of radiation therapy in addition to surgery for astrocytomas of the adult cerebrum. Cancer 55:919-927; 1985.

96. Laws, E.R.; Taylor, W.F.; Clifton, M.B.; Okazaki, H. Neurosurgical management of low-grade astrocytoma of the cerebral hemispheres. J. Neurosurg. 61:665-673; 1984.

97. Leibel, S.A.; Sheline, G.E.; Wara, W.M.; Boldrey, E.B.; Nielsen, S.L. The role of radiation theary in the treatment of astrocytomas. Cancer 35:1551-1557; 1975.

98. Levy, L.F.; Elvidge, A.R. Astrocytoma of the brain and spinal cord. J. Neurosurg. 13:413; 1956.

99. Muller, W.; Afra, D.; Schroder, R. Supratentonal Recurrences of Gliomas: Morphological Studies in Relation to Time Intervals with Astrocytomas. Acta Neurochir. 37:75-91; 1977.

100. Olmsted, C.M.; Plenk, H. Radiation therapy of astocytomas grades I-IV. Intl. J. Radiat. Oncol. Biol. Phys. 4(suppl. 2):229; 1978 (abstract).

100a. Shaw, E.G.; Dumas-Deport, C.; Scheithauer, B.W.; Gilbertson, D.T., et al. Radiotherapy in the management of low-grade supratentorial astrocytomas. J. Neurosur. 70:853; 1989.

101. Sheline, G.E. Radiation therapy of brain tumors. Cancer 39:873-881; 1977.

102. Stage, W.S. Stein, J.J. Treatment of malignant astrocytomas. Radiology 120:7-18; 1974.

Pediatric Tumors

103. Allen, J.C. Childhood brain tumors: current status of clinical trials in newly diagnosed and recurrent disease. Pediatr. Clin. N. Am. 32:633-651; 1985.

103a. Bloom, H.J.G.; Glees, J.; Bell, J. The Treatment and Long-Term Prognosis of Children with Intracranial Tumors: A Study of 610 Cases, 1950-1981. Int. J. Rad. Oncol. Biol. Phys. 18:723-746;1990.

104. Duffner, P.K.; Cohen, M.E. Recent developments in pediatric neuro-oncology. Cancer 58:561-568; 1986.

105. Finlay, J.L.; Goins, S.C. Brain tumors in children. I. Advances in diagnosis. Am. J. Pediatr. Hematol./Oncol. 9(3):246-255; 1987.

106. Finlay, J.L.; Goins, S.C. Brain tumors in children. III. Advances in chemotherapy. Am. J. Pediatr. Hematol./Oncol. 9(3):264-271; 1987.

107. Finlay, J.L.; Goins, S.C.; Uteg, R.; Giese, W.L. Progress in the management of childhood brain tumors. Hematol./Oncol. Clin. N. Am. 1:753-776; 1987.

108. Finlay, J.L.; Uteg, R.; Giese, W.L. Brain tumors in children. II. Advances in neurosurgery and radiation oncology. Am. J. Pediatr. Hematol./Oncol. 9(3):256-263; 1987.

109. Halperin, E.C.; Kun, L.E.; Constine, L.S.; Tarbell, N.J. Retinoblastoma and optic glioma. In: Halperin, E.C.; Kun, L.E.; Constine, L.S.; Tarbell, N.J., eds. Pediatric radiation oncology. New York, NY: Raven Press; 1989:108-133.

110. Halperin, E.C.; Kun, L.E.; Constine, L.S.; Tarbell, N.J. Supratentorial brain tumors. In: Halperin, E.C.; Kun, L.E.; Constine, L.S.; Tarbell, N.J. Pediatric radiation oncology. New York, NY: Raven Press; 1989:38-75.

111. Halperin, E.C.; Kun, L.E.; Constine, L.S.; Tarbell, N.J. Tumors of the posterior fossa of the brain an dthe spinal canal. In: Halperin, E.C.; Kun, L.E.; Constine, L.S.; Tarbell, N.J., eds. Pediatric radiation oncology. New York, NY: Raven Press; 1989:76-107.

111a. Jannoun, L.; Bloom, H.J.G. Long-term psychological effects in children treated for intracranial tumors. Int. J. Radiat. Oncol. Biol. Phys. 18:747-754; 1990.

112. Pendergrass, T.W.; et al. Eight drugs in one day chemotherapy for brain tumors: experience in 107 children and rationale for preradiation chemotheary. J. Clin. Oncol. 5:1221-1231; 1987.

Medulloblastoma

113. Berry, M.P.; Jenkin, R.D.; Keen, C.W.; Nair, B.D., et al. Radiation treatment for medulloblastoma. A 21-year review. J. Neurosurg. 55:43-51; 1981.

114. Bloom HJG: Adjuvant Therapy for Residual Disease in Children with Medulloblastoma. In, Bonadonna G, Mathe G, Salmon SE (eds): Recent Results in Cancer Research. Berlin, Germany: Springer-Verlag, 1979, pp. 412-422.

115. Bloom, H.J.G. Intracranial tumros: response and resistance to therapeutic endeavors, 1970-1980. Intl. J. Radiat. Oncol. Biol. Phys. 8:1083-1113; 1982.

116. Bloom, H.J.G. Medulloblastoma in children: increasing survival rates and further prospects. Intl. J. Radiat. Oncol. Biol. Phys. 8:2023-2027; 1982.

117. Bloom, H.J.G. Results of the SIOP medulloblastoma trial. Presented at the XVIIIth annual meeting of the International Society of Paediatric Oncology. Belgrade, Yugoslavia; 1986.

117a. Bloom, H.J.G. Bessell, G. Medulloblastoma in adults: a review of 47 patients treated between 1952 and 1981. Int. J. Radiat. Oncol. Biol. Phys. 18:755-762; 1990.

118. Brand, W.N.; Schneider, P.A.; Tokars, R.P. Long-term results of a pilot study of low-dose cranial-spinal irradiation for cerebellar medulloblastoma. Intl. J. Radiat. Oncol. Biol. Phys. 13:1641-1645; 1987.

119. Chan, C.; Housepian, E.M.; Herbert, C. Jr. Operative Staging System and a Megavoltage Radiotherapeutic Technique for Cerebellar Medulloblastomas. Radiology 93:1351-1359; 1969.

120. Cohen, A.; Cooper, P.R.; Kupersmith, M.J.; Flamm, E.S., et al. Visual recovery after transsphenoidal removal of pituitary adenomas. Neurosurgery 17:446-452; 1985.

121. Cumberlin, R.L.; Luk, K.H.; Wara, W.M.; Sheline, G.E., et al. Medulloblastoma. Tretment fresults and effect on normal tissues. Cancer 43:1014-1020; 1979.

122. Deutsch, M. Medulloblastoma: staging and treatment outcome. Intl. J. Radiat. Oncol. Biol. Phys. 14:1103-1107; 1988.

123. Harisladis, L.; Chang, C.H. Medulloblastomas in children: a correlation of staging of results of treatment. Intl. J. Radiat. Oncol. Biol. Phys. 9:833-842; 1977.

124. Hershatter, B.W.; Halperin, E.C.; Cox, E.B., et al. Medulloblastoma: the Duke University Medical Center experience. Intl. J. Radiat. Oncol. Biol. Phys. 12:1771-1777; 1986.

125. Hughes, E.N.; Shillito, J.; Sallan, S.E.; Loeffler, J.S., et al. Medulloblastoma at the Joint Center for Radiation Therapy between 1968 and 1984. Cancer 61:1992-1998; 1988.

126. Maor, M.H.; Fields, R.S.; Hogstrom, K.R.; van Eys, J. Improving the therapeutic ratio of craniospinal irradiation in medulloblastoma. Intl. J. Radiat. Oncol. Biol. Phys. 11:687-697; 1985.

127. Quest, D.O.; Brisman, R.; Antunes, J.L.; et al. Period of Risk for Recurrence in Medulloblastoma. J. Neurosurg. 48:159-163; 1978.

128. Silverman, C.L.; Simpson, J.R. Cerebellar medulloblastoma: the importance of posterior fossa dose to survival and patterns of failure. Intl. J. Radiat. Oncol. Biol. 8:1869-1876; 1982.

129. Smith, C.E.; Long, D.M.; Jones, T.K.; *et al.* Medulloblastoma: an analysis of time-dose relationship and recurrence patterns. Cancer 32:722-728; 1973.

Ependymoma

129a. Bloom, H.J.G.; Walsh, L. Tumours of the central nervous system. In: Cancer in Children - Clinical Management, H.J.G. Bloom, J. Lemerle, M.K. Neidhardt, P.A. Voute, eds. Berlin, Germany: Springer; 1975;93-119.
130. Kim, Y.H.; Fayos, J.V. Intracranial ependymomas. Radiology 124:805-808; 1977.
131. Marks, J.E.; Adler, S.J. A comparative study of ependymomas by site of origin. Intl. J. Radiat. Oncol. Biol. Phys. 8:37-43; 1982.
132. Pierre-Kahn; A.; Hirsch, J.F.; Roux, F.X.; Renier, D.; Sainte-Rose, C. Intracranial ependymomas in childhood: survival and functional results of 47 cases. Childs Brain 10:145-156; 1983.
133. Salazar, O.M.; Rubin, P.; Bassano, D.; *et al.* Improved Survival of Patients with Intracranial Ependymomas by Irradiation—Dose Selection and Field Extension. Cancer 35:1563-1574; 1975.
134. Shaw, E.G.; Evans, R.G.; Scheithauer, B.W.; Ilstrup, D.M.; Earle, J.D. Postoperative radiotherapy of intracranial ependymoma in pediatric and adult patients. Intl. J. Radiat. Oncol. Biol. Phys. 13:1457-1462; 1987.
135. Wollner, K.E.; Wara, W.M.; Sheline, G.E.; Davis, R.L. Intracranial ependymomas: results of treatment with partial or whole brain irradiation without spinal irradiation. Intl. J. Radiat. Oncol. Biol. Phys. 12:1937-1941; 1986.

Craniopharyngioma

136. Amacher, A.L. Craniopharyngioma: The Controversy Regarding Radiotherapy. Childs Brain 6:57-64; 1980.
137. Bucci, M.; Chen, L.; Hoff, J. Perioperative morbidity associated with operative resection of craniopharyngioma: a review of 10 years experience. Neurochiurgie 30:135-138; 1937.
138. Cavazzuti, V.; Fischer, E.G.; Welch, K.; Belli, J.A.; Winston, K.R. Neurological and psychophysiological sequelae following different treatment of craniopharyngioma in children. J. Neurosurg. 59:409-417; 1983.
139. Danoff, B.F.; Cowchock, F.S.; Kramer, S. Childhood craniopharyngioma: survival, local control, endocrine and neurologic function following radiotherapy. Intl. J. Radit. Oncol. Biol. Phys. 9:171-175; 1983.
140. Hoogenhout, J.; Otten, B.J.; Kazem I.; Stelinga, G.B.; Walder, A.H.D. Surgery and radiation therapy in the management of craniopharyngiomas. Intl. J. Radiat. Oncol. Biol. Phys. 10:2293-2297; 1984.
141. Katz, E.L. Late Results of Radical Excision of Craniopharyngioma in Children. J. Neurosurg. 42:86-90; 1975.
142. Kramer, S.; McKissock, W.; Concannon, J.P. Craniopharyngioma: Treatment by Combined Surgery and Radiation Therapy. J. Neurosurg. 18:217-226; 1961.
143. Matson, D.D.; Crigler, J.F. Management of Craniopharyngiomas in Childhood. J. Neurosurg. 30:377-390; 1969.
144. Pollack, I.F.; Lunsford, L.D.; Slamovits, T.L.; Gumerman, L.W., *et al.* Stereotaxic intracavitary irradiation for cystic craniopharyngiomas. J. Neurosurg. 68:227-233; 1988.
145. Stahnke, N.; Grubel, G.; Lagenstein, I.; Willig, R.P. Long-term follow-up of children with craniopharyngioma. Eur. J. Pediatr. 142:179-185; 1984
146. Wen, B.C.; Hussey, D.H.; Staples, J.; Hitchon, P.W., *et al.* A comparison of the roles of surgery and radiation therapy in the management of craniopharyngiomas. Intl. J. Radat. Oncol. Biol. Phys. 16:17-24; 1989.

Optic Gliomas

147. Alvord, E.C.; Lofton, S. Gliomas of the optic nerve or chiasm. J. Neurosurg. 68:85-98; 1988.
148. Danoff, B.F.; Kramer, S.; Thompson, N. The radiotherapeutic management of optic nerve gliomas in children. Intl. J. Radat. Oncol. Biol. Phys. 6:45-50; 1980.
149. Flickinger, J.C.; Torres, C.; Deutsch, M. Management of low-grade gliomas of the optic nerve chiasm. Cancer 61:635-642; 1988.
150. Hurst, R.W.; Newmann, S.A.; Cail, W.S. Multifocal intracranial MR abnormalities in neurofibromatosis. AJNR 9:293-296; 1988.
151. Packer, R.J.; Savino, P.J.; Bilanivk, L.T.; Zimmermann, R.A., *et al.* Chiasmatic gliomas of childhood. A reappraisal of natural history and effectiveness of cranial irradiation. Childs Brain 10:393-403; 1983.
152. Savoiardo, M.; Harwood-Nash, D.C.; Tadmor, R.; Scotti, G., *et al.* Gliomas of the intracranial anterior optic pathways in children. The role of computed tomography, angiography, pneumoencephalography, and radionuclide brain scanning. Radiology 138:601-610; 1981.
153. Tenny, R.T.; Laws, E.R., Jr.; Younge, B.R.; Rush, J.A. The neurosurgical management of optic glioma: results in 104 patients. J. Neurosurg. 57:452-458; 1982.
154. Weiss, L.; Sagerman, R.H.; King, G.A.; Chung, C.T., *et al.* Controversy in the management of optic nerve glioma. Cancer 59:100-1004; 1987.
155. Wong, J.Y.C.; Uhl, V.; Wara, W.M.; Sheline, G.E. Optic gliomas. A reanalysis of the University of California, San Francisco experience. Cancer 60:1847-1855; 1987.

Meningiomas

156. Barbaro, N.M.; Gutin, P.H.; Wilson, C.B.; Sheline, G.E., *et al.* Radiation therapy in the treatment of partially resected meningiomas. Neurosurgery 20:525-528; 1987.
157. Carella, R.J.; Ransohoff, J.; Newall, J. Role of radiation therapy in the management of meningioma. Neurosurgery 10:332-338; 1982.
158. Donnell, M.S.; Meger, G.A.; Donegan, W.L. Estrogen receptor protein in intracranial meningiomas. J. Neurosurg. 50:499-502; 1979.
159. Forbes, A.R.; Goldberg, I.D. Radiation therapy in the treatment of meningioma: the Joint Center for Radiation Therapy experience 1970 to 1982. J. Clin. Oncol. 2:1139-1143; 1984.
160. Glaholm, J.; Bloom, H.J.G.; Crow, J.H. The role of radiotherapy in the management of intracranial meningiomas: the Royal Marsden Hospital Experience with 186 patients. Int. J. Radiat. Oncol. Biol. Phys. 18:755-762; 1990.
161. Pertuiset, B.; Farah, S.; Clayes, L.; Goutorbe, J., *et al.* Operability of intracranial meningiomas. Personal series of 353 cases. Acta Neurochir. (Wien) 76:2-11; 1985.
162. Schregg, J.G.; Gomez, F.; Therese, L.M.B.; Tribolet, N. Presence of sex steroid hormone receptors in meningioma tissue. Surg. Neurol. 15:415-518; 1981.
163. Simpson, D. The recurrence of intracranial meningiomas after surgical treatment. J. Neurol. Neurosurg. Psychiat. 20:22-39; 1957.
164. Tilzner, L.L.; Plap, F.U.; Evans, J.P.; Stone, D.; Kelly, A. Steroid receptors in human meningiomas. Cancer 49:633-636; 1982.
165. Wara, W.M.; Sheline, G.E.; Newman, H.; Townsend, J.J.; Boldrey, E.B. Radiation therapy of meningiomas. Am. J. Roentgenol. Radium Ther. Nucl. Med. 123:453-458; 1975.

Oligodendrogliomas

166. Bullard, D.E.; Rawlings III, C.E.; Phillips, B.; Cox, E.B., *et al.* Oligodendroglioma—an analysis of the value of radiation therapy. Cancer 60:2179; 1987.
167. Chin, H.W.; Hazel, J.J.; Kim, T.H.; Webster, J.H. Oligodendrogliomas—a clinical study of cerebral oligodendrogliomas. Cancer 45:1448-1466; 1980.
168. Lindegaard, K.F.; Mork, S.J.; Eide, G.E., Halvorsen, T.B., *et al.* Statistical analysis of clinicopathological features, radiotherapy and survival in 170 cases of oligodendroglioma. J. Neurosurg. 67:224-230; 1987.
169. Mork, S.J. Oligodendroglioma—incidence and biologic behavior in a defined population. J. Neurosurg. 63:881; 1985.
170. Sheline, G.E.; Boldrey, E.; Karlsberg, P.; *et al.* Therapeutic Considerations of Tumors Affecting the Central Nervous System: Oligodendrogliomas. Radioiogy 82:84-89; 1964.
171. Shenkin, H.A. The Effect of Roentgen-ray Therapy on Oligodendrogliomas of the Brain. J. Neurosurg. 22:57-59; 1965.
172. Wallner, K.E.; Gonzales, M.; Shelina, G.E., *et al.* Treatment of oligodendrogliomas with or without postoperative irradiation. J. Neurosurg. 68:684-688; 1988.

Pituitary Adenomas

172a. af Trampe, E.; Lundell, G.; Lax, I.; *et al.* External irradiation of growth hormone producing pituitary adenomas: Prolactin as a marker of hypothalamic and pituitary effects. Int J Radiat Oncol Biol Phys. 20:655-660; 1991.

173. Ciric, I. Pituitary Tumors. Neurol. Clin. 3:751-768; 1985.
174. Kernohan, J.W.; Sayre, G.P. Tumors ot the Pituitary Gland and Infundibulum. Washington, D.C.: Armed Forces Institute of Pathology; 1956.
175. Sheline, G.E.; Boldrey, E.B.; Phillips, T.L. Chromophobe Adenomas of the Pituitary Gland. Am. J. Roentgenol. 92:150-173; 1964.
176. Wilson, C. Surgical management of endocrine-active pituitary adenomas. In: Walker, M.D., ed. Oncology of the nervous sytem. Boston, MA: Martinus Nijhoff Publishers; 1983:117-150.

Chordomas

177. Amendola, B.E.; Amendola, M.A.; Oliver, E.; McClatchey, K.D. Chordoma: role of radiation therapy. Radiology 158:839-843; 1986.
178. Falconer M, Bailey 1, Duchen L: Surgical Treatment of Chordoma and Chondroma of the Skull Base. J Neurosurg 29:261-275, 1968.
179. Heffelfinger MH, Dahlin DC, MacCarthy CS, et al: Chordomas and cartilaginous tumors at the skull base. Cancer 32:410-420, 1973.
180. Raffel, C.; Wright, D.C., Gutin, P.H., Wilson, C.B. Cranial chordomas. Neurosurgery 17:703-710; 1985.
181. Suit, H.D.; Goitein, M.; Munzenrider, J.; Verhey, L.; Davis, K.R.; Koehler, A.; Linggod, R.; Ojemann, R.G. Definitive radiation therapy for chordoma and chondrosarcoma of base of skull and cervical spine. J. Neurosurg. 56:377-385; 1982.

Tumors of the Pineal and Supra-sellar Region, Germinomas

182. Amendola, B.E.; McClatchey, K.; Amendola, M.A. Pineal region tumors: analysis of treatment results. Intl. J. Radiat. Oncol. Biol. Phys. 10:991-997; 1984.
183. Bradfield, J.S.; Perez, C.A. Pineal Tumors and Ectopic Pinealomas—Analysis of Treatment and Failures. Radiology 103:399-406; 1972.
184. Edwards, M.S.B.; Hudgins, R.J.; Wilson, C.B.; Levin, V.A.; Wara, W.M. Pineal region tumors in children. J. Neurosurg. 68:689-697; 1988.
185. Fields, J.N.; Fulling, K.H.; Thomas, P.R.M.; Marks, J.E. Suprasellar germinoma: radiation therapy. Radiology 164:247-249; 1987.
186. Jennings, M.t.; Gelman, R.; Hochberg, F. Intracranial germ-cell

tumors: natural history and pathogenesis. J. Neurosurg. 63:155-167; 1985.
187. Legido, A.; Packer, R.J.; Sutton, L.N.; D'Angio, G.; Rorke, L.B.; Burce, D.A.; Schutt, L. Suprasellar germinomas in childhood: a reappraisal. Cancer 63:340-344; 1989.
188. Linstadt, D.; Wara, W.M.; Edwards, M.S.B.; Hudgins, R.J.; Sheline, G.E. Radiotherapy of primary intracranial germinomas: the case against routine craniospinal irradiation. Intl. J. Radiat. Oncol. Biol. Phys. 15:291-297; 1988.
189. Rich, T.A.; Cassady, J.R.; Strand, R.D. Radiation therapy for pineal and suprasellar germ cell tumors. Cancer 55:932-940; 1985.

CNS Lymphomas

189a. Brada, M.; Deanaley, D.; Horwich, A.; Bloom, H.J.G. Management of primary cerebral lymphoma with initial chemotherapy: preliminary results and comparison with patients treated with radiotherapy alone. Int. J. Radiat. Oncol. Biol. Phys. 18:782-792; 1990.
190. Freeman, C.R.; Shustik, C.; Brisson, M.; et al. Primary malignant lymphomas of the central nervous system. Cancer 58:1106-1111; 1986.
191. Gonzalez, D.G.; Schuster, Uitterhoeve, A.L. Primary non-Hodgkin's lymphoma of the central nervous system. Results of Radiotherapy in 15 cases. Cancer 51:2048-2052; 1983.
192. Letendre, L.; Banks, P.M.; Reese, D.F.; Miller, R.H.; Scanlon, P.W.; Kiely, J.M. Primary lymphoma of the central nervous system. Cancer 49:939-943; 1982.
192a. Lindstadt, D.E.; Wara, W.M.; Leibel, S.A.; Gutin, P.H.; Wilson, C.B.; Sheline, G. Postoperative radiotherapy of primary spinal cord tumors. Int. J. Radiat. Oncol. Biol. Phys. 16:1397-1404; 1989.
193. Littman, P.; Wang, C.C. Reticulum cell sarcoma of the brain. A review of the literature and a study of 19 cases. Cancer 35:1412-1420; 1975.
194. Loeffler, J.S.; Ervin, T.J.; Mauch, P.; et al. Primary lymphomas of the central nervous sytem: patterns of failure and factors that influence survival. J. Clin. Oncol. 3:490-494; 1985.
195. Mendenhall, N.P.; Thar, T.L.; Agrr, O.F.; et al. Primary lymphoma of the central nervous system. Cancer 52:1993-2000; 1983.
196. Murray, K.; Kun, L.; Cox, J. Primary malignant lymphoma of the central nervous sytem. J. Neurosurg. 65:600-607; 1986.
197. Sagerman, R.H.; Collier, C.H.; King, G.A. Radiation therapy of microgliomas. Radiology 149:567-570; 1983.

Omar M. Salazar, M.D., F.A.C.R., Radiation Oncology
Sandra McDonald, M.B., Ch.B., Radiation Oncology
Paul Van Houtte, M.D., Radiation Oncology

Alex Yuang-Chi Chang, M.D., Medical Oncology
Richard H. Feins, M.D., Surgical Thoracic Oncology
Thomas Anderson, M.D., Medical Oncology

Chapter **31**

LUNG CANCER

Why do people smoke? The heart has its reasons which reason knows not.

Blaise Pascal (187)

PERSPECTIVE

Lung cancer accounts for 19% of all cancer in men, compared with 11% in women. It is responsible for 34% of cancer-related deaths in men and 21% in women. Furthermore, the overall 5-year survival rate is still below 15% (29a). Only one third of patients are eligible for surgical resection with curative intent, and among them, less than one third will be alive 5 years post surgery. Little progress has been made in the past decade to improve long-term survival significantly. Nevertheless, all disciplines involved in lung cancer management have advanced notably, and as a result, some small but significant improvements in survival have been noted (29a,145). Whereas the relative 5-year survival rate for whites and blacks were 10% and 7%, respectively, from 1970 to 73, they were 13% and 11%, respectively, from 1981 to 1986 (29a). Today, lung cancer is not considered to be a single disease entity, but to be composed of several diseases conditioned by histopathologic types that determine patterns of spread, treatment, and prognosis. Furthermore, the modern management of lung cancer requires, more than ever, cooperation between all specialties involved in diagnosis and therapy.

EPIDEMIOLOGY AND ETIOLOGY

Epidemiology

1. In 1991, there were about 101,000 new cases of lung cancer in men and 60,000 in women (29a) in the United States. According to the World Health Organization, 660,500 new cases of lung cancer are diagnosed annually worldwide (71).

2. In 1991, there were approximately 92,000 deaths from lung cancer in men and 51,000 in women (29a) in the United States. Worldwide, lung cancer results in one death every minute years round (71).

3. Most striking is the rising incidence among women during the last decade. The percentage of change in the rate of lung cancer incidence from 1947 to 1969 was 133% for men and 108% for women (145). The worldwide incidence in the period 1960 to 1980 was 76% for men and 35% for women.

4. A corresponding increase in cancer death rates has been seen from 1960 to 1985. In women it has practically tripled, going from less than 10/100,000 to a surprising 27/100,000, which was almost as high as that of breast cancer in 1985. In men, it has almost doubled, going from 40/100,000 to 75/100,000 (145). There will be 2 million cases of lung cancer annually in the year 2000, including 60% in developing countries (180).

5. Cigarette smoking increases the risk of developing and dying from lung cancer. The death rate increases with increase in exposure. For smokers of less than < 1/2, 1/2 to 1, 1 to 2, 2 and more than two packs/daily, the death rates in a recent study were 95, 108, 229, and 264 in 100,000, respectively (70).

6. There has been a decline in cigarette smoking in the U.S.A. In 1965 50.2% of men and 31.9% of women smoked; in 1987 these figures stand at 31.7% and 26.8% respectively (62a).

7. Cigarette smoking is more common in blacks (34%) than whites (28.8%) although whites smoke more cigarettes per day (62a).

8. The largest differences in smoking habits are seen among educated groups. In 1966, 36.5% of people with less than a high school diploma smoked as compared to 33.7% of college graduates. In 1987, these figures stand at 35.7% and 16.5% respectively. This represents a drop of more than 50% among college graduates. It is estimated that by the year 2000 only 22% of the adult population and a mere 10% of college graduates will be cigarette smokers (62a).

9. Today, through legislative efforts, there are several antitobacco health policies in effect in many western hemisphere countries. In the United States and some Scandinavian countries, the incidence of lung cancer among young males appears to be decreasing. Nevertheless, a major difference in mortality will only be seen during the next century.

10. The average age for onset for lung cancer is about 60 years (less than 1% of cases occur under aged 30 years).

645

Etiology

A variety of agents have been proven to be carcinogens in humans.

1. *Tobacco smoke* is the dominant agent and represents a complex mixture of physical and chemical carcinogens.

   There is a direct relationship between the amount of tobacco exposure and risk for developing lung cancer. In addition to the increased lung cancer risk, smoking is also associated with an increased risk of upper respiratory, genitourinary, and digestive tract cancer. The type of cigarettes seems to also influence the risk; that is, a filter apparently decreases the risk. Stopping smoking is associated with a gradual decrease in the risk, but a long period of time (> 6 years) is necessary before an appreciable diminution of risk occurs (169).

   Interestingly, in Asians, the proportion of cases attributable to active smoking may not be as high. The rate of smoking deaths has been reported as low as 4% to 44% among Chinese or Japanese women. Identification of nonsmoking risk factors in these patients include combustion by-products from cooking, heating stoves, and oil furnances.

2. *Asbestos* exposure is associated with the development of mesothelioma and also bronchogenic carcinoma. The risk from asbestos is particularly more pronounced when combined with cigarette smoking (141).

3. *Atmospheric pollution* has been implicated as a causative agent because of the higher incidence of lung cancer in urban than rural areas.

4. A more direct relationship has been shown also in cases of *pitchblende* miners who are involved with radioactive ores.

5. *Metals*, mostly nickel and silver, but also chromium, cadmium, beryllium, cobalt, selenium, and steel have been proven to be carcinogenic in animals and are occupational hazards, particularly when combined with other factors.

6. *Chemical products* such as chloromethyl ethers have been associated with the development of lung cancer, especially small cell lung cancers (SCLC) (15).

Lung Cancer Biology (35)

Biologic properties inherent within lung cancer cells may have prognostic importance and may be potentially useful in monitoring response to therapy or recurrence. Cell lines are established from a variety of organ sites, including the primary tumor, bone marrow aspirates, lymph node biopsies, malignant effusions, and other surgically resected sites. These allow detailed studies of the biologic properties of these tumor cells and permit clinical correlation with patients. Stability in culture is usually noted for these cell lines over prolonged periods.

SCLC lines are subclassified into classic (70%) and variant (30%) subgroups:

1. *Classic cell lines* (Table 31-1) (35) express elevated levels of levadopa decarboxylase, bombesin/gastrin-releasing peptide (BBS/GRP), neuron-specific enolase (NSE) and creatinine (CR) kinase BBS, have a relatively long doubling time and low cloning efficiency *in vitro* and are radiosensitive.

2. *Variant cell lines* have low or undetectable levels of levadopa decarboxylase, the marker of neuroendocrine differentiation. They lack BBS/GRP, but unlike non-small cell lung lines, express elevated levels of NSE and CR Kinase-BBS. They have more rapid growth than classic lines, are radioresistant, and morphologically more closely resemble large cell undifferentiated carcinoma. They also have 4 to 60 time DNA amplification of c-mycogene and show increased expression of the gene.

Data suggest that these properties are clinically relevant in predicting response to therapy and survival (82).

DETECTION AND DIAGNOSIS (32)

Clinical Detection

Clinical manifestations are varied and mimic other pulmonary conditions. A change of pulmonary habits is the most significant sign of lung cancer. Cough, chest pain, rust-streaked or purulent sputum production, hemoptysis, and dyspnea are common symptoms of lung cancer.

Table 31-1. Biologic Properties of Lung Cancer Cell Lines

Characteristic	SCLC		NSCLC
	Classic	Variant	
Growth Morphology	Suspension	Suspension	Attached
Cytology	SCLC	SCLC	NSCLC
Colony Forming Efficiency	2%	13%	6%
Doubling Time	72 hr	32 hr	40 hr
Dense Core Granules	+	-	-
DDC	++	-	-
BLI/GRP	++	-	-
NSE	++	+	-
CK BB	++	++	-
Neurotensin	++	-	-
Peptide Hormone	++	+/-	-
BLI Receptors	+	-	-
EGF Receptors	-	-	+
Chromosome 3, Del	+	+	-
Leu-7 Antigen	+	+	-
Radiation Sensitivity	Sensitive	Resistant	Resistant
C-myc Amplification	-	+	+/-

SCLC = small cell lung cancer; NSCLC = non-small cell lung cancer; DDC = L-dopa decarboxylase; BLI/GRP = bombesin/gastrin releasing peptide; NSE = neuron specific enolase; CKBB = creatine kinase.

From Carney and DeLeij (35), with permission.

Local complications depend on the location of the tumor and include:

- superior vena caval obstruction
- shoulder/arm pain with brachial plexus involvement by a superior sulcus by tumor
- recurrent pleural effusions and pneumonitis resulting from bronchial obstruction
- cardiac failure or arrhythmia from cardiac involvement
- hoarseness secondary to recurrent laryngeal nerve paralysis

Paraneoplastic syndromes: Extrapulmonary manifestations of lung cancer may be recognized before the lung cancer itself produces any symptoms. Approximately 2% of patients present with a paraneoplastic syndrome. These may be categorized as:

- *Metabolic*: Cushing's syndrome, hypercalcemia, excessive antidiuretic hormone, and carcinoid syndrome
- *Neuromuscular*: peripheral neuritis, cortical or cerebellar degenerations, and myopathy
- *Dermatologic*: acanthosis nigricans and dermatomyositis
- *Skeletal*: pulmonary hypertrophic osteoarthropathy including clubbing of fingers
- *Vascular*: migratory thrombophlebitis and nonbacterial verrucous endocarditis
- *Hematologic*: anemia and disseminated intravascular coagulopathy

An initial *metastatic* presentation may be cerebral metastases. A chest film is mandatory in suspected brain tumor to rule out a primary tumor in the lung. Bone and liver metastases are also possible.

Radiographic *screening procedures* or cytologic studies performed annually generally do not aid in early detection. Serial sputum cytologies can detect occult lesions. If cytology is positive and radiographs are negative, the patient requires fiber optic bronchoscopy and guided bronchial washout studies for localization. Three large-scale, randomized trials involving periodic applications of these two procedures to high-risk individuals failed to demonstrate any significant benefit in terms of survival even if the resectability of the lung cancer was higher in the intensively screened populations.

Therefore, mass radiologic and cytologic screening for lung cancer cannot be recommended at this time (23,61,103).

Immunologic depression is common and is more impaired in this cancer than others because of its advanced state at the time of diagnosis. This depression is reflected in skin tests to recall antigens (Candiolin, tuberculin, dinitrochlorobenzene) and absolute lymphocyte counts, in contrast to serum immunoglobulin levels and antibody synthesis, which are normal (91).

Diagnostic Procedures (3,4)

The management of clinically suspected lung cancer requires pathologic confirmation of a tumor, definition of its histology, determination of tumor extent, and evaluation of the host's physiological function in regard to the proposed treatment.

A careful *history and physical* examination are most important in establishing the diagnosis of pulmonary neoplasm.

Radiographic studies (Table 31-2) (5): Posterior-anterior and lateral chest films are the most valuable tools to establish the diagnosis when there is clinical suspicion of bronchogenic carcinoma. They may show a peripheral parenchymal tumor, the effects of bronchial obstruction (atelectasis), or regional metastases (hilar and mediastinal enlargement, rib erosion). When indicated, fluoroscopy, tomography, computed tomography (CT) scan, magnetic resonance imaging (MRI) scan, bronchography, and even angiography may be used to further define the nature and extent of involvement. CT scans are increasingly used for defining the disease extent (62,87).

Bronchoscopy yields positive histology only if the bronchogenic carcinoma is centrally located or has invaded centrally.

Cytologic studies include sputum examinations by Papanicolaou technique. In the hands of expert cytologists, positive results may be found in as many as 75% of cases of bronchogenic carcinoma after repeated examinations. Routine bronchial washings at the time of bronchoscopy yield results in only 44% of cases which is not as good as the sputum examinations performed after bronchoscopy. Selective bronchiolar washout techniques with fiber optic scopes can identify occult lesions (49).

Table 31-2. Imaging Modalities For Detection and Diagnosis of Lung Cancer

METHOD	CAPABILITY	RECOMMENDED FOR USE
Primary tumor and regional nodes work-up		
CT	Most useful of all modalities for determining characteristics of T and N in the thorax and M in the brain and liver	Yes
MRI	Not as good as CT	No
Percutaneous Needle Biopsy		
	Guided by flouroscopy or CT, accurate in establishing syologic diagnosis from T (particularly peripheral lung lesions); M (especially liver or bone); less experience with N	Yes
Metastatic work-up for clinically suspected metastases		
Chest Films		
Posteroanterior and Lateral		
	Baseline high resolution image to assiss T, less reliable for N and M	Yes
Previous	May establish change in T, N1/N2, or M	Yes

CT = computed tomography; MRI = magnetic resonance imaging; T = tumor; N = node; M = metastasis.
From Bragg et al. (5), with permission.

For a bronchial *brush biopsy*, an ingenious controllable brush and a new controllable guide have been developed. This procedure is applicable to small and peripheral nodules (97).

Percutaneous *needle biopsy* under videoscopic and CT scan control has been introduced to diagnose peripheral lesions. The risks of seeding the needle tract, pneumothorax, and hemorrhage are low in the hands of an experienced surgeon or radiologist. This technique has a high degree of accuracy.

Histologic confirmation of a diagnosis of bronchogenic carcinoma may be forthcoming only after exploration and direct biopsy of tumor or its metastases.

Scalene lymph node biopsy is often performed. It should be recognized that the right scalene fat pad drains the right lung and left lower lobe. The left scalene fat pad drains the lingula and the left upper lobe. If metastatic scalene lymph nodes are found, thoracotomy is contraindicated.

Mediastinoscopy is another test of operability. This method explores the mediastinal lymph nodes to the level of the carina and yields better results for the right side than the left where the exploration is limited by the aortic arch. If metastases to lymph nodes are found, thoracotomy is usually contraindicated (30,116).

Radioisotopic procedures include technetium-99, which is used for angiograms to detect superior vena caval obstruction and coupled with methyldiphosphonate to detect possible bone metastases. Routine lung scanning with macroaggregate or radioactive gas such as xenon yields information on lung perfusion or ventilation and are used to assess the pulmonary function. Gallium may be fixed by the tumor and gallium scans are advocated by some investigators as preoperative screens for mediastinal nodes.

A variety of *tumor markers*, including hormones, antigens, and proteins, have been identified in lung cancer. Their major role is in the monitoring of tumor response or to possibly detect early relapses. The carcinoembryonic antigen (CEA) remains the gold standard for non-small cell lung cancers (NSCLC). Its concentration correlates well with tumor extent: 50% to 60% of patients with metastatic disease have elevated CEA titers (45). In addition to CEA, the tissue polypeptide antigen and the immunoreactive calcitonin (CT) are two other possible markers for NSCLC. For SCLC, the best marker is certainly the neuron-specific enolase (NSE), an isoenzyme of the enolase that is a good marker for all neuroendocrine tumors. Elevated NSE titers are observed in 60% to 70% of patients with limited SCLC and in 80% to 95% of those with extensive small cell cancer. Furthermore, NSE is a good marker to monitor tumor response. CEA and CT may complement to NSE especially in patients with a normal NSE value.

Recommended Procedures (Table 31-2)

Conventional chest radiographic procedur*es* are limited, but are the most definitive determinants in staging of intrathoracic disease. The major question is whether the disease is confined to the lung, or if pleura, mediastinum, or other structures are invaded. For the nodal compartment, it is difficult to determine mediastinal and scalene involvement. Sixteen common radiographic presentations are shown in Fig. 31-1 and show how lung cancers can masquerade as benign or infectious disease problems (24).

Tomograms are helpful to determine the extent of the primary tumor within major bronchi, but their use is dimin-

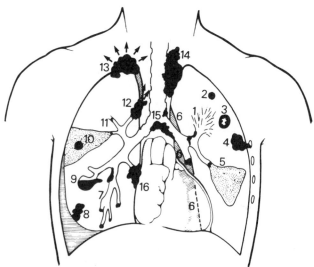

Fig. 31-1. The most frequent manifestations of bronchial carcinoma (after Grunze): (1) hilar lung cancer with endobronchial growth (relatively early elicitation of the cough reflex); (2) typical round focus; (3) tumor cavern (note the thick irregular walls); (4) subpleural focus infiltrating the chest wall; (5) obstructive segmental discontinuation with retention in pneumonia, in (10) already with abscess formation; (6) atelectasis, which is hidden behind the cardiac shadow (lateral X-ray); (7) secondary bronchiectasis due to partial stenosis; (8) focus near to the pleura, with effusion; (9) necrotising tumor with draining bronchus (abscess symptom); (11) obstruction emphysema due to valve occulusion; (12) and (13) outbreak of carcinoma into the mediastinum, e.g. in the direction of the vena cava (upper inflow congestion) or as Pancoast tumor; (14) lymph node involvement in the upper mediastinum and paratracheally, extending to the upper clavicular fossa. Detection by lymph node biopsy according to Daniels or by mediastinoscopy; (15) and (16) carcinoma spreading to the trachea and pericardium, respectively. Note, a bronchial carcinoma can be masked even in a normal X-ray. From Bates (24), with permission of Springer-Verlag.

ishing because of the availability of much more accurate procedures such as the CT scan or MRI.

CT is the most important and valuable radiologic procedure in the diagnosis, staging, and therapeutic planning of lung cancer (142).

1. Primary (T) staging with CT is preferred to MRI to delineate and diagnose most peripheral pulmonary nodules and central masses. Primary staging is difficult with CT or MRI because it is impossible to distinguish tumor from distal atelectasis or pneumonia. The disadvantage of chest film is the inability to determine chest wall, mediastinal, hilar, subcarinal involvement but unfortunately CT is also insensitive. MRI may improve specificity, but unless bone destruction is evident, it is limited in determining chest wall invasion; with vascular invasion it can possibly define mediastinal extension (3-5).

2. Nodal (N) staging is well established by CT and relates to identifying enlarged nodes which can be sampled by mediastinoscopy, transbronchial needle aspiration, or limited thoracotomy. CT accuracy improves with nodal size.

3. Metastases (M) staging often is part of CT of the thorax with liver and adrenal assessment. The adrenal is found variously to be abnormal in 10% to 40% of patients at

autopsy but 66% of CT-identified adrenal masses are found to be non-neoplastic and require needle biopsy. Percutaneous lung biopsy is reserved for advanced and metastatic disease confirmation, whereas thoracotomy is favored for small nodules. Seeding is not a major concern; there is a 20% to 30% risk of pneumothorax but only 5% of such patients require tubal thoracotomy. There are no significant advantages of MRI over CT with the possible exception of hilar assessments and definition of mediastinal invasion.

CT scanning can determine if the tumor is limited to the lung or has involved the chest wall or mediastinum. It is also valuable to search for distant metastases (brain, liver, adrenals). Compared with CT, MRI offers two advantages: multiplanar images can be obtained easily and great vessels can be identified without contrast media. It has also proven to be as accurate as CT in evaluating the hilus and the mediastinum for enlarged lymph nodes. When making the decision for surgery, it must be remembered that an enlarged lymph node seen on CT is not necessarily a metastatic deposit and, in general, histologic confirmation is recommended.

Mediastinoscopy assesses the status of mediastinal and scalene nodes. It is an important tool for diagnosis and tumor staging.

To find occult metastasis, *radioisotopic scans* are essential to determine the status of brain, liver, and skeleton.

If a *bone scan* is positive, then a search for specific targeted lesions should be made by specific site by detailed skeletal radiography, rather than doing skeletal surveys by conventional radiographs.

Bone marrow aspiration and biopsy are essential for small cell carcinoma (72).

Determination of the *immunologic status* of the patient may also be important to determine the outcome. CEA can be used to monitor treatment responses.

Laboratory studies include the complete blood cell count and sonogram liver test. Abnormal laboratory values should be further defined, especially in the event of a paraneoplastic syndrome.

Monoclonal antibodies. A promising new labeled monoclonal antibody technetium 99m NR-LU-10, compared with standard imaging, identifies 85% of patients with extensive small cell cancer in 77% of all organs involved, with a 95% accuracy. It upstaged 15% of limited-stage disease to extensive and may be comparable with a complete battery of tests to stage small cell cancer. (16)

CLASSIFICATION

Histopathology

There are four major histologic types of tumors: squamous cell carcinoma (SCC); adenocarcinoma (including the bronchoalveolar type); large cell anaplastic carcinoma; and small cell anaplastic carcinoma, which includes the oat cell type (63,101). Pathologic behavior varies with the different kinds of tumor, as indicated in Table 31-3 (7).

SCC: There have been reports (161) that the incidence of SCC (the commonest form of lung cancer worldwide) has undergone an absolute and relative decline in the United States. This has been accompanied by an absolute and relative increase in the incidence of adenocarcinoma. SCC arises from metaplastic bronchial epithelium; 50% to 60% are proximal or involve the hilus. It tends to grow into the bronchial lumen and to produce obstruction with associated pneumonitis. It is also less likely to metastasize early (43,111).

Adenocarcinoma tends to be located more in the periphery of the lung, but metastasizes widely and frequently to the other lung, liver, bone, kidney, and the central nervous system (CNS). Bronchoalveolar carcinoma, an unusual subtype of adenocarcinoma, appears to have a distinct presentation and biologic behavior (49a).

Small cell anaplastic carcinoma tends to be disseminated at the time of diagnosis. This is an aggressive and rapidly growing neoplasm. Disease is limited to the thorax at presentation in only 25% of patients. Metastases will be found in regional lymph nodes, lung, abdominal lymph nodes, liver, adrenal gland, bone, CNS, and also bone marrow. A bone marrow biopsy may be positive in one third of patients at presentation and is an absolute requirement in the management of this disease (43,72). Variant pathology of small cell carcinoma has not proven to be of different biologic behavior or chemotherapeutic response (19).

Large cell anaplastic carcinoma metastasizes in a pattern quite similar to adenocarcinoma with a predilection for mediastinal lymph nodes, pleura, adrenals, CNS, and bone.

Anatomic Staging

The definitions of tumor (T) and node (N) categories for carcinoma of the lung according to the American Joint Committee (AJC) for Cancer Staging are shown in Table 31-4 (109,110). This classification applies to NSCLC. For SCLC the definition of limited disease (LD) versus extensive disease (ED) is the most widely used with LD confined to the lung and regional nodes and ED denoting metastatic disease outside the lung and regional nodes. For staging diagram, see Fig. 31-2.

Differences Between Staging Systems

Differences between recent editions of AJC and International Union Against Cancer staging texts distinguish T3 from the T4 category. T3 is invasion of adjacent structures: pleura, pericardium, and diaphragm. T4 denotes invasion of surrounding structures: mediastinum, heart, great vessels,

Table 31-3. Staging of Lung Cancer: Histopathologic Classification	
	% INCIDENCE
Epidermoid carcinomas	25-30
Small cell anaplastic carcinomas	20-25
Adenocarcinomas	32-40
Large cell carcinomas	8-16
Adapted from World Health Organization (7).	

Table 31-4. TNM Classification and Stage Grouping of Lung Cancer

TNM Classification		Stage Grouping			
TX	Positive cytology	Occult carcinoma	TX	N0	M0
		Stage 0	Tis	N0	M0
	< 3 cm	Stage I	T1	N0	M0
T1	> 3 cm; extends to hilar region; invades visceral pleura; partial atelectasis		T2	N0	M0
		Stage II	T1	N1	M0
			T2	N1	M0
T2	Chest wall, diaphragm, pericardium, mediastinal pleura etc., total atelectasis	Stage IIIA	T1	N2	M0
			T2	N2	M0
			T3	N0,N1,N2	M0
T3	Mediastinum, heart, great vessels, trachea, esophagus etc., malignant effusion	Stage IIIB	Any T	N3	M0
			T4	Any N	M1
		Stage IV	Any T	Any N	
T4	Peribronchial, ipsilateral hilar				
	Ipsilateral mediastinal, subcarinal				
N1	Contralateral mediastinal, scalene or supraclavicular				

T = tumor; N = node; M = metastasis.
From AJC/UICC (2,9), with permission.

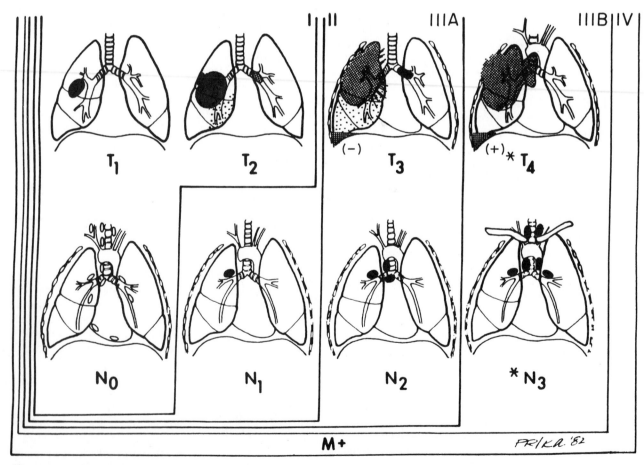

*New category

Fig. 31-2. Anatomic stage grouping: lung (see Table 31-4).

trachea, esophagus, vertebrae, pleural effusion (+ cell). Current chest wall with rib destruction distinguishes N2 from N3 ipsilateral mediastinal versus contralateral mediastinal nodes and supraclavicular nodes. T1 or T2 equivalent to node involvement indicating size is not an overriding factor.

Staging Work-up

There are three types of staging work-ups:
1. *Clinical and imaging evaluation* should be done before thoracotomy is performed.
2. *Pathologic* (postsurgical) *evaluation* is performed after thoracotomy and includes both biopsies and/or the entire resected specimen of lungs and regional nodes.
3. *Recurrent staging* is done at the time of recurrence for a previously staged lung tumor.

PRINCIPLES OF TREATMENT

Multidisciplinary Approach

The strategy for control of bronchogenic carcinoma is based on an individual selection of the treatment modality or combinations of these that can offer the maximum benefit for the patient. Several important prognostic factors are considered: histology, tumor extent, and patient's physical condition. Tables 31-5 and 31-6 are concise, multimodality treatment summaries of the role of surgery, radiation therapy, and chemotherapy according to disease stage.

Surgery (97,98,110,111,144,162,166)

For localized, non-small cell carcinomas (stages I and II), surgery is the treatment of choice because these lesions usually can be excised completely. The choice of the surgical procedure — lobectomy, pneumonectomy, segmental or

sleeve resection — depends on the extent of malignant disease and the patient's functional status. The procedure of choice is usually that which will encompass all existing disease and provide maximum conservation of normal lung tissue. On occasion, stage III disease may present borderline cases for surgery. Localized chest-wall or pericardium invasion, superior sulcus tumor, limited mediastinal nodal involvement, and phrenic involvement are not absolute surgical contraindications (115). Each case must carefully be evaluated and individualized. The primary aim is to achieve complete tumor resection and avoid an exploratory thoracotomy or an incomplete surgical resection. The presence of distant or extrathoracic metastasis is indicative of inoperability and a surgical procedure is an absolute contraindication. Achieving palliation by resection in the presence of metastasis is a myth. There is no proven place to date for debulking surgical procedures in lung cancer.

Immunotherapy (19,21,62,93,96,122,168)

A living vaccine, BCG (Bacille Calmette-Guerin stain of *Mycobacterium tuberculosis bovis*), levamisole, and *Corynebacterium parvum* have been used after surgery or radiotherapy without any apparent benefits. The early positive results of some studies (99,168) were not confirmed by large-scale trials carried out by other groups such as the Lung Cancer Study Group.

Radiotherapy (26,48,76,80,86,90,94,102,118,128, 139,159,160)

Irradiation is widely used in the management of bronchogenic carcinoma to achieve varying goals: (l) definitive irradiation of localized lung cancer; (2) as part of a combined treatment approach; and (3) palliation of symptoms.

Table 31-5. Multidisciplinary Treatment Decisions for Non-Small Cell Lung Cancer (12a,27,76a,132)

Stage	Surgery	Radiation Therapy	CT
I $T_1 T_2 N_0 M_0$	Segmental wedge/sleeve resection Lobectomy Pneumonectomy Plus hilar node resection	NR except for medically inoperable; DRT 60-70 Gy	NR
II $T_1 T_2 N_1 M_0$	Lobectomy Pneumonectomy Plus hilar node resection	ART postop optional 50 Gy/5-6 weeks	NR
III $T_3 N_{0-2} M_0$	Complete resection surgery and chest wall en bloc	ART postop 50-60 Gy/5-6 weeks	IC III
$T_{any} N_3 M_0$	Usually unresectable	DRT if unresectable 60-70 Gy/6 wks	IC III
IV $T_4 N_3 M_0$	NR	PRT 40-50 Gy/4-6 wks and/or split course	IC III
$T_{any} N_{any} M_+$	NR	PRT 5 Gy/wk for 10-12 and/or wks, to 50-60 Gy/ 10-12 wks	IC III

RT = radiation therapy; ART = adjuvant; DRT = definitive; PRT = palliative; NR = not recommended; CCR = concurrent chemotherapy and radiation; IC III = investigational chemotherapy, phase II/III clinical trials.

PDQ: NR - IC III = CisPt, ADRIA, CYT

Table 31-6. Multidisciplinary Treatment Decisions for Small Cell Lung Cancer (12b,27,132)			
Stage	Surgery	Radiation Therapy	Chemotherapy
$T_1T_2 N_0M_0$	Lobectomy (selected cases)	ART 50 Gy after CT	and/or	MAC CCR
$T_3T_4N_{1-3} M_0$	NR	Post-CT consolidation ART 50 Gy CNS prophylaxis 2 Gy x 15 (30 Gy)	and/or	MAC CCR
Metastatic	NR	PRT Selected sites - 30 Gy HBI - 6 Gy	MAC

RT = radiation therapy; ART = adjuvant; PRT = palliative; NR = not recommended; RCT = recommended chemotherapy; HBI = half-body irradiation; MAC = multiagent chemotherapy; CCR = concurrent chemotherapy and radiation.

PDQ: RCT - MAC = CAV, CAVP-16, VPP + other regimens

Definitive Irradiation

Local chest irradiation is an effective modality for locoregional control of lung cancer. It is generally used for unresectable intrathoracic cancer (stage III cancer) (118,119,120,126).

1. Optimum doses are in the range of 5,000 to 6,000 cGy delivered in 5 to 6 weeks. This represents a compromise between tumor dose requirement and normal tissue tolerance.
2. Thoracic irradiation is limited by the tolerance of vital organs that lie within the treatment field. The main complications: pneumonopathy, myelopathy, and to some extent, cardiomyopathy, are all time-dose-volume related events. Doses as low as 2,500 cGy will lead to severe radiation fibrosis with or without effusion and/or pneumonitis. A dose higher than 4,500 cGy delivered continuously to the spinal cord can also lead to a late, irreversible radiation myelopathy.
3. Recent technical developments have helped to improve the accuracy and delivery quality of radiation treatment. Among them are CT scan, computerized treatment planning, individually tailored (through cereobend shielding) fields of irradiation and highly sophisticated megavoltage therapy equipment. CT has brought two major advances: (l) precise information about tumoral extension and its relationship to surrounding structures that include dose-limiting organs; (2) cross-sectional data throughout the proposed treatment volume providing qualitative as well as quantitative information to use tissue-inhomogeneity correction factors. The additional information provided by chest CT scans has been shown to change the radiation-treated volume in one third of patients.
4. Recently, a dose-response relationship has been demonstrated for NSCLC (Fig. 31-3). Doses of 60 Gy give better responses and tumor control than lower doses; this is particularly true for tumors smaller than 6 cm (69,100). Further confirmation of a dose response in NSCLC was shown by Choi et al. (40) with regard to the locoregional failure rate, which decreased from 79% to 37% in 2 to 5 years for doses ranging from 30 to 50 Gy. Also, for SCLC, higher doses (50 to 60 Gy) yield the best results (27).
5. Distant metastases and locoregional relapses account for the vast majority of failures. Several approaches are

being explored, including increasing the total doses, modifications of the fractionation, radiation modifiers, and combined modality treatments.

a. *Intraoperative radiation*: One way to increase the total dose delivered to the tumor without exposing normal surrounding structures is by implanting radioactive sources or administering a single shot of external radiation at the time of surgery. Either one of these approaches requires close interaction and collaboration between surgeons and radiation oncologists. Additional external conventional radiation therapy after surgery is still necessary to treat all locoregional areas and boost the target volume. In a recent report, Calvo (34) stressed the real advantage for intraoperative radiation therapy (IORT) (10 to 15 Gy boost) was in resected bronchogenic cancers, with a frequency-following response (local progression) of 44%, but there was a high complication rate and only 10 to 15 Gy boost are recommended. For resected patients, IORT + x-ray therapy led to a 4-year, 28% survival rate versus a 7% survival rate for unresectable cases.

b. *Split-course schedules*: No significant improvement in survival has been achieved by split-course over continuous course (83). These schedules are generally used for palliation. Such schedules consist of two courses of radiation, each lasting 1 to 2 weeks with a 2 to 3 week rest period in between. Commonly used regimens are 4,000 to 5,000 cGy given in 250 to 400 cGy fractions (i.e., 2.5 Gy x 10 or 4.0 Gy x 5). The rest period allows for further tumoral reduction, repair of normal tissue damage, detection of metastatic disease, and overall assessment of the patient's condition. If the second course of irradiation is warranted, fields can be reduced to further decrease the possibilities of normal tissue damage. Split-course schedules deliver a higher-than-normal daily dose; this implies a much higher biologic dose, which must be kept in mind when normal tissue tolerance is considered. With the exception of a rapid split course consisting of five daily treatments of 4 Gy each repeated after 2 to 3 weeks of rest, most other split-course schedules seem to yield similar results as daily conventional (uninterrupted) therapy.

TREATMENT DECISIONS

RESPONSE RATE: RADIATION NSCLC

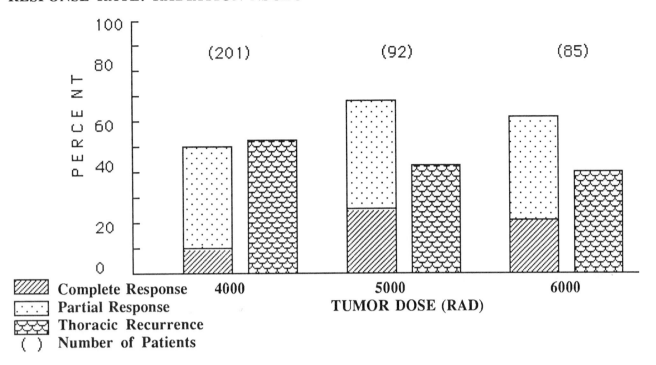

Complete Response
Partial Response
Thoracic Recurrence
( ) Number of Patients

Fig. 31-3. Tumor response rates of non-small cell carcinoma of the lung and thoracic recurrences correlated with different doses of irradiation. From Perez *et al.* (119), with permission.

c. *Hyperfractionation*: This implies the delivery of two to three fractions per day. It allows delivery of much higher total doses, thus enhancing the possibilities for success. It conveys more acute side effects but risks for the more dreaded late irradiation effects appear to be less. Currently, several studies are exploring doses in excess of 60 Gy delivered with hyperfractionated schemes. The most important recently completed hyperfractionation study is an Radiation Therapy Oncology Group (RTOG) randomized phase II trial, evaluating a dose range from 60 to 80 Gy, with 70 cGy yielding the best 1-year survival rate of 58% and minimal complications compared with those given lower and higher total doses. (47)

d. *Hypofractionation* implies delivery of one to two weekly high doses for a total of ten to 12 fractions. It allows patients treated for palliative purposes, those difficult to transport, or those living at great distances to be treated with a convenient schedule that appears to be as effective as conventional daily treatment (164-166,178). A recent randomized study comparing 5 Gy once a week for 12 weeks (60 Gy) with 2 Gy daily for 6 weeks (60 Gy) yielded identical results. Although hypofractionation seems to convey a much better acute tolerance and convenience, it can increase the potential for late complications such as pulmonary fibrosis. It is essential to cone down and reduce field size at the 30 Gy level approximately halfway through the treatment course.

Combined Approaches (158)

1. *Preoperative irradiation* is no longer advocated. Although radiation therapy can ablate gross tumors into microscopic deposits in 30% to 50% of instances and some tumors that initially were unresectable can be made operable, no improvements in survival have been noted. However, preoperative radiation therapy is still advocated for good-risk patients with a superior sulcus (Pancoast) tumor. When either a pathologic complete response (CR) or microscopic residual disease is found at surgery, there is a 53% chance for 5-year recurrence-free survival versus 17% probability of 5-year recurrence-free survival if there is gross residual disease found according to Reddy in a recent retrospective analysis of 74 stage III M0 non-small cell lung cancer patients (124).

2. *Postoperative radiation* has no role after complete resection of T1-T2, N0, M0 NSCLC tumors. Survival of these patients with surgery only is approaching 60% at 5 years. Nevertheless, it presupposes a thorough staging and confirmation of an early stage without nodal or distant metastases. In completely resected NSCLC with involvement of hilar and/or mediastinal nodes, postoperative irradiation decreases local relapses (165). However, its impact on survival is still not well established although some retrospective series have shown survival benefits. In fact, stage III non-small cell tumors have a high probability of subclinical metastatic disease that eventually will affect the overall survival of patients. Survival in lung cancer is a poor parameter with which

to judge a locoregional modality such as radiation therapy and to some extent surgery. Commonly, doses of 5,000 cGy are administered, avoiding the spinal cord after 40 to 45 Gy. Pulmonary function tests have shown minimal impairment despite loss of some lung volume due to irradiation. This was shown by Choi *et al.* (41) in a convincing serial prospective study conducted for ten to 12 years postoperatively.

In cases of incomplete resection, postoperative irradiation is always used. It is best to administer radiation doses immediately after surgery rather than awaiting overt recurrences. When a local failure is detected after surgery, salvage therapy with irradiation has less efficacy because of tumor burden and disease spread.

3. *Chemoradiotherapy approaches*: Distant metastases remain the most common failure pattern in lung cancer. Consequently, a systemic treatment could be a key factor to improve survival (22).

For NSCLC, chemotherapy has been used for many years as an adjuvant treatment to surgery or radiation therapy. Unfortunately, most studies have failed to demonstrate any benefits; this may reflect the inadequacy of the actual agents used rather than the concept itself.

During the last few years, the concept of neoadjuvant chemotherapy has been introduced. This consists of two to three cycles of chemotherapy given before radiotherapy. The cited advantages to starting with drugs are: (1) any tumor shrinkage achieved with drugs will enhance reoxygenation of hypoxic cells, which in turn increases radiosensitivity; (2) chemotherapy given after radiation therapy seems to be less effective due to a subsequent impairment of blood supply; and (3) evaluation of tumor responses allows selection of patients for possible maintenance chemotherapy. Disadvantages of this approach are: (1) tumor progression with more hypoxic and less effective radiosensitization; (2) potential interruption of radiation therapy course because of drug complications; and (3) exacerbation of acute toxicity with attendant need to reduce radiation doses that have been proven effective and necessary. Studies are ongoing and conflicting data are being generated.

Preoperative chemotherapy is used in some experimental protocols for stage III NSCLC patients. One study has reported a high response rate with improvements in resectability to almost 75% and a better 3-year survival (124). Nevertheless, preoperative chemotherapy needs further investigation and corroboration.

Chemotherapy plus irradiation, either given concomitantly or sequentially is being explored for regional disease. Most series show an increase in responses when the combined treatment is used. Some studies have even shown modest gains in survival (50). The optimal combination of these two modalities for regionally advanced NSCLC remains to be determined with respect to sequencing, dose, and duration of therapy.

For SCLA, chemotherapy has been the main therapeutic modality for the last 15 years. Because of the disseminated nature of the disease, surgery is no longer used, although it has been used recently for small lesions on an experimental basis. For metastatic disease (extensive disease), irradiation mainly retains a palliative role and is used exclusively with that aim. It is for limited SCLC that controversies persist over how to sequence the standard modalities for the primary

site (127a). Recent studies strongly suggest that minimal tumor dose of 50 cGy or more, standard fractionation is necessary to control the tumor in the thorax (PDQ).

Despite excellent responses and prolongation of median survival by chemotherapy in limited SCLC recurrences tend to occur in area of previous involvement even after a CR and long-term survival is still low. The high rate of local chest relapses seen with chemotherapy alone and the high degree of local control achieved with irradiation have led to the merging of these two modalities in an attempt to improve results. After much controversy and many studies, it appears that the best results occur when radiation therapy is given early in the course of disease, either concomitantly or alternating with chemotherapy. The latter yields better tolerance, and in some studies the results appear to be excellent (31,117,123,157) (Fig. 31-4).

Prophylactic (elective) brain treatment significantly decreases brain relapses in small cell cancer. This concept now is being applied also to both adenocarcinoma and large cell anaplastic carcinomas. The usual therapeutic schedule of 3 Gy daily for ten fractions has been changed by some coopera-

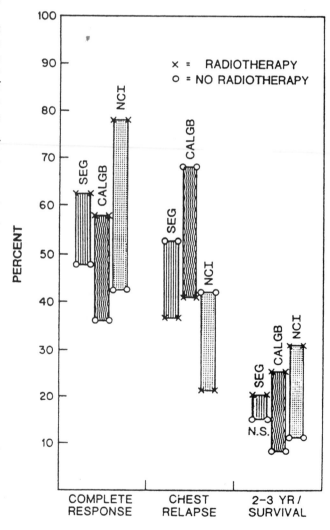

Fig. 31-4. The role of consolidation radiation therapy is vividly demonstrated in this figure, with improvement in complete response and survival and decrease in thoracic relapses. From Comis (44), with permission.

tive groups to 2 Gy daily for 18 fractions to improve on late morbidity. Results of elective brain therapy seem to be optimum when a CR has been achieved in the chest and/or locoregional disease is under control. There are increasing reports on significant neurological, mental, and psychometric deficits in long-term survivors treated with prophylactic cranial irradiation, and the optimal dose and schedule of PCI has not been defined (60a,91a,156a).

Palliative Irradiation

One of the primary goals of radiation therapy is to relieve distressing symptoms of lung cancer. Some symptoms may be due to the primary tumor (obstruction, hemoptysis, superior vena caval obstruction); others are due to advance of local disease (chest pain, bone involvement, cord compression); and others are due to metastatic disease (brain, bone, liver, and abdomen). (24,29,138)

When facing true *emergency situations*, it is better to start with three large daily fractions (4 Gy each) on consecutive days followed by normal fractions. Such an approach offers a rapid reversal of life-threatening signs and symptoms. More routine palliative situations are usually treated with 30 Gy in 2 weeks with or without a boost. This treatment provides effective palliation in two thirds of all patients, without need for retreatment. (139)

When *metastatic disease* is extensive, it is necessary to apply radiation fields to several areas. This carries an intrinsic danger of having to overlap radiation fields over previously treated areas. Such "chasing" of disease can be obviated with the use of large-body irradiation. Irradiation of the upper, lower, or midsection of the body (half-body irradiation) with either single doses (6 Gy to upper and 8 Gy to middle or lower half) or fractionated doses of radiation achieves rapid pain relief and offers the advantage of consolidating large symptomatic areas within a single radiation field; this is particularly true for multiple bone metastases. (60,129,131,132)

Recently, a *hypofractionated regimen* of 5 Gy weekly for ten to 12 fractions has offered excellent local palliation with reduced acute side effects. This schedule is convenient for patients with advanced lung cancer who are in poor general condition. (133,134)

For *relief of bronchial obstruction*, one can use high-dose-rate or low-dose-rate brachytherapy with a reported 84% and 67% (125,151) relief of symptoms, respectively, with confirmed widening of bronchi upon bronchoscopy. Some patients with intrinsic endobronchial obstructing lesions or extrinsic compression due to tumor have been palliated successfully with endobronchial laser and/or brachytherapy (laser is used only if the lesion is endobronchial) (104a).

Chemotherapy (17,46,59,65) (Tables 31-7 and 31-8)

Because of the frequency of metastases on presentation ($\geq$ 50%) and the inevitable development of metastases in the majority of patients (90%), chemotherapy is frequently used (38,46,67,108,127).

Despite the widespread application of single-agent and multiagent chemotherapy, only small gains have been made in non-small cell bronchogenic carcinomas. Small cell anaplastic cancers have, however, proven to be highly responsive to combination chemotherapy. The majority of the patients have partial response (30% to 50%) or CR (10% to 40%) with prolongation of survival (1,28).

SCC, adenocarcinomas, and large cell anaplastic carcinoma: (Table 31-7)

1. In non-small cell carcinomas, chemotherapy currently is restricted to progressive (recurrent or metastatic), advanced stage IV disease and may be accepted for palliation of inoperable symptomatic patients whose disease is beyond control by radiation therapy. Most recent data also suggest combination chemotherapy may be beneficial for patients with stage III disease (with mediastinal disease, or N2, N3) after surgery or radiotherapy (77,78,88,89,112). Neoadjuvant chemotherapy (chemotherapy followed by surgery) has also been reported to be promising (26), most likely due to better staging procedures and the use of cisplatin-containing regimens.

Table 31-7. Response Rates of Multiagent Chemotherapy in Non-Small Cell Lung Cancer

Chemotherapy	% Response Rate	Reference
MVP	87	33
MVP	74	66
Vincristine + cisplatin + etoposide	70	25
5-FU + etoposide + cisplatin	67	152
MVP + radiotherapy	65	150a
5-FU + cisplatin + radiotherpay	57	164
MVP	53	100
CAP + PT	53	146
5-FU + cisplatin + radiotherpay	56	155
MACC	46	52
CAP	39	92
EP	28	163

MVP = mitomycin C, vinblastine, and cisplatin; MACC = methotrexate, adriamycin, cyclophosphamide, CCNU; CAP + PT = cyclophosphamide, adriamycin, cis-Dichlorodiammineplatinum(II) + cisplatin; EP = etoposide and cisplatin; 5-FU = 5-flourouracil.

Table 31-8. Response Rates to Chemotherapy of Small Cell Carcinoma (Limited Disease)

THERAPY	% CR	MEDIAN SURVIVAL (WK)	% 2 YR NED
CAV	81	56	15
CAV	100	69.5	25
CAV + etoposide	42	67	20
CAV + etoposide + cisplatin	39	72	20
CAV	62	60	28
CAV	65	60	29
CAV + etoposide + cisplatin	65	90	33
Cyclophosphamide, lomustine, doxorubicin, vincristine	48	49	25
MACC	54	58	21

NED = no evidence of disease; CR = complete remission; CAV = cyclophosphamide, doxorubicin, vincristine; MACC = methotrexate, adriamycin, cyclophosphamide, lomustine.

2. The overall response rate for most widely used single agents has not been higher than 25% (the range varies from 0% to 35%); the net gain in survival for stage IV patients is virtually nil. The most active agents are cisplatin, vinca alkaloid (vinblastine or vindesine), mitomycin-C, and ifosfamide. The response rates reported in the old literature usually are not reliable by the current, more stringent response criteria. Most agents have a low objective response rate. Table 31-7 lists those agents that have been active in NSCLC and are most commonly incorporated into combination chemotherapy.

3. With a few exceptions (46,167), combination chemotherapy has failed to increase overall survival in patients with stage IV NSCLC, but can be palliative to relieve symptoms. In general, 25% to 35% responses rates can be expected. Higher response rates have been reported, but rarely substantiated. The majority of responding patients have symptomatic palliation.

4. Chemotherapy usually is not indicated for totally a-symptomatic patients with advanced NSCLC, but should be offered to patients with early symptoms which may progress rapidly if not treated. Ideally, all patients should be encouraged to participate in prospective clinical trials (112).

5. The use of new agents or new combination chemotherapy are under active investigation. The number of agents available and the diversity of possible therapeutic schedules have generated a great number of combinations that may include from two to seven drugs. The general impression is that using any combination of two to four drugs produces an equal result as long as the associated drugs have proven effective when used alone.

6. Although no regimen can be considered standard and none has been shown superior to the others, CAMP, CAP, MVP, and VP (etoposide and cisplatin, or vindesine or vinblastine and cisplatin) are commonly used and in general are well tolerated. (38,65,127) (Table 31-7).

7. Alternating chemotherapy regimens is slightly superior to single combination chemotherapy (105). The large variation of response rates to combination chemotherapy can be explained by such factors as patient selection, dose intensity of regimen, and tumor burden.

In general, patients with good performance status, minimal tumor burden, and higher-dose chemotherapy (at the expense of potentially more complications) have a higher response possibility. A Canadian Cooperative Group Study found two-drug combinations superior to best support care in prolonging survival in advanced stages, i.e., 25 to 32 weeks median survival for chemotherapy versus 17 weeks for the controls. (112)

8. Adjuvant chemotherapy: Surgical adjuvant chemotherapy has not shown evidence of increased survival over surgery alone in stage I or II operable cases. In ten controlled trials including more than 5,000 patients, chemotherapy showed no advantage, and two studies presented evidence of adverse effects (42). Agents used included cyclophosphamide, methotrexate, 5-FU, and vinblastine administered for short courses of months up to 2 years. Absence of effective chemotherapy with high response rates for non-small cell carcinoma limits its use as adjuvant therapy. The vast majority of prospective randomized studies of radiation therapy with adjuvant chemotherapy have been somewhat discouraging and occasionally more negative for combined modalities than for each one alone (42). However, the use of cisplatin-based chemotherapy has been shown to prolong disease-free survival and provide some survival benefit in patients with stage III disease either completely or incompletely resected. In comparison, radiotherapy only reduced local recurrence rate without prolonging survival (77,78,89).

9. Chemotherapy as a radiosensitizer: Chemotherapy can be used as a radiosensitizer to enhance local cell killing and could improve local tumor control. Schaake-Koning et al. (139a) produce evidence of radiosensitization using daily cisplatin plus radiation and demonstrated a significant improvement in overall survival compared to patients receiving irradiation alone. Radiosensitization is useful but not sufficient since non-small cell lung cancer becomes metastatic in a majority of cases (36a).

Small cell carcinoma: The most frequently used classification only makes distinctions between limited disease (i.e., confined to one hemithorax including ipsilateral positive scalene lymph nodes) or extensive disease (all remaining cases). During the last decade, chemotherapy has become the primary treatment for this disease (17), but nevertheless, other modalities (i.e., radiation therapy and/or surgery) play an important role in obtaining locoregional disease control (54).

1. Combination chemotherapy is now the accepted treatment for all stages, since this cancer is known to be widely disseminated in virtually all cases at the time of diagnosis (Table 31-8). Surgery is rarely justified except in patients with small primary tumor without clinical evidence of mediastinal lymph node or distant metastasis and who have had a CR to chemotherapy. In this case, chemotherapy followed by surgery may offer long-term disease-free survival (143).

2. Virtually every combination of active agents has been used in this disease. Regimens including three, four, or five drugs have been used without demonstrating clear superiority to any other regimens containing more than three drugs.

3. Several effective agents have been identified; cyclophosphamide, doxorubicin, vincristine, nitrosourea such as semustine and lomustine, etoposide, and cisplatin are the most commonly used, with individual response rates between 20% and 40%. Several combination regimens achieve a response rate of at least 80%. This response is usually achieved within the first 6 weeks of treatment (17,36) that usually continues for 6 months. Maintenance chemotherapy longer than 6 months is not beneficial to patients. Alternating combination chemotherapy has been reported to be better than single-combination chemotherapy, but not all investigators agree (56,57,59).

4. Toxicity usually increases when the number of drugs is increased. The challenge is to achieve and maintain a CR, since prolonged survivals are only seen in this group of patients (17,36,73). Although progress has been made in the management of this disease (better responses and increases in median survival), long-term survival (over 2 years) is still disappointingly low (up to 20% of patients with limited stage and 10% with extensive stage).

5. For patients with limited-stage disease, a combined approach of chemotherapy and radiotherapy to thoracic disease is likely to be better than chemotherapy alone (31,123). The best way to combine treatment seems to be to incorporate radiation therapy during the chemotherapy course (not before or after finishing chemotherapy), which can increase the median survival as well as the number of patients in long-term survival. Radiotherapy to the chest also decreases local relapse rate (31,53,123).

6. Patients with extensive disease, even in CR, continue to relapse. Local relapse and brain metastasis are of particular interest (17,36). Failure within the chest is a common finding with chemotherapeutic regimens; the major contribution of thoracic radiotherapy has been to increase locoregional control. (87,107)

7. The brain and leptomeninges are sanctuary sites for chemotherapy. Prophylactic brain irradiation has reduced the incidence of metastasis without influencing survival (which reflects the necessity for more effective treatment to control the disease in other sites) (17).

8. Today, there is no single curative treatment approach for small cell carcinoma. However, investigations continue with combination multiagent chemotherapy, radiation therapy to primary site or brain, or an even more experimental approach combining these modalities as well as using autologous bone marrow transplantation.

9. The evaluation of new drugs has many different strategies according to Ettinger et al. (55) and one of the most controversial is testing new agents in untreated new patients, rather than in previously treated patients with recurrent or metastatic disease. The response rates in nontreated patients can range from 80% for previously nontreated patients to 10% for prior drug therapy (55).

10. Dose Rate Intensity of Drugs: Controversy exists over the issue of whether increasing dose rate intensity of commonly used front-line regimens above levels that produce modest toxicity will produce improved survival. Retrospective studies are plagued by methodologic difficulties and show inconsistent results (85a). The issue is best settled by randomized trials. Preliminary results from a prospective randomized study in extensive stage disease do not suggest any advantage to higher than standard doses of etoposide plus cisplatin (80a).

RESULTS AND PROGNOSIS

Results: Non-Small Cell Cancers

The overall survival for all patients treated is 5% to 10%, with little impact made by current diagnostic screening procedures or newer multimodality approaches in the common adenocarcinomas and SCCs. With the rising incidence, as noted earlier, the mortality rate for this malignancy is such that respiratory cancers represent the major cancers for which the burden of premature death has increased and account for 25% of all years of life lost prematurely due to cancer (104).

Overall Survival

According to Surveillance, Epidemiology, and End Results Program (SEER) data based on 16,257 patients observed, relative 5-year survival is 8% to 10% and 10-year survival is 5% to 7%. For 5-year survivors, there is a small attrition, but 68% will be alive at 10 years. The survival is somewhat better for females than for males — 13% versus 10% 5-year survival (113). Some subsets of patients with metastatic disease live longer than others: good performance status, female gender, and age of 70 years or older appear to be associated with a modestly more favorable outcome (18a).

By Stage (Table 31-9) (135)

The AJC has revised staging criteria and there is an improvement in stage III — especially IIIa — patients, but this is due to the creation of a new T4 and N3 category that is different from the previous classification when very poor prognosis patients were included in the T3 category (Fig. 31-5).

1. For stage I disease, 50% 5-year actual survival occurs, for stage II the rate drops to 30% 5-year actual survival (Fig. 31-5). Node-negative patients do better than node-positive patients stage for stage: T1, N0 versus T1, N1 is 68.5% versus 54.1%, respectively (Table 31-9). Size of tumor is important to outcome (137) when postoperative radiation therapy is added to surgical resection, but there is a steady attrition, rather than a plateau in survival. (154)

Table 31-9. Surgical Results By Stage of Non-Small Cell Lung Cancer

| TNM | Clinical | | Surgical | |
	%	Median Survival	%	Median Survival
T1 N0 M0	61.9	60 +	68.5	60 +
T2 N0 M0	35.8	26	59.0	60 +
T1 N1 M0	33.6	20	54.1	60 +
T2 N1 M0	22.7	17	40.0	29
T3 N0 M0	7.6	8	44.2	26
T3 N1 M0	7.7	8	17.6	16
Any N2 M0	4.9	11	28.8	22
Any M1	1.7	6	-----	---
Total				-

T = tumor; N = node; M = metastasis.
From Mountain (109), with permission.

2. *For stage III disease* confined to lung (IIIa), the 5-year survival is 15%; it falls to less than 5% for stages IIIb and IV (Fig. 31-5). Most patients remain in advanced stages.

Histopathology

There is little difference in outcome for the common varieties of adenocarcinoma and SCC: 5-year survival ranges from 20% to 34% versus 26% to 43%, respectively, with the 10-year result being about 16% to 17% for both (Table 31-10) (165).

By Modality

The survival results presented are largely due to the successful resection of lung cancer.

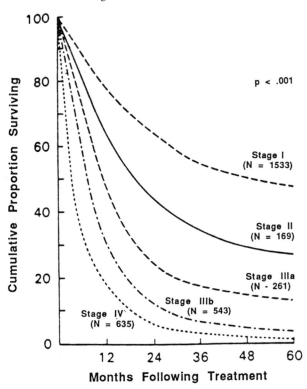

Fig. 31-5. Cumulative portion of patients surviving 5 years by clinical stage of disease. From Mountain (109), with permission.

1. *Surgical results* (Tables 31-9 and 31-10): In a large collation of approximately 3,000 cases from the literature, 5-year survival varies from 26% to 36% but at 10 years is 8% to 17%. If the lesion is found early and is localized to lung (T1, N0), approximately 50% will survive.

2. *Radiation therapy results — postoperative:* The addition of irradiation postoperatively (Table 31-11) has varied from a doubling in survival to no change or even a detrimental effect. Most nonrandomized studies (68,85,146a) show a gain in 5-year survival; however, randomized studies show no gain.

3. *Radiation therapy — unresectable:* For unresectable disease, irradiation alone with salvage chemotherapy yields less than 5% 5-year survival usually in well-differentiated carcinomas. Our experience at Strong Memorial Hospital (oral communication, S. McDonald, M.D., November 1989), confirms a less than 5% long-term survival. According to the RTOG, differences in clearance rates are reflected in median survivals, but there are no real gains in overall survival (Fig. 31-6). Complete responders live longer than partial responders. Different fractionation schedules using both hyperfractionation and accelerated franction indicate that improved regression rates and again in survival are possible.

   a. *Hyperfractionation:* The RTOG cooperative group reports an important observation in assessing an optimal hyperfractionation and dose levels schedule for non-small cell lung cancer by Cox *et al.* (47). Exploring five different dose levels ranging from 60.0–79.2 Gy, the best outcome was at 69.9 Gy with a 1-year and 3-year survival rate of 58% and 20%, respectively, better than standard daily fractionation of 60 Gy which in past RTOG protocols has yielded a 1- and 3-year survival rate of 30% and 7%, respectively.

   b. *Accelerated fractionation:* Saunders *et al.* (137a) worked with CHART (**C**ontinuous, **H**yperfractionated, **A**ccelerated, **R**adiotherapy) in head and neck as well as lung cancer. Further updating their experience in advanced T3T4 squamous cell cancers in the upper

Table 31-10. Survival Following Surgery by Histologic Type in Non-Samll Cell Lung Cancer

HISTOLOGIC TYPE	(%) SURVIVAL		% RESECTABLE
	5 YEAR	10 YEAR	
Squamous cell	33	17	60
Adenocarcinoma	26	16	38
Large cell	28	8	38
Bronchioalveolar	51	24	
Small cell	1	<0.5	11

From Weisenberger et al. (165). Reprinted with permission from The New England Journal of Medicine, *315:1377; 1986*

Table 31-11. Survival Following Postoperative Radiation Therapy in Non-Small Cell Lung Cancer

	RT DOSE	HISTOLOGY	5-Year Survival (%)	
			RT	CONTROL
Randomized studies:				
Van Houtte et al. (159)	60 Gy	All	24	43
Weisenberger et al. (165)	50 Gy	Epidermoid	38	38
Non-randomized studies:				
Green et al. (68)	50-60 Gy	Epidermoid	21	6
		Adenocarcinoma	50	14
Kirsch et al. (85)	(N/A)	Epidermoid	34	0
		Adenocarcinoma	12	0
Choi (39)	40-60 Gy	Epidermoid	33	33
		Adenocarcinoma	43	8

RT = radiotherapy; N/A = not applicable.
Adapted from DeVita (106).

aerodigestive passages, they note a 90% complete regression for primary and nodes compared to 62% using historical controls with conentional fractionation. This demanding regimen is given t.i.d. (8 a.m.,

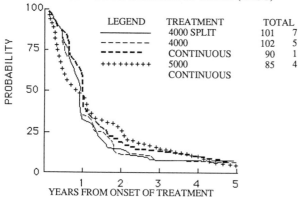

RESULTS - Benchmark

Fig. 31-6. RTOG survival rates according to various doses of irradiation delivered to primary tumor. From Perez *et al.* (119), with permission.

2 p.m., 8 p.m.) on 12 consecutive days at 1.4–1.5 Gy fractions to a total dose of 50.4 Gy–54 Gy.

4. *Chemotherapy results*: Although multiagent chemotherapy improves the response rate over single agents (Table 31-7), the CR rate remains low (i.e., < 10% to 15%), despite regressions in the majority of cancers (i.e., 53% to 87%), and the median survival for most advanced and metastatic disease (stages III and IV) usually is less than 1 year.

Results: Small Cell Cancers

The expectation of increasing curability for small cell cancer in proportion to its response rates (80% to 100%) has not been actualized in terms of survival. Median survival at 1 year (11 to 16 months) in limited-stage patients in most randomized clinical trials using multiagent chemotherapy alone increased by 3 months for combined modality approaches (13 to 16 months). Reports of 5-year survivors in mature studies range from 2% to 19% for chemotherapy alone and are no different than non-small cell cancers (Table 31-12) but increase to 14% to 35% for combined modality.

With incorporation of current chemotherapy regimens into the treatment program, however, survival is unequivocally prolonged, with at least a 4- to 5-fold improvement in median survival compared with patients who are given no therapy. Furthermore, about 10% of the total population of

Table 31-12. Results Using Combined Modalities (CT + RT) and Chemotherapy (CT) in Non-Small Cell Lung Cancer

Drugs	Median Survival (mo)		2-Year Disease-free or Overall Survival (actual or projected) (%)		Ref.
	CT	CMT	CT	CMT	
CML/VAP	11.6	15.0	12	28 (OS)	23
			6	23 (DFS)	
CAEV	13.6	I: 13.1	8	I:15 (DFS)	22
		II: 14.6		II:25	
CAV	11.2	14.0	19	28 (OS)	21
CAV	12.7	16.5	2	15 (DFS)	31
CMVL	11.5	10.5	8	5 (DFS)	32
AV/CM	R:12.0	13.0	12	14 (OS)	33
	NR: 7.0	8.5	12	4	
VMVAC	CR:16.0	CR:16.0	CR:25	CR:35 (OS)	34

CT = Chemotherapy; CMT = Combined modality (CT+RT); R = Responders; NR = Nonresponders;
CR = Complete responders; OS = overall survival; DFS = disease-free survival; C = cyclophosphamide;
A = doxorubicin; E = etoposide; V = vincristine; M = methotrexate; L = lomustine; P = procarbazine.

patients remain free of disease over 2 years from the start of therapy, a time period during which most relapses occur. However, even these patients are at risk of dying from lung cancer (both small and non-small cell types) (81).

Radiation therapy has been added to most treatment programs because of the high incidence of in-field thoracic failures. Then, the addition of irradiation to chemotherapy can increase median survival by 5 to 6 months and often double 2-year survival, but the figures are still disappointing because it does not translate into long-term survival. CR rates are greater with than without radiotherapy, (i.e., 40% to 50% versus 60% to 80%), chest relapses are less (i.e., 20% to 30% versus 50% to 60%), and 2 to 3-year survival improves from 10% to 15% to 20% to 30% .

Prophylactic cranial irradiation (PCI) has been widely advocated and used in numerous randomized studies because analogies were drawn to leukemias and there is a known high incidence of central nervous system metastases (≥ 50%) at autopsy, although regimens of 30 Gy fractionated doses have been successful in terms of decreasing or eliminating brain relapse, that is, 0% to 17% with PCI and 13% to 36% without PCI.

Long-term survival: Despite improved high response rates, long-term 5-year survival is dismal, ranging from 1% to 12%, with most series being less than 5%, similar to non-small cell cancers (Table 31-13) (81,140).

Adjuvant surgery: There may be a role for adjuvant surgery following chemotherapeutic CR in small cell carcinoma. If patients are rendered N0 and no pathologic evidence of tumor is seen, survival improves and outcome is best (79). One could argue that they did not have any residual tumor and surgery was of minor incremental value.

Prognosis

In a retrospective review of 410 patients, favorable prognostic factors for long-term survival after treatment for inoperable carcinoma of the lung were performance status, early stage, high total dose of radiation, large cell histology, and thoracotomy to determine resectability (19).

Table 31-13. Studies Reporting Small Cell Lung Cancer Patients Living 5 Years or Longer

Reference	Total No. Treated Patients	No. Survivors at 5 years	% Survivors at 5 Years (Both Stages)
Limited > Smith *et al.* (1981)	17	4	12
Extensive	25	1	
Limited > Livingston *et al.* (1984)	103	11	5
Extensive	270	6	
Limited > Vogelsang *et al.* (1985)	94	5	2
Extensive	131	0	
Limited > Johnson *et al.* (1985)	103	17	8
Extensive	149	4	
Limited > Jacobs *et al.* (1986)	102	2	1
Extensive	138	0	
Limited > Osterlind *et al.* (1986)	443	19	3
Extensive	431	3	
Totals by Stage	LD 862	LD 58	LD 7
Overall Totals	ED 1144	ED 14	ED 1
	2006	72	4

LD = limited disease; ED = extensive disease.
From Seifter and Ihade (140), with permission.

Karnofsky status: It is remarkable that using a measure such as patient mobility or ambulation can provide a stratification akin to the most sophisticated staging work-up. In both limited (median survival 10–16 months) and extensive (median survival 6–12 months) stage disease, ambulatory or performance status is an extremely important prognostic factor (123a). Furthermore, young women appear to have a more favorable prognosis (167a).

CLINICAL INVESTIGATIONS (1,5)

Prevention

Prevention of lung cancer must be one of the primary aims of research. Reduction and/or elimination of the respiratory carcinogen is conceptually the simplest method to improve the general outcome. Major efforts must be made to persuade patients to stop smoking, and the physician's role in tobacco control cannot be overemphasized. Self-help "quit kits," counseling, and nicotine replacement are helpful to induce patients to quit smoking (20,156). Chemoprevention using ß-carotene and retinol is being tested in the Seattle lung clinical trial with a recruitment goal of 13,000 smokers and 4,000 asbestos workers and a final goal of an efficacy value of 33% decrease in incidence (64).

Stages I and II SCC, adenocarcinoma, and large cell carcinoma. The failure of adjuvant radiation therapy, chemotherapy, and immunostimulation to increase overall survival has shifted interest to either specific immunostimulation, new drug combinations, or even chemoprevention of second cancers (a major challenge among long-term survivors). Furthermore, any adjuvant therapy trial must take into account the high proportion of patients with T1, N0, M0 tumors that are definitely cured by resection. The addition of an adjuvant treatment must always try to avoid an increase in morbidity or mortality. Elective beam irradiation is being considered for adenocarcinomas and large cell carcinomas.

For stage III tumors, the major search is for an optimal combination of different modalities to improve the current results. For stage IV tumors, new and more effective drugs are needed.

1. For radiation therapy, different schedules testing hyperfractionation with higher total doses and additional boosting with high-dose rate brachytherapy (154) and low-dose rate brachytherapy intraluminally (125) is being investigated. Radiosensitizers, radioprotectors, neutron beams, and high linear energy transfer particles are other approaches. Fluosol and atmosphere oxygen breathing suggest promise of improved response (95). To study the advantage of soe escalation, 3-dimensional radiotherapy planning is applied for the conformation therapy of a bronchial carcinoma (76a).
2. Multiagent chemotherapy and new drugs are still being explored in an attempt to achieve higher response rates, the primary aim when using chemotherapy in combined approaches or as an adjuvant to surgery and/or irradiation; it is hoped it will have a major impact on survival (88).
3. Immunostimulation with chemotherapy or radiation therapy programs is also under study.
4. Biologic response modifiers such as ß-interferon and irradiation are promising; pilot studies have reported a gain in median survival (37).

For *SCLC*, better drug combinations or new drugs and the best chemoradiation therapy schedule must be identified for limited disease. (87)

Recommended Reading

During the last few years, good reviews of the multidisciplinary approach in lung cancer have been published (1,6-8,10-15). These books are included in the general references section. We particularly recommend recent *Seminars in Oncology* series (1988), *Lung Cancer Workshop*, edited by Bleehen (27), and Minna's chapter in DeVita *et al.*, *Cancer: Principles and Practice of Oncology* (106). Some older but good books are *Lung Cancer* (11); and the European Organization for Research and Treatment of Lung Cancer's (EORTC) *Symposium on Progress* and *Perspectives in Lung Cancer Treatment* (6); Scarantino (138), and Bates (24) with emphasis on radiotherapy management.

REFERENCES

General References

1. Ackerman, L.V.; Del Regato, J.A. Cancer diagnosis, treatment, and prognosis, 4th ed. St. Louis, Mo.: C.V. Mosby, Co.; 1970:329-376.
2. American Joint Committee on Cancer, Manual for Staging. Philadelphia, PA: J.B. Lippincott Co., 1988.
3. Bragg, D.G. Imaging in primary lung cancer: the roles of detection, staging, and follow-up. Seminars in Ultrasound CT and MR 10:453; 1989.
4. Bragg, D.G.; Dodd, G.D. Imaging in Cancer. CA 37:130-185, 194-245, 1987.
5. Bragg, D.G.; Rubin, P., Youker, J.E. Oncologic Imaging. Elmsford, NY: Pergamon Press, 1985.
5a. del Regato; Spjut, H.J.; Cox, J.D.. In Ackerman & del Regato's Cancer: Diagnosis, Treatment and Prognosis. 6th ed. St. Louis, MO: C.V. Mosby Co.; 1985; 377-424.
5b. Emami, B.; Perez, C.A. Lung. In: Perez, C.A., Brady, L.W., eds. Principles and Practice of Radiation Oncology. Philadelphia, PA: JB Lippincott Co.; 1992; 806-838.
6. Henry, J.; Van Houtte, P., eds. EORTC symposium on progress and perspectives in lung cancer treatment. Intl. J. Radiat. Oncol. Biol. Phys. 6:977-1120; 1980.
7. International Histologic Classification of Tumors, Nos. 1-20. Geneva, Switzerland: World Health Organization, 1978.
8. International Union Against Cancer (UICC) Illustrated Tumor Nomenclature, 2nd ed. New York, NY: Springer-Verlag; 1969.
9. International Union Against Cancer (UICC). TNM Classification of Malignant Tumors, 4th ed. New York, NY: Springer-Verlag; 1987.
10. Israel, L.; Chahinian, A.P., eds. Lung cancer: natural history, prognosis, and treatment. New York: Academic Press; 1976.
11. Livingston, R.B., ed. Lung cancer. The Hague, the Netherlands: Martinus Nijhoff Publishers; 1981.
12. Muggia, F.M.; Rozencweig, M., eds. Lung cancer: progress in therapeutic research. New York, NY: Raven Press; 1979.
13. Salazar, O.M.; Creech, R.H.; Rubin, P.; *et al.* Oncologic multidisciplinary decisions in oncology: bronchogenic carcinoma. Elmsford, NY: Pergamon Press; 1981.
14. Selawry, O.S.; Strauss, M.J., eds. Lung cancer. Semin. Oncol. 1:161-286; 1974.
15. Strauss, M.J., ed. Lung cancer: clinical diagnosis and treatment, 2nd ed. New York, NY: Grune & Stratton; 1983.

Specific References

16. Abrams, P., Fer, M., Raubion, C., Hanley, M., *et al.* and a Multicenter Study Group. A new procedure for staging small cell lung cancer: gamma camera imaging using a technetium-99m labeled monoclonal antibody fab. Abstract. J. Clin. Oncol. 9:232, 1990.
17. Aisner, J.; Alberto, P.; Bitran, J.; *et al.* Role of chemotherapy in small cell lung cancer. Consensus report of the International

Association for the Study of Lung Cancer Workshop. Cancer Treat. Rep. 67:11-19, 37-43; 1983.

18. Aisner, S.C., Finkelstein, D.M., Ettinger, D.S., *et al.* The clinical significance of variant morphology small-cell carcinoma of the lung. J. Clin. Oncol. 8:402-409, 1990.

18a. Albain, K.S.; Crowley, J.J.; LeBlanc, M.; *et al.* Survival determinants in extensive-stage non-small lung cancer: The Southwest Oncology Group experience. J Clin Oncol. 9(9):1618-1626; 1991.

19. Amery, W.K. Final results of a multicenter placebo-controlled levamisole study of resectable lung cancer. Cancer Treat. Rep. 62:1677-1683; 1983.

20. Anda, R.F.; Remington, P.L.; Sienko, D.G.; *et al.* Are physicians advising smokers to quit? The patient's perspective. J. Am. Med. Assoc. 257:1916-1919; 1987.

21. Anthony, H.M.; Mearns, A.J.; Mason, M.K.; *et al.* Levamisole and surgery in bronchial carcinoma patients: increase in deaths from cardiorespiratory failure, thorax 34:4-12; 1979.

22. Arriagada, R.; Bertino, J.R.; Bleehan, N.M.; Brodin, O. Consensus report on combined radiotherapy and chemotherapy modalities in lung cancer. Antibiot. Chemother. Basel Karger. 41:232-241;1988.

23. Ball, W.; Frost, J.; Tockman, M.; Levin, M. Early lung cancer detection. Results of the initial radiologic and cytologic screening of the Johns Hopkins study. Am. Rev. Respir. Dis. 13L A84; 1984.

24. Bates, M., ed. Bronchial Carcinoma. An Integrated Approach to Diagnosis and Management. Berlin, Germany: Springer Verlag, 1984.

25. Bitran, J.D.; Golomb, H.M.; Hoffman, P.C.; *et al.* Protochemotherapy in non-small lung carcinoma. An attempt to increase surgical resectability and survival. A preliminary report. Cancer 57:44-53; 1986.

26. Bleehen, N.M. Role of radiation therapy and other modalities in the treatment of small cell carcinoma of the lung. In: Muggia, F.N.; Rozencweig, M., eds. Lung cancer: progress in therapeutic research. New York, NY: Raven Press; 1979:567-574.

27. Bleehen, N.M. Workshop on radiotherapy for lung cancer. Cancer treatment Symposia 2:1-149; 1985.

28. Bloedorn, F.G. Rationale and benefit of preoperative irradiation in lung cancer. J. Am. Med.Assoc. 196:340-341; 1966.

29. Borgelt, B.; Gelber, R.; Kramer, S. The palliation of brain metastases: final results of the first 2 studies by the radiation therapy oncology group. Intl. J. Radiat. Oncol. Biol. Phys. 6:1-9; 1980.

29a. Boring, C.C.; Squires, T.S.; Tong, T. Cancer statistics 1991 CA 41: 19-51; 1991.

30. Bowen, T. E.; Zastchuk, R.; Greene, D .C ; *et al.* The value of anterior mediastinoscope in bronchogenic carcinoma of the left upper love. J. Thorac. Carciovasc. Surg. 76:169-271; 1978.

31. Bunn, P.A. Jr.; Lichter, A.S.; Makuch, R.W.; Matthews, M.J.; Anderson, A.J.; Edison, M.; Cohen, M.H.; Glatstein, E.; Veach, S.R.; Minna, J.D. Chemotherapy alone or chemotherapy with chest radiation therapy in limited stage small cell lung cancer. Ann. Intern. Med. 106:655-662; 1987.

32. Burbank, F. U.S. Lung cancer rates begin to rise proportionately more rapidly for females than for males: a dose-response effect? J. Chronic. Dis. 25:473-479; 1972.

33. Burkes, R.; Ginsberg, R.F.; Shepherd, M.; *et al.* Phase II pilot program of neo-adjuvant chemotherapy for stage III (T1-3, N2, M0) unresectable non-small cell lung cancer (NSCLC) (abstract). Lung Cancer 4 (suppl.) A166; 1988.

34. Calvo, F.A., Ortiz de Urbina, D., Abuchaibe, O., Azinovic, W., Aristu, J., Santos, M., Escude, L., Herreros, J., Llorens, R. Intraoperative radiotherapy during lung cancer surgery: technical description and early clinical results. Int. J. Radiat. Oncol. Biol. Phys. 19:103-111, 1990.

35. Carney, D.N.; De Leij, L. Lung cancer biology. Semin. Oncol. 15:199-214; 1988.

36. Catane, R.; Lichter, A.; Lee, Y.J.; *et al.* Small cell lung cancer. Analysis of treatment factors contributing to prolonged survival. Cancer 48:1936-1943; 1981.

36a. Chabner, B.A.; Friedman, M.A. Progress against rare and not-so-rare cancers. N Engl J Med. 326:563-564; 1992.

37. Chang, A., McDonald, S., Kim, I.S., Sobel, S., Smith, J., Boros, L., Keng, P., Rubin, P., Wallenberg, J. Combination treatment of radiation and recombinant interferon beta ser in patients with inoperable or metastatic non-small cell lung cancer. In: Proceed-

ings of American Society of Clinical Oncology. J. Clin. Oncol. 9:247, 1990.

38. Chang, A.Y.C.; Kuebler, J.P.; Tormey, D.C.; *et al.* Phase II evaluation of a combination of mitomycin-C, vincristine and cisplatin in advanced non-small cell lung cancer. Cancer 51:54-59; 1986.

39. Choi, N.C. Reassessment of the role of postoperative radiation therapy in resected lung cancer. Int. J. Radiat. Oncol. Biol. Phys. 8:2015-2018; 1982.

40. Choi, N.C., Carey, R.W. Importance of radiation dose in achieving improved loco-regional tumor control in limited stage small-cell lung carcinoma: an update. Int. J. Radiat. Oncol. Biol. Phys. 17:307-311, 1989.

41. Choi, N.C., Kanarek, D.J., Grillo, H.C. Effect of postoperative radiotherapy on changes in pulmonary funtion in patients with Stage II and IIIA lung carcinoma. Int. J. Radiat. Oncol. Biol. Phys. 18: 95-101, 1990.

42. Cohen, M.H. Bronchogenic carcinoma. In: Staquet, M., ed. Randomized trials in cancer: a critical review by sites. New York, NY: Raven Press; 1978:297-330.

43. Cohen, M. H. Signs and symptoms of bronchogenic carcinoma. Semin. Oncol. 1:183-189; 1974.

44. Comis, R.L. Chemotherapy of small cell lung cancer. Updates in Cancer: Principles and Practice of Oncology. Devita, Jr., V.T. (ed). Philadelphia, PA.; J.B. Lippincott Co. 7: 13; 1987

45. Concannon, J.P.; Dalbow, M.H.; Liebler, G.A.; *et al.* The carcinoembryonic antigen assay in bronchogenic carcinoma. Cancer 34:184-192; 1974.

46. Cormier, Y.; Bergeron, D.; LaForge, J.; *et al.* Benefits of polychemotherapy in advanced non-small cell bronchogenic carcinoma. Cancer 50:845-849; 1982.

47. Cox, J.D., Azarnia, N., Byhardt, R.W., Shin, K.H., Emami, B., Perez, C.A. N2 (Clinical) non-small cell carcinoma of the lung: prospective trials of radiation therapy with total doses 60 Gy by the Radiation Therapy Oncology Group. Int. J. Radiat. Oncol. Biol. Phys. 20: 7-12; 1991.

48. Cox, J.D.; Byhardt, R.W.; Komaki, R. The role of radiotherapy in squamous large cell and adenocarcinoma of the lung. Semin. Oncol. 10: 81-94; 1983.

49. Dahlgren, S.; Find, B. Comparison between diagnostic results obtained by transthoracic needle biopsy and by sputum cytology. Acta Cytol. 16:53-58; 1972.

49a. Daly, R.C.; Trastek, V.F.; Pairolero, P.C.; *et al.* Bronchoalveolar carcinoma: Factors affecting survival. Ann Thor Surg. 51(3):368-377; 1991.

50. Dillman, R.O.; Seagren, S.L.; Propert, K.J. *et al.* A randomized trial of induction chemotherapy plus high-dose radiation versus radiation alone in stage III non-small cell lung cancer. N. Engl. J. Med. 323:940-945;1990.

51. Doyle, P.T.; Weir, J.; Robertson, E.M.; *et al.* Role of computed tomography in assessing "operability" of bronchial carcinoma. Br. Med. J. 292: 231-233; 1986.

52. Eagan, R.T.; Ingle, J.N.; Grytak, S.; *et al.* Platinum based poly chemotherapy versus dianhydrogalaticol in advanced non-small cell lung cancer. Cancer Treat. Rep. 61:1339-1345; 1977.

53. Einhorn, L.H.; Bond, L.H.; Hornback, N.; *et al.* Long-term results in combined modality treatment of small cell carcinoma of the lung. Semin. Oncol. 5: 309-313; 1978.

54. Eisert, D.R.; Cox, J.D.; Komaki, R. Irradiation for bronchial carcinoma: reasons for failure. I. Analysis of local control as a function of dose, time, and fractionation. Cancer 37:2665-2670; 1976.

55. Ettinger, D.S. Evaluation of new drugs in untreated patients with small-cell lung cancer: its time has come. J. Clin. Oncol. 8:374, 1990.

56. Evans, W.K.; Feld, R.; Murray. N.; Willan, A. *et al.* Superiority of alternating non-cross-resistant chemotherapy in extensive small cell lung cancer. A multicenter, randomized clinical trial by the National Cancer Institute of Canada. Ann. Intern. Med. 107:451-458; 1987.

57. Evans, W.K.; Shepherd, F.A.; Feld, R.; *et al.* VP-16 and cisplatin as first-line therapy for small cell lung cancer. J. Clin. Oncol. 3:1471-1477; 1985.

58. Feld, R.; Evans, W.K.; Coy, P.; *et al.* Canadian multicenter randomized trial comparing sequential and alternating administration of two non-cross-resistant chemotherapy combinations in

patients with limited small cell carcinoma of the lung. J. Clin. Oncol. 5:1401-1409; 1987.

59. Feld, R. Combined modality induction therapy without maintenance chemotherapy for small cell carcinoma of the lung. J. Clin. Oncol. 2:294-304; 1984.

60. Fitzpatrick, R.T.; Rider, W.D. Half-body radiotherapy. Intl. J. Radiat. Oncol. Biol. Phys. 1:197-208; 1976.

60a. Fleck, J.F.; Einhorn, L.H.; Lauer, R.C.; et al. Is prophylactic cranial irradiation indicated in small-cell lung cancer? J Clin Oncol (2):209-214; 1990.

61. Fontana, R.; Sanderson, D.; Woolner, L.; Taylor, W.; Miller, W.; Muhm, J. Lung cancer screening: the Mayo program. J. Occup. Med. 28:746-750; 1986.

62. Fox, R.M.;Woods, R.L.; Tattersall, M.H.; et al. A randomized study of adjuvant immunotherapy with levamisole and corynebacterium parvum in operable non-small cell lung cancer. Intl. J. Radiat. Oncol. Biol. Phys. 6:1043-1045; 1980.

62a. Garfinkel, M.A.; Silverberg, E. Lung cancer and smoking trends in the United States over the past 25 years. CA 41: 137-145; 1991.

63. Gazdar, A.F.; Linnoila, R.I. The pathology of lung cancer — changing concepts and newer diagnostic techniques. Semin. Oncol. 15:215-225; 1988.

64. Goodman, G.E., Omenn. G.S. Seattle lung cancer chemoprevention trial: caret-beta-carotene and retinol efficacy trial. In: Proceedings of American Society of Clinical Oncology. J. Clin. Oncol. 9:233, 1990.

65. Gralla, R.J.; Kris, M.G. Chemotherapy in non-small cell lung cancer: results of recent trials. Semin. Oncol. 15(suppl. 4):2-5; 1985.

66. Gralla, R.J.; Kris, M.G.; Martini, N.; Zaman, M. A neoadjuvant trial in stage IIIA non-small cell lung cancer in patients with clinically apparent mediastinal node involvement wit MVP chemotherapy (mitomycin + vinca alkaloid + cisplatin). Abstract. Lung Cancer. 4 (suppl); A161; 1988.

67. Greco, A. Rationale for chemotherapy for patients with advanced non-small cell lung cancer. Semin. Oncol. 13(suppl. 3):92-96; 1986.

68. Green, N.; Kurohara, S.S.; George, F.W. III; Crews, Q.E., Jr. Postresection irradiation for primary lung cancer. Radiology 116:405-407; 1975.

69. Haffty, B.G.; Goldberg, N.B.; Gerstley, J.; Fischer, D.b.; Peschel, R.E. Results of radical radiation therapy in clinical stage I, technically operable non-small cell lung cancer. Intl. J. Radiat. Oncol. Biol. Phys. 15:69-75; 1988.

70. Hammond, E.C.; Horn, D. Smoking and death rates — report on forty-four months of follow-up of 187,783 men. Cancer 38:28-58; 1988.

71. Hansen, H.H. Strategies against tobacco use. The physician's view. Lung Cancer 4: (suppl.):20; 1988.

72. Hansen, H.H.; Muggia, F.M. Staging of inoperable patients with bronchogenic carcinoma with special reference to bone marrow examination and peritoneoscopy. Cancer 30:1395-1401; 1972.

73. Hansen, M.; Hanson, H.H.; Dombernowsky, P. Long-term survival in small cell carcinoma of the lung. J. Am. Med. Assoc. 244:247-250; 1980.

74. Heelan, R.T.; Martini, N.; Westcott, J.W. Carcinomatous involvement of the hilum and mediastinum computed tomographic and magnetic resonance evaluation. Radiology 156:111-115; 1985.

75. Hilaris, B.S.; Martini, N.; Luomanen, R.K.; et al. The value of preoperative radiation therapy in apical cancer of the lung. Surg. Clin. North Am. 54:831-840; 1974.

76. Hilaris, B.S.; Nori, D.; Beattie, E.J.; et al. Value of perioperative brachytherapy in the management of non-oat cell carcinoma of the lung. Intl. J. Radiat. Oncol. Biol. Phys. 9:1161-1166; 1983.

76a. Hodapp, N.; Boesecke, R.; Schlegel, W.; Bruggmoser, G.; Wannenmacher, M. Three-dimensional treatment planning for conformation therapy of a bronchial carcinoma. Radiother. Oncol. 20:245-249; 1991.

77. Holmes, E.C.; Gail, M. Surgical adjuvant therapy for stage II and stage III adenocarcinoma and large-cell undifferentiated carcinoma. J. Clin. Oncol. 4(5):710-715; 1986.

78. Holmes, E.C.; Hill, L.E.; Gail, M. A randomized comparison of the effects of adjuvant therapy on resected stages II and III non-small cell carcinoma of the lung. Ann. Surg. 202:335-341; 1985.

79. Holoye, P.Y.; McMurtrey, M.J.; Mountain, C.F.; Murphy, W.K.; Dhingra, H.M., Umsawasdi, T., Glisson, B.S., Lee, J.S., Carr, D.T., Valdivieso, M., Hong, W.K. The role of adjuvant surgery in the combined modality therapy of small-cell bronchogenic carcinoma after a chemotherapy-induced partial remission. J. Clin. Oncol. 8:416-423, 1990.

80. Holsti, L.; Mattson, K. Long-term results of split-course radiation therapy of lung cancer: a randomized study. Intl. J. Radiat. Oncol. Biol. Phys. 6:977-982; 1980.

80a. Ihde, D.C.; Mulshine, J.L.; Kramer, B.S.; et al. Randomized trial of high vs. standard dose etoposide (VP16) and cisplatin in extensive stage small cell lung cancer (SCLS). Proc ASCO 10:A-819, 240; 1991.

81. Johnson, B.E., Grayson, J., Makuch, R.W., Linnoila, R.I., Anderson, J.J., Cohen, M.H., Glatstein, E., Minna, J.D., Ihde, D.C. Ten-year survival of patients with small-cell lung cancer treated with combination chemotherapy with or without irradiation. J. Clin. Oncol. 8:396-402; 1990.

82. Johnson, B.E.; Ihde, D.C.; Makuch, R.W.; et al. Myc family oncogene amplification in tumor cell lines established from small cell cancer patients and its relationship to clinical status and course. J. Clin. Invest. 79:1629-1634; 1987.

83. Katz, H.R.; Alberts, R.W. A comparison of high-dose continuous and split-course irradiation in non-oat-cell carcinoma of the lung. Am. J. Clin. Oncol. 6:445-457; 1983.

84. Kies, M.S.; Mira, J.G.; Livingston, R.B., et al. Multimodal therapy for limited small cell lung cancer: a randomized study of induction combination chemotherapy with or without thoracic irradiation in complete responders, and with wide field versus reduced volume radiation in partial responders. J. Clin. Oncol. 5:592-600, 1987.

85. Kirsh, M.M.; Rotman, H.; Argenta, L.; et al. Carcinoma of the lung: results of treatment over ten years. Ann. Thorac. Surg. 21:371-377; 1976.

85a. Klasa, R.J.; Murray, N.; Coldman, A.J. Dose-intensity meta-analysis of chemotherapy regimens in small-cell carcinoma of the lung. J Clin Oncol. 9(3):499-508; 1991.

86. Komaki, R.; Roh, J.; Cox, J.; et al. Superior sulcus tumors: results of irradiation of 36 patients. Cancer 48:1563-1568; 1981.

87. Kubota, K., Furuse, K., Kawahara, M., Fukuoka, M., Negoro, S. Randomized trial of chemotherapy (CT) with or without thoracic radiation therapy (RT) for treatment of locally advanced non-small cell lung cancer (NSCLC). In: Proceeding of American Society of Clinical Oncology. J. Clin. Oncol. 9:226, 1990.

88. Kudoh, S., Fukuoka, M., Negoro, S., Furuse, K., Kawahara, M. A randomized trial in advanced non-small cell lung cancer: cisplatin and vindesine vs. cisplatin, vindesine and mitomycin vs. cisplatin and etoposide alternating with vindesine and mitomycin. In: Proceedings of American Society of Clinical Oncology. J. Clin. Oncol. 9:228, 1990.

89. Lad, T.; Rubistein, L.; Sadeghi, A. The benefit of adjuvant treatment for resected locally advanced non-small cell lung cancer. J. Clin. Oncol. 6:9-17; 1988.

90. Levitt, S.H.; Bogarous, C.R.; Ladd, G., Jr. Split-dose intensive radiation therapy in the treatment of advanced lung cancer: a randomized study. Radiology 88:1159-1161; 1967.

91. Liebler, G.A.; Concannon, J.P.; Magovem, G.J.; et al. Immunoprofile studies for patients with bronchogenic carcinoma. 1. Correlation of pretherapy studies with survival. J. Thorac. Cardiovasc. Surg. 74:506-518; 1977.

91a. Lishner, M.; Feld, R.; Payne, D.G.; et al. Late neurological complications after prophylactic cranial irradiation in patients with small-cell lung cancer: The Toronto experience. J Clin Oncol. 8(2):215-221; 1990.

92. Livingston, R.B. Combination chemotherapy of bronchogenic carcinoma. 1. Non-oat cell. Cancer Treat. Rev. 4:153-165; 1977.

93. Lowe, J.; Shore, D.F.; Iles, P.B.; et al. Intrapleural BCG in operable lung cancer. Lancet 1:11-14; 1980.

94. Lung Cancer Study Group. Effects of postoperative mediastinal radiation on completely resected stage II and III epidermoid cancer of the lung. New Engl. J. Med. 315:1377-1381; 1986.

95. Lustig, R., Lowe, N., Prosnitz, L., Spaulding, M., Cohen, M., Stitt, J., Brannon, R. Fluosol and oxygen breathing as an adjuvant to radiation therapy in the treatment of locally advanced non-small cell carcinoma of the lung: results of a phase I/II study. Int. J. Radiat. Oncol. Biol. Phys. 19:97-103; 1990.

96. McKneally, M.F.; Maver, C.; Lininger, L.; et al. Four-year follow-

up on the Albany experience with intrapleural BCG in lung cancer. J. Thorac Cardiovasc. Surg. 81:485-492; 1981.

97. Martini, N.; McCormack, P. Therapy of stage III (non-metastatic disease). Semin. Oncol. 10:95-110; 1983.

98. Martini, N.; Beattie, E.J. Results of surgical treatment in stage I lung cancer. J. Thorac. Cardiovasc. Surg. 74:499-505; 1977.

99. Martini, N.; Kris, M.G.; Gralla, R.; *et al.* The effects of preoperative chemotherapy on the resectability of non-small cell lung carcinoma with mediastinal lymph node metastases (N2 M0) Ann. Thorac. Surg. 45:370-379; 1988.

100. Mason, B.A.; Catalano, R.B. Mitomycin, vinblastine, and cisplatin combination chemotherapy in non-small cell lung cancer (abstract). Proc. Am. Soc. Clin. Oncol. 21:477; 1980.

101. Matthews, M.J. Problems in morphology and behavior of bronchopulmonary malignant disease. In: Israel, L.; Chahinian, A.P., eds. Lung cancer: natural histology, prognosis, and therapy. New York, NY: Academic Press; 1976:471-476.

102. Mattson, K.; Holsti, L.; Jakobsson, M.; *et al.* Inoperable non-small lung cancer: radiation with or without chemotherapy. Eur. J. Cancer Clin. Oncol. 24:477-482; 1988.

103. Melamed, M.; Flehninger, B.; Zaman, M.; Heelan, R.; Perchick, W.; Martini, N. Screening for early lung cancer: results of the Memorial Sloan-Kettering study in New York: Chest 86:44-53; 1984.

104. Mettlin, C. Trends in years of life lost to cancer: 1970-1985. Ca-A Cancer J. Clin. 39:33-39'; 1989.

104a. Miller, J.I.; Phillips, T.W. Neodymium: YAG laser and brachytherapy in the management of inoperable bronchogenic carcinoma. Ann Thor Surg. 50(2):190-196; 1990.

105. Miller, T.P.; Chen, T.T.; Coltman, C.A.; *et al.* Effect of alternating combination chemotherapy on survival of ambulatory patients with metastatic large cell and adenocarcinoma of the lung. A Southwest Oncology Group Study. J. Clin. Oncol. 4:502-508; 1986.

106. Minna, J.D.; Pass, H.; Glatstein, E.; Ihde, D.C. Cancer of the lung. In: DeVita, V.T., Jr.; Hellman, S.; Rosenberg, S.A., eds. Cancer: principles and practice of oncology, 3rd ed. Philadelphia, PA: J.B. Lippincott Co.; 1989:591-705.

107. Mornex, F., Trillet, V., Chauvin, F., Ardiet, J.M., Schmitt, T., Romestaing, P., Carrie, C., Mahe, M., Mornex, J.F., Fournel, P., Souquet, P.J., Boniface, E., Vincent, M., Piperno, D., Rebattu, P., Gerard, J.P., the Groupe Lyonnais d'Oncologie Thoracique. Hyperfractionated radiotherapy alternating with multidrug chemotherapy in the treatment of limited small cell lung cancer (SCLC). Int. J. Radiat. Oncol. Biol. Phys. 19:23-31, 1990.

108. Morstyn, G.; Ihde, D.C.; Lichter, A.S.; *et al.* Small cell lung cancer 1973 to 1983: early progress and recent obstacles. Intl. J. Radiat. Oncol. Biol. Phys. 10:515-539; 1984.

109. Mountain, C.F. A new international staging system for lung cancer. Chest 89:2255-2335; 1986.

110. Mountain, C.F. Prognostic implications of the international staging system for lung cancer. Semin. Oncol. 15:236-245; 1988.

111. Mountain, C.F.; McMurtrey, M.J.; Frazier, D.H. Regional extension of lung cancer. Intl. J. Radiat. Oncol. Biol. Phys. 6:1013-1020; 1980.

112. Murray, N., Coppin, C., Rapp, E., Pater, J., Cormier, Y., Evans, W., Hodson, D., Clark, D., Feld, R., Arnold, A., Ayoub, J., Wilson, K., Latreille, J., Wierzbicki, R., Hill, D. The Canadian multicenter trial in non-small-cell lung cancer (NSCLC): an analysis of drug delivery. Abstract. In: Proceedings of American Society of Clinical Oncology 9:225, 1990.

113. Myers, M.H.; Gloeckler Ries, L.A. Cancer patient survival rates: SEER program results for 10 years of follow-up. Ca-A Cancer J. Clin. 39:21-32; 1989.

114. Osterlind, K.; Hansen, H.H.; Hansen, H.S., *et al.* Chemotherapy versus chemotherapy plus irradiation in limited small cell lung cancer. Results of a controlled trial with 5 years of follow-up. Br. J. Cancer 54:7-17, 1986.

115. Paulson, D.I. Carcinoma of the superior pulmonary sulcus. Ann. Thorac. Surg. 28:3-4; 1979.

116. Pearson, F.G. An evaluation of mediastinoscopy in the management of presumably operable bronchogenic carcinoma. J. Thorac. Cardiovasc. Surg. 55:617-624; 1968.

117. Perez, C.A.; Einhorn, L.; Oldham, R.K. Randomized trial of radiotherapy to the thorax in limited small cell carcinoma of the lung treated with multi-agent chemotherapy and elective brain irradiation: a preliminary report. J. Clin. Oncol. 2:1200-1208; 1984.

118. Perez, C.A.; Pajak, T.F.; Rubin, P.; Simpson, J.R.; Mohiuddin, M.; Brady, L.; Rerez, T.R.; Rotman, M. Long-term observations of the patterns of failure in patients with unresectable non-oat cell carcinoma of the lung treated with definitive radiotherapy. Report by the Radiation Therapy Oncology Group. Cancer 59:1874-1881; 1987.

119. Perez, C.A.; Stanley, K.; Grundy, G., *et al.* Impact of irradiation technique and tumor extent in tumor control and survival of patients with unresectable non-oat cell carcinoma of the lung. RTOG 73-01. Cancer 50:1091-1099, 1982.

120. Perez, C.A.; Stanley, K.; Rubin, P.; *et al.* Patterns of tumor recurrence after definitive irradiation for operable non-oat cell carcinoma of the lung. Intl. J. Radiat. Oncol. Biol. Phys. 6:987-996; 1980.

121. Perez, C.A.; Stanley, K.; Rubin, P.; *et al.* Prospective randomized study of various irradiation doses and fractionation schedules in the treatment of inoperable non-oat cell carcinoma of the lung. Preliminary report of the radiation therapy oncology group. Cancer 45:2744-2753; 1980.

122. Perlin, E.; Oldham, R.K.; Weese, J.L.; *et al.* Carcinoma of the lung: immunotherapy with intradermal BCG and allogeneic tumor cells. Intl. J. Radiat. Oncol. Biol. Phys. 6:1033-1039; 1980.

123. Perry, M.C.; Eaton, W.L.; Propert, K.J.; Chahinian, A.P.; Skarin, A.; Carey, R.W.; Ware, Ware, J.H.; Kreisman, H.; Zimmer, B.; Faulkner, C. Chemotherapy with or without radiation therapy in limited small cell carcinoma of the lung. New Engl. J. Med. 316:912-918; 1987.

123a. Rawson, N.S.; Peto, J. An overview of prognostic factors in small cell lung cancer: A report from the subcommittee for the management of lung cancer of the United Kingdom Coordinating Committee on Cancer Research. Br J Canc 61(4):597-604; 1990.

124. Reddy, S., Penfield Faber, L., Baumann, L.A., Lee, M.S., Jensik, R.J., Kittle, F.C., Bonomi, P.D., Taylor, S.G., Hendrickson, F.R. Preoperative radiation therapy in regionally localized Stage III non-small cell lung carcinoma: long-term results and patterns of failure. Int. J. Radiat. Oncol. Biol. Phys. 19: 287-292; 1990.

125. Roach, M.; Leidholdt, M., Tatera, B.S., Joseph, J. Endobronchial radiation therapy (EBRT) in the management of lung cancer. Int. J. Radiat. Oncol. Biol. Phys. 18:1449-1455, 1990.

126. Roswit, B.; Patno, M.E.; Rapp, R.; *et al.* The survival of patients with inoperable lung cancer. A large-scale randomized study of radiation therapy vs. placebo. Am. J. Roentgenol. 90: 688-697; 1968.

127. Ruckdeschel, J.C.; Finkelstein, D.M.; Ettinger, D.S.; *et al.* A randomized trial of the four most active regimens for metastatic non-small cell lung cancer. J. Clin. Oncol. 4:14-22; 1986.

127a. Salazar, O.M. Combined modalities treatment of small cell lung cancer. Chest 96:745-785; 1991.

128. Salazar, O.M. Tumor control and radiation toxicity in the treatment of lung cancer: an analysis of time-dose-volume factors. In: Muggia, F.; Rozencweig, M.; eds. Lung cancer: progress in therapeutic research. New York: Raven Press; 1979:267-278.

129. Salazar, O.M.; Creech, R.H.; Rubin, P.; *et al.* Half-body and local chest irradiation as consolidation following response to standard induction chemotherapy for disseminated small cell lung cancer. An Eastern Cooperative Oncology Group Pilot Report. Intl. J. Radiat. Oncol. Biol. Phys. 6:1093-1102; 1980.

130. Salazar, O.M.; Rubin, P.; Brereen, J.C.; *et al.* Predictors of radiation response in lung cancer — a clinicopathological analysis. Cancer 37:1636-1650; 1976.

131. Salazar, O.M.; Rubin, P.; Keller, B.E.; *et al.* Systemic (half-body) radiation therapy: response and toxicity. Intl. J. Radiat. Oncol. Biol. Phys. 4: 937-950; 1978.

132. Salazar, O.M.; Scarantino, C.W.; Rubin, P.; *et al.* Total (half-body) systemic irradiation for occult metastases in non-small cell lung cancer: an eastern cooperative oncology group pilot Report Cancer 46:1932-1944; 1980.

133. Salazar, O.M.; Slawson, R.G.; Poussin-Rosillo, H.; *et al.* A prospective randomized trial comparing once-a-week vs. daily radiation therapy for locally advanced non-metastatic, measurable lung cancer: preliminary report. Intl. J. Radiat. Oncol. Biol. Phys. 12: 779-787; 1986.

134. Salazar, O.M.; Van Houtte, P.; Rubin, P. Once-a-week radiation

therapy for locally advanced lung cancer: final report. Cancer 54: 71 9-725; 1984.

135. Salazar, O.M.; Van Houtte, P.; Rubin, P. Once-a-week treatment for lung cancer. Intl. J. Radiat. Oncol. Biol. Phys. 9:923-930; 1983.

136. Salazar, O.M.; Zagars, G. "Radiation therapy — new approaches". In: Livingston, R.B., ed. Lung cancer, vol. 1. The Hague, the Netherlands: Martinus Nijhoff; 1980.

137. Sandler, H.M., Curran, W.J., Turrisi, A.T. The influence of tumor size and pre-treatment staging on outcome following radiation therapy alone for Stage I non-small cell lung cancer. Int. J. Radiat. Oncol. Biol. Phys. 19:9-15, 1990.

137a. Saunders M.I.; Dische, S.; Grosch, E.J.; et al. Experience with CHART. Int J Radiat Oncol Biol Phys. 21:871; 1991.

138. Scarantino, C.W., ed. Lung Cancer. Diagnostic Procedures and Therapeutic Management — With Special Reference to Radiotherapy. Berlin, Germany: Springer-Verlag; 1985.

139. Scarantino, C.; Salazar, O.M.; Rubin, P.; et al. The optimum radiation schedule in treatment of superior vena caval obstruction: importance of technetium-99m scintiangiograms. Intl. J. Radiat. Oncol. Biol. Phys. 5:1987-1995; 1979.

139a. Schaake-Koning, C; van den Bogaert, W.; Dalesio, O.; et al. Effects of concomitant cisplatin and radiotherapy on inoperable non-small-cell lung cancer. N Engl J Med. 326:524-530; 1992.

140. Seifter, E.J.; Ihade, D.C. Therapy of small cell lung cancer: a perspective on two decades of clinical research. Semin. Oncol. 15:278-299; 1988.

141. Selikoff, I.J.; Hammond, E.C. Asbestos-associated diseases in United States shipyards. CA 28:87-99; 1978.

142. Seydel, H.G.; Kutcher, G.J.; Steiner, R.M.; et al. Computed tomography in planning radiation therapy for bronchogenic carcinoma. Intl. J. Radiat. Oncol. Biol. Phys. 6:601-606; 1980.

143. Shields, T.W. Surgery of small cell lung cancer. Chest 89(suppl.):2645-2675; 1986.

144. Shields, T.W.; Yee, J.; Conn, S.H.; et al. Relationship of cell type and lymph node metastasis to survival after resection of bronchial carcinoma. Ann. Thorac. Surg. 20:501-510; 1975.

145. Silverberg, E. Cancer statistics. CA 39:3-21; 1989.

146. Skarin, A.; Sheldone, T.; Malcolm, A.; et al. Neoadjuvant chemoradiotherapy of non-small-cell lung cancer. Long-term follow-up. Abstract. Lung Cancer. 4 (suppl.): A166; 1988.

146a. Slater, J.D.; Ellerbroek, N.A.; Barkley Jr., H.T.; et al. Radiation therapy following resection of non-small cell bronchogenic carcinoma. Int J Radiat Oncol Biol Phys. 20:945-952; 1991.

147. Slawson, R.G.; Salazar, O.M.; Poussin-Rosillo, H.; et al. Once-a-week vs. conventional daily radiation treatment for lung cancer: final report. Intl. J. Radiat. Oncol. Biol. Phys. 15:61-68; l988.

148. Spain, R.; Anderson, P.; Speer, J.; et al. Improved survival with mitomycin-C, cis-platinum stage III limited, initally inoperable, non-small cell lung cancer (abstract). In: Proceedings of the IV World Conference on Lung Cancer, August 25-30, 1985. Toronto, Canada; 1985:33.

149. Smith, J.; Hansen, H.H. Current status of research into small cell carcinoma of the lung: summary of the second Workshop of the International Association for the Study of Lung Cancer (IASLC). Eur. J. Cancer Clin. Oncol. 21:1295-1298, 1985.

150. Souhami, R.L.; Geddes, D.M.; Spiro, S.G.; et al. Radiotherapy in small cell cancer of the lung treated with combination chemotherapy: a controlled trial. Br. Med. J. 288:1643-1646, 1984.

150a. Spain, R.; Anderson, P.; Speer, J. et al. Improved survival with mitomycin-C cisplatinum stage III limited, initially inoperable, non-small cell lung cancer (abstract). In: Proceedings of the IV World Conference on Lung Cancer, Toronto, Canada, 33:1985.

151. Speiser, B.; Spratling, L. Intermediate dose rate remote afterloading brachytherapy for intraluminal control of bronchogenic carcinoma. Int. J. Radiat. Oncol. Biol. Phys. 18: 1443-1449, 1990.

152. Sridhar, K.S.; Thurer, R.J.; Raskin, N.; Beattie, E.J. Pre-operative FED chemotherapy (CT), surgery and radiation therapy (RT) in non-small cell lung cancer (NSCLC) (abstract). Lung Cancer 4 (suppl.) A160; 1988.

153. Strauss, M.B., ed. Familiar medical quotations. Boston, Mass.: Little, Brown, and Co.; 1968.

154. Talton, B.M., Constable, W.C., Kersh, C.R. Curative radiotherapy in non-small cell carcinoma of the lung. Int. J. Radiat. Oncol. Biol. Phys. 19:15-23, 1990.

155. Taylor, S.R.; Trybula, M.; Bonomi, P.O.; et al. Simultaneous cisplatin fluorouracil infusion and radiation followed by surgical resection in regional localized stage III NSCLC. Ann. Thorac. Surg. 43:87-91; 1987.

156. Tennesen, P.; Fryd, V.; Hansen, M.; et al. Effect of nicotine chewing gum in combination with group counseling on the cessation of smoking. New Engl. J. Med. 318:15-18; 1988.

156a. Turrisi, A.T. Brain irradiation and systemic chemotherapy for small-cell lung cancer: Dangerous liaisons? J Clin Oncol 8(2):196-199; 1990.

157. Turrisi, A.T.; Glover, D.J.; Mason, B.; et al. Concurrent twice daily multifield radiotherapy and platinum-etoposide chemotherapy for limited small cell lung cancer update 87 (abstract). Proc. Am. Soc. Clin. Oncol. 6:172; 1987.

158. Van Houtte, P.; Henry, J. Preoperative and postoperative radiation therapy in lung cancer. Cancer Treatment. Symposia 2:57-62; 1985.

159. Van Houtte, P.; Rocmans, P.; Smets, P.; et al. Postoperative radiation therapy in lung cancer: a controlled trial after resection of curative design. Intl. J. Radiat. Oncol. Biol. Phys. 6:983-986; 1980.

160. Van Houtte, P.; Salazar, O.; Henry, J. Radiotherapy in non-small cell lung cancer: present progress and future prospectives. Eur. J. Cancer Clin. Oncol. 20:997-1006; 1984.

161. Vincent, R.G.; Pickren, J.W.; Lane, W.W.; et al. The changing histopathology of lung cancer. Cancer 39:1647-1655; 1977.

162. Vincent, R.G.; Takita, H.; Lane, W.E.; et al. Surgical therapy of lung cancer. J. Thorac. Cardiovasc. Surg. 71:581-591; 1976.

163. Vogl, S.E.; Hemta, C.R.; Cohen, M.H. MACC chemotherapy for adenocarcinoma and epidermoid carcinoma of the lung. Cancer 44:864-868; 1979.

164. Weiden, P.; Piantadosi, S. Preoperative chemotherapy in stage III non-small cell lung cancer: a phase II study of the lung study group (abstract). Proc Am Soc Clin Oncol 7:197; 1988.

165. Weisenberger, T.H. and Gail, M. et al. (LCSG) effects of postoperative mediastinal radiation on completely resected stage II and stage III epidermoid cancer of the lung (LCSG). New Engl. J. Med. 315:1377-1381;1986.

166. Wilkins, E.W.; Scannell, G.; Craver, J. Four decades of experience with resections for bronchogenic carcinoma at the Massachusetts General Hospital. J. Thorac. Cardiovasc. Surg. 76:364-368; 1978.

167. William, A.; Cormier, Y.; Murray, N.; et al. Chemotherapy can prolong survival in patients with advanced non-small cell lung cancer. Report of a Canadian multicenter randomized trial. J. Clin. Oncol. 6:633-641; 1988.

167a. Wolf, M.; Holle, R.; Hans, K.; et al. Analysis of prognostic factors in 766 patients with small cell lung cancer (SCLC): The role of sex as predictor for survival. Br J Canc. 63(6):986-992; 1991.

168. Wright, P.; Feld, R.; Mountain, C.; et al. A prospective double-blind clinical trial of intrapleural bacillus calmette-guerin (BCG) in patients with stage I non-small cell lung cancer. In: Salmon, S.E.; Jones, S.E., eds. Adjuvant therapy of cancer III. New York, NY: Grune & Stratton; 1981:265-276.

169. Wynder, E.L. Etiology of lung cancer: reflections on 2 decades of research. Cancer 30:1332-1339; 1972.

Charles D. Sherman, Jr., M.D., Surgical Oncology
Craig S. McCune, M.D., Medical Oncology

Philip Rubin, M.D., Radiation Oncology
Christopher B. Caldwell, M.D., Surgical Oncology

Chapter 32

MALIGNANT MELANOMAS

The analysis of many a success or failure (in cancer management) often reveals the important role played by the physician or physicians who dealt with the case in its inception and their decisive influence on the eventual result. Where temporizing guesswork, amateurish approaches, and defeatist attitudes may fail, intelligent understanding, prompt skillful treatment, and a hopeful, compassionate attitude may succeed.

Ackerman and del Regato (1)

PERSPECTIVE

Melanomas develop from melanocytes, which are derived from neural crest cells that migrate to the skin, eye, central nervous system, and occasionally elsewhere during fetal life. The relationship between pre-existing benign nevi and melanoma is not clear.

Although the average person has 20 moles on the body, each year only seven people out of every 100,000 develop a melanoma. Yet the incidence is rising rapidly, and because some 30% to 40% of these people will die (2), it is a serious problem. These lesions are clearly visible to patients and physicians alike, even in their earliest stages, and should be diagnosed long before they begin to metastasize. However, our education of both the public and professionals is not good, and late diagnosis is fairly common. Each physician must learn which of those 20 moles seen on the average patient who comes into the office may be malignant. The physician must also teach patients to recognize suspicious lesions (see Detection and Diagnosis section).

Treatment of early lesions by adequate excision carries minimal morbidity, and can result in near 100% cures. Treatment of late lesions is relatively ineffective for cure. Students should realize that the widely varying mortality reports found in the literature depend more on stage at diagnosis than variations in surgical and treatment technique (2).

EPIDEMIOLOGY AND ETIOLOGY

Data from Queensland, Australia (23) show clearly that there is an increase in melanoma in body sites that are exposed to the sun. The vast majority of melanomas seem to arise from preexisting benign nevi. This emphasizes the importance of watching for any changes in existing lesions. Recent epidemiologic studies (22) show that exposure to sunlight is a major risk factor for the development of malignant melanoma and that the incidence (in whites) increases steadily as one approaches the equator. Melanomas occur in all races. However, in blacks, they are rare, and are confined to nonpigmented skin, such as the palms and soles. There are minor differences in occurrence between males and females. Mela-

nomas rarely occur before puberty; they are most common during middle age. Fair-skinned and red-haired people are particularly prone. It has been estimated that 5% to 10% of all cases of malignant melanoma occur in a hereditary pattern. Two types of precursor lesions have been identified, the dysplastic nevus and the congenital nevus. Patients with these types are particularly identified by the familial dysplastic nevus syndrome (25), in which the risk of melanoma approaches 100% for some individuals. Those with dysplastic nevi in a nonfamilial pattern also have an increased risk for melanoma. Congenital nevi occur in approximately 1% of newborn children. It has been estimated that there is a 5% to 20% risk of melanoma in patients with large (> 2 cm) congenital nevi (22). The incidence of melanoma continues to rise, doubling every 15 years since 1925 (43) (Hollub, A., M.D. American Cancer Society, written communication, 1981).

DETECTION AND DIAGNOSIS

Early Detection

Educating the Physician and Patient

Early detection is possible in almost every case and depends on a knowledgeable physician and alert patient (32). To educate both physician and patient, there is no substitute for an atlas of photographs of early suspicious changes. In Queensland, Australia, a program of public and professional education on early detection has led to the remarkably high 5-year survival rate of 81% (23). Biopsy of any questionable lesion should be performed.

History

Melanoma developing in a pre-existing nevus may cause itching, or may bleed. Changes in size, thickness, color, or contour are important signs.

Physical Examination

Margins and surfaces are often irregular. Color of lesions varies from black to tan and translucent gray to red. Small dermal nodules nearby may be satellites. Complete examinations should include a search for satellite lesions, enlarged regional nodes, and hepatomegaly. Nodularity indicates vertical spread through the skin, an ominous sign.

Typical Appearances

There are three typical appearances (Table 32-1) (33).

1. *Lentigo maligna melanoma:* Lentigo maligna melanoma also refers to melanoma in Hutchinson's melanotic freckle (benign pigmented lesion), and tends to be on sun-exposed surfaces. This lesion grows radially, produces complex colors, and eventually penetrates focally in a vertical phase.

2. *Superficial spreading melanoma:* This is the most common type, constituting 60% to 70% of most series (2). It has a disorderly appearance in color and outline, and tends to have biphasic growth horizontally and vertically, presenting a "breaking up" appearance to the patient. It tends to ulcerate and bleed with growth.

3. *Nodular lesions* initially grow vertically, are of a uniform blue-black color, and are sharply delineated. To the patient they may look like blood blisters.

Atypical Sites

1. In blacks, cutaneous melanomas are usually seen only on the soles of the feet (usually the heel).

2. Nailbed melanoma can be confused with paronychia, pyogenic granuloma, and traumatic subungual hemorrhage.

3. Mucosal melanomas can be amelanotic, or can vary in color from tan to black. They are located in conjunctivae, nasal, vaginal, oral, and rectal mucosa.

4. Giant hairy nevi or blue nevi occasionally undergo malignant change.

5. Distant metastatic spread (as to the liver) with unknown primaries should lead to a search for choroid melanoma in the eye.

6. Initial presentation as a metastatic lesion, particularly in lymph nodes, without any evident primary site, occurs in approximately 10% of melanoma patients.

Diagnostic Procedures

Excisional biopsy with a margin of normal skin is recommended. Shave biopsies are to be discouraged, as this limits the pathologists' ability to determine the depth of penetration by the tumor (T-stage).

Some biopsy specimens are suspected to be melanoma, but cannot be diagnosed firmly by histopathologic appearance. *Monoclonal antibodies* such as S-100 are highly specific for melanoma antigens and can assist in this differential. Special stains for the presence of melanin are also useful when there is uncertainty.

CLASSIFICATION

T-Stage: Anatomic Staging (Table 32-2, Fig. 32-1) (1,4)

Melanoma is an excellent example of the usefulness of a method of classifying tumors that allows one to estimate the chance of regional node involvement and of ultimate distant metastases and death (3). This classification should lead to conclusions about the best treatment for each subclass when it is combined with the use of different treatment options for each subclass (27). Clark *et al.* (20) made an important contribution when they showed that the risk of node metastases and ultimate death were directly related to the depth of penetration of the various layers of the skin. In Clark's level I (20), the melanoma is confined to the epidermis, never metastasizes, and has a 100% cure rate. In level V the melanoma has penetrated through to the subdermal fat, has a 60% to 70% chance of regional node metastases, and only a 10% cure rate. Clark's level II is determined by microscopic analysis of penetration of epidermal basement membrane into the papillary dermis; level III by build-up of tumor at the interface between the papillary and reticular dermis; and level IV by extension of cells between the bundles of collagen fibers in the reticular dermis.

There was significant inconsistency among pathologists in accurately classifying the same lesion. Because of this, Breslow

---

Table 32-1. Differential Clinical and Histologic Features of Malignant Melanomas

Type of Melanoma	Location	Median Age (years)	Sex / Race Predilection	Duration *	Margin of Lesion	Color	% Incidence
Lentigo-maligna	Exposed surfaces-especially head and neck	70	None/Caucasian	5-15	Flat, irregular	Shades of brown, black; hypopigmentation (regression)	15
Superficial spreading	All body surfaces	56	Lower extremity/predominate in female / Caucasion	1-5	Palpable, irregular	Shades of brown, black; gray, pink; central or halo depigmentation	50
Nodular	All body surfaces	49	None /Caucasion	1-24 mo	Palpable	Uniform bluish black;	30
Palmar-Plantar-Mucosal	Palms, soles, mucous membrane	61	M:F=2:1/black	1-24 mo	Palpable nodule, irregular	Black nodules, irregularly colored	5

*Figures present common durations of various types; we have encountered neoplasms of each type with much shorter and much longer durations.

From Nihm et al. (33). Reprinted by permission of the New England Journal of Medicine.

Table 32-2. TNM Classification and Stage Grouping for Skin Melanoma

TNM	Classification	Clark Level		Stage	Grouping		
pT1	≤ 0.75 mm	Level II		Stage I	pT1	N0	M0
pT2	> 0.75 to 1.5 mm	Level III			pT2	N0	M0
pT3	> 1.5 to 4 mm	Level IV		Stage II	pT3	N0	M0
pT4	> 4.0 mm/satellites	Level V		Stage III	pT4	N0	M0
					Any pT	N1,N2	M0
N1	Regional ≤ 3 cm			Stage IV	Any pT	Any N	M1
N2	Regional > 3 cm and/or in-transit metastasis						

T = tumor; N = node; M = metastasis
From AJC/UICC (1,4).

adopted the technique of direct measurement of the thickness of the tumor in millimeters (17). Most pathologists have adopted the Breslow modification and find that it is reproducible and accurately separates melanomas into subgroups with increasing risk of nodal metastasis and poorer prognosis. Melanoma may spread within the dermal lymphatics and form new growths near the primary (satellites).

Differences

There are differences in the tumor T3-T4 category of tumor classification. Tumors of more than 1.5 mm but less than 3 mm in thickness and pT3b tumors of more than 3 mm but not

more than 4 mm in thickness. Instead of 3 mm, pT4 is 4 mm or greater and pT4b is inclusive of satellites within 2 cm of the primary. The (N) nodal categories have also changed so that there is now an N2a and b. The N2 catetory includes nodes greater than 3 cm, and N2b addresses intrinsic metastases in lymphatics; N2c encompasses both.

Staging Work-up

After excisional biopsy of a melanoma, the Clark-Breslow analysis gives one an immediate estimate of the likelihood of regional lymph node metastases as well as a reasonably clear long-range prognosis. For lesions less than 0.75 mm thick,

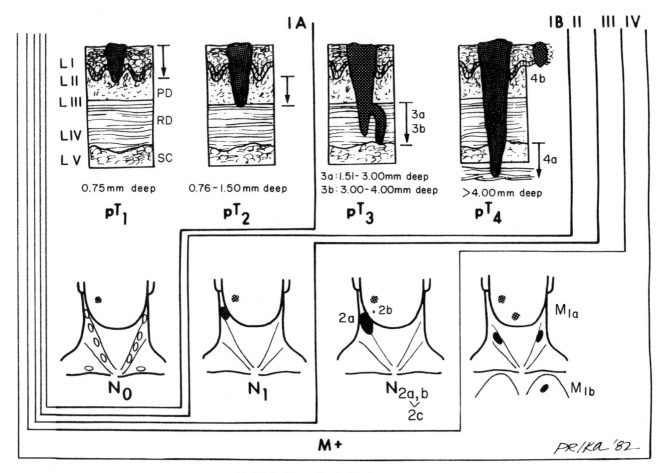

Fig. 32-1. Anatomic staging for melanoma.

there is a minimal risk of metastases and almost 100% curability. As the thickness of the lesion increases, the risk of regional node involvement and distant metastases increases steadily; the need to consider additional tests to evaluate the extent of the disease likewise increases. Routine radiographs and radioisotopic scans are advised to search for metastatic disease if the lesion is advanced and complaints suggest bone, brain, or liver metastases.

Recommended Procedures

1. History and physical examination as indicated above.
2. Routine laboratory data, including liver enzyme measurement.
3. Chest x-ray.
4. Computerized tomography: If advanced disease is probable, radioisotopic scans of bone, brain, and liver may be useful.

PRINCIPLES OF TREATMENT (Table 32-3)

Surgery

Melanoma remains essentially a surgically treated disease. Surgical resection should be used for both the primary tumor and any localized metastasis. Even distant metastasis (e.g. in brain) should be resected if it appears to be unifocal.

Primary Excision

Adequate resection of the primary lesions remains by far the most important chance for cure. For thin lesions (<1.5 mm thick) wide local excision with a 1-3 cm margin of grossly normal tissues is adequate (45). In some body areas, these defects can be closed primarily (28).

Therapeutic Node Dissection

Regional lymph node dissection should be considered for all patients who have clinically palpable regional lymph nodes, since approximately 30% of these patients can be cured by the regional lymphadenectomy (18). For patients who have clinically enlarged nodes and thick lesions (> 4.0 mm) the risk for distant metastases is high and the potential curative benefit of lymph node dissection is slim. The number of patients who are cured is probably small enough to not be statistically significant. Node dissection should be considered for locoregional control and palliation of any symptoms since it carries essentially no mortality. Since there are no effective alternative treatments, node dissections should be done in such patients unless there is clinical evidence of distant metastases.

Prophylactic Node Dissection

Regional lymph node dissection is recommended if there is a significant chance of node involvement (i.e., lesions > 1.5 mm thick) and no evidence of distant disease. There is controversy over this point (46,47), but this author (Charles D. Sherman) believes that the data show an increased survival in those patients treated by node dissection who have a significant risk of node involvement but are at a stage before there is any clinical evidence of such involvement. Patients with melanomas in sites with more than one drainage area (i.e., to neck, axilla, groin) are usually not considered for prophylactic node dissection, but should be watched carefully (every 1 to 2 months) and surgery should be done if nodes enlarge.

Hyperthermic Isolation Perfusion

Hyperthermic isolation perfusion consists of isolating the extremity with a tourniquet, inserting cannulas in the main artery and vein, and then perfusing the limb with highly concentrated chemotherapeutic agents using a pump oxygenator and thermal blanket to elevate the temperature of the limb. Stehlin *et al.* (40) are among the principal advocates of adding such perfusions to the primary treatment. For upper extremity melanomas, node dissections for levels III, IV, and V (> 1.5 mm thick) are done. If the lesion is distal to the elbow and frozen section shows node metastases, a perfusion also is done. For lower extremity melanomas, perfusion is done for all levels III, IV, and V lesions, but prophylactic node dissection is done only if the primary lesion is near the groin. Stehlin *et al.* (40) note that survival is significantly better using hyperthermic perfusions for extremity lesions—adding hyperthermia gives much better results than perfusion alone.

			(13,23,23a,28,35a,38a,46,47)
Table 32-3. **Multidisciplinary Treatment Decisions: Malignant Melanomas**			
Stage	**Surgery**	**Radiation Therapy**	**Chemotherapy**
I	Adequate resection	NR	IC II or IM
	2-3 cm margin	NR	
	No elective node dissection		
II	Radical resection	NR	IC II or IM
	3-5 cm margin	NR	
	Elective node dissection, optional		
III	3-5 cm margin	NR	IC II or IM
	Therapeutic node dissection		
IV	As above if feasible and few metastases	If unresectable, PRT 30-60 Gy and hyperthermia	IC II
Recurrence	Re-excision if possible with margin	If recurrence and resect post-op ART 30-50 Gy	IC II

RT = radiation therapy; ART = adjuvant; PRT = palliative; NR = not recommended;
IM = immunotherapy; IL-2 = interleukin-2; LAK = lymphokine activated killer cells;
IC II = investigational chemotherapy, phase I/II clinical trials.

PDQ: NR - IC II = DTIC/ McCCNU IL-2/LAK

Perfusion can produce regression of recurrent melanoma on extremities; however, an alternative approach, surgical resection, may be equally efficacious and have a lower complication rate. As an adjuvant to standard surgical approaches, for newly diagnosed primary melanoma lesions, this approach remains investigational.

Head and Neck Melanomas

Because of anatomic restrictions, smaller margins of normal tissues are sometimes justified, but because surgery gives essentially the only chance for cure, adequate excisions are necessary. Resection of enlarged nodes in front of the ear, in the parotid, and in the neck may be necessary.

Complications of surgery include an increased incidence of wound complications and often permanent edema from ilioinguinal dissection, necessitating support stockings.

Subungual melanomas require amputation of the digit.

Radiation Therapy (26,35,42)

Most melanomas are considered radioresistant. Radiation therapy in general is not recommended for treatment for primary or regional nodes, or as adjuvant therapy.

There is interest in exploring high daily fractional doses for recurrent locoregional disease or metastasis. Doses of 600 cGy delivered once or twice a week to moderate levels of 2,000 to 3,000 cGy are more effective than smaller fractional doses of 200 to 500 cGy to similar or even higher dose levels of 3,000 to 5,000 cGy (44). Although the radiobiologic mechanism for this response is presumed to be a result of a large shoulder on an irradiation dose-response curve (25), there are numerous variations in the *in vivo* response. Most controlled clinical trials have not shown this advantage for fractional doses which can be compensated by greater total doses. In an RTOG study by Sause *et al.* (38a), using large fractionated doses of 8.0 Gy x 20, no difference in the local control rates were found.

Chemotherapy (Table 32-4 and Table 32-5)

There is no successful chemotherapeutic agent or combination that has consistently yielded regressions in metastatic melanomas (30).

Response rates for most agents have been low. Dacarbazine has proven to be the most active agent and yields responses in 20% to 25% of patients (16,23). The mean duration of response, however, is only 4 to 5 months.

Many unsuccessful attempts have been made to combine active single agents in the treatment of melanoma. Recently, some newer combinations have shown more promise. Two groups have achieved a 50% response rate with dacarbazine, cisplatin, carmustine, and tamoxifen (29).

When deciding whether chemotherapy is appropriate for a particular patient, the likelihood of a response and its probable duration must be weighed against the toxicity of the regimen chosen. Patients with poor performance status and those with liver or brain metastases rarely respond.

Immunotherapy

In recent years, four developing immunologic therapies have been applied to the treatment of melanoma with some degree of success.

1. *Interleukin-2/lymphokine-activated killer cells*: This treatment involves removing and separating a large number of a patient's lymphocytes by leukapheresis. These cells are then incubated in the laboratory with their growth factor, interleukin-2 (IL-2). This produces growth of a population of cells called lymphokine-activated killer cells (LAK). After preparation of these cells in the laboratory, they are transfused back to the same patient, along with high doses of the IL-2 to support the survival of the lymphocytes. Responses were seen in 23% of melanoma patients; however, comparison with administration of IL-2 alone suggests that this is equally effective (38). Durable remissions have been reported in a small subset of patients (8%) after being treated with IL-2 and LAK, with a 24-month follow-up, however, there is high toxicity—34% to 52% (14). Although continuous infusion high-dose IL-2 + LAK may be less toxic than bolus high-dose IL-2 + LAK, the continuous infusion schedule appears to be less effective (23a).

2. Monoclonal antibodies directed at melanoma cell surface antigens are also under investigation. Some responses have been observed in clinical trials (39). Allergic reactions are a problem that may be overcome in the transition to human monoclonal antibodies.

3. Vaccines for the induction of active specific immunotherapy are under investigation. In this approach, melanoma tumor cells are incorporated into a vaccine and injected intradermally. Responses have been seen in vaccines using the patient's own tumor cells (16) and in those using melanoma cells from cultured lines (31).

Table 32-4. Metastatic Melanoma: Responses to Chemotherapy			
Group	**Treatment**	**(%) Response Rate**	**Reference**
	DTIC	12-28	
ECOG	DTIC	14	13a
	DTIC + Methyl-CCNU	14	
	Methyl-CCNU	15	
COG	DTIC	17	38a
	DTIC + CCNU	18	
	DTIC + BCNU + VCR	22	
	DTIC + BCNU + HU	10.9	

DTIC = dacarbazine; VCR = vincristine; HU = hydroxyurea; ECOG = Eastern Cooperative Oncology Group; COG = Central Oncology Group.
Adapted from Constaza et al. (21).

Table 32-5. Results Adjuvant Therapy for Melanoma			
Group	**No. Patient**	**Treatments Evaluated**	**Results**
COG	174	DTIC Control	No benefit of DTIC
WHO/Melanoma Group	761	DTIC BCG DTIC + BCG Control	No difference
NCI	181	Methyl-CCNU BCG BCG+TCV Control	No difference
SEG	136	C. Parvum DTIC + C. Parvum	No difference
GIF, France	248	BCG BCG + CCNU, DTIC, VM-26	No difference
SWOG	217	BCNU, hydroxyurea, TIC (BHD)	BHD alone better than combined with BCG
EORTC	200	DTIC Levamisole Control	No difference
SEG	260	C. parvum Control	Survival benefit for melanomas > 3 mm (p=0.01)
SEG	237	BCG C. parvum	No difference
ECOG	98	BCG Control	No difference

COG = Central Oncology Group; WHO = World Health Organization; NCI = National Cancer Institute; SEG = Southeastern Cancer Study Group; GIF = ; SWOG = Southwestern Cancer Study Group; EORTC = European Organization for Research and Therapy of Cancer ; ECOG = Eastern Cooperative Oncology Group; DTIC = dacarbazine; BCG = bacillus Calmette-Guerin; TCV = ; VM-26 = vincristine; BHD = carmustine (BCNU), hydroxyurea, dacarbazine; CCNU = Lomustine; C.parvum = Corynebacterium parvum.
Adapted from DeVita et al. (9).

The response duration for some of these patients is beyond 3 years.

4. The interferon preparations have been evaluated extensively for melanoma. Although responses occur, they are only in about 15% of patients and are not long-lasting (19).
5. Intralesional Bacille Calmette-Guerin achieves complete local control of advanced melanoma in 67% of patients and may lead to long-term survival in 27% of complete responders with recurrent melanoma consisting of intransit or subcutaneous foci (15).

SPECIAL TREATMENT CONSIDERATIONS

Recurrence and spread: Melanoma may run an unpredictable course; therefore, it is worthwhile to be aggressive in treating recurrences. Skin nodules, nodes, and soft tissue metastases may be re-excised if they are solitary and localized (34).

Metastases: Virtually all organs are at risk and metastases can spread to such sites as brain, lung, and liver. As noted above, if metastases can be resected without leaving residual disease, that is, by far, the treatment of choice (34). Resection of metastases to the gastrointestinal tract (especially if there is bleeding) may be indicated.

For multiple recurrences limited to an extremity, isolation perfusion can give effective long-term local control.

Uveal melanomas are highly curable by proton beam irradiation. This method avoids cataract production, and saves the eye and vision. Tumor control is as high as 90% (24).

Mucosal melanomas tend to be more radiosensitive and radiocurable. In accessible sites, irradiation is often combined with surgery preoperatively or postoperatively.

RESULTS AND PROGNOSIS

Survival by stage. Typical 10-year survival curves are illustrated by stage, survival is reported at higher than 80% for stage I, 50% or higher for stage II, 25% or higher for stage III, and 10% or higher for stage IV. (Fig. 32-2)

Survival after treatment for cutaneous melanoma depends on the biology of the particular lesion, the degree to which it has penetrated the skin and spread to other tissues or organs, the patient's sex, and the primary site (13). In Australia, where melanoma is more common and the public is alerted, age-adjusted survival figures for 5 years are over 80% for an entire series of 1,187 patients (23). Women have a 5% to 10% higher survival rate than do men.

For *superficial melanomas* (≤ 1.5 mm thick), 5- and 10-year survival rates are 95% or higher. Survival rates of patients whose lymph nodes are already involved at the time of first diagnosis drop to 30% to 40% at 5 years.

For *invasive melanomas*, the level and vertical thickness determine the 10-year survival (Fig. 32-3). The presence of ulceration reduces the 5-year survival in stage II patients from 55% to 15% (17).

For *nodal metastases* (5) the 5-year survival drops from 73% (negative nodes) for stage I patients to 24% (positive nodes)

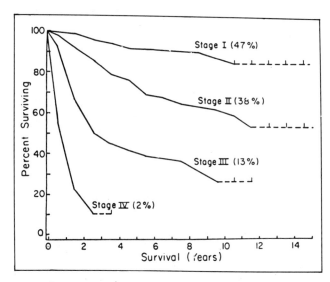

Fig. 32-2. Results by Stage: Fifteen-year survival results for more than 4000 melanoma patients treated at the University of Alabama in Birmingham and the Sydney Melanoma Group who are subgrouped according to the new four-stage system proposed by the American Joint Commission on Cancer. The distribution of patients is shown in parentheses. Note that the patients with clinically localized melanoma (Stage I by the original three-stage system) have now been divided into two stages according to tumor thickness and level of invasion (newly designated Stages I and II). From Ketcham *et al.* (27), with permission.

for stage II patients. For patients in clinical stage I but also pathologic stage II (as a result of nodal involvement found histologically), the 5-year survival is 48%.

1. For synchronous versus metachronous nodes, the delay in appearance of metastases until 3 years is a more favorable prognostic sign; that is, 60% versus 37% survival for simultaneous nodes and primary. Both groups ultimately metastasize and patients die; the 10-year survival is less than 20% (6).
2. The number of involved nodes affects outcome; if one node is involved, the 5-year survival is 60%, versus about 10% if four or more nodes are involved (6).

For *elective nodal (prophylactic) dissections*, the controversy lies in the report of Veronesi *et al.* (46) of a randomized trial in which no significant advantage was found for nodal dissections for extremity lesions (Fig. 32-4). For subgroups such as those with level IV lesions, a difference was found in favor of nodal dissections, that is, 70% 5-year survival for patients having excision with nodal dissection versus 58% for patients having excision alone, but it was not statistically significant. Many historical controls show a distinct advantage for elective node dissections: Balch *et al.* (6) found 100% vs 25% survival in level IV.

CLINICAL INVESTIGATIONS

1. High-dose chemotherapy combined with autologous bone marrow transplants is under study (41).
2. Optimal fractionation of radiation dose (high dose versus standard dose) is also being studied. Some of the more frequently advocated schedules are:
   - 3 x 800 cGy/wk to 2,400 ccGy
   - 6 x 600 cGy/biweekly to 3,600 cGy
   - 20 x 200 cGy/d to 4,000 cGy

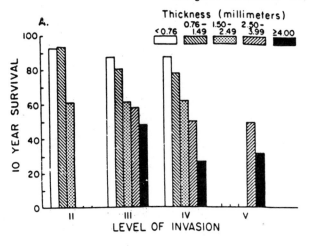

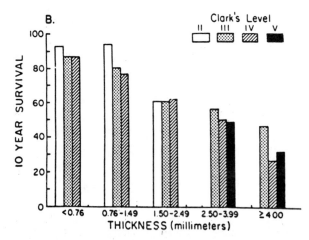

Fig. 32-3. Results: Comparison of two microstaging methods (tumor thickness versus level of invasion. Top. Ten-year survival rates for Stage I melanoma patients according to levels of invasion subgrouped by tumor thickness. There were statistically significant differences in survival rates for patients with lesions of various thicknesses within levels III, IV, and V. Bottom. Ten-year survival rates for Stage I melanoma patients according to tumor thickness subgrouped by levels of invasion. There were no statistically significant differences in survival rates for patients with lesions of various levels of invasion within each thickness subgroup. From Balch *et al.* (13), with permission.

3. Treatment with monoclonal antibodies conjugated to toxins or radioisotopes, infusions of laboratory-cultured, tumor-infiltrating lymphocytes with IL-2 (14,36), and administration of vaccines for active specific immunotherapy are immunologic areas under investigation.
4. Phase II trials with Taxol are in progress (27a).

Recommended Reading

Recent review and update can be found as chapters in major oncologic textbooks such as Balch *et al.* in DeVita (9). Some of the classic references are noted: Clark *et al.* (2) present a well-illustrated collection of scientific and clinical writings on human malignant melanoma. This is partially presented in *Seminars in Oncology* (5). The modification of Clark's levels (20) to thickness of lesion by Breslow (17) and Balch *et al.* (11) constitutes the basis for current classification schema and

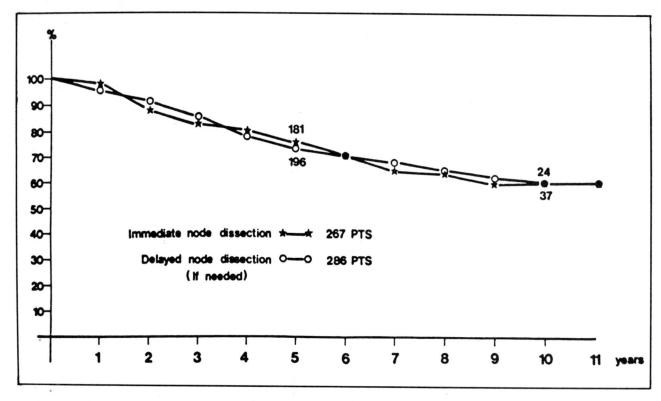

Fig. 32-4. Results: Immediate versus Delayed Node Dissection. Survival of 553 patients with Stage I and Stage II melanoma of the extremities (World Health Organization WHO Melanoma Group Study Trial #1), analyzed according to initial surgical treatment. There was no survival advantage for elective immediate node dissection in this group of patients overall. From Veroniesi *et al.* (47), with permission.

determines incidence of lymph node metastases, distant spread, and 5-year survival. The Australian study by Davis *et al.* (23) is essential from the educator's point of view. For the pros and cons of surgical dissection, refer to the writings of Balch (6,10-12) and Veronesi (46,47).

REFERENCES

General References

1. American Joint Committee on Staging and End-Results Reporting (AJC) Manual for Staging of Cancer. Chicago, IL: AJC; 1978.
2. Clark WH Jr.; Goldman LI; Mastrangelo MJ. Human Malignant Melanoma. New York, NY: Grune and Stratton; 1979.
3. International Histologic Classification of Tumors, Nos. 1-20. Geneva: World Health Organization; 1978.
4. International Union Against Cancer. TNM Classification of Malignant Tumors, 4th ed. New York, NY: Springer-Verlag: 83-88; 1987.
5. Yarbro JW; Clark WH Jr.; Bornstein RS, *et al.*, eds. Human cutaneous malignant melanoma. Semin Oncol. 2:81-188; 1975.

Specific References

6. Balch CM. Surgical management of regional lymph nodes in cutaneous melanoma. J Am Acad Dermatol. 3:511-524; 1980.
7. Balch CM. The role of elective lymph node dissection in melanoma: rationale, results, and controversies. J Clin Oncol. 6:163-172; 1988.
8. Balch CM, Hersey P. Current status of adjuvant therapy. In: Balch CM, Milton GW, eds. Cutaneous Melanoma: Clinical Management and Treatment Results Worldwide. Philadelphia, PA: J.B. Lippincott Co: 197; 1985.
9. Balch CM, Houghton A, Peters L. Cutaneous melanoma. In: DeVita VT Jr, Hellman S, Rosenberg SA, ed. Cancer: Principles and Practice of Oncology, 3rd ed. Philadelphia, PA: J.B. Lippincott Co: 1499-1542; 1989.
10. Balch CM, Murad TM, Soong S, *et al.* A multifactorial analysis of melanoma. Ann Surg. 188:732-742; 1978.
11. Balch CM, Murad TM, Soong S, *et al.* Tumor thickness as a guide to surgical management of clinical stage I melanoma patients. Cancer. 43:883-888; 1979.
12. Balch CM, Soong S, Murad TM, *et al.* A multifactorial analysis of melanoma. Prognostic factors in melanoma patients with lymph node metastases (stage III). Ann Surg. 193:377-388; 1981.
13. Balch CM, Soong SJ, Shaw HM, *et al.* An analysis of prognostic factors in 4,000 patients with cutaneous melanoma. In: Balch CM, Mildon GW, eds. Cutaneous Melanoma: Clinical Management and Treatment Results Worldwide. Philadelphia, PA: J.B. Lippincott Co: 332; 1985.
14. Bar MH, Sznol M, Atkins MB, *et al.* Metastatic malignant melanoma treated with combined bolus and continous infusion of interleukin-2 and lymphokine-activated killer cells. J Clin Oncol. 8(7):1138-1147; 1990.
15. Bauer R, Kopald K, Lee J, Wong J, Morton D. Long term results of intralesional *BCG* for locally advanced recurrent melanoma. Proc Am Soc Clin Oncol. (Abstract); 9:276; 1990.
16. Berd, D.; Maquire, H.C.; Mastrangelo, M.J. Induction of cell-mediated immunity to autologous melanoma cells and regression of metastases after treatment with a melanoma cell vaccine preceded by cyclophosphamide. Cancer Res. 46:2572-2577; 1986.
17. Breslow, A. Thickness, cross-sectional areas, and depth of invasion in the prognosis of cutaneous melanoma. Ann Surg. 172:902-908; 1970.
18. Calabro, A.; Singletary, S.E.; Balch, C.M. Patterns of relapse in 1001 consecutive patients with melanoma nodal metastases. Arch Surg. 124:1051-1055; 1989.
19. Clark JW, Longo DL. Interferons in cancer therapy. In: DeVita VT, Hellman S, Rosenberg SA, eds. Updates. Philadelphia, PA: J.B. Lippincott Co: 1-16; 1987.
20. Clark WH Jr, From L, Bernardino EA, *et al.* The histogenesis and biologic behavior of primary human malignant melanomas of the skin. Cancer Res. 29:705-726; 1969.
21. Constanza ME, Nathanson L, Schoenfeld D, *et al.* Results with

methyl-CCNU and DTIC in metastatic melanoma. Cancer. 40:1010-1015;1977.

22. Cutler SJ, Young JL, eds. Third National Cancer Survey. Incidence Data. NCI Monogr. 41:1-454; 1975.

23. Davis NC, McLeod GR, Beardmore GL, *et al*. Primary cutaneous melanoma: a report from the Queensland melanoma project. CA. 26:80- 107; 1976.

23a. Dutcher, J.P.; Gaynor, E.R.; Boldt, D.H.; *et al*. A phase II study of high-dose continuous infusion interleukin-2 with lymphokine-activated killer cells in patients with metastatic melanoma. J Clin Oncol. 9(4):641-648; 1991.

24. Gragoudas ES, Goiten M, Verhey L, *et al*. Proton beam irradiation: an alternative to enucleation for intraocular melanomas. Ophthalmology. 87:571-581; 1980.

25. Greene MH, Clark WH, Tucker MA, Elder DE, Kraemer KH, Guerry D, Witmer KW, Thompson J, Matozzo I, Fraser MC. Acquired precursors of cutaneous malignant melanoma. The familial dysplastic nevus syndrome. N Engl J Med. 213:91-97; 1985.

26. Habermaiz, H.J.; Fischer, J.J.; Radiation therapy of malignant melanoma: experience with high individual treatment doses. Cancer. 38:2250-2262; 1976.

27. Ketcham AS, Balch CM. Classification and staging systems. In: Balch CM, Milton GW, eds. Cutaneous Melanoma: Clinical Management and Treatment Results Worldwide. Philadelphia, PA: J.B. Lippincott Co: 55, 216; 1985.

27a. Legha, S.S.; Ring, S.; Papadopoulos, N.; *et al*. A phase II trial of taxol in patients with malignant melanoma. Invest New Drugs 9(1):59-64; 1991.

28. Mastrangelo JH, Baker AR, Katz HR. Cutaneous melanoma. In: DeVita VT, Hellman S, Rosenberg SA, eds. Cancer: Principles and Practice of Oncology. 2nd ed. Philadelphia, PA: JB Lippincott Co: 1371-1422; 1985.

29. McClay ER, Mastrangelo MJ, Bellet RE, Berd D. Combination chemotherapy and hormonal therapy in the treatment of malignant melanoma. Cancer Treat Rep. 71:465-469; 1987.

30. McCune CA. Malignant melanoma. In: Rosenthal SN, Bennett JM, eds. Practical Cancer Chemotherapy. New York, NY: Medical Examination Publishing Co: 373-384; 1981.

31. Mitchell MS, Kan-Mitchell J, Kempf RA, Harel W, Shau H, Lind S. Active specific immunotherapy for melanoma: phase I trial of allogeneic lysates and a novel adjuvant. Cancer Res. 48:5883-5893; 1988.

32. Nathanson L. Etiology, detection, and diagnosis of melanoma. Curr Concepts Oncol. 5:1-7; 1982.

33. Nihm MC, Clark WH, From L. The clinical diagnosis, classification, and histogenic concepts of the early stages of cutaneous malignant melanomas. N Engl J Med. 284:1078-1082; 1971.

34. Overett TK, Shiu MH. Surgical treatment of distant metastic melanoma: Indications and results. Cancer. 56:1222-1230; 1985.

35. Overgaard J. Radiation treatment of malignant melanoma. Intl J Radiat Oncol Biol Phys. 6:41-44; 1980.

36. Quirt IC, Tannock IF. Interleukin-2 for metastatic melanoma: Treating polyuria with insulin. J Clin Oncol. 8(7):1125-1127; 1990.

37. Rige DS, Koof AW, Friedman R. The rate of malignant melanoma in the U.S.: are we making an impact? J Am Acad of Dermatol. 17(6):1050-1053; 1987.

38. Rosenberg RA, Lotze MT, Muul LM, *et al*. Progress report on the treatment of 157 patients with advanced cancer using lymphokine-activated killer cells and interleukin-2 or high-dose interleukin-2 alone. N Engl J Med. 316:879-905; 1987.

38a. Sause, W.T.; Cooper, J.S.; Rush, S.; Ago, C.T.; Cosmatos, D.; Coughlin, C.T.; JanJan, N.; Lipsett, J. Fraction size in external beam radiation therapy in treatment of melanoma. Int J Radiat Oncol Biol Phys. 20:429-432; 1991.

39. Spitler LE, de Rio M, Khentigan A, *et al*. Therapy of patients with malignant melanoma using monoclonal antimelanoma antibody-ricin A chain immunotoxin. Cancer Res. 47:1717-1723; 1987.

40. Stehlin JS Jr, Giovanella BC, de Ipolyi PD, *et al*. Results of hyperthermic perfusion for melanoma of the extremities. Surg Gynecol Obstet. 140:339-348; 1975.

41. Stitt JA, Neidhart JA, Stidley C. Effects of radiation therapy on patients receiving dose intensive chemotherapy with granulocyte-colony stimulating factor (G-SCF) and granulocyte-monocyte stimulating factor (GM-CSF). Abstract. Proc Am Soc Clin Oncol. 9:284;1990.

42. Strauss A, Dritschilo A, Nathanson L, *et al*. Radiation therapy of malignant melanomas: an evaluation of clinically used fractionation schemes. Cancer. 47:1252-1256; 1981.

43. Straus SMB, ed. Familiar Medical Quotations. Boston, MA: Little Brown and Co; 1968.

44. Trott KR, von Lieven H, Kummermehr J, *et al*. The radiosensitivity of malignant melanomas, part I: experimental studies. Intl J Radiat Oncol Biol Phys. 7:9-13; 1981.

45. Urist, MM, Balch CM, Soong SJ, *et al*. The influence of surgical margins and prognostic factors predicting the risk of local recurrence in 3445 patients with primary cutaneous melanoma. Cancer. 55:1398-1402; 1985.

46. Veronesi U, Adamus J, Bandiera DC, *et al*. Inefficacy of immediate node dissection in stage I melanoma of the limbs. N Engl J Med. 297:627-630; 1977.

47. Veronesi U, Adamus J, Bandiera DC, Brennhoud O, Caceres E, Cascinelli M, Claudio F, Ikonopisov RL, Javorski VV, Morabito A, Rode I, Sergeev S, Van Slooten E, Szczygiel K, Trapeznikov NN, Wagner RI. Delayed regional lymph node dissection in stage I melanoma of the skin of the lower extremities. Cancer. 49: 2420; 1982.

Charles W. Scarantino, M.D., Ph.D.,
  Radiation Oncology
LeRoy G. Hoffman, M.D., Radiation Oncology

Robert D. Ornitz, M.D., Radiation Oncology
David S. Enterline, M.D., Radiology

Chapter **33**

METASTASES AND DISSEMINATED DISEASE

Omnis cellula e cellula.

Virchow (93)

PERSPECTIVE

The American Cancer Society estimates there will be one million new cases of cancer diagnosed in 1989 (81). Approximately 30% of patients will have detectable metastases at the time of first diagnosis (excluding skin other than melanoma) and 60% to 70% will develop metastatic disease at some time prior to death.

The patient with metastatic disease poses one of the most challenging problems in oncology, as it involves therapeutic and supportive disciplines. Current therapeutic maneuvers, in general, have been ineffective in eliminating overt disease (1). Therefore, most patients will need palliative and supportive care. The therapeutic approach will vary according to tumor burden, presence of symptoms, performance status, and temporal development of progressive disease. The relief of symptoms caused by the presence of metastatic disease will become a paramount clinical priority. In addition, nutritional and psychosocial support needs will have to be addressed to maintain a reasonable quality of life.

Clearly, each aspect must be evaluated and focused to familiarize personnel involved in the care of the cancer patient if a multidisciplinary treatment approach of the whole patient is to be used.

Epidemiology

1. The four most favored sites of metastatic disease are bone, lung, brain, and liver. The most common malignancies responsible for metastases to four major organs are summarized in Table 33-1.
2. The temporal identification of metastases differs significantly between time of diagnosis and autopsy (Table 33-2). This may be related to either inadequate screening methods or actual increase in metastatic deposits occurring with time.
3. Bone metastases arise commonly from carcinoma of the prostate, thyroid, lung, breast, and kidney, as 50% or more patients show this dissemination pattern.
4. Lung metastases are seen most commonly in carcinoma of the breast and kidney (50% incidence), followed by melanomas, sarcomas, and probably the gastrointestinal (GI) tract.

5. Liver metastases are common in carcinoma of the GI tract, pancreas, lung, and breast.
6. Brain metastases may frequently present as solitary lesions and most commonly arise from the lung, colon, and kidney.

Etiology

In the last 2 decades there has been an increase in our knowledge of the pathogenesis of metastases without concomitant improvement in treatment results. The majority of deaths from cancer are probably related to the inherent resistance of tumor cells to cytotoxic therapies (22). The single most important property of tumor cells responsible for the lack of response is the biologic heterogeneity of the primary tumor and its metastases. Heterogeneity is not limited to one property, but is a manifestation of a number of cellular properties, including karyotypes, receptors, morphology, cell surface enzymes, growth properties, and finally the ability to invade and produce metastases.

The mechanism of metastases is a complex function that transcends the humoral theory (tumor disseminating through humoral substances) and mechanical theory (the release of cells by simple pressure phenomena). Rather, current interest centers on more active mechanisms by which tumors can cross specific host barriers. Liotta (51) suggested that metastasis "results from a complex cascade of active biochemical and cellular processes" (Table 33-3).

Suggested Steps in Development of Metastases

Premetastatic: Genetic alterations of DNA result from oncogene activation and amplification with production of autocrine growth factors and autonomy from host microenvironment. The resultant cell population may manifest or exhibit many enzymatic metabolic and molecular perturbations that result in critical membrane-associated changes (61), such as the activation of c-erb genes which codes a receptor for epidermal growth factor and transforming growth factor alpha which is secreted by tumor cells (29).

Metastases: The constant tumor-host interactions within the tumor microenvironment result in a breakdown of

677

Table 33-1. Primary Clinically Important Metastatic Patterns

Primary Site	Lung	Liver	Bone	Brain
Rectum	+	+		
Melanoma	+	+		
Wilm's	+	+		
Ovary	+	+		
Ewing's	+		+	
Thyroid	+		+	
Breast	+		+	+
Bladder	+	+	+	
Unknown primary	+	+	+	
Lung	+	+	+	+
Neuroblastoma	+			
Head and Neck	+			
Testis	+			
Kidney	+			
Sarcoma	+			
Uterus	+			
Cervix	+			
Colon		+		
Stomach		+		
Pancreas		+		
Prostate			+	

constraints inherent in normal tissue architecture and in the formation of malignant cells capable of surviving in a normal milieu.

1. Angiogenesis: Formation of blood supply by tumor through release of an angiogenic factor(s) (26).
2. Invasion into host stroma accompanied by lysis of host basement membrane and connective tissue through the release of enzymes such as cathepsin B, plasminogen activator, and collagenase (42,52,82).
3. Intravasation: Cells gain access to the lymphatic and blood vessel systems and disseminate: experimental evidence indicates that 24 hours after gaining access to circulation less than 1% of all cells are viable and less than 0.1% of the cells will survive to form metastases (21).

Table 33-3. Summary of Development of Metastases*

Premetastatic
    Oncogene activation and amplification
Metastases
    Angiogenesis
    Invasion—lysis of host basement membrane
    Intravasation—cell gain access to vascular system
    Arrest—escape or discharge of tumor cells
    Extravasation—selective adherence to endothelial cells

*See text for details.

4. Arrest: Nonspecific arrest of cell emboli and formation of adhesion between tumor cells and small vessel endothelial cells (60).
5. Extravasation: Escape or discharge of metastasized tumor cells from circulation occurs by mechanisms similar to those responsible for invasion (see (b), above). Tumor cells (1) may recognize tissue specific motility factors, (2) may respond to organ-specific factors (64), or (3) produce their own growth factors (autocrine stimulation) (29). They also show affinity for a type IV collagen and may secrete collagenase to facilitate invasion (52).

Several additional factors relate to tumor metastases. For example, tumor cell populations are heterogeneous with respect to their metastatic capabilities (7); tumor metastases are probably clonal in origin and arise from a single progenitor (88,65); the subpopulation of cells with the greatest metastatic potential can change following perturbation (67); and the predilection of the primary tumor for specific organ sites seems to be selective and as such may rely on a match of the seed (tumor) and soil (organ) for growth (40,57). Finally Muschel and Liotta discuss the role of oncogenes in metastases (58a).

DETECTION AND DIAGNOSIS

The detection and confirmation of metastatic disease are the most important determinants in clinical decision-making regarding appropriate therapy, including choice of modality(s), intensity of therapy, and duration. Metastatic work-up is mandatory for appropriate and accurate staging. Data accession from staging allows for reliable reporting of tumor incidence by codification of presenting disease burden as well as the scientific assessment of efficacy of any given treatment strategy. An obvious corollary is that it is imperative for the

Table 33-2. Incidence of Metastases At Diagnosis and Autopsy*

	Metastatic Site							
	% BONE		% BRAIN		% LUNG		% LIVER	
Site of Primary	DIAGNOSIS	AUTOPSY	DIAGNOSIS	AUTOPSY	DIAGNOSIS	AUTOPSY	DIAGNOSIS	AUTOPSY
Lung	16 (38)+	20–36	18–28 (8–14)+	18–37 (42)+		21–60	17	25–48 (74)+
Breast	20–40	44–73	15	9–20		59–69		56–65
Prostate	20–40	50–70	<1	2	5.0	15–53	1	5–13
Kidney	6–10	24–50	4	7–8	5–30	50–75	13	27–40
Bladder	5	12–25	<1	<1	5–10	25–30	>5	30–50
Testis (germinal)	<1	20	<1	<10	2–12	70–80	<1	50–80
Colon-rectum	<1	22	4	8	<5	25–40	20–24	60–71
Cervix	<1	8–20	<1	2–3	<5	20–30	<1	20–35
Ovary	<1	9	<1	<1	<5	5–10	<5	10–15
Uterus	<1	5–12	<1	<5	<1	30–40	<1	10–30

*Numbers represent estimates from several sources (1,53,59).
†Represents values for small cell carcinoma.

oncologist to have a firm understanding of the natural history of a given tumor as well as the pathophysiologic mechanisms by which it disseminates. The behavior of a verrucous carcinoma of the floor of mouth will not parallel that of a poorly differentiated squamous carcinoma of the tonsillar fossa or a mantle zone lymphoma of the pharyngeal tongue.

A somewhat more pragmatic and current concept regarding metastatic evaluation transcends the purity of scientific medicine and relates to the current medicoeconomic crisis facing all practicing physicians. With the exponential growth of medical knowledge, the development of sophisticated procedures bestows the inexorable concomitant of rising medical costs. Recently published data relating to Medicare reimbursement confirmed that a majority of expenditure occurs during the last 3 months of a patient's clinical course. In such cases when a tumor burden is catastrophically overwhelming, each physician must decide on an individual and personal level when it no longer is cost-effective or humane to submit a patient to complex and expensive treatment strategies that have negligible probability of palliating or improving quality of life. Unfortunately, some common tumors, such as malignant melanoma, when widely disseminated are still largely untreatable even with the most aggressive biologic and combined therapies.

The astounding developments in oncogenetics, dating back to the original work of Jacob and Monod (41) have begun to open the door to our understanding of the genetic control of tumor induction and growth. Our preliminary understanding of the molecular basis of malignant transformation will undoubtedly lead to new concepts in biologic therapy, but as importantly, to newer and more refined means to use existing modalities such as sequencing of radiation and cytotoxic drug interface, development of new agents (chemotherapy), genetic engineering of new biologics to regulate oncogene expression or repression, and refinement in the use of such physical agents as thermal radiotherapy. The art of medicine will not necessarily yield to the science of medicine, but rather a more balanced understanding will lead to improved cure rates, disease-free survival, and quality of life. However, with all the future holds in terms of scientific discovery, the traditional methodologies of medical evaluation will still play a paramount role in diagnosis.

Clinical Detection

There is simply no substitute for the classical medical history and physical examination to provide initial narrative data and findings to focus a staging (metastatic) work-up. Often one needs only the time to listen carefully to allow a patient to essentially self-diagnose. As John Milton observed that "he also serves who stands and waits," so the astute oncologist need only incorporate historical information from the patient or family member to chart an initial diagnostic course. This information, integrated with physical findings such as the presence of palpable lymphadenopathy, organomegaly, cutaneous exanthems, and localizing neurologic signs can often lead almost immediately to either an initial diagnosis of malignancy or suspected pattern of metastatic dissemination.

The importance of the classical history and physical examination becomes even more relevant if one is to not only consider the classical description of tumor pathophysiology (e.g., lung cancer most commonly disseminates to bone, liver, central nervous system (CNS), or adrenal glands), but

how this behavior has been modified with the advent of successful systemic therapy that allows patients to survive long enough to express highly unusual patterns of metastatic involvement. Such examples personally observed have been colon cancer metastases to bone marrow as the first site of dissemination and breast cancer biopsy-proven to involve the bilateral pharyngeal tonsils and head of the pancreas. While it cannot be argued that common dissemination patterns occur most commonly, it is probably equally true that the unusual is becoming more common.

The search for metastases is a principle goal of staging malignancies. While careful history and physical examination are imperative, the use of laboratory and imaging tests is necessary for confirmation of clinical suspicions and for finding occult metastasis. The detection of occult malignancies has tremendous impact on therapy and patient longevity.

Detection of metastases is a balance between the sensitivity and specificity of a given test, the medical necessity of detection, and the cost-effectiveness of each test.

Diagnostic Procedures

Choosing the correct test or tests to evaluate for metastasis requires assessment of the advantages and disadvantages of each modality for a given area of interest. The summary of available tests by body area follows.

1. Pulmonary metastasis:
   a. Chest radiograph is a fundamental method of detecting lung and chest pathology. The two-view examination is low-cost and relatively sensitive to disease. Scanning equalization radiography techniques are being developed that improve sensitivity over conventional chest radiographs (95,96).
   b. Chest computerized tomography (CT) has become the next test of choice. Detection of parenchymal nodules a few millimeters in size is feasible and the evaluation includes the mediastinum, pleura, and soft tissue of the chest. The major disadvantage is examination cost and the nonspecific pathologic features of the lesions. Inflammatory disease, atelectasis, or large pleural effusions may mask underlying malignancy. CT has largely replaced whole lung tomography for detection (48).
   c. Magnetic resonance imaging (MRI) of the lung is a helpful supplemental examination in assessing mediastinal or vascular involvement or in defining extension of a mass, such as in superior sulcus tumors (28,35).
2. Hepatic metastasis:
   a. CT of the abdomen is the method of choice for detection of hepatic metastasis and to evaluate the rest of the abdomen. While some tumors, such as colon metastases, can be seen without intravenous (IV) contrast enhancement, enhanced examinations with bolus technique are the standard. Dynamic scanning can better define questionable areas (7,64).
   b. Ultrasound of the liver is limited in most instances. Sensitivity is less than CT and it is more difficult to assess therapeutic response.
   c. MRI of the liver may detect more lesions than will CT. However, the remainder of the abdomen is less visible and respiratory artifacts may compromise the liver images. MRI can differentiate some lesions,

such as hemangiomas, and define vascular patency (46,71).

 d. Nuclear medicine liver-spleen scans using sulfur colloid tagged technetium is much less sensitive and specific than CT and MRI. Size threshold for detection is 2 cm or greater depending on the depth of the lesion (8). Single photon emission computed tomography of the liver does improve resolution.

 e. Angiography of metastasis is usually reserved for more specific occurrences, including therapy planning, delineating vascular anatomy for infusion pumps, resection, or transplantation. Liver function tests may be elevated with large lesions, particularly lactic dehydrogenase. In a patient with normal liver enzymes that subsequently become elevated, metastases should be suspected (45).

3. Bone metastasis:

 a. Skeletal radiographs are targeted to clinical symptomatology and correlating abnormalities found on radioisotope bone scan. Approximately 30% to 50% of the bone must be destroyed before metastasis is detected. Skeletal surveys are necessary for some tumors, such as multiple myeloma, because of the high incidence of false-negative bone scans in these tumors. Radiographs are more specific, but less sensitive than bone scan.

 b. Technetium 99-labelled diphosphonate radiopharmaceutical bone scans demonstrate areas of increased or decreased metabolic bone activity. Sensitivity is high, but specificity is low. Occasionally aggressive metastasis and some treated or reparative lesions are not detected on bone scan.

 c. MRI and CT are useful for treatment planning when surgery or more detailed anatomy is needed. The strength of MRI is assessment of marrow replacement and soft tissue extension while CT gives superior details of cortical bone destruction (63,90,92).

4. Lymph node metastasis: CT accurately assesses lymph node size. As size and number of nodes increase, suspicion of malignancy rises. Lymphangiography is useful in certain cases such as evaluation of Hodgkin's disease, as it may detect disease in normal-sized nodes negative by CT criteria (48). Gallium scanning may be useful in assessing areas of active residual lymphomas versus fibrosis following treatment (40a). Radioisotope-labeled monoclonal antibodies are a potential method of detecting metastases currently under study (49,70).

5. Brain metastasis: CT of the brain is useful for delineating metastatic disease. Intravenous contrast assesses for abnormality of the blood-brain barrier. While multiple lesions are relatively specific for metastatic disease, the solitary lesion raises a differential, including primary malignancy, infection, and, occasionally, infarction. MRI is more sensitive and specific than CT, but more expensive (13,17). Gadolinium enhanced MRI also evaluates the blood-brain barrier and is the most sensitive detection modality (17a,34, 87a). Lesions in the posterior fossa are better visualized due to the lack of bone artifacts and multiplanar evaluation.

6. Spinal cord metastasis:

 a. Metastases usually present with extradural compression of the thecal sac and spinal cord or nerves extending from involved vertebra or paravertebral metastases. When symptoms can be localized, MRI is the best overall assessment because it demonstrates extent of canal compression and images the location of soft tissue masses and bone destruction. It is relatively time-consuming and requires a patient who can remain motionless. Analgesia or sedation is frequently required in this patient population. Intradural and intramedullary metastases may also be detected, but are better seen with enhanced sequences.

 b. Myelography directly visualizes the subarachnoid space and assesses for extradural defects and cord block. Cervical puncture may be needed for assessing total blockage because the upper extent of a block must be defined and multiple levels may occur. Cerebral spinal fluid for cytology, protein, glucose, and cell count is obtained during the procedure. Postmyelographic CT is useful to delineate soft tissue components and bone destruction (17,20).

7. Metastasis of unknown primary: Evaluation for the primary source is usually unproductive. Breast and prostate evaluation and examination directed by clinical history are indicated, but the yield is low (86).

8. Other metastasis:

 a. Recurrent breast carcinoma is evaluated by regular mammography, physical examination, and monthly self-examination (86a).

 b. Metastatic disease to the kidney is usually encountered in evaluation of the abdomen by CT. Ultrasound, renal scan, IV pyelogram, and retrograde pyelogram may detect these lesions.

 c. Adrenal metastases are best seen with CT. Chest CT should include the adrenal glands due to the 15% metastatic incidence of lung primary metastases. MRI of the adrenals may be able to separate metastasis from adenoma due to significantly longer T2 relaxation time (3).

 d. Pleural effusions are detected on chest radiograph and by CT and ultrasound. Decubitus radiographs of the chest may show small effusions and assess for loculation.

Biologic Markers

The generic definition of a tumor marker is any substance synthesized by a tumor and released into the general circulation or body fluids. Clinical usefulness is enhanced when it is ordinarily not present in healthy controls, and is found to be proportionally increased with an enlarging tumor compartment. The marker ideally should be detectable with tumor cell burdens below the threshold of common imaging techniques and normalize with effective therapy.

Some tumor markers may not actually be produced by the malignant cell population, but may represent the biomolecular response of the host to the tumor. A critical aspect in the clinical usefulness of tumor markers involves an appreciation that very few markers clinically used today are truly tumor-specific, but are rather tumor-associated. A recent review by Jacobs and Haskell discusses the biologic properties of the tumor markers and their role in cancer management (40b). Bates et al. (4) have conveniently classified tumor markers into six major categories:

1. Oncofetal antigens:
   - carcinoembryonic antigen (CEA)
   - alphafetoprotein (AFP)
2. Ectopic hormone:
   - adrenocorticotropic hormone
   - antidiuretic hormone
   - parathormone
   - calcitonin
3. Placental proteins:
   - human chorionic gonadotropin (HCG)
   - human placental lactogen
   - regan isozyme (of alkaline phosphatase)
4. Enzymes:
   - prostatic acid phosphatase
   - lactic dehydrogenase
   - neuron-specific enolase
5. Serum proteins:
   - immunoglobulins
6. Miscellaneous:
   - polyamines
   - ferritin
   - hydroxyproline
   - catecholamine metabolites

Many tumor markers are entirely unsuitable as cancer screening tests, not due to poor sensitivity but rather to lack of specificity. Pragmatically, the clinical usefulness of a tumor marker rests with its return to normal following effective therapy. Markers are certainly becoming more heavily relied on to serve as bioindices to assess response to therapy.

Applied Concepts of Oncomarkers

Some examples of tumor markers used in patients with metastatic disease are discussed below.

1. CEA:
   a. Colon: Found to be elevated in 19% to 40% of patients with stage A and 100% of patients with metastatic disease (98); rising titer following resection, usually associated with recurrence, particularly metastasis, since only 19% to 30% colon cancers recur locally (38).
   b. Breast: Elevated in 30% to 50% of patients, including 70% with advanced disease (14).
   c. Lung: Rising level may correlate with relapse.
2. AFP: Most commonly elevated in patients with hepatocellular (72%) and testicular teratocarcinoma or embryonal cell cancer (75%); also elevated in pancreatic (23%) and gastric cancer 18% (96).
3. HCG: Germ cell tumors—Elevation in patients with pure seminoma suggests presence of nonseminomatous elements (69); found elevated in 58% of patients with stage II and 87% of those with stage III (12).
4. Acid phosphatase: Prostate—Found elevated in up to 80% of patients with stage D disease (31); may be associated with less-differentiated tumors.
5. Prostate-specific antigen: Expressed independently of prostatic acid phosphatase; elevated levels found in 63% to 86% of patients with various stages of prostate cancer; may be used to monitor recurrence (44).
6. CA 19-9: Detected by radioimmunoassay incorporating a monoclonal antibody raised against a human colorectal carcinoma line; found elevated in 21% to 42% of patients with gastric cancer, 20% to 40% with

colorectal, and 71% to 93% of pancreatic cancer patients (33).

The detection of metastases is not an academic exercise, but rather the most important aspect of initial diagnosis; it dictates appropriateness of care. It identifies patient subsets that might be eligible for phase II or III clinical trials. Moreover, it precludes recommendation for locoregional therapy alone, which may carry significant morbidity and could not be justified unless it were administered with true curative intent. A pneumonectomy could not be supported in the face of a malignant pleural effusion or a Whipple's resection for a pancreatic lesion associated with bulky celiac adenopathy and liver metastases. A patient with an endolaryngeal tumor associated with a fixed vocal cord and invasion of the preepiglottic space is certainly not a definitive external beam radiation candidate. Conversely, the patient with non-small cell lung cancer associated with a solitary pulmonary nodule should not be precluded from potential resection unless CT-directed fine-needle aspiration biopsy confirms metastases as opposed to an incidental granuloma. The holistic care of the cancer patient, including recruitment of paramedical support services, depends on the metastatic (M) status of the patient. The M0/M1 condition is indeed the melody to which the therapeutic lyrics are cast.

CLASSIFICATION AND STAGING

The most commonly used system for staging metastases is that suggested by the American Joint Committee (AJC) (5). The M classification simply designates the presence or absence of metastases.

- MX: the presence of metastatic disease is not assessed
- M0: no evidence of metastatic disease
- M1: distant metastases are present. Specific sites for metastatic disease should be individually noted

A more detailed classification based on the criteria of number of metastases, number of organ systems involved, and the degree of functional impairment has been suggested by Rubin (74) (Table 33-4) (74). Although cure is rare in patients with metastases, it has been observed in patients with solitary metastasis. However, as our understanding of the mechanisms of metastases improves and new therapeutic maneuvers become more effective, more patients with favorable prognosis will be identified and categorized accordingly.

Table 33-4. Classification Schema

M0:	No evidence of metastases
M1a:	Solitary, isolated metastasis confined to organ system or one anatomic site
M1b:	Multiple metastatic foci confined to one organ system or one anatomic site, i.e., lungs, skeleton, liver, etc., no functional to minimal functional impairment.
M1c:	Multiple organs involved anatomically, no or minimal to moderate functional impairment of involved organs
M1d:	Multiple organs involved anatomically, moderate to severe functional impairment of involved organs
Mx:	No metastatic workup done
M*:	Modified to show viscera involved by letter subscript: pulmonary metastases (Mp), hepatic (Mh), osseous (Mo), skin (Ms), brain (Mb), etc.
M+:	Microscopic evidence of suspected metastases, confirmed by pathologic examination

*Visceral involvement by direct extension is not considered a metastasis.
From Rubin (74), with permission.

PRINCIPLES OF TREATMENT

The concept of individualized therapy is no more apparent than in the treatment of a patient with metastatic disease. The presentations range from the patient with a single asymptomatic focus of disease to the patient with multiple symptomatic sites affecting one or several organ systems. Therapeutic aggressiveness will be tempered by numerous objective factors, including the temporal onset of the metastasis, site of the primary, potential response of the tumor, organ system involved, age, and subjective findings that include degree of pain, presence of anorexia, cachexia, and nausea and vomiting, all of which affect the performance status. The influence of objective factors on the therapy has been considered in each chapter dealing with the primary tumor sites. Therefore, the subjective findings will be discussed in more detail below as they affect not only the tolerance of the patient, but also the natural history of the disease. The important point is that all factors must be considered in each patient and the question should be asked, "What will the treatment add to the quality and/or quantity of life of the individual?"

Etiology and Treatment of Pain

Pain—Etiology: The type of pain that results can vary and has been categorized as somatic, visceral, and deafferentation (24,25).

1. Somatic: Activation of nociceptors in the cutaneous or deep tissue. This results in dull or aching well-localized pain (e.g., metastatic bone pain or postsurgical incision pain).

2. Visceral: Activation of nociceptors caused by stretching, infiltration, and compression of the viscera (e.g., bone or pancreas metastases). The pain is poorly localized, but can be described as a squeezing and pressure-like sensation. If acute in onset, it can be associated with nausea and vomiting.

3. Deafferentation: Results from infiltration, compression, or iatrogenic injury caused by surgery, irradiation, or chemotherapy. It can be described as burning or viselike (as in radiotherapy-induced brachial plexopathies, postherpetic neuralgia, or cisplatin neuropathy).

Pain—Treatment: The approach to pain relief has become more complex and important because of the need for a compassionate assessment of the quality of life of a cancer patient. There is no need to deny pain medication to the patient with severe pain while considering cytoxic therapies. The most important consideration is a stepwise use of analgesics until the goal of pain relief has been achieved. Some suggested approaches are listed below.

1. Mild to moderate pain: Nonopiod analgesics with potency similar to or greater than aspirin are the drugs of choice. They may be important in patients with bone metastases because they decrease the prostaglandin release and the role of the latter in bone resorption (43). Failure to control pain has led to more common use of combined narcotic and non-narcotic drugs, such as codeine, oxycodone, and propoxyphene. A suggested protocol includes one to two tablets of the narcotic medications every 3 to 4 hours. Nonrelief after adequate trial (3 to 4 days) will require opiates.

2. Moderate to severe pain: Those most commonly used include morphine (prototype), hydromorphone,

levorphanol, methadone, and oxymorphone. These produce their effects by combining with the opiate receptors in the peripheral and CNS.

Individualization is necessary as is, to some extent, physician comfort and familiarity with various analgesics. Equianalgesic doses are given in Table 33-5 (24,25).

Cachexia: In the normal host, caloric intake and metabolic needs are balanced. The predominant source of energy in the tumor cell is glucose, which is metabolized to lactic acid via the Cori cycle. The lactate is then reconverted to glucose with expenditure of energy. In the cancer patient with a hypermetabolic state, the increased glucose production will therefore lead to increased expenditure of energy by at least 10% (97). Recent studies in animals indicate that circulating factors such as cytokines, tumor necrosis factor alpha (TNFα), and interleukin IL-1 ß to be associated with the cachexic-anorexic syndrome (7). TNFα is identical to cachectin, which inhibits lipoprotein lipase activity and may influence the metabolic changes leading to cachexia-anorexia (91).

Cachexia and the complications thereof are among the most common causes of death in patients with cancer. Weight loss in patients with cancer can occur as a result of the disease or the therapy. DeWys *et al.* (19) found a relationship between the primary lesion and the degree of weight loss. Lymphoma affected the weight loss less than colon, lung, and gastric cancers. Grosevenor and Bulcavage (32) evaluated food intake and weight loss in a group of cancer patients. He found a significant correlation between the symptoms of abdominal fullness, taste changes, dry mouth, constipation, nausea and vomiting, and greater than 5% weight loss. He noted no difference between patients who had previous chemotherapy and those who had no treatment.

Therefore, weight loss is not only due to the effects of cytotoxic therapy, but can be the result of tumor effect. In addition, Marton *et al.* (56) found that weight loss tended not to be present to a great degree in breast and prostate cancer, whereas in lung and pancreas, weight loss can be a prominent symptom.

Additional salient features associated with cachexia of malignancy include:

1. Delayed gastric emptying: This may be related to gastric paresis. The latter may be associated with altered

Table 33-5. Equianalgesic Doses of Selected Opioid Agonists*

Drug	Equianalgesic Dose+ (mg)	Starting Oral Dose (mg)
Morphine	10 IM	30–60
	60 PO	30–60
Hydromorphone	1.5 IM	
	7.5 PO	4–8
Methadone	10 IM	
	20 PO	5–10
Codeine	130	
	200	60
Meperidine	75 IM	
	300 PO	75

*Important when changing drugs or routes of administration. Values compared with standard dose of 10 mg morphine.

+Relative potency of a drug = $\dfrac{\text{dose of A}}{\text{dose of B}}$ to produce same effect.

IM = intramuscular; PO = orally.

glucose metabolism (47,78). Metoclopramide has been shown to improve gastric emptying.

2. Altered glucose metabolism: This results from hyporesponsiveness to insulin release by islet cell or "simply" resistance to insulin (85). The prolonged elevation of blood glucose may act to suppress appetite and explain the lack of enthusiasm for meals other than breakfast.

3. Alterations in taste: Cancer patients can experience a metallic or bitter taste especially associated with meats and other protein-containing foods. DeWys (18) found a correlation between lowered threshold for bitter taste and aversion to meat while there was an elevated threshold for sweet substances. In addition, these alterations were associated with tumor burden.

Just as there may be several underlying mechanisms associated with cachexia-anorexia, several therapeutic maneuvers can be considered. Metoaclopramide can aid in promoting gastric emptying, and may be suggested in patients complaining of abdominal fullness (early satiety). Meats may be substituted with other high-protein foods such as eggs, milk, and/or sweeter nutritional supplements to relieve this symptom.

Anabolic steroids have been used as appetite stimulants. A short course of dexamethasone (8 mg/d) has been associated with improved appetite and a feeling of well-being. Prolonged use is discouraged because of unacceptable side effects. Tchekmedyian *et al.* (89) recently reported the effect of megestrol acetate (160 mg/d) on appetite stimulation in 33 patients with advanced cancer, including lung and colon. Fourteen (42%) of the patients experienced an improved sense of well-being, while nine (27%) had greater than 2.3 kg weight gain. Sixteen patients had a sustained subjective improvement for more than 2 months. Although only a few patients were studied, the characteristics of these patients—all with metastatic disease refractory to conventional therapy and greater than 10% loss of body weight—suggests that megestrol acetate may favorably affect the sense of well-being and potentially improve appetite and weight gain.

Hydrazine sulfate is an inhibitor of gluconeogenesis and prevents conversion of lactate to glucose. It has been studied in patients with malignancy with more than 10% weight loss and found to be associated with increased caloric intake, weight gain, and glucose tolerance (15).

Whether the amelioration of cachexia will affect survival directly is not known. However, in a subgroup of patients, reversal of the cachexia-anorexic syndrome will enable the patient to receive and tolerate cytotoxic therapy and, therefore, may indirectly affect survival. In other patients with widely disseminated disease, the quality of life becomes as important as the quantity of life and therefore, an important consideration when evaluating the patient for anticachectic maneuvers.

Nausea: Nausea in malignant disease is usually associated with the treatment (chemo-radiotherapy) and secondarily as a consequence of disease. The latter is most prominent in patients with brain metastases and secondarily the GI tract.

The act of vomiting is thought to be regulated by the vomiting center located in the medulla oblongata. The vomiting center receives stimuli from the chemoreceptor trigger zone (CTZ) and the GI tract (via the vagus nerve). Knowledge of the different receptors in the CTZ and GI tract will lead to a better understanding and more rational use of specific agents:

1. Agents that act by blocking dopamine receptors:
   - Metoclopramide (substituted benzamides): Found to be very effective for cisplatin-induced emesis (30) as well as other agents (87).
   - Butyrophenones (haloperidol and droperidol): Both found to be effective (59), but probably not as potent as metoclopramide.
   - Phenothiazines (prochlorperazine, chloropromazine).

2. Agents that block serotonin receptors: Hydroxy tryptamines have been identified in both GI and CNS. The best studied agent so far is odansetron (GR-507/75). In addition to having antiemetic properties, it has not been associated with dystonic reaction (16,16a).

3. Corticosteroids: antiemetic mechanism of these remains unclear, but effectiveness has been established (55).

4. Cannabinoids: Dronabinol (∂-9-tetrahydrocannabinol) has been found to be better than placebo and at least equivalent to oral prochlorperazine (27).

The treatment and control of nausea requires a knowledge of the agents available, clinical experience, and familiarity with the particular agents. The general opinion is that several agents may be necessary to ease the symptoms associated with metastatic disease itself or the side effects of treatment. As in all other aspects of oncology, most successful results come from the total team approach.

Psychosocial Issues

Holland and Wellisch (39) wrote "psychological and social issues arise in the care of all patients with cancer, irrespective of the type of cancer or the type of treatment. It is important to integrate these crucial aspects of care into the treatment plan. With effective intervention, clinicians can help to recognize troublesome and disturbing problems, reduce their negative impact, and enhance the quality of life for patients and those close to them." The two most important aspects are the integration of psychosocial issues into the overall care of the patient and the influence of the negative impact. Delinquency in considering the important psychosocial factors may detract from patient tolerance of effective therapy, thereby affecting survival or the quality of life.

Aside from the stress caused by the disease and therapeutic intervention, emotional and behavioral issues persist in most patients once the diagnosis of cancer is made. Some of the more prevalent issues are addressed below.

Anxiety

In managing anxiety, provide information to the patient at a rate that he or she can assimilate most comfortably; set aside uninterrupted time to listen to the patient; provide anxiolytic drugs (e.g., diazepam 5 mg or short-acting oxazepam 15 mg) if necessary.

Sleep Disturbance

The prevalence of this issue is not known, but studies indicate cancer patients achieve less restful sleep than controls; temazepam 30 mg, diazepam 10 mg, or diphenhydramine 50 to 100 mg may be helpful (80).

Depression

This is the most common psychiatric illness in cancer patients (50). However, it is difficult to diagnose because some of the symptoms may be related to disease process or treatment (e.g., loss of appetite, sleep disturbance, and decreased energy). Other signs include tearfulness, decreased ability to concentrate, feeling of guilt, helplessness, and suicidal thoughts. Management may require expert pyschotherapy and use of antidepressants.

Sexual Dysfunction

As the number of patients achieving long-term survival increases, sexual function is becoming more important in the assessment of quality of life. Sexual dysfunction can occur (a) as part of the disease process; (b) as a side effect of therapeutic intervention; and (c) as psychologic stress. To establish a more rational approach to understanding the problems associated with sexual dysfunction, Shover et al. (79) suggested the use of the sexual response cycle, which includes three phases: desire, arousal, and orgasm, each with subjective objective, and physical evaluations. The treatment plan has many components: sexual counseling, attitudinal change, physical handicaps, and adjusting body imagery.

Confronting the problems associated with sexuality (loss of sexual desire and feelings of sexual attractiveness and the range of sexual activities) is often neglected in cancer patients. Addressing these problems early may help reduce some of the anguish that accompanies the diagnosis of cancer and its treatment.

Surgery

The role of surgery in patients with metastatic disease is usually diagnostic (2). However, there are limited palliative and curative applications. The need to prove that a specific lesion is metastatic is important, especially if the lesion appears years after the primary tumor was controlled. In particular instances, debulking procedures are necessary, for example, after an unresectable breast tumor has been made resectable by chemotherapy or radiotherapy. In other situations, palliative surgery may be indicated to control bleeding.

Radiation Therapy

The effectiveness of radiotherapy for palliation of pain secondary to metastatic disease has been well established. For patients who have multiple areas of symptomatic pain, hemibody irradiation has recently been incorporated within the radiotherapeutic armamentarium.

The clinical application of a single high-dose, large field irradiation (hemibody irradiation,) for the palliation of multiple areas of cancer-related pain was first reported by Fitzpatrick and Rider in 1976 (23). Since that time, numerous investigators have reported on the subjective and objective responses obtained after hemibody irradiation (53,68,72,73). Salazar (75) reported on Radiation Therapy Oncology Group (RTOG) study which tested the efficacy of escalating doses of hemibody irradiation. The three major tumor types included breast (36%), prostate (35%), and lung (18%); 77 experienced pain relief (21% having complete relief of pain), 50% of these within 2 days and 80% within 1 week. The study also suggested that doses of 600 to 800 cGy were effective, while increasing the dose above 800 cGy was not associated with improved response.

More recently, interest has centered around the ability of hemibody irradiation to affect occult or asymptomatic overt disease thereby raising the idea of hemibody irradiation as a systemic agent (66,66a). All patients received standard palliative treatment and were then randomized to receive hemibody irradiation or no further therapy. Four hundred ninety-nine patients were randomized and 45% of those randomized to hemibody irradiation required new treatment in the hemibody field, versus 57% not receiving hemibody irradiation, while progressive disease occurred in 20% receiving hemibody irradiation versus 38% not receiving it. The difference was most notable in patients with prostate or breast cancer. Thus, it appears that the potential for hemibody irradiation may not only be in the rapid relief of pain, but also in its ability to delay disease progression.

Chemotherapy

The emergence of new agents and techniques for the treatment of systemic disease as single modalities or in combination with irradiation and surgery will impact on the use of such agents in the management of systemic disease. They include cytotoxic and hormonal agents, growth and differentiation factors, monoclonal antibodies, and bone marrow transplants.

Therapeutic Management of Metastases

Since the majority of patients with cancer other than skin will develop metastases at some time during their disease course, appropriate management will be extremely important. The improvement in quality of life due to relief of symptoms from metastasis can be a most rewarding experience to the patient and physician. It is of utmost importance for the physician to be aware of all therapy modalities so that good palliation can be provided in each case. The performance status of the patient, type of symptoms, location of metastasis, histology, life expectancy, disease tempo, and patient wishes are factors to be considered in choosing appropriate palliative therapy.

Palliative treatment should relieve symptoms as quickly as possible for as long as possible without significant acute side effects or risk of long-term complications, if appropriate. For some patients bedridden with widely metastatic disease and who have run the gamut of therapeutic programs, good supportive care at home or in a hospital can relieve suffering during the final days. Others with symptoms from a solitary metastasis to a vital organ may become symptom-free for several years with surgical treatment. It is the responsibility of the physician to evaluate all factors in the disease process and to develop an individualized program that will give the best palliation.

Surgery can be very effective in quickly relieving symptoms or preventing further loss of function from spinal cord compression. Prophylactic surgical stabilization of a metastasis to a weight-bearing bone can prevent fracture while receiving radiation therapy. Chemotherapy or hormonal therapy can sometimes relieve symptoms due to widespread metastases. Radiation therapy can often relieve symptoms of pain, swelling, respiratory insufficiency, bleeding, or neurologic problems due to metastasis. The appropriate choice of nonnarcotic or narcotic medication, dose, and route of administration can control pain in the majority of patients. Often a combination of therapies will provide the best results.

RESULTS AND PROGNOSIS

Brain Metastases

Surgery can be very effective at quickly relieving the symptoms associated with a solitary metastasis in more than 80% of patients or provide a tissue diagnosis in others (69). The symptoms of nausea, vomiting, and ataxia associated with a cerebellar metastasis will be relieved in nearly all patients after tumor resection with very little risk of morbidity from surgery. Long-term survival greater than 48 months has been demonstrated in 18% to 33% of patients when the primary is controlled and no other metastases exist. Surgery should be followed by whole brain irradiation to prevent the development of other brain metastases (58,83). Recently Patchell, *et al.* conducted a randomized study of surgery plus radiotherapy versus radiotherapy only in treatment of single metastases to the brain. Patients who received surgery and radiotherapy had longer survival (40 weeks versus 15 weeks) and a better quality of life (63a).

Radiation therapy has been proven effective in relieving symptoms from solitary or multiple metastases in 60% to 80% of patients (37). Improvement occurs within 2 to 3 weeks in most cases with little acute or chronic toxicity. The RTOG compared different treatment schedules of whole brain irradiation—2,000 cGy/x 4; 3,000 cGy/x 10, and 4,000 CGy/x 15 or 20—and found them as effective as more protracted schedules without increased toxicity (10). Because patients receiving brain irradiation often have extensive disease elsewhere, median survival is only 4 to 6 months. Some subsets of patients with good performance status, controlled primaries, and solitary brain lesions have median survivals of around 12 months (15a,36,54).

Stereotactic radiosurgery was a technique first developed in the early 1950s by a Swedish neurosurgen for the delivery of a very large fraction of ionizing radiation to a small intracranial target using stereotactically directed narrow beams. More recently, stereotactic radiosurgery has been used in several centers for the treatment of small solitary radiographically defined brain metastases. It appears that control rates of greater than eighty percent can be obtained with minimal risk of serious complications. The large dose per fraction may be more effective than conventional radiation therapy in more resistant tumors, such as renal cell carcinomas, sarcomas, and melanomas. Because patients often develop systemic or other intracranial metastases, survival advantage of this technique has not been demonstrated. It does appear that this technique may have a role to play as does surgical excision of a solitary brain metastases (52a).

Chemotherapy given by intrathecal or intraventricular route may be effective in sterilizing the CNS fluid and relieving symptoms. Intravenous lomustine or intra-arterial cisplatin have been used in patients with progressive high-grade gliomas. Corticosteroids (dexamethasone and prednisone) can relieve symptoms due to swelling in 24 hours. Doses of 20 mg/d are often adequate, but on occasion doubling the dose is more effective.

Bone Metastases

Local treatment for a bone metastasis will usually relieve pain and prevent loss of function, but does not address the systemic disease, which may require hormonal or chemotherapy depending on histology of the primary. The pathophysiology and options for the management of bone metastases are reviewed thoroughly in a recent report by Nielsen *et al.* (62a).

1. Surgery should be considered for stabilization of a weight-bearing long bone if significant cortical destruction exists and the patient is ambulatory. This often is accomplished by an intramedullary rod and cement although a hip prosthesis may be necessary if the hip is involved. Removal of extradural bone fragments, debulking of tumor, and stabilization of vertebrae are effective in relieving pain due to pathologic vertebral body compression if a patient otherwise is in good medical condition.

2. Radiation therapy has been very effective for relieving pain and improving function either alone or after surgical stabilization of bone metastasis. The following moderate dose schedules were evaluated by RTOG: 2,000 cGy x 5; 3,000 cGy x 10; 4,000 cGy x 15; all were found to be effective (97). For patients with diffuse bone metastasis, upper or lower hemibody irradiation with single fractions of 600 to 800 cGy with lung transmission correction can relieve pain within 24 to 48 hours (4a,76).

   The radiotherapeutic considerations for metastatic tumors to several common sites are discussed below:

   a. Proximal femur (hip): Radiation portals should include all involved areas while avoiding the knee joint if possible. If stabilization has been performed, radiotherapy should be started as soon as the wound heals, and portals should include the fixation device to encompass micrometastases dislodged by the surgery. A strip of soft tissue should be left unirradiated to preserve lymphatic drainage.

   b. Pelvis: Portals should encompass area involved by tumor, yet avoid uninvolved bone to spare bone marrow. Pelvic fields will probably include small bowel; therefore the dose and fractionation of irradiation should be within tolerance of the small bowel.

   c. Spine: Portals should include symptomatic vertebrae with a one vertebral body margin; spinal cord tolerance should not be exceeded.

   d. Chemotherapy can improve the quality of life in patients with widespread bone metastases. Diffuse metastatic breast or prostate cancer will often stabilize and improve after removing the estrogen or testosterone stimulation.

3. A reawakening of radioisotopic therapy (RIT) is occurring with recent excellent results in bone pain relief by the iv use of Strontium 89 (64a).

Lung Metastases

Surgery can remove solitary lung metastasis for diagnostic or therapeutic purposes without significant morbidity. If the primary is controlled and there are no other metastatic sites, long-term survival may be possible, especially in renal cell, thyroid, colon, and osteosarcoma.

Radiation therapy can relieve or prevent symptoms of hemorrhage, obstruction, and pain associated with metastases. Often small fields and abbreviated treatment courses may be used. Irradiation to the whole lung is limited by the sensitivity of normal lung tissue to 1,500 cGy. A more practical approach is the use of small boost fields to involved sites to doses from 3,000 to 5,000 cGy at 180 cGy/fraction. In addition, high single doses (600 cGy) can used. Symptoms related to recurrent obstructing endobronchial lung cancer will often resolve with endobronchial debulking by laser treatment and endobronchial brachytherapy.

Chemotherapy can be curative in sensitive tumors such as germ cell, choriocarcinoma, and Hodgkin's disease. Iodoantipyrine is effective in metastatic thyroid tumors that demonstrate uptake. Improvement in symptoms related to multiple pulmonary metastases from other cancers have occurred with chemotherapy and hormone therapy. Chest tube drainage and insertion of a sclerosing agent such as tetracycline or single-agent chemotherapy is effective in preventing recurrence of a malignant pleural effusion.

Liver Metastases

The prognosis for patients with extensive liver metastases is quite poor in most cases. The symptoms associated with liver metastases include anorexia, nausea, pyrexia, malaise, and a failure to thrive.

Surgery can remove a solitary metastasis and some patients are cured without other metastatic disease. More extensive involvement of a single lobe can also be resected in certain cases with good palliation but with less chance of cure. Survival after resection of hepatic metastases in the absence of extrahepatic disease is related to a number of factors, including:

1. Number of metastases: The five-year survival in patients with less than four lesions is 37% and 23% with more than four lesions.
2. Disease-free interval (DFI): The 5-year survival in patients with DFI of less than 1 month is 27% and 42% with a DFI more than 1 year.
3. CEA level before liver resection: Patients with a CEA level less than 5 ng/mL had a 47% 5-year survival, while patients with a CEA level higher than 30 ng/mL had a 28% 5-year survival.

Radiation therapy can relieve pain due to a diffusely involved, massively enlarged liver with very little acute toxicity. The limiting factor in treating hepatic metastases is the tolerance of the normal liver. The incidence of radiation hepatitis is low after doses less than 3,000 cGy. Dose schedules from 600 cGy x 1, 300 CGy x 7, 250 cGy x 10 and 200 cGy x 15 are all effective and well tolerated. The RTOG treated patients with 3,000 cGy in 15 fractions and found a 55% improvement in pain without hepatic toxicity (11); others studied 2,100 to 2,400 cGy in 300 cGy fractions and reported pain relief in 90% of patients and a median survival of 4.5 months (77).

Chemotherapy: The rationale for hepatic arterial infusion is to achieve high drug levels in the intrahepatic tumor, while maintaining low systemic levels. The most commonly used drug is 5-flurouracil; the average response rates from several studies were 51% (84). Monoclonal antibodies have been successful in treatment of primary hepatomas and may have a role in treatment of metastatic disease of other cancers.

CLINICAL INVESTIGATIONS

The challenge for the health professional in caring for the patient with metastatic disease will be to determine the best therapeutic plan for the patient after careful evaluation of all available subjective and objective findings. The information

provided above should serve as a guide to formulating a therapeutic plan because each patient, by definition, presents with his or her own set of complex variables.

From the time-honored patient history and physical examination using newer diagnostic procedures and careful subjective evaluation, one should begin to formulate a treatment plan that should lead to the use of a modality efficacious in achieving the desired goal. Implicit in the management of the patient with metastatic disease is the concern for improving the quality of life or minimizing the adverse effects of the disease or treatment. For the First International Consensus Workshop on RT in the Treatment of Metastases, Hanks *et al.* (33a) provide a thought-provoking and soul-searching statement critically examining the crisis in health care costs in the U.S. (540 billion dollars in 1988).

A more efficient means of palliation of metastases in general and bone metastases in particular is addressed by Poulter *et al.* (66a) in their RTOG study dealing with the addition of single dose hemibody irradiation (HBI) to standard local field irradiation.

Bates *et al.* (4b) provide an overview of the management of bone metastases and its compression. It is evident in their report and in the consensus statement that treatment decisions are based more on one's training and local custom than clinical trials.

The role of radiotherapy in the management of brain metastases is comprehensively discussed by Coia (15a) particularly with regard to endpoints of response and prognostic factors as a basis for choosing a fractionation schema.

The concluding report by Maher *et al.* (53a) focuses on differences in attitude between U.S., Canada, and Europe on treatment strategies in advanced and metastatic cancer. In spite of broad agreement that the progress in metastatic management has been poor, there was disagreement as to whether or not the treatment was considered radical or palliative. The author notes this study gives limited support to the view that method of reimbursement may be directly or indirectly related to the therapy proposed. To compare the benefits of different treatments, it is necessary to consider the long-term control rate, life expectancy of patients, and the financial and human cost of treatment.

Recommended Reading

The student will find an excellent introduction to metastases in *Principles of Metastases* by Weiss (2b). Schirrmacher's article (2a) provides experimental and treatment approaches. A recent and worthwhile book on metastases is *Mechanisms of Invasion and Metastasis* by Mareel *et al.* (1a) and Hill's chapter on "Metastasis" (1) is an excellent up-to-date summary on the subject.

REFERENCES

General References

1. Hill, R.P. Metastasis. In: Tannock, I.F., Hill, R.P., (eds). The Basic Science of Oncology, 2nd ed. New York, NY: McGraw-Hill, Inc. 1992; 178-195.
1a. Mareel, M.M.; DeBaetselier, P.; Van Roy, R. Mechanisms of Invasion and Metastasis. Boca Raton, FL: CRC Press; 1991.
2. Rosenberg, S.A., ed. Surgical Treatment of Metastatic Cancer. Philadelphia, PA: J.B. Lippincott Co.; 1987.
2a. Schirrmacher, V. Cancer metastasis: Experimental approaches, theoretical concepts and impacts for treatment strategies. Adv Cancer Res 43:1-73; 1985.

2b. Weiss, L. Principles of Metastases. Orlando, FL: Academic Press; 1985.

2c. Wright, D.C.; Delaney, T.F. Treatment of Metastatic Cancer. In: DeVita, V.T.; Hellman, S.; Rosenberg, S.A., eds. Cancer: Principles and Practice of Oncology, 3rd ed. Philadelphia, PA: J.B. Lippincott Co.; 1989; 2245-2332.

Specific References

3. Baker, M.E.; Blinder, R.; Spritzer, C. MR evaluation of adrenal masses at. 1.5 T. A.J.R. 3:307-312; 1989.

4. Bates, S.E.; Longo, D.L. Use of serum tumor markers in cancer diagnoses and management. Semin. Oncol. 14:102-138; 1987.

4a. Bates, T. A review of local radiotherapy in the treatment of bone metastases and cord compression. Int J Radiat Oncol Biol Phys 23:217-221; 1992.

4b. Bates, T.; Yarold, J.R.; Blitzer, P.; Nelson, O.S.; Rubin, P.; Maher, J. Bone metastasis consensus statement. Int J Radiat Oncol Biol Phys. 23:215-216; 1992.

5. Beahrs, O.H.; Henson, D.E.; Hutter, R.V.P. Manual for staging of cancer/American Joint Committee on Cancer. 3rd ed. Philadelphia, PA: J.B. Lippincott Co. 6-10; 1988.

6. Beck, S.A.; Tisdale, M.J. Production of lipolytic and proteolytic factors by a murine tumor producing cachexia in the host. Cancer Res. 47:5919-5923; 1987.

7. Berland, L.L. Screening for diffuse and focal liver disease: the case for hepatic computed tomography. JCU. 12:83-89; 1984.

8. Bernardino, M.E.; Thomas, J.L.; Barnes, P.A. Diagnostic approaches to liver and spleen metastases. Radiol Clin North Am. 20:469-485; 1982.

9. Beutler, B.; Greenwald, D.; Holmes, J.D. Identity of tumor necrosis factor and the macrophage-secreted factor cachectin. Nature. 316:552-554; 1985.

10. Borgelt, B.; Gelber, R. The palliation of brain metastases: final results of the first two studies by the R.T.O.G. Int J Radiat Oncol Biol Phys. 6:1-8; 1980.

11. Borgelt, B.; Gelber, R.; Brady, L. The palliation of hepatic metastases: results of the radiation therapy oncology group pilot study. In J Radiat Oncol Biol Phys. 7:587-591; 1981.

12. Bosl, G.J.; Lange, P.H.; Fraley, E.E. et al. Human chorionic gonadotropin and alphafetoprotein in staging of nonseminomatous testicular cancer. Cancer. 47: 328-332; 1981.

13. Bradley, W.G.; Waluch, V.W.; Yadley, R. A. et al. Comparison of CT and MR in 400 patients with suspected disease of the brain and cervical spinal cord. Radiology.152:695-702; 1984.

14. Caffier, Y.; Brandau, H. Serum tumor markers in metastatic breast cancer and course of disease. Cancer Detect Prev. 6:451-457; 1983.

15. Chlebowski, R.T.; Bulcavage, L.; Grosvenor, R.D. Hydrazine sulfate in cancer patients with weight loss: a placebo-controlled clinical experience. Cancer. 59: 436-410; 1987.

15a. Coia, L.R. The role of radiation therapy in the treatment of brain metastases. Int J Radiat Oncol Biol Phys. 23:229-238; 1992.

16. Cunningham, D.; Popli, A.; Ford, I.T. et al. Prevention of emesis in patients receiving cytotoxic drugs by GR38032F, a selective 5-HT3 receptor antagonist. Lancet. i.1461-1462; 1987.

16a. Cubeddu, L.X.; Hoffman, I.S.; Fuenmayor, N.T.; et al. Efficacy of Ondansetron (GR 38032) and the role of Serotonin in Cisplatin-induced nausea and vomiting. N Engl J Med 322:810-816; 1990.

17. Davis, J.M.; Zimmerman, R.A.; Bilaniuk, L.T. Metastases to the central nervous system. Radiol Clin North Am. 20:417-435;1982.

17a. Davis, PC; Hudgins, PA; Peterman, SB et al. Diagnosis of cerebral metastasis: Double-dose delayed CT versus contrast enhanced MR imaging. AJNR 12: 293-300, 1990.

18. DeWys, W.D. Abnormalities of taste as a remote effect of a neoplasm. Ann. N.Y. Acad Sci. 230:427-434; 1974.

19. DeWys, W.D.; Begg, C.; Lavin, P.T. Prognostic effect of weight loss prior to chemotherapy in cancer patients. Am J Med. 69:491-497; 1980.

20. Dillon, W.P.; Norman, D.; Newton, T.H. et al. Intradural spinal cord lesions: Gd-DTPA-enhanced MR imaging. Radiology. 170:229-237; 1989.

21. Fidler, I.J. Metastasis: Quantitative analysis of distribution and fate of tumor emboli labeled with 125 I-5-iodo-2' deoxyuridine. JNCI. 45:773-782; 1970.

22. Fidler, I.J.; Balch, C.M. The biology of cancer metastases and implications for therapy. Curr Probl Surg. 24:130-209; 1987.

23. Fitzpatrick, P.J.; Rider, W.D. Half-body radiotherapy. Int J Radiat Oncol Biol Phys. 1:197-207; 1976.

24. Foley, K.M. The treatment of cancer pain. N Engl J Med. 313:84-95; 1985.

25. Foley, K.M.; Arbit, E. Management of cancer pain. In: DeVita, V.T.; Hellman, S.; Rosenberg, S., eds. Principles and practice of oncology. 3rd ed. Philadelphia, Pa: J.B. Lippincott Co.; 2064-2087; 1989.

26. Folkman, J.; Klagsburn, M. Angiogenic factors. Science. 235:442-447; 1987.

27. Frytak, S.; Moertel, C.G.; O'Fallon, J. et al. Delta 9-tetrahydro cannabinol as an antiemetic in patients treated with cancer chemotherapy: a double blind comparison with prochlorperazine and a placebo. Ann Intern Med. 91:825-830; 1979.

28. Gefter, W.B. Chest applications of magnetic resonance imaging: an update. Radiol Clin North Am. 26(3):573-588; 1988.

29. Goustin, A.S.; Leof, E.B.; Shipley, G.D. Growth factors and cancer. Cancer Res. 46:1015-1029; 1986.

30. Gralla, R.J.; Itri, L.M.; Pisko, S.E.; et. al. Antiemetic efficacy of high dose metoclopramide; randomized trials with placebo and prochlorperazine in patients with chemotherapy induced nausea and vomiting. New Engl J Med. 305:905-909: 1981.

31. Griffiths, J.C. Prostatic-specific acid phosphatase: reevaluation of radioimmunoassay in diagnosing prostatic disease. Clin. Chem. 26:433-436; 1980.

32. Grosvenor, M.; Bulcavage, L.; Chlebowski, R.T. Symptoms potentially influencing weight loss in a cancer population. Cancer. 63:330-334; 1989.

33. Gupta, M.K.; Arciaga, R.; Bocci, L. Measurement of a monoclonal-antibody-defined antigen (CA 19-9) in the sera of patients with malignant and nonmalignant diseases. Cancer. 56:227-283; 1985.

33a. Hanks, G.E.; Maher, E.J.; Coia, L. The first international consensus workshop on radiation therapy in the treatment of metastatic and locally advanced cancer. Int J Radiat Oncol Biol Phys. 23:201; 1992.

34. Healy, M.E.; Hesselink, J.F.; Press, G.A et al. Increased detection of intracranial metastases with intravenous Gd-DTPA. Radiology. 165:619-624; 1987.

35. Heelan, R.T.; Demas, B.E.; Caravelli, J.R. et al. Superior sulcus tumors: CT and MR imaging. Radiology. 170:637-641;1989.

36. Hendrickson, F.R. Radiation therapy of metastatic tumors. Sem in Oncol. 2:43-46; 1975.

37. Hendrickson, F.R.; Lee, M.S. The influence of surgery and radiation therapy on patients with brain metastases. Int J Radiat Oncol Biol Phys. 9:623-627;1983.

38. Hine, K.R.; Dykes, P.W. Serum CEA testing in postoperative surveillance of colorectal carcinoma. Br J Cancer. 49:689-693;1984.

39. Holland, J.; Wellisch, D. Psychosocial issues and cancer. CA. 38: 130-132; 1988.

40. Horak, E.; Darling, D.L.; Tarin, 0. Analysis of organ-specifc effects on metastatic tumor formation by studies in vitro. JCNI. 76:913-922; 1986.

40a. Israel, O; Front, D; Epelbaum, R; et al. Residual mass and negative gallium scintigraphy in treated lymphoma. J Nucl Med. 31: 365-368, 1990.

40b. Jacobs, EL and Haskell, CM. Clinical use of tumor markers in oncology. Current Problems in Cancer, Nov/Dec: 299-350, 1991.

41. Jacob, F.; Monod, J. On the regulation of gene activity. Cold Spring Harbor Symp. Quant Biol. 26:193-206; 1961.

42. Jones, P.A.; DeClerck, Y.A. Extracellular matrix destruction by invasive tumor cells. Cancer Metastasis Rev. 1: 289-319; 1982.

43. Kantor, T.G. Control of pain by non-steroidal anti-inflammatory drugs. Med Clin North Am. 66:1053-1059; 1982.

44. Killian, C.S.; Yang, N.; Emrich, L.J.; et al. Prognostic importance of prostate-specific antigen for monitoring patients with stages B2 to Dl prostate cancer. Cancer Res. 45:886-891; 1985.

45. Kim, N.K.; Yasmineh, W.G.; Freier, E.F.; et al. Value of alkaline phosphatase, 5-Nucleotidase, Y-glutamytransferase and glutamate dehydrogenase activity measurements (single and combined) in serum in diagnosis of metastases to the liver. Clin Chem. 23:2034-2038; 1977.

46. Kressel, H.Y. Strategies for magnetic resonance imaging of focal liver disease. Radiol Clin North Am. 26:607-615; 1988.

47. Kris, M.G.; Yeh, S.D.J.; Gralla, R.S. et al. Symptomatic gastroparesis in cancer patients: a possible cause of cancer associ-

ated anorexia that can be improved with oral metochlopramide. Abstract. Proc Am Soc Clin Oncol. 4:267; 1985.

48. Lee, J.K.T.; Sagel, S.S.; Stanley, R.J. eds. Computed body tomography with MRI correlation. 2nd edition. New York, NY: Raven Press; 1989.

49. LeRoy, M.; Teillac, P.; Rain, J.D.; *et al.* Radioimmunodetection of lymph node invasion in prostatic cancer. Cancer. 64:1-5; 1989.

50. Levine, P.M.; Silberfarb, P.M.; Lipowski, Z.J. Mental disorders in cancer patients: study of 100 psychiatric referrals. Cancer 42:1385-1391; 1978.

51. Liotta, L.A. Tumor invasion and metastases. Monographs in Pathology. 4: 183-192;1986.

52. Liotta, L.A.; Rao, C.N.; Barksy, S.H. Tumor invasion and the extracellular matrix. Lab Invest. 49:636-649; 1983.

52a. Loeffler, J.S.; Alexander, E.; Kooy, H.M.; Wen, P.Y.; Fine, H.A.; Black, P.M. Radiosurgery for brain metastases. Prin and Prac Onc. 5: 3-12, 1991.

53. Lombardi, F.; Lattuada, A.; Gasparini, M. *et al.* Sequential half-body irradiation as systemic treatment for progressive Ewings sarcoma. Int Radiat Oncol Biol Phys. 8:1679-1682; 1982.

53a. Maher, E.J.; Coia, L.; Duncan, G.; Lawton, P.A. Treatment strategies in advanced and metastatic cancer: Differences in attitude between the USA, Canada, and Europe. Int J Radiat Oncol Biol Phys. 23:239-244; 1992.

54. Mandell, L.; Hilaris, B. The treatment of single brain metastasis from non-oat cell lung carcinoma. Cancer. 58:641-648;1986.

55. Markman, M.; Sheidler, V.; Ettinger, D.S. Antiemetic efficacy of dexamethasone: randomized, double blind, crossover study with prochlorperazine in patients receiving cancer chemotherapy. New Engl J Med. 311-549-552; 1984.

56. Marton, K.I.; Sox, H.C.; Krupp, J.R. Involuntary weight loss: diagnostic and prognostic signficance. Ann Intern Med. 95:568-574; 1981.

57. McLemore, T.L.; Eggleston, J.C.; Shoemaker, R.H.; *et al.* Comparison of intrapulmonary, percutaneous, intrathoracic and subcutaneous models for the propagation of human pulmonary and nonpulmonary cell lines in athymic nude mice. Cancer Res. 48:2880-2886; 1988.

58. Moser, R.P.; Johnson, M.L. Surgical management of brain metastaes. Oncology. 3:123-127; 1989.

58a. Mushel, R. and Liotta, LA. Role of oncogenes in metastasis. Carcinogenesis 9: 705-710, 1988.

59. Neidhart, J.; Gayer, M.; Metz, E. Halidol is an effective antiemetic for platinum and mustard induced vomiting when other agents fail. Proc Am Soc Clin Oncol Abstract. 21:365; 1980.

60. Nicholson, G.L. Organ colonization and the cell surface properties of malignant cells. Biochem Biophys Acta 695: 113-176; 1982.

61. Nicholson, G.L. Transmembrane control of the receptors on normal and tumor cells II. Surface changes associated with t.ransformation and malignancy. Biochem Biophyt Acta 458:1-72;1976.

62. Nicholson, G.L.; Dulski, K.; Basson, J.C.; *et al.* Preferential organ attachment and invasion in vitro by B-16 melanoma cells selected for differing metastatic colonization and invasive properties. Invasion Metastasis. 5:144-158; 1985.

62a. Nielson, O.S.; Munro, A.J.; Tunnock, I.F. Bone metastases: Pathophysiology and management policy. J Clin Oncol 9:509-524; 1991.

63. Pagani, J.J.; Libshitz, H.I. Imaging bone metastases. Radiol Clin North Am. 27:545-567; 1982.

63a. Patchell, RA; Tibbs, P.A.; Walsh, J.W. *et al.* A randomized trial of surgery in the treatment of single metastases to the brain. New Eng J of Med 322: 494-500.

64. Paushter, D.M.; Zeman, R.K.; Scheibler, M.L. *et al.* CT evaluation of suspected hepatic metastases: comparison of techniques for IV contrast enhancement. A.J.R. 152:267-271; 1989.

64a. Porter, A.T.; McEwan, A.J.B.; and Members of the Canadian strontium 89 Group. First results of a phase III study to determine whether the addition of Strontium 89 therapy to standard fractionated local field irradiation is more efficacious than local field iradiation alone in the management of endocrine resistant metastatic prostate cancer. Int J Radiat Oncol Biol Phys. In press, 1992.

65. Poste, G.; Tzeng, J.; Doll, J. Evolution of tumor cell heterogeneity during progressive growth of individual lung metastases. Proc Natl Acad Sci. USA. 79:6574-6578; 1982.

66. Poulter, C.A.; Cosmatos, D.; Rubin, P. *et al.* A preliminary report of RTOG 82-06 phase II study of whether the addition of single dose hemibody irradiation to standard fractionated local field irradiation is more effective than local field irradiation alone in the treatment of symptomatic osseous metastases. Abstract 147. Int J Rad Oncol Bio Phys. 17 (suppl 1) 192; 1989.

66a. Poulter, C.A.; Cosmatos, D.; Rubin, P.; *et al.* A report of RTOG 82-06: A phase III study of whether the addition of single high dose hemibody irradiation to standard fractionated local field irradiation is more effective than local field irradiation alone in the treatment of symptomatic osseous metastases. Int J Radiat Oncol Biol Phys 23:207-214; 1992.

67. Pritchett, T.R.; Skinner, D.G.; Selser, S.F. Seminoma with elevated human chorionic gonadotropin. The case for retroperitoneal lymph node dissection. Urology. 25:344-346; 1985.

68. Quasim, M.M. Halfbody irradiation (HBI) in metastatic carcinomas. Clin Radiol. 32:215-219; 1981.

69. Ransohoff, J. Surgical management of metastatic tumors. Semin Oncol. 2:21-27; 1985.

70. Raventos, A.; DeNardo, S.J.; DeNardo, G. Prospects for radiolabeled monoclonal antibodies in metastatic disease. J. Thorac. Imag. 44-49; 1987.

71. Reinig, J.W.; Dwyer, A.J.; Miller, D.L. *et al.* Liver metastasis detection: comparative sensitivities of MR imaging and CT scanning. Radiology. 162:43-47; 1987.

72. Rowland, C.G.; Bullimore, J.A.; Smith, P.J. Halfbody irradiation in treatment of metastatic prostate carcinoma. Br J Urol. 53: 628-629; 1981.

73. Rowland, C.G.; Garrett., M.S.; Crowley, F.A. Halfbody radiation in plasma cell myeloma. Clin Radiol. 34:507-510; 1983.

74. Rubin, P. A unified classification of tumor: an oncotaxonomy with symbols. Cancer. 31:963-982; 1973.

75. Salazar, O.M.; Rubin, P.; Hendrickson, F.R. *et al.* Single-dose halfbody irradiation for the palliation of bone metastasis from solid tumors: a preliminary report. Int J Radiat Oncol Biol Phys. 7:773-787; 1981.

76. Salazar, O.M.; Rubin, P.; Hendrickson, F.R. *et al.* Single-dose halfbody irradiation for palliation of multiple bone metastases from solid tumors: final radiation therapy oncology group report. Cancer 58:29-36; 1986.

77. Sherman, D.M.; Weichselbaum, R.; Order, S.E. *et al.* Palliation of hepatic metastasis. Cancer. 41:2013-2017; 1978.

78. Shivshanker, K.; Bennett, R.W.; Haynie, T.P. Tumor-associated gastroparesis: correction with metaclopramide. Am J Surg. 145: 221-225; 1983.

79. Shover, L.B.; Schain, W.S. *et al.* Psychological aspects of patients with cancer: sexual problems of patients with cancer. In: DeVita, V.T.; Hellman, S.; Rosenberg, S. eds. Principles and practice of oncology. 3rd ed. Philadelphia, PA: J.B. Lippincott Co; 2206-2215;1989.

80. Silberfarb, P.M.; Hauri, P.J.; Oxman, T.E. Insomnia in cancer patients. Soc Sci Med. 20:849-850; 1985.

81. Silverberg, E.; Lubera, J.A. Cancer statistics, 1989. CA. 39: 3-20; 1989.

82. Sloane, B.F.; Honn, K.V. Cysteine proteinase and metastasis. Cancer Metastasis Rev. 3: 249-265; 1984.

83. Smalley, S.R.; Sehray, M.F. Adjuvant radiation therapy after surgical resection of solitary brain metastasis: association with pattern of failure and survival. Int J Radiat Oncol Biol Phy. 13:1611-1616; 1987.

84. Smiley, S.; Schouten, J.; Chang, A. *et al.* Intrahepatic arterial infusion with 5-FU for liver metastases of colorectal carcinoma. Proc Am Soc Clin Oncol. 22:391; 1981.

85. Smith, F.D.; Kisner, D.; Schein, P.S. Nutrition and cancer: prospects for clinical research. Nutr Cancer. 2(1): 34-39; 1980.

86. Steckel, R.J.; Kagan, A.R. Evaluation of the unknown primary neoplasm. Radiol Clin North Am. 20:601-605; 1982.

86a. Stomper, P.C.; Recht, A.; Berenberg, A.L.; *et al.* Mammographic detection of recurrent cancer in the irradiated breast. AJR 148: 39-43, 1987.

87. Strum, S.B.; McDermed, J.E.; Opfell, R.W. *et al.* Intravenous metoclopramide. An effective antiemetic in cancer chemotherapy. JAMA. 247: 2683-2686; 1982.

87a. Sze, G.; Milano, E.; Johnson, C. *et al.* Detection of brain metastases: Comparison of contrast enhanced MR with unenhanced MR and enhanced CT. AJNR 11: 785-791, 1990.

88. Talmadge, J.E.; Wolman, S.R.; Fidler, I.J. Evidence for the clonal origin of spontaneous metastasis. Science. 217:361-363; 1982.

89. Tchekmedyian, N.S.; Tait, N.; Moody, M. *et al.* Appetite stimulation with megestrol acetate in cachectic cancer patients. Semin Oncol. 13 (suppl 4):37-43; 1986.

90. Thrall, J.H.; Ellis, B.I. Skeletal metastases. Radiol Clin North Am. 25:1155-1170; 1987.

91. Tong, D.; Gillich, L.; Henderson, F.R. The palliation of symptomatic osseous metastases: final results of the study by the radiation therapy oncology group. Cancer. 50:893-899; 1982.

92. Totty, W.G.; Murphy, W.A.; Lee, J.K.T. Soft tissue tumors: MR imaging. Radiology. 160:135-141; 1986.

93. Virchow, R. Die Cellular Pathologie in ihrer Begrundung auf Physiologische und Pathologische Gewebelebre. Berlin: Hirschwald, 1858.

94. Waldmann, T.A.; McIntire, K.R. The use of radioimmunoassay for alpha-fetoprotein in the diagnosis of malignancy. CA. 34:1510-1515; 1974.

95. Wandthe, J.C.; Plewes, D.B. Chest equalization radiography. J Thorac Imag. 1(1)14-20; 1985.

96. Wandthe, J.C.; Plewes, D.B. Comparison of scanning equalization and conventional chest radiography. Radiology. 172:641-645; 1989.

97. Young, V.R. Energy metabolism and requirements in the cancer patient. Cancer Res. 37:2336-2347; 1977.

98. Zamcheck, N. Carcinoembryonic antigen. Quantitative variations in circulating levels in benign and malignant digestive tract diseases. Adv Intern Med. 19:413-433; 1974.

Edgar C. Henshaw. M.D., Medical Oncology
Paul R. Schloerb, M.D., Surgery

Chapter **34**

NUTRITION AND THE CANCER PATIENT

Other men live to eat while I eat to live.

Socrates (61)

PERSPECTIVE

Weight loss can be the presenting symptom in cancer patients, and most patients begin to lose weight at some point in the disease. This weight loss, which in many patients becomes severe, is referred to as cachexia (1,4,8,10,12,13). It is usually accompanied by anorexia and early satiety, weakness and fatigue, and anemia (109). A 10% weight loss is often considered to constitute cachexia, although there is no universally accepted defining value. Weight loss in the cancer patient is usually caused in part by anorexia and the consequent decreased food intake, and in part by a poorly understood alteration in patient metabolism caused by the stress of the malignancy. Thus, the cachexia of the cancer patient differs greatly from simple undernutrition. These patients have abnormalities in the metabolism of carbohydrate, lipid, and protein, and in the body content of water and electrolytes, as well as alterations in hormonal and immunologic function that may be secondary to the wasting syndrome.

It has been found consistently that among patients who will eventually die of a particular cancer (e.g., lung cancer), at a given stage of disease those with weight loss will survive for a shorter time than those without (39). It is impossible to determine to what degree survival is affected because more aggressive cancer is more likely to cause weight loss, and because weight loss is itself a detrimental symptom. In either case, cachexia is an undesirable syndrome. This chapter will discuss the causes of wasting, and will provide a guide to the indications for, as well as the newer approaches to, nutritional treatment. The relationship of diet to carcinogenesis is another important aspect of nutrition, and is covered in some individual disease site chapters in the sections on etiology.

NUTRITIONAL PROBLEM IN CANCER

Normal Body Composition

The body of the young adult male is normally composed of about 20% fat by weight and 80% lean body mass. In the female these values are about 30% and 70% respectively. Water is the largest single component of the lean body mass (73%), and makes up about 50% (female) to 60% (male) of total body weight (96). As fat increases with aging, body water and lean body mass decrease as a fraction of body weight. Extracellular fluid, which includes plasma volume, is about 20% of body weight. Blood volume is about 7% of body weight in normal men and 6.5% in normal women. These values are about 0.5% less in obese individuals, and are increased proportionately in thin persons (1). Total exchangeable body sodium is about 3,000 mEq in normal individuals, and total exchangeable potassium is about 3,500 mEq with approximately 2,000 mEq of chloride in the body.

The second major contributor to lean body mass is protein, with small contributions from carbohydrates, minerals, and nucleic acids. Fig. 34-1 (2) illustrates the carbohydrate, fat, protein, and water composition, by weight, of a normal 71.5 kg man, and the caloric equivalents of these components. The tumor itself may differ slightly from normal body tissue in mineral and water content (33).

The preservation of the lean body mass, as well as of nutritional support, is a major objective of day-to-day food intake in disease. Lean body mass is sacrificed in states of undernutrition, especially because of the need for glucose. The central nervous system requires glucose at a rate of 120 to 140 g/d (32), and once liver glycogen is depleted, body proteins must be degraded to provide the carbon for this glucose. Body stores of glycogen are depleted within 24 hours of food deprivation, and thereafter protein and fat stores become the major source of carbon and energy (32). As shown in Fig. 34-1 (2), the body proteins are limited, the largest source being 5.2 kg of protein in skeletal muscle.

Alterations in Body Composition

The effects of cancer vary from patient to patient. Some patients maintain a good nutritional state until late in the disease. Most patients, however, undergo changes, sometimes dramatic, in body composition. Changes in composition similar to those of cancer cachexia occur in severe trauma, chronic infection, and starvation.

The most striking changes are (1) a decrease in total body protein, (2) a decrease in body fat, and (3) a relative expansion of extracellular, sodium-containing fluid (ECF). Protein is the major source of nitrogen in the body, and nitrogen balance (i.e., the intake versus output of nitrogen) has traditionally been measured to assess whether body protein stores are increasing or decreasing. Thus, the loss of protein in cancer patients is often referred to as negative nitrogen balance. Negative nitrogen balance is also prominent after severe trauma, major surgery, infections, and starvation. The expansion in ECF often occurs in the absence of obvious collections of ECF. When obvious changes in ECF occur, as

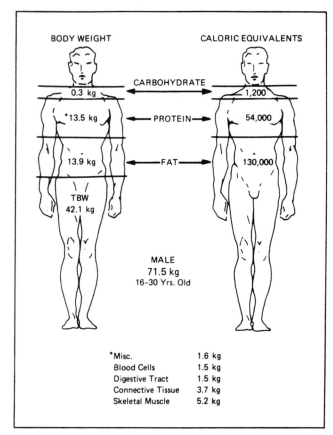

BODY WEIGHT

CALORIC EQUIVALENTS

CARBOHYDRATE

0.3 kg   1,200

*13.5 kg   PROTEIN   54,000

13.9 kg   FAT   130,000

TBW
42.1 kg

MALE
71.5 kg
16-30 Yrs. Old

*Misc.	1.6 kg
Blood Cells	1.5 kg
Digestive Tract	1.5 kg
Connective Tissue	3.7 kg
Skeletal Muscle	5.2 kg

Fig. 34-1. The left-hand figure shows the total body weight (TBW) of carbohydrate, protein, fat, and total body water in a 71.5 kg man. The inserted table, denoted by an asterisk, shows the distribution of protein among organ systems. The right-hand figure indicates the caloric equivalents of the components. From Brennan (2). Reprinted with permission from *The New England Journal of Medicine,* 304:375-382; 1981.

in malignant ascites or pleural effusion, the retention of sodium-containing and protein-rich ECF may be marked. In fact, redistributions of body fluid resulting from malignancy or from associated complications, such as peritonitis, intestinal obstruction, and thrombophlebitis, may produce fluid electrolyte derangements as severe as any seen as a result of external losses.

Because of wide variations in lean body mass, body water, and body fat, a cancer patient's body weight alone may be a poor reference for calculating the dosage of therapeutic agents.

Causes of Cancer-induced Alterations

Cancer promotes loss of fat and lean body mass by affecting the host in two major ways: decreasing nutrient intake and altering host metabolism.

Decreased Nutrient Intake

The most common cause of decreased intake is a loss of appetite. This is seen in almost all cancer patients in the course of the illness, as well as in most animals with tumors (4,41,77). Although the cause of anorexia is not understood, anorexia apparently can be a direct effect of the tumor. Experiments with parabiotic rats demonstrate the presence of a circulating anorectogenic factor in a rat tumor (86). There is clear-cut evidence in animals that loss of normal feeding responses (appetite) can be an early manifestation of

a particular tumor, while the tumor is small and before any evidence of weight loss or cachexia has appeared (77,78). Similarly, there are some patients in whom anorexia is the presenting symptom of cancer (37,92). However, the effect varies strikingly among tumors, both human and animal (106). There are patients who eat well until late in the course of their disease.

Anorexia may be caused secondarily by or aggravated by psychologic factors (23,54). In addition, patients with advanced disease may suffer a change in taste sensation, such that sensitivity to sweetness is reduced (40). Attempts to increase these patients' appetites by adding more sweeteners to food, however, have met with limited success. It has been demonstrated in both animals and humans that cancer symptoms and treatment side effects can lead, by association, to learned food aversions (24), and the importance of this mechanism to the anorexia of cancer requires further study. Finally, there is sometimes direct interference with food intake or absorption by head and neck or gastrointestinal (GI) cancers.

Alterations of Host Metabolism

The second major cause of wasting in the cancer patient is an often profound effect of the tumor on the host's metabolism of nutrients.

Energy expenditure: With animal tumors, energy expenditure is generally elevated in tumor-bearing animals (64,76,79). This is probably the case with many human cancer patients as well. However, as noted above, cancer patients are not a homogeneous population and in different series, and in different patients within series, measurements of resting energy expenditure (REE) have been reported to be low, normal, and high compared with normal controls. However, in people who have lost weight through simple malnutrition, REE is reduced as a compensatory mechanism. In patients who have lost weight because of cancer, measurements have usually indicated elevated rates compared with noncancer patients who are equally physically wasted even when they are not elevated, compared with healthy controls of the same height and weight (63,65,67,89,115). That is, the cancer patients' REE's often are not reduced as much as would be expected for the weight lost and decreased amount of food consumed, and those patients are therefore in abnormally negative energy balance.

The regulation of energy expenditure is poorly understood under normal conditions, and the cause of the abnormality in cancer patients is completely unknown.

Protein metabolism: The fractional rate of protein synthesis is often reduced in muscle of cancer-bearing animals (9,46,71,83,107,116) and humans (21,68,71), although the measurement is difficult in humans. Muscle wasting indicates that the protein degradation rate is not comparably reduced; limited data do not suggest an increased degradation rate (21,46,66,67,70). In liver of tumor-bearing animals, the rate of protein synthesis may be decreased (46) or increased (71,83,116,117) (presumably stimulated by elevated glucocorticoid hormone levels). Flux of isotopically-labeled amino acids is increased in some cancer patients (59,60,84); this has been interpreted to indicate increased total body protein synthesis. This indirect measurement must be interpreted with caution, however, and it is not clear what tissues would be responsible for an increased rate of protein synthesis.

The regulation of protein synthesis is not understood and the cause of the decreased rate in cancer patients is unknown. Protein synthesis is inhibited in states of dietary deficits, and this is presumably a factor in cancer cachexia. However, the negative nitrogen balance caused by cancer, and by a number of other stresses such as major surgery, severe trauma, burns, and infections, is not solely a matter of decreased nutrient availability (70,72). Studies of total parenteral nutrition show that given equal amounts of nutrients, cancer patients improve much less in measures of nutritional status than do normal, malnourished patients (29,82,88). Surgeons have consistently been frustrated in their attempts to prevent the obligatory nitrogen loss after surgery, and there are some patients with far-advanced cancer who cannot be repleted or even maintained despite high nutrient inputs (82,108). There are likewise some animal tumors in which forced feeding of the animal, even with supranormal quantities of food, does not prevent the loss of carcass (nontumor) weight (106). Nevertheless, in less extreme cases host nutrition status can usually be maintained or at least improved by proper alimentary therapy. This improvement may, however, require larger quantities of nutrient than would simple starvation (28).

Glucose metabolism: While fasting blood glucose and insulin levels are generally normal in cancer patients, a sizable proportion of patients have an abnormal response to a glucose load (glucose tolerance test), with slow glucose clearance, insulin resistance, and lower than normal insulin response to elevated blood glucose concentration (66,85,94,98). The cause of this abnormality is not clear and the incidence in cancer patients is not precisely known, but it is a fairly common finding and has been demonstrated in early cancer patients before any weight loss was apparent.

A further abnormality is an increased rate of glucose turnover, that is, an increased rate of synthesis and utilization of glucose (55). Glucose is synthesized primarily in the liver (and also the kidney) from lactate and alanine, and, to a small extent, glycerol. In cancer patients, synthesis from lactate and alanine are increased (30,43,51,52,56,57,69,72). Much of the lactate is derived from glucose through the Cori cycle, in which glucose is converted to lactate in peripheral tissues (e.g., during muscular activity) and lactate is converted to glucose in the liver. This is a net energy-requiring cycle, since more adenosine 5'-triphosphate is required to synthesize glucose in the liver than is yielded through glycolysis in the periphery, and the increased cycling is apparently futile. The tissues that generate the lactate in the Cori cycle is unknown. Glycolysis in large tumors occasionally may explain the lactate source, but the tumors are generally too small to account for the high lactate production. The increased synthesis of glucose from alanine may be driven by increased alanine production from tissues in negative protein balance.

Lipid metabolism: Utilization of body fat is a physiologic response in humans and animals during adaptation to negative energy balance, and loss of body fat is characteristic in tumor-bearing animals and human cancer patients in negative energy balance. In addition to this adaptation, however, there appear to be abnormalities in lipid metabolism. Cancer patients frequently demonstrate hyperlipidemia, with elevations of triglycerides and low-density lipoproteins (103). Glycerol and free fatty acid turnover are increased (45,63,98). In some weight-loss patients, glucose infusion has failed to suppress lipolysis normally. Serum lipoprotein lipase is im-portant for the transfer of triglycerides into fat cells, and is decreased in starvation and states where fat must be mobilized. Enzyme activity has been reported to be low compared with healthy controls in the serum of weight-losing cancer patients and has been considered to be abnormal, but values have not been compared with those of similarly malnourished noncancer patients (113).

Mechanism of Tumor Effect on Host

The mechanism of the detrimental effects of the tumor on host nutrient metabolism is not known (110). Although in some patients the tumor's use of energy sources, such as glucose, might account for the deprivation of normal tissues, in most patients the amount of tumor tissue is much too small (119). The likely explanation is that tumors often stimulate the host to secrete, or secrete themselves, hormones that induce a stress reaction in the host. Recently there have been discovered a number of immunologically and metabolically active polypeptide hormones that are secreted in response to various stresses by lymphocytes, monocytes, and other tissues. Examples are interleukins (IL) 1 through 6; interferons alpha, ß, and gamma; tumor necrosis factor (TNF); lymphocytotoxin; the hemopoietic growth and differentiation factors; and many less well-defined factors that are presently being characterized. IL-2, interferons, and TNF each have been administered to patients, and in high doses each produces a debilitating flu-like syndrome with symptoms that seem an exaggeration of those of the cachectic cancer patient: severe anorexia, severe weakness and fatigue, dramatic increase in ECF (at least with IL-2), and almost certainly negative nitrogen balance. Continuously elevated levels of any of these hormones might be anticipated to produce cachexia. In a fascinating model case, a transplantable tumor that secretes large amounts of TNF because it has been transfected with a plasmid containing the TNF gene caused severe cachexia in the host mouse (87). With spontaneous human tumors, it is perhaps more likely that the tumors induce the host to release the stress hormones. For instance, in what might be an analogous situation, a majority of patients with leishmaniasis and malaria have high serum levels of TNF (97), presumably produced by trypanosome-infected macrophages. TNF has been called "cachectin" (25) because it is postulated to be responsible for the severe wasting in these diseases. TNF/cachectin itself is probably not responsible for cachexia in the majority of cancer patients because serum TNF levels are elevated in only a minority of cancer patients (97,101), but this example provides a model illustrating how lymphokines could be responsible for cancer cachexia. This hypothesis is being investigated. Perhaps another analogous situation is seen in patients with severe burn injuries, in whom long-lasting elevation of catecholamines has been demonstrated (118).

Abnormal Regulation of Nitrogen Balance in Tumors

Malignancies continue to grow in patients whose normal tissues are in negative nitrogen balance. In fact, normal tissues themselves vary in response to starvation and stress. In starving rats, skeletal muscle consistently and extensively loses protein while brain and testes do not lose protein even in rats starving to death (19). It appears that a cancer develops a high priority for net positive protein balance even if its tissue of origin, such as muscle, has a low priority. Protein metabolism is controlled by presently unknown hormonal mechanisms. Presumably, malignant cells are less responsive to the hormonal signals than are most normal tissues.

Experimental Therapies

Hydrazine: Hydrazine is an inhibitor of phosphonenol pyruvate carboxykinase, an enzyme in the gluconeogenesis pathway. Since this pathway appears to be overactive in cancer patients, as noted above, and is wasteful of energy, hydrazine has been administered to inhibit this process. Chlebowski and co-workers (34,35) have shown in careful studies that 60 mg. hydrazine sulfate three times a day given over 1 month decreases glucose utilization and REE modestly and slows or prevents weight loss with no apparent detrimental effects. It is not yet clear whether these effects on metabolism are large enough to be translated into real benefit for the patients.

Megestrol acetate: Preliminary studies indicate that high doses of this progesterone analog can cause weight gain in weight-losing cancer patients (20). This regimen is expensive and it has not yet been established that the weight gain is protein rather than simply fluid and fat or that real symptomatic improvement results, but this experimental therapy appears hopeful.

Alanyl-glutamine dipeptide: Glutamine and alanine are two of the most physiologically important products of protein and amino acid catabolism in muscle (81), and administration of the two as a dipeptide is being investigated because the dipeptide offers advantages of greater stability and lower osmolarity compared with the individual amino acids (18). Recent evidence suggests that supplementation of total parenteral nutrition with this dipeptide inhibits muscle protein loss (108).

Ketogenic diet: A ketogenic diet, based on a high proportion of medium-chain triglycerides and added 3-hydroxybutyrate, is being investigated as an approach to inhibiting protein catabolism in muscle and inhibiting gluconeogenesis in liver in cancer patients (90,99). In a small series of patients, the performance score of patients was improved on this diet compared with a standard diet (47). Whether such diets will prove practical is not known.

NUTRITIONAL SUPPORT IN CANCER TREATMENT (3,5)

Loss of weight, especially fat, is not necessarily a bad thing. Loss of muscle and other lean tissue, on the other hand, may be detrimental, associated as it is with loss of physical strength, loss of respiratory strength, and decreased resistance to infection. Consequently, in the management of the cancer patient, the physician must be concerned with accurately assessing the patient's nutritional status—his need for nutritional support, his losses, both internal and external, which may be related to the malignancy, and his need for an adequate replacement of nutrition by enteral or parenteral means.

Nutritional Assessment

Studies by different groups over a period of many years have used techniques for measuring nitrogen balance to assess nutritional status. Although these techniques have proved useful in determining the fraction of ingested protein or nitrogen that is retained and excreted, it must be emphasized that this rather gross external measurement provides no indication of the fate of protein within the body (8). Protein requirements for wound healing, immunologic response, cellular response to injury and infection, protein turnover, and other needs are not necessarily revealed by measurement of nitrogen balance.

Clinical judgment and common sense should prevail in the nutritional assessment of cancer patients (73). For example, if an elderly man with a 4-month history of progressive dysphagia and a 18 kg weight loss is found to have a carcinoma of the esophagus, the cause and effect is obvious, as is the need for nutritional support. It is not necessary to mobilize computer resources and a battery of diagnostic tests to know that extensive supplementation is required. Less obvious is the case of an individual of average weight and previously good health, who develops intestinal obstruction or a ruptured viscus or a malignant effusion. Acute translocation of protein stores may represent an acute nutritional deficiency that, although not always obvious, may require correction.

Nutritional Evaluation Parameters and Harris-Benedict Equations

Nutritional evaluation: Evaluation of nutrition can be carried out with minimal difficulty (27). Dietary history is helpful and should include height and actual weight, as well as ideal weight, age and usual dietary habits. The Harris-Benedict equations (50) use age, height, and weight to calculate basal energy expenditure (BEE) as follows:

Men: BEE (kcal) = 66 + [13.7 x wt (kg)] + [5 x ht(cm)] - [6.8 x age (yr)]

Women: BEE (kcal) = 655 + [9.6 x wt (kg)] + [1.7 x ht (cm)] -[4.7 x age (yr)]

Serum albumin: Measurement of the serum albumin is helpful as an indicator of visceral protein stores. Hypoalbuminemia may be present in as many as half of hospitalized patients and has been used to define so-called hospital malnutrition. At the University of Rochester's Strong Memorial Hospital, a decrease of serum albumin concentration below 3.5 g/dL was found in about 20% of patients over a period of 6 months. This figure represents all patients, including those with end-stage cancer as well as patients with acute, remediable diseases, such as burns. The serum albumin concentration is only one indicator of protein calorie malnutrition. Since the turnover of albumin is approximately 20 days, better indicators are proteins with shorter turnover times, such as transferrin or prealbumin. Normal values at the Strong Memorial Hospital Clinical Laboratory are: serum transferrin, 180 to 365 mg/dL; serum prealbumin, 15 to 40 mg/dL.

Urine Creatinine: Measurement of 24-hour urine creatinine makes possible the calculation of the creatinine/height index (26,114). Urine creatinine excretion is proportional to body muscle mass and lean body weight. Based on the fact that patients lose weight but not height as the result of illness, measurement of the 24-hour urinary creatinine can keep track of changes in lean body weight. The creatinine/height index is compared with that of a group of healthy individuals of comparable heights. This index can be valuable when dealing with malnutrition states that last long enough to produce body weight loss and, therefore, to create sufficient changes in the index. The normal creatinine/height index group does not take into account some of the normal extremes, such as individuals who are tall and thin or short and fat, but otherwise in perfect health.

Immunocompetence: Assessment of immunocompetence may be useful in nutritional assessment as well as in predicting risk of infection and mortality. Immunocompetence is measured by skin tests using different antigens such as streptokinase/ streptodornase, mumps, purified protein derivative, *Candida* and others. As reported by Meakins *et al.* (74) the relationship among anergy (no reaction to skin test antigens), infection, and mortality is striking. In surgical patients with immunocompetence, as evidenced by local reaction to skin test antigens, the mortality in more than 900 patients was approximately 3%, while 36% of the patients with anergy died. In anergic patients, approximately half developed serious infections. At least as important was the demonstration by this group that adequate nutritional support could reverse the anergy and reduce the incidence of sepsis and mortality.

Prognostic nutritional index. A prognostic nutritional index based upon nutritional assessment data, complications, and clinical outcome in more than 160 patients has been developed to attempt to assess the relative importance of various factors used for nutritional assessment (31). In this study, it was found that a prognostic nutritional index correlated best with serum albumin, serum transferrin, delayed hypersensitivity (skin tests), and triceps skinfold thickness.

Anthropometric indices: Use of anthropometric indices, such as the triceps skinfold thickness and arm muscle circumference, have been advocated. These are relatively simple, noninvasive measurements that can be performed by the dietician. Their value in nutritional assessment of hospitalized patients in this country remains to be determined (75).

To provide a consistent and rapid form of nutritional assessment and to maintain uniform records, small computer programs are available for calculation of basal energy requirements, as well as nutritional needs for both enteral and parenteral nutritional support (95).

Nutritional Support

Urinary urea nitrogen (UUN): Provision of adequate calories and protein is the key to promoting recovery and survival (42,49,100,118). Protein requirements are dictated not only by body size, but by severity of trauma or infection, and by both external and internal losses. Caloric needs similarly are influenced by severity of trauma, body temperature, sepsis, and by fluid losses.

Some indication of protein requirements can be obtained by measurement of UUN. Direct measurement of total urine nitrogen content is cumbersome. An alternate method, sufficiently accurate for most purposes, is measurement of the UUN. UUN accounts for about 70% of the total urine nitrogen (27). If 2 g of nitrogen are added to the 24-hour UUN, an approximation of the total 24-hour UUN excretion may be obtained (27). Approximately another 2 g may be added for nonurinary loss to obtain an approximation of total 24-hour UUN excretion. Multiplication of this value by 6.25 gives an indication of protein equivalence per day. Calories should be provided at a ratio of about 150 kcal/g of nitrogen (36,61). About one third of the administered calories should be given as fat (80).

Parenteral and enteral routes. Nutritional support is indicated in malnourished patients, including those who cannot, will not, or should not take sufficient food orally, or who cannot take sufficient nutriments to fulfill nutritional requirements. Nutritional support is provided by enteral or parenteral routes (Fig. 34-2) (49) when the stomach and intestinal tract are available and functioning normally (105,112).

Although it is time-consuming, encouraging patients to eat and providing acceptable nutritional supplements will be rewarding.

1. For enteral nutrition: Use of nasogastric tube, cervical esophagostomy (48), feeding gastrostomy or jejunostomy will provide access to the GI tract. Availability of several products for enteral nutrition has expedited nutritional management in this form.

   Some general principles should be followed, as noted by Benotti and Blackburn (22). Continuous administra-

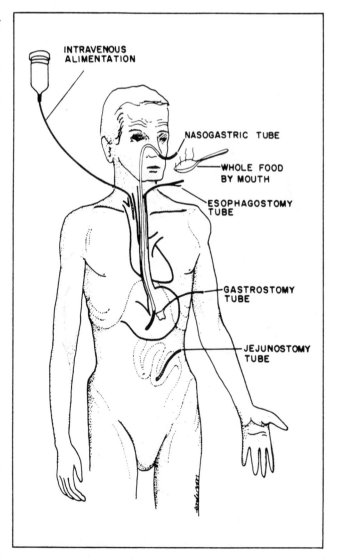

Fig. 34-2. Enteral and parenteral routes of nutrition. Nutritional support is a major feature of effective cancer management. From Hardy (49), with permission.

tion of nasogastric or jejunostomy feeding is preferable. Initially, these are administered as half-strength dilutions at a rate of 50 cc/h. Every 4 hours, aspiration is done and if the residual is greater than 100 mL, the rate is decreased. The tubing is flushed at that time. Gradually, the concentration is increased to full strength and the rate is increased to that required (about 100 cc/h). If the patient is to be sent home on tube feedings, intermittent administration every few hours is acceptable and well tolerated. A feeding gastrostomy is helpful for patients with head, neck, or esophageal cancer who are receiving radiation therapy. The gastrostomy can be done under local anesthesia and, if necessary, is available indefinitely for nutritional support.

2. A needle jejunostomy may be fashioned at the conclusion of laparotomy if indicated (38,58). Feedings may be started in the recovery room because the functioning of the intestine, unlike the stomach, remains normal immediately after operation. As shown by Hoover *et al.* (58), this procedure has been remarkably free of complications. When it has served its nutritional purpose, the jejunostomy catheter is simply withdrawn.

3. *For parenteral nutrition* (2,6,7), several options are available. For peripheral intravenous (IV) nutritional support, amino acid solutions containing only 10% glucose may be used. Additional calories are supplied with fat emulsions. It is not possible to use higher than 10% glucose in a peripheral vein because of the high incidence of thrombophlebitis that is a limiting factor even with the use of 10% glucose. Use of peripheral nutrition is beneficial for nutritional support involving less than 1 week of therapy.

To avoid the adverse consequences of infusion of a hypertonic solution in a peripheral vein, central venous cannulation, usually through the subclavian vein, is used. The current technique was developed by Dudrick *et al.* (42) and Wilmore *et al.* (118) at the University of Pennsylvania. It has made possible long-term nutritional support in both infants and adults. Inserting the subclavian catheter is a meticulous, sterile procedure that, if not properly done, can lead to serious complications such as pneumothorax, arterial hematoma, and sepsis.

For the patient who requires long-term nutritional support, use of a Hickman or Broviac catheter may be useful (93). These catheters are also available for IV cancer chemotherapy. Insertion of this type of catheter (Fig. 34-3) (93) is accomplished via the cephalic vein at the deltopectoral groove or percutaneously into the subclavian vein using a local anesthetic. The catheter exits through a point on the lower anterior chest wall as shown in Fig. 34-3. The smaller siliconized rubber portion of the catheter is inserted and advanced a distance so that the top lies in the region of the right atrium. X-ray or fluoroscopy is used to confirm accurate placement. These catheters have proved satisfactory (111) and are ideal for home parenteral nutrition.

Treatment of Intestinal Fistula

An important area of nutritional support in cancer patients involves treatment of intestinal fistula. This is a distressing complication of surgery or of the tumor itself and is frequently associated with intestinal obstruction, which must be relieved if the fistula is to close. Administration of parenteral

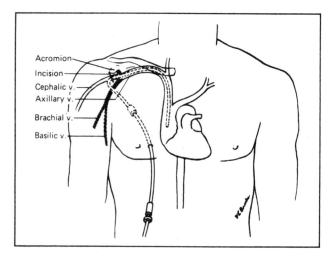

Fig. 34-3. The Hickman or Broviac catheter used for long-term or home parenteral nutrition. V = vein. From Riella and Scribner (93); by permission of Surgery, Gynecology & Obstetrics.

nutritional support which allows the patient to abstain from oral intake, greatly diminishes the volume of fistula drainage (102). This reduction in fistula drainage facilitates management of the patient and reduces the need for fluid and electrolyte replacement. In the absence of obstruction the fistula will close usually. A trial of several weeks of parenteral alimentation is justified to accomplish this objective.

Conclusion

The role of nutritional support in the management of the cancer patient and in the treatment of cancer rests with maintenance of body strength and well-being. There is no conclusive evidence that provision of adequate nutritional support will preferentially feed the tumor or that it will enhance tumor growth. Although some reports suggest that provision of adequate nutritional support is associated with improved response to radiation therapy or chemotherapy, there is no definitive evidence based on an adequate, prospective, randomized study to provide an answer to this question (62).

The catabolic effects of cancer are well known. The possible role of nutritional support in promoting improved survival is not fully understood.

Recent work studying body composition and survival in the chemotherapy of lymphoma in those patients receiving parenteral nutrition revealed some weight gain with chemotherapy. These body composition studies, however, suggested that this weight gain was either water or fat (91). No improvement in survival accompanied nutritional support in this reported experience. The severe metabolic insult associated with cancer chemotherapy has been studied by Herrmann *et al.* (53) who concluded that aggressive nutritional support was justified by the deleterious effects of chemotherapy.

According to our present knowledge, it appears unlikely that any striking improvement in survival or effective therapy is to be expected from use of nutritional support. In terms of patient well-being and maintenance of strength, however, nutritional support is probably justified.

Objectives of nutritional support include preservation of body cell mass and muscle strength, normal cell composition and organ function, replacement of "third space" losses, prevention of mineral and vitamin deficiencies, and preservation of normal hemodynamics and protein kinetics.

Indications for parenteral nutrition in cancer (49,82) include extensive surgery, short bowel syndrome resulting from extensive small bowel resection, radiation enteritis, GI obstruction, enteric fistula, peritonitis or other major sepsis, and renal or hepatic failure.

Use of minimum amounts of essential L-amino acids in renal failure is associated with decreased uremia. Branched-chain amino acids have been investigated in patients with hepatic failure and with sepsis. Results are conflicting and do not support general use of branched-chain amino acid solutions.

Nutritional support, by enteral or parenteral means, represents a valuable therapeutic modality for the management of cancer patients. Although complications may include mechanical and catheter placement problems as well as metabolic, fluid electrolyte, hydration, and septic complications, increasing experience has reduced such incidents and has further defined the indications and usefulness of these techniques.

Recommended Reading

The volume of *Cancer Research* devoted to "Nutrition and Cancer Therapy" (13) provides an excellent practical and theoretical background, and is all-inclusive through 1987. Recent texts by Kinney *et al.* (11), Rombeau and Caldwell (14,15), Dietel (5), Silberman and Eisenberg (17), and Fischer (6) present important background information as well as practical approaches to both enteral and parenteral nutrition. For a more general understanding of nutrition not specifically related to cancer, see *Nutritional Support of Medical Practice* edited by Schneider *et al.* (16).

REFERENCES

General References

1. Ballinger, W.F.; Collins, J.A.; Drucker, W.R.; *et al.* Manual of surgical nutrition. Philadelphia, Pa.: W.B. Saunders Co., 1975.
2. Brennan, M.R. Total parenteral nutrition in the cancer patient. New Engl. J. Med. 304:375-382; 1981.
3. Committee on Diet, Nutrition, and Cancer. Assembly of Life Sciences, National Academy of Sciences, National Academy Press; Washington, D.C.; 1982.
4. Costa, G. Cachexia, the metabolic component of neoplastic diseases. Cancer Res. 37:2327-2335; 1977.
5. Deitel, M. (Ed.). Nutrition in clinical surgery. Baltimore, Md.: Williams & Wilkins Co.; 1985.
6. Fischer, J.E. Surgical Nutrition. Boston, Mass.: Little, Brown, and Co., 1983.
7. Grant, J.P. Handbook of Total Parenteral Nutrition. Philadelphia, Pa.: W.B. Saunders Co., 1980.
8. Heber, D.; Byerly, L.O.; Chi, J.; Grosvenor, M.; Bergman, R.N.; Coleman, M.; Chlebowski, R.T. Pathophysiology of malnutrition in the adult cancer patient. Cancer 58:1867-1873; 1986.
9. Henshaw, E.C. Nutritional control of protein synthesis. In: Clemens, M.J., ed. Gene expression, Boca Raton, Fla: CRC Press; 1980:119-157.
10. Kern, K.A.; Norton, J.A. Cancer cachexia. J. Parenteral Enteral Nutrition 12:286-298; 1988.
11. Kinney, J.M.; Jeejeebhoy, K.N.; Hill, G.L.; Owen, O.E. Nutrition and metabolism in patient care. W.B. Saunders Co., Philadelphia, PA; 1988.
12. Milder, J.W. (ed): Nutrition and Cancer Therapy (Conference). Cancer Res 37:No. 7:1977.

Specific References

13. Norton, J.A.; Peacock, J.L.; Morrison, S.D. Cancer cachexia. CRC Critical Rev. Oncol. Hematol. 7:289-327; 1987.
14. Rombeau, J.L.; Caldwell, M.D. Enteral and tube feeding. W.B. Saunders Co., Philadelphia, PA; 1984.
15. Rombeau, J.L.; Caldwell, M.D. Parenteral Nutrition. W.B. Saunders Co., Philadelphia, PA; 1986.
16. Schneider, H.A.; Anderson, C.E.; Coursin, D.B. (eds) Nutritional support of medical practice. New York, NY: Harper and Row Publishers, 1983.
17. Silberman, H.; Eisenberg, D. Parenteral and enteral nutrition for the hospitalized patient. Appleton-Century-Crofts, East Norwalk, CT; 1982.

Specific References

18. Addis, T.; Poo, L.J.; Lew, W. The quantities of protein lost by the various organs and tissues of the body during a fast. J. Biol. Chem. 115-116; 1936.
19. Adibi, S.A. Experimental basis for use of peptides as substrates for parenteral nutrition: A review. Metabolism 36:1001-1011; 1987.
20. Aisner, J.; Tchekmedyian, N.S.; Tait, N.; Parnes, H.; Novak, M. Studies of high-dose megestrol acetate: potential applications in cachexia. Seminars in Oncology 15 (Suppl. 1) 68-75; 1988.
21. Bennegard, K.; Lindmark, L.; Eden, E.; Svaninger, G.; Lundholm, K. Flux of amino acids across the leg in weight-losing patients. Cancer Res. 44:386-393; 1984.
22. Benotti, P.; Blackburn, G.L. Protein and caloric or macronutrient metabolic management of the critically ill patient. Critical Care Med. 7:520-525; 1979.
23. Bernstein, I.L. Physiological and psychological mechanisms of cancer anorexia. Cancer Res. 42:715s-720s; 1982.
24. Bernstein, I.L.; Bernstein, I.D. Learned food aversions and cancer anorexia. Cancer Treatment Rep. 65(suppl. 5):43-47; 1981.
25. Beutler, B.; Cerami, A. Tumor necrosis, cachexia, shock and inflammation: A common mediator. Ann. Rev. Biochem. 57:505-518; 1988.
26. Bistrian, B.R.; Blackburn, G.L.; Sherman, M; *et al.* Therapeutic index of nutritional depletion in hospitalized patients. Surg. Gynecol. Obstet. 141:512-516; 1975.
27. Blackburn, G.L.; Bistrian, B.R.; Miani, B.S., *et al.* Nutritional and metabolic assessment of the hospitalized patient. J. Parenteral Enteral Nutr. 1:11-22; 1977.
28. Blackburn, G.L.; Miani, B.S.; Bistrian, B.R., *et al.* The effect of cancer on nitrogen electrolyte and mineral metabolism. Cancer Res. 37:2348-2353; 1977.
29. Brennan, M.R. Metabolic response to surgery in the cancer patient. Consequences of aggressive multimodality therapy. Cancer 43:2053-2064; 1979.
30. Burt, M.E.; Lowry, S.F.; Gorschboth, C.; Brennan, M.R. Metabolic alterations in a noncachectic animal tumor system. Cancer 47:2138-2146; 1981.
31. Buzby, G.P.; Mullen, J.L.; Matthews, D.O.; *et al.* Prognostic nutritional index in gastrointestinal surgery. Am. J. Surg. 139:160-167; 1980.
32. Cahill, G.F., Jr. Starvation in man. New. Engl. J. Med. 222:668-675; 1970.
33. Cameron, I.L.; Smith, N.K.R.; Pool, T.B.; *et al.* Intracellular concentration of sodium and other elements as related to mitogenesis and oncogenesis in vivo. Cancer Res. 40:1493-1500; 1980.
34. Chlebowski, R.T.; Bulcavage, L.; Grosvenor, M.; *et al.* Hydrazine sulfate in cancer patients with weight loss. A placebo-controlled experience. Cancer 59:406-410; 1987.
35. Chlebowski, R.T.; Heber, D.; Richardson, B.; Block, J.B. Influence of hydrazine sulfate on abnormal carbohydrate metabolism in cancer patients with weight loss. Cancer Res. 44:857-861; 1964.
36. Coon, W.W.; Kawalczyk, R.S. Protein metabolism. In: Ballinger, W.R., Collins, J.A., Drucker, W.R., (eds). Manual of surgical nutrition. Philadelphia, Pa.: W.B. Saunders Co.; 1975; 50-72.
37. Costa, G.; Land, W.W.; Vincent, R.G.; et al Weight loss and cachexia in lung cancer. Nutr. Cancer 2:98-103; 1980.
38. Delany, H.M.; Carnevale, N.; Garvey, J.W.; *et al.* Postoperative nutritional support using needle catheter feeding jejunostomy. Ann. Surg. 186:165-170; 1977.
39. DeWys, W.D. Anorexia in cancer patients. Cancer Res. 37:2354-2358; 1977.
40. DeWys, W.D.; Begg, C.; Lavin, P.T.; *et al.* Prognostic effect of

weight loss prior to chemotherapy in cancer patients. Am. J. Med. 69:491-497;1980.

41. DeWys, W.D.; Walters, K. Abnormalities of taste sensation in cancer patients. Cancer 36:1888-1896;1975.

42. Dudrick, S.J.; Wilmore, D.W.; Vars, H.M.; *et al.* Long-term total parenteral nutrition with growth, development, and positive nitrogen balance. Surgery 64:134-142;1968.

43. Eden, E.; Edstrom, S.; Bennegard, K.; Schersten, T.; Lundholm, K. Glucose flux in relation to energy expenditure in malnourished patients with and without cancer during periods of fasting and feeding. Cancer Res. 44:1718-1724;1984.

44. Eden, E.; Edstrom, S.; Bennegard, K.; Lindmark, L.; Lundholm, K. Glycerol dynamics in weight-losing cancer patients. Surgery. 97:176-184;1985.

45. Eden, E.; Ekman, L.; Bennegard, K.; Lindmark, L.; Lundholm, K. Whole-body tyrosine flux in relation to energy expenditure in weight-losing cancer patients. Metabolism 33:1020-1027;1984.

46. Emery, P.W.; Lovell, L.; Rennie, M.J. Protein synthesis measured in vivo in muscle and liver of cachectic tumor-bearing mice. Cancer Res. 44:2779-2784;1984.

47. Fearon, K.C.H.; Borland, W.; Preston, T.; Tisdale, M.J.; Shenkin, A.; Calman, K.C. Cancer cachexia: influence of systemic ketosis on substrate levels and nitrogen metabolism. Am. J. Clin. Nutr. 47:42-48;1988.

48. Graham, W.P., III; Royster, H.P. Simplified cervical esophagostomy for long-term extra-oral feeding. Surg. Gynecol. Obstet.25:127-128;1967.

49. Hardy, J.D. Nutrition and cancer. In: Ballinger WF, Collins JA, Drucker WR, et al (eds): Manual of Surgical Nutrition. Philadelphia,Pa.: W.B. Saunders Co;1975.

50. Harris, J.A.;Benedict, F.G. A Biometric Study of Basal Metabolism in Man. Washington D.C., Carnegie Institution of Washington, 90:1919.

51. Heber, D.; Byerly, L.O.; Chlebowski, R.T. Metabolic abnormalities in the cancer patient. Cancer 55:225-229;1985.

52. Heber, D.; Chlebowski, R.T.; Ishibashi, D.E.; Herrold, J.N.; Block, J.B. Abnormalities in glucose and protein metabolism in noncachectic lung cancer patients. Cancer Res. 42:4815-4819;1982.

53. Herrmann, V.M.; Garnick, M.B.; Moore, F.D.; *et al.* Effect of cytotoxic agents on protein kinetics in patients with metastatic cancer. Surgery 90:381-387;1981.

54. Holland, J.C.; Rowland, J.; Plum, M. Psychological aspects of anorexia in cancer patients. Cancer Res. 37:2425-2428;1977.

55. Holroyde, C.P.; Galrezda, T.G.; Putnam, R.C. *et al.* Altered glucose metabolism in metastatic carcinoma. Cancer Res. 35:2710-2714;1975.

56. Holroyde, C.P.; Reichard, G.A. Carbohydrate metabolism in cancer cachexia. Cancer Treatment Repts. 65(suppl. 5);55-59;1981.

57. Holroyde, C.P.; Skutches, C.L.; Boden, G.; Reichard, G.A. Glucose metabolism in cachectic patients with colorectal cancer. Cancer Res. 44:5910-5913;1984.

58. Hoover, H.C., Jr.; Ryan, J.A.; Anderson, E.F.; *et al.* Nutritional benefits of immediate postoperative jejunal feeding of an elemental diet. Am. J. Surg. 139:153-159;1980.

59. Jeevanandam, M.; Lowry, S.F.; Brennan, M.F. Effect of the route of nutrient administration on whole-body protein kinetics in man. Metabolism 36:968-973;1987.

60. Jeevanandam, M.; Lowry, S.F.; Horowitz, G.D.; Brennan, M.F. Cancer cachexia and protein metabolism. Lancet (v) 1423-1426;1984.

61. Kinney, J.M. Energy requirements of the surgical patient. In: Ballinger, W.F.; Collins, J.A.; Drucker, W.R.; *et al.* eds. Manual of surgical nutrition. Philadelphia, Pa.: W.B. Saunders Co.; 1975;223-235.

62. Koretz, R.L. Parenteral nutrition: Is it oncologically logical. J. Clin. Oncol. 2:534-538;1984.

63. Legaspi, A.; Jeevanandam, M.; Starnes H.F., Jr.; Brennan, M.F. Whole body lipid and energy metabolism in the cancer patient. Metabolism 36:958-963;1987.

64. Lindmark, L.; Bennegard, K.; Eden, E.; Ekman, L.; Schersten, T.; Svaninger, G.; Lundholm, K. Resting energy expenditure in malnourished patients with and without cancer. Gastroenterology. 87:402-408;1984.

65. Lindmark, L.; Edstrom, S.; Ekman, L.; Karlberg, I.; Lundholm, K. Energy metabolism in nongrowing mice with sarcoma. Cancer-Res.43:3649-3654;1983.

66. Lundholm, K.; Bennegard, K.; Eden, G.; Svaninger, G.; Emery, P.W.; Rennie, M.J. Efflux of 3-methylhistidine from the leg in cancer patients who experience weight loss. Cancer Res. 42:8407-8411;1982.

67. Lundholm, K.; Bylund, A.-C.; Holm, J.; Schersten, T. Skeletal muscle metabolism in patients with malignant tumor. Eur. J. Cancer 12:465-473;1976.

68. Lundholm, K.; Edstrom, S.; Ekman, L; Karlberg, I.; Bylund, A.-C.; Schersten, T. A comparative study of the influence of malignant tumor on host metabolism in mice and man. Cancer 42:453-461;1978.

69. Lundholm, K.; Edstrom, S.; Karlberg, I.; *et al.* Relationship of food intake, body composition, and tumor growth to host metabolism in nongrowing mice with sarcoma. Cancer Res. 40:2516-2522;1980.

70. Lundholm, K.; Edstrom, S.; Karlberg, I.; Ekman, L.; Schersten, T. Glucose turnover, glyconeogenesis from glycerol, and estimation of net glucose cycling in cancer patients. Cancer 50:1142-1150;1982.

71. Lundholm, K.; Holm, G.; Schersten, T. Insulin resistance in patients with progressive malignant disease. Cancer Res. 39:1968-1972;1979.

72. Lundholm, K.; Karlberg, I.; Ekman, L.; Edstrom, S.; Schersten, T. Evaluation of anorexia as the cause of altered protein synthesis in skeletal muscles from nongrowing mice with sarcoma. Cancer Res. 41:1989-1996;1981.

73. Malt, R.A. Keep it simple. Nutr. Today 6:30-33;1971.

74. Meakins, J.L.; Peitsch, J.B.; Bubenick, O. *et al.* Delayed hypersensitivity: Indication of acquired failure of host defenses in sepsis and trauma. Ann. Surg. 186:241-250;1977.

75. Michel, L.; Serrano, A.; Malt, RA. Nutritional support of hospitalized patients. New. Engl. J. Med. 304:1147-1152;1981.

76. Mider, G.B.; Fenninger, L.D.; Haven, F.L. *et al.* The energy expenditure of rats bearing walker carcinoma 256. Cancer Res. 11:731-736;1951.

77. Morrison, S.D. Generation and compensation of the cancer cachectic process by spontaneous modification of feeding behavior. Cancer Res. 36:228-233;1976.

78. Morrison, S.D. Partition of energy expenditure between host and tumor. Cancer Res. 31:98-107;1971.

79. Morrison, S.D. Origins of anorexia in neoplastic disease. Am. J. Clin. Nutr. 21:1104-1107;1978.

80. Mueller, C.B.; Thomas, E.J. Nutritional needs of the normal adult. In: Ballinger, W.F., Collins, J.A., Drucker, W.R., *et al.* eds. Manual of surgical nutrition. Philadelphia, Pa.: W.B. Saunders, Co.; 1975;142-165.

81. Newsholme, E.A.; Newsholme, P.; Curi, R.; Challoner, M.A.; Ardawi, M.S. A role for muscle in the immune system and its importance in surgery, trauma, sepsis and burns. Nutrition 4:261-268;1988.

82. Nixon, D.W.; Lawson, D.H.; Hutner, M. *et al.* Hyperalimentation of the cancer patient with protein-calorie undernutrition. Cancer Res. 41:2038-2045;1981.

83. Norton, J.A.; Maher, M.; Wesley, R.; White, D.; Brennan, M.F. Glucose intolerance in sarcoma patients. Cancer 54:3022-3027;1984.

84. Norton, J.A.; Moley, J.R.; Green, M.V.; Carson, R.E.; and Morrison, S.D. Parabiotic transfer of cancer anorexia/cachexia in male rats. Cancer Res. 45:5547-5552;1985.

85. Norton, J.A.; Schamberger, R.; Stein, T.P.; Milne, G.W.A; Brenna, M.F. The influence of tumor-bearing on protein metabolism in the rat. J. Surg. Res. 30:456-462;1981.

86. Norton, J.A.; Stein, T.P.; Brennan, M.F. Whole body protein synthesis and turnover in normal man and malnourished patients with and without known cancer. Ann. Surg. 194:123-128;1981.

87. Oliff, A.; Defeo-Jones, D.; Boyer, M.; Martinez, D.; Kiefer, D.; Virocolo, G.; Wolfe, A.; Socher, S.H. Tumors secreting human TNF/cachectin induced cachexia in mice. Cell 50:555-563;1987.

88. Ota, D.M.; Copeland, E.M.; Strobel, H.W. *et al.* The effect of protein nutrition on host and tumor metabolism. J. Surg. Res. 22:181-188;1977.

89. Peacock, J.L.; Inculet, R.I.; Corsey, R.; Ford, D.B.; Rumble, W.F.; Lawson, D.; Norton, J.A. Resting energy expenditure and body cell mass alterations in noncachectic patients with sarcoma. Surgery 102:465-472; 1987 .

90. Phinney, S.D.; Bistrian, B.R.; Wolfe, R.R.; Blackburn, G.L. The

human metabolic response to chronic ketosis without caloric restriction: Physical and biochemical adaptation. Metabolism 32:757-768;1983.

91. Popp, M.B.; Fisher, R. I.; Wesley, R.; *et al.* A prospective randomized study of adjuvant parenteral nutrition in the treatment of advanced diffuse lymphoma: influence on survival. Surgery 90:195-203;1981.

92. Rabinovitz, M.; Pitl ik, S.D.; Leifer, M.; Garty, M.; Rosenfeld, J.B. Unintentional weight loss. A retrospective analysis of 154 cases. Arch. Intern. Med. 146:186-187;1986.

93. Riella, M.C.; Scribner, B.H. Five years' experience with a right atrial catheter for prolonged parenteral nutrition at home. Surg. Gynecol. Obstet . 143:205-208;1976 .

94. Schein, P.S.; Kisner, D., Haller, D.; Blecher, M.; Hamosh, M. Cachexia of malignancy: Potential role of insulin in nutritional management. Cancer 43:2070-2076; 1979 .

95. Schloerb, P.R. Computer-assisted nutritional support in surgery. Contemporary Surgery 25:53-57;1984.

96. Schloerb, P.R.; Friis-Hansen, B.J.; Edelman, I.S. *et al.* The measurement of total body water in the human subject by deuterium oxide dilution . J. Clin Invest. 29:1296-1310;1950 .

97. Scuderi, P.; Lam, K.S.; Ryan, R.J.; Petersen, E.; Sterling, K.E.; Finley, P.R.; Ray, C.G.; Slyman, D.J.; Salmon, S.E. Raised serum levels of tumor necrosis factor in parasitic infections. Lancet ii:1364-1365; 1986 .

98. Shaw, J.H.F.; Wolfe, R.R. Fatty acid and glycerol kinetics in septic patients and in patients with gastrointestinal cancer. Ann. Surg. 205 ;368-376;1987 .

99. Sherwin, R.S.; Hendler, R.G., Fel ig, P. Effect of ketone infusions on amino acid and nitrogen metabolism in man. J. Clin. Invest. 55:1382-1390; 1975 .

100. Shizgal, H.M.; Forse, R.A. Protein and calorie requirements with total parenteral nutrition . Ann. Surg. 192:562-569; 1980 .

101. Socher, S.H.; Martinez, D.; Craig, J.B.; Kuhn, J.G.; Oliff, A. Tumor necrosis factor not detectable in patients with clinical cancer cachexia. J. Natl. Cancer Inst. 80:595-598;1988.

102. Soeters, P.B.; Ebeid, A.M.; Fischer, J. Review of 404 patients with gastrointestinal fistulas (impact of parenteral nutrition). Ann. Surg. 190:189-202;1979.

103. Spiegel, R.J.; Schaefer, E.J.; Magrath, I.T.; Edwards, B.K. Plasma lipid alterations in leukemia and lymphoma. Am. J. Med. 72:775-782;1982.

104. Stehle, P.; Mertes, N.; Puchstein, C., *et al.* Effect of parenteral glutamine peptide supplements on muscle glutamine loss and nitrogen balance after major surgery. Lancet (i):231-233;1989.

105. Stephens, R.V.; Randall, H.T. Use of a concentrated, balanced, liquid elemental diet or nutritional management of catabolic states. Ann. Surg. 170: 642-667;1969.

106. Stewart, A.G.; Begg, R.W. Systemic effects of tumors in force-fed rats. III. Effect on the composition of the carcass and liver and plasma lipids. Cancer Res. 13:560-565;1953.

107. Svaninger, G.; Bennegard, K; Ekman, L.; Ternell, M.; Lundholm, K. Lack of evidence for elevated breakdown rate of skeletal muscles in weight-losing, tumor-bearing mice. JNCI 71:341-346;1983.

108. Terepka, A.R.; Waterhouse, C. Metabolic observations during the forced feeding of patients with cancer. Am. J. Med. 20:225-238;1956.

109. Theologides, A. The anorexia-cachexia syndrome: a new hypothesis. Ann. N.Y. Acad. Sci . 230:14-22;1974

110. Theologides, A. Cancer cachexia . Cancer 43:2004-2012;1979 .

111. Thomas, J.H.; MacArthur, R.I.; Pierce, G.E. *et al.* Hickman-Broviac catheters (indications and results). Am. J. Surg. 140:791-796;1980.

112. Tompkins, R.K.; Kraft, A.R.; Zollinger, R.M. Alternate routes of surgical fluid administration. J. Surg. Res. 9:397-403;1980.

113. Viteri, F.E.; Alvarado, J. The creatinine height index: its use in the estimation of the degree of protein depletion and repletion in protein calorie malnourished children. Pediatrics 46:696-706;1970.

114. Vlassara, H.; Spiegel, R.J.; Doval, D.S.; Ceramie, A. Reduced plasma lipoprotein lipase activity in patients with malignancy-associated weight loss. Horm. Metabol. Res. 18:698-703;1986.

115. Warnold, I.; Lunkholm, K.; Schersten, T. Energy balance and body composition in cancer patients. Cancer Res. 38:1801-1807;1978.

116. Warren, R.S.; Jeevanandam, M.; Brennan, M.F. Protein synthesis in the tumor-influenced hepatocyte. Surgery 98:275-281;1985.

117. Warren, R.S.; Jeevanandam, M.; Brennan, M.F. Comparison of hepatic protein synthesis ln vivo versus in vitro in the tumor-bearing rat. J. Surg. Res. 42:43-50;1987.

118. Wilmore, D.W.; Long, J.M.; Mason, A.D. *et al.* Catecholamines: mediator of the hypermetabolic response to thermal injury. Ann. Surg. 180:653-669;1974.

119. Young, V.R. Energy metabolism and requirements in the cancer patient. Cancer Res. 37:2336-2347;1977.

Linda S. Jones, M.S., R.N. Nursing Oncology
Jean E. Johnson, Ph.D., R.N. Nursing Oncology

Chapter **35**

THE NURSE AND CANCER CARE

Apprehension, uncertainty, waiting, expectation, fear of surprise, do a patient more harm than any exertion. Remember, he is face to face with his enemy all the time, internally wrestling with him.... "Rid him of his adversary quickly," is the first rule with the sick.

Florence Nightingale (1860)

PERSPECTIVE

The purpose of this chapter is to introduce the reader to the nature and scope of the practice of nursing oncology and the roles nurses perform in the specialty, and to give examples of areas of research relevant to nursing practice. Professional issues are discussed in the first section of this chapter, followed by a summary of research on the problem of chemotherapy-induced nausea and vomiting and the impact of informational interventions on cancer patients.

DOMAIN OF NURSING ONCOLOGY

For many years, there were nurses who concentrated their practice on the care of cancer patients. The recent, rapid development of cancer nursing as a special area of concentration paralleled the development of oncology as a specialty in medicine. Of particular significance was the impact of the introduction of chemotherapeutic agents for treatment of cancer. Soon after such therapies were incorporated into clinical practice, nurses became responsible for the administration of the agents and the care of patients receiving them. The organizations formed to meet needs of physicians who specialized in oncology practice provided support for nurses who cared for oncology patients to form an organization to meet their needs. The Oncology Nursing Society became a national organization in 1975. With a current membership of 25,000, it is the largest of the professional oncology organizations.

In spite of the numbers of nurses in all areas of practice, including oncology, the questions "What is nursing?" and "What are the unique contributions of nursing?" continue to be asked. The practice of oncology nursing has the same nature and scope as all nursing; it is health oriented. Such an orientation is broader than the patient's disease or medical condition. It requires a focus on the individual as a functioning human within a social context and consideration of the various factors that at any one time may be threatening the person's biologic and behavioral integrity. Prevention of illness, promotion of healthy life-styles, and maximization of functional status and quality of life during all phases of illness are of specific concern to nurses; that concern is evident in their practice. The practice of nursing reflects the high value nurses place on the role of the patient and family as active participants in the health care process.

Nurses are especially concerned about their working relationships with other health professionals, because they view those relationships as essential to the achievement of their patient care goals. Nurses believe that the most productive relationship is collaborative, based on valuing the power on both sides, recognizing and accepting separate and combined spheres of activity and responsibility, safeguarding the legitimate interests of each party, and by both parties recognizing common goals (2).

The American Nurses' Association, in the booklet *Nursing: A Social Policy Statement* (2), proposed a definition of nursing that has become widely accepted by the members of the profession: *Nursing is the diagnosis and treatment of human responses to actual or potential health problems.*

This definition specifies the phenomena that are the focus of nursing practice. There are a wide range of health-related responses by sick and well persons addressed by nurses. The diagnosis and treatment of *responses* to actual or potential health problems is uniquely different from diagnosing and treating health problems. Nurses focus on helping patients and their families manage symptoms and changes in their lives created by a health problem. That difference explains how nursing's focus is unique but complementary to that of medicine.

Nurses use the same types of resources and aids to their practice that other practice professions use. Nurses draw on theories and knowledge from a variety of scientific disciplines as the basis of their practice, use a logical and systematic process to assess and reach a diagnosis, plan and execute action, and evaluate the effects in terms of outcomes. Nursing differs from other practice professions in its focus; that is, it uses the resources and methods to assist people with their responses to actual or potential health problems so that adaptive outcomes are obtained.

PREPARATION AND ROLES FOR CANCER NURSES

The roles and responsibilities of the nurse in cancer care are as diverse as the many diseases labelled cancer. As do medical specialists, nurses use a sophisticated and rapidly changing knowledge base to plan and deliver nursing care. Many subspecialties in oncology nursing have evolved because of the special needs of different cancer patient populations. By virtue of increased educational preparation and expertise in oncology, the registered professional nurse has assumed responsibilities beyond the clinical care of the patient and family. The clinical, research, education, and administrative roles of nurses are described in this section.

BASIC LEVEL

The basic preparation of the registered professional nurse is education in a 2-year associate degree program, a 3-year diploma hospital-associated nursing program, or a 4-year baccalaureate program. Graduates of each program are eligible to sit for the examination that leads to a license for the practice of professional nursing. Educational programs differ in the amount and type of content on the care of cancer patients and families. The Oncology Nursing Society's Education Committee (12) recommended that all student nurses have content in their basic curriculum on the physical and psychosocial aspects of cancer nursing care at all stages of the disease and application of the nursing process to individuals with cancer. Students are expected to demonstrate principles of cancer nursing care that reflect up-to-date knowledge and skills and meet pre-established guidelines for delivery of nursing care (10). Students in any of the three basic programs also should be taught to apply concepts from other sciences to cancer nursing, use interdisciplinary approaches in care delivery, and apply research in their oncology nursing practice. As the roles of cancer nurses continue to be delineated, nursing students assimilate information about current and future trends and issues in cancer nursing and cancer care.

Despite the emphasis on providing cancer content in nursing school curricula, it is recognized that cancer nursing requires a knowledge base and clinical expertise beyond that acquired in a basic nursing program. The majority of the special knowledge developed in cancer nursing is learned in practice or provided through continuing education programs. Because the care of patients is so specialized and the knowledge base is constantly changing and expanding, nurses must constantly update their knowledge and skills. The definition and development of cancer nursing as a specialty has been orchestrated by the Oncology Nursing Society (ONS). The ONS, in collaboration with the American Nurses' Association, assumed the leadership in defining the scope of cancer nursing practice, the credentials and qualifications for cancer nurses, and the standards for patient care (4). Roles were defined for nurses in the prevention, detection, diagnosis, treatment, and rehabilitation of cancer patients and their families.

By 1991, more than 10,000 nurses were certified as possessing the skill and knowledge required for the practice of oncology nursing. Certification was developed by the nursing profession to measure continuing competence in a discrete area of nursing. The cancer nursing certification examination was developed to test nursing skills and knowledge of cancer nursing practice, characteristics of major cancers, treatment, issues and trends in cancer care, prevention and detection, diagnosis and staging, pathophysiology, cancer epidemiology, and historical perspectives in cancer care. The expertise developed in practice is recognized and emphasized by the examination's eligibility requirements of 30 months practice as a registered nurse with a minimum of 1,000 hours of that practice in oncology nursing (11).

Nurses with basic preparation provide the majority of direct patient care for cancer patients. Nurses oversee the patient's care, plan and implement appropriate nursing interventions, and evaluate the patient's responses to that care. The nurse has a defined role in assisting patients and families to deal with the physical and psychosocial impact of cancer and its treatment across all health care settings and cancer stages. Based on an understanding of the stages and progression of cancer and individuals' responses to the disease, the nurse can anticipate patients' needs and reduce their physical and psychologic vulnerability through deliberate interventions to diminish the impact of cancer and the trauma of its treatment.

The nurse has an important role in coordinating the efforts of the multidisciplinary team involved in cancer care. The nurse structures his or her practice so there are frequent contacts between patient and nurse. This places the nurse in a unique position to evaluate the impact of the various disciplines involved in the care. The nurse forms an important link in maintaining communication with all members of the multidisciplinary team and assists the patient and family to understand the role of each team member. As goals are mutually established with the patient and family, the nurse validates the relevance of these goals and the acceptability of plans for achieving them. By viewing the experience of cancer from the patient's perspective, the nurse can help the individual adapt in the most realistic and healthy manner.

ADVANCED LEVELS

In 1977, there were five master's degree programs in the United States offering a specialty in cancer nursing (1). Ten years later, 42 nursing programs offered master's degrees in cancer nursing (38). These programs were developed in response to increasing demands for nurses who were expert in the cancer field, had in-depth knowledge and skills, and who would be able to provide leadership to advance and improve the quality of patient care. Advanced oncology practice is characterized by "expert competency and leadership in the provision of care to individuals with an actual or potential diagnosis of cancer" (37).

The master's-prepared nurse assumes many different roles in advanced practice. Along with direct patient care in a variety of settings, the nurse may direct other nurses as a coordinator or consultant. The advanced nursing degree prepares nurses to synthesize and apply sophisticated cancer nursing knowledge with theory and research derived from many disciplines. The results of this application of knowledge within the framework of the nursing process are improved understanding of the cancer problem and its impact on patients and families, improved clinical problem solving, and enhanced patient outcomes (36).

Master's-prepared nurses are also educators, administrators, and researchers. Cancer nursing educators teach nursing students, medical students, practitioners of various disciplines, allied health personnel, patients and families, and consumers of health care. Their contributions include the development of patient education materials, presentation of continuing education programs, and classroom and clinical teaching of oncology content in degree-granting programs. The nurse-educator must demonstrate advanced clinical knowledge and skills along with expert use of teaching and learning principles.

Oncology nurse-managers assume the varied administrative roles that occur in any health care setting. The major focus is on using resources in an efficient and cost-effective manner to produce the highest level of care. As health care settings and fiscal management become more complex, a special body of knowledge in nursing administration is needed to complement cancer nursing skills. The nursing administrator's highest priority is to create an environment conducive to and supportive of a professional nursing practice that meets the health needs of patients.

The research role of the master's-prepared nurse is closely aligned with the advanced practice of nursing and the care of patients and families. Drawing from practice, the nurse identifies and redefines practice problems to allow application of scientific knowledge and methods in a search for solutions. In addition to identifying clinical problems suitable for research, the nurse collaborates in the conduct of research, evaluates available research for its practice implications, and implements research findings that have the potential to improve cancer nursing and the care of cancer patients (3). Another important research role of the master's-prepared nurse is quality assurance investigations to monitor the quality of nursing care delivery. Through this role the nurse with advanced preparation identifies practice problems, measures their impact, and makes changes in practice to improve patient care.

The major goal for nurses obtaining the doctoral degree is the acquisition of research skills that can be used to develop scientific knowledge related to nursing. Although developing the knowledge base of the practicing nurse is an important role for nurses with doctorate degrees, this is not their only contribution to oncology nursing. The cadre of doctorally-prepared nurses in oncology nursing have degrees representing many different disciplines; this expertise has contributed to the development of a wide range of skills and responsibilities in cancer nursing. It also has allowed the research base of cancer nursing to evolve from a broad understanding and perspective of human nature and disease.

Today, more nurses are entering doctoral programs in nursing. As a result, there are academic programs tailored to cancer nurses. Doctorally prepared nurses have an important role in teaching and administering these programs. Although the majority of doctorally prepared nurses in cancer care are employed in nursing schools to teach and do research in cancer nursing, the next decade will see a shift as more doctorally prepared nurses are employed to provide direct nursing care to patients and families, and their research will be closely aligned with the problems encountered in clinical settings. Doctorally prepared nurses have the major responsibility for providing leadership that ensures the growth and stability of the profession. This role is assumed within the education, administration, practice, and research roles filled by nurses with doctoral degrees.

SUMMARY OF NURSING'S ROLE IN CANCER CARE

Integrating the various roles of nurses in cancer care enhances and improves the care of patients and their families. Nursing experts cooperate to plan and execute clinical care, educate patients and families, and research clinical problems in nursing. A progressive-care setting employs nurses with different preparation levels and provides an environment wherein their diverse skills can maximize patient outcomes and they can develop further expertise and knowledge in oncology nursing. Frequent changes in the medical management of cancer demand that nurses adapt their care and develop new standards to support changes in patient responses and outcomes. As new treatment modalities are developed, nurses revise the model for multidisciplinary care delivery and generate appropriate standards for clinical care, patient and family education, and generate ideas for investigation.

Combining the expertise of nurses at all levels helps shape care delivery to the needs of patients and families. As clinical issues are encountered, the nurse can draw on a variety of perspectives and proficiencies for problem solving. Most important, the research derived from clinical problems encountered in practice has the greatest chance of generating solutions that have a positive impact on care. As the scientific base for medical management of the patient grows, the need for refined nursing knowledge becomes imperative. The knowledge being developed by cancer nurse researchers has the potential to improve care and reshape the role of the nurse. Fernsler, et al (22) noted that the proliferation of nursing research reflects the evolution of cancer nursing as a distinct specialty. Although nurses are involved in the investigation of many clinical problems, developing a body of knowledge that directs clinical practice is a particular challenge. The unique contributions of research to the practice of oncology nursing are exemplified by the research findings on chemotherapy-induced nausea and vomiting, and by nurses providing information to patients and their families.

CHEMOTHERAPY-INDUCED NAUSEA AND VOMITING

Nausea and vomiting are frequently experienced side effects of a number of chemotherapeutic agents, and can have significant negative effects on patients' quality of life. The symptoms not only cause acute discomfort but can also interfere with a patient's usual life activities. These side effects cause patients to dread chemotherapy sessions and can result in patients being unable to participate in a complete treatment course that could be life saving. Nausea and vomiting occur following the administration of chemotherapeutic drugs and also as an anticipatory response to receiving therapy. The mechanism by which the drugs cause nausea and vomiting is not completely understood (24). Receptors in both the central nervous system and the gastrointestinal tract are probably involved. Posttreatment nausea and vomiting can occur at the time of administration of the therapeutic agent or be delayed by 24 hours or more. The psychologic process of conditioning may be implicated in anticipatory as well as posttreatment reactions. Characteristics of drugs and patients have been found to be related to both anticipatory and posttreatment nausea and vomiting.

The measurement of nausea and vomiting has been problematic. Nausea especially (and perhaps some responses labelled vomiting) is a subjective experience most directly evaluated by patients' perceptions of their experience. Patient reports are used to measure such subjective experiences. Vomiting can be measured objectively by counting the number of episodes or measuring the amount of vomitus. Objective measures of vomiting can become important when electrolyte balance and/or nutritional status are of concern. However, objective measures do not necessarily reflect patients' subjective evaluations of the experience. Both objective and subjective measures are needed for a comprehensive assessment. Drawing on various sources, Grant (25) classified chemotherapeutic agents into categories of mild, moderate, or severe based on their emetic potential. Patient characteristics associated with posttreatment nausea and vomiting are prior experience with nausea and vomiting from chemotherapy (23), a history of heavy alcohol intake (18,41) and age — children experience more nausea and vomiting than do adult patients (24). Delayed emesis is vomiting that begins or persists 24 hours or more after administration of chemotherapy (24). Delayed emesis occurs less often in patients who do not vomit on the day of chemotherapy. Patients most likely to experience delayed vomiting are those who receive high-dose cisplatin (31).

The patient characteristics found in multiple studies to be associated with anticipatory vomiting are being younger as opposed to older, receiving higher dosages or more emetogenic chemotherapy drugs, and experiencing higher levels of anxiety (16). Other characteristics found in at least one study to be associated with anticipatory nausea and/or vomiting included sensations of itching, taste, and odor during chemotherapy, a history of motion sickness, and an inhibitive rather than facilitating coping style (16). Several of these factors are known to facilitate conditioning to symptoms. When nausea and vomiting elicited by chemotherapeutic agents becomes associated with stimuli in the environment, then the environmental stimuli can independently elicit nausea and vomiting. Patients can experience nausea and vomiting as a conditioned response when they come in contact with any number of stimuli associated with receiving chemotherapy, such as sight of the clinic, thoughts about receiving therapy, and smells that resemble those of the drugs. Andrykowski, et al. (13) found that all of the patients studied who experienced anticipatory nausea and/or vomiting experienced nausea during or after treatment. Therefore, the most important factor in preventing anticipatory nausea and vomiting is the prevention of or reducing awareness of nausea and vomiting during chemotherapy administration.

Most of the research on the control of nausea and vomiting has been done relatively recently; most articles and books were published in the 1980s. Much of the research has been conducted by multidisciplinary teams, which reflects the shared responsibility of physicians and nurses for controlling nausea and vomiting in the clinical setting. Several reviews of this research have been published recently (8,24,42,43). Because only the main conclusions will be presented here, the reader is referred to these reviews for more thorough discussions.

It has been demonstrated repeatedly that appropriate combinations of the more active antiemetic drugs have resulted in the best pharmacologic control of nausea and vomiting associated with chemotherapeutic agents (24). Triozzi and Laszlo (42) emphasized the importance of preventing nausea and vomiting. They stated that effective therapy with any antiemetic regimen must be initiated before nausea and vomiting have begun and that antiemetics given after nausea and vomiting occur will not stop the response. They recommended that antiemetic therapy begin hours before chemotherapy and be continued around the clock for as long as the patient can be expected to experience problems. The as needed schedule is discouraged because that schedule will allow nausea and vomiting to occur. If nausea and vomiting

can be prevented, environmental stimuli will not be associated with them, and patients will be at much lower risk of developing anticipatory nausea and vomiting.

Gralla et al. (24) set forth the following guidelines for effective combination antiemetic regimens: (a) combine agents with different mechanisms of activity and non-overlapping toxicities; (b) individual drugs should have demonstrated efficacy when used singly; and c) agents may be added if they lessen the side effects of the regimen or if they reduce other toxicities of the chemotherapy.

Antiemetics research has shown that agents that block dopamine receptors are effective. These include: (l) phenothiazines (prochlorperazine and chlorpromazine); (2) substituted benzamides (metoclopramide); and (3) butyrophenones (haloperidol and droperidol). Corticosteroids (dexamethasone and methylprednisolone) have been found to be useful, as have benzodiazepines (lorazepam and diazepam) and cannabinoid. The addition of antihistamines (diphenhydramine) to the regimen can be useful for controlling some of the side-effects of the antiemetic drugs, especially those from metoclopramide. The newest class of antiemetic agents, the serotonin antagonists (ondansetron, granisetron, batanopride), are effective in the management of cisplatin-induced emesis. The serotonin antagonists are not only highly effective; they do not cause the side effects often found with other antiemetics.

Research on psychological aspects of nausea and vomiting associated with chemotherapy also appeared in literature during the 1980s. Studies on anticipatory nausea and vomiting dominated that research, but there was interest also in the effects of psychologic interventions on posttreatment responses. Reviews of that literature have been published (15-17). Behavioral interventions were tested most frequently. They included hypnosis, progressive muscle relaxation training, systematic desensitization, biofeedback, and stress inoculation training. Results of well-controlled studies suggest that hypnosis, progressive muscle relaxation training, and systematic desensitization can reduce conditioned nausea and vomiting. Other behavioral techniques have received less rigorous study. Comparisons among the various behavioral interventions with respect to their efficacy have not been a major thrust of past research. These techniques should be considered as additions to the combination-antiemetic regimens for the control of chemotherapy-related nausea and vomiting. The mode of action of the behavioral interventions, weakening the conditioned association between nausea and vomiting and neutral stimuli in the environment and/or reduction in anxiety, is complementary to the use of pharmacologic agents found to be effective antiemetics. Behavioral interventions may be especially useful complements to the antiemetic regimens for patients who fail to respond to appropriate combinations of pharmacologic agents.

NURSING ACTIONS

The goal for management of chemotherapy-induced nausea and vomiting is prevention. If prevention cannot be achieved, then one should try to minimize the number of episodes and length of time over which nausea and vomiting occur and/or patients' memory of the experience.

The most effective approaches to management of chemotherapy-induced nausea and vomiting are combination antiemetic drugs, starting drugs prior to administering chemotherapy, and continuing drug therapy posttreatment for as long as necessary to prevent delayed nausea and vomiting. Management principles are affected by the specific chemotherapy drugs used and by the patient's unique responses to the chemotherapy and antiemetic drugs. The nurse and oncologist cooperate to achieve the best antiemetic regimen for individual patients. Nurses are responsible for administering, or instructing patients to self-administer the antiemetic drugs on an appropriate schedule prior to chemotherapy. This is a key factor in the prevention of nausea and vomiting. Nurses must adhere to a sometimes complex schedule for administration of the antiemetic drugs. This requires the nurse to insure that the drugs are administered at the appropriate time and that the patient has the drugs and knows how and when to take them after discharge from the direct care of the nurse. The nurse's assessments of the patient's responses during treatment and after, when the patient may be at home, are critical to adjusting the antiemetic regimen so that each patient achieves the best possible control of nausea and vomiting with minimal side effects from the antiemetic drugs. The nurse and oncologist jointly should review the patient's response during and following each episode of chemotherapy. Adjustments to the regimen are based on that review.

Behavioral techniques should be considered for patients who are at high risk for anticipatory vomiting. These patients experience nausea and vomiting during and after treatment that is not eliminated by antiemetics, are receiving high dosages of the more emetogenic chemotherapy drugs, are young, and are especially anxious. Training is required to learn how to teach patients the use of behavioral techniques. Most clinical psychologists have been trained in these techniques and can either train patients in the use of such skills or train nurses so they in turn can teach patients to use the behavioral techniques. Progressive muscle relaxation is the least complicated of the techniques. Tape recorded training sessions for progressive muscle relaxation are available or can be made locally. Patients can use the tape to assist them in achieving a high level of relaxation in self-directed sessions at home as well as in the clinic setting.

INFORMATIONAL INTERVENTIONS

Assessment of the type of information that cancer patients find important showed that patients wanted information in two domains (33). One had to do with diagnosis and the plan of treatment; the other consisted of descriptions of experiences, self-care, and how to accommodate to home life and work.

The first domain has to be assimilated before patients and families are receptive to additional information. Oncologists are responsible for explaining the diagnosis, treatment plan, and prognosis to patients and families. Nurses often contribute additional explanations and assist the patient and family to understand the disease and treatment options. It is accepted that patients have a right to this type of information and therefore no further research has been deemed necessary to demonstrate its worth to patients and families.

Nurses are responsible for transmitting information that falls in the second domain. This includes expected responses to the disease and its treatment, instruction about activities that increase abilities to cope with the experience, and how to perform self-care. This information includes descriptions of the symptoms patients may experience, treatment side effects, self-care activities, coping techniques, and resources available to assist with problems patients and families may encounter.

Providing patients with information is often called patient education. The patient education orientation emphasizes methods of presenting information and the degree of knowledge gained by patients. The literature used by professionals to keep informed about their practice has often been the basis for decisions about the information to be included (19,26). A consistent finding is that patients learn the material presented, as shown by their answers on tests of their knowledge. It often has been assumed that patients benefited if they learned the material presented (21,26) even though the impact on patients' well-being was not assessed.

In other studies, investigations have gone beyond patient learning to assess the impact of the information on patients' behavior. In a study of patients receiving chemotherapy, Dodd (20) evaluated the effects of three types of informational interventions by testing patients' knowledge of chemotherapy, the use of and effectiveness of self-care activities for ameliorating side effects, and patients' mood state. The 48 patients studied were randomized into four informational intervention groups. The first was told the names of the chemotherapeutic agents and their potential side effects. The second was given information on side-effect management techniques. The third group was given a combination of the information on drugs and side-effect management. Subjects in a control group received the usual care in the clinic. Consistent with previous research, patients who were given information about the chemotherapeutic agents they were receiving had higher knowledge scores than those who were not informed. Patients who were made aware of side-effect management had significantly better performance scores for self-care than those who did not receive that information. There was no significant effect on patients' moods from either type of intervention. This study of chemotherapy patients suggests that providing instruction in self-care activities for the management of side effects can increase patients' ability to care for themselves, but that learning about the chemotherapeutic agents may not affect patients' behavior or emotional responses.

Dodd (19) also has studied the effects of instruction in self-care activities for the management of side effects in radiation therapy patients. The 60 patients studied received external radiation therapy for treatment of limited disease (n = 27) or advanced disease (n = 33). Patients were randomized to two groups: (1) an experimental group received information about self-care management techniques that were developed from the literature and reviewed by a radiation oncologist and oncology clinical nurse specialists; and (2) a control group received the usual suggestions from the radiation therapy staff on side-effect management. The outcome measures, taken 6 weeks after the time of the intervention, were performance of self-care activities, anxiety, and perceptions of personal control. The experimental group performed significantly more of the self-care behaviors that were perceived to be of low efficacy than did the control group. However, there were no significant differences between groups for total amount of self-care behaviors performed and efficacy of these activities, delay of initiating self-care behavior, perception of the severity and distress from experienced side effects, anxiety, or perceptions of personal control. These discouraging results may have been due in part to the experimental intervention not being specific to the side effects associated with the part of the body irradiated.

Rainey (34) evaluated the effect of a slide presentation of information that (1) introduced the personnel of the radiation department; (2) showed radiation therapy equipment; (3) outlined the sequence of treatment procedures; (4) explained patients' experiences; (5) explained how radiation therapy works; (6) dispelled misconceptions; and (7) encouraged questions. A control group of patients (n = 30) was evaluated before the experimental intervention (n = 30) was introduced. All patients were assessed on outcome variables during the first 3 days of therapy and again during the final 5 days of therapy. The patients who saw the slide presentation had higher knowledge scores after viewing the presentation than did the control group, but by the last week of therapy there were no differences between groups on knowledge about radiation therapy. The last week of therapy, patients who viewed the slide presentation had lower anxiety and less mood disturbance than did the control group. Thus, an information intervention that included material that could have helped patients understand aspects of their impending experience was associated with reduced emotional response. However, the effect on emotional response was probably not due to a gain in factual knowledge, because there were no differences between groups on factual knowledge scores at the time differences in emotion were observed. It should be noted that patients in Rainey's study were not randomly assigned to groups and the sample included patients with a variety of diagnoses, all stages of disease, and varying treatment histories.

Theories about coping with physical illness can provide a focus for the developing body of research on the effect of information on patients' ability to cope with their physiologic and psychologic responses caused by their cancer treatment. Using theory and research on coping with physical illness other than cancer, Johnson *et al.* (29) evaluated the effectiveness of a preparatory information intervention on patients' ability to cope with radiation therapy. Previous research with surgical patients demonstrated that various preparatory informational interventions were associated with a reduction in negative emotional responses following surgery (27). However, concrete, objective information was superior to other types of information with respect to the speed with which patients resumed their presurgery activities.

The specific characteristics of concrete, objective information are descriptions of: (1) the physical sensations experienced by most individuals, that is, what can be expected to be seen, heard, felt, smelled, and tasted; (2) the environment in which treatment will take place; and (3) the length of time required for procedures and sequence of events. Concrete, objective information is believed to bolster patients' ability to cope because it helps them form an accurate cognitive representation of the impending experience that facilitates their understanding of their experience (34). Attention is focused on the concrete or factual dimensions (e.g., diarrhea occurs most often in the morning, or the treatment table is narrow) of their experience instead of the emotional or evaluative dimensions (e.g., diarrhea is severe, or the treatment table is uncomfortable). Focusing attention on the concrete, factual dimensions of the experience can bolster patients' ability to draw effectively on their existing coping strategies and to use resources in the environment so that the potential adverse impact of the treatment experience is minimized.

A randomized clinical trial was conducted to evaluate the usefulness of this theory, referred to as the self regulation theory, for bolstering patients' ability to cope with radiation therapy (29). The sample was restricted to patients receiving radiation treatments for early-stage prostate cancer. The intervention consisted of four taped messages. The first message described the treatment planning experience; the second described the experience of receiving a radiation treatment; the third described the experiences that could be expected to occur during the weeks of treatments, including possible therapy side effects; and the fourth described the experiences that could be expected to occur following radiation therapy. The specific content of the messages was derived from interviews with other patients during and following radiation treatments for prostatic cancer (30). In addition to concrete, objective descriptions of the usual side effects, the last two messages included suggestions for activities that could be used by patients to manage side effects they experienced. All patients were instructed by physicians and nurses to use these activities.

The control patients received the usual care provided to patients in the department, and in addition were seen by the research staff at the same points in the treatment process as the experimental patients. Patients were engaged in conversation about general topics; they were not given specific information about the experience of therapy by the research staff.

The disruption of patients' usual activities due to receiving radiation therapy was evaluated by using the Sickness Impact Profile (14) and patients' emotional response was assessed with the Profile of Mood States (9). These outcome measures were taken during the weeks of radiation therapy and at 1 and 3 months posttherapy. The experimental group patients had significantly less disruption in their usual activities both during and following radiation therapy than the control patients. The intervention did not significantly reduce the level of emotional response. Consistent with Dodd's (20) findings, patients reported low emotional response overall, making it difficult to show further reduction.

The theory-based intervention of concrete, objective information has been shown to bolster patients' ability to cope with a number of experiences associated with physical illness. That contributes to the confidence in the finding that the intervention bolstered radiation therapy patients' ability to cope with their experiences. The hypothesis that the intervention had its effect because it reduced ambiguity about the impending experience and helped patients acquire a sense of understanding their experience was also supported (28).

It can be observed readily that people differ with respect to preference for information and, therefore, some people should benefit more than others from informational interventions. Systematic investigation has just begun on how individual characteristics, such as informational preference, modify the effectiveness of informational interventions on patients' responses to cancer and cancer treatment.

Rainey's (40) study of radiation therapy patients, in addition to assessing the effects of an informational intervention, evaluated the influence of two individual characteristic coping styles. One was avoidant-vigilant coping and the other was repression-sensitization coping. Sensitizers and vigilant copers were characterized as typically seeking information about threatening or stressful events while repressors and avoiders shut out of awareness of threatening and anxiety-producing stimuli and thoughts. Rainey found that neither way of measuring the individual characteristic interacted with the informational intervention for an effect on the outcome of emotional response measures. The trends in the data suggested that repressors or avoiders were not worse off when they received the experimental information. The sensitizers who did not receive the experimental information had the highest emotional response scores. These findings suggest that certain types of patients may be helped more than others by informational interventions, but that such informational interventions are not likely to be disruptive to other types of patients. This same conclusion was drawn from research on coping with the experience of having surgery (44).

SUMMARY OF RESEARCH ON INFORMATION INTERVENTIONS

Patients' experiences with radiation therapy have been the focus of the majority of studies of the effects of informational interventions on cancer patients' ability to cope and manage their self-care. The assessments of the studies have included patients' ability to manage their self-care, to control their emotional response, and to maintain their usual activities. The studies by Dodd (19), Rainey (40), and Johnson et al. (29) suggest that radiation therapy patients benefit from instruction about management of side effects and descriptions of their impending experience that help them focus on the factual components versus the emotional and evaluative components of the experience. Johnson and Lauver (28) provided support for the explanation that intervention helps patients to cope because it fosters a sense of understanding of the experience as it unfolds, which may in turn bolster the ability to use problem-solving coping methods. Problem-solving approaches for coping with radiation therapy could enhance patients' ability to manage their side effects, minimize the disruption to their usual activities, and help them to maintain a relatively low level of negative emotional reaction.

NURSING ACTIONS

This body of research supports the conclusion that cancer patients benefit from the type of informational interventions nurses are responsible for providing patients and their families. Some guidelines for selecting the types of information most likely to be beneficial can be derived from the research. The guidelines for type of information to select are: (1) information that focuses on activities that patients can perform that may have a positive impact on their specific side effects; (2) factual descriptions of the specific side effects they may experience such as time of day they are most apt to be experienced, when in the treatment process they are most apt to appear, and when they can be expected to go away; (3) factual descriptions of the treatment rooms and treatment machines, including physical sensations that may be experienced; and (4) sequence of diagnostic and treatment procedures. Information that focuses patients' attention on how

upsetting or distressing the experience is should be avoided. Information about how chemotherapy and radiation therapy works has not been demonstrated to help patients cope with the experience or to enhance their self-care behaviors. Such information does not seem to be essential. Its inclusion could distract patients' attention from the beneficial information.

The goals to be achieved by providing cancer patients with information are: (1) facilitating their ability to anticipate their experience over all phases of the treatment process and recovery period; (2) focusing their attention on factual components instead of the emotional components of the experience; and (3) enhancing their use of problem-solving coping strategies and use of self-care activities. These goals and the guidelines for selecting types of information to include provide a structure for informational interventions that are based on knowledge derived from clinical research.

FUTURE OF CANCER NURSING

As the care of patients and families becomes more sophisticated and complex, the need for intensified collaboration within the multidisciplinary team is emphasized. The role of the nurse in cancer care is likely to grow more critical as changes occur, including the use of more toxic drugs, increased outpatient care, and multimodality treatment. Effective responses to these pressures from society and the health care system require increased numbers of nurses with advanced preparation for practice and research. The last decade has witnessed dramatic changes in cancer nursing and recognition from other disciplines and the public of the unique and important services nurses provide cancer patients and their families. Continued growth of the scientific base for care delivery and refinements in nursing management of the cancer patient and family will bring about changes in the care delivered by nurses and the structure in which nurses practice.

Recommended Reading

The most comprehensive nursing oncology textbooks are Groenwold's *Cancer Nursing: Principles and Practice* (7) and Baird's *Cancer Nursing: A Comprehensive Textbook* (6). Additional information on symptom management is offered in Baird's *Decision Making in Oncology Nursing* (5) and *McNally et al.'s Guidelines for Oncology Nursing Practice* (10). The journals "Oncology Nursing Forum," "Cancer Nursing," and "Seminars in Nursing Oncology" are also excellent sources of current clinical and research knowledge in cancer nursing.

REFERENCES

General References

1. American Cancer Society and Oncology Nursing Society. The Master's Degree with a Specialty in Cancer Nursing: Role Definition and Curriculum. New York, NY: American Cancer Society; 1988.
2. American Nurses' Association. Nursing: A Social Policy Statement. Kansas City, MO: American Nurses' Association; 1980.
3. American Nurses' Association Commission on Nursing Research. Guidelines For the Investigative Function of Nurses. Kansas City, MO: American Nurses' Association; 1981.
4. American Nurses' Association and Oncology Nursing Society. Standards of Oncology Nursing Practice. Kansas City, MO: American Nurses' Association; 1987.

5. Baird, SB, ed. Decision Making in Oncology Nursing. St Louis, MO: CV Mosby & Co; 1988.

6. Baird, SB; McCorkle, R.; Grant, M., eds. Cancer Nursing: A Comprehensive Textbook. Philadelphia: WB Saunders; 1991.

7. Groenwald, SL; Frogge, MH; Goodman, M; Yarbro, CH; eds. Cancer Nursing: Principles and Practice. 2nd ed. Boston, MA: Jones & Bartlett; 1990.

8. Laszlo, J, ed. Antiemetics and Cancer Chemotherapy. Baltimore, MD: Williams & Wilkins Co; 1983.

9. McNair DM, Lorr M, Doppleman LF. Manual for the Profile of Mood States. San Diego, CA: Educational and Industrial Testing Service; 1971.

10. McNally, J.C.; Miaskowski, C.; Rostad, M.; Somerville, E.T. Guidelines for Oncology Nursing Practice. Philadelphia: W.B. Saunders; 1991.

11. Oncology Nursing Certification Corporation. Oncology Nursing Certification Corporation Bulletin and Application. Pittsburgh, PA: Oncology Nursing Certification Corporation; 1991.

12. Oncology Nursing Society Education Committee. Standards of Oncology Nursing Education: the Generalist and Advanced Practice Levels. Pittsburgh, PA: Oncology Nursing Society; 1989.

Specific References

13. Andrykowski MA, Redd WH, Hatfield AK. Development of anticipatory nausea: prospective analysis. J. Consult. Clin. Psych. 53:447-454; 1985.

14. Bergner, M.; Bobbitt, R.A.; Carter, W.B.; Gilson, B.S. The sickness impact profile: development and final revision of a health status measure. Med. Care 19:787-805; 1981.

15. Burish, T.G.; Carey, M.P. Conditioned aversive responses in cancer chemotherapy patients: theoretical and developmental analysis. J. Consult. Clin. Psych. 54:593-600; 1986.

16. Burish, T.G.; Carey, M.P. Conditioned responses to cancer chemotherapy: etiology and treatment. In: Fox, B.H.; Newberry, B.H., eds. Impact of Psychoendocrine Systems in Cancer and Immunity. Toronto, Canada: Hogrefe: 147-178; 1984.

17. Burish, T.G.; Redd, W.H.; Carey, M.P. Conditioned nausea and vomiting in cancer chemotherapy: treatment approaches. In: Burish, T.G.; Levy, S.M.; Meyerowitz, B.E., eds. Cancer Nutrition and Eating Behavior: A Biobehavioral Perspective. Hillsdale, NJ: Erlbaum: 205-224; 1985.

18. D'Acquisto, R.W.; Tyson, L.B.; Gralla, R.J.; *et al.* The influence of a chronic high alcohol intake on chemotherapy-induced nausea and vomiting. Proc. Am. Soc. Clin. Oncol. 5:257; 1986.

19. Dodd, M.J. Efficacy of proactive information on self-care in radiation therapy patients. Heart Lung 16:538-544; 1987.

20. Dodd, M.J. Measuring informational intervention for chemotherapy knowledge and self-care behavior. Res. Nurs. Health 7:43-50; 1984.

21. Dodd, M.J.; Mood, D.W. Chemotherapy: helping patients to know the drugs they are receiving and their possible side effects. Cancer Nurs. 4:311-318; 1981.

22. Fernsler, J.; Holcombe, J.; Pulliam, L. A survey of cancer nursing research January 1975-June 1982. Oncol. Nurs. Forum 11:46-52;1984.

23. Gralla, R.J.; Braun, T.J.; Squillante, A.; *et al.* Metoclopramide: initial clinical studies of high dosage regimens in cisplatin-induced emesis. In: Poster, D., ed. The Treatment of Nausea and Vomiting Induced by Chemotherapy. New York, NY: Masson Publishing; 1981:167-176.

24. Gralla, R.J.; Tyson, L.B.; Kris, M.G.; Clark, R.A. The management of chemotherapy-induced nausea and vomiting. Med. Clin. N. Am. 71:289-301; 1987.

25. Grant, M. Nausea, vomiting, and anorexia. Semin. Oncol. Nurs. 3:277-292; 1987.

26. Israel, M.J.; Mood, D.W. Three media presentations for patients receiving radiation therapy. Cancer Nurs. 5:57-63.; 1982.

27. Johnson, J.E. Coping with elective surgery. In: Werley, H.H.; Fitzpatrick, J.J., eds. Annual Review of Nursing Research, vol. 2. New York, NY: Springer-Verlag; 1984:107-132.

28. Johnson, J.E.; Lauver, D. Alternative explanations of coping with stressful experiences associated with physical illness. Adv. Nurs. Sci. 39-52; 1989.

29. Johnson, J.E.; Nail, L.M.; Lauver, D.; King, K.B.; Keys, H. Reducing the negative impact of radiation therapy on functional status. Cancer 61:46-51; 1988.

30. King, K.B.; Nail, L.M.; Kreamer, K.; Strohl, R.; Johnson, J.E. Patients' descriptions of the experience of receiving radiation treatment. Oncol. Nurs. Forum 12:55-61;1985.

31. Kris, M.G.; Gralla, R.J.; Clark, R.A.; *et al.* Incidence, course, and severity of delayed nausea and vomiting following the administration of high-dose cisplatin. J. Clin. Oncol. 3:1379-1384;1985.

32. Laszlo, J., ed. Antiemetics and Cancer Chemotherapy. Baltimore: Williams & Wilkins; 1983.

33. Lauer, P.; Murphy, S.P.; Powers, M.J. Learning needs of cancer patients: a comparison of nurse and patient perceptions. Nurs. Res. 31:11-16; 1982.

34. Leventhal, H.; Johnson, J.E. Laboratory and field experimentation: development of a theory of self-regulation. In: Wooldridge, P.J.; Schmitt, M.H.; Skipper, J.K, Jr.; Leonard, R.C., eds. Behavioral Science and Nursing Theory. St. Louis: C.V. Mosby; 1983:189-262.

35. McNair, D.M.; Lorr, M.; Doppleman, L.F. Manual for the Profile of Mood States. San Diego: Educational and Industrial Testing Service; 1971.

36. Oncology Nursing Society. Scope of advanced oncology nursing practice. ONS News 2(2):1; 1987.

37. Oncology Nursing Society. Scope of oncology nursing practice. Oncol. Nurs. Soc. News 3(6):1-2; 1988.

38. Oncology Nursing Society Education Committee. Survey of graduate programs in cancer nursing. Oncol. Nurs. Forum 15: 825-831; 1988.

39. Perez, E.A.; Heleth, P.J., Gandara, D.R. Serotonin antagonists in the management of cisplatin-induced emesis. Semin. Oncol. 18 (suppl. 3): 73-80; 1991.

40. Rainey, L.C. Effects of preparatory patient education for radiation oncology patients. Cancer 56:1056-1061;1985.

41. Sullivan, J.R.; Leyden, M.J.; Bell, R. Decreased cisplatin induced nausea and vomiting with alcohol ingestion. New Engl. J. Med. 309:796;1983.

42. Triozzi, P.L.; Laszlo, J. Optimum management of nausea and vomiting in cancer chemotherapy. Practical Therapeutics 34:136-149;1987.

43. Wickham, R. Managing chemotherapy-related nausea and vomitting: The state of the art. Onc. Nurs. Forum 16: 563-574; 1989.

44. Wilson, J.F. Behavioral preparation for surgery: benefit or harm? J. Behav. Med. 4:79-102;1981.

Richard B. Patt, M.D., Anesthesiology, Psychiatry, and Oncology

Chapter 36

BASIC AND ADVANCED METHODS OF PAIN CONTROL

We must all die. But that I can save him from days of torture, that is what I feel is my great and ever new privelege. Pain is a more terrible lord of mankind than even death himself.

Albert Schweitzer (161a)

PERSPECTIVE

Overall, pain is one of the most common symptom associated with cancer (171a,180) (Table 36-1) and often produces greater anticipatory distress than other features of the disease. Cross-cultural epidemiologic studies indicate that about one-third of patients in active therapy and more than two-thirds of patients with advanced disease experience significant pain (31,167). Historically, cancer pain has been treated inadequately (14) and funding available for research has been negligible compared with that allocated to study cancer prevention and treatment (27). Recognition of the gravity and scope of the global cancer pain problem is increasing in association with the appearance of new specialty journals and heightened activity by professional groups, regulatory agencies, the World Health Organization, governments, and the pharmaceutical industry (72).

Patients with pain related to cancer or cancer therapy present to their physicians with varying degrees of urgency, in proportion to the severity and complexity of their pain problems. Comprehensive management involves individualization of therapy, close follow-up, and a proactive approach to treatment. The frequency of uncontrolled pain and requirements for emergency care are reduced when problems are anticipated and symptoms are monitored and treated promptly.

TYPES OF PAIN

Definition

Pain, as defined by the International Association for the Study of Pain, is an unpleasant sensory and emotional experience associated with actual or potential tissue damage or described in terms of such (108). Pain is a subjective phenomena, measured by subjective tools such as a visual analogue scale (Fig. 36-1) and other devices (21a,31a,46a). Assessment and treatment depend on the clinician's willingness to believe the patient's report of pain.

Classification of Cancer Pain

A number of schemata for classifying cancer pain have been suggested that, when applied, have the potential to aid in diagnosis and management (146a). One such classification is based on chronicity of symptoms. Acute pain is frequently associated with signs of sympathetic hyperactivity and heightened distress. Acute pain often is manifest at the onset of disease, and while analgesics may be required on a transient basis, symptoms often revolve as antitumor therapy progresses (49). In contrast, assessment and management of patients with chronic pain tends to be more complex. With time, biologic and behavioral adjustment to symptoms occurs and corroborating signs of tachycardia, hypertension, and diaphoresis are often absent. Various pain behaviors (alterations in facial expression, gait, posture, and mood) may be observed (54) and may persist throughout treatment. Premorbid chronic nonmalignant pain sometimes precedes the diagnosis of cancer and can complicate management. Pain due to cancer usually signals tumor progression with actual injury to tissue, and as a result, response to intervention is somewhat predictable. In contrast, chronic nonmalignant pain, even in the cancer patient, is more often associated with drug seeking behavior, symptom magnification, and pain on the basis of somatic delusion or depression (133), and symptoms often persist despite intervention.

Classification of cancer pain based on its intensity determines where the patient is likely to fall along the "analgesic ladder" (Fig. 36-2). A general classification by pathophysiology distinguishes among somatic, visceral, and neuropathic pain, each of which has different characteristics and requires different approaches to treatment (see below). Finally, Foley has devised a classification scheme, summarized in Table 36-2, based on patient characteristics and stage of disease that she suggests is predictive of patients' response to therapy (52).

Patterns of Pain

Despite efforts at classification, pain in the cancer patient is still an individual phenomena and successful treatment requires that efforts at management be tailored to meet the needs of the individual patient. Pain may be constant and unremitting, in which case it is most amenable to an around-the-clock dosing schedule contingent on time rather than symptoms. This approach to management endeavors to prevent pain rather than treat it retroactively, and is best accomplished by the proper use of long acting analgesics or, in selected cases, infusions of analgesics.

Table 36-1. Common Symptoms in Patients with Advanced Cancer Symptom

Symptom	Percent	Symptom	Percent
Weight Loss	77	Insomnia	29
Pain	71	Urinary Symptoms	23
Anorexia	67	Dysphagia	23
Dyspnea	51	Decubitus Ulcer	19
Cough	50	Hemorrhage	14
Constipation	47	Drowsiness	10
Weakness	47	Paralysis	8
Nausea/Vomiting	40	Jaundice	6
Edema, Ascites,		Colostomy	4
Pleural Effusion	31	Diarrhea	4

From Twycross (171a), with permission.

Despite the establishment of an effective preventative schedule, breakthrough pain is still a common phenomenon that must be anticipated and addressed. Breakthrough pain refers to intermittent exacerbations of pain that can occur spontaneously or in relation to specific activity. Breakthrough pain that is related to specific activity, such as eating, defecation, socializing, or walking, is referred to as incident pain. Breakthrough pain is best managed by supplementing the preventative regimen with analgesics with a rapid onset of action and a short duration. Once a pattern of incident pain is established, "rescue" or "escape" doses of analgesics can be administered in anticipation of the pain-provoking activity. When treatment by infusion therapy (subcutaneous, intravenous, epidural) has been elected, the addition of patient controlled analgesia (PCA), which permits patients to administer a preset amount of narcotic at preset intervals, is an effective means to manage breakthrough and incident pain in selected patients.

Pain that is intermittent and unpredictable in onset represents a a further challenge to management. Around-the-clock dosing is likely to be unsatisfactory because analgesia is often inadequate during painful episodes and sedation usually supervenes during pain-free intervals. Pain that occurs intermittently is usually best managed by the prn administration of an appropriately potent analgesic of rapid onset and short duration. When intermittent pain is well-localized, there may be a role for nerve block therapy as well.

ASSESSMENT

Purposes and Tools

The evaluation of the patient presenting with cancer-related pain serves multiple purposes. The initial encounter should be broadly based; rather than limiting inquiry to the pain

Table 36-2. Classification of Cancer Pain by Patient Type

Pain Syndrome	Patient Characteristics
Acute cancer-related pain	Patients tend to be hopeful
Related to diagnosis	Endure pain readily, often without seeking treatment
Related to treatment	Recurrence of pain can be devastasting (identified with recrudescence of disease)
Chronic cancer-related pain	Psychological adaption/maladaption established
Associated with treatment	Disease quiescent; Overriding concern is with reestablishment of functional lifestyle
Associated with progression	Hopelessness, helplessness often predominate
Patients with preexisting chronic pain	Require intensive intervention and support; Pain behavior established; Accurate diagnosis essential
Patients with history of drug abuse	Difficult to evaluate and treat; Risk of inadequate treatment Coordinate rehabilitation, social work
Dying patients	Adequacy of treatment has greatest impact on patient and family; Assure comfort at all costs

Adapted from Foley (52). Reprinted with permission from The New England Journal of Medicine, 313:84–95; 1985.

syndrome per se, the process should encompass evaluation of the person, their feelings and attitudes about pain and disease, family concerns, and the patient's premorbid psychologic history (i.e., pre-existing depressive or anxiety disorders, personality disorder, substance abuse). A compassionate but

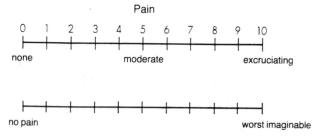

Fig. 36-1. An example of a typical visual analogue scale (VAS), a tool used commonly to elicit self reports of pain severity. From Rowlingson *et al.* (146a), with permission.

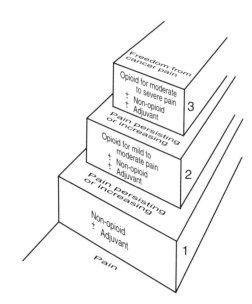

Fig. 36-2. World Health Organization-advocated three-step ladder approach to the pharmacologic management of cancer pain. From World Health Organization (187), with permission.

objective approach to assessment instills confidence in the patient and family that will be of value throughout treatment. Thorough review of the patient's records and a detailed pain history serve both to help delineate the source of pain and to distinguish the degree to which the patient's complaints are related to nocioceptive mechanisms versus psychological modulators. The primary care physician who has known the patient over time is a source of valuable information and should be consulted personally. Psychological testing is of value, although in selected cases it must be abbreviated in consideration of poor physical and emotional condition (27). Table 36-3 summarizes the components of a comprehensive evaluation of the patient with cancer pain.

Since pain is regarded as a subjective experience, quantitative measurement necessarily depends on subjective tools. The tool used most frequently is some variant of a unidimensional visual analogue scale (VAS), which commonly consists of a horizontal line evenly "anchored" or divided into 10 segments numbered consecutively between 0 and 10 (Fig. 36-1). Patients are instructed that 0 represents "total absence of pain" and 10 denotes the "most severe pain they can imagine." Patients are then instructed to simply mark the number that best describes the level of pain they are experiencing at some given point in time. Ideally, a 0–10 score is elicited not only for the current level of pain, but also pain at its least worst and on average. Modified VAS's for use with children substitute a continuum of smiling to crying faces for numbers (see Fig. 36-3) or may utilize colors or a pain "thermometer" (8a,110).

Of the multiple pain questionnaires developed to obtain additional information, the McGill Pain Questionnaire is widely used (106). It employs a five-point scale labelled "no pain," "mild pain," "moderate pain," "severe pain," and "intolerable pain," as well as instructions for patients to select from

Table 36-3. Initial Evaluation of the Patient with Cancer Pain

Review of medical record
Pain questionnaire
Psychological questionnaires
Thorough medical history, including review of systems
Thorough psychological history
Cultural background
Pain history
    Onset
    Duration
    Progression
    Location
    Radiation
    Characteristics
    Factors that decrease pain
    Factors that increase pain
    Prior pain medications, efficacy, side effects
    Current pain medications, efficacy, side effects
    Effect of pain and pain medications on:
        Activity
        Mood
        Sleep
        Appetite
        Posture
        Sexuality
Thorough physical examination
Review of radiologic studies

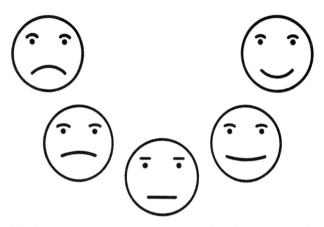

COMPARISON OF VAS AND SAS ANALOG SCALES

Fig. 36-3. An example of an assessment tool used to measure pain intensity in pediatric patients.

a list of 78 adjectives commonly used to describe pain. Part of the McGill Pain Questionnaire is illustrated in Fig. 36-4. Schematic representations of the body to be shaded to indicate where pain is located are often included as components of the evaluation. Recently, the Wisconsin Brief Pain Inventory (21a,31a) and the Memorial Pain Assessment card (46a) were introduced and validated. These instruments are easily understood by patients, require a minimum of time to complete, and seem reliable, suggesting that they will play an important role in the standardization of cancer pain assessment.

Diagnostic maneuvers are pursued to determine the underlying cause of pain so that, when possible treatment can be directed at alleviating the source of pain in preference to relying on a purely symptomatic approach to treatment. Direction of treatment at the source of pain permits more focused, specific care, reducing the likelihood of complications from overtreatment of symptoms. Identification of psychological factors that may exacerbate and/or maintain the pain may suggest specific cognitive behavioral interventions, counseling, or medications directed at modifying these factors. Escalations of pain usually signal progressive injury to tissue, and anatomic localization of a painful lesion through radiologic studies or diagnostic nerve blocks may suggest additional treatment options. For example, the identification of spinal cord impingement or impending vertebral collapse may warrant mechanical or surgical stabilization to forestall paraplegia. Pain of unknown etiology may be an early symptom of recurrent disease or undiagnosed malignant neoplasm. This is particularly true for herpes zoster. The pain consultant should not be dissuaded from ordering additional tests because the patient has already been "worked up" or because antineoplastic treatment has been abandoned. Nevertheless, often only symptomatic treatment is warranted, particularly when expectancy of life is limited.

TYPES OF PAIN

Somatic Pain

Somatic pain occurs as a result of activation of nocioceptors in cutaneous and deep tissues. Pain is typically well localized, and is often characterized as aching or gnawing, and tends to be opioid-responsive.

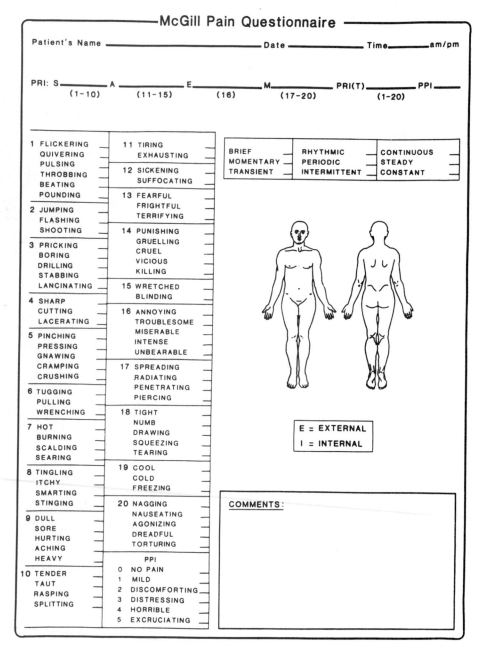

Fig. 36-4. Components of the McGill Pain Questionnaire (MPQ), one of the more commonly used tools for assessing pain.

Visceral Pain

Visceral pain results from distention or chemical irritation of visceral end-organ structures. In contrast to somatically mediated pain, it is characteristically described as vague in distribution and deep, dull, aching, dragging, squeezing, or pressure-like. When acute, it may be paroxysmal and colicky and can be associated with nausea, vomiting, diaphoresis, and alterations in blood pressure and heart rate.

Neuropathic Pain

Neuropathic pain (138b) results from injury to elements of the peripheral or central nervous system and includes, respectively, deafferentation and central pain. Neuropathic pain is typically characterized by spontaneous burning dysesthesia, hyperpathia and hyperalgesia in the absence of peripheral tissue damage. Pain is diffuse, is often excruciating, and may be accompanied by exaggerated skeletal muscle and autonomic responses. Patients may report symptoms consistent with alterations in sensory threshold including anesthesia and allodynia (pain in response to a stimulus that usually does not provoke pain, such as light stroke). An additional characteristic is persistence despite standard analgesic therapy and a tendency in some instances towards favorable response to tricyclic antidepressants, anticonvulsant drugs, and mexilitene. Central pain syndromes may result from primary cortical, thalamic, and spinal cord lesions. In addition, the concept of central pain has been used to explain the occurrence of symptoms in association with disruption of neural pathways (deafferentation). Examples include phantom limb pain, spinal cord transection, postherpetic neuralgia, and pain following chemical or surgical neurolysis.

CANCER PAIN SYNDROMES

Finally, the patient's history, physical findings, and the results of radiologic studies aid the practitioner in determining the specific pathologic process that is present. Numerous distinct cancer pain syndromes have been recognized and described (51,122a). Mechanisms include obstruction of lymphatic and vascular channels, distention of a hollow viscus, edema and tissue inflammation or necrosis. Severe symptoms are most often related to invasion of pain sensitive structures by tumor mass.

Osseous Invasion

Infiltration of bone is the most common cause of cancer pain (58). Since up to 50% decalcification must be present before osseous lesions are visible on plain roentgenograms, scintigraphy (isotope scanning) is preferred for detecting most bone metastases (58). Exceptions include primary bone tumors, thyroid cancer and multiple myeloma (41). Abnormal findings on scintigrams are not specific for malignant disease, and it is essential that they be interpreted together with other radiologic studies in the context of clinical findings. Neoplastic involvement must be differentiated from changes related to infection, trauma or degeneration because treatment differs. Although the majority of skeletal metastases do not produce pain (58), pain from bony metastases can produce a variety of symptoms. When present, pain is usually constant but may be greatest at night and is often worse with movement or weight bearing. Patients may report a dull ache or deep, intense pain, and there may be referred pain, muscle spasm, or paroxysms of stabbing pain, particularly when bony lesions are accompanied by nerve compression. Knee pain associated with metastatic involvement of the hip is an important example of referred bony pain.

Spinal Cord Invasion

Malignant involvement of the vertebral column is frequently associated with localized spinal and/or radicular pain, and often weakness and tingling in a dermatomal pattern. Pain almost always precedes neurologic changes by weeks or days, and tends to be dull, steady, and aching, and increases gradually over time. Pain may be exacerbated when lying down, and partially relieved by sitting or standing. Rapid progression of neurologic deficit, particularly of motor weakness, or the appearance of urinary or fecal incontinence signals progressive epidural-spinal cord compression and warrants urgent intervention. In a review of 130 cases of spinal cord compression from tumor, 96% of patients were found to have increased pain as their presenting symptom, and in 10% of patients pain was the only abnormal clinical finding (60). Plain films and CT scanning are sensitive screening procedures used to evaluate suspected cord compression, but myelography remains the definitive diagnostic procedure. The role of MRI is still being defined (153b). Treatment is either with immobilization and high dose corticosteroids and/or radiation or decompressive laminectomy. Surgery is not advisable when overall clinical condition is poor or spinal metastases are present at multiple levels. A further indication for surgery is when the source of the primary tumor is unknown and laminectomy could be expected to provide a tissue diagnosis. Although invasion of the upper lumbar vertebrae is usually heralded by dull backache and radicular signs, it should be noted that pain may be localized to the sacroiliac joints or iliac crests, and that radiologic investigations of the lumbar spine should not be overlooked when these symptoms are present.

Neural Invasion

Invasion or compression of somatic nerves by tumor is generally associated with constant, burning dysesthetic pain, often with an intermittent lancinating component. Diffuse hyperesthesia and localized paresthesia are not uncommon, and muscle weakness and atrophy may be present if the affected structure is a mixed or motor nerve bundle.

Brachial plexus invasion (Pancoast's or superior sulcus syndrome) is associated most commonly with carcinoma of the lung (primary or metastatic) and breast, and the lower cord of the plexus (C8-T1) is affected most frequently. Horner's syndrome may accompany infiltration of the brachial plexus by either tumor or radiation fibrosis. Suspected brachioplexopathy requires a complete radiologic evaluation, which may include myelography if epidural extension is suspected. Differentiating brachial plexus abnormalities due to radiation fibrosis versus tumor invasion can be difficult because clinical findings are similar. In a large study comparing patients with radiation injury versus tumor involvement, Horner's syndrome and severe pain and weakness (C8-T1) were more common in the tumor group while weakness of shoulder abduction and arm flexors and the presence of lymphedema were more common in the radiation group (50).

Invasion of the lumbar plexus is associated with radicular lower extremity pain, characteristically described as aching or pressure-like. In a large retrospective study (n = 85) of patients with lumbosacral plexopathy (70), pain was the presenting symptom in 90% of patients, and about one-half of patients went on to develop significant weakness and numbness weeks or months after the initial appearance of pain. Abnormalities in reflexes and straight leg raising were common findings. Computerized tomography investigations of the pelvis and lumbar spine and diagnostic nerve blocks are helpful to corroborate clinical findings.

Invasion of the sacral plexus is most often associated with severe constant lower backache and radiation of pain down the posterior thigh, often with progression to perineal sensory loss and bowel or bladder dysfunction. Plain films, tomography and scintigrams frequently demonstrate bony invasion of the sacral plates.

TREATMENT OF CANCER PAIN

Antitumor Therapy

A detailed discussion of the role of palliative antineoplastic therapy is beyond the scope of this chapter. In many cases, the pathologic process responsible for pain can be altered with radiotherapy (5a,100), chemotherapy (43,78a,181), hormonal treatment (78a,105) and even whole-body hyperthermia (43,44), and these options should be considered when new symptoms develop or a major intervention is being planned to relieve pain.

It is important to recognize that palliative antitumor measures have definite limitations related to efficacy, patient acceptance, side effects and complications. Finally, the decision to pursue antitumor therapy does not imply that analgesic drugs and other supportive therapy should be discontinued.

Pharmacologic Management

Oral analgesics are the mainstay of therapy for patients with cancer pain. An estimated 70-90% of patients can be rendered relatively free of pain when rational principles of pharmacologic management are applied in a thorough, careful manner (107,122b,128,145). The World Health Organization has adopted a "ladder" approach to cancer pain management that relies exclusively on the administration of oral agents (Fig. 36-2) (187) Although simplistic, this approach is applicable to most patients, is readily exportable to developing nations, and its application has produced positive preliminary results in pilot studies (167,177).

While pain can be managed in most patients with oral agents alone, even through the terminal stages of illness, a significant proportion of patients require alternative forms of therapy. The introduction of transdermal fentanyl represents an alternate route that has utility both in patients with early and advanced disease. A survey of 138 patients with advanced cancer and pain conducted at Memorial Sloan Kettering Hospital indicated that a majority needed at least two routes for the administration of analgesics, and that up to one third of patients require three to four routes (30). The role of more interventional forms of analgesia, such as neural blockade, CNS opioid therapy and stimulation analgesia is currently not well defined, but these modalities are often successful when traditional therapy has failed.

The oral route should be maintained as long as possible to preserve independence and mobility (64a). Treatment has been simplified by the recent introduction of slow release preparations of morphine (MS Contin, Oramorph) transdermal formulations of fentanyl and the widespread recognition of rational principles of therapy, summarized below (128).

PRINCIPLES OF PHARMACOLOGIC MANAGEMENT OF CANCER PAIN

1. Comprehensive assessment ideally precedes initiation of therapy. Treatment strategy should be directed toward relief of "total pain;" (148) concomitant functional disability (disturbance of sleep, appetite, mood, activity, posture and sexuality) should be determined and addressed by the treatment plan. Concrete goals, acceptable to the patient, family and treating physicians should be established.
2. As with less potent analgesics, opioid therapy should be individualized or "tailored" to suit the patient's needs (46). Dose response and side effects vary widely based on a number of physiologic and behavioral factors (such as age and previous drug history) (23,74,122b).
3. Once an acceptable drug regimen has been established adequacy should be periodically reassessed. Patients are often reluctant to request more potent analgesics. Increased drug requirements related to progression of disease and the development of physical tolerance should be anticipated. Tolerance is most frequently manifested by decreased duration of analgesics.
4. When NSAIDs provide insufficient relief of pain, or are poorly tolerated, the addition or substitution of a codeine or oxycodone-type preparation is usually recommended as an analgesic of intermediate potency.
5. When combinations of codeine or oxycodone and NSAIDS or either alone are insufficient, therapy should progress to include more potent oral opioid analgesics

in a "ladder" fashion (Fig. 36-2) (52,187). Less potent analgesics should not be summarily excluded, since NSAIDs may provide additive or synergistic analgesia, and codeine or oxycodone-type preparations may be useful for breakthrough or incident pain. Opioids should initially be introduced in low doses since the early appearance of side effects will influence compliance.

6. Patient and family education is an essential element of a successful pain relief program and is ideally accomplished through the combined efforts of physicians and nurses. Patients frequently maintain deeply rooted cultural fears of addiction. The distinction among psychological addiction, physical dependence and drug tolerance should be explained (Table 36-4). Concepts and details of side effects, tolerance, overdosage, and withdrawal should be explored (Table 36-5). The treatment plan should anticipate and avoid these problems.
7. A time-contingent analgesia schedule is more effective than symptom-contingent administration:if analgesics are withheld until pain becomes severe, sympathetic arousal occurs and even potent analgesics may be ineffective. Once established, patterns of anticipation and memory of pain contribute to suffering, even during periods of adequate analgesia. Around-the-clock administration of appropriate analgesics maintains therapeutic blood levels and decreases the likelihood of

Table 36-4. Characteristics of Tolerance vs Dependency vs Addiction vs Withdrawal

TOLERANCE   Larger doses of narcotic are required over time to maintain the original analgesic effect. Tolerance is usually associated with physical dependence, but neither implies addiction. It is usually first manifest by decreased duration of analgesic activity. Efforts at countering tolerance include combining narcotic and nonnarcotic analgesics, substituting an alternative narcotic analgesic (because cross tolerance may be incomplete), and maintenance of the oral route. Ultimately, management is usually effectively accomplished with dose increases that are usually well-tolerated since tolerance also occurs to the side effects of narcotic analgesics.

PHYSICAL   Occurs with chronic use of narcotics, but is not a
DEPENDENCE   psychological phenomenon, and as such is distinct from addiction. When present, physical symptoms (abstinence syndrome, withdrawal) occur when narcotic administration is stopped abruptly or if an antagonist is administered. Management is with the continued administration of narcotics, but in gradually decreasing doses. One regimen involves daily reduction by 10-25% of the total daily dose.

ADDICTION   Psychological dependence characterized by compulsive drug use, drug seeking behavior, and the use of narcotics for purposes other than control of pain. Addiction and physical dependence usually coexist, but addiction is not implied by physical dependence. Iatrogenic drug addiction is vanishingly rare and the fear of narcotic addiction should not be a major factor in treating cancer pain.

WITHDRAWAL   Occurs in physically dependent patients when narcotics are suddenly withdrawn or a narcotic antagonist is administered. Abstinence syndrome is manifest by anxiety, irritability, alternating chills and hot flashes, excessive salivation, lacrimation, and rhinorrhea, diaphoresis, piloerection, nausea, vomiting abdominal cramps, insomnia and, rarely, multifocal myoclonus. The time course of withdrawal is a function of the half life of the narcotic. Treatment is with the administration of narcotics in small increments. Prevention is preferred.

Table 36-5. Comparison of Opioids Used in Cancer Pain Management

Generic Name	Trade Name	Dose	Route	Schedule	Peak
PURE AGONISTS					
Morphine	MSIR	20-30 mg	ORAL	2-4 hr	1.5-2 hr
	Roxanol	10 mg	IM/IV	1-4 hr	0.5-1 hr
Controlled Release Morphine	MS Contin, Oramorph	30 mg	ORAL	12-8 hr	3-4 hr
Hydromorphone	Dilaudid	7.5 mg	ORAL	2-4 hr	1-2 hr
		1.5 mg	IM	2-4 hr	0.5-1 hr
Oxymorphone	Numorphan	1 mg	IM	3-6 hr	0.5-1 hr
		5-10 mg	RECTAL	3-6 hr	1.5-3 hr
Meperidine	Demerol	300 mg	ORAL	3-4 hr	1-2 hr
		75 mg	IM	3-4 hr	0.5-1 hr
Heroin	Diamorphine	5 mg	IM	4-12 hr	
Methadone	Dolophone	20 mg	ORAL	4-12 hr	.5-1.5 hr
		10 mg	IM	4-6 hr	.5-1.5 hr
Oxycodone	Roxycodone	20-30 mg	ORAL	3-6 hr	1 hr
Transdermal Fentanyl	Duragesic	0.1 mg	TD	72 hr	8-12 hr
AGONIST/ANTAGONISTS					
Buprenorphine	Bupronex	0.4 mg	IM	4-6 hr	0.5-1 hr
		0.8 mg	SL	5-6 hr	2-3 hr
Pentazocine	Talwin	60 mg	IM	3-4 hr	0.5-1 hr
		180 mg	ORAL	3-4 hr	1-2 hr
Nalbuphine	Nubain	10 mg	IM	3-6 hr	0.5-1 hr
Butorphanol	Stadol	2 mg	IM	3-4 hr	0.5-1 hr

intolerable pain (120). Compliance is enhanced by the prescription of long-acting agents (levorphanol, methadone), slow-release formulations of morphine (MS Contin, Oramorph) or transdermal fentanyl systems.

8. Selected patients benefit from the addition of adjunctive drugs, including tricyclic antidepressants, anticonvulsants, steroids, amphetamines, phenothiazines, oral local anesthetics, and antihistamines. Almost all patients receiving opioid analgesics will require a laxative, and up to two-thirds will benefit from the regular administration of an antiemetic at least transiently (62).

9. When possible, analgesics should be administered orally to promote independence and mobility. Transdermal systems (fentanyl) have the same advantages.

10. When pain control is inadequate with oral analgesics or the oral route is contraindicated, consideration should be given to alternative means of drug delivery. Oxymorphone hydrochloride (Numorphan) rectal suppositories provide 4 to 6 hours of potent analgesia. Other options include transdermal systems, continuous subcutaneous or intravenous infusions of opioids by means of a portable pump, patient-controlled analgesia (intravenous or subcutaneous), and intrathecal or epidural opioids administered via an externalized catheter or internalized pump. New means of administering narcotics are being explored and include mucous membrane (sublingual and transnasal) and inhaled absorption (68). A report describing the successful administration of nitrous oxide to a series of dying adolescents is a further example of innovative care (56).

11. Maintain familiarity with the pharmacologic profiles of a variety of drugs (Table 36-5). Consider drug substitution when a patient exhibits tolerance to the analgesic effects or intolerance to the side effects of medications. Half or two-thirds the calculated equianalgesic dose of the new drug is recommended as a starting dose, which is then titrated upwards as needed (52).

12. Avoid chronic administration of meperidine, particularly when renal function is impaired. Accumulation of normeperidine, a metabolite, is associated with CNS excitation and seizures (73).

13. Avoid the use of agonist-antagonist drugs. These agents may precipitate withdrawal, and their administration complicates the transition to pure agonist agents. Pentazocine (Talwin), the only oral agent currently available in the United States, is associated with a high incidence of hallucinations and confusion.

14. Adequate pain relief cannot always be achieved through pharmacologic means alone. Initial screening should identify patients in whom behavioral or psychological modalities may be employed successfully. When comprehensive trials of pharmacologic therapy have failed, consideration should be given to alternative modalities including additional antitumor therapy, neural blockade, CNS opioid therapy, neurosurgery, and electrical stimulation.

NONOPIOID ANALGESICS

These agents are effective when administered as the sole drug treatment for mild pain, and when combined with opioids to treat moderate to severe pain. Less potent analgesics are often ignored in favor of opioids for the treatment of cancer pain because of the mistaken assumption that all cancer pain is equally severe. Likewise, when cancer pain is refractory to nonopioid analgesics, there is a tendency to replace these drugs with opioids, ignoring the potential for additive or synergistic analgesia (159,159a). Though no analgesics are free of the potential for side effects, the practice of reducing opioid requirements by the continued administration of nonopioid analgesics is effective in limiting the adverse effects associated with higher doses of opioids, as well as delaying the development of tolerance. It is noteworthy that the "mild opioids" (codeine, dihydrocodeine, oxycodone, propoxyphene, pentazocine) have not been shown to be more analgesic than aspirin or acetaminophen, and that the mild opioids are more effective when they are administered concommitantly with aspirin, acetaminophen or nonsteroidal anti-inflammatory agents (7).

The nonopioid analgesics are a heterogeneous group of drugs often considered together because of common indications for their use rather than similarity of structure or uniformity of pharmacologic action (7). Of the nonopoid analgesics, the nonsteroidal antiinflammatory drugs (NSAIDs) are particularly useful because, in addition to providing pain relief, these agents reduce stiffness, swelling and tenderness. Simple pain relief accompanies intermittent use. A few days to weeks of regular use are required before their anti-inflammatory actions fully exert themselves. A ceiling effect has been demonstrated, above which no further analgesia can be expected, but the dosage at which this is observed clinically varies among patients and as a result authorities have suggested a role for dose titration (138a). Tolerance and physical dependence do not occur.

A variety of NSAIDs are available. Since most clinicians believe that these drugs are interchangeable, the most useful classification may be on the basis of dosage schedule, side effects, toxicity, and prior experience (Fig. 36-5). The common problems associated with the use of NSAIDS in cancer patients are related to gastric irritation, prolonged bleeding time, and masking of fever. Phenylbutazone should be avoided because of the uncommon but grave occurrence of agranulocytosis and aplastic anemia.

The NSAIDs, as well as steroids, are particularly effective for the treatment of metastatic bone pain. A biochemical mechanism is attractive to explain how even very small bone metastases are sometimes associated with severe pain. Osseous metastases elaborate PGE2, which probably contributes to pain by sensitization of peripheral nociceptors to various substances including bradykinin, histamine, and hydroxytriptamine (6). The NSAIDs act peripherally, potentially reducing pain and inflammation through inhibition of the cyclo-oxygenase pathway of arachidonic acid breakdown

(119). Inhibition of the enzyme cyclo-oxygenase decreases the formation of prostaglandin PGE2 (57). As tumor deposits enlarge, stretching of periosteum, pathologic fracture, and perineural invasion contribute to pain, and requirements for more potent analgesics increase.

OPIOID ANALGESICS

Opioid analgesics are the mainstay of therapy for moderate to severe cancer pain. Historically, the optimal use of the opioids has been hampered by improper prescribing patterns (98) and patient and physician misconceptions about addiction liability (128). Recently there has been widespread acknowledgement that, in the great majority of cases, cancer pain can be significantly relieved with opioid analgesics as the main form of treatment when rational principles of therapy are applied consistently (128).

Morphine remains the standard of reference to which other analgesics are commonly compared (Table 36-5). The pharmacokinetic and pharmacodynamic profile of a single 10 mg dose of morphine administered intramuscularly forms the basis of most tables and charts compiled to describe the pharmacologic characteristics of other analgesics administered by various routes (Table 36-5).

In general, the various opioids produce analgesia by similar mechanisms and, when administered in comparable doses, the quality of analgesia and spectrum of side effects are similar. Nevertheless, individuals vary in their sensitivity to the analgesic effects and toxicity of the various drugs, forming the basis for the clinical use of morphine alternatives. Other reasons for selecting alternate opioids, preparations, and routes include convenience of dosing, variable patterns of pain, gastrointestinal dysfunction, incomplete cross-tolerance, the need for concentrated formulations, and prior favorable experience.

Transdermal Fentanyl

Fentanyl is an ultra-short acting opioid analgesic, about 100 times more potent than injected morphine, that has been used as a component of anesthesia for more than 20 years. Recently, a transdermal system (similar to that used for the delivery of nitroglycerine, scopolamine, and clonidine) has been developed that effectively converts fentanyl to a long-acting agent. Once treatment has been established, a single application of the patch sustains consistent plasma levels of analgesic for 72 hours, requiring that most patients change the system only once every three days. This convenience factor may translate into improved comfort, especially for patients with compliance problems or for whom the need to take pills regularly represents an insidious reminder of their disease. It is also a boon for patients with poor alimentary function who would otherwise require treatment with expensive and relatively bulky subcutaneous pumps. In most studies of transdermal fentanyl, patients have been extremely satisfied with treatment (110a,153a).

Although low levels of fentanyl can be detected in the bloodstream just 1 hour after administration, a consistent, near-peak level is not obtained for a period of 12-18 hours. Patients need to be cautioned that pain relief will accrue over the first day of treatment and need to be provided with rescue doses of short-acting analgesics during this time. In addition, as a result of the formation of a skin depot of drug, effects

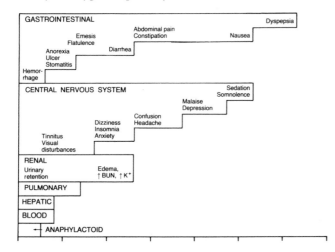

Fig. 36-5. Relative frequency of potential toxicities of nonsteroidal antiinflammatory agents. From Stambaugh (159), with permission.

persist for 12-18 hours following removal of the patch. Side effects are similar to those that have been observed with other opioids (nausea, sedation, constipation, respiratory depression), but because of the system's latency, will need to be managed for a prolonged period even after removal. Topical irritation is uncommon. The patch is available in four sizes designed to release 25,50,75,or 100 micrograms hourly for 3 days, and multiple patches may be used to obtain the correct dosage. The patch should be applied to intact, non-irradiated skin, preferably over the upper body. A hairless area like the shoulder is preferred and clipping is preferable to shaving if hair must be removed. Skin may be prepared by rinsing with plain water and drying, but soap, oils, or alcohol that might alter skin permeability should not be applied. Patches usually adhere well despite bathing, but if dislodged may be reinforced with micropore tape. If a patch must be removed because of side effects, the skin beneath should not be scrubbed or stimulated.

The dose recommendations promulgated by the patch's manufacturer are conservative (Table 36-6). As a result, serious side effects like respiratory depression are extremely unlikely but about 50% of patients will require that their dose be incremented early in the course of therapy. The company recommends that dosage should not be increased more frequently than every 72 hours, but experience has shown that 24 hours is a sufficient interval. Respiratory depression is responsive to stimulation or the administration of naloxone, but should it occur, treatment for up to 24 hours in a supervised setting is required because of the drug's latency. As with management of cancer pain with other long-acting analgesics, a supplementary prescription of a short-acting opioid analgesic should be provided to counter breakthrough pain. Heightened activity and fever can theoretically increase transdermal absorption, although this has not emerged as a clinically important problem.

CONTINUOUS SUBCUTANEOUS INFUSION (CSCI) OF OPIOIDS

The continuous subcutaneous infusion (CSCI) of opioids is now commonly used and represents an excellent option for patients whose medical condition precludes the use of the oral route or in whom pain is poorly controlled despite large doses of oral opioids (16,101). In one representative study of 40 patients with advanced cancer pain, CSCI of opioids was effective in 80% of patients and the incidence of side effects was low (175). Treatment is best initiated in the hospital setting, but is readily adaptable to the home. A variety of infusion pumps are commercially available which, overall, are portable, battery-driven, inexpensively-leased and feature sophisticated alarm systems. The potential advantages of CSCI are listed in Table 36-7. An example of a pump suitable for continous subcutaneous, intravenous, or intraspinal administration, with or without patient controlled analgesic, is shown in Fig. 36-6.

Initiating Therapy

To initiate a CSCI of opioid, the 24 hour dose of parenteral drug is summed. If the patient's drug regimen includes oral analgesics, conversion tables are utilized (Table 36-5) to calculate the equianalgesic parenteral dose of opioid. The total daily dose of parenteral drug is divided by 24 and the pump is set accordingly. The pump's tubing is primed with drug and it is attached to a 27g pediatric butterfly needle which is inserted subcutaneously and taped flush to the patient's skin. Any subcutaneous site can be used, although the infraclavicular fossa and chest wall are frequently selected to aid easy ambulation (Fig. 36-7). The infusion site is checked twice daily for signs of irritation, and is changed on an as needed basis. The tubing, needle, and site are changed routinely at least weekly.

Maintenance of Therapy

Absorption of subcutaneously administered opioids is rapid and steady state plasma levels are generally approached within 1 hour (116). Absorption is related to the vascularity of the infusion site, the ionization and lipid solubility of the drug, and the volume of injectate. Most parenteral narcotics are suitable for CSCI. Meperidine, methadone, and pentazocine are associated with excessive tissue irritation and should be avoided.

Table 36-6. Dosage Equivalency for Transdermal Fentanyl (Based on daily morphine equivalence*)

Oral 24 Hour Morphine (mg/day)	IM 24 Hour Morphine (mg/day)	Transdermal Fentanyl (mg/day)
45-134	8-22	25
135-224	23-37	.75
225-314	38-52	75
315-404	53-67	100
405-494	68-82	125
495-584	83-97	150
585-674	98-112	175
675-764	113-127	200
765-854	128-142	225
855-944	143-157	250
945-1034	158-172	275
1035-1124	173-187	300

A conservative analgesic activity ratio of 10 mg IM morphine to 60 mg oral morphine was also used. As a result, about 50% of patients converted from oral to transdermal fentanyl will require rapid upward dose titration. Thus, a 10 mg IM or 60 mg oral dose of morphine every 4 hr for 24 hr (total 60 mg/day IM or 360 mg/day oral) was considered approximately equivalent to transdermal fentanyl 100 ug/hr.

Courtesy: Janssen Pharmaceutica (modified).

Table 36-7. Advantages of Continuous Subcutaneous Opioid Infusions

1. Avoids repetitive intramuscular or subcutaneous injections.

2. Avoids necessity for intravenous access.

3. Eliminates delays in the administration of analgesics.

4. When effective, provides continous level pf pain relief without peak level side effects or trough level breakthrough pain.

5. Can be modified with addition of patient controlled analgesia.

6. Readily accepted and managed by patients and their families in the home.

7. Potential for earlier discharge home without compromising pain control.

Adapted from Mauskop (101), with permission.

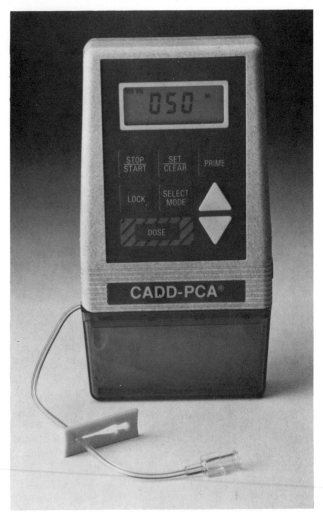

Fig. 36-6. An example of a portable drug infusion pump suitable for subcutaneous, intravenous, epidural, or intrathecal administration, with or without patient controlled analgesia (PCA). Courtesy: Pharmacia Deltec, Inc.

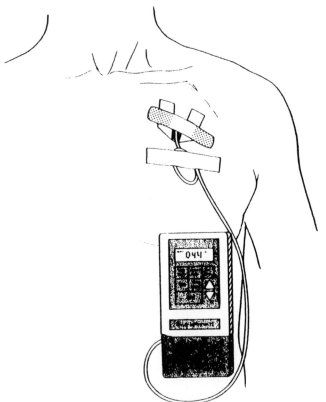

Fig. 36-7. System for administering a continuous subcutaneous infusion of analgesic. From Bruera and Ripamonti (17b), with permission.

Physician orders should provide for rescue doses of drug adequate to counter incomplete analgesia. One method involves ordering subcutaneous injections equal to the hourly dose, to be administered every 1-2 hours, prn. At the end of 24 hours the infusion is increased by the sum of the recorded rescue doses. If analgesia is adequate but side effects are prominent (usually oversedation), the infusion rate may be halved and titrated upwards, as needed.

Breakthrough pain may be related to underdosage, unrecognized tissue irritation, tumor progression, or psychological factors (101). Screening for psychological contributions to complaints of pain should be undertaken early on and treated specifically. Inadequate dosing can be confirmed and resolved by upward titration. Tissue irritation may result in decreased drug absorption, and requires that injection sites be inspected and rotated more frequently. Ideally, the concentration of the infusate is calculated to allow a maximum infusion rate of 1–2 ml/hour. Increased pain associated with tumor progression is the most frequent cause for discontinuing CSCI in favor of intravenous or intraspinal analgesia.

CONTINUOUS INTRAVENOUS INFUSION (CII) OF OPIOIDS

The administration of opioid analgesics by continuous infusion occupies an important and accepted role as an alternative management approach for carefully selected patients with cancer pain (137). Indications for opioids administered by continuous intravenous infusion (CII) are similar to the indications for CSCI. Indications include intolerance of the oral route because of gastrointestinal obstruction, malabsorption, narcotic-induced emesis, dysphagia, or the requirement for large numbers of pills. Other indications include a prominent "bolus-effect" with intermittent injections (Fig. 36-8), the necessity for rapid titration, and requirements for bolus injections that exceed nursing capabilities. Although CII is used frequently during the terminal phases of illness (77), imminence of death is not a valid indication for its use (137). In the presence of anxiety, CII should not be used as a substitute for counseling or sedation.

Anecdotal reports suggest that once treatment is stabilized, home infusion therapy is safe and effective (52,53; Patt, R., Unpublished data, October 1991; Oral communication, Portenoy, R., October 1990), and this practice is likely to become more common in association with increasingly sophisticated home care support. Continuous intravenous infusion is, however, less suitable than CSCI for the home environment because of requirements for maintenance of intravenous access and is generally preferred only when a permanent venous access device is already present. Otherwise, the current use of CII is predominantly restricted to

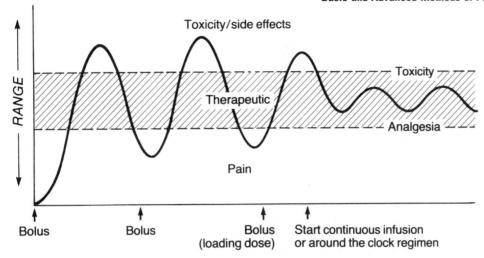

Fig. 36-8. Intermittent (prn) versus continuous or "by-the-clock" drug administration. Note wide swings in plasma levels of drug ("rollercoaster effect") associated with intermittent (symptom-contingent) administration as contrasted with the smoother sine wave pattern of continuous or time-contingent administration. From Bruera and Ripamonti (17b), with permission.

patients who are expected to die within the hospital setting or in whom rapid titration of analgesics is necessary. One further distinction between CII and CSCI that may influence decision making is the inability to sufficiently concentrate subcutaneous formulations of opioids to control pain when dosage requirements increase.

Experience with CII of opioids is best documented for the control of acute postoperative pain. Further research in cancer patients is still needed (137). In studies of postoperative patients comparing CII and bolus opioid therapy, relief of acute pain has been shown to be superior with lower doses administered continuously (20,147). Despite unproven convictions that CII represents a panacea for chronic cancer pain, studies indicate that CII is ineffective in up to one third of patients (21,139). This dissonance introduces the danger that unless the apparent limitations of CII are realized, the complaints of patients whose pain control is inadequate despite treatment will not be taken seriously. Therapy with CII can be accomplished successfully with a variety of opioids, although the bulk of experience is with morphine. Meperidine should be avoided because of the possibility of central nervous system toxicity related to accumulation of normeperidine (73). The theoretical risk of increased sedation due to accumulation of chlorobutanol, a preservative found in most commercial formulations of morphine, becomes actual only when very high doses are used (16). A flow-calibrated infusion device with alarm features is used to deliver medications. Patient-controlled analgesia is an option reserved for patients with the capacity to understand and use this modification correctly.

Recommended procedures for the selection of drugs and dosage are essentially the same as with CSCI therapy (see above), except that it is recommended that loading boluses be used when therapy is initiated and again each time that dosage is incremented (137). Portenoy recommends that the loading dose be selected empirically, using the hourly rate as a rough guide. As with opioids administered by other routes, dosage must be individualized. Accordingly, during titration the infusion rate is incremented, either by 10-20% several times daily or by the sum of the previous time period's "rescue" doses. In this way, dosage is adjusted upward until

pain relief is adequate or side effects become intolerable. There is no ceiling dose, and indeed the administration of hourly doses as high as 500 mg morphine equivalents have been documented without problems (139). Escape doses of a short acting opioid with rapid onset should be used to counter breakthrough pain, and adjuvant drugs (antiemetics, laxatives, amphetamines) should be prescribed judiciously to counter opioid-mediated side effects. Nursing requirements are stringent and consist mainly of frequent monitoring of vital signs, particularly after the administration of loading boluses.

ADJUVANT MEDICATIONS

This heterogeneous grouping consists predominantly of medications originally developed for purposes other than relief of pain, but that have been found to have analgesic properties or are acknowledged to have a complementary role in the management of patients with pain (17a).

Antidepressants

Depression may be related to the presence of pain and in some cases depressive symptoms decrease when pain control improves (160). Classically, antidepressants are used in cancer patients when depression persists despite improved pain control. The tricyclic antidepressants are also useful adjuncts to modify anxiety and disturbances in sleep. Recently, observers have noted their potential to produce analgesia independent of psychological effects (102,182). A recent survey of oncologic centers in Italy indicated that 63% of 35 respondents used antidepressants in a total of 44% of patients, and that 98% of patients appeared to benefit from treatment (97).

In support of a distinction between modulation of pain and affect, most clinicians using amitriptyline and its analogues for pain relief do so in doses usually inadequate to combat depression (10-100 mg nightly). While most controlled studies have documented analgesic efficacy in patients with noncancer pain (102,182), clinical experience suggests that the tricyclics constitute a useful treatment for pain of central, deafferentation or neuropathic origin, particularly when pain has a prominent dysesthetic or burning character. Specific applications include postherpetic neuralgia, postsurgical pain, postablative anesthesia dolorosa, posttreatment neuritis and neuropathy, and invasion of neural structures by tumor. A thorough trial of tricyclic antidepressants may be useful in any patient whose pain has responded inadequately to standard pharmacologic management.

Initial treatment is usually with low nighttime doses that are gradually increased as tolerated (amitriptyline 10-100 mg, trazadone 50-150 mg). Patients are cautioned that relief of pain is often not well-established until 1 to 3 weeks of treatment have elapsed. The common adverse effects of tricyclics, dry mouth, and morning drowsiness are uncommon in the low dosage range and usually resolve over the course of 1 to 2 weeks of regular administration. If adverse effects occur with amitriptyline, dosage should be reduced in the elderly or the infirm, or in the presence of increased confusion. Other reported side effects include tachyarrhythmias, hypotension, hypertension, blurred vision, urinary retention, and constipation.

The restoration of a normal pattern of nighttime sleep is an essential step toward the return to normal functional capacity, and in this regard tricyclic antidepressants administered in low nighttime doses may be extremely useful. Sleep deprivation forms part of a vicious cycle of daytime fatigue and decreased activity, resulting in an inordinate focus on pain.

Anticonvulsants

Carbamezepine, phenytoin, valproic acid, and clonazepam, alone or in combination with the tricyclic antidepressants, have been used successfully to treat pain of neuropathic origin (166). On the basis of well-documented efficacy for the treatment of trigeminal neuralgia (tic douloureux) (163), considerable anecdotal experience has accumulated for the use of these agents for neuropathic cancer pain syndromes, including neural invasion by tumor, radiation fibrosis or surgical scarring, herpes zoster, and deafferentation (63,166). Improvement can be expected in a proportion of patients whose predominant complaint is pain of a lancinating, burning, or hyperesthetic nature (128,166).

Side effects of therapy are potentially serious and can include bone marrow depression, hepatic dysfunction, ataxia, diplopia, and lymphadenopathy. Periodic monitoring of CBC and liver function tests are recommended, as is caution in the prescence of hepatic dysfunction and reduced count

Oral Local Anesthetics

There is now good preliminary evidence from small controlled trials for an analgesic effect for the oral local anesthetics (sodium channel blocking or membrane stabilizing drugs) mexiletine (33a) and tocainide (85a). They are currently considered as second line drugs for neuropathic pain that has proven to be resistant to treatment with the antidepressants and anticonvulsants (17a). Doses are started low (mexilitene 150 mg bid) and titrated upwards as tolerated to achieve pain relief.

Other Pharmacologic Adjuncts: Antihistamines, Antipsychotics, Amphetamines, Steroids, Laxatives, Antiemetics

Antihistamines, steroids, amphetamines and antipsychotics have been recommended as coanalgesics in selected patients with cancer pain (52,128), although clinical trials are lacking. Phenothiazines have been used in the past but with the exception of methotrimeprazine, which has been shown to produce analgesia comparable to morphine (81), evidence to support their efficacy is minimal (103), and their use for pain treatment should be discouraged because side effects (e.g., Parkinson-like symptoms) can be troublesome. In contrast, hydroxyzine and amphetamines have demonstrated coanalgesic properties (55,61), although their roles in clinical management are controversial. Amphetamines often have decided beneficial effects on mood and alertness and have also been used successfully to counter the drowsiness associated with opioid administration (17).

Oral steroids have been administered for a variety of cancer pain syndromes as well as for the management of nausea. Pain relief is presumably related to reduced peritumoral edema and inflammation with consequent relief of pressure and traction on nerves and other pain-sensitive structures. It is difficult to quantify the degree to which the beneficial effects of steroids on mood, appetite, and weight (111) contribute to improved subjective pain reports. The efficacy of steroids in the control of symptoms associated with spinal cord compression raised intracranial pressure and carcinomatous meningitis has been demonstrated conclusively. Their use in other pain problems is more empirically based. For example, steroids administered over short time periods to patients with tumor invasion of the brachial and lumbosacral plexus have been anecdotally reported to reduce pain (53).

Used chronically, potential side effects of steroids include weight gain, Cushing's syndrome, proximal myopathy, avascular bone necrosis, and gastrointestinal bleeding (especially when combined with the NSAIDs). An open trial involving 280 patients suggests that the potential benefits of steroids in terminal cancer patients outweighs their potential risks (149).

Local and perilesional injections of water soluble steroids have a time-tested role in the treatment of nonmalignant back pain (183) and have been reported as providing good temporary relief in various neuropathic cancer pain syndromes (1). The comparative effects of oral versus intralesional steroid administration have not yet been investigated.

The regular administration of opioid analgesics by any route is associated with side effects, notably constipation, nausea, vomiting and sedation. Preventive, regular and aggressive treatment with antiemetics and laxatives is recommended, particularly since constipation can exacerbate pain and discomfort (62,138).

NONPHARMACOLOGIC MANAGEMENT

PSYCHOLOGIC AND BEHAVIORAL INTERVENTION

Psychological Aspects of Cancer Pain

Depression, anxiety and other psychological disorders occur in a high proportion of patients with cancer, even independent of symptoms (34). Inadequate pain control has been cited as one of several factors that predispose to depression (66), and in a representative study of cancer patients matched for disease site and progression, those with pain were more depressed, anxious, and hostile than their counterparts in whom pain was absent (3). Pain and psychological well being are closely-linked: psychological disturbances often resolve once pain is adequately controlled (160), and alternatively, once psychological factors are effectively addressed pain management is often simplified (11).

While feelings traditionally regarded as unhealthy (sadness, anger, guilt, regret) are common in cancer patients, their expression may represent a natural and important step in the process of coming to terms with disease (78,134). When, despite reassurance and support, these reactions are not self-limited, brief psychotherapy is often helpful, and when clinical depression or anxiety persists, psychopharmacotherapy is indicated (15a,66).

Treatment of patients with poorly controlled pain and psychological distress represents a challenge to the treatment team. Each aspect of patient suffering needs to be specifically addressed, and the importance of pain management should not be minimized because of the presence of psychological problems.

Behavioral Pain Management

A variety of behavioral pain management techniques (hypnosis, relaxation, biofeedback, sensory alteration, guided imagery, and cognitive strategies) have been used in patients with cancer (15a,109a,113). Although controlled studies documenting the efficacy of these modalities in patients with cancer are lacking, they play an accepted role in the management of pain of both malignant and nonmalignant origin.

Most behavioral interventions involve instruction in specific skills that, with practice the patient can use independently or with supervision to enhance the effectiveness of intercurrent methods of pain relief.

As early as 1914, Behan in his textbook *Pain* (8), noted that "violent anger or great joy preempts the sensorium to such an extent that sense perception is dulled and may become absolutely negated." Many of the modern behavioral techniques of pain and symptom control use similar strategies to distract the subject from pain.

Specifically, the various forms of relaxation training endeavor to focus the patients' concentration away from pain and on the quality of their breathing or on progressive contraction-relaxation of muscle groups. Treatment may be facilitated by the use of prerecorded tapes and/or biofeedback that correlate the body's physiologic responses to objective measures (temperature, electromyography). In addition to a simple reduction in awareness of pain sensation and an improved sense of self control, these techniques may actually reduce nociception by attenuating muscle spasm and traction on pain-sensitive structures and by decreasing sympathetic arousal. Cognitive measures focus on facilitating alterations in the meaning and significance of pain. They reinforce patients' ability to cope with persistent pain and to remain active and hopeful despite its presence. Preliminary reports on hypnosis, with and without group therapy, suggest a moderate degree of efficacy in selected patients (18,157).

According to Cleeland (22,23), patients whose pain is well controlled are not good candidates for behavioral pain management because motivation may be lacking, while at the opposite extreme patients with severe pain are also typically not good candidates because of functional limitations in their capacity to learn new skills (22,23). Cleeland goes on to suggest that behavioral pain management training is probably most effective for patients in whom significant psychological problems are absent.

Patient acceptance improves when the distinction between behavioral pain management and psychotherapy is clear, and when the decision to institute behavioral methods is understood not to reflect belief that pain is psychogenic. Treatment is more difficult when confusion is present or when concentration is impaired due either to the primary disease or intercurrent drug therapy.

Like with other specialized techniques for pain management, the availability of trained experts is a limiting factor. Nurses, volunteers, and hospice workers have adopted behavioral pain management techniques, and investigators have shown that in other areas of symptom control (i.e., nausea) when properly trained, nonpsychologists can use these modalities successfully (Morrow,G., Oral communication, October 1989).

NERVE BLOCKS

Nerve blocks, like other invasive modalities, are considered when pain persists despite aggressive pharmacologic management, or when drug therapy produces unwanted side effects that are persistent (125a). Nerve blocks play an important role in the treatment of intractable cancer pain and remain a primary focus of the anesthesiologist with specialized training in pain management. The role of neural blockade is complemented by the support offered by the multidisciplinary pain management team.

Local Anesthetic Blockade

Local anesthetic injections can be broadly classified as being applicable for diagnostic, prognostic or therapeutic purposes (13). Diagnostic nerve blocks help to characterize the underlying mechanism of pain and to define the anatomic pathways involved in pain transmission. Diagnostic nerve blocks can help distinguish between pain of somatic, sympathetic, central, or psychogenic origin, and their main use is as a preliminary step prior to the performance of a therapeutic nerve block or other definitive therapy. The results of the same diagnostic nerve block may be interpreted for prognostic purposes to affect a rough simulation of the effects expected to accompany more prolonged blockade with the injection of a neurodestructive (neurolytic) substance. Careful interpretation of the results of prognostic blocks helps the anesthesiologist determine the potential for a subsequent neurolytic block to relieve pain, and also provides an opportunity for the patient to experience, in advance, the side effects that sometimes accompany neurolytic blockade.

While local anesthetic blocks are widely used in the treatment of pain of nonmalignant origin they play a more limited therapeutic role in patients with cancer pain (113,141a). The main limitation of local anesthetic blockade as a therapeutic tool in patients with cancer pain is that pain relief tends to be transient.

In selected cases of myofascial pain, therapeutic injections of local anesthetics into "trigger points," subcutaneous foci of localized muscle spasm, in conjunction with physical therapy may provide persistent relief of pain (170). When intralesional or perineural injections of steroids are planned, local anesthetics are often added to verify anatomic placement and to temporarily interrupt pain and muscle spasm. Local anesthetic injections administered in a series have been shown to produce long standing pain relief in acute reflex sympathetic dystrophy (RSD), a poorly understood disorder of the sympathetic nervous system associated with burning pain, and fluctuating vasomotor disturbances (127). When similar symptoms result from tumor invasion of nervous structures (pancoast syndrome, lumbosacral plexopathy), local anesthetic blockade of the stellate ganglion or lumbar sympathetic chain has been utilized to relieve pain with some success (59).

Neurolytic Blockade

Neurolytic blockade (chemical neurolysis) involves the injection of alcohol or phenol near a nerve or nerves for the purpose of destroying a portion of the targeted nerve to interrupt the transmission of impulses for a prolonged period of time. Nervous structures are affected indiscriminately, and great care must be exercised to relieve pain without producing unwanted motor sensory or autonomic dysfunction.

Neither chemical nor surgical interruption of nerves reliably produce permanent relief of pain because of axonal regrowth and/or the development of deafferentation pain. These limitations, together with the risk of accidental damage to nervous and non-nervous structures limit the application of ablative procedures to patients with severe intractable pain and a limited expectancy of life (125,125a). Careful selection of the proper procedure and attention to technical detail will limit the incidence of side effects and unwanted neurologic deficit (125a).

In general, neurolytic blocks are more effective for pain that is well localized, occupies a limited topography, and that is of somatic or sympathetic origin. While well controlled studies are lacking, large clinical series report significant relief of pain in an average of 50-80% of patients, with the best results obtained when studies include patients who have recieved multiple blocks (64,129,172). Overall, significant complications are reported in less than 5% of patients (64,122,125,129). Optimal results are insured by the judicious use of fluoroscopic and CT guidance to verify needle localization, as well as the application of simple adjuncts such as careful aspiration, the use of a nerve stimulator, the administration of test doses of local anesthetic, and eliciting paresthesias.

Peripheral Nerve Blocks

Peripheral nerve blocks have a limited but important role in the management of cancer pain (37,124a). Multiple blocks are often required because of overlapping sensory fields. Careful patient selection is essential to avoid motor weakness when mixed nerves are targeted.

Neoplastic head and neck pain remains a therapeutic challenge, because of the tendency for tumors in these regions to invade locally and because of the rich innervation of rostral structures. Physiologic splinting, a strategy that is normally adopted unconsciously, is often ineffective in cases of craniocervical pain because many symptoms that aggravate pain (swallowing, eating, coughing, and movement of the head) are involuntary. Treatment success may be adversely affected by anatomic distortion induced by prior surgery or radiotherapy, and the potential for tumor invasion or radiation fibrosis to reduce contact between the neurolytic and targeted nervous tissue. Nevertheless, in selected patients, blockade of the involved cranial and/or upper cervical nerves is of great value. Blockade of the trigeminal nerve within the foramen ovale at the base of the skull or of its branches may be sufficient treatment for localized pain. If

tumor progression is anticipated, it is preferable to prophylactically extend the field of analgesia by blocking the gasserian ganglion in its entirety (95). In other cases, blockade of the ninth or tenth cranial nerve or upper cervical nerves may be required for complete relief.

Bilateral destruction of the glossopharyngeal and vagus nerves is not recommended because of potential intereference with swallowing mechanisms and protective airway reflexes (13,95). When intractable craniocervical pain is not amenable to nerve block therapy, intraspinal opioid therapy by means of an implanted cervical epidural catheter (178) or intraventricular opioid therapy may be considered (89). Intractable hiccoughs (singultus) is also amenable to nerve block therapy. Unilateral phrenic nerve block has been used under these circumstances with excellent results (13). Prior to performing a neurolytic phrenic nerve block, the results of a prognostic block with local anesthetic are evaluated to assure that ventilatory function will not be compromised.

Pain originating in the thoracic wall, abdominal wall, or parietal peritoneum can be treated with multiple intercostal blocks (13,37) or paravertebral somatic nerve root injections. Careful attention to the depth of needle insertion makes pneumothorax uncommon. In patients with normal urinary and gastrointestinal function, injections of the appropriate sacral nerve roots within their foramina provide a means of relieving perineal pain with minimal risk of sphincter disturbance (146). Neurolytic injections of other peripheral nerves are sometimes attempted, but generally only after local anesthetic injection has confirmed that reduction in pain is possible without decriment in motor function. When preexisting motor dysfunction is present or the involved limb is rendered useless by intractable pain (plexus invasion, pathologic fracture), neurolytic block of the brachial plexus or its branches is a further option (75,114).

Central (Neuroaxial) Nerve Blocks

Subarachnoid (intrathecal) injections of alcohol or phenol (164a) (Fig. 36-9) continue to play an important role in the management of intractable cancer pain in selected patients. Their advantages include: (1) a high proportion of good results in selected patients; (2) ease of performance with minimal requirements for equipment; (3) minimal or no requirements for hospitalization; (4) duration of pain relief that is generally adequate for the preterminal state; (5) ease of repetition when necessary; (6) suitability for aged or debilitated patients, and (7) a low complication rate when proper technique is observed.

These procedures produce pain relief by chemical rhizotomy. Since alcohol and phenol destroy nervous tissue indiscriminately (130,154), exquisite attention to selection of the injection site, volume, and concentration of injectate, and selection and positioning of the patient are essential to avoid neurologic complications. Most authorities agree that neither alcohol nor phenol offers a clear advantage, except insofar as variations in baricity facilitate patient positioning (76,85b,164).

Dozens of reports of large uncontrolled series of patients treated with chemical rhizolysis have appeared in the medical literature. Results are difficult to compare because of variations in patient selection, extent, and type of underlying neoplasm, injection techniques, and criteria for success. Swerdlow (165) has analyzed the results of 13 published series

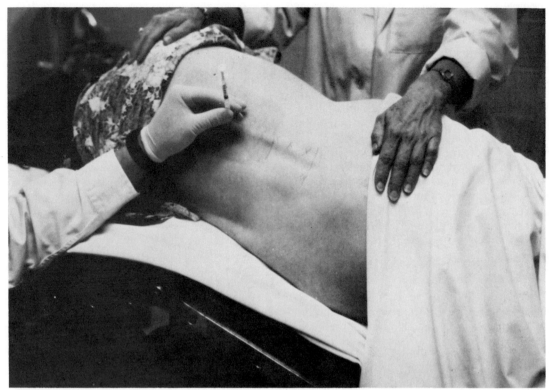

Fig. 36-9. Photograph of patient receiving a midthroacic intrathecal alcohol block. Note position of table to facilitate localization of alcohol to involved dermatomes and anterior tilt intended to localize injection of hypobaric alcohol to posterior sensory roots. From Swerdlow (164a), with permission.

documenting the treatment of over 2500 patients. In 58% of the patients "good" relief was obtained, "fair" pain relief was observed in an additional 21%, and in 20% of patients "little or no relief" was noted. Average duration of relief is difficult to estimate but generally is regarded by authorities to be 3 to 4 months (13), with a wide range of distribution. Reports of analgesia persisting 1 to 2 years are not infrequent (165).

Complication rates should be low with proper attention to detail and when repeated blocks with small volumes are selected over a single treatment with a large volume of drug. In representative series using alcohol (n = 252) and phenol (n = 151), a total of 407 and 313 blocks were performed respectively (64,161). In these two series, no instance of fecal incontinence was observed and of eight patients with transient urinary dysfunction, only one persisted.

Chemical rhizolysis can be performed at any level up to the mid-cervical region, above which the spread of drug to medullary centers carries significant risk of cardiorespiratory collapse (65). Blocks in the region of the brachial outflow are best reserved for patients with pre-existing compromise of upper limb function. Similarly, lumbar injections are avoided in ambulatory patients, as are sacral injections in patients with normal bowel and bladder function. Hyperbaric phenol saddleblock is relatively simple and is particularly applicable in patients with colostomy and urinary diversion.

Epidural neurolysis with phenol is an alternative for patients with pain of moderately extensive anatomic distribution (36). Until recently, epidural neurolysis was used infrequently. Results were inferior to those obtained with subarachnoid blockade (165), presumably because the dura acts as a barrier to diffusion, resulting in limited contact between the drug and targeted nerves. There has been a resurgence of interest in epidural neurolysis related to improved results associated with modifications in technique (140). Modifications require inpatient admission and consist of placement of an indwelling catheter for serial neurolysis performed over several days. In contrast to the subarachnoid route, epidural instillation of neurolytics may be associated with lower incidences of motor weakness, headache, and meningeal irritation (76,165).

Sympathetic Blockade

Unlike somatic nerve blocks, repeated local anesthetic injections of the sympathetic system may produce prolonged relief of pain by interrupting reflex mechanisms (59,127,141a). When local anesthetic blocks provide only temporary relief or when clinical findings are suggestive of visceral or sympathetically-mediated pain, consideration of chemical sympathectomy is warranted (134b).

Celiac Plexus Block

Celiac plexus block continues to be one of the most efficacious and common nerve blocks used to provide prolonged relief of cancer pain. It has great potential for relieving upper abdominal and referred back pain secondary to malignant neoplasms involving structures derived from the embryonic foregut. The most common indication for celiac axis block is pancreatic cancer which, contrary to traditional teaching, is frequently associated with painful rather than painless jaundice (169).

Celiac axis block is most commonly performed by positioning needles bilaterally within the retroperitoneum by a posterior, percutaneous approach (13). Despite the proximity of major organs (including aorta, vena cava, kidneys, and pleura), and the requirements for a large volume of neurolytic (50 cc of 50% alcohol), complication rates are uniformly low (15,169). Radiologic guidance is mandatory to verify needle placement. Traditionally, fluoroscopy has been used but CT guidance is increasing in popularity because vascular structures and viscera can be visualized. Alternative approaches include injection under direct vision at the time of laparotomy (48), transaortic injection (69), and an anterior approach similar to that used for pancreatic biopsy (99).

An 85 to 94% incidence of good to excellent relief of pain has been obtained in large series of patients undergoing one or more neurolytic celiac plexus blocks for pain from pancreatic cancer (15), or a variety of intra-abdominal neoplastic conditions (71,169). In a series of 136 patients, analgesia was present until the time of death in 75% of cases, and in an additional 12.5% pain relief was maintained for more than 50% of survival time (15).

Lumbar Sympathetic and Superior Hypogastric Block

When trials of local anesthetic blockade have been shown to provide temporary relief of pain, neurolysis of the lumbar sympathetic chain with phenol may be undertaken. The most common indications are pelvic pain of urologic, gynecolgic or rectal origin, although pain in the lower extremities due to lymphadema or reflex sympathetic imbalance are also amenable to treatment (13). In contrast to subarachnoid injection, risks of bowel, bladder and motor dysfunction are virtually nil, particularly when radiologic, guidance is used. The recent introduction of hypogastric plexus block (presacral neurotomy) provides another excellent option for pelvic pain of visceral origin (134a,134b).

Cervocothoracic (Stellate Ganglion) Block

Repeated local anesthetic injections of the sympathetic-outflow to the head, neck, and arm often provide persistent relief of pain and, because of their documented ease and safety, these injections are preferred to neurolytic injection. Stellate neurolysis is hazardous because of the close proximity of other important structures (brachial plexus, innervation to larynx, epidural space, and vertebral artery) and the potential for inaccurate needle localization. If local anesthetic injections have been documented to provide temporary relief of pain, surgical extirpation of the ganglia may be considered or neurolysis may be performed cautiously using radiologic guidance and small volumes of injectate (141).

INTRASPINAL OPIOID THERAPY

While local anesthetic-induced epidural anesthesia plays an important role in the management of the acute pain associated with labor, surgery, and postoperative recovery, it has only occasionally been used to manage chronic cancer pain (132). Pain relief associated with local anesthetics administered by the epidural route is nonspecific and is accompanied by motor weakness, sensory anesthesia, and intereference with sympathetic activity. In contrast, the hallmark and main advantage of epidural and intrathecal opioid analgesia is its selectivity; motor, sensory, and sympathetic systems are unaffected (29).

Intraspinal opioid analgesia involves the delivery of minute quantities of narcotics in close proximity to their sites of action (substantia gelatinosa of the spinal cord) (155). Analgesia is often superior to that achieved when opioids are administered by other routes (178a) because drug concentrations at the opioid receptors is high (29). Since the absolute amount of drug administered is reduced, side effects are minimized (172).

Indications and Screening

As with nerve blocks and neurosurgery, the most accepted indication for intraspinal opioid therapy is pain that is inadequately controlled despite aggressive efforts at conservative management, or for patients in whom the occurence of persistent side effects impedes pharmacologic control (28,153). In contrast to nerve blocks and neurosurgery, intraspinal opioid therapy more often provides effective relief of generalized pain as well as pain that is bilateral or midline, particularly in the trunk or lower limbs (28). While the bulk of experience is with catheters placed in the lumbar region, and there have been anecdotal reports of rostral analgesia from morphine administered in the lumbar region (162), the treatment of more cephalic pain is facilitated by catheter implantation at thoracic or cervical levels (178).

The institution of intraspinal opioid therapy requires the participation of an anesthesiologist or neurosurgeon familiar with techniques of screening, implantation, and mainte-

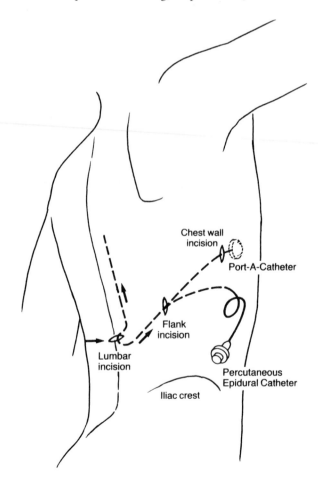

Fig. 36-10. Diagram illustrating an implanted intrathecal/epidural silastic catheter with its proximal end near the spinal canal and its distal end externalized (percutaneous) or alternatively attached to a port (subcutaneous). From Waldman et al. (178a), with permission.

nance, as well as a home care system that is adaptable and innovative. Screening can generally be accomplished on an outpatient basis by observing the patient's response to morphine administered through a temporary epidural catheter which is inserted percutaneously (153).

Epidural versus Subarachnoid (Intrathecal) Administration

The field of CNS opioid therapy is sufficiently new that guidelines for administration and selection of route, drug, and protocol are still emerging. Controlled studies are lacking. The epidural route requires that higher doses of opioids be administered than does subarachnoid administration because the dura acts as a barrier to diffusion of drug into the CSF and to receptor sites in the spinal cord. By either route, though, the equianalgesic dose of opioids is a fraction of that required for oral, subcutaneous, intramuscular or intravenous administration (172). Starting doses for epidural and subarachnoid morphine are in the range of 5-10 mg and 0.5-2 mg, respectively, with a 12-24 hour duration of effect (28,29).

The most accepted means of long-term administration is epidurally via a surgically implanted silastic catheter (Fig. 36-10) which is, in many respects, similar to a Hickmann or Broviac catheter (Fig. 36-8) (28,39,153). Morphine is usually administered in initial doses of 5-10 mg once or twice daily. Alternatively, continuous administration of morphine via a battery-powered portable pump (Fig. 36-6) such as the Pharmacia Deltec or Cormed II or III, eliminates peak and trough effects (Fig. 36-8) and may delay the development of tolerance (153). Continuous administration also reduces nursing requirements and handling that might predispose to infection. A pump with reliable alarm systems is preferred, and in some cases a patient-controlled-analgesia feature is desirable. In addition, physician prescription of an oral or parenteral "escape" dose of opioid is essential to counter breakthrough or incident pain.

Subarachnoid catheter placement is an alternative to epidural administration. Opioid requirements are less than with epidural administration because of more direct access to the CNS. Morphine may be administered via an implanted subcutaneous port or an infusion device implanted within the subcutaneous tissue of the anterior abdominal wall. One system (Infusaid, Shiley) (Fig. 36-11) utilizes a freon-driven pump, initially developed for intra-arterial hepatic chemotherapy, which is about the size and shape of a hockey puck. A 50 ml reservoir is filled percutaneously every 14-21 days, and a constant volume of drug (2-4 ml/day) is infused continuously (24). Alterations in dosage are accomplished by replenishing the reservoir with an opioid of the appropriate concentration, or by bolus administration through a separate port. More sophisticated systems (Synchromed, Medtronics) (see Fig. 36-12) incorporate microprocessor technology to facilitate alterations in infusion rates noninvasively via a laptop computer and telemetry (128a). For either system equipment costs, independent of surgical fees, are estimated range between $6,000-8,000 (136). While subarachnoid infusion devices offer advantages to the patient because the apparatus is completely internalized, the cost is difficult to justify in the preterminal patient, and additional surgery is required. The risk:benefit ratio shifts in favor of these systems for patients with more indolent disease and a life expectancy of 3–6 months or more (7a).

Although subarachnoid infusion techniques offer advantages to the patient because the apparatus is completely internalized, they are costly, and involve additional surgery. While subarachnoid and epidural drug delivery systems have not been compared in a controlled fashion, the potential for leakage of cerebrospinal fluid, chronic headache, meningitis, and equipment malfunction are greater with subarachnoid administration (19,28,96,153).

Side Effects, Tolerance

Side effects (pruritus, nausea, vomiting, urinary retention, respiratory depression) are uncommon in patients in whom narcotics have been prescribed chronically (28,29). Treatment of adverse effects is generally symptomatic and may include an antihistamine for pruritus, standard antiemetics, and temporary bladder catheterization. Side effects that are persistent or severe may be countered with intravenous or intramuscular naloxone, often with preservation of analgesia (142). Epidural hematoma, a rare complication of epidural anesthesia (84) has not been reported with implanted or

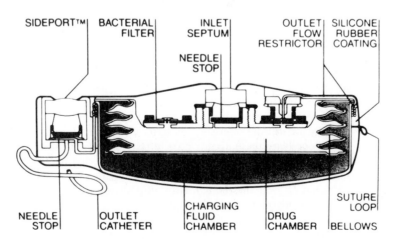

Fig. 36-11. Implantable infusion pumps for the administration of intrathecal morphine. Schematic of freon-driven Infusaid pump: freon in charging fluid chamber expands at a constant rate compressing diaphragm, resulting in continuous drug administration at a constant, fixed rate. Courtesy: Infusaid, Inc.

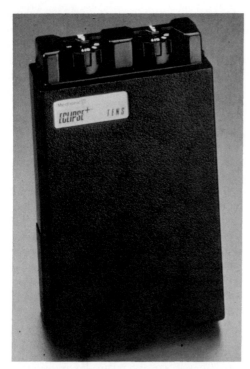

Fig. 36-12. Implantable infusion pumps for the administration of intrathecal morphine. Microprocessor-controlled Synchromed pump: telemetry-mediated external programming permits variable rates of infuson with options for pre-programmed boluses and nocturnal/diurnal variations in drug delivery. Courtesy: Medtronic, Inc.

silastic catheters, although patients with bleeding disorders or who are taking anticoagulants are theoretically at risk.

Tolerance to the analgesic effects of intraspinal opioids eventually occurs, and is similar to tolerance observed with the administration of opioids by other routes. Researchers have reported on a number of experimental methods of reversing and slowing tolerance (25), but in general the most accepted form of treatment is with the administration of higher doses of opioid.

Alternatively, if tolerance persistently interferes with effective analgesia, more potent opioids (fentanyl, sufentanil) have been substituted for morphine (10,185). These agents have not been approved by the FDA for epidural use, and experience in chronic home-based therapy is limited (10), but based on extensive experience with parturients and surgical patients, starting doses in the range of 50-100 ug and 25-50 ug/4 hours, respectively, are effective and safe (126). Fentanyl and sufentanil are, respectively, about 100 and 1000 times as potent as morphine (Table 36-6). Standard commercial formulations of fentanyl and sufentanil are free of preservative, but because of their marked lipophilicity these drugs must be diluted in saline (in volumes of about 1:10) to promote a sufficiently wide distribution in the epidural space. The addition of a dilute concentration of local anesthetic (0.125-0.25% bupivicaine) has also been advocated for patients with breakthrough pain that persists despite increased narcotic administration (38). In a series of terminal patients treated with combined epidural morphine and bupivicaine, pain was consistently reduced and significant hypotension did not occur (38).

INTRAVENTRICULAR OPIOIDS

Clinical experience with small doses of morphine administered through Ommaya reservoirs suggests that this is an effective and practical method of relieving pain in selected patients. Access to the ventricular system is usually through a coronal burr hole made under local anesthesia, although an alternative technique involving passage of a percutaneous catheter through a 14 gauge Touhy needle into the cisterna magna has been described (150). The goal of most practitioners is ongoing outpatient administration by a family member or visiting nurse (82,83,89,118).

The quality of analgesia is excellent in most cases and is apparently unaffected by the site of pain. The majority of treatment has been rendered for patients with cervicofacial pain because more conservative or traditional techniques frequently prove inadequate. Other candidates include patients with cervicobrachial pain, bilateral or midline pain or unremitting pain in any body part that persists despite neurosurgery or which is not amenable to surgery. A trial of lumbar or cisternal morphine generally preceedes implantation (89,118). Optimum life expectancy is on the order of about 6 months. Premature initiation increases risks of sepsis, tolerance, and respiratory depression. In imminently preterminal patients, tolerance may already exist, which, together with a high incidence of mental confusion, complicates management (83,89).

Various hardware, drug preparations, and dosing schedules have been devised. Doses of morphine between 0.2 mg and 4 mg are used most commonly, and duration of analgesia averages 24 hours (83,118). Minor side effects, similar to those associated with the administration of intraspinal opioids (see above), have been reported. Dose-related respiratory depression and infection, potentially serious sequelae, are extremely rare in published series (9,83).

NEUROSURGICAL INTERVENTION

Ready access to neurosurgical opinion and intervention is an important component of a comprehensive cancer pain control program. Advances in pharmacologic management, the introduction of intraspinal opioids, improved multidisciplinary care are among developments that have resulted in a restricted but more clearly defined role for analgesic neurosurgery (42,168a). As with chemical neurolysis and intraspinal opioid therapy, neurosurgical intervention is primarily reserved for patients who have failed thorough attempts at pharmacologic and other means of conservative control, either because of insufficient analgesia or intolerance of side effects.

Over a 75 year period, a variety of neurosurgical procedures have been introduced with the intention of providing safe, effective, and reliable pain relief (Fig. 36-13). Most have been abandoned because these goals have not been adequately satisfied (121). The spectrum of analgesic neurosurgical operations has been extensively reviewed by this author (123,124) and by others (91,184). Because of its extreme clinical relevance percutaneous cordotomy is discussed in detail. Percutaneous pituitary ablation, while it is performed in a limited number of centers, is mentioned because of its potential to relieve widespread bony metastatic pain.

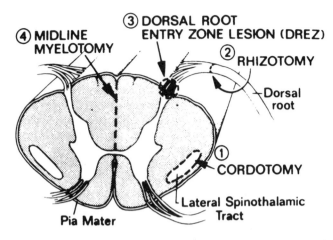

④ MIDLINE MYELOTOMY
③ DORSAL ROOT ENTRY ZONE LESION (DREZ)
② RHIZOTOMY
Dorsal root
① CORDOTOMY
Lateral Spinothalamic Tract
Pia Mater

Fig. 36-13. Schematic of spinal cord illustrating potential sites of lesioning for neurosurgical interventions to control severe pain.

Percutaneous Cordotomy

Percutaneous cordotomy has become the most frequently used neurosurgical procedure performed to relieve cancer pain (91). It is particularly well-suited for unilateral pain confined to the trunk or lower limb. The prototype procedure, open cordotomy, is performed under general anesthesia and involves thoracic or cervical laminectomy and near-complete section of the anterolateral quadrant of the spinal cord (158) Percutaneous cordotomy has largely supplanted the open approach, extending the relevance of spinothalamic tractotomy to patients too ill to undergo the open procedure safely (80,168). The percutaneous approach is commonly employed even when predicted life expectancy is limited to a few weeks (86). It is a simple, safe and effective operation accompanied by minimal surgical and psychological trauma (80,86,91).

Percutaneous cordotomy produces a stereotactically guided thermal lesion in the lateral spinothalamic tract within the cord's anterolateral quadrant, most commonly at the C1-2 level. The targeted fibers transmit pain and temperature sensation originating distally from the opposite side of the body. The procedure is performed in an equipped radiologic suite under local anesthesia.

Cordotomy is ideally suited for the treatment of intractable unilateral lower extremity pain because preservation of proprioception, tactile sensation, and motor strength result in a minimum of dysfunction. When more extensive lesioning is performed to produce higher levels of analgesia, the incidence of both inadequate pain relief and complications increases (87,184). Perineal and abdominal wall pain can usually be treated effectively without significant problems (87,184). As reviewed by Ventafridda *et al.*, results are only fair for unilateral low brachial plexus and chest wall pain (174). The role of cordotomy is limited for upper extremity pain because of a high failure rate and the increased incidence of respiratory and other neurologic complications. Pain involving both lower extremities or pelvic or back pain that crosses the midline is technically amenable to bilateral cordotomy, but bilateral procedures are currently performed with much less frequency because of increased risks of paraparesis and bladder and respiratory dysfunction (80,86).

Results are difficult to compare because of variations among series in patient selection, surgical technique, and

follow-up. Immediate relief of malignant pain is usually cited as ranging between 60% and 80%. When failures are subject to repeat cordotomy, overall success rate is 86% to 96% (85,87). In one typical series of cancer patients treated with percutaneous cordotomy, 75% were pain-free until their death, an additional 8% had significant pain relief, 8% had partial, transient relief, and 9% were considered failures (86).

Careful patient screening is essential since pain relief is transient, rarely persisting in excess of 1 to 2 years (86). The risks of neurologic and respiratory impairment are modest in well selected patients (85,86). Extensive lesioning for rostral or bilateral pain sites may result in Ondine's Curse, a sleep apnea syndrome which, once established, has a high rate of mortality (135).

Pituitary Ablation

Surgical hypophysectomy was first advocated to reduce tumor spread in 1953 (93). The observation that some patients experienced postsurgical pain relief led Moricca (112) to suggest pituitary destruction by percutaneous injection of absolute alcohol as a primary treatment for oncogenic pain. Alcohol ablation is preferred to surgical removal because it is comparatively simple, safe, and inexpensive, and entails only a brief hospitalization. The incidence and severity of complications have been further reduced by technical modifications that permit selective destruction of the anterior hypophysis (40,88). While pituitary ablation is performed in a limited number of centers, in part because of its technical demands, sufficient clinical experience has accumulated for it to be regarded as a well-accepted pain-relieving modality.

Pituitary destruction is considered to treat intractable bilateral pain due to widespread bony metastases when life expectancy is moderate. Previously, selection of patients had been restricted to individuals with hormone-sensitive tumors. More recent reports suggest efficacy in patients with other malignant neoplasms, particularly when complaints are of head and neck pain (40,79).

The technical aspects of the procedure have been carried out variously by neurosurgical or anesthesiology teams, or in collaboration, with apparently similar results (109). General anesthesia is induced and a 16 gauge needle is passed through one nostril toward the pituitary fossa by the transphenoidal route. The needle tip is localized within the anterior bony margins of the pituitary fossa. A 20 gauge needle is passed through the introducer a few millimeters into the substance of the gland, and after the injection of a minute quantity of contrast medium, a total of 0.8-1.0 ml of absolute alcohol is injected in 0.1 ml increments over 10-15 minutes. During the process, anesthesia is lightened to facilitate detection of pupillary movement or dilation that may signal damage to the optic chiasm.

Results vary among studies owing in part to differences in patient selection and technique. In a review of six clinical series, complete or almost complete pain relief was achieved in 42% to 98% of patients (123), some of whom were injected more than one time, with other patients experiencing lesser degrees of relief. In at least one case, analgesia was so profound as to allow a patient previously immobile from pain to return to work for an extended period (94). In the series reviewed, the median duration of pain relief ranged between 7 weeks and 4 months. Some patients remained free of pain for up to 2 years, and a significant number of patients died painlessly. Pain relief usu ally develops gradually over the first 24-48 hours following the procedure, but in some cases is immediate and in others accrues over more prolonged periods.

Miles (109) reported six procedure-related deaths in an early series of 250 patients, but in a recent, more representative study there was no mortality attributed to the procedure (79). The most frequent complications in a large series were self-limited headache (17%), diabetes insipidus (17%), and nausea (9%) (40). Visual disturbance, a potentially serious complication, occurs infrequently. Hospitalization for a minimum of 48 hours is required for observation and routine steroid replacement is indicated in all patients not already receiving steroids.

ELECTRICAL STIMULATION

Electrical stimulation has been applied at various levels of the nervous system to relieve pain through interaction with endogenous neuromodulatory mechanisms (168a). Advantages of stimulation-analgesia include decreased dependence on narcotic drugs, avoidance of the sequelae sometimes associated with neuroablative procedures and an enhanced sense of control by patients. Electrical stimulation of the nervous system requires a pulse generator, an amplifier and paired electrodes. Depending on the targeted site, the technique and complexity of instituting stimulation vary. Most systems are designed to enable patients to control the frequency and intensity of stimulation within preset limits in response to varying analgesic requirements.

Transcutaneous Electrical Nerve Stimulation

Transcutaneous electrical nerve stimulation (TENS) is the most commonly used stimulation modality. Rapid bursts of low-voltage electrical current are transmitted through a pair of electrodes applied to the skin overlying the painful region. At the proper settings, the stimulus is experienced as repeated painless paresthesias. Most systems use a rectangular wave form and permit regulation of current, frequency, and pulse width. Commercially available units are compact, safe, simple to use, and are relatively inexpensive.

Numerous controlled studies of TENS have shown reduction of acute pain in over 60% of subjects and a long term efficacy of about 30% in reducing chronic pain (151). Other stimulation modalities have not been studied as thoroughly. Acute pain syndromes that respond well to TENS include rib fractures (115), postoperative incisional pain (5,26,131,156), labor and dental pain (5). For chronic pain, TENS is used in combination with other modalities (pharmacologic, psychologic, anesthetic), since the characteristic response is reduction rather than elimination of pain. Examples of chronic pain syndromes in which TENS has been used include peripheral nerve injury, neuralgia, radiculopathy, and compression syndromes (186).

Reports of results of TENS for pain related to malignant neoplasm are less encouraging. Ventafridda *et al.* (176) obtained good to excellent results in 43% of patients with cancer pain but noted significant reduction in efficacy with the passage of time, a characteristic observation (186). In a follow-up study, 96% of 37 patients with cancer pain noted marked reductions in pain intensity during the first 10 days of treatment, but by the end of 30 days this number had declined to 27% (176).

Localized pain is more likely to respond than is vague, generalized pain (117,179). Pain that is of central, psychogenic, or visceral origin is unlikely to respond well (117). The individual response to stimulation varies. Trials for several weeks are necessary in some patients before maximum pain relief is realized (179). Transcutaneous electrical nerve stimulation is extremely safe and warrants trial as an adjunctive modality in patients with cancer pain. The main limitation of peripheral stimulation is a tendency for loss of effect with time (176).

Spinal Cord (Epidural) Stimulation

Spinal cord stimulation involves the placement of stimulating electrodes in proximity to the spinal cord in the epidural space. Historically, laminectomy was required to implant electrodes, exposing patients to the rigors of general anesthesia, major surgery, and prolonged hospitalization. New systems have been devised that are implantable through a standard 15 gauge epidural needle. Percutaneous insertion is accomplished by an anesthesiologist or neurosurgeon and has the advantage of enabling a trial of stimulation before the unit's pulse generator (battery) is implanted subcutaneously. The main indications for dorsal column stimulation have been chronic back and leg pain, particularly for the "failed back" or postlaminectomy syndrome (33). Patients with multiple sclerosis, diabetic neuropathy, herpes zoster peripheral vascular disease, and stump neuromata have also been treated with some success (45,47,144).

Strict guidelines for patient selection are still not established. Authors suggest that patients who demonstrate excessive pain behavior are less likely to benefit, and psychological screening is strongly recommended (90,92). Effective epidural stimulation, like peripheral stimulation, requires that stimulation generate paresthesias over the painful region, although preliminary response to TENS is not predictive of response to spinal cord stimulation (90).

There has been considerable experience with spinal stimulation instituted for the relief of cancer pain. Although many instances of success have been reported, overall results have been poor (90,104,152). Pooled results should not be interpreted too strictly since criteria for implantation technique, follow-up and success vary considerably, but a review of 16 series reporting on spinal stimulation for 88 patients with cancer pain indicates that treatment was successful in only 48% of patients (90,104). Increasing use of percutaneous methods of implantation, which are associated with reduced morbidity may, in the future, permit sufficient trials in cancer patients to determine reliable screening criteria (168a).

Deep Brain Stimulation

Chronic stimulation of deep brain structures is a form of neurosurgical intervention introduced recently for the control of generalized pain. In the future, deep brain stimulation is expected to play a prominent role in the management of widespread intractable cancer pain and may be of use for selected cases of nonmalignant pain, as well. Reports are promising, although an insufficient number of patients have been treated to determine long-term efficacy.

Interest has focused on two distinct areas of the brain which, when stimulated seem to produce pain relief by different mechanisms.

Periventricular and Periaqueductal Grey Stimulation

Stimulation of these regions, as well as the medial posterior thalamus, is associated with the release of endogenous opioidlike substances (endorphins) into the third ventricle (4,143). Endorphins are hypothesized to activate a descending pain-inhibitory system originating in the central brain stem and terminating in the substantia gelatinosa, where suppression of pain transmission is postulated to occur.

Pain relief resembles that which accompanies exogenous opioid administration, in that analgesia is reversed by naloxone administration and tolerance can occur with chronic stimulation. Tolerance can sometimes be reversed with the administration of disulfiram, tryptophan or tricyclic compounds (35).

The main advantage of periventricular stimulation over ablative procedures is the prospect of pain relief without the risks associated with major surgery or denervation procedures. Analgesia tends to be widespread and bilateral, rather than limited to a distinct area subserved by a single nerve. These characteristics make periventricular stimulation an attractive alternative for the treatment of intractable pain that crosses the midline or involves the head, neck or upper extremities. Destructive procedures designed to relieve these syndromes have low success rates, are associated with high incidences of mortality and morbidity, and may be accompanied by functional loss.

According to Young and Brechner's (189) review of periventricular and periaqueductal grey stimulation for noncancer and malignant pain, 65 to 70% of carefully selected patients experience pain relief sufficient to allow discontinuation of opioid use and resumption of normal activities.

Stimulation of the Posterior Internal Capsule/ Sensory Thalamus

Stimulation of the internal capsule and discrete thalamic centers is being investigated for relief of central pain disorders. In contrast to stimulation of the periaqueductal and periventricular regions, endorphins are not released when these areas are stimulated, nor does tolerance occur. Pain relief is strictly contralateral and is not reversed when naloxone is administered. Distinct thalamic sensory nuclei are targeted for facial versus body pain. Studies indicate that long-term pain control can be expected in greater than 50% of patients (67,171,190). Painful conditions that have been successfully treated include thalamic syndrome, anesthesia dolorosa, postherpetic neuralgia, spinal cord injury, brachial plexus avulsion and phantom limb pain (188). Despite promising results, the mechanism for pain relief is poorly understood. Theories include restoration of disrupted inhibitory impulses, increased sensory input to partially denervated areas of the somatosensory cortex, and interference with spontaneous neuronal hyperactivity (2).

CONCLUSION

Pain associated with cancer and its treatment has the potential to disrupt the well being of patients and their family along multiple dimensions. Poorly controlled pain may have a negative impact on activity, mood, socialization, appetite, sleep, posture and sexuality. Injudicious treatment may produce equally troublesome side effects.

Cancer pain is variable in its causation, presentation, impact, and responsiveness to treatment, and hence careful assessment is a most important first step in effective management. Despite well-documented historical inadequacies in the medical management of cancer pain and the need for further scientific investigation, currently available treatment modalities have the potential for producing significant relief of pain in most, if not all patients. Since practitioners in a variety of medical specialties can expect to become involved in the care of patients with cancer, it is imperative that medical students and residents learn principles of cancer pain management including familiarity with commonly used modalities and indications for alternative treatment.

REFERENCES

1. Abram SE. The role of nonneurolytic blocks in the management of cancer pain. In: Abram SE. (ed). Cancer Pain. Boston, MA: Kluwer Academic Publishers; 1988; pp 67-75.
2. Adams JE. Electrical stimulation of the internal capsule for the control of central pain. In: Morley TP. (ed). Current Controversies in Neurosurgery. Philadelphia, PA: W.B. Saunders Co.; 1976; 83:510-514.
3. Ahles TA, Blanchard EB, Ruckdeschel JC. Multidimensional nature of cancer pain. Pain 1983; 17:277-288.
4. Akil H, Richardson DE, Hughes J, et al. Elevations in levels of enkephalin-like materials in the ventricular CSF of pain patients upon analgetic focal stimulation. Science 1979; 201:463-465.
5. Ali JA, Yaffee CS, Serretti C. The effect of transcutaneous electrical nerve stimulation on postoperative pain and pulmonary function. Surgery 1981; 89:507-512.
5a. Ashby M. Palliative radiotherapy. In: Patt RB (ed). Cancer Pain. Philadelphia, PA: J.B. Lippincott Co; 1993; pp 235-250.
6. Baines M, Kirkham SR. Carcinoma involving bone and soft tissue. In: Wall PD, Malzack R. (eds). Textbook of Pain. New York, NY: Churchill Livingstone; 1984; pp 453-459.
7. Beaver WT. Maximizing the benefits of weaker analgesics. In: IASP Refresher Course on Pain Management. Vol. 1. Hamburg, Germany: International Association for the Study of Pain. 1987; pp 1-25.
7a. Bedder MD, Burchiel KJ, Larson A. Cost analysis of two implantable narcotic delivery systems. J Pain Symptom Mngmt. 1991; 6:368.
8. Behan RJ. Pain: Its Origin, Conduction, Perception and Diagnostic Significance. New York, NY: D. Appleton; 1921.
8a. Beyer JE, Wells N. Assessment of cancer pain in children. In: Patt RB (ed). Cancer Pain. Philadelphia, PA: J.B. Lippincott Co; 1993; pp 57-84.
9. Black P. Neurosurgical management of cancer pain. Semin Oncol. 1985; 12:438-444.
10. Boersman FB, Noorduin H, Vanden Bussche G. Continuous epidural sufentanil infusion for relief of cancer pain on outpatient basis. 2nd International Symposium on Regional Anesthesia. Williamsburg, Virginia, May 28-30, 1988.
11. Bond MR. Psychological and emotional aspects of cancer pain. In: Bonica JJ, Ventafridda V. (eds). Advances in Pain Research and Therapy. vol. 2. New York: Raven Press; 1979; pp 81-88.
12. Bonica JJ. Cancer Pain: A Major National Health Problem. Cancer Nursing. 1978; 1:313-316.
13. Bonica JJ. Management of Pain. Philadelphia, PA: Lea and Febiger, 1953.
14. Bonica JJ. Treatment of cancer pain. Current status and future needs. Semin Anesth. 1985; 9:589-616.
15. Brown BL, Bulley CK, Quiel EC. Neurolytic celiac plexus block for pancreatic cancer pain. Anesth Anala. 1987; 66:869-873.
15a. Breitbart W. Diagnosis and treatment of psychiatric complications in the cancer patient with pain. In: Patt RB (ed). Cancer Pain. Philadelphia, PA: J.B. Lippincott Co; 1993; pp 209-233.
16. Bruera E, Brenneis C, Michaud M, et al. Continuous infusion of narcotics using a disposable device in patients with advanced cancer. Cancer Treatment Rep. 1987; 71:635-637.
17. Bruera E, Chadwick S, Brenneis C, et al. Methylphenidate associ-

ated with narcotics for the treatment of cancer pain. Ca Treat Rep 1987; 71:67-70.

17a. Bruera E, Ripamonti C. Adjuvants to opioid analgesics. In: Patt RB (ed). Cancer Pain. Philadelphia, PA: J.B. Lippincott Co; 1993; pp 143-159.

17b. Bruera E, Ripamonti C. Alternate routes of administration of opioids for the management of cancer pain. In: Patt RB (ed). Cancer Pain. Philadelphia, PA: J.B. Lippincott Co; 1993; pp 162-167.

18. Butler B. The use of hypnosis in the care of the cancer patient. Cancer. 1954; 7:1-14.

19. Cherry DA, Gourlay GK. The spinal administration of opioids in the treatment of acute and chronic pain: Bolus doses, continuous infusion, intraventricular administration and implanted drug delivery systems. Palliative Med. 1987; 1:89-106.

20. Church JJ. Continuous narcotic infusions for the relief of postoperative pain. Br Med J 1979; 1:977-979.

21. Citron ML, Johnson-Early A, Fossieck BE, et al. Safety and efficacy of continuous intravenous morphine for severe cancer pain. Am J Med 1984; 77:199-204.

21a. Cleeland CS. Assessment of pain in cancer. In: Foley KM, Bonica JJ, Ventafridda V (eds). Advances in Pain Research and Therapy, vol.16. New York, NY: Raven Press; 1990; p 47.

22. Cleeland CS. The impact of pain on the patient with cancer. Cancer 1984; 54:2635-2641.

23. Cleeland CS, Tearnan BH. Behavioral control of cancer pain. In: Holzman AD, Turk DC (eds): Pain Management. New York, Pergamon Press; 1986; pp 193-212.

24. Coombs DW, Saunders RL, Harbaugh R, et al. Relief of continuous chronic pain by intraspinal narcotics infusion via an implanted reservoir. JAMA 1983; 250:2336-2339.

25. Coombs DW, Saunders RL, LaChance D, et al. Intrathecal morphine tolerance: Use of intrathecal clonidine, DADLE, and intraventricular morphine. Anesthesiology 1985; 62:358-363.

26. Cooperman, AM, Hall B, Mikalacki K, et al. Use of transcutaneous electrical stimulation in control of postoperative pain. Results of a prospective randomized study. Am J Surg 1977; 133:185-187.

27. Copp LA, Anderson VC, Brown MJ, et al. National institutes of health concensus panel: Integrated approach to the management of pain. J Pain Symptom Management 1987; 2:35-44.

28. Cousins MJ, Cherry DA, Gourlay GK. Acute and Chronic Pain: Use of Spinal Opioids. In: Cousins MJ, Bridenbaugh PO (eds). Neural Blockade, 2nd ed. Philadelphia, PA: JB Lippincott; 1988; pp 955-1029.

29. Cousins MJ, Mather LE. Intrathecal and epidural administration of opioids. Anesthesiology 1984; 61:276-310.

30. Coyle N, Adelhardt J, Foley KM. Changing patterns in pain, drug use, and routes of administration in the advanced cancer patient. Pain 1987; 339.

31. Daut RL, Cleeland CS. The prevalence and severity of pain in cancer. Cancer 1982; 50:1913-1918.

31a. Daut, RL; Cleeland, CS; Flanery, RC. Development of the Wisconsin brief pain questionnaire to access pain in cancer and other diseases. Pain 1983; 17:197.

32. DeChristoforo R, Corden BJ, Hood JC, et al. High-dose morphine infusion complicated by chlorobutanol-induced somnolence. Ann Int Med 1983; 98:335-336.

33. De La Porte C, Siegfried J. Lumbosacral spinal fibrosis (spinal arachnoiditis): Its diagnosis and treatment by spinal cord stimulation. Spine 1983; 8:593-603.

33a. Dejgard A, Petersen P, Kastrup J. Mexiletine for treatment of chronic painful diabetic neuropathy. Lancet i:9-11; 1988.

34. Derogatis LR, Morrow GR, Fetting J, et al. The prevalence of psychiatric disorders among cancer patients. JAMA 1983; 249:751-757.

35. Dieckmann G, Witzmann A. Initial and long-term results of deep brain stimulation for chronic intractable pain. Appl Neurophysiol 1982; 45:167-172.

36. Dobrogowski J, Marian K. Epidural neurolytic block in cancer patients. In: Erdmann W, Oyama T, Pernack MJ (eds). Pain Clinic I. Utrecht, The Netherlands: VNU Science Press; 1985; pp 51-54.

37. Doyle D. Nerve blocks in advanced cancer. Practitioner 1982; 226:539-544.

38. Du Pen SL. After epidural narcotics: What next for cancer pain control. Anesth Analg 1987; 66:546.

39. Du Pen SL, Peterson D, Bogosian A, et al. A new permanent exteriorized epidural catheter for narcotic self-administration to control cancer pain. Cancer 1987; 59:986-993.

40. Duthie AM, Ingham V, Dell AE, et al. Results of treatment using a transsphenoidal cryoprobe. Anaesthesia 1983; 38:448-451.

41. Edeiken J, Karasick D. Imaging in cancer. CA: A Journal for Clinicians 1987; 37:239-245.

42. Epstein JA. Changing trends in the neurosurgical management of chronic pain. Spine 1985; 10:100-101.

43. Estes NC, Morphis JG, Hornback NB, et al. Intraarterial chemotherapy and hyperthermia for for pain control in patients with recurrent rectal cancer. Am J Surg 1986; 152:597-601.

44. Faithfull NS, Reinhold HS, Van Den Berg AP, et al. The effectiveness and safety of whole body hyperthermia as a pain treatment in advanced malignancy. In: Erdmann W, Oyama T, Pernak MJ (eds). Pain Clinic. Utrecht, The Netherlands: VNU Science Press; 1985.

45. Feeney DM, Gold GN. Chronic dorsal stimulation: Effects on H reflex and symptoms in a patient with multiple sclerosis. Neurosurgery 1980; 6:564.

46. Ferrer-Brechner T. Rational management of cancer pain. In Raj PP (ed): Practical Manaaement of Pain. Chicago, IL: Yearbook Medical Publishers; 1986; pp 312-328.

46a. Fishman B; Pasternak S, Wallenstein S. et al. The Memorial pain assessment card: A valid instrument for the evaluation of cancer pain. Cancer 60:1151;1987.

47. Fiume D. Spinal cord stimulation in peripheral vascular pain. Appl Neuro Physiol 1983; 46:290-294.

48. Flanigan DP, Kraft R. Continuing experience with palliative chemical splanchnicectomy. Arch Surg 1978; 113:509-511.

49. Foley KM. Cancer pain syndromes. J Pain Symptom Management 1987; 2:513-17.

50. Foley KM. Overview of cancer pain and brachial and lumbosacral plexopathy. In: Foley KM (ed). Management of Cancer Pain. New York, NY: Memorial Sloan Kettering Cancer Center; 1985; pp 25-63.

51. Foley KM. Pain syndromes in patients with cancer. In: Bonica JJ, Ventafridda V (eds). Advances in Pain Research and Therapy, vol 2. New York, NY: Raven Press; 1979; pp 59-75.

52. Foley KM. Treatment of cancer pain. N Engl J Med 1985; 313:84-95.

53. Foley KM, Inturrisi CM. Analgesic drug therapy in cancer pain: Principles and practice. Med Clin North Am 1987; 71:207-232.

54. Fordyce WE. Behavioral Methods for Chronic Pain and Illness. St. Louis, MO: C.V. Mosby; 1976.

55. Forrest WH Jr, Brown BM Jr, Brown CR. Dextroamphetamine with morphine for the treatment of postoperative pain. N Engl J Med 1977; 296:712-715.

56. Fosburg MF, Crone RK. Nitrous oxide analgesia for refractory pain in the terminally ill. JAMA 1983; 250:511-514.

57. Galasko CSB. Mechanisms of bone destruction in the development of skeletal metastases. Nature 1976; 263:507-510.

58. Galasko CSB. Skeletal Metastases. London, UK: Butterworths; 1986; pp 99-124.

59. Gerbershagen HU. Blocks with local anesthetics in the treatment of cancer pain. In: Bonica JJ, Ventafridda V (eds). Advances in Pain Research and Therapy, vol 2. New York, NY: Raven Press; 1979; pp 311-323.

60. Gilbert RW, Kim JH, Posner JB. Epidural spinal cord compression from metastatic tumor: Diagnosis and treatment. Ann Neurol 1978; 3:40-51.

61. Halpern LM. Psychotropics and Ataratics and Related Drugs. In: Bonica JJ, Ventafridda V (eds). Advances in Pain Research and Therapy, vol 2. New York, NY: Raven Press; 1979; pp 275-283.

62. Hanks GW. Antiemetics for terminal cancer patients. Lancet 1982; 1:1410.

63. Hatangdi VS, Boas RA, Richard EG. Postherpetic Neuralgia: Management with Antiepileptic and Tricyclic Drugs. In: Bonica, JJ, et al. (eds). Advances in Pain Research and Therapy, vol 1. New York, NY: Raven Press; 1976; pp 583-587.

64. Hay RC. Subarachnoid alcohol block in the control of intractable pain: report of results in 252 patients. Anesth Analg 1962; 41:12-16.

64a. Hill CS. Oral opioid analgesics. In: Patt RB (ed). Cancer Pain. Philadelphia, PA: J.B. Lippincott Co; 1993; pp 129-142.

65. Holland AJC, Youssef M. A complication of subarachnoid phenol blockade. Anaesthesia 1979; 34:260-262.

66. Holland J. Managing depression in the patient with cancer. Ca - A Cancer Journal for Clinicians 1987; 37:366-371.

67. Hosobuchi Y. Subcortical electrical stimulation control of intractable pain. Report of 122 cases. J Neurosura 1986; 64:543-553.

68. Inturrisi CE. Newer methods of opioid drug delivery, in IASP Refresher Courses on Pain Management Book of Abstracts, vol 1. Hamburg, International Association for the Study of Pain, 1987; pp 27-39.

69. Ischia S, Luzzani A, Ischia A, et al. A new approach to the neurolytic block of the coeliac plexus: The transaortic technique. Pain 1983; 16:333-341.

70. Jaeckle KA, Young DF, Foley KM. The natural history of lumbosacral plexopathy in cancer. Neurology 1985; 35:8-15.

71. Jones J, Gough D. Coeliac plexus block with alcohol for relief of upper abdominal pain due to cancer. Ann R Coll Surg Engl 1977; 59:46-49.

72. Joranson DE, Dahl JL, Engber D. Wisconsin initiative for improving cancer pain management: Progress report. J Pain Symptom Management 1987; 2-114.

73. Kaiko RF, Foley KM, Grabinski PY, et al. Central nervous system excitatory effects of meperidine in cancer patients. Ann Neurol 1983; 13:180-185.

74. Kaiko RF, Wallenstein SL, Rogers AG, et al. Sources of variation in analgesic responses in cancer patients with chronic pain receiving morphine. Pain 1983; 15:191-200.

75. Kaplan R, Aurellano Z, Pfisterer W. Phenol brachial plexus block for upper extremity cancer pain. Reg Anesth 13:58-61.

76. Katz J. The current role of neurolytic agents. Adv Neurol 1974; 4:471-476.

77. Kellar M. A retrospective review of patients receiving continuous morphine infusion. PRN Forum 1984; 3:5-6.

78. Kubler-Ross E. On Death and Dying. New York, NY: MacMillan; 1969.

78a. Kurman M. Palliative chemotherapy. In: Patt RB (ed). Cancer Pain. Philadelphia, PA: J.B. Lippincott Co; 1993; pp 251-276.

79. Lahuerta J, Lipton S, Miles J, et al. Update on percutaneous cervical cordotomy and pituitary alcohol neuroadenolysis: An audit of our recent results and complications. In Lipton S, Miles J (eds): Persistent Pain, vol 5. New York, Grune & Stratton; 1985; pp 197-223.

80. Lahuerta J, Lipton S, Wells JCD. Percutaneous cordotomy: Results and complications in a recent series of 100 patients. Ann R Coll Surg Engl 1985; 67:41-44.

81. Lasagna RG, DeKornfeldt TJ. Methotrimeprazine: A new phenothiazine derivative with analgesic properties. JAMA 1961;178:887-890.

82. Lazorthes J, Verdie JC, Bastide R, et al. Spinal versus intraventricular chronic opiate administration with implantable drug delivery devices for cancer pain. Appl Neurophysiol 1985; 48:234-241.

83. Lenzi A, Galli G, Gandolfini M, et al. Intraventricular morphine in paraneoplastic painful syndrome of the cervicofacial region: Experience in 38 cases. Neurosurgery 1985; 17:6-11.

84. Lerner SM, Gutterman P, Jenkins F. Epidural hematoma and paraplegia after numerous lumbar punctures. Anesthesiology 1973; 39:550-551.

85. Levin AB. Techniques and results of cordotomy in patients with pain of benign and malignant origin. In: Rizzi R, Visentin M (eds). Pain Therapy. Amsterdam, The Netherlands: Elsevier Science Publishers; 1983.

85a. Lindstrom P, Lindblom U. The analgesic effect of tocainide in trigeminal neuralgia. Pain 28:45-50; 1987.

85b. Lipton S. Neurolysis: Pharmacology and drug selection. In: Patt RB (ed). Cancer Pain. Philadelphia, PA: J.B. Lippincott Co; 1993; pp 343-358.

86. Lipton S. Percutaneous cordotomy. In: Wall PD, Melzack R (eds). Textbook of Pain. New York, NY: Churchill Livingstone; 1984; pp 632- 638.

87. Lipton S. Percutaneous cervical cordotomy. In: Bonica JJ, Ventafridda V (eds). Advances in Pain Research and Therapy, vol 2. New York, NY: Raven Press; 1979; pp 425-437.

88. Lloyd JW, Rawlinson WAL, Evans PJD. Selective hypophysectomy for metastatic pain: A review of ethyl alcohol ablation of the anterior pituitary in a regional pain relief unit. Br J Anaesth 53:1129-1132; 1981.

89. Lobato RD, Madrid JL, Fatela LV, et al. Intraventricular morphine for intractable cancer pain: Rationale, methods, clinical results. Acta Anaesthesiol Scand 31:68-74; 1987.

90. Loeser JD. Dorsal column and peripheral nerve stimulation for relief of cancer pain. In: Bonica JJ, Ventafridda (eds). Advances in Pain Research and Therapy, vol 2. New York, NY: Raven Press; 1979; pp 499-507.

91. Long DM. Surgical therapy of chronic pain. Neurosurgery 6:317-326; 1980.

92. Long DM, Erickson D, Campbell J, et al. Electrical stimulation of the spinal cord and peripheral nerves for pain control: A 10 year experience. Appl Neuro Physiol 44:207-217; 1981.

93. Luft R, Olivecrona H. Experiences with hypophysectomy. J Neurosurg 10:301-316; 1953.

94. Madrid JL. Chemical Hypophysectomy. In: Bonica JJ, Ventafridda V (eds). Advances in Pain Research and Therapy, vol 2. New York, NY: Raven Press; 1979; pp 381-392.

95. Madrid JL, Bonica JJ. Cranial Nerve Blocks. In: Bonica JJ, Ventafridda V (eds): Advances in Pain Research and Therapy vol 2. New York, NY: Raven Press, 1979; pp 463-468.

96. Madrid JL, Fatela LV, Alcorta J, et al. Intermittent intrathecal morphine by means of an implantable reservoir: A survey of 100 cases. J Pain Symptom Management 3:67-71; 1988.

97. Magni G, Arsie D, De Leo D. Antidepressants in the treatment of cancer pain: A survey in Italy. Pain 29:347-353; 1987.

98. Marks RM, Sachar EJ. Undertreatment of medical inpatients with narcotic analgesics. Ann Intern Med 78:173-181; 1973.

99. Matamala AM, Lopez FV, Martinez LI. Percutaneous approach to the celiac plexus using CT guidance. Pain 4:285-288; 1988.

100. Mauch PM, Drew MA. Treatment of metastatic cancer to bone. In: Devita VT (ed). Cancer: Principles and Practice of Oncology, ed 2, Philadelphia, PA: JB Lippincott Co; 1985; pp 2132-2141.

101. Mauskop A. Continuous subcutaneous infusions of narcotics. In: Foley KM (ed). Management of Cancer Pain. New York, NY: Memorial Sloane-Kettering Cancer Center; 1985; pp 189-203.

102. Max MB, Culnane M, Schafer SC, et al. Amitriptyline relieves diabetic neuropathy pain in patients with normal or depressed mood. Neurology 37:589-596; 1987.

103. McGee JL, Alexander MR. Phenothiazine analgesia: Fact or fantasy. Am J Hosp Pharm 36:633-650; 1979.

104. Meglio M, Cioni B. Personal experience with spinal cord stimulation in chronic pain management. Appl Neurophysiol 45:195-200; 1982.

105. Mellette SJ. Management of malignant disease metastatic to the bone by hormonal alterations. Clin Orthop 73:73-78; 1970.

106. Melzack R. The McGill pain questionairre: major properties and scoring methods. Pain 1:357-373; 1975.

107. Melzack R, Mount BM, Gordon JM. The Brompton mixture vesus morphine solution given orally: Effects on pain. CMA Jnl 120:435-438; 1979.

108. Merskey H. Classification of chronic pain. Pain (Suppl 3). 1986; p 226.

109. Miles J. Pituitary destruction. In: Wall PD, Melzack R (eds). Textbook of Pain. New York, NY: Churchill Livingstone, 1984; pp 656-665.

109a. Millard RW. Behavioral assessment of pain and behavioral pain management. In: Patt RB (ed). Cancer Pain. Philadelphia, PA: J.B. Lippincott Co; 1993; pp 85-97.

110. Miser AW. Assessment and treatment of children with pain. Anesth Prog 34:116-118; 1987.

110a. Miser AW, Narang PK, Dothage JA, et al. Transdermal fentanyl for pain control in patients with cancer. Pain 37:15; 1989.

111. Moertel CG, Schutt AG, Reitemeir RJ, et al. Corticosteroid therapy of preterminal gastrointestinal cancer. Cancer 33:1607-1609; 1974.

112. Moricca G. Pituitary neuroadenolysis in the treatment of intractable pain from cancer. In: Lipton S (ed): Persistent Pain: Modern Methods of Treatment, vol 1. New York, NY: Academic Press; 1977; pp 149-173.

113. Mount BM. Psychological and social aspects of cancer pain. In: Wall PD, Melzack R (eds). Textbook of Pain. Edinburgh, UK: Churchill Livingstone: 1984; pp 460-471.

114. Mullin V. Brachial plexus block with phenol for painful arm associated with Pancoast's syndrome. Anesthesiology 53:431-433; 1980.

115. Myers, RA, Woolf CJ, Mitchell D. Management of acute traumatic pain by peripheral transcutaneous electrical stimulation. S Afr Med J 52:309-312; 1977.

116. Nahata MC, Miser AW, Miser JS, *et al.* Analgesic plasma concentrations of morphine in children with terminal malignancy receiving a continuous subcutaneous infusion of morphine sulfate to control severe pain. Pain 18:109-114; 1987.

117. Nielzen S, Sjolund BH, Eriksson BE. Psychiatric factors influencing the treatment of pain with peripheral conditioning stimulation. Pain 13:365-371; 1982.

118. Obbens EAMT, Stratton-Hill C, Leavens ME, *et al.* Intraventricular morphine administartion for control of chronic cancer pain. Pain 28:61-68; 1987.

119. Osteolytic metastases, editorial. Lancet 2:1063-1064; 1976.

120. Paalzow LK. Pharmacokinetic aspects of optimal pain treatment. Acta Anaesthesiol Scand Suppl 74:37-43; 1982.

121. Pagni CA. General comments on ablative neurosurgical procedures. In: Bonica JJ, Ventafridda V (eds). Advances in Pain Research and Therapy. New York, NY: Raven Press, 1979; pp 405-423.

122. Papo I, Visca A. Phenol subarachnoid rhizotomy for the treatment of cancer pain: A personal account of 290 cases. In: Bonica JJ, Ventafridda V (eds). Advances in Pain Research and Therapy, vol 2. New York, NY: Raven Press; 1979; pp 339-346.

122a. Patt RB. Classification of cancer pain and cancer pain syndromes. In: Patt RB (ed). Cancer Pain. Philadelphia, PA: J.B. Lippincott Co; 1993; pp 3-22

122b. Patt RB. General principles of pharmacotherapy. In: Patt RB (ed). Cancer Pain. Philadelphia, PA: J.B. Lippincott Co; 1993; pp 101-104.

123. Patt R. Neurosurgical Interventions for Chronic Pain Problems. In: Frost EAM (ed). Anesthesiol Clin North Am 5:609-638; 1987.

124. Patt R. Pain therapy. In: Frost EAM (ed). Clinical Anesthesia in Neurosurgery. 2nd ed. Butterworths; In press.

124a. Patt RB. Peripheral neurolysis. In: Patt RB (ed). Cancer Pain. Philadelphia, PA: J.B. Lippincott Co; 1993; pp 359-376.

125. Patt R, Jain S. Recent advances in the management of oncologic pain. In: Stoelting RK, Barash PG, Gallagher TJ (eds): Advances in Anesthesiology, vol 6. Chicago, IL. Yearbook Medical Publishers, 1989; pp 355-414.

125a. Patt RB. Jain S. Therapeutic decision making for invasive prodecures. In: Patt RB (ed). Cancer Pain. Philadelphia, PA: J.B. Lippincott Co; 1993; pp 275-384.

126. Patt R, Potenza V, White E. Epidural sufentanil as the sole anesthetic for extracorporeal shock wave lithotripsy. Anesth Analg 68:5221; 1989.

127. Payne R. Neuropathic pain syndromes, with special reference to causalgia and reflex sympathetic dystrophy. Clin J Pain 2:59-73; 1986.

128. Payne R, Max M, Inturrisi C, *et al.* (eds). Principles of Analgesic Use in the Treatment of Acute Pain and Chronic Cancer Pain. Washington, D.C., American Pain Society, 1986.

128a. Penn RD, Paice JA, Gottschalk W, et al. Cancer pain relief using chronic morphine infusions: Early experience with a programmable implanted drug pump. J Neurosurg 61:302; 1984.

129. Perese DM. Subarachnoid alcohol block in the management of pain of malignant disease. Arch Surg 76:347-354; 1958.

130. Peyton Wt, Semansky EJ, Baker AB. Subarachnoid injection of alcohol for relief of intractable pain with discussion of cord changes found at autopsy. Am J Cancer 30:709; 1937.

131. Pike PM. Transcutaneous electrical stimulation. Its use in management of postoperative pain. Anaesthesia 33:165-171; 1978.

132. Pilon RN, Baker AR. Chronic pain control by means of an epidural catheter. Cancer 37:903-905; 1976.

133. Pilowsky I. Pain and illness behavior. In: Wall, PD, Melzack R: Textbook of Pain. Edinburgh, UK: Churchill Livingstone; 1984; pp 767- 775.

134. Pilowsky I, Spence ND. Pain, anger and illness behavior. Psychosom Res 20:411-416; 1976.

134a. Plancarte RB, Amescua C, Patt RB, *et al.* Superior hypogastric plexus block for pelvic cancer pain. Anesthesiology 73:236; 1990.

134b. Plancarte RB, Valasquez R, Patt RB. Neurolytic blocks of the sympathetic axis. In: Patt RB (ed). Cancer Pain. Philadelphia, PA: J.B. Lippincott Co; 1993; pp 377-426.

135. Polatty RC, Cooper KR. Respiratory failure after percutaneous cordotomy. South Med J 79:897-899; 1986.

136. Pope K. A service station for nervous disorders. NY Acad Sci Focus 2:1; 1987.

137. Portenoy RK. Continuous intravenous infusion of opioid drugs. Med Clin North America 71:233-241; 1987.

138. Portenoy RK. Constipation in the cancer patient. Med Clin North Am 71:303-311; 1987.

138a. Portenoy RK. Drug therapy for cancer pain. Am J Hospice Care 7:10; 1990.

138b. Portenoy RK. Issues in the management of neuropathic pain. In: Basbaum A, Besson JM (eds). Towards a New Pharmacotherapy of Pain. New York, NY: John Wiley & Sons; 1991, p 393.

139. Portenoy RK, Moulin DE, Rogers A, *et al.* Intravenous infusions of opioids in cancer pain: Clinical review and guidelines for use. Cancer Treat Rep 70:575-581; 1986.

140. Racz GB, Heavner J, Haynsworth R. Repeat epidural phenol injections in chronic pain and spasticity. In: Lipton, S, Miles, J (eds). Persistent Pain, vol 5. Orlando, FL: Grune & Stratton; 1985; pp 157-179.

141. Racz GB, Holubec JT. Stellate ganglion phenol neurolysis. In Racz GB (ed): Techniques of Neurolysis. Boston, Kluwer Academic Publishers, 1989; pp 133-143.

141a. Raj PP. Local anesthetic blocks. In: Patt RB (ed). Cancer Pain. Philadelphia, PA: J.B. Lippincott Co; 1993; pp 329-342.

142. Rawal N, Schott U, Dahlstrom B. Influence of naloxone infusion on analgesia and respiratory depression following epidural morphine. Anesthesiology 64:194-201; 1986.

143. Richardson DE. Long-term follow-up of deep brain stimulation for relief of chronic pain in the human. In: Brock, M (ed). Modern Neurosurgery. New York, NY: Springer-Verlag; 1982; pp 449-453.

144. Richardson, RR, Sigueira EB, Cerullo LJ. Spinal epidural stimulation for treatment of acute and chronic intractable pain: Initial and long-term results. Neurosurgery 5:344; 1979.

145. Richlin DM, Jamron LM, Novick NL. Cancer pain control with a combination of methadone, amitriptyline, and non-narcotic analgesic therapy: A case series analysis. J Pain Symptom Management 2:89-94; 1987.

146. Robertson DH. Transsacral neurolytic nerve block: An alternative approach to intractable perineal pain. Br J Anaesth 55:873-875; 1983.

146a. Rowlingson JC, Hamill RJ, Patt RB: Comprehensive assessment of the patient with cancer pain. In: Patt RB (ed). Cancer Pain. Philadelphia, PA: J.B. Lippincott Co; 1993; pp 23-39.

147. Rutter PC, Murphy F, Dudley HA. Morphine: Controlled trial of different methods of administration for postoperative pain relief. Br Med J 1:12-13; 1980.

148. Saunders C. The Management of Terminal Illness. London, UK: London Hospital Medical Publications; 1967.

149. Schell HW. The risk of adrenal corticosteroid therapy in far advanced cancer. Am J Med Sci 252:641-644; 1966.

150. Schoeffler PF, Haberer JP, Monteillard CM, *et al.* Morphine injections in the cisterna magna for intractable pain in cancer patients. Anesthesiology 67:A246; 1987.

151. Schomburg FL, Carter-Baker SA. Transcutaneous electrical nerve stimulation for postlaparotomy pain. Phys Ther 63:188-193; 1983.

152. Shealy CN, Mortimer JT, Reswick JB. Electrical inhibition of pain by stimulation of the dorsal columns: A preliminary report. Anesth Analg 46:489-491; 1967.

153. Shetter AG, Hadley MH, Wilkinson E. Administration of intraspinal morphine sulfate for the treatment of intractable cancer pain. Neurosurgery 18:740-747; 1986.

153a. Simmonds MA, Payne R, Richenvauvher J, *et al.* TTS (fentanyl) in the management of pain in patients with cancer. Proc Am Soc Clin Oncol (abstract) 8:324; 1989.

153b. Smith JL. Oncologic emergencies. In: Patt RB (ed). Cancer Pain. Philadelphia, PA: J.B. Lippincott Co; 1993; pp 527-542.

154. Smith MC. Histological findings following intrathecal injections of phenol solutions for relief of pain. Br J Anaesth 36:387-406; 1963.

155. Snyder SH. Opiate receptors in the brain. N Engl J Med 296:266-271; 1977.

156. Solomon RA, Viernstein C, Long DM. Reduction of postoperative pain and narcotic use of transcutaneous electrical nerve stimulation. Surgery 87:142-146; 1980.

157. Spiegel D, Bloom JR. Group therapy and hypnosis reduce metastatic breast carcinoma pain. Psychosom Med 45:333-339; 1983.

158. Spiller WG, Martin E. The treatment of persistent pain of organic origin in the lower part of the body by division of the antero-lateral column of the spinal cord. JAMA 58:1489; 1912.

159. Stambaugh JE. Role of nonsteroidal antiinflammatory drugs. In: Patt RB (ed). Cancer Pain. Philadelphia, PA: J.B. Lippincott Co; 1993; pp 105-118.

159a. Stambaugh JE, Drew J. The combination of ibuprofen and ocycodone acetaminophen in the management of chronic cancer pain. Clin Pharmacol Ther 44:665; 1988.

160. Sternbach RA, Timmermans G. Personality changes associated with reduction of pain. Pain 3:177-181; 1975.

161. Stovner J, Endresen R. Intrathecal phenol for cancer pain. Acta Anaesthesiol Scand 16:17-21; 1972.

161a. Strauss MB (ed). Familiar Medical Quotations. Boston, MA: Little, Brown and Co.; 1968; p 356b.

162. Sullivan SP, Cherry DA. Pain from an invasive facial tumor relieved by lumbar epidural morphine. Anesth Analg 66:777-779; 1987.

163. Sweet WH. Treatment of trigeminal neuralgia (tic douloureux). N Engl J Med 315:174-177; 1986.

164. Swerdlow M. Intrathecal neurolysis. Anaesthesia 33:733-740; 1978.

164a. Swerdlow M. Neurolytic blocks of the neuraxis. In: Patt RB (ed). Cancer Pain. Philadelphia, PA: J.B. Lippincott Co; 1993; pp 427-442.

165. Swerdlow M. Subarachnoid and extradural blocks. In: Bonica JJ, Ventafridda V: Advances in Pain Research and Therapy, vol 2. New York, NY: Raven Press; 1979; pp 325-337.

166. Swerdlow M. The use of anticonvulsants in the management of cancer pain. In: Erdmann W, Oyamma T, Pernak MJ (eds): The Pain Clinic. Utrecht, Netherlands, VNU Science Press; 1985.

167. Takeda F. Preliminary report from Japan on results of field testing of WHO draft interim guidelines for relief of cancer pain. Pain Clin 1:83-89; 1986.

168. Tasker RR. Merits of percutaneous cordotomy over the open operation. In: Morley TP (ed): Current Controversies in Neurosurgery. Philadelphia, PA: WB Saunders and Co.; 1976; pp 496-501.

168a. Tasker R. Neurosurgical and neuroaugmentative intervention. In: Patt RB (ed). Cancer Pain. Philadelphia, PA: J.B. Lippincott Co; 1993; pp 471-500.

169. Thompson GE, Moore DC, Bridenbaugh PO, et al. Abdominal pain and celiac plexus nerve block. Anesth Analg 56:1-5; 1977.

170. Travel JG, Simons DG. Myofascial Pain and Dysfunction: The Triger Point Manual. Baltimore, MD: Williams and Wilkins; 1983.

171. Turnbull JM, Shulman R, Woodhurst WB. Thalamic stimulation for neuropathic pain. J Neurosurg 52:486-493; 1980.

171a. Twycross RG. Symptom control in terminal cancer: Lecture notes. Oxford, UK: Sir Michael Sobell House; 1988.

172. Vainio A, Tigerstedt. Opioid treatment for radiating cancer pain: Oral administration vs. epidural techniques. Acta Anaesthesiol Scand 32:179-185; 1988.

173. Vander Ark GD, McGrath KA. Transcutaneous electrical stimulation in treatment of postoperative pain. Am J Surg 130:338-340; 1975.

174. Ventafridda V, De Conno F, Fochi C. Cervical percutaneous cordotomy. In: Bonica JJ, et al. (eds). Advances in Pain Research and Therapy, vol 4. New York, NY: Raven Press; 1983; pp 185-198.

175. Ventafridda V, Spoldi E, Caraceni A, et al. The importance of continuous subcutaneous morphine administration for cancer pain control. In: Erdmann W, Oyama T, Pernak MJ (eds): Pain Clinic, vol 1. Utrecht, Netherland: VNU Science Press; 1986; pp 47-55.

176. Ventafridda V, Sganzerla EP, Fochi C, et al. Transcutaneous nerve stimulation in cancer pain, in Bonica JJ, Ventafridda V (eds): Advances in Pain Research and Therapy, vol 2. New York, NY: Raven Press; 1979; pp 509-515.

177. Ventafridda V, Tamburini M, Caraceni A, et al. A validation study of the WHO method for cancer pain relief. Cancer 59:850-856; 1987.

178. Waldman SD, Feldstein GS, Allen ML, et al. Cervical epidural implantable narcotic delivery systems in the management of upper body pain. Anesth Anala 66:780-782; 1987.

178a. Waldman SD, Leak DW, Kennedy LD, Patt RB. Intraspinal opioid therapy. In: Patt RB (ed). Cancer Pain. Philadelphia, PA: J.B. Lippincott Co; 1993; pp 285-328.

179. Wall PD, Sweet WH. Temporary abolition of pain in man. Science 155:108-109; 1967.

180. Walsh TD. Oral morphine in chronic cancer pain. Pain 18:1-13; 1984.

181. Walsh TD. The role of the oncologist in cancer pain management. In, Burrows GD, Elton D, Stanley GV (eds): Handbook of Chronic Pain Management. Amsterdam: Elsevier; 1986.

182. Watson CPN, Evans RJ, Reed K, et al. Amitriptyline vs. placebo in postherpetic neuralgia. Neurology 32:671-673; 1982.

183. White Ah, Derby R, Wynne G. Epidural injections for diagnosis and treatment of low-back pain. Spine 5:78-86; 1980.

184. White JC, Sweet WH. Pain and the Neurosurgeon. A Forty Year Experience. Springfield, IL: Charles C Thomas; 1969.

185. Wolfe MJ, Davies GK. Analgesic action of extradural fentanyl. Br J Anaesth 52:357-358; 1980.

186. Woolf CJ. Transcutaneous and Implanted nerve Stimulation. In: Wall PD, Melzack R (eds). Textbook of Pain. Edinburgh, UK: Churchill Livingstone; 1984; pp 679-690.

187. Cancer pain relief and palliative care. Report of a WHO Expert Committee. Geneva, World Health Organization, 1990 (Technical Report Series No. 804).

188. Young RF. Surgical role in relief of pain. Semin Anesth 4:323-331; 1985.

189. Young RF, Brechner T. Electrical stimulation of the brain for relief of intractable pain due to cancer. Cancer 57:1266-1272; 1986.

190. Young RF, Kroening R, Fulton W, et al. Electrical stimulation of the brain in the treatment of chronic pain: Experience over 5 years. J Neurosurg 62:389-396; 1985.

Philip Rubin, M.D., Radiation Oncology
Louis S. Constine III, M.D., Radiation Oncology

Diana F. Nelson, M.D., Radiation Oncology
George W. Casarett, Ph.D., Pathologist

Chapter **37**

LATE EFFECTS OF CANCER TREATMENT:
RADIATION AND DRUG TOXICITY

The problems of radiation therapy are in vivo problems which involve dynamic and interacting components of organized tissues, organs and systems of the body . . . A knowledge of the normal cell, its structures and its functions, is essential to an understanding of the complexities of radiation cytopathology and the more gross manifestations of radiation pathology.

George W. Casarett (178)

PERSPECTIVE

Much of the mystery and fear surrounding the use of radiation in cancer therapy evolves from concerns regarding the potential for late injury that can occur after the treatment has been completed. This is particularly true for tissues with slow cell renewal kinetics in which acute or immediate radiation reactions are absent. A substantial body of clinical experience and pathologic data have established the progression in time of tissue injury triggered by a course of irradiation. The temporal sequence of events that occurs on the cellular level ultimately express themselves as tissue and organ structural and functional impairments. Depending on how vital the organ is, severe morbidity or even mortality can occur. A dose effect or dose response of a normal tissue needs to be evaluated in time. The "time course paradigm" (35,36) has been postulated in most normal tissues as a sequence of clinical events based upon a series of histopathologic alterations following irradiation. Such a schema can also be applied to chemotherapy.

A major difference between chemotherapy and radiotherapy is believed to be the absence of late effects after exposure to drugs; the concern for tolerance of chemotherapy regimens is their acute and subacute toxicity (104). However, this difference is illusory, resulting from a paucity of data on the late toxicities of chemotherapy. The increasing documentation of late somatic changes in organs attributable to chemotherapy alone has dispelled the view that there are few late effects associated with the prolonged use of drugs (52). In fact, seemingly safe cyclic doses of chemotherapy can result in severe and life-threatening toxicities in a variety of organs.

The basis for radiation changes is parenchymal cellular hypoplasia of stem cells and alterations in the fine vasculature and fibroconnective tissues. The late effects of chemotherapy are postulated to predominately result from parenchymal cellular depletion of both non-cycling and cycling cells also, but with sparing of the microcirculation and fibroconnective tissue stroma. The evidence for this hypothesis will be pre-sented based upon documented histopathologic changes in clinical situations and in vivo and *in vitro* laboratory modeling. A modification of the radiation time course paradigm (175) will be made to accommodate the late effects of cytotoxic drugs.

GENERAL CONCEPTS OF RADIOSENSITIVITY AND CHEMOSENSITIVITY

Radiosensitivity or Responsiveness Based on Cell Mitotic Behavior and Potential

Cellular radiosensitivity: The sequential changes following irradiation that occur in tissue are based upon the mitotic behavior of the component cells and potential for either staying in cycle or differentiating (175). The original description used to illustrate cellular radiation sensitivity is reinterpreted in current cellular kinetic terminology (4,99). The vegetative and differentiating intermitotic cell described by Cowdry (50) is supplanted by the undifferentiated stem cell (USC) and the committed stem cell (CSC). The maturation of the cell into a fixed post mitotic cell is referred to as the functional mature cell (FMC). The difficult cell to define is the reverting mature cell (RMC), since it may appear to be a non-cycling functional mature cell but, under appropriate stimulus, has the capacity to dedifferentiate and proliferate. The classic example is the conversion of hepatocytes into hepatoblasts when a major portion of the normal liver is resected. The basic tenet of this concept is that cellular radiosensitivity is directly related to mitotic behavior and severity of the radiation changes to the mitotic potential of the cell. The dividing or cycling cell (USC or CSC) is more vulnerable to radiation than the non-dividing cell, particularly if it is a functional mature cell (FMC) or a reverting mature cell (RMC). That is, radiation cell death is expressed as a mitotically-linked death and occurs only when the cell divides — with a few exceptions such as the small lymphocyte.

Cell cycle correlation to radiosensitivity: The radiosensitivity of cells is based on their progression through the cell cycle. Undifferentiated stem cells are mainly a reserve compartment with only a small percent moving from G_0 to G_1. In bone marrow, these comprise less than 1% of all cells in the reserve pool. Committed stem cells are committed to differentiate and form the largest percentage of cycling cells from G_1 to S to G_2 M. Reverting mature cells can slowly proliferate and are in G_0 to G_1 and the length of G_1 increases as a function of increasing cell cycle time. Functional mature cells are in G_0 and have no potential for division (e.g., neurons). Proliferating cells are more radiosensitive than quiescent cells, particularly in early S phase and G_2 M.

Organization of tissues according to cell renewal: The parenchymal cell compartments of the various organs in the body can be considered as either rapid or slow renewal systems. The epithelial tissues lining mucosal surfaces in the upper aerodigestive passages, gastrointestinal (GI) tract, urinary systems, and bone marrow are examples of rapid renewal tissues. These tissues tend to have uncommitted (USC) or committed stem cell (CSC) compartments that rapidly proliferate and differentiate. The functional cell is usually differentiated and is a fixed, mature cell (FMC), essentially incapable of further mitotic activity. Slow renewal tissues are characterized by a parenchymal cell compartment that turns over slowly but often has the capacity, when challenged by injury, to respond by dedifferentiating and proliferating. That is, a mature-appearing parenchymal cell may revert to a stem cell and regenerate or repopulate the lost parenchymal cells. Examples of tissues that are conditionally proliferative include the liver after partial resection, bone on fracturing, the microcirculation in wound healing, the endocrine gland to increased trophic hormone stimulus, and the bone marrow (protected areas) following irradiation of a large segment. Many adult organs have little or no capacity to restore their parenchymal cells in that proliferation primarily occurs early in life and is fixed. Examples of this type of tissue or organ are the central nervous system, heart, kidney, and muscle, where lost cells are replaced by fibrosis.

Chemosensitivity Based on Cell Mitotic Behavior and Potential

Drug action as phase or cycle specific: Cell cycle kinetics has been classically used to describe the response of cells to chemotherapeutic agents (226). Drug action is described either as *phase* or *cycle* specific, referring to cell killing either in S phase or elsewhere in the cycle (166,226). The expression of cell lethality at time of mitosis in rapidly proliferating tissues appears clinically as an acute injury. The cells most vulnerable are those actively cycling or dividing stem cells, in contrast to those cells in G_0 or prolonged G_1, which are protected particularly from S phase-specific drugs such as hydroxyurea or methotrexate (18,40,225). The relationship between cell kill, dosage of the cytotoxic agent, and the proliferation rate is such that rapidly proliferating cells are more sensitive than slowly proliferating cells, and cell killing is an exponential function of drug dose (40). Those cells that are post-mitotic have been previously thought to be insensitive to drugs and their tissues resitant to late effects. It is now known that this may apply to tumor effects, but not necessarily normal tissues. The best illustration is the effect of Adriamycin on cardiac muscle or myocytes (212). The vulnerability of cells to drugs is dependent upon the cell's

capacity to absorb, concentrate, or metabolize these agents or their derivatives and may be both dependent and/or independent of cell mitotic behavior and maturation.

Drug action on stem cell depletion: The dose limiting organ(s) is a function of drug targeting in a specific tissue. The experimental evidence of Botnik *et al.* (25) in a variety of tissues shows that, despite the normal appearance of regenerated cells and tissues after chemotherapy insult, some of their proliferative reserve capacity has been lost. For example, when chemotherapeutically treated bone marrow is further challenged to repopulate by serial transplantation using the Till and McCullough model (220), the loss of stem cells is uncovered. That is, more nucleated cells are required to give rise to a similar number of spleen colonies as in nontreated animals. This phenomenon of stem cell depletion has been found in other tissues, such as skin or hair follicles. The term *stem cell senescence* (183) was introduced to describe the concept of depletion of stem cell reserve or loss of normal mitotic potential of reserve stem cells. Radiation acts in a similar fashion, but the late effects are always associated with vascular changes. An underlying endarteritis of small arterioles, and thickening of capillaries occurs following fractionated schedules of irradiation as practiced in clinical tumor treatment. Both drugs and radiation can lead to accelerated aging due to stem cell senescence (25,102).

Chemoresistance and Radiation Resistance

Mechanisms of drug resistance: The concept of drug radioresistance has been thoroughly explored and is either a primary or acquired resistance, which represents an adaptive change by the tumor cell. The mechanisms that lead to drug resistance are generally considered to be:

- Insufficient drug uptake by cancer cell;
- Insufficient activation of drug;
- Increased inactivation of drug;
- Increased activation of a target enzyme;
- Decreased requirement for specific metabolic product;
- Increased use of an alternative biochemical pathway — "salvage;"
- Rapid repair of a drug-induced lesion;
- Spontaneous mutation to drug resistant cells as expressed in the Goldie and Coleman hypothesis.

Mechanisms of radiation resistance, intrinsic and extrinsic factors: The major determinants of cell survival curves relate to the shoulder (D_q) and slope (D_o) and refer to its "intrinsic radiosensitivity." The wider the shoulder and the shallower the slope, the more radioresistant the cell. To review this subject in detail, the reader should review Chapter 5, "Basic Concepts of Radiobiology." Extrinsic factors, such as oxygenation, pH, and as alluded to, cell cycle, affect radioresistance of cell. Poorly oxygenated or hypoxic cells and cells in late S or early G_1 are more resistant to irradiation. The ability of cells to repair radiation injury is important and both sublethal repair and potentially lethal repair capacities determine cell radioresistance.

Radioresistance as a relative concept: Radioresistance is a relative term in that all tissues, if exposed to excessive high doses beyond tolerance, will ultimately become necrotic, because of parenchymal and/or vascular cell damage. The higher the fractional and total dose and the shorter the time of exposure, the more rapid the onset of tissue necrosis with many cellular compartments destroyed. In this regard, there is always a dose-limiting tissue in the radiation field, and most universally it is the vasculoconnective tissue component. Although direct parenchymal cellular depletion of an organ occurs after irradiation, it is often the fine arterio-capillary circulation that either rapidly occludes and infarcts tissue leading to necrosis or a slower sclerosis which triggers fibrosis. This produces a histochematic barrier blocking transport of vital metabolites and, in turn, contributes to the parenchymal cell depletion and hypoplasia and an eventual late effect. The distribution of many of the late radiation lesions reflects primarily vascular injury and cannot be explained simply as an indirect effect of parenchymal cell loss resulting in underlying vascular injury. Devastating late effects due to this process can occur in both rapidly and slow proliferating normal tissues without a clinically recognizable acute phase.

Clonogenic tumor cell depletion as a model for late effects: Whereas all forms of radiation are additive when delivered to the same tissue volume, this is not true for combinations of agents particularly when chosen to avoid overlapping toxicity in specific organs. If the diagramatic presentation of reduction of the number of tumor cells (147) were applied to normal tissues, theoretical models for late effects due to chemotherapy could be developed. Also, cell killing by drugs is similar to that developed for radiotherapy and is based upon first order kinetics or exponential cell kill.

The assumption is made that active drugs provide a degree of tumor cell log kill. In most multidrug regimens, the number of tumor cells is progressively reduced as the induction, consolidation and maintenance phases of regimens are completed. If the tumor clonogenic cells are reduced to zero, then cure results. If drug resistance appears, then the tumor can recur. The early or late reappearances are often a function of the time at which drug resistance developed. Parallels between the phases of drug treatment and the radiotherapy regimen can be drawn. The radiation boost field and boost dose may be compared to the consolidation phase. In the current practice of radiation treatment, there is no equivalent to prolonged and cyclic maintenance dose schedules as in chemotherapy.

Stem cell depletion as a basis for normal tissue late effects: When this concept of stem cell depletion is applied to normal tissues, a similar set of events can be pictured. For the cancer treatment to be successful, a differential degree tumor and normal tissues cell kill must occur. Either an extremely large number of stem cells must exist in normal tissue or a greater capacity to repair and repopulate vital parenchyma must exist as compared to tumors. As drugs or radiation regimens deplete these stem cells, first reversible or then irreversible injury occurs. A major conceptual difference is that there is no known radio- or chemoresistance in normal tissues as there is with tumors (58).

Role of Microvascular Injury and Late Effects

The role of vascular effects in late radiation injury: The prime importance of radiation induced changes in the fine microcirculation and connective tissues as compared to parenchymal cell hypoplasia is well documented by Rubin and Casarett (178). As previously stated, hypoplasia of rapidly and continually self-repopulating parenchymal tissues or organs are caused largely through direct mechanisms such as cell death at mitosis with resultant parenchymal cell loss and atrophy. In slowly repopulating or nonrepopulating tissues, the production of parenchymal hypoplasia is due both to direct cell

effects and indirect effects on the fine vasculoconnective tissue stroma. In both circumstances, the slowly progressive arteriolar fibrosis and interstitial fibrosis after irradiation contribute to the delayed parenchymal hypoplasia and cause the late effects of radiation. Because of the universal distribution of fine vessels and capillaries in all organs and tissues, the consequences of this damage will vary depending upon the relationship of parenchymal cells to vessels, the reserve of vasculature, degree of circulatory blood flow impairment, collateral circulation, capacity for vascular regeneration and the functional demands placed upon the circulatory apparatus in situations of pathologic and physiologic stress.

The essential lesion occurs in the endothelium of small vessels such as arterioles, capillaries, and venules as compared to larger vessels. The resulting lesion is a consequence of inherent radiosensitivity of the relevant cells, lumenal compromise due to smaller diameter of the vessels for a given tissue, or direct organ damage from parenchymal cell injury. The swelling of endothelial cells leads to a narrowing obstruction which impedes blood flow. This leads to thrombosis and regenerative attempts by the endothelial cells. The early changes are spotty in their distribution along the course of vessels, rather than uniform and continuous (178). Consequently, in any one histologic section, thorough and competent examination of fine vessels may reveal relatively few sites of prominent changes, since focal narrowing of an arteriole supply to a capillary network is often distal to the site of parenchymal necrosis. Hopewell (105,106) stresses the need for serial sections to appreciate these lesions. Alternately, microangiography allows for fuller viewing of the fine circulation of tissues because of the loss of detail in regular microsections which are 5-10 microns (μ). It is understandable why the observer, without proper training, can conclude that the apparent absence of such vascular lesions in a microsection is proof of their insignificance.

The progression of vascular damage and the cicatrization process interstitially leads to more and more points along the couse of the affected small blood vessels that show degenerative and fibrotic change, so that more sections of small blood vessels per unit area of tissues readily reveal the changes.

Numerous investigations have substantiated one consistent change after irradiation of tissues: the appearance of irregularly spaced vascular constrictions, particularly in the walls of arterioles (35,36,105,106,140). The possible development of such constrictions, because of slow depopulation of damaged endothelial cells and reactive hyperplasia to regenerate the loss, can lead to clones of cells at irregularly spaced intervals along the vessel wall, producing a "sausage segment" effect (105). The basis for these observations is provided by the 3H-thymidine labeling studies of endothelial cells (105,106). In all sites studied to date, the labeling index for normal endothelial cells is low — less than 1%. This explains why the manifestation of endothelial injury, which is expressed months later, is associated with a phase of increased labeling or compensatory hyperplasia that is focal in distribution. The only other lesion that could account for these "sausage segments" would be smooth muscle that has an even lower rate of labeling — that is, less than 0.1% (105,106). The endothelial cells in labeling studies are more depressed and tend to show proliferative phases more than smooth muscle.

The evidence for focal constriction includes an autoradiographic correlation with histologic observations showing that these constrictions represent thickening of the arteries due to endothelial hyperplasia, resulting in partial or total occlusion of the vascular lumen. This has been observed in a variety of tissues such as heart, kidney, lung, brain, and dermis. Hopewell (106) in particular, using pig dermis, has confirmed that cells in these occlusive lesions are synthesizing DNA. Three phases of this vascular injury occur in time: early, intermediate, and late. It is the intermediate lesions mediated through depletion of endothelial cells which are associated with reduction in blood flow. Tissue atrophy reestablishes the normal vascular density. The tissue atrophy can be as a result of direct cell hypoplasia or, secondarily, to a hyponutritional state in the tissue because of poor blood circulation. The late changes greater than one year observed in blood vessels are mainly characterizd by arteriole changes that include hyaline, fibrinoid, and collagenous thickening of vessel walls.

Pathologic and clinical illustrations of the type of radiation vascular damage are (178):

- Lignous fibrosis subcutaneously and telangiectasia of the skin.
- Sclerosis of the renal arterioles and glomeruli.
- Ulceration and infarction necrosis or fibrosis of bowel due to obliterative arteritis.
- Ischemic necrosis of the brain.
- Intersitial capillary injury of the myocardium.
- Veno-occlusive thrombosis of central veins of the liver.
- Choroidal vasculitis and hemorrhage (12).
- Pulmonary interstial fibrosis.
- Bone necrosis.
- Bladder ulcers, telangiectasia, and contracted bladder.

Sparing of the microvasculature and late chemotherapy effects: Similar studies with cytotoxic chemotherapeutic agents will be required by investigators who have studied radiation changes in the microcirculation. The absence of vascular effects, which is suggested in some of the systems studied to date, indicates a major difference between these therapeutic modes in their production of late effects. This may also provide new insights to explain previously unexplained, enhanced effects of combining drugs and radiation.

Time-course Paradigm

Clinical pathologic course of events: The expression of injury in time after irradiation allows for identification of an early or acute injury which is often reparable, and a later component, which is irreparable. The mechanisms of action, according to Casarett (35,36) are presented both as a parenchymal cell loss and injury and alteration of the vasculoconnective tissue. The initial recovery on the tissue level is predominately due to parenchymal cellular repopulation. The progressive component is the arteriocapillary fibrosis which predominates in the late irreparable injury and accentuates the cellular depletion of the parenchyma. A clinical pathologic course for most normal tissues and organs has been presented by Rubin and Casarett (178) in a paradigm based on documented histopathophysiologic events in humans and in vivo laboratory animals. The clinical pathologic course of events is illustrated in terms of subclinical and clinical damage with a threshold which can be expressed as a radiation tolerance dose (Fig. 37-1a). A similar clinical pathologic course(s) is postulated following chemotherapy administration (Fig. 37-1b). Precise quantification of pathophysiologic injury is often

difficult to define and needs solution in order to provide the data that can be clinically useful. The search for predictive biochemical, metabolic, or physiologic parameters in terms of early events following irradiation and/or chemotherapy is a major direction of research and hopefully can be used to monitor the more permanent pathologic damage that will occur, or is occurring, on a subclinical level (174). The current inability to detect such changes in a variety of tissues should not lead to the false conclusion that immediate cellular and ultrastructural changes are not occurring.

Dose-limiting organs and tissues in radiation oncology have been segregated into three classes according to their tolerance doses (123). The minimal tolerance dose ($TD_{5/5}$) and the maximal tissue tolerance dose ($TD_{50/5}$) refer to a severe to life-threatening complication of 5 and 50%, occurring within five years of therapeutic radiaiton treatment. The different categories of tissues stress the vital importance of the organ or tissue for survival. In the first category are those organs and tissues which, if injured irreparably, lead to death or severe morbidity; in the second category are those that are associated with moderate morbidity, and in exceptional circumstances, death; in the third category are those with mild transient and reparable consequences with little to no morbidity occurring (181).

Kinetics of cell radiation and chemopathology: The clinical pathologic course of events following radiation exposure can be complicated by the addition of chemotherapy, which can augment these changes. Similarly, chemotherapy followed by irradiation can result in a parallel set of events. Depending upon which mode is employed first (Figs. 37-1a and 37-1b), the evidence suggests that both leave residual injury when large enough doses of either agent are used. This can result in subclinical residuum that may be uncovered by the subsequent use of a seemingly safe dose of the other mode. Thus, classically, when radiation therapy precedes chemotherapy (Fig. 37-1a), the introduction of the second mode can lead to the expression of subclinical damage; when frank injury is already present, increased morbidity or even fatality can result. The same is true of chemotherapy preceding radiation therapy (Fig. 37-1b). In addition to such complications (dashed lines) caused by the addition of the second mode alone, associated infection, trauma or stress can exacerbate the situation. This will be further illustrated under the specific normal tissue sections.

Combined effects of drugs and radiation: Radiation acts both on the microcirculatory sysems and parenchymal cells of tissues and organs; chemotherapy acts predominately on the cellular parenchymal component. In rapid renewal systems, the same stem cell population is affected and the increased acute toxicity of both modes combined can usually be reduced by applying them sequentially. In slow renewal tissues, their additive effects are often due to entirely different target cell populations in same organ system. However, the late effects may not be avoided since chemotherapy, even when applied at delayed times (in prolonged maintenance schedules), can result in additional stem cell kill and lead to expression of subclinical radiation effects. Thus distinct cell compartments due to the heterogeneity of tissue within an organ are being affected by each mode resulting in an additive pathophysiologic effect. There is a need to be aware of these iatrogenic syndromes secondary to cancer treatment so that they are not confused with recurrent or metastatic disease (26,52). These iatrogenic

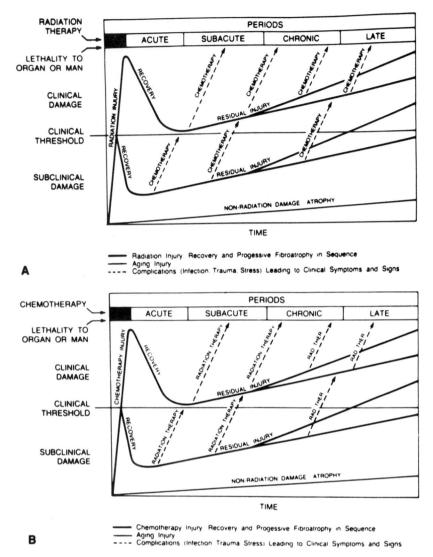

Fig. 37-1. *The clinicopathologic course of events following radiation exposure combined with chemotherapy.* The clinicopathologic course of events following radiation exposure can be complicated by the addition of chemotherapy, which can augment these changes. Similarly, chemotherapy can result in a parallel set of events. Depending on which mode is employed first, evidence suggests that both leave residual injury when large enough doses of either agent are used. This can result in subclinical residuum, which may be uncovered by the addition of subsequent use of a seemingly safe dose of the other mode. (a) Classically, when radiation therapy precedes chemotherapy, the introduction of the second mode can lead to the expression of subclinical damage or when injury is present, can lead to death. (b) The same is true of chemotherapy preceding radiation therapy. In addition to complications (broken lines) caused by the addition of the second mode alone, associated infection, trauma, or stress can lead to overt syndromes of injury. Modified from Rubin and Casarett (178), with permission.

entities can be further aggravated if more cytotoxic treatment is administered due to such confusion. In the pediatric setting, the many proliferating tissues are even more vulnerable than in adults in which when many normal organs are in a mature steady state with slow cell renewal kinetics. The differences and similarities of late effects following radiation therapy and chemotherapy will be illutrated in a number of specific organ systems. These late effect sydromes are occurring at different times and their time course of expression needs to be appreciated so that they can be recognized clinically.

The new hypothesis for explaining the late effects due to chemotherapy and irradiation stems from the different mechanisms of action. There has been a tendency to refer to

clinical drug-radiation reactions as "recall" phenomenon of radiation injury or an enhancement of radiation injuries. The evidence accumulating in the literature is that many chemotherapcutic agents are either effecting different target cell populations as compared to irradiation, or similar cell populations through entirely different pathophysiologic mechanisms. The effect on organ physiology may be additive, but is not a simple stem cell depletion of a similar population by the two different modes (4). Furthermore, the regional administration of radiation results in focal injury to the vasculo-connective tissue stroma, whereas chemotherapeutic administration does not. This differential effect on the microvasculature is an important aspect of the altered pathophysiology of drug-radiation interactions.

ORGAN TOLERANCE: DOSE-LIMITING TISSUES

Organ tolerance is determined by the radiosensitivity of the relevant stem cell subpopulations, which may not always be proliferating or dividing (99). The functional capacity of cells is often distinct from the regenerative capacity and permits organ physiology to be preserved in the face of injury and allows for recovery or repair of the insult. Most organ systems are composed of many cell subpopulations, that is, 20-40 or more, each performing an important activity (178). The most radiosensitive vital cell population determines organ tolerance and organ failure just as the degree of importance of an organ that has been irradiated determines the survival of an organism.

There are many vital organs and tissues in the body but not all of them are dose-limiting. The focus of the next section will be directed to those organs that can result in fatalities when tolerance is exceeded and have been referred to as category I organ systems. These organ systems are heart, lung central nervous system, liver, kidney, GI tract, and bone marrow organ. Each will be assessed in terms of their clinical syndromes, pathopysiology, radiation dose/time/volume factors, chemotherapy factors, and combined modality considerations.

Heart and Cardiac Effects

The functional and structural complexity of the heart is mirrored by the variety of radiation injuries that can occur. A classification system modified from Fajardo and Stewart (77)

includes: (1) acute pericarditis during radiation (rare, and associated with juxtapericardial cancer); (2) delayed pericarditis which can present abruptly or as chronic pericardial effusion; (3) pancarditis which includes pericardial and myocardial fibrosis with or without endocardial fibroelastosis (only after large doses); (4) myopathy in the absence of significant pericaridal disease; (5) coronary after disease (uncommon), usually involving the left anterior descending artery; (6) functional valvular injury; and (7) conduction defects. The histologic hallmark of these injuries is fibrosis in the interstitium, with normal-appearing mycocytes and capillary and arterial narrowing (77).

Several parameters must be considered in the evaluation of these injuries, including (1) relative weighting of the radiation portals and thus the amount of radiation delivered to different depths of the heart; (2) the presence of juxtapericardial tumor; (3) the volume and specific areas of the heart irradiated; (4) the total and fractional irradiation dose; (5) the presence of other risk factors in each individual patient such as age, weight, blood pressure, family history, lipoprotein levels, and habits such as smoking; and (6) the use of specific chemotherapeutic agents.

Clinical Syndromes (Fig. 37-2)

Pericarditis: Delayed acute pericarditis can be symptomatically occult or present suddenly with fever, dyspnea, pleuritic chest pain, friction rub, ST and T wave chanbges and decreased QRS voltage (7,213). Up to 30% of patients treated for Hodgkin's disease with a mean midplane heart dose of 46

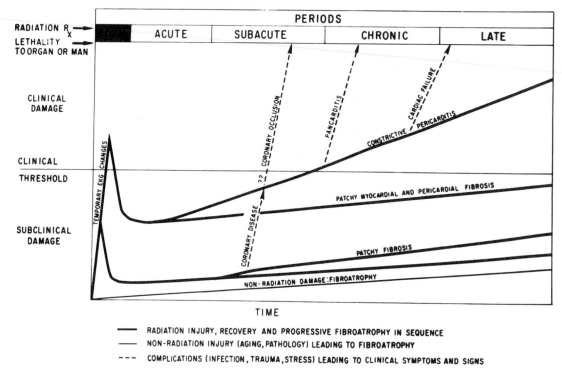

Fig. 37-2. *Clinicopatholgic course: The heart.* The heart is usually considered a moderately radioresistant structure. Temporary electrocardiographic changes, usually a reversal of T waves, are the only manifestation seen during the acute period despite large fractionated doses. These changes are of little clinical significance. Although occlusion of the fine vessels occurs months after irradiation, the caliber of the coronary arteries is sufficiently large that myocardial infarction from coronary occlusion is rarely attributable to radiotherapy per se. Pericardial reactions such as chronic pericarditis or effusions have been documented, usually in cases of mediastinal node disease or after excessive irradiation. From Rubin and Casarett (178), with permission.

Gy will be affected. With equally weighted anterior and posterior fields and the use of subcarinal blocking, the frequency decreases to 2.5% (34). A report by Stewart on 25 patients who developed cardiac damage, primarily pericarditis, shows the relevance of radiation dose and cardiac volume to the type of injury (210). The onset of delayed acute pericarditis averages 6 months and 92% of effusion occur within 12 months. Although the effusion usually resolves in 1-10 months, it may persist for years. Up to 50% of patiets will develop some degree of tamponade (paradoxical pulse, Kussmaul's sign) occasionally requiring percardiocentesis. Chronic effusive-constrictive pericardiitis develops in 10-15% of patients and may require pericardectomy. Alternately, constriction may present 5-50 years following irradiation with no antecedent acute disease (7,33,213). Diuretics are sometimes necessary to control peripheral edema or ascites.

Pancarditis: This development is both rare and severe and probably requires doses of at least 60 Gy (213). Intractable congestive heart failure can result. Restrictive hemodynamics are demonstrated by catheterization.

Myocardiopathy: This injury is highly potentiated by Adriamycin (Table 37-1), but occurs in its absence. An autopsy study of patients who were treated with at least 35 Gy, many with anterior-only portals (mean dose of 56 Gy to anteror heart surface) showed myocardial fibrosis in 50%, fibrous thickening of the mural endocardium in 75%, and pericardial thickening in over 90% (29). Right ventricular endioastolic function may also be reduced by up to 25% in asymptomatic patients (32). Ejection fractions may be decreased in up to 33%.

Valvular disease: Fibrous valvular endocardial thickening occurs in 80% of autopsied patients treated with high radiation doses. The mitral, aortic, and tricuspid valves were most frequently affected (29).

Arrhythmia: High degree atrio-ventricular conduction abnormalities are rarely seen and have been attributed to fibrosis of the AV node conducting branches (45).

Coronary artery disease (CAD): The incidence and extent of this sequelae is unclear. Both autopsy and patient series have documented the occurence of CAD after doses as low as 24 Gy and after higher doses (29,63,129). At autopsy patients treated with anterior weighted radiation techniques had narrowing of up to 75%, most frequently involving the proximal portion of the arteries. The media and adventitia were thickened or replaced by fibrosis tissue, either diffusely

Table 37-1. Agents Causing Cardiac Toxicity

Agents	Toxicity
Adriamycin, daunorubicin	Cardiomyopathy
5-florouracil	Myocardial infarction + ischemia
Actinomycin D	Acute hemorragic necrosis
Mithromycin	Cardiomyopathy
Cyclophosphamide (H.D.)	Diffuse myocardial necrosis + CHF
Mitomycin C	Cardiomyopathy
Imidazole carboxamide	Cardiomyopathy
VP-16-213 (+RAD)	Myocardial ischemia
MOPP (±RAD)	Myocardial ischemia + infarction
BCNU	Cardiomyopathy

Reprinted from Rubin, P. The Franz Buschke lecture. Late effects of chemotherapy and radiation therapy: a new hypothesis. Intl. J. Radiat. Oncol. Biol. Phys. 10:5-34; 1984; with permission from Pergamon Press Ltd, Headington Hill Hall, Oxford OX3 0BW, UK.

or focally. Bizarre fibroblasts, hyalination, intimal thickening with collagen, endothelial cells, and histiocytes are seen (29). A recent study of patients irradiated for Hodgkin's disease did show a statistically significant increase in myocardial infarction beyond that in a control population (20). However, the increased relative risk is small. The use of modern radiotherapy techniques and appropriate cardiac shielding may afford a decrease in any adverse cardiac sequelae.

Pathophysiology

The *severe cardiomyopathies* encountered as a late effect of cancer treatment demonstrates the additive effects of both radiation and drugs through the action on two different populations of cells.

Radiation alters the fine vasculoconnective stroma of the myocardium (75,76,77,97,130). The histopathologic and ultrastructural changes of Adriamycin alone, radiation alone, and both radiation and Adriamycin dramatically show these independent and additive organ effects (see Figs. 37-3a, b, and c) (66,67,68,73).

Radiation changes in the heart are typical in man and are experimentally reproducible and similar in rabbits and some primates (14,75,76,212). The hallmark is a pericardial effusion clinically and fibrosis pathologically involving a thickened collagenous pericardium and an extensive fibrinous exuate. When the myocardium is involved, there is a diffuse interstitial fibrosis that follows the pattern of septae in the myocardium. With therapeutic doses of radiation, direct damage to myocytes in humans and animals does not occur (212).

The coronary arteries are large enough not to be the main focus of radiation lesions, and coronary thrombosis is a relatively infrequent occurrence; that is, less than 5% of all patients treated. It does not differ from spontaneous arteriosclerosis in unirradiated patients (126,211), and therefore, is difficult to establish without a matched cohort of patients managed by other means.

In a variety of radiation schedules, serial sacrifice of rabbits yielded a predictable and identifiable sequence of lesions in the myocardial microvasculature (75). Severe alterations in myocardial capillaries, including irregularities of the endothelial cell membranes, cytoplasmic swelling, thrombosis and rupture of the walls, have all been reported (76). Quantitative studies showed the ratio of capillaries to myocytes was reduced by approximately 50% over unirradiated controls at 120-540 days. By pulse labeling with tritiated thymidine, a peak incorporation entirely within capillary endothelial cells was noted. Fajardo and Stewart's hypothesis is that radiation insult results in latent damage to the capillary endothelial cells. A compensatory burst of endothelial cell proliferation occurs and the cells die at the time of mitosis. The resulting reduction in capillaries leads to ischemia, and in turn, myocardial fibrosis (76).

Lung and Pulmonary Effects

Clinical Syndromes (Fig. 37-4)

The lung is one of the most sensitive organs to cancer treatment. Radiation has long been known to produce dramatic effects in lung, both relatively acute and early, as well as late (148,153,187,221,222). The sequence of morphologic changes have been well documented and intensively studied at the microscopic and ultrastructural level (158,159). Radiation pneumonitis and radiation fibrosis are the two major

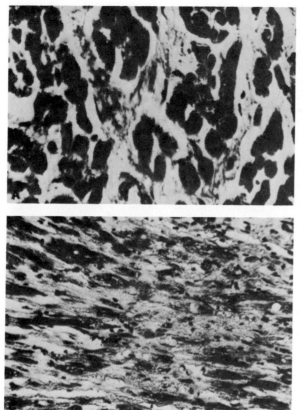

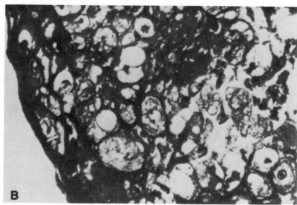

Fig. 37-3. (A) Radiation therapy effects. The myocardium or cardiac myocytes are normal in appearance, with increased fibrosis in the interstitium with capillary and arterial narrowing. (B) Chemotherapy effects. The effect of doxorubicin (Adriamycin) is dramatic, with vacuolization selectively localized to the cardiac myocytes. The interstitium is normal in appearance, showing vascular sparing, despite dramatic cellular changes. (C) Combined radiation and chemotherapy effects illustrates damage to both the vascular connective tissue stroma and the cardiac myocyte. From Eltringham *et al.* (67), with permission.

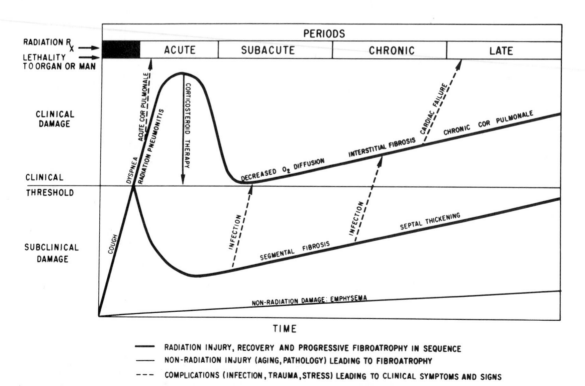

Fig. 37-4. *Clinicopatholgic course: the lung.* Pulmonary radiation reaction is usually manifested clinically after a course of irradiation is completed. With low doses, as portrayed by lower heavy line, pathologic changes are subtle and consist of some segmental fibrosis or septal thickening. Large doses given to more than half of the total lung volume can lead to dyspnea and in severe cases to acute cor pulmonale. Corticosteroid therapy can reverse this acute phase, but interstitial fibrosis continues, leading to altered pulmonary physiology. In the chronic period, chronic cor pulmonale and cardiac failure can eventuate. From Rubin and Casarett (178), with permission.

manifestations of radiation injury. The pneumonitis phase occurs 1-3 months later and the fibrotic phase 2-4 months after a course of irradiation is completed.

There are two distinct, delayed lung injuries following irradiation in contrast to chemotherapy. Acute pneumonitis, seen after irradiation exposure of both lungs, occurs with single doses exceeding 7.5 Gy with a steep dose response up to 10 Gy, resulting in high lethality (182). This radiation lesion is attributuable to ablation of type II alveolar cells and results in early surfactant release into the alveoli. In contradistinction, bleomycin effects type I cells with secondary alterations in type II alveolar cells (Table 37-2). A different but distinct early release of surfactant occurs with bleomycin toxicity and when combined with radiation, leads to a shift of the radiation dose response curve to the left (230). The true late effects of pulmonary fibrosis can be seen both with and without an acute phase. The role of vascular injury is an important aspect of interstitial fibrosis and occurs following irradiation. Septal changes are also seen after drug injury, but these may be secondary in nature, following the alveolitis they produce.

Table 37-2. Antitumor agents with Pulmonary Toxicity

Agent	Toxicity
Bleomycin (±RRad) (±O2)	Acute/late pneumonitis/fibrosis
BCNU	Late pulmonary fibrosis
Procarbazine	Hypersensitivity
Actinomycin D (+RAD)	Acute/late pneumonitis
Cyclophosphamide	Penumonopathy
Busulfan	Penumonopathy
Prednisone (+RAD)	Acute/late pneumonopathy
Chlorambucil	Acute/late pneumonopathy
Mitomycin C	Acute/late pneumonopathy
VM 26	Acute/late pneumonopathy

Reprinted from Rubin, P. The Franz Buschke lecture. Late effects of chemotherapy and radiation therapy: a new hypothesis. Intl. J. Radiat. Oncol. Biol. Phys. 10:5-34; 1984; with permission from Pergamon Press Ltd, Headington Hill Hall, Oxford OX3 0BW, UK.

Pathophysiology

The first event, and rather startling discovery made, after *lung irradiation*, was the immediate injury to the alveolar type II cell as detected by electron microscopy and the early release of surfactant (187) (see Fig. 37-5). These two events are readily detected within minutes to hours and have no

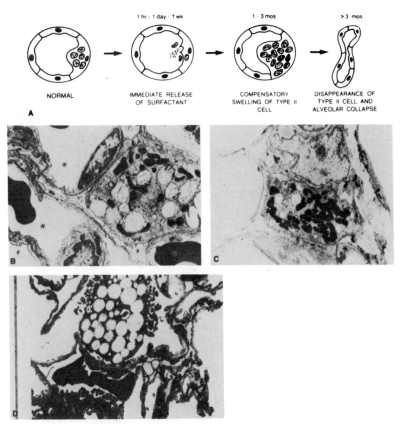

SURFACTANT & TYPE II PNEUMOCYTE

RADIATION PNEUMONITIS AS AN ALVEOLITIS SEQUENCE OF CHANGES IN ALVEOLAR TYPE II CELLS

Fig. 37-5. *Radiation pneumonitis (A) is an alveolaritis with dramatic sequential changes in the alveolar Type II cells following irradiation shown diagrammatically. Detailed in the diagram, from left to right, and elucidated by photographs are: the normal cell (B), showing the large surfactant-containing globules in the cytoplasm of the Type II cell, distinguishing it from the flattened Type I cell. The dramatic release of the surfactant globules immediately after radiation from one hour to weeks later is shown in (C) an in (D), the compensatory accumulation of surfactant globules in the cytoplasm of the Type II cell is demonstrated, occurring months later. The last step is postulated in the line diagram (A) and remains to be substantiated in studies: The Type II cell attempts to divide and dies. Acute pneumonitis results from the loss of sufficient numbers of alveolar Type II cells which maintain alveolar potency.*

evident manifestations, clinically or radiographically (83). If a biopsy were done, no histopathologic changes would be seen at the microscopic level, but ultrastructural changes demonstrate that a dramatic sequence of changes are occurring. The latent period is often 1-3 months before detectable pathologic or clinical syndromes occur as a result of alveolar type II cell injury and eventual loss (83). The next phase is a proliferative one for type II pneumonocytes, occurring between 1-3 months and there is compensatory hypertrophy of lamellar bodies (Fig. 37-5) (183). The late fibrotic phase begins at 3-6 months and is recognized by sclerosis of the alveolar wall and extensive endothelial damage with loss and replacement of some capillaries, and eventual replacement of alveolar spaces, by fibrosis with loss of function (183). With single doses of 10-20 Gy, a greater proportion of endothelial injury was noted (158) and less alveolar cell damage, but this was based on conventional H and E sections and light microscopy (158). Radiation produces a blistering of the capillary endothelial cells and plays an independent role in leading to both early and late pulmonary effects.

Sequential ultrastructural studies (163) have identified endothelial cell changes in alveolar capillaries within five days of irradiation, leading to platelet thrombi and lumenal obstruction. Recanalization occurs months later and is reflected in decreased pulmonary blood flow, arterial hypoxia, particularly after exercise and altered CO diffusion. The relationship between alveolar type II cell injury and capillary damage needs to be better elucidated. Travis (221) has studied the histologic changes in CBA mice, describing three consecutive phases (acute, intermediate and late), and has related both the acute and the fibrotic histologic changes to a progressive increase in breathing frequency. Although detailed analysis of the morphology of radiation injury is recorded, the cause and effect and temporal manifestations are not completely understood.

There are numerous pulmonary function parameters which include: pulmonary ventilation tests, nuclear medicine techniques for aeration and blood flow, diffusion capacities and alveolar lavage for surfactant release and collagenase, as well as biopsy analyses for hydroxyproline content and cellular alterations. Radiographic studies include CT using density and pixel numbers, and NMR promises to distinguish normal from abnormal irradiated tissues in the intact organ. Serial studies are possible and predictive parameters for sequencing modes and determining pulmonary tolerance may be feasible in the future using surfactant release (187).

The potential use of alveolar surfactant lavage to detect later pneumonitis is shown in our experimental work on mice (187). The steep dose response curve for surfactant release is identical to that for lethality of the mice at 200 days.

Renal Effects

Clinical Syndromes (Fig. 37-6)

Rubin and Casarett combined autopsy and clinical data to define different periods in the progression of renal dysfunction following irradiation (178). the acute period (up to 6 months) is rarely symptomatic and a decreased glomerular

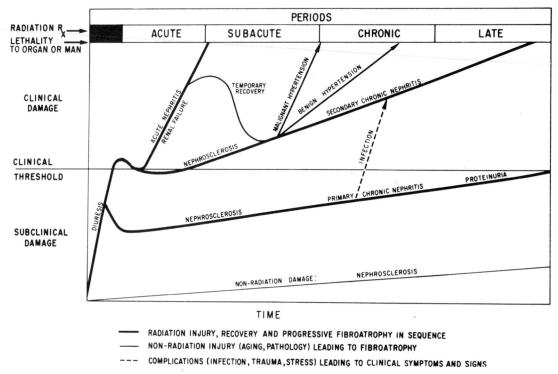

Fig. 37-6. *Clinicopathologic course in the kidney.* The immediate acute period following fractionated therapeutic irradiation is silent clinically. The pathologic changes are subtle and spotty initially and are seen mainly in the vascular bed. The essential lesion is an arteriolar nephrosclerotic process which is progressive. Its rate of progression is usually determined by volume, dose and time factors. The manifestations of clinical radiation nephritis may appear as a variety of syndromes which, depending on the rate and degree of the arteriolar nephrosclerotic process, lead to the insidious clinical onset of one or any combination of the following: acute renal failure, malignant hypertension, primary or secondary chronic nephritis, benign hypertension, proteinuria or anemia. Recovery from the acute renal failure does not alter the underlying pathologic picture, and the prognosis remains poor. From Rubin and Casarett (178), with permission.

filtration rate may be present. In the subacute period (6-12 months) the signs and symptoms include dyspnea on exertion, headaches, ankle edema, lassitude, anemia, hypertension, albuminuria, papilledema, elevated blood urea, and urinary abnormalities (granular and hyalin casts, red blood cells). Death might occur from chronic uremia or left ventricular failure, pulmonary edema, pleural effusion, and hepatic congestion. In the chronic period (generally after 18 months) either benign or malignant hypertension is seen, depending on the severity of the renal insult. Chronic radiation nephropathy in its mildest forms may not be diagnosed until 10 to 14 years following therapy. Abnormalities may include only proteinuria and azotemia with urinary casts and mild or no hypertension. A contracted renal size (mild atrophy) is seen on IVP. When chronic nephropathy is severe, death may result.

The immediate acute period following fractionated therapeutic irradiation is silent clinically. The initial pathologic changes are subtle and spotty and are seen mainly in the vascular bed. The essential lesion is an arteriolar nephrosclerotic process which is progressive. Its rate of progression is usually determined by volume, dose and time factors. The manifestations of clinical radiation nephritis may appear the a variety of syndromes previously denoted, depending on the rate and degree of the arteriolar nephrosclerotic process. Recovery from the acute renal failure does not alter the underlying pathologic picture, and the prognosis remains poor.

Pathophysiology

The *initial injury* is clinically silent and the major focus of change is in the arteriolar-glomerular area rather than tubular epithelium (Fig. 37-7). The cortical tubules rather than the medullary tubules are involved, and usually follow rather than precede the vascular alterations. Microangiography dramatically indicates glomerulosclerosis as a function of increasing dose, so that complete obliteration of glomeruli occur at single doses above 5-20 Gy (140).

In the sequential morphologic study of Glatstein *et al.* (92), radiation-induced lesions in the kidney were detected by light microscopy and occurred as a progressive replacement of capillary walls and lumena leading to glomerular sclerosis which preceded tubular atrophy. Larger arteries were not affected while glomeureli were being lost. These observations were corroborated by 86 Rb extraction techniques (91), which estimate total capillary blood flow within the kidneys which was reduced significantly but was still reversible 2-3 months after irradiation. Prior to any histologic identification of tubular depletion (4 months or later), the evidence suggests that a functional lesion is occurring in glomenular capillaries and precedes tubular depletion (165). This observation may, however, be related to other factors in the experimental design of the relevant studies such as use of nephrectomized animals where renal hypertrophy may be occurring.

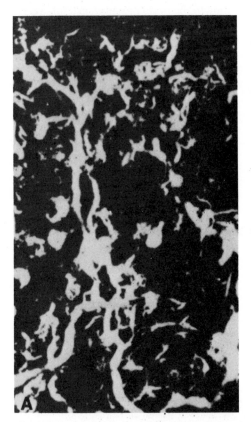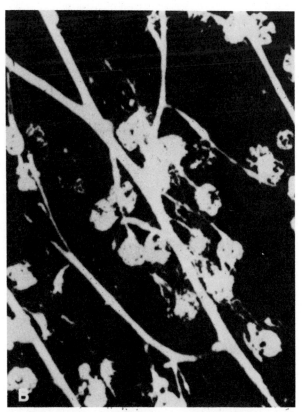

Fig. 37-7. *Radiation nephropathy.* The underlying pathology in the various radiation syndromes is a result of the severity of the microvascular lesions, which is related to both the total dose and the volume of kidney exposed. In (A), a microangiographic view of the normal renal cortex indicating normal afferent and efferent arterioles with full rounded glomerular tufts is demonstrated. Following an exposure dose of 2000 cGy (B), a dramatic change is seen in the afferent and efferent arterioles, with scattered areas of segmental narrowing that are spotty in nature and an entire disruption of the glomerular apparatus with a variety of defects and fragmentation indicating damage to their fine vasculature. From Maier and Casarett (140), with permission.

Liver: Hepatic Effects

Clinical Syndromes

Since the hepatic cells are relatively resistant to the direct cytocidal actions of radiation and since relatively large doses are required to cause marked acute inflammation in the liver, the acute clinical period tends to be relatively silent clinically. However, the progressive damage in the fine vasculature of the liver may eventually lead to clinically significant secondary degeneration of liver during the later part of the acute clinical period or even later, depending upon the dose and the rate of progression of vascular damage (Fig. 37-8) (Table 37-3).

The relative sensitivity of the liver to irradiation injury precludes the eradication of infiltrating tumours from this organ by high doses to its entirety. Following such doses a series of pathological changes occur including hyperemia, an increase in volume, dilatation and congestion of sinusoids, atrophy of hepatocytes, and veno-occlusive lesions appearing as early as 2.5-6 months (178). The patient develops ascites, and there is an increase in hepatic size and a rise in bilirubin and alkaline phosphatase levels.

Pathophysiology

The basic lesion of radiation hepatopathy consists of central vein thrombosis at the lobular level and results in retrograde congestion leading to hemorrhage and secondary alterations in surrounding hepatocytes (109,131) (Fig. 37-9). Severe acute changes often progress to progressive fibrosis or cirrhosis and liver failure (111). This unique venoocclusive lesion is unlike the usual radiation-induced fine arteriolar-capillary damage seen in most other tissue (174) and may represent an endothelial platelet agglutination phenomenon (199).

Central Nervous System Effects

Clinical Syndromes (Fig. 37-10)

The initial response of the central nervous system to iradiation may be increased intracranial pressure due to radiation edema but this is a complex event to analyze. This is usually incidental to radiotherapy of brain tumors, in which unfavorable circumstances for cerebral edema may exist before radiation treatment is undertaken. Toward the end of the acute period, transitory myelitis may develop with electrical parethesia associated with neck flexion. It is not until the subacute period that the severe manifestations of infarction and gliosis show themselves as brain necrosis or the Brown-Sequard syndrome with transection of the cord. In children in the chronic clinical period poor cerebration and mental retardation may follow total-brain irradiation, as for medulloblastoma. However, pre-existing hydrocephalus due to posterior fossa tumors cause cerebral atrophy and poor mentation independant of and augmenting the radiation effect. Repeated courses of irradiation tend to exceed tolerance, further obliterate the vasculature and increase the risk of brain necrosis. The addition of chemotherapy can enhance the effects of irradiation (Table 37-4).

Radiation necrosis (RN) occurs in 0.1-1.0% of cases after 50-60 fractionated over 6 weeks. Above this rather narrow dose range the likelihood of RN substantially increases. In one of the few prospective studies, Marks reported a 5% incidence in patients treated with 45 Gy or more in 1.8-2.0 Gy fractions (141). Although the onset of symptoms can be as early as 6 months after treatment, the peak time of presentation is 1-2 years. Seventy-five percent of cases are apparent by 3 years. Headache and other expressions of increased intracranial pressure are frequently present in addition to focal deficits.

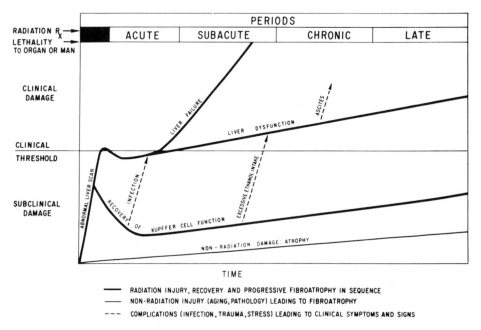

Fig. 37-8. *Clinicopathologic course: the liver.* Since the hepatic cells are relatively resistant to the direct cytocidal actions of radiation and since relatively large doses are required to cause marked acute inflammatin in the liver, the acute clinical period tends to be relatively silent clinically. However, the progressive damage in the fine vasculature of the liver may eventually lead to clinically significant secondary degeneration of liver during the latter part of the acute clinical period or later, depending upon the dose and the rate of progression of vascular damage. From Rubin and Casarett (178), with permission.

Table 37-3. Chemotherapeutic Agents Producing Hepatic Toxicity

Drug	Effect
Nitrosoureas	
BCNU	Elevated liver enzymes
CCNU	Elevated liver enzymes
Streptozotocin	Elevated liver enzymes
Antimetabolites	
Methotrexate	Fibrosis, cirrhosis
6 mercaptopurine	Cholestasis,k necrosis
Azathioprine	Cholestasis, necrosis
Cytosine arabinoside	Elevated liver enzymes
Antibiotics	
Mithramycin	Acute necrosis
Enzymes	
L-asparaginase	Fatty metamorphosis

From Perry et al. (161), with permission.

Radiation necrosis is visualized on CT as a mass lesion with surrounding edema (192). Angiography may show areas of avascularity, as compared to neovascularity in a recurrent tumor. Magnetic resonance has recently been shown to identify a spectrum of radiation changes with great sensitivity (48). Differentiation of RN from recurrent tumor generally requires pathologic documentation, although metabolic PET scans may be helpful. Radiation necrosis is often progressive and fatal. Surgical debulking is performed when possible (240a). Corticosteroids may offer transient relief.

Reducing the volume of irradiation is presumed to decrease the risk for RN. Although Kun's data support such a relationship in children, other reports do not (54,127).

Necrotizing leukoencephalopathy and mineralizing microangiopathy (Fig. 37-11): Leukoencephalopathy is characterized by multiple noninflammatory necrotic foci in the white matter with demyelinization and reactive astrocytosis. The demyelinization of the white matter contributes to cerebral atrophy and ventricular enlargement. Mineralizing microangiopathy may accompany the process. The clinical

Table 37-4. CNS: Late Effects and Chomotoxic Agents

Acute encephalopathies	Mineralizing microanigiopathy
IT MTX — XRT	XRT ± IT MTX
XRT ± IT MTX	
HDMTX ("strokelike")	Cerebral atrophy
Asaraginases (early and late)	IT MTX ± XRT
HMM/PMM	IT ARA-C ± XRT
Ftorafur (IV)	
Procarbazine	Pontine myelinolysis
BCNU (intracarotid)	XRT ± IT MTX
cis-DDP (intracarotid)	
Cyclophosphamide (?)	Neuropathies
5-azacytidine	Vincas (VCR, VDS, VBL) also
PALA	cranial cic-DDP (also cranial
Spirogermanium	and VIII)
Misonidazole	HMM/PMM
High-dose ARA-C	Procarbazine
	5-azacytidine
Chronic encephalopathies	VP-16-213; VM-26
	Misonidazole (also VIII)
Necrotizing leukoencephalopathy	Methyl-G
XRT → IT MTX	
IT or IV MTX	
IT ARA-C	

From Evans et al. (70), with permission.

features include lethargy, seizures, spasticity, paresis, and ataxia. Almost all patients who have developed this complication have received greater than 20 Gy whole brain irradiation, usually as prophylaxis for CNS leukemia in which methotrerate is also administered. Following doses of greater than 35 Gy or IT Mtx of 150 mg for established CNS leukemia or lymphoma, as many as 50% of patients are affected (175). Mineralizing microangiopathy has rarely been reported following radiation doses below 20 Gy (168).

Neuropsychologic and intellectual deficits: The incidence and extent of cognitive and emotional dysfunction among patients treated with irradiation are difficult to define. Variables include the underlying disease (brain tumor or

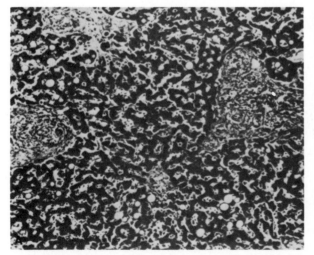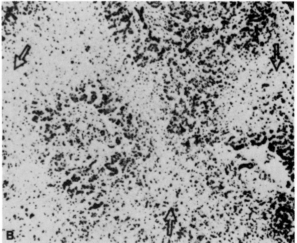

Fig. 37-9. *Radiation hepatopathy.* There is a difference in distribution in radiation-induced and chemotherapy-induced lesions. Chronic radiation hepatitis (a), showing isolated scattered islands of fibrosis surrounding the central lobular veins and secondary atrophy of surrounding hepatocytes. The rest of the lobule appears normal. Chemotherapy(methotrexate) (b), showing a diffuse necrosis of hepatocytes and fatty replacement with a few zones of hepatic cell viability surrounding the central protal veins. The arrows point to a peripheral location of the severe hepatocyte necrosis. From Minow *et al.* (145), with permission.

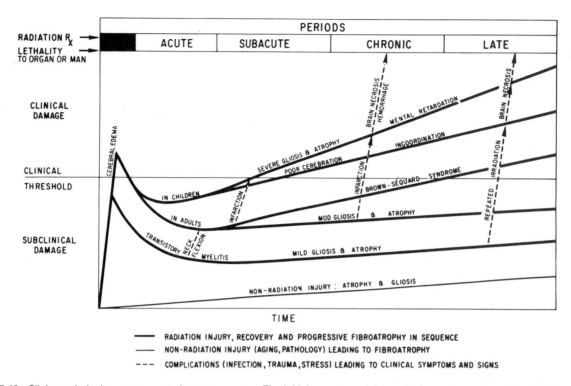

Fig. 37-10. *Clinicopathologic course: central nervous system.* The initial response of the central nervous system to irradiation may be increased intracranial pressure as a result of radiation edema, but this is a complex event to analyze. It is usually incidental to irradiation of brain tumors, in which unfavorable circumstances for cerebral edema may exist before radiation treatment is undertaken. Toward the end of the acute period, transitory myelitis may develop with electrical paresthesia associated with neck flexion. It is not until the subacute period that the severe manifestations of infarction and gliosis show themselves as brain necrosis or the Brown-Sequard syndrome with transection of the cord. In children in the chronic clinical period poor cerebration and mental retardation may follow total-brain irradiation, as for medulloblastoma. However, preexisting hydrocephalus because of posterior fossa tumors cause cerebral atrophy and poor mentation independent of and augmenting the radiation effect. Repeated courses of irradiation tend to exceed tolerance, further obliterate the vasculature and increase the risk of brain necrosis. From Rubin and Casarett (178), with permission.

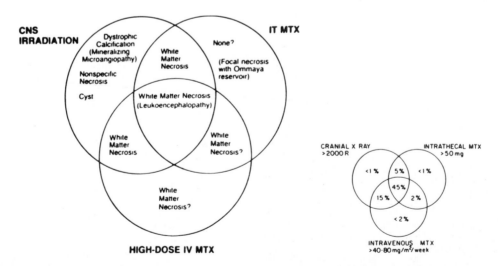

Fig. 37-11. *Encephalopathies.* Encephalopathies are induced by both radiation and chemotherapy and can be both acute and chronic. The first Venn diagram (a) illustrates the pathophysiology of delayed neurotoxic sequelae months to years later, associated with CNS irradiation, intrathecal methotrexate, and high-dose intravenous methotrexate, alone or in combination. The second Venn diagram (b) shows the incidence is greatest for all modes combined. In this diagram, the incidence is shown to be very low with either radiation or chemotherapy alone, but rises considerably (to 45% of patients) when all these modes are combined. The mechanism for this is believed to be attributable to the alteration of the blood-brain barrier by irradiation followed by entry of methotrexate into the central nervous system, causing this diffuse necrosis and damage. From Evans *et al.* (70), with permission.

leukemia) and associated pathology (such as hydrocephalus or increased intracranial pressure), and other therapies (surgery and chemotherapy). Several studies of children treated for brain tumors demonstrate an adverse neurocognitive effect of therapy. The extent of the contribution of irradiation to these dysfunctions is unclear. LeBaron (128) documented effects in children treated without irradiation which were almost as severe as those treated with irradiation. Those patients who required irradiation might have more risk factors for adverse neurocognitive effects (such as a tumor with a worse prognosis and a higher risk of CNS relapse).

Myelopathy: The spectrum of radiation injuries to the spinal cord inludes both transient and irreverisible syndromes (94). A rapidly evolving permanent paralysis can rarely be seen. This is presumed to result from an acute infarction of the cord. The most common syndrome is a transient myelopathy seen at 2-4 months following irradition. A shocklike sensation along the spine and tingling or pain in the hands is brought on by neck flexion or stretching of the arms. This L'Hermitt's sign has most commonly been described after 40-45 Gy mantle irradiation for Hodgkin's disease (114). The mechanism is presumably a transient demyelinization.

Chronic progressive radiation myelitis (CPRM) is rare. Intramedullary vascular damage that progresses to hemorrhagic necrosis or infarction is the likely mechanism, although extensive demyelinization that progresses to white matter necrosis is an alternative explanation. The initial symptoms are usually paresthesias and sensory changes that start 9-15 months following therapy and progress over the subsequent year (198). Much longer intervals to initial symptomatology have occasionally been seen. Since a definitive diagnosis of myelitis requires pathology, which cannot be obtained except at autopsy, the diagnosis rests on supportive information. The neurologic lesion must be within the irradiated volume. Recurrent or metastatic tumor must be ruled out. CSF protein may be elevated, and myelography can demonstrate cord swelling or atrophy. Magnetic resonance and CT imaging provide additional supportive information.

The frequency of CPRM and radiation dose causing this event are poorly defined. This is due to the diagnostic difficulties and the variety of radiation techniques (with uncertian dosimetries). Wara's review suggests that 42 Gy in 25 fractions carries a 1% risk, 45 Gy a 5% risk, and 61 Gy a 50% risk (237). Cohen's data indicate the 5% risk to be at 49 Gy (44).

An increased risk of myelopathy is associated with higher individual fraction sizes, shorter overall treatment time, higher total doses, and long lengths of the cord treated (especially > 10 cm) (94). Children may be more sensitive to CPRM, developing it after lower radiation doses and with shorter latency periods (198). Actinomycin D may decrease the dose threshold (133).

Pathophysiology (Fig. 37-12)

In the *central nervous system*, the neurons and neuro-ganglions are considered in their mature state to be some of the most resistant cells in the human. These cells are fixed post-mitotic cells and are not able to divide (174). The vulnerable portions of the system are proliferating cells such as the oligodendrogliocytes which produce myelin, and the fine vasculature which, in essence, composes the interstitium along with astrocytes in the brain. Most radiation injuries reflect events occurring, not in functioning mature nerve cells, but the vasculoconnective tissue stroma. The radiopathologic literature is the classic "chicken and egg" argument, since the biassociation of cerebral and spinal cord necrosis and vessel thickening is evident (174). Most of the recent literature (19,38) on the cerebral atrophy following neutron therapy suggested a new mechanism of action for high LET irradiation directly on neurons due to high lipid content of the brain and increased energy absorption. However, careful studies of late effects in the brain by Brady (26), and on the spinal cord by van der Kogel and Barendsen (229) confirm the importance of damage to the interstitium and vasculature as the major target of injury for both neutrons and photons.

In the first weeks following irradiation, early demyelinating changes are generally limited to scattered astocytic or microglial reactions with occasional perivascular collections of mononuclear cells. Subsequently, neural tissue begins to break down with the appearance of regions of myelin destruction, proliferative and degenerative changes in glial cells, and vascular changes including endothelial cell loss, proliferation, capillary occlusion, degeneration, and hemorrhagic exudates. When a critical mass of capillary endothelial cells fail, then vasogenic edema develops in response to the loss of essential support of dependent neurons reflecting cerebral cortical atrophy. Intracerebral calcifications are sometimes present and presumably represent lesions of mineralizing microangiopathy.

The basic mechanisms underlying the pathologic changes are not precisely known for any particular syndrome of irradiation damage. The three most commonly proposed mechanisms may act alone or in combination. The endothelial cell is essential for potency of the microcirculation. This cell is radiosensitive and damage is expressed as cell death or endothelial hyperplasia. Since endothelial cell turnover is slow, injury based on these cells occurs over a prolonged time interval. The oligodendrocyte maintains myelin. These cells show a decrease in numbers within weeks following irradiation. Damage in individual nerve fibers can be demonstrated quantitatively by electron microscopy as early as 2 weeks after irradiation and preceding vascular damage (227). Effects on myelin synthesis and maintenance may be especially important in childhood since myelogenesis is most active in the first year of life. An immunologic response to glial cell antigens (as suggested by an increase in myelin basic protein levels in the CSF after irradiation) may also contribute to CNS injury. Support for this hypothesis remains speculative.

Gastrointestinal Effects

Clinical Syndromes

1. The radiosensitivity of the gastric mucosa is reflected in the early depression of HCl and pepsinogen secretion after modest doses of 15 to 20 Gy. Although there is some recovery of cellular structure, suppression continues for a longer time in many cases, yet complete recovery of function can take place at one year (as shown by the line returning toward the normal aging line in Fig. 37-13). A more serious course of events is illustrated by the upper line, generally at levels at or above 50 Gy. Cellular and functional recovery is never complete and the chance of developing a radiation ulcer is

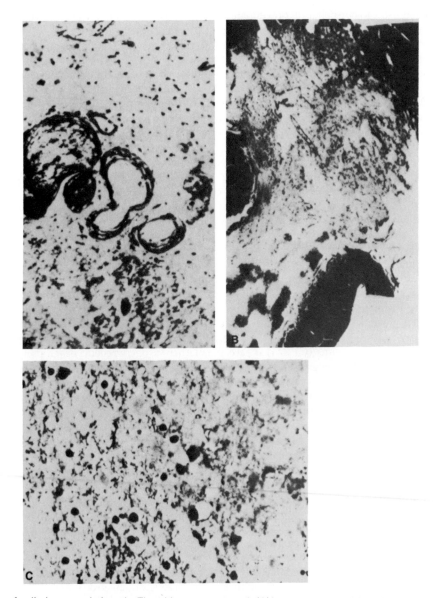

Fig. 37-12. *Pathology of radiation encephalopathy.* The white matter necrosis (A) is very common with methotrexte and is diffuse, unrelated to vascularization. In contrast, in (B), the radiation-induced lesions are oriented around vessels that are damaged, such as the dystrophic calcification of fine vessels, referred to as mineralizing microangiopathy. (A) and (B) From Lindgren (131a), with permission.

high. An ulcer in this anatomic setting allows for hemorrhage and perforation, an event which can be fatal. A chronically atrophic and contracted stomach may develop. The zone between the heavy lines defines the clinical range generally encountered, but the lines define the most common courses.

2. The early onset of malabsorption of fat and hypermotility after modest doses illustrates the radiosensitivity of the small intestine (Fig. 37-13). Generally, recovery at lower dose levels is without stigmata although some persistence of small bowel dysfunction and mesenteric cramping can be noted. Surgical intervention and adhesions could precipitate a more serious course of events. With higher doses, the clinical threshold is crossed, with diarrhea, malabsorption of fat and leakage of albumen into the bowel. The risk of infarction and perforation remains despite recovery if an obliterative arteritis develops. The underlying lesion is one of ulceration and segmental enteritis which can lead to stenosis

of the bowel lumen, with varying degrees of obstruction during the chronic period being a complication. The zone between the two heavy lines represent the clinical spectrum.

3. The manifestations of radiation injury in the colon and rectum are less than that in the small intestine after similar doses (Fig. 37-14). The initial reaction of hypermotility at modest levels of 10-20 Gy rapidly disappears. If constipation is a later complication, roughage can traumatize the bowel surface mucosa. The onset of tenesmus may be obscured by the simultaneous onset of diarrhea if a large segment of small bowel is being treated, in addition to the rectum. The higher dose (heavy line) can cause painless rectal bleeding 6-12 months after irradiation which rarely is fatal. Segmental colitis and rectal strictures are major concerns. Fortunately, severe bowel injury is not common owing to improved radiation techniques and the monitoring of radium applications. The clinical range is between the

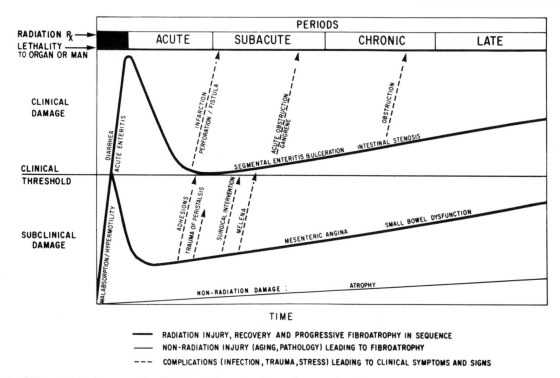

Fig. 37-13. *Clinicopathologic course: irradiated small intestine.* The early onset of malabsorption of fat and hypermotility after modest doses illustrates the radiosensitivity of the small intestine. Generally, recovery at lower dose levels is without stigmata although some persistence of small bowel dysfunction and mesenteric cramping can be noted. Surgical intervention and adhesions could precipitate a more serious course of events. With higher doses, the clinical threshold is crossed, with diarrhea, malabsorption of fat and leakage of albumen into the bowel. The risk of infarction and perforation remains despite recovery if an obliterative arteritis develops. The underlying lesion is one of ulceration and segmental enteritis which can lead to stenosis of the bowel lumen, with varying degrees of obstruction during the chronic period being a complication. The zone between the two heavy lines represents the clinical spectrum. From Rubin and Casarett (178), with permission.

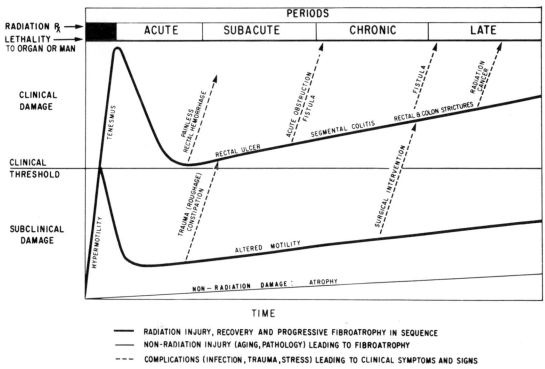

Fig. 37-14. *Clinicopathologic course: irradiated colon and rectum.* The manifestiations of radiation injury of the colon and rectum are less than that of the small intestine to similar doses. The initial reaction of hypermotility at modest levels of 1000 to 2000 R rapidly disappears. If constipation is a later complication, the roughage could traumatize the bowel surface mucosa. The onset of tenesmus may be obscured by the simultaneous onset of diarrhea if a large segment of small bowel is being treated, in addition to the rectum. The higher dose (heavy line) shows painless rectal bleeding 6 to 12 months after irradiation which rarely is fatal. Segmental colitis and rectal strictures are major concerns; but fortunately, severe bowel injury is not common owing to improved techniques and the monitoring of radium applications. The clinical range is between the two heavy lines. From Rubin and Casarett (178), with permission.

two heavy lines. Chemotherapy given in conjunction or sequentially with irradiation may augment gastrointestinal injury (Table 37-5).

Pathophsyiology (Fig. 37-15)

Progressive endoarteritis is the critical radiation lesion for late effects in the alimentary tract. This results in either ulceration and infarction necrosis with more rapid obliteration of vessels, or an increasing slow fibrosis and stricture of bowel with gradual narrowing of the fine vasculature (178). Unlike the acute mucosal loss and gradual return of regenerative epithelial clonogenic clusters in bowel crypts after irradiation, late ulceration is spotty and focal. The long axis of the ulcer is transverse, similar to ulcers that occur in obliterative vasculitis of other origins (178). Fistulas and perforation are focal and transmural, representing geographic loss of a segment of mucosa and its smooth musculature. The etiology for this occurrence cannot be explained by simultaneous cellular hypolasia of two different cells, that is, mucosa and smooth muscle. The association of obliterative endoarteritis in zones of necrosis and perforation indicate infarction necrosis of supplying vessels as the essential mechanism (178). Surgical handling of bowel and freeing of adhesions months to years after irradiation interfers with a tenuous blood supply and can percipitate alterations in hemodynamics. This may lead to repeated operations for infarction necrosis which often results in fatality (178). Mucosal surfaces are intact with endoarteritis as an underlying defect requiring an event such as surgical handling or trauma to result in a clinical manifestation (120).

Bone Marrow Effects

Clinical Syndromes

The elements of the blood and bone marrow respond to irradiation by progressively decreasing in number due to the destruction of primitive radiosensitive precursor cells (Fig. 37-16). The neutropenia seen in the first week is due to a cessation of production and a rapid turnover of these cells. This is followed in 2-3 weeks by thrombocytopenia and in 2-3 months by anemia. Recovery is related to the degree of initial response and generally begins with a regeneration of the depleted stem cells (Table 37-6). If large volumes of bone marrow have been irradiated, a hypoplastic marrow can persist and occaisionally become aplastic. This latter event may also be due to cancer infiltrating the marrow and should be suspected if the depression in blood count does not occur at a predictable time or if only a limited volume of the bone

Table 37-5. Gastrointestinal Chemotoxic Agents and Late Effects

Agents	Late Effects
5-fluorouracil	Enteritis
Adriamycin (+RAD)	Esophagitis
Actinomycin D (+RAD)	Enteritis
Cic-platinum (+RAD)	Enteritis
Methotrexate	Enteritis
Cyclophosphamide (+RAD)	Esophagitis
Hydroxyurea	Enteritis
Procarbazine	Enteritis
5-FU + meCCNU (+RAD)	Fistulas, perforation

Reprinted from Rubin, P. The Franz Buschke lecture. Late effects of chemotherapy and radiation therapy: a new hypothesis. Intl. J. Radiat. Oncol. Biol. Phys. 10:5-34; 1984; with permission from Pergamon Press Ltd, Headington Hill Hall, Oxford OX3 0BW, UK.

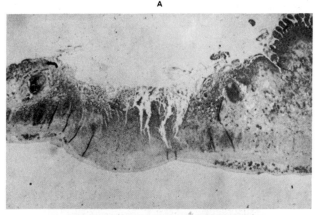

A

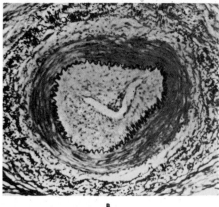

B

Fig. 37-15. *Radiation pathology of subacute clinical period: radiation ulcer of small intestine.* (A) Section of a region of small bowel with ulceration 6 months after radiation therapy (about 6000 R) (low magnification). From Rubin and Casarett (178), with permission. (B) Cross section of a small artery underlying the ulcer shown in (A), showing obstruction of the lumen by marked endothelial proliferation (endarteritis obliterans) and other changes in the arterial wall (high magnification). From Rubin and Casarett (178), with permission.

marrow has been irradiated. In Fig. 37-16, the upper heavy lines represent the course after the exposure of large volumes of bone marrow; the lower heavy lines, after localized bone marrow irradiation.

The bone marrow is the major dose-limiting organ, in terms of its acute toxicity, when radiation and chemotherapy are combined. Following the sequential use of these modes, damage may persist, despite normal appearing peripheral blood counts after aggressive treatment by each modality separately. The effects of chemotherapy on bone marrow are readily reflected by the peripheral blood counts with the nadir occurring 2-3 weeks after treatment (102). Schemas for monitoring blood values and modifying drug administration are in wide practice. In contrast, the effects of radiation therapy are more varied in that the compenstory mechanisms for regeneration vary both with dose and volume exposed. The repopulation and recovery of irradiated bone marrow is further confounded by the volume dependent nature of their compensatory mechanisms and the lack of correlation between the hemogram, which is often normal, and bone marrow injury (187). Future refinement in assay systems for progenitor cells such as CFU-GM, BFU-E, CFU-Mega, and CFU-GEMM will allow study of different cell lineages (82).

Table 37-6. Bone Marrow Regeneration (BMR) Patterns and Compensatory Mechanisms

	Regeneration				
TECHNIQUES OF IRRADIATION	EXPOSED BONE MARROW	UNEXPOSED BONE MARROW	EXTENSION	DOSES (RAD) DAILY	TOTAL
Small field	0	Local-regional ↑ BMR	$\overline{0}$		
Large field	0	Generalized ↑↑ BMR	$\overline{0}$		
Segmental filed	Suppresses BMR and recovers BMR	Generalized ↑↑ BMR	↑↑		
Total body	Active	——	$\overline{0}$	5–10	>100

$\overline{0}$ = Normal; ↑ = increased activity; ↑↑ = very increased activity.

Reprinted from Rubin, P. The Franz Buschke lecture. Late effects of chemotherapy and radiation therapy: a new hypothesis. Intl. J. Radiat. Oncol. Biol. Phys. 10:5-34; 1984; with permission from Pergamon Press Ltd, Headington Hill Hall, Oxford OX3 0BW, UK.

In addition, assay systems for the connective tissue stroma (CFU-F) of bone marrow allows for a means to study the microenvironment essential for normal hematopoesis (142).

Pathophysiology

The late effects of bone marrow regeneration after cancer treatment have become a focus of intense research. Both radiation dose and volume need to be studied in order to appreciate the dynamic events that are occurring after irradiation. Furthermore, it is essential to view the entire bone marrow organ as a functional whole unit rather than simply examining the irradiated marrow and the peripheral blood counts.

TOTAL BODY IRRADIATION

Total body irradiation in these settings, and with a low dose and dose rate as an incidental exposure during space travel, has stimulated a renewed interest in the biological effects of TBI. The lethal syndromes that follow high-intensity irradiation are related to the doses which the whole of specific sensitive organs receive (72). Different threshold dose levels exist for irreversible injury to the stem cell populations of various organs or tissues. Once exceeded, the result is loss of the organ's functional integrity coupled with an inability to repopulate or repair (99). The degree of importance of the

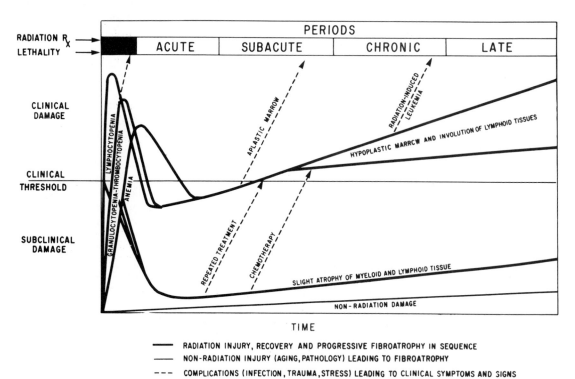

Fig. 37-16. *Clinicopathologic course: the blood (total-body irradiation).* The elements of the blood and bone marrow follow a response pattern of decreased number after irradiation owing to their cell kinetics after destruction of primitive radiosensitive precursor cells. The neutropenia seen in the first week is caused by a cessation of production and a rapid turnover of these cells. This is followed in 2 to 3 weeks by thrombocytopenia and in 2 to 3 months by anemia. Recovery is related to the degree of initial response and generally begins with a regeneration of the depleted stem cells. If large volumes of bone marrow have been irradiated, a hypoplastic marrow can persist and occasionally become aplastic. This latter event may be caused by cancer infiltrating the marrow and should be suspected if the depression in blood count does not occur at a predictable time and only if a limited volume of bone marrow has been irradiated. The upper heavy lines represent the course after the exposure of large volumes of bone marrow; the lower heavy lines, after localized bone marrow irradiation. From Rubin and Casarett (178), with permission.

organ determines the survival of the individual, and the time course of the expression of injury relates to the cell kinetics and cycle time of the stem cell. The classic radiation lethality syndromes relating to bone marrow, GI and central nervous system failure each have a tolerance dose and time course to fatality (Table 37-7) (178). When the whole body is irradiated intensively with single exposures, death will occur within minutes to months as a function of dose and the organ system affected. Damage to other organs, not directly leading to death, will additionally contribute qualitatively or quantitatively to the syndrome. The prominent acute syndromes and modes of death after single-dose TBI are, in the order of occurrence and decreasing threshold dose, the central nervous system (CNS) syndrome, the GI syndrome and the haemopoietic syndrome (178). Table 37-7 summarizes a variety of parameters of the acute radiation syndromes in man. Animal data available on these syndromes are generally consistent with observations in man. For example, haemopoietic death occurs in 50% of humans in 30-60 days following single doses of 2.4-7.5 Gy (22). Similarly, the hemopoietic $LD_{50/30-60}$ is 6-7 Gy in rodents, 6 Gy in rabbits, 2.5 Gy in pigs and goats, and 6 Gy in the macaque monkey (22). For any particular organ-related syndrome the actual threshold dose may not be clinically relevant because the adverse effects resulting from injury to another organ system may predominate. Thus, when the dose is at the threshold for the CNS syndrome, it is far above the threshold for the GI and haemopoietic syndromes. Clear differences exist in the timing of the development of the pathology which leads to functional impairment from the loss of relevant cells in the determining organs. Thus, the CNS syndrome becomes apparent within a few minutes to hours after irradiation and continues to express itself during the early parts of the latent periods for the GI and haemopoietic syndromes. Similarly, when the dose permits survival of the individual through the period of the CNS syndrome but exceeds the threshold for the GI syndrome, then this syndrome becomes apparent during the latent period for the haemopoietic syndrome. It should be noted that the median acute lethal dose ($LD_{50/60}$) for man for brief, intensive TBI is not precisely known, nor is the influence of age or sex. However, this dose has been estimated to be between 3 and 5 Gy, with deaths primarily associated with the haemopoietic and GI syndromes.

Survival after TBI intentionally administered as preparation for bone marrow transplantation (BMT) results from the infusion of viable bone marrow and intensive supportive care. Patients so treated will demonstrate delayed adverse effects dependent on the tolerance of individual organs to irradiation of their entirety. Since TBI for BMT is currently administered in both single and fractionated doses, the tolerance of whole organs to these two ablative strategies must be considered.

PARAMETERS OF THERAPY TOLERANCE DOSES AND TOLERANCE VOLUMES

THE CHANGING ORDER OF RADIOSENSITIVITY: DOSE /TIME /VOLUME FACTORS

In this multimodality era, there are many factors affecting our concepts of radiosensitivity. The rapid advances of radiation oncology and its science of radiation biology and radiation physics, and accumulating information on the interaction of other therapeutic modalities (e.g., chemotherapy, biologic response modifiers) with radiation, impact on our understanding of normal tissue toxicities. Thus, previously defined radiation tolerance doses (TD_5 and TD_{50}) remain as valuable guides (Table 37-8), but their applicability has changed — radiation doses customarily demed "safe" may no longer be so. When combined with another mode, such doses can lead to severe late effects with regards to different vital organs (154). Factors relevant to defining tolerances doses include those due to therapy, the host, and the tumor.

Therapy Factors

1. Dose: There is no absolute or fixed dose that ablates a normal tissue because the $TD_{5/5}$ and $TD_{50/5}$ are dependent on dose, time, and volume factors.
2. Fractionation: The fraction size of radiation and time interval are major determinates of both early and late effects. With alternate fractionation regimens under investigation, the $TD_{5/5}$ and $TD_{50/5}$ will shift for different organs. Hyperfractionation, accelerated fractionation, and hypofractionation will have different effects on tolerance doses.

Table 37-7. Some Aspects of the Acute Radiation Syndromes in Man (After Whole Body Irradiation)

Aspects	Acute Syndromes in Whole Body Irradiation		
	CENTRAL NERVOUS SYSTEM (CNS) SYNDROME	*GASTROINTESTINAL (GI) SYNDROME*	*HAEMOPOIETIC SYNDROME*
Chief determining organ	Brain	Small intestine	Bone marrow
Syndrome threshold	20 Gy	5 Gy	1 Gy
Syndrome latency	1/4–3 hours	3–5 days	2–3 weeks
Death threshold	50 Gy	10 Gy	2 Gy
Death time	Within 2 days	3 days to 2 weeks	3 weeks–2 months
Characteristic signs and symptoms	Lethargy, tremors, convulsions, ataxia	Malaise, anorexia nausea, vomiting, diarrhoea GI malfunction, fever, dehydration, electrolyte loss, circulatory collapse	Malaise, fever, dyspnea on exertion, fatigue, leukopenia, thrombopenia purpura
Major underlying pathology	Vasculitis (CNS), encephalitis, meningitis, oedema (CNS) infections	Depletion of intestinal epithelium, neutropenia (marrow damage),	Bone marrow atrophy, pancytopenia, infection, haemorrhage, anaemia

From Rubin and Casarett (178), with permission.

Table 37-8. Parameters of Therapy:
Tolerance Doses (TD 5/5 - TD 50/5)

Single Dose (Gray)			Fractionated Dose (Gray)		
Lymphoid	2	- 5	Testes	1	- 2
Bone Marrow	2	- 10	Ovary	6	- 10
Ovary	2	- 6	Eye (Lens)	6	- 12
Testes	2	- 10	Lung	20	- 30
Eye (Lens)	2	- 10	Kidney	20	- 30
Lung	7	- 10	Liver	35	- 40
Gastro Intestinal	5	- 10	Skin	30	- 40
Colo-rectal	10	- 20	Thyroid	30	- 40
Kidney	10	- 20	Heart	40	- 50
Bone Marrow	15	- 20	Lymphoid	40	- 50
Heart	18	- 20	Bone Marrow	40	- 50
Liver	15	- 20	Gastro Intestinal	45	- 50
Mucosa	5	- 20	VCTS*	50	- 60
VCTS*	10	- 20	Spinal Cord	50	- 60
Skin	15	- 20	Peripheral Nerve	65	- 77
Peripheral Nerve	15	- 20	Mucosa	65	- 77
Spinal Cord	15	- 20	Brain	60	- 70
Brain	15	- 25	Bone and Cartilage	> 70	
Bone and Cartilage	> 30		Muscle	> 70	
Muscle	> 30				

*vasculo-connective tissue systems
From Rubin (176), with permission.

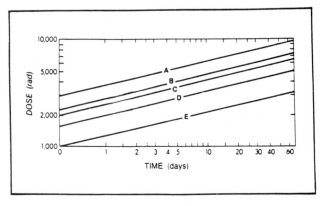

Fig. 37-17. *Strandqvist lines: defined radiation tolerance doses.* The dose-time isoeffect line relates total dose delivered and total time independent of fractionation for different tissue end points: A, skin necrosis; B, cure of skin carcinoma; C, moist desquamation of skin; D, dry desquamation of skin; and E, skin erythema. From Hall (99), with permission.

3. Volume: A major factor in determining a tolerance dose is whether the whole organ or partial organ is exposed to irradiation. With the more widespread use of TBI, IORT, and radiosurgery, single or brief radiation exposures with various dose rates to various volumes will create a different set of normal tissue toxicities.

4. Time: the interval between fractions and the overall duration of therapy effect tolerance doses. The time to expression of the effect is related to the cell kinetics of different subpopulations within a tissue/organ.

5. Chemotherapy: Of the various modalities, the addition of chemotherapy and timing of its delivery relative to irradiation has a major impact on organ sensitivity. The use of an agent may dramatically effect either the same cell or a different cell subpopulation, which leads to lower threshold doses for organ injury. The most common factor altering the tolerance dose concepts of normal tissues is the widespread use of drugs.

6. Innovations: The new modalities, hyperthermia, radiosensitizers and radioprotectors, immunological and biologic response modifiers may all or each alter late effects.

Dose Factors

The concept of an optimal dose that will provide maximal curability and minimal toxicity is the basis of varying fractionation schedules (65,173,175,178). The Strandqvist lines or isoeffect plots based upon varying dose-time regimens suggested that an optimal zone could be found, yielding a favorable therapeutic ratio (Fig. 37-17) (209). Although these lines were drawn with parallel slopes, it became apparent to many investigators that tumors may respond differently than normal tissues and a divergence of the isoeffect slopes occurs (231). The importance of the volume of normal tissue (137) and dose-time factors needs to be stressed in considering tolerance of normal tissue or organ effects. In

reexamining and revising the tolerance doses for different vital dose limiting tissues and organs, the volume factor is even more relevant today in view of the increasing use of total body irradiation in which whole organ systems are exposed. More time concentrated schedules are in use which vary from single exposure to short intense fractionation schedules. Another new modality — intraoperative radiation therapy — has lead to the use of large single doses to large tissue volumes and has provided new insights to the tolerance dose. Accordingly, a tabulation of the changing order of radiosensitivity is mainly based upon dose, but volume is also considered.

Currently, the prescribed tolerance dose is at best a calculated estimate of the TD_5 and TD_{50} based upon recorded human and animal data (72,99,178). The complication probability for either 5% (TD_5) and 50% (TD_{50}) assumes uniform irradiation of all or part of an organ, conventional fractionation schedules (1.8-2.0 Gy per fraction and five fractions per week), relatively normal organ function as a baseline, no adjuvant drugs or surgical manipulations, and age ranges which exclude children and the elderly. In ordering the organ radiosensitivity according to dose level, a variety of factors are considered including: the endpoint chosen (late more than acute effects), the use of single or fractionated regiments, and the volume of the organ. Since the literature is not always complete or precise (72,178), extrapolation is inevitably involved in using either clinical or experimental animal data. The dose levels are rounded off rather than offering doses to one or two decimals as is occasionally reported. Such accuracy can be as misleading as the general estimates of tolerance doses offered.

Single Doses Whole Organ (Table 37-9) (17)

- *Two to ten gray (200-1,000 cGy):* At doses less than 10 Gy, the cells most affected are those of lymphoid tissue, lymphocytes, bone marrow, hematopoetic stem cells, lens epithlium, ovarian oocyte, testes spermatogonia, lung type II cells and GI epithilium and villi. Most of these include highly radiosensitive, rapidly dividing stem cells and are directly effected without injury to the microvasculature or connective tissue stroma.

- *Ten to twenty gray (1,000-2,000 cGy):* At doses between 10 and 20 Gy, the majority of other organ systems respond

Table 37-9. Parameters of Therapy: Tolerance Doses (TD 5/5 - TD 50/5)

Target Cell	Complication Endpoint	Dose Range (Gray) TD5 - TD50
Range: 100 - 1000 cGy - SD / WO:		
Lymphoid and Lymphocytes	Lymphopenia	2 - 5
Bone Marrow Hematopoetic Stem Cells	Aplasia	2 - 10
Lens Epithelium	Cataract	2 - 8
Ovarian Oocytes	Sterility	2 - 6
Testes Spermatogonia	Sterility	2 - 6
Lung Type II Cells	Pneumonitis	7 - 10
Gastro Intestinal Epithelial Cells	Enteritis	5 - 10
Range: 1000 - 2000 cGy - SD / WO:		
Colo-Rectal Epithelial Cells	Colitis	10 - 20
Upper Aero-Digestive Mucosa	Mucositis	15 - 20
Kidney	Nephritis	11 - 19
Heart	Carditis	18 - 20
Liver	Hepatitis	15 - 20
Peripheral Nerve	Neuropathy	15 - 20
Spinal Cord	Myelopathy	15 - 20
Brain	Encephalopathy	15 - 20
Microcirculation	Vasculitis	15 - 20
Connective Tissue Stroma	Inflamation	15 - 20
Range: >2000 cGy - SD / WO:		
Bone and Cartilage	Osteitis / Gracture	> 20
Muscle	Myositis / Myopathy	> 20
Endocrines: Pituitary/Adrenals	Hypopituitarism	> 20
Pancreas	Pancreatitis / Diabetes	> 20

to irradiation, including the upper aerodigestive mucosa, kidney, heart, liver, peripheral nerves, spinal cord and brain. Skin probabaly would be effected as well. These are deliberately listed as organs with effects related to both radiation damage to microcirculation and connective tissue interstitium as well as parenchymal cells. Due to the large single doses used, it is difficult to distinguish between the impact of indirect vascular injury as distinct from direct effects on parenchymal cells that are often slowly cycling.

- *Twenty gray or more (> 2,000 cGy):* At doses greater than 20 Gy, a number of otherwise radioresistant structures may be affected, including: bone and cartilage, muscle, endocrine organs such as the pituitary and adrenals, reproductive organs such as the uterus and prostate, and other organs such as the pancreas and biliary system.

Fractionated Doses, Whole and Partial Organ Volumes (49,178,188) (Table 37-10)

The greatest clinical experience, with limited field irradiation to part of an organ, has provided insights into tissue/organ radiation sensitivity. Many dose ranges have been avoided in human situations and only animal data exist as a guide. Unfortunately, large fraction sizes and shorter time intervals are often employed in experiments and are different from conventional clinical schedules where 2 Gy daily and 10 Gy weekly are the standard. Despite these limitations, an ordering of radiation sensitivity according to fractionated regimens illustrates a shifting in relative position as compared to single exposures for these same tissues/organs.

- *Two to ten gray (200-1,000 cGy):* With fractionated doses of less than 10 Gy, the testes spermatogonia, ovarian oogonia and lens epithilium are injured. The testes spermatogonia are very sensitive to smaller fractional doses and are more efficiently destroyed than ovarian tissue. Lymphocytes and lymphoid tissues also will be suppressed with trivial doses.

- *Ten to twenty gray (1,000-2,000 cGy):* With fractionated doses of 10 to 20 Gy, the normal bone marrow will be depressed but with limited volumes larger doses will be required for this effort. In disease states, small fractional doses, even < 10 Gy, may ablate the bone marrow. Growing cartilage and growing bone will also be arrested within this dose range.

- *Twenty to thirty gray (2,000-3,000 cGy):* Between 20 and 30 Gy, a number of vital organs reach their radiation threshold and decompensate despite fractionation. This is most apparent when an entire organ is so treated. The kidneys and lungs are both vulnerable at this dose level and reflect a combination of injury to the microvasculature and epithelial cells.

- *Thirty to forty gray (3,000-4,000 cGy):* The liver becomes vulnerable. For many organs, there are little data on whole organ fractional therapy schedules but skin and oropharyngeal mucosa can become acutely reactive. The liver displays a special veno-occlusive event secondary to platelet adhesion to central veins at or somewhat above this dose level.

- *Forty to fifty gray (4,000-5,000 cGy):* At this dose level, the heart and GI organs are likely to manifest severe (life threatening) injury particularly with large or entire organ irradiation.

- *Fifty to sixty gray (5,000-6,000 cGy):* The majority of organs are vulnerable to fractionated schedules in the 50 to 60 Gy range. Gastrointestinal injury is significant and the colo-rectal tissues become vulnerable. The spinal

Table 37-10. Parameters of Therapy: Tolerance Doses TD5-TD50 (Fractionated Dose - Whole or Partial Organ)

Target Cell	Complication Endpoint	Dose Range (Gray) TD5-TD50
Range: 200 - 1000 cGy - FD/W or PO:*		
Lymphocytes and Lymphoid	Lymphopenia	2 - 10
Testes Spermatogonia	Sterility	1 - 2
Ovarian Oocytes	Sterility	6 - 10
Diseased Bone Marrow	Severe Leukopenia	
(CLL or Multiple Myeloma)	and Thrombocytopenia	3 - 5
Range: 1000 - 2000 cGy - FD/W or PO:*		
Lens	Cataract	6 - 12
Bone Marrow stem cell	Acute aplasia	15 - 20
Range: 2000 - 3000 cGy - FD/W or PO:*		
Kidney: Renal Glomeruli	Arterionephrosclerosis	23 - 28
Lung: Type II: VCTS	Pneumonitis / Fibrosis	20 - 30
Range: 3000 - 4000 cGy - FD/W or PO:*		
Liver Central Veins	Hepatopathy	35 - 40
Bone Marrow	Hypoplasia	25 - 35
Range: 4000 - 5000 cGy - FD/W or PO:*		
Heart / Whole Organ	Pericarditis and Pancarditis	43 - 50
Bone Marrow Microenvironments, Sinusitis	Permanent Aplasia	45 - 50
Range: 5000 - 6000 cGy - FD/W or PO:*		
Gastrointestinal	Infarction Necrosis	50 - 55
Heart / Partial Organ	Cardiomyopathy	55 - 65
Spinal Cord	Myelopathy	50 - 60
Brain	Encephalopathy	50 - 60
Range: >6000 - 7000 CGy - FD/W or PO:*		
Mucosa (VAD)	Ulcer	65 - 75
Rectum	Ulcer	65 - 75
Bladder	Ulcer	65 - 75
Mature Bones	Fracture	65 - 75
Pancreas	Pancreatitis	

*FD = fractionated dose
W or PO = whole or partial organ
From Rubin (176), with permission.

cord and brain may become demyelinated. Vasculo-connective tissue stroma is effected in this dose range and is a major consequence even in partial organ irradiation. Thus in lung, liver, kidney and bone marrow, long-term fibrosis occurs even if small volumes are irradiated.

• *Sixty to seventy gray (6,000-7,000 cGy):* In this range, the brain is more likely to react to irradation by undergoing demyelination at the TD_{5-50} levels. The rectum and bladder become vumerable to major injury at the TD_5 level. Mature bone and cartilage are able to withstand these dose as are the pancreas, peripheral nerves and muscle.

Volume Factors (137)

The volume of an irradiated organ or tissue may be as important as the fractionation effect in determining the total dose prescribed. Patterson (156) first quantified the impact of volume on radiation response of normal skin, showing an inverse relationship of dose and volume using similar fractionation schemas. Von Essen (231) demonstrated that an increase in the volume of tumor and normal skin leads to an adverse therapeutic ratio since the slopes for tumor curability

and normal tissue tolerance were different (Fig. 37-18). Fractionation of dose resulted in favorable therapeutic ratios for skin tumors less than 3 cm² but were virtually impossible to achieve for large volumes exceeding 100 cm². A three-dimensional model relating dose-time and volume indicated the balance required for an uncomplicated cure.

The concept of a "tolerance volume" needs to be defined similar to a "tolerance dose." The volume is most critical to the outcome of injury (Fig. 37-19). Generally, it is clinically safe to obliterate a certain volume of a vital organ with large doses, that is, exceeding the TD_{90-100}, similar to surgical resection. Loss of the volume does not affect organ survival since the organ can offer compensation for such loss through regeneration or hypertrophy and remain functional for survival despite being impaired. The following definitions are used.

• *Tolerance volume (TV) 5-25%:* When 5-25% of the organ volume irradiated can result in a life threatening or lethal complication.

• *Tolerance volume (TV) 50-90%:* When 50-90% of the organ volume irradiated can result in a life threatening or lethal complication.

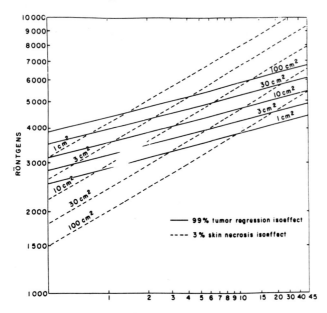

Fig. 37-18. *Strandqvist lines: isoeffect slopes for tumor regression and skin necrosis.* Isoeffect lines for tumor and skin (normal tissue) are no longer parallel. Despite increasing fractionation, it is not possible to achieve a favorable therapeutic ratio for larger skin cancer (100 cm²). From Von Essen(231), with permission.

1. These are generally the two levels of critical volumes for the dose-limiting or vital organs defined as class I (essential for survival). Only the GI tract and the central nervous system can have disastrous outcomes after small volumes (TV 5-25%) are exposed to doses exceeding tolerance (TD 5-50%). It is important to note that necrotic bowel can be resected and on occasion necrotic foci can be successfully resected in brain. For the majority of organs often considered dose limiting, such as the bone marrow, the lung, the kidney and in all probability the heart and the liver, high doses to smaller volumes are tolerated. Such organs may decompensate when more than 50% of the total volume (as applied to paired organs) is exceeded. When organ decompensation begins clearly depends upon the potential compensatory

regnerative mechanisms that follow significant organ volume loss. For example, there are numerous mechanisms that exist in the bone marrow when a certain percentage of the volume is ablated (179,184). Paradoxically, there is in-field regeneration of bone marrow after "ablative doses," that is > 3,000 cGy, when more than 50% of its volume is irradiated. For example, in Hodgkin's disease, irradiation of mantle fields (25% of the bone marrow organ volume) leads to permanent aplasia or hypoplasia of sternal marrow due to compensatory hyperplasia of the unirradiated bone marrow. However, with total nodal irradiation, which effects more than 50% of the bone marrow organ, compensating mechanisms lead to extension of bone marrow into the femoral shafts and humeri and a return of in-field vertebral bone marrow regeneration.

2. The dose volume histogram is being adopted by numerous investigators to predict unfavorable outcomes as a result of volume loss in a critical structure (137) (Fig. 37-20). Thus, the dose response curves for an individual organ will change as a function of volume and dose. With computerized 3-D dosimetry programs, each patient's customized radiation therapy should be considered as a complete dose-response curve (DRC), rather than as one point on a DRC. The data in the clinical and experimental literature can be divided into four categories:

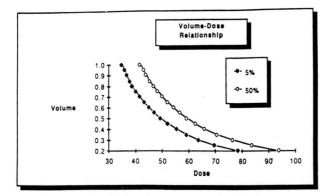

Fig. 37-19. *Volume-Dose Relationship.* As the volume of an organ irradiated decreases, the dose to produce 5% or 50% complications increases. This illustrates there is no "fixed" safe dose or tolerance dose TD$_5$ and TD$_{50}$, but it varies. From Rubin (176), with permission.

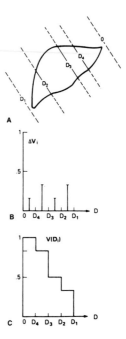

Fig. 37-20. *Creation of a Dose Volume Histogram.* (A) Representation of the three-dimensional distribution of doses within a planar isodose map for the organ; dashed lines show isodose lines outside the organ under consideration. Note the convention that the index i on D$_i$ increases with decreasing dose. (B) Differential dose-volume histogram derived from a complete set of such maps. (C) The equivalent integral, or dose-cumulative-volume, histogram. V(D$_i$) refers to the fraction of the organ receiving dose D$_i$ or more. From Lyman (137), with permission.

- Whole organ — single doses
- Whole organ — fractionated doses
- Partial organ — single doses
- Partial organ — fractionated doses

3. From this type of analysis it is possible to generate a modifying factor derived from dose and volume, but the data required is incomplete for many organ sites. Restated, the range of tolerable total doses used in the clinic varies with the volume and dose fractionation. Volume modifying factors (VMF) and dose modifying factors (DMF), therefore, can be approximated for different vital organs. Although it is beyond the scope of this presentation to present an accurate analysis of this data, the basis for such a determination is provided. These modifying factors are defined:

- Volume modifying factors (VMF):

$$\text{VMF} = \frac{\text{Tolerance Dose (TD) 5-50 for partial organ irradiation}}{\text{Tolerance Dose (TD) 5-50 for whole organ irradiation}}$$

- Dose modifying factors (DMF):

$$\text{DMF} = \frac{\text{Tolerance Dose (TD) 5-50 for fractionated irradiation}}{\text{Tolerance Dose (TD) 5-50 for single dose irradiation}}$$

Generally, the VMF for most organ systems allows for an increment in tolerance dose from one to five times as one decreases the volume used for whole organ irradiation. More often, this increment is only 2 to 3 times the dose. The DMF for most organ systems is similar. That is, the tolerance dose increases by a factor of 2 to 3 times when the ratio of single doses is compared to conventional daily dose fractionation.

According to Lyman (137,138), many authors have offered a simple model for dependence of dose on irradiated volume to cause a specified complication. This is a power-law relationship of the form:

$$\text{TD(V)} = \text{TD(1)V}^n \qquad (1)$$

where TD = tolerance dose, V = the fraction of the volume (or the ratio of the size of irradiated tissue to some reference size), and n = a size dependent parameter. Further, Lymann presented a three-parameter model which connects the three variables of interest: complication probability (P), dose (D), and volume (V), expressed as follows:

$$P = \frac{1}{\sqrt{2\pi}} \int_{-\infty}^{t_{max}} e^{-t^2/2} \, dt \qquad (2)$$

where $t = (D-TD_{50}(V)/(V))$ and $(V) = m*TD_{50}(V)$. Equation 1 is used to obtain $TD_{50}(V)$, and m is the third free parameter which is to be determined by the data. This formula is a combination of the power law dose-volume relationship (equation 1) and an error function representation of the complication-dose relationship, and gives back these equations if complication probability or volume, respectively are held constant.

The 3-D display relating dose and volume with the probability of complications is important to this clinical concept (138) (Fig. 37-21). The dose response curve and its steepness varies as a function of volume and organ tolerance should not be viewed or expressed simply as a function of dose. That is,

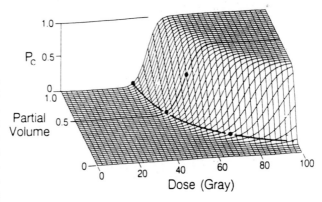

Fig. 37-21. *Modification of Dose Response Curves by Volume factor.* Each organ has a spectrum of dose-response curves as a function of volume irradiated. A three-dimensional surface representation of the probability of complication for the heart as a function of the dose and the partial volume that is uniformly irradiated. From Lyman (137), with permission.

there are a large number of dose response curves to express organ tolerance according to the volume of the irradiated organ.

Uniform Toxicity Scoring

To conclude on an important pragmatic note, there is a need to develop a uniform toxicity scoring for late effects (180,190). The introduction of mutlimodal management to cancer treatment has resulted in differences in reporting toxicity to treatment. The radiation oncologist is more aware of the importance of late effects once the acute phase of the reaction has been managed, in contrast to medical oncologists. However, chemotherapy produces late effects similar to irradiation and these complications have been increasingly documented in the literature. Yet the focus still remains on relatively acute and subacute effects. As a result, two different scoring and grading systems for toxicity have emerged. The radiation scores have been oriented toward specific pathologic lesions, whereas chemotherapy grades usually reflect functional and physiologic changes. Toxicity reporting of multiagent chemotherapy combinations and their interaction with radiation effects has stimulated national cooperative groups to form committees to assess acute effects and develop appropriate scoring and grading systems. A recommendation for a uniform system is the desired end product based upon "consensus criteria." In September 1985, a conference on toxicity was held in Baltimore, MD. A subcommittee, comprised of representatives from several cooperative groups and the National Cancer Institute, was formed at this meeting with the aim of addressing the question of standardized toxic effects criteria. Conclusions and recommendations made by the committee are summarized below (190).

1. There is a need for uniform toxicity scoring, both for acute and late effects but particularly with regard to late effects in vital organs.
2. The toxicity scale should consist of five grades including mild, moderate, severe, life-threatening, and fatal. The emphasis should be on grades 3, 4, and 5 with consideration for both peak grade and time in developing an appropriate index
3. In addition to the major modalities of radiation therapy and chemotherapy which are known to produce such

late toxicities, the effects of host co-factors, other modalities and recurrent tumor need to be carefully considered.

4. Endpoints need to be clearly defined in terms of somatic and genetic effects and second malignant tumors with appropriate time scales set, preferably more than 6 months following the introduction of treatment. There is a need for a working committee on late effects representing all major modalities including a radiation oncologist, a medical oncologist, and a surgical oncologist, depending upon the site.

5. Protocols for longitudinal studies of key dose limiting normal tissues and organs, using appropriate standard diagnostic laboratory and imaging tests, need to be developed. These should include CT, MRI, and PET scans.

6. Actuarial risk reporting and recall of long-term survivors should be done initially in select patients cohorts, namely survivors beyond 2 years. Although malignancies in which there is 50% survival have been considered most appropriate for such studies, this requirement may be too stringent and instead the assessment of adverse effects should be done in all survivors beyond 2 years. This is particularly true for highly fatal cancers where intensive regimens of combined modalities are used.

7. Publications should routinely present therapeutic ratios and use standard toxicity and late effects scoring along with tumor response rates (190).

Further efforts were made at Williamsburg in 1987 to develop precise criteria for category I/II organ toxicity by defining the late effect pathologic lesion, evaluative diagnostic tests, medical and surgical interventions and the character of the acute and late effects according to organ site (180). Most recently, Wittes has circulated a standardized system for acute toxicity scoring derived at an NCI consensus meeting which was recommended by the national cooperative groups and to all investigators involved in clinical trials (RE Wittes: personal written communication, 1988). A similar standardized late effects classification needs to be more widely adopted and should be based upon the available RTOG - EORTC late effects system. Protocols needs to be developed prospectively to accurately document late effects in all long term survivors, that is, more than 2 years survival (180).

Conclusions: Specific Organs TD_5 - TD_{50}

1. There is a shifting of the order of organ radiosensitivity depending on different critical cell subpopulations in the organ, in addition to differences in repair, repopulation and regeneration capacities of the critical cell.

2. There is a wide range of radiosensitivity of organ failure depending on volume and dose-time factors.

3. A thorough understanding of radiation pathophysiology of the multiple cell populations interacting is required to understand late effects in this multimodal era.

4. The tolerance doses $TD_{5/5}$ - $TD_{50/5}$ for specific organs serve as a guide but are not "safe doses" due to the impact of drugs and other innovations.

5. Volume is perhaps more critical as a clinical guide, that is, a certain percentage of a critical volume is lost with high doses — akin to surgical resection — but is within tolerance for survival.

6. Volume modifying factors need better definition and data similar to tolerance doses TD_{5-50} such as tolerance volume 5-25 and 50-90 must be generated.

7. Tolerance scoring needs to be uniform both for acute and late effects and be adopted both by radiation oncologists and medical oncologists.

8. Chemotherapy has altered concepts of "early" and "late" effects and produces late effects itself.

9. Predictive assays using serum biochemical markers are possible.

10. Corrective and preventative maneuvers are possible to avoid late effects. Late radiation damage should not be viewed as permanent and irreversible.

REFERENCES

1. Ahlgren, J.D., Smith, F.P., Kerwin, D.M., Sikic, B.I., Weiner, J.H., Schein, P.S. Pulmonary disease as a complication of chlorozotocin chemotherapy. Cancer Treat. Rep. 65: 223-229, 1981.
2. Alexander, J., Dainiak, N., Berger, H.J., Goldman, L., Johnstone, D., Reduto, L., Duffy, T., Schwartz, P., Gottschalk, A., Zaret, B.L. Serial assessment of doxorubicin cardiotoxicity with quantitative radionuclide angiocardiography. New Engl. J. Med. 300:278-283, 1979.
3. Alpert, H. Veno-occulsive disease of the liver associated with oral contraceptives: case report and review. Hum. Pathol. 7:709-718, 1976.
4. Alpes, T. Cellular radiobiology. London: Cambridge University Press, 1979.
5. Andrews GA (1967) Radiation accidents and their management. Radiat Res [Suppl] 7:390-397.
6. Ang K, Van der Kogel A, Van der Schueren E. Lack of evidence for increased tolerance of rat cord with decreasing fraction doses below 2 Gy. Intl. J Radiat Oncol Biol Phys 11:105-110, 1985.
7. Applefeld M, Cole J, Pollock S, et al. The late appearance of chronic pericardial disease in patients treated by radiotherapy for Hodgkin's disease. Ann. Intern. Med. 94:338-341, 1981.
8. Aronim, P.A., Mahaley, M.S., Rudnick, S.A., Dudka, L., Donahue, J.F., Selker, R.B., Moore, P. Prediction of BCNU pulmonary toxicity in patients with malignant gliomas — an assessment of risk-factors. New Engl. J. Med. 303:183-188; 1980.
9. Aso, Y., Yoneda, K., Kikkawa, Y. Morphologic and biochemical study of pulmonary changes induced by bleomycin in mice. Lab. Invest. 35: 558-568; 1976.
10. Avner, E.D., Ingelfinger, J.R. Special considerations relating to the pediatric cancer patient. In: Rieselbach, R.E.; Garnick, M.B., eds. Cancer and the kidney. Philadelphia: Lea and Febiger, 1981.
11. Berg, N.O.; Lindgren, M. Relation between field size and tolerance of rabbit's brain to roentgen irradiation (200 kV) via a slit-shaped field. Acta Radiol 1:147-168, 1963.
12. Berge, G.; Brun, A.; Hakansson, C.H.; Lindgren, M.; Nordberg, U.-B. Sensitivity to irradiation of the brain stem. Irradiation myelitis in the treatment of a nasopharynx carcinoma. Cancer 33:1263-1268, 1974.
13. Bergsagel, D.E. Total body irradiation for myelomatosis. Br. Med. J. ii:325-327; 1971.
14. Bieber, C.P., Jamieson. S., Raney, A., Burton, N., Bogarty, S., Hoppe, R., Kaplan, H.S., Strober, S., Stinson, E.B. Cardiac allograft survival in Rhesus primates treated with combined total lymphoid irradiation and rabbit antithymocyte globulin. Transplantation 28:347-350, 1979.
15. Billingham, M.E. Endocardial changes in anthracycline treated patients with and without irradiation. Front. Radiat. Ther. Oncol. 13: 67-81, 1979.
16. Billingham, M.E., Bristow, M.R., Glatstein. E., Mason. J.W., Masek, M.A., Daniels. J.R. Adriamycin cardiotoxicity: endomyocardial biopsy evidence of enhancement by irradiation. Am. J. Surg. Pathol. 1(1):17-23; 1977.
17. Bleyer, W.A. Neurologic sequelae of methotrexate ionizing radiation: a new classification. Cancer Treat. Rep. 65: 89-98; 1981.
18. Bleyer, W.A., Griffin, T.W. White matter necrosis, mineralizing microangiography, and intellectual abilities in survivors of child-

hood leukemia: associations with central nervous system irradiation and methotrexate therapy. In: Gilbert, H.A.; Kagan, A.R., eds. Radiation damage to the nervous system. New York: Raven Press; 1980:155-174.

19. Bloom, H.J.G., Wallace, E.N.K., Henk, J.M. The treatment and prognosis of medulloblastoma in children. A study of 82 verified cases. Mer. J. Roentgen. 105:43-62; 1969.

20. Boivin, J-P, Hutchison, G.B., Lubin, J., Mauch, P. Coronary artery disease mortality in patients treated for Hodgkin's disease. Cancer 69:1241-1247; 1992.

21. Bonadonna, G., Valagussa, P. Chemotherapy of breast cancer. Current views and results. Intl. J. Radiat. Oncol. Biol. Phys. 9: 279-297; 1983.

22. Bond, V.P.; Fludner, T.M.; Archambeau, J.O. Mammalian radiation lethality. New York: Academic Press; 1965.

23. Borch, R.F., Pleasants, M.E. Inhibition of cis-platinum nephrotoxicity by diethyldithiocarcamate rescue in a rat model. Proc. Natl. Acad. Sci. USA 76(12):6611-6614; 1979.

24. Botnik, L.E., Hannon, E.C., Hellman, S. Multisystem stem cell failure after apparent recovery from alkylating agents. Cancer Res. 38:1942-1947; 1978.

25. Botnik, L.E., Hannon, E.C.M., Hellman, S. Late effects of cytotoxic agents on the normal tissue of mice. Front. Radiat. Ther. Oncol. 13:36-47; 1979.

26. Brady, L.W., Ed. Long-term normal tissue effects of cancer treatment. Can. Clin. Trials 4(Suppl): 7:9-71; 1981.

27. Bristow, M.R., Mason, J.W., Billingham, M.E., Daniels, J.R. Doxorubicin cardiomyopathy: evaluations by phonocardiology, endomyocardial biopsy, and cardiac catheterization. Ann. Intern. Med. 88:168-175; 1978.

28. Britten, M., Halman, K., Meredith, W. Radiation cataract—new evidence on radiation dosage to the lens. Br. J. Radiol. 39:612-617; 1966.

29. Brosius, F.C. III, Waller, B.F., Roberts, W.C. Radiation heart disease. Analysis of 16 young (aged 15-33 years) necropsy patients who received over 3,500 rads to the heart. Am. J. Med. 70:519-530; 1981.

30. Bundey, S., Evans, K. Survivors of neuroblastoma and ganglioneuroma and their families. J. Med. Genet. 19:16-21; 1982.

31. Burger, P.C., Kamenar, E., Schold, S.C., Fay, J.W. Phillips, G.L.; Herzig, G.P. Encephalomyelopathy following high-dose BCNU therapy. Cancer 48: 1318-1327; 1981.

32. Burns, R.J., Bar-Shlomo, B., Druck, M. Detection of radiation cardiomyopathy by gated radionuclide angiography. Am J Med 74:297-302; 1983.

33. Byhardt, R., Brace, K., Ruckdeschel, J. Dose and treatment factors in radiation related pericardial effusion associated with the mantle technique for Hodgkin's disease. Cancer 35:795; 1975.

34. Carbell SC, Chaffey JT, Rosenthal DS et al. Results of total body irradiation in the treatment of advanced non-Hodgkin's lymphoma. Cancer 43:994-1000; 1979.

35. Casarett, G.W. Aging. In: Vaeth, J.M., ed. Frontiers of radiation therapy and oncology, vol. 6. New York: S Karger; 1972:479-485.

36. Casarett, G.W. Similarities and contrasts between radiation and time pathology. In: Strehler, B., ed. Advances in gerontological research. New York: Academic Press, 1964:109-163.

37. Cassady, J.R. Carabell, S.C., Jaffe, N. Chemotherapy irradiation related hepatic dysfunction in patients with Wilms' tumor. In: Vaeth, J.M., ed. Frontiers of radiation therapy and oncology, vol. 13. Combined effects of chemotherapy and radiotherapy on normal tissue tolerance. New York, S. Karger; 1979:147-160.

38. Catterall, M., Bloom, H.C.J., Ash, D.V., Walsh, L., Richardson, A., Uttley, D., Gowing, N.F.C., Lewis, P., Chaucer, B. Fast neutrons compared with megavoltage X rays in the treatment or patients with supratentorial blioblastoma: a controlled pilot study. Intl. J. Radiat. Oncol. Biol. Phys. 6: 261-266; 1980.

39. Ch'ien, L.T., Rhomes, J.A., Aur, J.A., Stagner. S., Cavallo, K., Wood, A., Geff, J., Pitner, S., Huster, H.O., Seifert, M.J., Simone, J.V. Long-term neurological implications of somnolence syndrome in children with acute lymphocytic leukemia. Ann. Neurol. 8:273-277; 1980.

40. Chabner, B.A., Myers, C.E., Oliverio, V.T. Clinical pharmacology of anticancer drugs. Semin. Oncol. 4: 217-226; 1977.

41. Chaffey, J.T., Hellman. S. Radiation fractionation as applied to murine colony forming cells in differing proliferative states. Radiology 93:1167-1172, 1969.

42. Chen, G.T.Y., Austin-Seymour, M., Castro, J.C., Collier, J.M., Lyman, J.T., Pitluck, S., Saunders, W.M., Zink, S.R. Dose volume histograms in treatment planning evaluation of carcinoma of the pancreas. In: Proceedings Eighth International Conference on Uses of Computers in Radiation Therapy; 1984:264-268.

43. Choi, N.C.; Kanarek, O.J.; Kazemi, H. Physiologic changes in pulmonary function after thoracic radiotherapy for patients with lung cancer and role of regional pulmonary function studies in predicting postradiotherapy pulmonary function before radiotherapy. Cancer Treat. Symp. 2:119-130; 1985.

44. Cohen, L., Creditor, M. Isoeffect tables for tolerance of irradiated normal human tissues. Intl. J. Radiat. Oncol. Biol. Phys. 9:233-241; 1983.

45. Cohen, S.; Bharati, S.; Glass, J.; et al. Radiotherapy as a cause of complete atrioventricular block in Hodgkin's disease: an electrophysiological-pathological correlation. Arch. Intern. Med. 141:676-679; 1981.

46. Concannon, J.P., Summers, R.E., Cole, C., Weill. C. Effects on renal function. X-radiation combined with systemic actinomycin D. Am. J. Roentgenol. 108: 141-147; 1970.

47. Constine LS, Donaldson SS, McDougall IR et al. Thyroid dysfunction after radiotherapy in children with Hodgkin's disease. Cancer 53:878-883; 1984.

48. Constine, L. S., Konski, A., Ekholm, S., McDonald, S., Rubin, P. Adverse effects of brain irradiation correlated with MR and CT imaging. Intl. J. Radiat. Oncol. Biol. Phys. 15:319-330; 1988.

49. Constine, L.S., Rubin, P.: Total body irradiation: normal tissue effects. In: Bleehen, N.M., ed. Radiobiology in radiotherapy. Springer-Verlag; 1987:95-121.

50. Cowdry, E.V. Textbook of histology, 4th ed. Philadelphia: Lea and Febiger; 1950.

51. Croizat, H., Friendel, E., Tubiana, M. Proliferative activity of stem cells in the bone marrow of mice after single and multiple irradiations (total and partial body). Intl. J. Radiat. Biol. Phys. 18: 347-358; 1970.

52. D'Angio, G., ed. Delayed consequences of cancer therapy: proven and potential. Cancer 37:979-1236; 1976.

53. Danjoux, C.E., Catton, G.E. Delayed complications in colorectal carcinoma treated by combination radiotherapy and 5-fluorouracil — Eastern Cooperative Oncology Group (ECOG) Pilot Study. Intl. J. Radiat. Oncol. Biol. Phys. 5: 311-316, 1979.

54. Danoff, B. F., Cowchock, S., Marquette, C., Mulgrew, L., Kramer, S. Assessment of the long-term effects of primary radiation therapy for brain tumors in children. Cancer 49:1580-1586; 1982.

55. Deeg HJ, Flounoy N, Sullivan K et al. Cataracts after total body irradiation and marrow transplant: a sparing effect of dose fractionation. Intl J Radiat Oncol Biol Phys 10:957-964; 1984.

56. Dethlefsen, L.A. Cellular recovery kinetic studies relevant to combined modality research and therapy. Intl. J. Radiat. Oncol. Biol. Phys. 5: 1175-1184;.1979.

57. DeVita, V.T. Principles of chemotherapy. In: Cancer: principles and practice of oncology. DeVita, V.T., Hellman, S., Rosenberg, S.A., eds. Philadelphia: J.B. Lippincott; 1982:132-155.

58. DeVita, V.T. The relationship between tumor mass and resistance to chemotherapy: implications for surgical adjuvant treatment of cancer. The James Ewing Lecture delivered at the 35th annual meeting of the Society of Surgical Oncology, April; 1982.

59. Devney RB, Sklar CA, Nesbit ME et al. Serial thyroid function measurements in children with Hodgkin's disease. J. Pediatr. 105:225-227; 1984.

60. Doll R, Smith PG. The long-term effects of X-irradiation in patients treated for metropathia haemorrhagica. Br. J. Radiol. 41:362-368; 1968.

61. Donaldson, S.S., Moskowitz, P.S., Canty, E.L., Efron, B. Radiation-induced inhibition of compensatory renal growth in the weanling mouse kidney. Radiology 128:491-495, 1978.

62. Donaldson, S.S., Moskowitz, P.S., Fajardo, L.F. Combination radiation-adriamycin therapy: renoprival growth, function, and structural effects in the immature mouse. Intl. J. Radiat. Oncol. Biol. Phys. 6: 851-859; 1980.

63. Dunsmore LD, LoPonte MA, Dunsmore RA. Radiation-induced coronary artery disease. J. Am. Coll. Cardiol. 8:239-244; 1986.

64. Edwards, M.S., Wilson, C.B. Treatment of radiation necrosis. In: Gilbert, H.A., Kagan, H. R., eds. Radiation damage to the nervous system. New York: Raven Press, 1980:129-144.

65. Ellis, F. Is NSD-TDF useful to radiotherapy? Intl. J. Radiat. Oncol. Biol. Phys. 11:1685-1699, 1985.

66. Eltringham, J.R. Cardiac response to combined modality therapy. Front. Radiat. Ther. Oncol. 13:161-174, 1979.

67. Eltringham, J.R., Fajardo, L.F., Stewart, J.R. Adriamycin cardiomyopathy: enhanced cardiac damage in rabbits with combined drug and cardiac irradiation. Radiology 115:471-472, 1975.

68. Eltringham, J.R., Fajardo, L.F., Stewart, J.R., Klauber, M.R. Investigation of cardiotoxicity in rabbits from adriamycin and fractionated cardiac irradiation: preliminary results. Front. Radiat. Ther. Oncol. 13: 21-35; 1979.

69. Ercan, M.T., Or, I.S., Bekdik, C.F., Sarizi, T., Yazicioglu, A. 99mTC-Methyl CCNU for the static imaging of kidneys. Eur. U. Nucl. Med. 5:109-114, 1980.

70. Evans, A., Bleyer, A., Kaplan, R., Meadows, A.T., Poplack, D., Sheline, G. Central nervous system workshop. Cancer Clin. Trials 4(Suppl):31-35; 1981.

71. Evans, R.G. Radiobiologic considerations in magna-field irradiation. Intl. J. Radiat. Biol. Phys. 9:1907-1912; 1983.

72. Fajardo, L.F. Pathology of radiation injury. New York: Masson Publishing USA Inc.; 1982.

73. Fajardo, L.F., Eltingham, J.R., Stewart, J.R. Combined cardiotoxicity of adriamycin and x-radiation. Lab. Invest. 34(1):89-96, 1976.

74. Fajardo, L.F., Eltingham, J.R., Stewart, J.R., Klauber, M.R. Adriamycin nephrotoxicity. Lab. Invest. 43:242-253, 1980.

75. Fajardo LF, Stewart J.R. Experimental radiation-induced heart disease. 1. Light microscopic studies. Am. J. Pathol. 59:299-316; 1970.

76. Fajardo, L.F.; Stewart, J.R. Pathogenesis of radiation-induced myocardial fibrosis. Lab. Invest. 29:244-257; 1973.

77. Fajardo, L.F., Stewart, J.R., Cohn, K.E. Morphology of radiation-induced heart disease. Arch. Pathol. Lab. Med. 86: 512-519, 1968.

78. Field, S.B., Michalowski, A. Endpoints for damage to normal tissues. Intl. J. Radiat. Oncol. Biol. Phys. 5:1185-1196; 1979.

79. Filler, R.M., Maddock, C.I., Tefft, M., Vawter, G., Brown, B.: Effects of actinomycin D and x-ray on partially hepatectomized rats. Surgical Forum 19:358-360; 1968.

80. Frei, E. Summary and prospective statement concerning the Genitourinary workshop. Cancer Clin. Trials 4: 25-29; 1981.

81. Friedman, M.A., Bozdeck, M.J., Billingham, M.E., Rider, A.K. Doxorubicin cardiotoxicity: serial endomyocardial biopsies and systolic time intervals. J. Am. Med. Assoc. 15:1603-1606, 1978.

82. Frindel, E., Croizat, H., Vassont, F. Stimulating factors liberated by treated bone marrow: In vivo effect on CFU kinetics. Exp. Hematol. 4: 56-61; 1976.

83. Fryer, C.J.; Fitzpatrick, P.J.; Rider, W.D.; Poon, P. Radiation pneumonitis: experience following a large single dose of irradiation. Intl. J. Radiat. Oncol. Biol. Phys. 4:931-936; 1978.

84. Fukushima, S., Araio, M., Cohen, S.M., Jacobs, J.B., Friedell, G.H. Scanning electron microscopy of cyclophosphamide induced hyperplasia of the rat urinary bladder. Lab Invest. 44:89-96, 1981.

85. Gangji, D., Reaman, G.H., Cohen, S.R., Bleyer, W.A., Poplack, D.G. Leukoencephalopathy and elevated levels of myelin basic protein in the cerebrospinal fluid of patients with acute lymphoblastic leukemia. New Engl. J. Med. 303:19-21; 1980.

86. Garnick, M.B., Mayer, R.J., Abelson, H.T. Renal failure associated with cancer chemotherapy. In: Acute Renal Failure, Brenner, B.M., Lazarus, J.M. and Myers, B.D., eds. Philadelphia, W.B. Saunders, 1981.

87. Gavin, P.R.; Gillette, E.L. Radiation response of the canine cardiovascular system. Radiat. Res. 90[Suppl]:489-500; 1982.

88. Ghione, M. Cardiotoxic effects of antitumor agents. Chemother. Pharmacol. 1: 25-34, 1978.

89. Gilladoga, A.C., Tan, C.T.; Phillips, F.C., Sternberg, S.S.; Tang, C., Wollner, N., Murphy, M.L. Cardiac status of 40 children receiving adriamycin over 495 mg/m^2 and animal studies. Proc. Am. Assoc. Cancer Res. 15:107; 1974.

90. Ginsberg, S.J., Comis, R.L. The pulmonary toxicity of antineoplastic agents. Semin. Oncol. 9:34-51, 1982.

91. Glatstein, E. Alterations in 86 Rubidium extraction in normal mouse tissues after irradiation. An estimate of long-term blood flow changes in kidney, lung, liver, skin and muscle. Radiation Res. 53: 88-101, 1973.

92. Glatstein E, Fajardo LF, Brown JM. Radiation injury in the mouse kidney. 1. Sequential light microscopic studies. Intl. J Radiat Oncol Biol Phys 2:933-943; 1977.

93. Glatstein E, McHardy-Young S, Brast N et al. Alterations in serum thyrotropin (TSH) and thyroid function following radiotherapy in patients with malignant lymphoma. J. Clin. Endocrinol. Metab. 32:833-841; 1971.

94. Goldwein, J.W. Radiation myelopathy: a review. Med. Pediatr. Oncol. 15:89-95; 1987.

95. Gonzalez-Vitale, J.C., Hayes, D.M., Cvitkovic, E., Sternberg, S.S. The renal pathology in clinical trials of cisplatinum (II) diamminedichloride. Cancer 39:1362-1371; 1977.

96. Goorin, A.M., Borow, K.M., Goldman, A., Williams, R.G., Henderson, I.C., Sallan, S.E., Cohen, H., Jaffe, N. Congestive heart failure due to adriamycin cardiotoxicity: its natural history in children. Cancer 47:2810-2816; 1981.

97. Greenwood, R.D., Rosenthal, A., Cassady, R., Jaffe, N., Nadas, A.S. Constructive pericarditis in childhood due to mediastinal irradiation. Circulation 50:1033-1039; 1974.

98. Griffin, T.V., Rasey, J.S., Bleyer, W.A. The effect of photon irradiation on blood-brain barrier permeability to methotrexate in mice. Cancer 40:1109-1111, 1977.

99. Hall, E.J. Radiobiology for the radiologist. New York: Harper and Row; 1978.

100. Harmon, W.E., Cohen, H., Schneeberger, E.E., Grupe, W.E. Chronic renal failures in children treated with methyl CCNU. New Engl. J. Med. 300:1200-1203, 1979.

101. Heller, C.G. Effects on the germinal epithelium of radiobiological factors in manned space flight. In: Langham, W.H., ed. NRC Publication 1487. Washington, D.C.: National Academy of Sciences, National Research Council; 1967:124-133.

102. Hellman, S., Botnik, L.E. Stem cell depletion: an explanation of the late effects of cytotoxins. Intl. J. Radiat. Oncol. Biol. Phys. 2:181-184, 1977.

103. Hindo WA, De Trana F, Lee M-S; et al. Large dose increment irradiation in treatment of cerebral metastases. Cancer 26:138-141; 1970.

104. Holland, J.F., Frei, E. Cancer medicine. Philadelphia: Lea and Febiger, 1973.

105. Hopewell, J.W. Early and late changes in the functional vascularity of the hamster cheek pouch after local irradiation. Radiation Res. 63:157-164; 1975.

106. Hopewell, J.W.: Radiation effects on vascular tissue. The non-neoplastic late effects session. Brussels. ICR, 1981.

107. Hornsey, S., Morris, C.C., Myers, R., White, A. RBE for damage to the CNS by neutrons. Intl. J. Radiat. Oncol. Biol. Phys. 1983.

108. Hornsey, S.; White, A. Isoeffect curve for radiation myelopathy. Br. J. Radiol. 53:168-169; 1980.

109. Hresnchyshyn, M.M. Results of the Gynecologic Oncology Group trials on ovarian cancer: preliminary report. In: Symposium on ovarian carcinoma. NCI Monograph 42:155-165, 1975.

110. Hubmann, F.H. Effect of X-irradiation on the rectum of the rat. Br. J. Radiol. 54:250-254; 1981.

111. Ingold, J.A.; Reed, G.B.; Kaplan, H.S.; Bagshaw, M.A. Radiation hepatitis. Am. J. Roentgenol. 93:200-208; 1965.

112. Jaffe, J.P.; Bosch, A.; Raich, P.C. Sequential half-body radiotherapy in advanced multiple myeloma. Cancer 43:124-128; 1979.

113. Jeneke, R.S., Dalbow, D.G., Bartuska, B.M., Deprez-De Campenere, D.: Comparative inhibition of myocardial RNA synthesis by anthracycline antibiotics. Cancer Treat. Rep. (In press).

114. Jones, A.M. Transient radiation myelopathy (with reference to L'Hermitt's sign of electrical paresthesia). Br. J. Radiol. 37:727-744; 1964..

115. Jongejan, H., Van der Kogel, A., Provoost, A. et al. Radiation nephropathy in young and adult rats. Intl. J. Radiat. Oncol. Biol. Phys. 13:225-232; 1987.

116. Kaplan, R.S., Wiernik, P.H.: Neurotoxicity of antineoplastic drugs. Semin. Oncol. 9: 103-130, 1982.

117. Keane, T.J.; Van Dyk, J.; Rider, W.D. Idiopathic interstitial pneumonia following bone marrow transplantation: the relationship with total body irradiation. Intl. J. Radiat. Oncol. Biol. Phys. 7:1365-1370; 1981.

118. Keizer, M.J. Protection of hematopoetic stem cells during cytotoxic treatment. Rijswijk, Netherlands: Radiobiological Institute; 1976:92.

119. Kemper T, O'Neill R, Caveness W. Effects of single dose

supervoltage whole brain radiation in *Macaca mulatta*. J. Neuropathol. Exp. Neurol. 36:916-940; 1977.

120. Ketcham, A., Withers, H.R. Gastrointestinal workshop. Cancer Clin. Trials 4: 15-18, 1981.

121. Kim TH, Khan FM, Galvin JM. A report of the work party: comparison of total body irradiation techniques for bone marrow transplantation. Intl J Radiat Oncol Biol Phys 6:775-784; 1980.

122. Kim TH, Panakon AM, Friedman M. Acute transient radiation hepatitis following whole abdominal irradiation. Clin Radiol 27:449-454; 1976.

123. Kline, L., Kim, J., Ceballos, R. Radiation optic neuropathy. Ophthalmology 92:1118-1126; 1985.

124. Knopse WH, Blom J, Crosby WH. Regeneration of locally irradiated bone marrow. II. Induction or regeneration in permanently aplastic medullary cavities. Blood 31:400-405; 1968.

125. Kolmer, J.A., Lucke, B. A study of the histologic changes produced experimentally in rabbits by arsphenamine. Arch. Dermatol. Syphilol. 3:483-514, 1921.

126. Kopelson, G., Herwig, K.J. The etiologies of coronary artery disease in cancer patients. Intl. J. Radiat. Oncol. Biol. Phys. 4:895-906, 1978.

127. Kun, L. E., Mulhern, R. K., Crisco, J.J. Quality of life in children treated for brain tumors: intellectual, emotional and academic functions. J. Neurosurg. 58:1-6; 1983.

128. LeBaron, S., Zeltzer, P., Zeltzer, L., Scott, S., Marlin, A. Assessment of quality of survival in children with medulloblastoma and cerebellar astrocytoma. Cancer 54:135-138; 1988.

129. Lederman, G., Sheldon, T., Chaffey, J., Herman, T., Gelman, R., Coleman, N. Cardiac disease after mediastinal irradiation for seminoma. Cancer 60:772-776; 1987.

130. Leith JT, DeWyngaert K, Glicksman A. Radiation myelopathy in the rat: an interpretation of dose relationships. Intl. J. Radiat. Oncol. Biol. Phys. 7:1673-1677; 1981.

131. Lewin, K., Millis, R.R. Human radiation hepatitis. A morphologic study with emphasis on the late changes. Arch. Pathol. 96: 21-26, 1973.

131a. Lindgren, M. On tolerance of brain tissue and sensitivity of brain tumor to irradiation. Acta. Radiol. Suppl. 170; 1958.

132. Littman, P., Meadows, A.T., Polgar, G., Borns, P. F., Rubin, E. Pulmonary function in survivors of Wilms' tumor. Cancer 37: 2773-2776; 1976.

133. Littman, P., Rosenstock, J., Bailey, C. Radiation myelitis following craniospinal irradiation with concurrent actinomycin D therapy. Med. Pediatr. Oncol. 5(1):145-151; 1978.

134. Lockhart, S.F.; Down, J.D.; Steel, G.G. The effect of low dose rate and cyclophosphamide on the radiation tolerance of the mouse lung. Intl. J. Radiat. Oncol. Biol. Phys. 12:1437-1440; 1986.

135. Lushbaugh CG, Casarett GW. The effects of gonadal irradiation in clinical radiation therapy: a review. Cancer 37:1111-1120; 1976.

136. Lushbaugh, C.G.; Rider, R.C. Some cytokinetic and histopathologic considerations of irradiated male and female gonadal tissues. Front Radiat. Ther. Oncol. 6:224-248; 1972.

137. Lyman, J.T. Complication probability as assessed from dose-volume histograms. Radiat. Res. 104 [Suppl. 8]:S-13 - S-19; 1985.

138. Lyman, J.T., Wolbarst, A.B. Optimization of radiation therapy III: a method of assessing complication probabilities from dose-volume histograms. Intl. J. Radiat. Oncol. Biol. Phys. 14:103-109, 1987.

139. Maier JG Effects of radiations on kidney, bladder and prostate. Front. Radiat. Ther. Oncol. 6:196-227; 1972.

140. Maier, J.G., Casarett, G.W. Pathophysiologic aspects of radiation nephritis in dogs. University of Rochester Atomic Energy Commission Report, UR-626; 1962.

141. Marks, J E., Wong, J. The risk of cerebral radionecrosis in relation to dose, time and fractionation. A follow-up study. In: Hamburger, F., ed. Progress in experimental tumor research, vol . 29. Karger, Basal; 1985.

142. Marsh, J.C.: The effects of cancer chemotherapeutic agents on normal hematopoietic precursor cells: a review. Cancer Res. 36: 1853-1882, 1976.

143. Meacham, G.C., Tillotson, F.W., Heinle, R.W. Liver damage after prolonged urethane therapy. Am. J. Clin. Pathol. 22: 22-27, 1952.

144. Merriam GR Jr, Focht EF A clinical study of radiation cataracts and the relationship to dose. Am J Roentgenol 77:759-785; 1957.

145. Minow, R.A.; Stern, M.H.; Casey, J.H.; Rodriguez, V.; Luna, M.A. Clinicopathologic correlation of liver damage in patients treated with 6-mercaptopurine and adriamycin. Cancer 38:1524-1528; 1976.

146. Mitchell, E.P., Schien, P.S. Gastrointestinal toxicity of chemotherapeutic agents. Semin. Oncol. 9: 52-64; 1982.

147. Monterdini, S., ed. Manual of cancer chemotherapy, 3rd ed., vol 56, UICC Technical Reprint Series. Geneva: UICC, 1981.

148. Moosavi, H., McDonald, S., Rubin, P., Cooper, R., Stuard, I.D., Penney, D.P.: Early radiation dose response in lung: an ultrastructural study. Intl. J. Radiat. Oncol. Biol. Phys. 2:921-932, 1977.

149. Morandet, N., Paramentier, C., Flamant. R.: Etude par le fer 59 des effets de la radiotherapie etendue des hematosarcomes sur l'erythropoiese. Biomedicine 18: 228, 1973.

150. Moskowitz, P.S., Donaldson, S.S. The clinical spectrum of radiation/chemotherapy nephropathy in children treated for Wilms tumor. Am. J. Radiol. (In press).

151. Moskowitz, P.S., Donaldson, S.S., Canty, E.L. Chemotherapy-induced inhibition of compensatory renal growth in the immature mouse. Am. J. Radiol. 134:491-496, 1980.

152. Nelson DF, Reddy KV, O'Mara RE *et al*. Thyroid abnormalities following neck irradiation for Hodgkin's disease. Cancer 42:2553-2562; 1978.

153. Nichols, W.C., Moertel, C.G. Nephrotoxicity of methyl CCNU (Letter). New Engl. J. Med. 301: 1181, 1979.

154. Orton, C.G., Cohen, L. A unified approach to dose-effect relationships in radiotherapy. I: Modified TDF and linear quadratic equations. Intl. J. Radiat. Oncol. Biol. Phys. 14: 549-557, 1988.

155. Parsons, J.J., Fitzpatrick, C.R., Hood, C.T., Ellingwood. K.E., Bova, F.J., Million, R.R. The effects of irradiation on the eye and optic nerve. Intl. J. Radiat. Oncol. Biol. Phys. 9:609-622, 1983.

156. Paterson, R. The treatment of malignancy by radium and X-rays. Being a practice of radiotherapy. London: Edward Arnold and Co., 1947.

157. Pedrick TJ, Hoppe RT. Recovery of spermatogenesis following pelvic irradiation for Hodgkin's disease. Intl. J. Radiat. Oncol. Biol. Phys. 12:117-121; 1986.

158. Penney, D.P.; Rubin, P.: Specific early fine structural changes in lung following irradiation.Intl. J. Radiat. Oncol. Biol. Phys. 2: 1123-1132; 1977.

159. Penney, D.P., Shapiro, D.L., Rubin. P. Finkelstein, J. Long-term effects of radiation on the mouse lung and potential induction of radiation pneumonitis. Intl. J. Radiat. Oncol. Biol. Phys. (To be published).

160. Perez CA, Korba A, Zwnuska F *et al*. ^{60}Co moving strip technique in the management of carcinoma of the ovary: analysis of tumor control and morbidity. Intl. J. Radiat. Oncol. Biol. Phys. 4:379-388; 1978.

161. Perry, M.C.: Hepatoxicity of chemotherapeutic agents. Semin. Oncol. 9: 65-74, 1982.

162. Phillips R, Karnofsky D, Hamelton L *et al*. Roentgen therapy of hepatic metastases. Am. J. Roentgenol. 71:826-834; 1984.

163. Phillips, T.L. An ultrastructural study of the development of radiation injury in the lung. Radiology 87: 49-54; 1966.

164. Phillips, T.L. Tissue toxicity of radiation-drug interactions. In: Sokal, G.H. and Maickel, R.P.,eds. Radiation-drug interactions in the treatment of cancer. Wiley Series in Diagnostic and Therapeutic Radiology. New York: John Wiley and Son, 1980:175-200.

165. Phillips, T.L., Ross, G. A quantitative technique for measuring renal damage after irradiation. Radiology 109: 457-462, 1973.

166. Pratt, W.B., Ruddon, R.W. The anticancer drugs. New York: Oxford University Press, 1979.

167. Price, R.A., Birdwell, D.A. The central nervous system in childhood leukemia III. Mineralizing microangiopathy and dystrophic calcification. Cancer 42:717-728; 1978.

168. Price, R.A., Jamieson, P.A. The central nervous system in childhood leukemia. H subacute leukoencephalopathy. Cancer 35:306-318, 1975.

169. Probert, J.C., Parker, B.R., Kaplan, H.S.: Growth retardation in children after megavoltage irradiation of the spine. Cancer 32: 635-639, 1973.

170. Prosnitz, L.R., Farber, L.R., Fisher, J.J., Bertino, I.R., Fischer, D.B. Long-term remissions with combined modality therapy for advanced Hodgkin's disease. Cancer 37:2826-2833, 1976.

171. Reactor safety study. Appendix VI. USNRC, Washington 1400 (NUREG 75/014); 1975.

172. Roswitt B, Malsky S, Reid C Radiation tolerance of the gastrointestinal tract. Front. Radiat. Ther. Oncol. 6:160-181; 1972.

173. Rubin, P. Radiation effect and tolerance, normal tissue. In: Vaeth, J. M., ed. Frontiers of radiation therapy and oncology, vol. 6. Baltimore: University Park Press, 1972.

174. Rubin P. Radiation toxicology: quantitative radiation pathology for predicting effects. Cancer 39[Suppl]:21:729-736; 1977.

175. Rubin, P. The Franz Buschke lecture. Late effects of chemotherapy and radiation therapy: a new hypothesis. Intl. J. Radiat. Oncol. Biol. Phys. 10:5-34; 1984.

176. Rubin, P. The law and order of radiation sensitivity, absolute vs relative. In: Vaeth, J.M., ed. Clinical radiation pathology, vol. 22. Baltimore: University Park Press; 1988.

177. Rubin P, Bennett JM, Begg C et al. The comparison of total body irradiation versus chlorambucil and prednisone for remission induction or active chronic lymphocytic leukemia: an ECOG study. I. Total body irradiation, response and toxicity. Intl. J. Radiat. Oncol. Biol. Phys. 7:1623-1632; 1981.

178. Rubin, P.; Casarett, G.W. Clinical radiation pathology, vols. I and II. Philadelphia: W.B. Saunders Co.; 1968.

179. Rubin P, Constine LS, Scarantino CW. The paradoxes in patterns and mechanisms of bone marrow regeneration after irradiation. II. Total body irradiation. Radiother. Oncol. 2:227-233; 1984.

180. Rubin, P., Constine, L.S., Van Ess, J. Late effects of toxicity scoring. NCI Monog. 6:9-18; 1988.

181. Rubin, P.; Cooper. R.A.; Phillips, T.L., eds. Radiation biology and radiation pathology syllabus. Chicago: American College of Radiation Publications; 1978.

182. Rubin P, Finkelstein JN, Siemann DW et al. Predictive biochemical assays for late radiation effects. Intl. J. Radiat. Oncol. Biol. Phys. 12:469-476; 1984.

183. Rubin, P.; Keys, H.; Poulter, C.A. Changing concepts in the tolerance of radioresistance and radiosensitivity of normal tissue/organs. In: Biological basis and clinical importance of tumor radioresistants. New York: Masson Publishing Co., 1983.

184. Rubin P, Landman S. Mayer E et al. Bone marrow regeneration and extension after extended field irradiation in Hodgkin's disease. Cancer 32:699-711; 1973.

185. Rubin, P., Nabila, A., Elbadawi, A., Thomson, R.A.E., Cooper, R.A. Bone marrow regeneration from cortex following segmental fractionated irradiation. Intl. J. Radiat. Oncol. Biol. Phys. 2: 27-38, 1977.

186. Rubin, P., Scarantino, C.W. The bone marrow organ and the critical structure in radiation-drug interaction. Intl. J. Radiat. Oncol. Biol. Phys. 4: 3-23, 1978.

187. Rubin, P., Shapiro, D., Finckelstein, J., Penney, D. The early release of surfactant following lung irradiation of alveolar type II cells. Intl. J. Radiat. Oncol. Biol. Phys. 6:75-77, 1980.

188. Rubin, P., Siemann, D. Principles of radiation oncology and cancer radiotherapy. In: Rubin, P., ed. Clinical oncology. A multidisciplinary approach, sixth edition. New York, American Cancer Society; 1983:58-72.

189. Rubin, P., Siemann, D.W., Shapiro, D., Finkelstein, J., VanHoutte, P., Penney, D. Surfactant release as an early measure of radiation pneumonitis. Intl. J. Radiat. Oncol. Biol. Phys. 9:1669-1673; 1983.

190. Rubin, P., Wasserman, T.H. The late effects of toxicity scoring. Intl. J. Radiat. Oncol. Biol. Phys. 14(1):S29-S28; 1988.

191. Rubin, P., Whitaker, J.N., Bryant, R.G., Herman, P.K., Ceckler, T.L., Gregory, P.K., Constine, L.S., Baggs, R.B. Myelin basic protein and magnetic resonance imaging for diagnosing radiation myelopathy. Preliminary report. Intl. J. Radiat. Oncol. Biol. Phys. 15:1371-1381; 1988.

192. Safadari, G. H., Fuentes, J. M., Dubois, J. M., Alirezai, M., Castan, P., Viahovitch, B. Radiation necrosis of the brain: time of onset and incidence related to total dose and fractionation of radiation. Neuroradiology 27:44-47, 1985.

193. Salazar OM, Van Houtte P, Rubin P Once-a-week radiation for locally advanced lung cancer: final report. Cancer 54:719-725; 1984.

194. Scarantino CE, Rubin P, Constine LS The paradoxes in patterns and mechanisms of bone marrow regeneration after irradiation. I. Different volumes and doses. Radiother. Oncol. 2:215-225; 1984.

195. Schacht, R.G., Feiner, H.D., Gallo, G.R., Lieberman, A., Baldwin, D.S. Nephrotoxicity of nitrosoureas. Cancer 48:1328-1334, 1981.

196. Schenken, L.L., Burdolt, D.R., Kovacs, C.J. Adriamycin radiation induced combinations: drug induced delayed gastrointestinal radiosensitivity. Intl. J. Radiat. Oncol. Biol. Phys. 5:1265-1270, 1979.

197. Schilsky, R.L. Renal and metabolic toxicities of cancer chemotherapy. Semin. Oncol. 9:75-83, 1982.

198. Schullheiss, T. E., Higgins, E. M., El-Mahdi, H. M. The latent period in radiation myelopathy. Intl. J. Radiat. Oncol. Biol. Phys. 10:1109-1115; 1984.

199. Schultz, H.P.; Glatstein, E.; Kaplan, H.S. Management of presumptive or proven Hodgkin's disease of the liver. A proven radiotherapy technique. Intl. J. Radiat. Oncol. Biol. Phys. 1:1-8; 1975.

200. Shalet SM, Beardwell CG, Jacobs HG et al. epubertal testis. Clin. Endocrinol. 9:483-490; 1978.

201. Shalet SM, Horner A, Ahmed JR. Leydig cell damage after testicular irradiation for acute lymphoblastic leukemia. Med. Pediatr. Oncol. 13:65-68; 1985.

202. Shapiro E, Kinsella T, Makuch R et al. Effect of fractionated irradiation on endocrine aspects of testicular function. J Clin Oncol 3:1232-1239; 1985.

203. Sheline GE, Wara, WM, Smith V. Therapeutic irradiation and brain injury. Intl. J. Radiat. Oncol. Biol. Phys. 6:1215-1228; 1980.

204. Siemann, D.W.; Hill, R.P.; Penney, D.P. Early and late pulmonary toxicity in mice evaluated 180 and 420 days following localized lung irradiation. Radiat. Res. 89:396-407; 1982.

205. Sklar CA, Kim TH, Ramsay NKC Thyroid dysfunction among long-term survivors of bone marrow transplantation. Am. J. Med. 73:688-694; 1982.

206. Sklar CA, Kim TH, Williamson IF et al. Ovarian function after successful bone marrow transplantation in post-menarcheal females. Med. Pediatr. Oncol. 11:361-364; 1983.

207. Sorokin, S.P. The cell of the lungs. In: Morphology of experimental respiratory carcinogenesis, proceedings of the biology division, Oak Ridge National Laboratory.

208. Speiser B, Rubin P, Casarett G. Aspermia following lower truncal irradiation in Hodgkin's disease. Cancer 32:692-698; 1973.

209. Standqvist, M. Studienuber die Kumulative Wirkung der Rontgenstrahlen bei Fraktionierung. Acta Radiologica 55:1-300, 1944.

210. Stewart, J.R., Cohen, K.E., Fajardo, L.F., Hancock, W., Kaplan, H.S. Radiation-induced heart disease. A study of twenty-five patients. Radiology 89(2):302-310; 1967.

211. Stewart, J.R., Fajardo, L.F.: Cancer and coronary artery disease. Editorial comment. Intl. J. Radiat. Oncol. Biol. Phys. 4: 915-916, 1978.

212. Stewart, J.R., Fajardo, L.F.: Dose response in human and experimental radiation-induced heart disease. Radiology 99(2):403-408, 1971.

213. Stewart JR, Fajardo LF (1984) Radiation-induced heart disease: an update. Prog Cardiovasc Dis 27:173-194.

214. Takahashi, I., Nagai, T., Miyaishi, K., Maehara, Y., Niibe, H. Clinical study of the radioprotective effects of amifostine (Ym-08310, WR-2721) on chronic radiation injury. Intl. J. Radiat. Oncol. Biol. Phys. 12: 935-939, 1986.

215. Tefft, M.: Radiation related toxicities in National Wilms' Tumor Study Number 1. Intl. J. Radiat. Oncol. Biol. Phys. 2:455-464, 1977.

216. Tefft, M.; Mitus, A.; Das, I.; Vawter, G.F.; Filler, R.M. Irradiation of the liver in children: review of experience in the acute and chronic phases, and in the intact normal and partially resected. Am J Roentgenol 108:365-385; 1970.

217. Tefft, M., Traggis, J.D., Miller, R.M. Liver irradiation in children: acute changes with transient leukopenia and thrombocytopenia. Am. J. Roentgenol. 4: 750-764, 1969.

218. Thomas ED, Storb R, Buckner CD Total body irradiation in preparation for bone marrow engraftment. Transplant Proc 8:591-593; 1976.

219. Thomas ED, Storb R, Clift RA et al. Bone marrow transplantation. New Engl J Med 292:832-843, 895-902; 1975.

220. Till, J.E., McCullough, E.A. A direct measurement of the radiation sensitivity of normal mouse bone marrow cells. Radiat. Res. 14:213-222, 1961.

221. Travis, E.L. The sequence of histological changes in mouse lungs after single doses of x-rays. Intl. J. Radiat. Oncol. Biol. Phys. 6:345-347; 1980.

222. Travis, E.L., Harley, R.A., Fenn, J.O., Klobukowski, C.J., Hargrove, H.B.: Pathologic changes in the lung following single and multiple fraction irradiation. Intl. J. Radiat. Oncol. Biol. Phys. 2:475-490, 1977.

223. Trott K-R Chronic damage after radiation therapy: challenge to radiation biology. Intl. J. Radiat. Oncol. Biol. Phys. 10:907-913; 1984.

224. Tubiana, M., Bernard, C.I., Lalanne, C. Modification de l'erythropoiese aupres radiotherapie pelvienne. Acta Radiol. 52:321; 1959.

225. Tubiana M, Friendel E, Croizat H Effects of radiation on bone marrow. Pathol. Biol. (Paris) 27(6):326-334; 1979.

226. Valeriote, F.A., Edelstein, M.B. The role of cell kinetics in cancer chemotherapy. Sem. Oncol. 4: 217-226, 1977.

227. Van der Kogel, A.J. Mechanisms of late radiation injury in the spinal cord. In: Radiation biology in cancer research. New York: Raven Press, 1980:461.

228. Van der Kogel AJ Radiation tolerance of the spinal cord: time-dose relationships. Radiology 122:505-509; 1977.

229. Van der Kogel, A.J., Barendsen, G.W. Late effects of spinal cord irradiation with 300 kV x-rays and 15 MeV neutrons. Brit. J. Radiol. 47: 393-398, 1974.

230. Van Houtte, P., Rubin, P., Finkelstein, J., Siemann, D.. Penney, D., Shapiro, D. The effect of bleomycin alone or in combination with radiation on surfactant release in the lung. Submitted to American Radium Society, 1982.

231. Von Essen, C. F. Roentgen therapy of skin and lip carcinoma: factors influencing success and failure. Am. J. Roentgenol. 83: 556-570; 1960.

232. Von Hoff, D.D., Layard, M.W., Basa, P., Davis, H.L., Jr.; Von Hoff, A.L., Rozencweig. M., Muggia, F.M. Risk factors for doxorubicin-induced congestive heart failure. Ann. Intern. Med. 91: 710-717,1979.

233. Von Hoff, D.D., Rozencweig, M., Piccart, M. The cardiotoxicity of anticancer agents. Semin. Oncol. 9 23-33,1982.

234. Wachholz BW, Casarett GW Radiation hypertension and nephrosclerosis. Radiat. Res. 41:39-56; 1970.

235. Wara, W.; Irvine, A.; Neger, R.; Howes, E.; Phillips, T. Radiation retinopathy. Intl. J. Radiat. Oncol. Biol. Phys. 5:81-83; 1979.

236. Wara WM, Phillips TL, Margolis LW, et al. Radiation pneumonitis: a new approach to the derivation of time-dose factors. Cancer 32:547-552; 1973.

237. Wara, W., Phillips, T., Sheline, G., Schwade, J. Radiation tolerance of the spinal cord. Cancer 35:1558-1562; 1975.

238. Weiss, B.R., Muggia, F.M. Cytotoxic drug-induced pulmonary disease: update 1980. Am. J. Med. 68: 259-266, 1980.

239. Willett C, Tepper J, Orlow E, et al. Renal complications secondary to radiation treatment of upper abdominal malignancies. Intl. J. Radiat. Onco.l Biol. Phys. 12:1601-1604; 1986.

240. Wolf EL, Berdon WE, Cassady JR, Baker DH, Freiberger R, Pavlov H. Slipped capital femoral epiphysis as a sequela to childhood irradiation for malignant tumors. Radiology 125:781-784; 1977.

240a. Woo E, Lam K, Yu Y: Cerebral radionecrosis: Is surgery necessary? J Neurosurg Psych 50:1407-1414, 1982.

241. Woods W, Dehner L, Nesbit M. Fatal veno-occlusive disease of the liver following high-dose chemotherapy, irradiation and bone marrow transplantation. Am. J. Med. 68:285-290; 1980.

242. Xu, G.Z., Cai, W. M., Qin, D.X., Yan, J.H., Wu, X.L., Hu, Y.H., Zhu, X., Zhang, H.X. Chinese herb destagnation series I: Combination of radiation and destagnation in the treatment of nasopharyngeal carcinoma (NPC) — a prospective randomized trial on 188 cases. Intl. J. Radiat. Oncol. Biol. Phys. 16(2):297-300; 1989.

GLOSSARY OF DRUG TERMS

NONPROPRIETARY NAME	TRADE NAME	NONPROPRIETARY NAME	TRADE NAME
Acetaminophen	Tylenol	Gallium Nitrate	Ganite
Acetylsalicylic Acid	Aspirin	G-CSF	Neupogen
Actinomycin D	Cosmegen	GM-CSF	Prokine
Allopurinol	Zyloprim	Goserlin Acetate	Zoladex
Amphotericin B	Fungizone		
Azathioprine	Imuran	Haloperidol	Haldol
		Hydroxydaunomycin	Adriamycin
BCNU	Bicnu	Hydroxyprogesterone Caproate	Delalutin
Bleomycin	Blenoxane	Hydroxyurea	Hydrea
Bromocriptine	Parlodel		
Busulfan	Myleran	Idarubicin	Idamycin
		Ifosfamide	Ifex
Carboplatin	Paraplatin	Interferon Alfa-2	Roferon/Intron-A
Carmustine (BCNU)	BiCNU	Interleukin-2	Proleukin
CCNU (Lomustine)	CeeNU		
Chlorambucil	Leukeran	L-Asparaginase (E. Coli)	Elspar
Chlorpromazine	Thorazine, Promapar	L-Phenylalanine mustard	Alkeran
Cisplatin	Platinol	Leuprolide	Lupron
Citrovorum Factor	Leucovorin	Levamisole	Ergamisol
Conjugated Estrogens	Premarin	Lidocaine HCL	Xylocaine
Cyclophamide	Cytoxan	Lomustine	CeeNU
Cyproheptadine	Periactin		
Cytarabine HCL	Cytosar	Mechlorethamine	Mustargen
Cytosine Arbinoside	Cytosar U	Medroxyprogesterone acetate	Depo-Provera
		Megestrol acetate	Megace
DTIC	Dacarbazine	Melphalan	Alkeran
Dactinomycin	Cosmegen	Mercaptopurine	Purinethol
Daunorubicin	Cerubidine	Mesna	Mesnex
Dexamethasone	Decadron, Hexadrol	Methenamine	Cystamin, Cystogen, Hexamine
Diamminedichloroplatinum	Platinol		
Diethylstilbestrol	DES	Methotrexate	Methotrexate, Mexate
Dinitrochlorobenzene	DNCB	Methyl CCNU	Semustine
Doxorubicin	Adriamycin	Methylprednisolone	Medrol
		Metoclopramide	Reglan
Erythropoitein	Epogen/Procrit	Methoxsalen	Oxsoralen
Estramustine phosphate	EMCYT	Mithramycin	Mithracin
Ethinyl Estradiol	Estinyl	Mitomycin C	Mutamycin
Etidronate disodium	Didronel	Mitotane	Lysodren
Etoposide	VePesid	Mitoxantrone	Novantrone
Fludarabine	Fludara	Nitrogen Mustard	Mustargen
Fluorouracil (5FU)	Adrucil, Efudex	Nystatin	Mycostatin
Fluoxymesterone	Halotestin		
Folinic Acid	Leucovorin	Octreotide acetate	Sandostalin
		Ondansetron HCl	Zofran
		O,p'-DDD	Lysodren

NONPROPRIETARY NAME	TRADE NAME	NONPROPRIETARY NAME	TRADE NAME
Pamidronate disodium	Aredea	Taxol	Taxol
Pentostatin	Nipent	Tamoxifen Citrate	Nolvadex
Phenylalanine Mustard (L-Pam)	Alkeran	Testosterone Propionate	Oral-Oreton; Inj-Neo-Hombreol
Phenytoin	Dilantin		
Platinum	Platinol	Tetracycline	Achromydin, Sumycin
Prednisone	Deltasone, Orasone	6-Thioguanine	Thioguanine
Procarbazine	Matulane	Triethylenemelamine	Tretamine
Prochlorperazine	Compazine	Triethylenethiophosphoramide	Thiotepa
Pyrimethamine	Daraprim	Trimethoprim	Proloprim, Trimpex
Quinacrine	Atabrine	VM-26	Teniposide
		Vinblastine	Velban
Streptozotocin	Zanosar	Vincristine	Oncovin
Sulfamethoxazole	Gantanol		
		Zinc Oxide	Calamine preparation

GLOSSARY OF DRUG PROGRAMS

ABBREVIATION	SPECIFIC DRUGS IN PROGRAM
ABVD	Doxorubicin/bleomycin/vinblastine/dacarbazine
AC	Doxorubicin/cyclophosphamide
ACOP	Doxorubicin/cyclophosphamide/vincristine/prednisone
APO	Doxorubicin/prednisone/vincristine
AV/CM	Doxorubicin/vincristine plus cyclophosphamide/methotrexate
BACOP	Bleomycin/doxorubicin/cyclophosphamide/vincristine/prednisone
BCD	Bleomycin/cyclophosphamide/dactinomycin
BCNU	Carmustine
Budr	Bromodeoxyuridine
BVCPP	Carmustine/vinblastine/cyclophosphamide/procarbazine/prednisone
BVCPP	BCNU/vinblastine/cyclophosphamide/procarbazine/prednisone
CAF	Cyclophosphamide/doxorubicin/5-FU
CAMP	Cyclophosphamide/doxorubicin/methotrexate/procarbazine
CAP	Cyclophosphamide/doxorubicin/cisplatin
CBDCA	Carboplatin
CBVM	Cytarabine/bleomycin/vincristine/methotrexate
CHAD	Cyclophosphamide/hexamethylmelamine/doxorubicin/diamminedichloroplatinum
CHOP	Cyclophosphamide/doxorubicin/vincristine/prednisone
CISCA	Cisplatin/cyclophosphamide/doxorubicin
CMC	Cyclophosphamide/methotrexate/CCNU
CMF	Cyclophosphamide/methotrexate/5-FU
CMFP	Cyclophosphamide/methotrexate/5-FU/prednisone
C-MOPP	Cyclophosphamide/vincristine/procarbazine/prednisone
COMP	Cyclophosphamide/vincristine/methotrexate/prednisone
COP-BLAM	Cyclophosphamide/vincristine/prednisone/bleomycin/doxorubicin/procarbazine

ABBREVIATION	SPECIFIC DRUGS IN PROGRAM
CYVADIC	Cyclophosphamide/vincristine/doxorubicin/dacarbazine
DTIC	Dacarbazine
DDMP	Diamino-dichlorophenylmethyl-pyrimidine
FAC	5-FU/doxorubicin/cisplatin
FAM	5-FU/doxorubicin/mitomycin-C
FAMMe	5-FU/doxorbicin/mitomycin/semustine
5-FU	Fluorouracil
FUDR	Floxuridine
HDMTX	High-dose methotrexate
Hexa-CAF	Hexamethylmelamine/cyclophosphamide/methotrexate/5-FU
IUDR	Idoxuridine
L-PAM	Melphalan
M-BACOD	Cyclophosphamide/doxorubicin/vincristine bleomycin/methotrexate/dexamethanone
MAC	Methotrexate with/without leukovorin rescue/actinomycin D/cyclophosphamide
MACOP-B	Methotrexate with leucovin rescue/doxorubicin/cyclophosphamide vincristine/prednisone/bleomycin
MOPP	Nitrogen mustard/also known as mechlorethamine/vincristine/procarbazine/prednisone
MOPP/ABV Hybrid	Nitrogen mustard/vincristine/procarbazine/prednisone/doxorubicin/vinblastine bleomycin
ProMACE-CytaBOM	Cyclophosphamide/doxorubicin/VP-16/cytarbine/bleomycin/methotrexate/prednisone
VAC	Vincristine/actinomycin-D/cyclophosphamide/doxorubicin
VACA	Vincristine/actinomycin D/cyclophosphamide/doxorubicin
VACOP-B	Vincristine/prednisone/bleomycin
VAP	Vincristine/doxorubicin/procarbazine
VACOP-B	VP-16/doxorubicin/cyclophosphamide/vincristine/prednisone/bleomycin

Index

Page numbers in *italics* refer to illustrations; numbers followed by t indicate tables.

Abdomen, acute, in neutropenic patient, 47–48
  computed tomography of, limitations and applications of, 171t
  germ cell tumor of, 277
    prognosis in, 279
  ultrasound scanning of, limitations and applications of, 171t
Absorption of chemotherapeutic agents, 108
Abstinence syndrome, 714t
ABVD regimen, for Hodgkin's disease, 225
Accuracy, 171
Acetic acid, in vulvar carcinoma detection, 404
Achalasia, esophageal cancer and, 558
Acid phosphatase, prostatic (PAP), in metastatic disease, 681
  in prostate cancer, 434
  serum (SAP), in prostate cancer, 434
Acquired immune deficiency syndrome. See *AIDS (acquired immunodeficiency syndrome)*.
Acromegaly, 544
  paraneoplastic, 139
  treatment of, 549, 550
    results of, 550t, 551
ACTH. See *Corticotropin (ACTH)*.
Actinic keratosis, 179
Actinomycin D (dactinomycin), cardiac toxicity of, 739t
  for gestational trophoblastic neoplasia, 382, 383t
  for Wilms' tumor, 264–265
  gastrointestinal toxicity of, 750t
  late effects of, 253t
  radiation-induced myelopathy and, 747
Acutarius, Johannes, quoted, 419
Acyclovir, for herpesvirus infection, 151–152
Addiction, 714t
Adenocarcinoma, clear cell, of ovary, 389
  endometrioid, of endometrium, 374
    of ovary, 389
  of anus, 588
  of cervix, 365, 366t. See also *Cervical carcinoma*.
    endometrial carcinoma vs., 374
  of endometrium. See also *Endometrial carcinoma*.
    endometrial hyperplasia vs., 374
    histologic subtypes of, 374, 375, 375t
  of esophagus, 559
    chemotherapy for, 563
  of gallbladder, 611
  of kidney, 421
    treatment of, 421–424
  of lung, 649, 649t. See also *Lung cancer*.
  of pancreas, 599. See also *Pancreatic cancer*.

Adenocarcinoma *(Continued)*
  of prostate, 434–435, *435*, 435t. See also *Prostate cancer*.
  of small intestine, 574, 574t, 575
  of stomach, 568–569. See also *Stomach cancer*.
  of vagina, 400. See also *Vaginal carcinoma*.
Adenoma(s), pituitary. See *Pituitary tumor(s)*.
Adenovirus 2, 26
ADH (antidiuretic hormone), inappropriate secretion of. See *Syndrome of inappropriate antidiuretic hormone secretion*.
Adrenal(s). See also *Adrenal cortex*.
  imaging of, 540–541, 540t
  metastasis to, diagnosis of, 680
Adrenal cortex, cancer of, 539–543
  complications of, 542–543
  diagnosis of, 540–541, 540t
  epidemiology of, 539–540
  etiology of, 540
  histopathology of, 541–542
  prognosis in, 543
  recommended reading on, 551
  results of treatment of, 543, 543t
  staging of, 542t
  treatment of, 542–543
  tests of function of, in adrenocortical cancer diagnosis, 541
  in pituitary tumor diagnosis, 545
Adrenalectomy, medical, for breast cancer, 202
Adrenocorticotrophic hormone. See *Corticotropin (ACTH)*.
Adriamycin. See *Doxorubicin (Adriamycin)*.
Aflatoxin(s), hepatocellular cancer and, 603
AFP. See *Alpha-fetoprotein (AFP)*.
Age-response function, in radiation therapy, 76, 77
AIDS (acquired immunodeficiency syndrome), 129–133
  Kaposi's sarcoma in, 130–132, 131t, 504
  recommended reading on, 133
Air pollution, lung cancer and, 646
Airway obstruction, 155
Alanyl-glutamine dipeptide, for cachexia, 694
Albinism, skin cancer in, 178
Albumin, serum, in nutritional assessment, 694
Alcohol, cancer due to, 4
  injection of, for neurolysis, 721–723, *723*
  pituitary ablation using, for pain, 727
Alimentary cancer, 557–589. See also specific sites, e.g., *Esophageal cancer*.
Alkylating agent(s). See also specific drugs.
  for chronic lymphocytic leukemia, 475

Alkylating agent(s) *(Continued)*
  for Langerhans cell histiocytosis, late effects of, 282
  for ovarian cancer, 394–395
  second malignancy due to, 4, 130
ALL. See *Leukemia(s), acute lymphocytic (ALL)*.
Allodynia, 712
Alopecia, due to chemotherapy, 113
Alpha interferon. See under *Interferon(s) (IFN)*.
Alpha ion, properties of, 92t
α/β ratio, in fractionation models, 86–87, 87
Alpha-fetoprotein (AFP), as tumor marker, 141
  in germ cell tumor, 276
  in hepatocellular cancer, 604
  in malignant liver tumors in children, 289
  in metastatic disease, 681
  in testicular cancer, 442, 448
Amino acid(s), branched-chain, for nutritional support, 697
Aminoglutethimide, for adrenocortical cancer, 542
  for breast cancer, 202, 202t
Amitriptyline, for pain, 719
AML. See *Leukemia(s), acute myelogenous (AML)*.
Amphetamine(s), for pain, 720
Amputation, for bone tumor, 516–517, *517*
  for soft tissue sarcoma, 494
Amyloid deposition, paraneoplastic, 140–141
Anal carcinoma, 587–589, 587t
  treatment of, 583t, 588–589, 588t, 589t
Analgesia. See also *Analgesic(s)*; *Pain management*; specific drugs.
  patient-controlled, 719
Analgesic(s), for pain in disseminated disease, 682, 682t
  nonopioid, 715–716
  opioid. See *Opioid analgesic(s)*.
  oral, 713–714
    alternatives to, 714–715
Analgesic ladder, 709, *710*, 713, 714
Anaplasia, 24, 30
Androgen(s), for breast cancer, 202, 202t
Androgen blockage, for prostate cancer, 439
Anergy, nutritional status and, 695
Anesthetic(s), local, nerve block using, 721–722
  oral, for pain, 720
  with intraspinal opioid therapy, 725
Aneuploidy, 31
  prognosis and, 35
Aneurysmal bone cyst, treatment of, 516, 523

771